Volume I

Principles and Practice of
EMERGENCY MEDICINE

Edited by

GEORGE R. SCHWARTZ, M.D.

Director of Emergency Medicine
University of New Mexico Medical Center;
Associate Professor of Community,
Family and Emergency Medicine
University of New Mexico School of Medicine
Albuquerque, New Mexico

Formerly, Director, Northeastern Emergency
Medical Services (a multi-hospital group);
Clinical Assistant Professor of Emergency Medicine
The Medical College of Pennsylvania
Philadelphia, Pennsylvania

PETER SAFAR, M.D., Dr. h.c.

Distinguished Service Professor
Resuscitation Research Institute
University of Pittsburgh; Past Chairman
Department of Anesthesiology/Critical Care Medicine
University of Pittsburgh
School of Medicine

JOHN H. STONE, M.D.

Professor of Medicine (Cardiology) and
Director, Emergency Medicine Residency
Grady Memorial Hospital/
Emory University School of Medicine, Atlanta, Georgia

PATRICK B. STOREY, M.D.

Professor of Medicine and Associate Dean
University of Pennsylvania School of Medicine, Philadelphia, Pennsylvania

DAVID K. WAGNER, M.D.

Professor of Surgery and Emergency Medicine
Associate Professor of Pediatrics
The Medical College of Pennsylvania, Philadelphia, Pennsylvania

1978

W. B. SAUNDERS COMPANY
Philadelphia, London, Toronto

W. B. Saunders Company: West Washington Square
Philadelphia, PA   19105

1 St. Anne's Road
Eastbourne, East Sussex BN21 3UN, England

1 Goldthorne Avenue
Toronto, Ontario M8Z 5T9, Canada

Library of Congress Cataloging in Publication Data

Main entry under title:

Principles and practice of emergency medicine.

Includes index.

1. Medical emergencies.   I. Schwartz, George R.
   II. Title: Emergency medicine. [DNLM: 1. Emergencies.
   2. Emergency medicine.   3. Critical care.
   WB105 P957]

RC86.7.P74   616'.025   75–25277

ISBN 0–7216–8031–3 (v.-1)

Principles and Practice of Emergency Medicine

Volume I   ISBN 0-7216-8031-3
Volume II   ISBN 0-7216-8033-X
Set   ISBN 0-7216-8034-8

Last digit is the print number: 9   8   7   6   5   4   3   2   1

CONTRIBUTORS

ELLEN E. ANDERSON, M.D.

Instructor of Surgery, The Medical College of Pennsylvania, Philadelphia, Pennsylvania

Abdominal Procedures

JAY MORRIS ARENA, M.D.

Professor of Pediatrics and Director of the Poison Control Center, Duke Medical Center, Durham, North Carolina

Poisonings

SUBHASH C. BANSAL, M.D.

Associate Professor of Surgery and Director of Surgical Research, The Medical College of Pennsylvania, Philadelphia, Pennsylvania

Immunologic Alterations in Acute Illness and Injury

BÉLA BENCZE, M.D.

General Director, Hungarian National Emergency and Ambulance Service, Budapest, Hungary

EMS in Hungary

GARRETT E. BERGMAN, M.D.

Assistant Professor of Pediatrics, The Medical College of Pennsylvania, Philadelphia, Pennsylvania

Pediatric Emergencies

ROBERT E. BINDA, JR., M.D.

Assistant Professor, Department of Anesthesiology, University of Pittsburgh School of Medicine; Staff Anesthesiologist, Children's Hospital, Pittsburgh, Pennsylvania

Renal Failure and Fluid-Electrolyte Imbalance

WILLIAM FRANCIS BOUZARTH, M.D.

Clinical Professor of Neurological Surgery, The Medical College of Pennsylvania; Deputy Director, Department of Neurosurgery, Episcopal Hospital, Philadelphia, Pennsylvania

Neurosurgical Procedures; Head and Spinal Injuries; Disaster Preparedness

EDWARD L. BRADLEY, III, M.D.

Associate Professor of Surgery, Emory University School of Medicine; Attending Surgeon, Emory University Hospital; Attending Surgeon, Grady Memorial Hospital; Consultant, Atlanta Veterans Administration Hospital, Atlanta, Georgia

Alimentary Tract Obstruction

GARRY L. BRIESE

Executive Director, Florida Chapter, American College of Emergency Physicians, Jacksonville, Florida

EMS Transportation

RICHARD A. BROSE, Ph.D.

Associate Professor of Medicine, University of Missouri–Kansas City School of Medicine; Director, Emergency Medical Services Training and Research Center, University of Missouri–Kansas City School of Medicine, Kansas City, Missouri

Categorization of Emergency Facilities

JOHN BULETTE, M.D.

Assistant Professor, Department of Psychiatry, The Medical College of Pennsylvania, Philadelphia, Pennsylvania

Evaluation of the Potentially Suicidal Patient

FRANK M. CALIA, M.D.

Professor of Medicine, University of Maryland School of Medicine; Chief, Medical Service, Veterans Administration Hospital, Baltimore, Maryland

Infectious Diseases

GEORGE J. CARANASOS, M.D.

Associate Professor of Medicine, University of Florida, College of Medicine; Chief, Division of General Medicine, Shands Teaching Hospital, Gainesville, Florida

Drug Reactions

RICHARD WAYNE CARLSON, M.D., Ph.D.

Assistant Professor of Medicine and Assistant Director, Shock Research Unit and the Center for the Critically Ill, University of Southern California School of Medicine, Los Angeles County/USC Medical Center and the Hollywood Presbyterian Medical Center, Los Angeles, California

Cardiovascular System Failure

NANCY L. CAROLINE, M.D.

Medical Director, Magen David Adom, Tel Aviv, Israel

Acute Respiratory Insufficiency; Respiratory Care Techniques and Strategies

ELSIE R. CARRINGTON, M.D.

Professor and Chairman, Department of Obstetrics and Gynecology, The Medical College of Pennsylvania and Hospital of The Medical College of Pennsylvania, Philadelphia, Pennsylvania

Obstetric and Gynecologic Procedures

C. GENE CAYTEN, M.D., M.P.H.

Assistant Professor of Surgery, University of Pennsylvania School of Medicine; Director, Center for the Study of Emergency Health Services; Attending Surgeon, Hospital of the University of Pennsylvania, and Veterans Administration Hospital, Philadelphia, Pennsylvania

Traumatology; EMS Planning and Evaluation

YOGINDER K. CHITKARA, M.D.

Research Associate, Alma D. Morani Laboratory of Surgical Immunobiology, The Medical College of Pennsylvania, Philadelphia, Pennsylvania

Immunologic Alterations in Acute Illness and Injury

STEPHEN D. CLEMENTS, JR., M.D.

Assistant Professor of Medicine, Emory University School of Medicine; Attending Physician, Emory University Hospital, Atlanta, Georgia

Disorders Caused by Coronary Atherosclerotic Heart Disease;
Effect of Electrolyte Abnormalities on the Electrocardiogram

LEONARD A. COBB, M.D.

Professor of Medicine, University of Washington; Director, Division of Cardiology, Harborview Medical Center, Seattle, Washington

Sudden Death

ERRIKOS CONSTANT, D.D.S., M.D., F.A.C.S.

Assistant Clinical Professor of Surgery, Michigan State University College of Human Medicine, East Lansing; Staff Surgeon (Plastic Surgery), Michigan State University Olin Health Center, East Lansing; Staff Surgeon (Plastic Surgery), Sparrow Hospital, St. Lawrence Hospital, Ingham Medical Center, Lansing, Michigan

Facial Trauma

MILTON CORN, M.D.

Professor of Internal Medicine, Georgetown University School of Medicine; Director, Emergency Department, Georgetown University Hospital, Washington, D.C.

Bleeding Disorders

R ADAMS COWLEY, M.D.

Professor of Thoracic and Cardiovascular Surgery, University of Maryland School of Medicine; Director, Maryland Institute for Emergency Medical Services, Baltimore, Maryland

Specialized Patient Care Units; Operating Rooms

ROBERT H. DAILEY, M.D.

Clinical Associate Professor of Medicine and Community and Ambulatory Medicine (Emergency Medicine), University of California at San Francisco; Chief, Department of Emergency Medicine, Valley Medical Center, Fresno, California

Difficulty in Breathing

JOHN K. DAVIDSON, M.D., Ph.D.

Professor of Medicine, Emory University School of Medicine; Director of Diabetes Unit, Grady Memorial Hospital, Atlanta, Georgia

Diabetic Ketoacidosis; Hyperglycemic States

WILLIAM E. DeMUTH, JR., M.D.

Professor of Surgery, The Pennsylvania State University College of Medicine, Philadelphia; General Surgeon, The Milton S. Hershey Medical Center, Hershey, Pennsylvania

Neck Trauma

ROBERT L. DONALD, M.D.

Clinical Assistant Professor of Medicine, University of Texas Medical School, Houston, Texas; former Chairman, Committee on Emergency Medical Services, American Medical Association, Texas Medical Association, and Harris County Medical Society; former Delegate from the AMA to the Commission on Emergency Medical Services; charter member of the American College of Emergency Physicians

EMS Transportation

MICHAEL E. ERVIN, M.D.

Assistant Clinical Professor, Wright State University School of Medicine; Director of Emergency Services, Miami Valley Hospital; Medical Director of Western Ohio Emergency Medical Services, Dayton, Ohio

Minor Surgical Procedures

RICHARD L. FABIAN, M.D.

Instructor in Otolaryngology, Harvard Medical School, Boston; Chief of Plastic Service and active staff member, Massachusetts Eye and Ear Infirmary, Boston; Chief of Surgery, E. K. Shriner Center for Mental Retardation, Waltham; Active Staff, N. E. Deaconess Hospital, Boston; Consultant in Otolaryngology, Veterans Administration Hospital, W. Roxbury, Massachusetts

Otolaryngologic Procedures

ALAN O. FEINGOLD, M.D.

Assistant Professor of Clinical Medicine, Emory University Medical School, Atlanta; Staff Physician, Dekalb General Hospital and Grady Memorial Hospital, Decatur, Georgia

Disorders of the Red Blood Cells; Splenomegaly

ROBERT DAVID FINK, M.D.

Clinical Associate Professor, Department of Psychiatry, University of Tennessee, Center for the Health Sciences; Superintendent, Memphis Mental Health Institute; Consulting Psychiatrist, Alcohol and Drug Dependence Clinic, Memphis Mental Health Institute, Memphis, Tennessee

Intoxication and the Alcohol Abstinence Syndrome

GERALD F. FLETCHER, M.D.

Professor of Internal Medicine (Cardiology), Emory University School of Medicine; Director of Internal Medicine, Georgia Baptist Hospital, Atlanta, Georgia

Insertion of a Temporary Transvenous Pacemaker

URI FREUND, M.D.

Hadassah Medical Center, Jerusalem, Israel

Cardiovascular System Failure

ARNOLD P. FRIEDMAN, M.D., F.A.C.P.

Professor of Neurology, University of Arizona Medical School; Attending Neurologist, Tucson Medical Center and St. Joseph's Hospital, Tucson, Arizona

Headache

AURÉL A. GÁBOR, M.D. (deceased)

Hungarian National Emergency and Ambulance Service, Budapest, Hungary

EMS in Hungary

JOHN T. GALAMBOS, M.D.

Professor of Medicine, Emory University School of Medicine; Chief of Gastroenterology, Grady Memorial Hospital; Associate Physician, Gastroenterology, Emory University Hospital, Atlanta, Georgia

Hepatic Disease

DONALD S. GANN, M.D.

Professor of Emergency Medicine, The Johns Hopkins University School of Medicine; Director, Division of Emergency Medicine, and Surgeon, The Johns Hopkins Hospital, Baltimore, Maryland

General Body Response to Trauma

JAMES G. GARRICK, M.D.

Head, Division of Sports Medicine, and Associate Professor, Department of Orthopedics, University of Washington, Seattle, Washington

Emergencies in Sports

JAMES E. GEORGE, M.D., J.D.

Emergency Physician, Underwood Memorial Hospital, Woodbury, New Jersey; Board Member, American College of Emergency Physicians

Medicolegal Problems

JAMES E. GERACE, M.D., Maj., M.C.

Chief, Pulmonary Disease Service, Tripler Army Medical Center; Associate Clinical Professor of Medicine, University of Hawaii; Visiting Pulmonologist, University of Hawaii and Queens Medical Center, Honolulu, Hawaii

Near-Drowning

GEOFFREY GIBSON, Ph.D.

Associate Professor, The Johns Hopkins University School of Medicine and The Johns Hopkins University School of Hygiene and Public Health, Baltimore, Maryland

Utilization of EMS

RAY W. GIFFORD, JR., M.D.

Head, Department of Hypertension and Nephrology, The Cleveland Clinic Foundation, Cleveland, Ohio

Hypertensive Crises

LEON GOLDMAN, M.D.

Professor and Chairman, Department of Dermatology; Director, Laser Laboratory, University of Cincinnati Medical Center; Director, Dermatology, Cincinnati General Hospital and Children's Hospital Medical Center, Cincinnati, Ohio

Laser and Microwave Injuries

ROBERTA BECKMAN GONZALEZ, M.D.

Clinical Associate in Medicine, University of Pennsylvania Medical School, Presbyterian University of Pennsylvania Hospital, and Graduate Hospital, Philadelphia, Pennsylvania

Endocrinologic Problems

GARY J. GRAD, M.D.

Clinical Assistant Professor, Downstate Medical Center; Acting Director, Child and Adolescent Outpatient Department, Kings County Hospital Center, Brooklyn, New York

Psychiatric Emergencies

BARBARA HARTLEY GREENE, M.D.

Assistant Professor of Medicine, Emory University School of Medicine; Staff Physician, Grady Memorial Hospital, Atlanta, Georgia

Porphyrias; Pheochromocytoma

ARTHUR H. GRIFFITHS

Communications Specialist, Division of Emergency Medical Services, Public Health Service, U.S. Department of Health, Education, and Welfare, Washington, D.C.

EMS Communications

WILLIAM F. HAMILTON, Ph.D.

Associate Professor of Decision Sciences and Management, Wharton School, University of Pennsylvania; Associate Director, Leonard Davis Institute of Health and Economics, University of Pennsylvania, Philadelphia, Pennsylvania

Financing the EMS

LINTON C. HOPKINS, M.D.

Assistant Professor of Neurology, Emory University School of Medicine; Attending Neurologist, Emory University Hospital and Grady Memorial Hospital, Atlanta, Georgia

Neuromuscular Diseases

J. WILLIS HURST, M.D.

Professor and Chairman, Department of Medicine, Emory University School of Medicine, Atlanta, Georgia

Chest Pain

LOREN A. JOHNSON, M.D.

Instructor in Emergency Medical Technology, Orange Coast College, Costa Mesa; Emergency Physician, Saint Francis Hospital, Lynwood, California

Trauma Due to Cold; Toxic Bites and Stings

E. JEFF JUSTIS, JR., M.D.

Clinical Assistant Professor of Orthopaedic Surgery, University of Tennessee College of Medicine; Consultant in Hand Surgery to Tennessee and Mississippi Crippled Children Services; Active Staff, The Campbell Clinic, Baptist Memorial Hospital, City of Memphis Hospital; Consulting Staff, LeBonheur Hospital and Arlington Hospital, Memphis, Tennessee

Trauma to the Hand

ALAN S. KAPLAN, M.D., M.P.H.

Director, Professional Programs, Office of the Assistant Commissioner for Professional and Consumer Programs, Food and Drug Administration, Rockville, Maryland

Legislative Aspects of Emergency Care

LESTER KARAFIN, M.D., F.A.C.S.

Professor of Urology, The Medical College of Pennsylvania; Clinical Professor of Urology, Temple University Medical Center; Chief, Section of Urology, Hospital of The Medical College of Pennsylvania; Attending Urologist, Temple University Hospital and St. Christopher's Hospital for Children, Philadelphia, Pennsylvania

Genitourinary Injuries

DOROTHY KARANDANIS, M.D.

Assistant Professor of Medicine, Emory University School of Medicine, Atlanta, Georgia

Diseases of Veins

JAMES W. KELLER, M.D.

Assistant Professor of Medicine, Emory University School of Medicine; Attending Hematologist and Medical Oncologist, Emory University Hospital and Grady Memorial Hospital, Atlanta, Georgia

Disorders of Leukocytes

ROBERT R. KELLY, M.D.

Emergency Physician, Salem Memorial Hospital, Salem, Oregon

Pericarditis

A. RICHARD KENDALL, M.D.

Professor and Chairman, Department of Urology, Temple University School of Medicine; Clinical Professor of Urology and Attending Urologist, The Medical College of Pennsylvania; Attending Urologist, St. Christopher's Hospital for Children, Philadelphia, Pennsylvania

Genitourinary Injuries

THOMAS C. KENNEDY, M.C.P.

Staff Associate, Center for the Study of Emergency Health Services, University of Pennsylvania, Philadelphia, Pennsylvania

Accident Prevention, Consumer Education and Community Involvement in EMS

YEHEZKIEL KISHON, M.D.

Lecturer in Internal Medicine, University of Tel-Aviv Medical School; Associate Director, Heart Institute, Sheba Medical Center, Tel-Hashomer, Israel

EMS in Tel-Aviv

NATHAN S. KLINE, M.D., F.A.C.P., F.R.C.Psych.

Director, Rockland Research Institute, Orangeburg; Clinical Professor of Psychiatry, College of Physicians and Surgeons, Columbia University, New York; Attending Physician, Lenox Hill Hospital, New York, New York

Psychiatric Emergencies

DAVID HOWARD KNOTT, M.D., Ph.D.

Clinical Associate Professor, Department of Psychiatry, University of Tennessee Center for the Health Sciences; Medical Director, Alcohol and Drug Dependence Clinic, Memphis Mental Health Institute; Assistant Superintendent, Research and Training, Memphis Mental Health Institute, Memphis, Tennessee

Intoxication and the Alcohol Abstinence Syndrome

WILLIAM G. LAVELLE, M.D.

Instructor in Otolaryngology, Harvard Medical School, Boston; Chief of Otolaryngology, Whidden Memorial Hospital, Everett; Active Staff, Massachusetts Eye and Ear Infirmary and Children's Hospital Medical Center, Boston, Massachusetts

Otolaryngologic Procedures

JEFFREY A. LEONARD, M.D.

Clinical Associate Professor, Department of Psychiatry, University of Pennsylvania, Attending Psychiatrist, Institute of Pennsylvania Hospital, Philadelphia, Pennsylvania

Headache

ROBERT L. LEOPOLD, M.D.

Professor of Psychiatry, School of Medicine; Professor of Health Care Systems, Wharton School; University of Pennsylvania, Attending Psychiatrist, Hospital of the University of Pennsylvania; Associate Neurologist, Psychiatrist, Graduate Hospital of the University of Pennsylvania; Attending Psychiatrist, Institute of Pennsylvania Hospital, Philadelphia, Pennsylvania

Crisis Intervention Services

DAVID G. LEVINE, M.D.

Assistant Clinical Professor of Psychiatry, School of Medicine, University of California, San Francisco; Mental Health Director and Program Chief, Community Mental Health Services, Marin County, California

Alcohol and Drug Abuse

JEAN-PIERRE LINDENMAYER, M.D.

Assistant Professor of Psychiatry, State University of New York; Acting Director, Psychiatric Inpatient Service, University Hospital, Downstate Medical Center, Brooklyn, New York

Psychiatric Emergencies

JOSEPH LINDSAY, JR., M.D.

Professor of Medicine, Division of Cardiology, The George Washington University School of Medicine; Director of Coronary Care Unit, George Washington University Hospital, Washington, D.C.

Aorta and Peripheral Arteries

GEORGE I. LITMAN, M.D.

Chairman, Sub-council of Cardiology, Northeastern Ohio Universities College of Medicine; Chief, Cardiology Service, Akron General Medical Center, Akron, Ohio

Use of Flow-Directed Balloon Tipped Catheter

GERALD L. LOONEY, M.D., M.P.H.

Assistant Professor, Department of Emergency Medicine, University of Southern California School of Medicine; Attending Staff, LAC-USC Medical Center; Director of Emergency Department, Glendale Adventist Medical Center, Glendale, California

EMS Manpower and Training; Education in the Emergency Department

MILTON N. LURIA, M.D.

Professor of Medicine and Health Services, University of Rochester School of Medicine and Dentistry; Physician, Strong Memorial Hospital, Rochester, New York

Syncope

WILLIAM R. MacAUSLAND, JR., M.D.

Associate Clinical Professor in Orthopaedic Surgery, Harvard Medical School; Assistant Clinical Professor in Orthopaedic Surgery, Tufts University Medical School, Boston, Massachusetts

Orthopedic Procedures; Trauma to Extremities and Soft Tissues

JAMES ROBERTSON MACKENZIE, M.D., F.R.C.S.(C.), F.A.C.S.

Assistant Clinical Professor of Surgery, McMaster University; Active Staff, Hamilton General Hospital; Chief of Emergency Department and active staff member, Chedoke General Hospital; Associate Staff Member, McMaster University Medical Center, Hamilton, Ontario, Canada

Abdominal Trauma

KARL G. MANGOLD, M.D.

Clinical Instructor, University of California, San Francisco; Vice President, American College of Emergency Physicians; Director, Department of Emergency Medicine, Vesper Memorial Hospital, San Leandro, California

Financing the Emergency Department

BENEDICT S. MANISCALCO, M.D.

Assistant Professor of Medicine (Cardiology), University of South Florida College of Medicine, Tampa, Florida

Cardiogenic Shock

JOHN P. MARIANO, B.S.

Emergency Medical Services Coordinator, Philadelphia Department of Public Health, Philadelphia, Pennsylvania

Disaster Preparedness

FRANK I. MARLOWE, M.D.

Associate Professor of Otolaryngology, The Medical College of Pennsylvania; Staff, Hospital of The Medical College of Pennsylvania; Staff, Presbyterian–University of Pennsylvania Medical Center; Consultant, Naval Regional Medical Center, Philadelphia, Pennsylvania

Vertigo

KENNETH L. MATTOX, M.D.

Assistant Professor of Surgery, Cora and Webb Mading Department of Surgery, Baylor College of Medicine; Deputy Surgeon-in-Chief and Director of Emergency Surgical Services, Ben Taub General Hospital, Houston, Texas

Hemoptysis

LEON MENZER, M.D.

Instructor in Neurology, Harvard Medical School; Instructor in Neurology, Tufts University Medical School; Assisting Physician in Neurology, Boston City Hospital, Boston, Massachusetts

Convulsions

SYLVIA H. MICIK, M.D.

Associate Professor, Clinical Pediatrics and Community Medicine, University of California School of Medicine, La Jolla; Director of Emergency Medical Services, San Diego; Attending Physician, University of California Medical Center, San Diego, California

Poison Control Centers

JAMES DeWITT MILLS, JR., M.D.

Clinical Instructor in Medicine, Georgetown University, Washington, D.C.; Chairman, Emergency Department, Mt. Vernon Hospital, and Emergency Department, Alexandria Hospital, Alexandria, Virginia

Organization and Staffing of the Emergency Department

JOHN A. MONCRIEF, M.D.

Professor of Surgery, Medical University of South Carolina, Charleston, South Carolina

Burns

WILLIAM W. MONTGOMERY, M.D.

Professor of Otolaryngology, Harvard Medical School; Senior Surgeon in Otolaryngology, Massachusetts Eye and Ear Infirmary; Chief, Head and Neck Tumor Clinic, Massachusetts General Hospital and Massachusetts Eye and Ear Infirmary; Consultant in Otolaryngology, Children's Hospital Medical Center, Boston, Massachusetts

Otolaryngologic Procedures

JACK COLBERT MORGAN, M.D.

Clinical Instructor, Department of Psychiatry, University of Tennessee Center for the Health Sciences, Memphis, Tennessee

Intoxication and the Alcohol Abstinence Syndrome

GARY G. NICHOLAS, M.D.

Assistant Professor of Surgery, The Pennsylvania State University College of Medicine, Philadelphia; General Surgeon, The Milton S. Hershey Medical Center, Hershey, Pennsylvania

Trauma to the Neck

EDDY D. PALMER, M.D.

Clinical Professor of Medicine, Rutgers Medical School, Piscataway; Attending Physician, Hackettstown Community Hospital, Hackettstown, New Jersey

Hematemesis and Melena

LEONARD F. PELTIER, M.D., Ph.D.

Professor of Surgery, University of Arizona College of Medicine; Chief, Orthopedics, Arizona Medical Center, Veterans Administration Hospital, Tucson, Arizona

Fat Embolism

THOMAS N. PERLOFF, M.Sc.

Associate Director, Urban Health Services Center, University of Pennsylvania, Philadelphia, Pennsylvania

The Health Maintenance Organization; National Health Insurance

ROBERT PAUL PROULX, M.D.

Associate Professor, Los Angeles County/USC Medical Center; Emergency Department Physician, St. Joseph Medical Center, Burbank, California

Heart Distress

JOHN JOSEPH PURCELL, JR., M.D.

Assistant Clinical Professor of Ophthalmology and Director of Cornea Service, Saint Louis University School of Medicine; Director of Cornea and External Disease Service, Saint Louis University Hospitals and Saint Mary's Hospital, Saint Louis, Missouri

Examination of the Eye and Its Adnexa; Ocular Trauma

JONATHAN E. RHOADS, JR., M.D.

Assistant Professor of Surgery and Attending Surgeon, The Medical College of Pennsylvania; Chief of Surgery, Philadelphia Veterans Administration Hospital, Philadelphia, Pennsylvania

Vascular Procedures

ARTHUR E. RIKLI, M.D., M.P.H.

Professor, Department of Community Health and Medical Practice, University of Missouri, Columbia, Missouri

Tokyo EMS

JAMES R. ROBERTS, M.D.

Instructor of Emergency Medicine, The Medical College of Pennsylvania; Attending Physician, Department of Emergency Medicine, Frankfort Hospital, Philadelphia, Pennsylvania

Snakebites

PETER ROSEN, M.D.

Director, Division of Emergency Medicine, Department of Health and Hospitals, Arizona Medical Center, Veterans Administration Hospital, Tucson, Arizona

Hypovolemic Shock

CONSTANTINE C. ROUSSI, M.D.

Chairman, Department of Emergency Medicine, Akron General Medical Center, Akron, Ohio

Diarrhea

ROBERT BARRY RUTHERFORD, M.D.

Associate Professor of Surgery, University of Colorado Medical School; Associate Professor of Surgery, Colorado General Hospital, Denver, Colorado

Trauma to the Peripheral Vascular System

G. ANTHONY RYAN, M.D., B.S., M.P.H.

Senior Lecturer, Department of Social and Preventive Medicine, Monash University, Melbourne, Australia

EMS in Australia

THOMAS D. SABIN, M.D.

Associate Professor of Neurology, Boston University; Director, Neurologic Unit, Boston City Hospital, Boston, Massachusetts

Coma; Confusion; Convulsions; Neurologic Emergencies

ALFRED M. SADLER, JR., M.D.

Clinical fellow in medicine at Harvard Medical School, Department of Internal Medicine; Resident Physician, Department of Medicine, Massachusetts General Hospital, Boston, Massachusetts

Emergency Medical Services in Perspective

BLAIR L. SADLER, J.D.

Vice President, Scripps Clinic and Research Foundation; Director, Green Hospital of Scripps Clinic, California

Emergency Medical Services in Perspective

ARTHUR P. SAFRAN, M.D.

Assistant Professor of Medicine, Instructor in Neurology, Boston University; Instructor in Neurology, Tufts University; Lecturer on Neurology, Harvard University, Boston; Staff, The Framingham Union Hospital, Framingham; Staff, Neurological Unit, Boston City Hospital, Boston, Massachusetts

Confusion

ATEF A. SALAM, M.D.

Associate Professor of Surgery, Emory University School of Medicine; Director of Vascular Surgery Service, Grady Memorial Hospital, Atlanta, Georgia

Upper Gastrointestinal Bleeding

HERBERT STANLEY SHUBIN, M.D. (deceased)

Associate Professor of Medicine and Associate Director, Shock Research Unit and the Center for the Critically Ill, University of Southern California School of Medicine, Los Angeles County/USC Medical Center and the Hollywood Presbyterian Medical Center, Los Angeles, California

Cardiovascular System Failure

HARVEY M. SILVERMAN, M.D.

Emergency Physician, Springfield Hospital, Springfield, Vermont

Smoke Inhalation

MARK E. SILVERMAN, M.D.

Associate Professor of Medicine (Cardiology), Emory University School of Medicine; Attending Cardiologist, Grady Memorial Hospital and Piedmont Hospital, Atlanta, Georgia

Arrhythmias

THEODORE E. WOODWARD, M.D.

Professor and Head, Department of Medicine, University of Maryland School of Medicine, Baltimore, Maryland

Infectious Disease

MOHAMMED T. YOUNIS, M.D., M.S. (surgery)

Assistant Professor of Surgery, The Medical College of Pennsylvania; Attending Surgeon and Director of the Surgical Intensive Care Unit, Hospital of The Medical College of Pennsylvania; Consultant, Veterans Administration Hospital, Philadelphia, Pennsylvania

Evaluation of Acute Abdominal Pain

PREFACE

Before the book there is the Preface. But before either book or Preface, there is the idea of the book. Dr. George Schwartz, himself an emergency physician and teacher, recognized in the early 1970s that there was a need for a comprehensive textbook of emergency medicine. The literature of this burgeoning discipline had, up to that point, consisted largely of manuals, handbooks, and periodicals. What was needed was far different: a book that would of necessity be large; a book that would begin with pathophysiology and end with the patient; a book that would address itself to the entire spectrum of care in the emergency department: minor and major, undifferentiated and clear-cut, medical and surgical. Epidemiologic, administrative, and legal aspects would also be covered. In short, it was to be a book that would help codify this rapidly growing field.

The editorial staff first met almost five years ago to plan in detail the contents of such a book. In view of the diversity of subject matter, it seemed wise to engage the efforts of diverse editors, all intimately involved in emergency medicine, each with his special area of expertise: an emergency physician, an anesthesiologist/critical care physician, who established the first physician fellowship program in critical care medicine, an internist/cardiologist, an internist with special knowledge of emergency medical care systems, and a surgeon who had established one of the first emergency medicine residencies in the United States. Each editor then took responsibility for selection of contributors from across the country.

The overall outline of the text deserves mention. Part I analyzes mechanisms of vital organ failure and death. It addresses the pathophysiology of such problems and the therapeutic methods for reversal. Part II is devoted to the fundamental procedures and techniques needed for effective care of the seriously threatened patient. Part III is divided into three sections: the first considers some common patient presentations, chosen because of their frequency and importance in everyday practice; the second section is concerned with management of the traumatized patient and special problems of trauma; the third describes the management of the patient who becomes suddenly and seriously ill for reasons other than trauma. Part IV describes the organizational aspects of providing appropriate emergency care: the out-of-hospital services, the epidemiology, information flow, communications, transportation, and the systems development needed to "take the health services system to the patient." Also addressed in this section is the organization of the acute care capacity of the hospital itself; in addition there is a brief description of foreign models of emergency medical service. The book concludes with a consideration of the legal and legislative issues in emergency medicine and with a broad view of the psycho-socio-economic aspects of the field.

Although the book is written for physicians with varied training and experience working in emergency departments, some concepts conveyed apply also to the short-term management of patients with acutely life-threatening conditions in prehospital settings. Some procedures which, for safe performance, require skills beyond those taught in emergency medicine are not covered.

In one sense, a Preface is a misnomer: though it is placed before the rest of the book, it is always written after the book is ready. Nevertheless, what we wanted to say before, we are quite happy to be able to say afterward.

THE EDITORS

ACKNOWLEDGMENTS

To the Contributors go our special thanks for many things. Their individual aims were on target and came out of many physician years of concern with the problems of the patient in the emergency department. Many of the contributors are deeply involved in the education of residents in emergency medicine. Others are no less committed, by way of the traditional disciplines, to improving the care of the patients in the emergency department.

Appreciation is certainly due Brian Decker, Medical Editor at W. B. Saunders Company, for his sensitive guidance and trust during the development of this book. John Dyson of Saunders copyedited the manuscripts and his experienced hand aided greatly. In addition, thanks are due Andrew J. Piernock, Jr., and the Saunders production crew, whose skill can be seen on every page.

Many persons were involved in the joyful labor of bringing forth this textbook. In acknowledgment of some of the people who helped and without whom this book would not have been possible, Dr. George Schwartz thanks his secretaries, Valerie McDaniels, Kathleen McNamee, and particularly Pat Fredericks; his family—Loretta, Ruth, and Rebecca; Dr. Waldo Nelson and Dr. Howard Kirz for their inspiration; and in the final stages Patricia Parkinson. Dr. Peter Safar is grateful to Eva, Philip, and Paul. Dr. John Stone thanks his secretary, Mae Nelson, and his family: Lu, Johnny, and Jim, who understood. The section on emergency medical systems, together with the organizational, legislative, and legal aspects of emergency care, could not have been done without the inspired help of Dr. Joseph A. Fortuna, who knew where everybody was and what they were doing. The complexity of managing the entire transaction with the multiple contributors to this section was resolved through the organizing capability of Nancy J. Wink, M.S.N. Also, Dr. David Wagner gratefully acknowledges the residents—wherein the future begins.

CONTENTS

VOLUME 1

Section 2 — Traumatic Emergencies

VOLUME 2

SECTION 3 — NONTRAUMATIC MEDICAL AND SURGICAL EMERGENCIES

Chapter I

THE DEVELOPMENT OF EMERGENCY MEDICINE

George R. Schwartz

"In the first place, in the physician or surgeon no quality takes rank with imperturbability. . . . Imperturbability means coolness and presence of mind under all circumstances, calmness amid storm, clearness of judgment in the moments of grave peril, immobility, impassiveness, or to use an old expressive word, phlegm."

William Osler, M.D.
from "Aequanimitas," 1889,
Philadelphia, Pennsylvania.

Rather like the slow maturing of a child until neurologic readiness makes possible major developmental advances, concentration on emergency care remained relatively dormant until the past two decades, during which time myriad forces led to an accentuated concern about caring for sudden illness and injury. Technology, public needs, and the demands and needs of the medical community melded to produce a kind of environmental readiness. The rapid emergence of Emergency Medicine was certainly foreseen and, through important studies (such as the NAS Report, 1966), stimulated. Constant pressure exerted by outspoken leaders brought increased Federal interest in Emergency Medical Systems, beginning in the 1950s and gaining momentum as the activities and numbers of workers in this field increased, culminating in such Federal responses as the EMS Systems Act of 1973.

Postgraduate training programs in Emergency Medicine are becoming more numerous throughout the United States, and many young physicians are electing to enter this form of medical practice as a primary career choice.

When Dr. James Mills, then President of the American College of Emergency Physicians, listed the steps to specialization in 1973, he described 11 key steps. By 1976, eight of these had been taken. Such a movement occurs slowly, and in February 1976 Dr. James Haviland forecasted that a minimum of two years or, more likely, four or five years would be required before full accreditation and recognition could be achieved. Patience has been a necessary attribute in those who chose this undeveloped field as their primary career commitment, but time also allows an increasingly solid foundation to be established for a new field—particularly one in which the service and education components have dominated while the research arm lagged. Finding a secure place in medical schools, where most research is done, has further slowed the needed clinical and basic investigation involving the earliest physiologic changes seen in acute illness and injury.

It is most significant, however, that the question in 1970 was "Will Emergency Medicine become a specialty?", whereas in 1976 the question has become "When?"

Some of the answers explaining the change from a status of uncertain viability of Emergency Medicine as a separate field to the present certainty—even though patience is still required—are reflected in the final vector of complex forces that have been acting and interacting sometimes to encourage and sometimes to discourage the development of the specialty. It is worthwhile to analyze some of these forces because they relate not only to changes within the medical care system, but in fact reflect significant changes within our society.

1

Three important elements can be identified as major stimulants to the growth of the field:

(1) Patients need and demand Emergency Medical Services (Walker, 1976; Satin, 1972).

(2) Hospitals and modes of medical practice have changed (Lee, 1960; Southwick, 1973; DeHoff, 1972).

(3) Technologic developments have expanded greatly the opportunities for *rapid* diagnosis and initiation of sound therapy (Gross, 1970).

Each of these factors has exerted complementary stimulation from different directions, i.e., from the patient, from the hospital medical community, and from physicians.

The first of these determinants, the needs and demands of patients, reflects the changes that have occurred in American society, particularly during the past three decades. The art and science of medicine involve intimate and extensive working with people, and the needs of society modify and shape the development of medical techniques and practice.

As travel around this country became easier and as people became ever less dismayed at the prospect of uprooting themselves and their families, a breakdown consequently took place in the traditional orientation toward a family doctor. People in unfamiliar surroundings tended to seek medical attention when they became ill, and came to expect medical service for acute illness and injury to be available around the clock. In addition, the ever-increasing hazards of modern life—especially the automobile—caused more trauma, much of it serious and requiring immediate and, at times, life-saving medical care. These factors, coupled with increased household and industrial injuries, 24-hour industries, and the general orientation of the population toward expecting medical services to be available stimulated the development of 24-hour emergency facilities.

The convenience and the feelings of security and protection that such facilities engendered answered a public need. Patients confirmed this need by using Emergency Departments in increasing numbers (Satin, 1972; Huntley, 1966). This trend was demonstrated throughout the country (Gibson, 1974). In fact, Emergency Medicine is, without doubt, the first medical specialty area whose development received substantial impetus from public demand, reflecting a deep-felt public need for prompt medical care when it was urgently needed. Perhaps this feeling of security was more needed in a country in flux—particularly when it is recognized that the tumultuous 60s and 70s have seen the most dramatic growth in numbers of patients using Emergency Department facilities—the same years when the words "future shock" began to have meaning (Toffler, 1972).

The second major stimulating factor was the changing role of the modern hospital and simultaneous changes in modes of medical practice. The hospital's increased social and community concerns, responding both to patient demand and to self-interest, led to the creation of "emergency rooms." What began as single rooms soon, with increased demand, became larger, more complex departments. Hospitals recognized that beds are filled by having a viable Emergency Department, that existing ancillary services are used more extensively, and that a hospital in a marginal financial situation could "move into the black" through their emergency unit.

In some areas, a receiving nurse simply called a physician when a patient arrived. Thus full-time staffing was not needed until the number of patients rose—which occurred with amazing rapidity in many areas. In hospitals located in heavily populated areas, it soon became evident that full 24-hour coverage of the Emergency Department by physicians was essential.

PHYSICIAN STAFFING OF EMERGENCY DEPARTMENTS—1950s AND EARLY 1960s

For the most part, the first full-time emergency physicians came from a background of general practice. They found that they enjoyed the structured working hours, and the ready availability of laboratory and x-ray facilities proved highly desirable. Some of these pioneers were older physicians who sought such work as they neared retirement; others saw the Emergency Department as a practice opportunity that could provide a stable income. Also, a number of foreign-born and foreign-trained physicians were attracted. For them, practice-building in the United States proved more difficult, and, since many were older, they neither wished nor could afford to spend the years necessary to build a private practice.

The part-time staffing was mixed. "Moonlighting" residents saw service in the Emergency Department as a good way to earn extra income. No tests of skills were needed; no demonstration of training other than a license was required. Some physicians new to an area worked part-time as they built their own practices. Early staffing therefore was provided by physicians with varied backgrounds and abilities. The lack of established standards for physicians in emergency practice led to inevitable variability in quality of care, depending on the extent and type of training and experience of the individual physicians.

CHANGES IN MEDICAL PRACTICE

At the same time "emergency rooms" were being established, medical practice in the United States was undergoing profound changes. More and more specialists were being trained and ever fewer general practitioners (Spiro, 1974). Role models for family physicians or primary care physicians were absent, and students reflected the specialty-oriented environment in which they generally trained.

The solo practitioner was, in fact, being replaced in many areas by partnerships and groups, the latter composed of diverse medical specialists and some general practitioners. The movement to recruit young physicians into careers in family practice was just beginning, and to the medical student trying to emulate and please his professors training for a specialty was the route to prestige and acceptance.

Although extremely long working hours were routine for most physicians, many realized that sleepless nights were associated with performance decrements and lowered over-all efficiency. The specialists' life-style afforded more structured hours as well as superior economic advantages. As the development and training of specialists peaked, an Emergency Department that was staffed by physicians for the full 24 hours proved to be a distinct advantage, and in some areas the hospital's medical staff provided the motivating force behind the development of a modern facility for emergency care. Even as the family practice movement gained momentum, the Emergency Departments complemented this development by providing night-time and off-hours coverage for emergency service.

Thanks to these developments the needs of both the patient and the community's physicians could be served. Community practitioners, specialists, and family physicians increasingly appreciated the role that a well-staffed emergency facility could play in providing care for their patients—and permitting them more time for other activities. Although still working longer hours, owing to the demand for their services, physicians were not immune to the life-style changes occurring within American and other industrialized societies. Also, the variety of cases and frequent requirements for immediate medical action led to the development of emergency physicians whose more sharply honed skills complemented the skills of other local physicians who could not keep up with advances in emergency treatment because of the demands and advances within their own specialties.

THE ROLE OF TECHNOLOGY

Important as these patient and physician factors were, the third determinant—advances in technology—proved to be the most important in the development of emergency medicine as a specialty. These advances made it possible to provide more and better immediate care for the acutely ill and injured. New techniques, sophisticated monitoring devices, and new-found skills in managing acute disease processes and injuries began to provide the type of skeletal structure from which physicians with vision could see the shaping of a new specialty field. Through continued education and enhancement of their skills and experience, emergency physicians won new respect from their colleagues.

Current debates about criteria for "brain death" and determining when patients actually "die" are, in fact, direct reflections of technologic developments that allow organ systems to be maintained through the use of external devices. Such devices and new resuscitative equipment also could be used successfully to save the lives of patients for whom heretofore the only pronouncement would have been death.

Technologic growth contributed still further to the expansion of emergency medicine by reducing the delays that limited diagnostic capabilities. Laboratory tests that once required a full day became automated, and results could be made available within minutes. Modern radiographic equipment and developing devices made roentgen diagnosis both more precise and far less time-consuming. Techniques of cardiopulmonary resuscitation were developed and improved.

Equipment needed to sustain life came within the financial reach of any hospital. For example, ventilators have become standard equipment; sophisticated monitoring devices are now available to community hospitals, not just to university centers; new pharmacologic agents have been introduced, and packaging techniques have improved startlingly. One has only to recall how long it once took a physician to prepare a single bottle of intravenous fluid to recognize the remarkable improvements in efficiency. Prepackaging of medications used for resuscitation also eliminated life-threatening delays.

Today's use of computers, although primitive in terms of their projected capabilities, serves to provide a glimpse of the future use of "electronic brains" as well as demonstrating immediate value for data retrieval and aid in diagnosis (Gorry, et al., 1968, 1973). Although the use of the computer to calculate and display a large range of physiologic variables immediately is as yet seen only in a few centers for the critically ill, the technology *is* available and will be applied more in the future—perhaps importantly in facilitating early diagnosis. But even now the Emergency Department has come to offer more help for the acutely ill or injured than is available in any other setting.

EARLY PROBLEMS

For minor problems, the Department can provide simple treatment on an outpatient basis and direct the patient into suitable channels when follow-up or continuing care is needed. However, staffing in the 1950s and 1960s often was difficult, primarily because of *(a)* lack of interest among physicians and *(b)* inadequate contractual and financial arrangements.

Furthermore, in this early period, the dearth of primary care physicians led to the use of emergency facilities for many non-acute illnesses. Faced by large patient volumes the emergency physician did not have time to deal with more serious, more challenging problems. In many hospitals, the emergency physician performed primarily a triage function, and sometimes was looked upon as a sort of perennial intern. Their status, already low in the eyes of many peers, was clouded further because, in general, physicians in Emergency Departments had no special training in the management of critically ill patients and learned their craft by experience and what few courses were available. In this age of certification, there was no certificate to acquire as proof of expertise in the management of emergency medical problems. Some physicians who were not so highly motivated or committed to their own re-education felt more at ease with the patient with minor problems, not with the critically ill. As experience and education acted to develop skilled emergency physicians, the nature of some practices made the application of such special abilities difficult—e.g., heavy loads of patients with nonacute conditions prevented concentration on more acute problems. Yet, a paradox existed: i.e., by treating such critically ill patients with care and skill, the practice was more gratifying and peer respect was won.

The basic motivations for most physicians, as for almost any other profession, are *(a)* prestige and peer respect, *(b)* adequate remuneration, *(c)* security. A persistent difficulty has been the maintenance of a balance between volume of patients and exercise of special, although time-consuming, skills. In such high patient volume settings, complex procedures are left for the "specialist." This attitude and the need to refer the difficult problems brought reduced peer respect as well as disagreeable economic problems. The specialist was on a fee-for-service basis, whereas his colleague in the Emergency Department often was salaried. Expansion of the responsibilities of the emergency physician was slowed by such economic pressures. This picture was altered radically when emergency physician groups began charging for their services.

In other instances, limited physician capabilities and, sometimes, staff by-laws made delays in extending the range of the Department inevitable. Many staff rules limiting what emergency physicians could do within their Department, often based on territorial considerations, also resulted in diminished peer acceptance and respect. Moreover, with a pressing service requirement, clinical research and development activities were difficult.

Nevertheless, medicine remains a field where the astute and able clinician is highly respected. There can be no separation between the growth of Emergency Medicine as a specialty and the growth in numbers of skilled emergency physicians. Regardless of how strong the political pressures exerted, the key to peer respect in Emergency Medicine is found in the demonstrable daily skills of those practicing in the field.

In the late 1960s and early 1970s, more physicians entered full-time emergency practice. Many had been in other fields and thus were termed "second-career" physicians. Relatively few had made Emergency Medicine their primary professional choice. Many of the "second-career" emergency physicians recognized their need for re-education in the management of acute illness and life-threatening injury.

The initial emphasis of these re-education studies was on trauma and on manipulative skills in surgery. The American College of Surgeons, which initiated many programs, was important, but the growth of the American College of Emergency Physicians, which later spearheaded such educational programs, was vital. The leaders who started the ACEP saw it grow rapidly and recognized that a major function of the College was the education of its members. The leaders also saw that specialty status was essential for the future growth of Emergency Medicine in order to attract young physicians and encourage a consistently high standard of care.

THE EMERGING SPECIALTY

By 1972, when postgraduate training programs were in their infancy, a meeting convened that resulted in a definition of an Emergency Medicine specialist as, "a physician who specializes in the immediate recognition and response to acute pathophysiology and in the administration, teaching and research of all systems related to any patient seeking emergency services."

The founders and early members of ACEP also brought to their task an additional element—pride and an awareness of the value of their work. This was later to have a substantial and positive influence on younger physicians choosing a specialty field. The "second-career" emergency physicians who were highly versed in patient evaluation and in performing life-saving treatment served as role models for their younger colleagues and medical students. Those physicians who had chosen Emergency Medicine as their primary career choice were often bright, enthusiastic young physicians committed to developing their field as a new specialty area.

Guided by the ACEP, pressures were exerted on the AMA and on the specialty groups, the goal being to provide the emergency physician with full recognition as a specialist. Shortly thereafter, the University Association for Emergency Medical Services, whose members were based at medical schools and university hospitals, joined the campaign.

In 1970, the Society for Critical Care Medicine was founded by academicians and scientists of varying specialty backgrounds. Most had intensive care units as their clinical base, but some demonstrated keen interest in the total emergency and critical care delivery system. The Society, together with the ACEP and the UAEMS, formed a federation that recognized some common objectives, one of which was the development of capable emergency physicians through residency programs. This was seen as a vital link in the medical care system.

OBJECTIONS TO SPECIALTY DEVELOPMENT

There were objections to the development of specialty and residency programs in Emergency Medicine. The basic argument was that because the emergency physician dealt with acute conditions involving organ systems usually cared for by other specialists, he could not be thought of as pursuing a specialty of his own. Further, it was argued that the care of a large patient population presenting a wide range of acute ailments required such extensive knowledge and so many skills that it would be impossible to define a specialty content. *Nevertheless, at the core of the developing specialty were skills involved in initial patient management and resuscitation not claimed by other medical specialties and subspecialties.* Furthermore, a serious need was present that could be met only by the presence of an emergency physician in the Department around the clock. When an acutely ill or severely injured patient arrived, evaluation and treatment had to be initiated by the emergency physician. Delay in such cases obviously was dangerous if the patient's welfare was the foremost consideration.

The other major objection to the recognition of Emergency Medicine as a specialty was related to the role of family physician frequently played by the Emergency Department in medically underserviced areas. In many emergency facilities, management of life-threatening conditions accounts for only a small percentage of the total medical problems treated. This situation, however, is changing somewhat as more family physicians enter active practice and as clinics and HMO's proliferate, with expanded evening hours for the care of routine illnesses. In some areas there is a relative decrease in total number of patients presenting at Emergency Departments when more family physicians open practices. At the same time, there has been an increase in the percentage of patients with more serious conditions seen in Emergency Departments—more ambulance arrivals, which tend to bring more serious conditions. Despite these trends, patients with so-called "non-urgent" conditions will always account for an appreciable part of the practice of Emergency Medicine. It should be remembered that what may not be an emergency in the eyes of the physician may well be an emergency to the patient, e.g., chest pain perceived by a patient as a "heart attack" is a true emergency— even if the final diagnosis is "anxiety reaction."

Even though relatively few life-threatening conditions may be treated each day by emergency physicians, once "boards" are established, Emergency Medicine will be a specialty with as much justification as any other specialized branch of medicine. It is too often forgotten that physicians are overtrained for what they usually do (i.e., the "routine problems"), but this hardly negates the need for extensive education and training. For example, the neurosurgeon usually spends most of his time dealing with conditions that do not require major neurologic surgery; similarly, most orthopedic problems do not require operative treatment—only routine management. To take another example, a gastroenterologist may be exquisitely

trained in endoscopic procedures and the management of serious gastroenterologic disease, but most of his patients do not require these finely tuned skills.

A similar situation obtains in Emergency Medicine. Some practitioners of this developing specialty are based in urban areas where knife and gun injuries are daily occurrences and where they are frequently called upon to treat critical illness. Others, particularly those in suburban community hospital settings, treat less dramatic trauma and spend more time evaluating patients who present with chest or abdominal pain. Nevertheless, all emergency physicians *must* have the core knowledge and the skill to initiate life-saving resuscitative measures and to provide prompt and correct evaluation in an emergency setting. These functions are pivotal in their influence on both prehospital care and subsequent critical care and on ambulance care. Regardless of whether two patients per day or 20 have serious disease, recognition of their condition is vital and requires both depth of knowledge and an understanding of the dynamics of the condition.

The persistent lack of standards for physicians who practiced Emergency Medicine became a thorn in the side of those committed to expertise in the field; moreover, the patient had no assurance. Although medical societies set down guidelines for who could practice surgery, who could give anesthesia, etc., the only requirement for assignment to an Emergency Department remained a license to practice in the state involved. Yet the emergency physician was responsible for life and death decisions and had to master the myriad skills required for resuscitation. Rarely did nomedical administrators inquire about a physician's special training or competence in acute care. A well-publicized study in 1969 showed that only one-third of American medical schools offered training in emergency care (Stephenson, 1969). The AMA and local Medical Societies provided no professional guidelines or standards. In fact, even as late as 1976, when such deficiencies were pointed out, one state medical society, rather than attempting to deal with these deficiencies, instead set out to castigate the physician who spoke up about its lack of standards. This sort of blindness, in the ancient tradition of killing the bearer of ill tidings, does not encourage high standards. Despite such occasional episodes of provincialism, the national organizations with broader perspective actively recognized the deficiencies and encouraged the development of specialty boards.

MODES OF PRACTICE ORGANIZATION

The concept of full-time emergency physicians with no other practice (the so-called "Alexandria Plan," named from where it originated) proved to be an effective way to organize an emergency group. However, despite such group development in the 1960s, insufficient full-time physicians often necessitated using part-time physicians or "moonlighting residents."

The senior editor of this textbook was a moonlighting resident during that period. Armed with his license and internship, he had been hired as the sole night-time physician in a busy city Emergency Department. There he was expected frequently to provide life-saving treatment and to handle difficult medical and surgical problems. On many mornings, following particularly rigorous nights, he asked himself whether he had a right to serve as emergency physician to the community. With so little training and experience, he was expected to make complex medical decisions and institute treatments where success frequently meant life for the patient.

Because the growth of Emergency Departments had exceeded the physician supply, staffing needs did not allow strict selection procedures; but without strict standards regarding training or experience for physicians providing emergency care, the variability in quality of treatment was substantial.

OTHER METHODS OF EMERGENCY DEPARTMENT STAFFING

Rotation of medical staff has been tried, as in the so-called "Pointiac Plan," but this was hardly an improvement. The disparities in skill are too great as each staff member takes his turn in the rotation. Certainly it offers no substitute for rigorous professional standards.

Multi-Hospital Groups

An important step may involve a newer mode of organization—the large multi-hospital emergency physician group. Important advantages already have been seen in those large groups with progressive leadership. Continuing education is improving, and quality of care review has been accomplished more readily. New programs can be initiated and special services offered by tapping a staff of 50 or 60 physicians rather than five or six at one hospital. Research activities can be accomplished more readily, thanks to a much expanded patient population. The problems of administration can be handled centrally, allowing physicians to focus more on patient care. Such groups also have the capability to try innovative techniques. And, of course, one important component is the security they offer to members, since Emergency Medicine is hospital-based and contractually established—often from year to year.

The aspect of increased security deserves special emphasis because, unlike a private practice of medicine where a physician can develop his own patients, regardless of how diligent the emergency physician is, he does not have his own practice. His work instead builds the hospital Emergency Department practice, which is contingent upon contract renewal by hospital administrators, a drawback that is at least partly overcome by being part of a large group. Non-renewal of one hospital contract is buffered by the existence of 10 or more hospitals under contract in the general vicinity.

Such large groups also can develop grants for research—a necessity if the field is to grow—and a facet hindered by the slow acceptance of departments of Emergency Medicine into most medical schools. Unfortunately, some of the multi-hospital groups are not taking advantage of their potential.

TIME AS A FURTHER FACTOR DEFINING EMERGENCY MEDICINE

In addition to resuscitation and initial patient management, another factor helps establish a meaningful definition for the field—the aspect of *time*. To "specialize," after all, really means to narrow one's focus of attention. For the emergency physician, this focus is on pathophysiologic alterations that occur within the first minutes or hours after the patient is seen and their progress or correction in that patient up to and including the first 24 hours of observation and treatment. That relatively few data exist dealing with the earliest changes in disease and trauma is in itself evidence of the lack of research attention given to this important time period by other specialties. Yet recognition and suitable treatment in the earliest stage of critical illness often have the most important beneficial effect on long-term outcome. For example, a successful resuscitation that keeps the brain viable during subsequent medical procedures has the greatest long-term significance for that patient.

The recognition of the *temporal limitation* is crucial in delineating specialty field content and in allowing the emergency physician to gain the knowledge in depth that is the hallmark of expertise. The depth is then defined and limited by time (e.g., 12 or 24 hours). This provides sufficient boundaries for researchers to gain a vast amount of information about the changes that occur during the initial period of acute illness of injury.

IDENTIFICATION OF SPECIAL SKILLS IN EMERGENCY MEDICINE

As training programs evolved, the need to focus on education to improve particular intellectual skills became evident. One function stood out as essential for the practice of Emergency Medicine—the decision-making ability. And, although leading educators do not know how best to educate physicians in this aspect (or even whether it is an ability that lends itself to an educational process), there is general agreement about its desirability.

The need for astute decision-making—frequently within the restrictions of a limited data base and necessarily brief periods of patient observation—presents complex intellectual tasks, the nature of which requires more study. Although prompt and accurate decision-making has always been an integral part of medicine, the Emergency Department is a site where this skill is constantly called upon. Patients frequently present with an undifferentiated symptom. To proceed from that point to a clinical impression or a diagnosis in the shortest possible time necessitates many clinical choices and the rapid integration of a wide array of inputs. It is critical to the patient's welfare that these functions be performed with the lowest possible risk of error. Implicit in the postgraduate training programs is application of this concept on a day-to-day basis.

EMERGENCY DECISION-MAKING UNIT

What was formerly termed a holding or observation area is changing to a newer concept of an Emergency Decision-making Unit. In such a facility, the patient's clinical course can be studied closely and monitored to improve the precision of early diagnosis. Such a unit provides the site for needed clinical investigation and the development of new diagnostic tests. Other intellectual-clinical skill areas also have been identified as goals in Emergency Medicine training. These are:

(*a*) Immediate response in particular critical situations.

(*b*) Stabilization of disrupted body systems and maintenance of failing organ systems.

(*c*) Triage abilities; i.e., to assess in a very brief time the relative severity of presenting problems.

Of course, there also has been continued concern with technical, surgical/manipulative abilities.

The identification of such particular goals in Emergency Medicine residency programs and the development of evaluative techniques serve further to define the specialty nature of the field.

CLINICAL PRACTICE OF THE EMERGENCY MEDICINE SPECIALIST

To apply to the fullest extent the special skills of the Emergency Medicine specialist sometimes may prove difficult; e.g., many Emergency Departments have a large patient volume. To treat large numbers of patients daily requires efficient organization, but even with the maximum efficiency the emergency physician with a pressing service load too often would be forced to refer the more challenging and complex patient problems to others, even though he is able to treat such patients with great skill.

Such a situation may not be the best environment for all specialists in Emergency Medicine. Above all, the emergency physician must be a superior clinician in the traditional sense: a diagnostician and a humanist. This takes time. There must be time to spend with the patients, time to deal with families enduring a crisis, and time to devote to resuscitation and stabilization. Sometimes a successful resuscitation requires hours. Facilities with high patient volume therefore can represent only one aspect of Emergency Medicine.

Reputations are never built on quantity. Expert resuscitation and precise decision-making both require time and depth of knowledge, and it is on performing such tasks well that the reputation of the Emergency Medicine specialist must rest. The development of the specialty of Emergency Medicine rests on the specialist emergency physician having a proper environment in which to apply his special skills.

THE CONSULTATIVE ROLE OF THE EMERGENCY SPECIALIST

As decision-making skills become finely tuned, patients will be referred to the emergency specialist by other physicians for emergency evaluation, diagnosis, and management. The development of this aspect of emergency practice is still, by and large, in its early stages. Nevertheless, it has proved successful in some instances—e.g., in the treatment of poisoning, cold injury, and snake bites, on which subjects certain emergency physicians have become expert.

The development of new emergency diagnostic instruments employing ultrasound, laser technology, and other scientific principles will encourage further use of the emergency physician as a consultant. Accuracy of diagnosis will be enhanced through wider use of mathematical models, computers, and the newer tests for stress and provocation. Techniques of decision analysis will make possible a fuller understanding of the sensitivity of diagnostic tests employed (Gorry, et al., 1973; Ginsberg, 1968; Ingelfinger, 1975; etc.).

ACCEPTANCE OF THE SPECIALTY

Concepts change slowly, and a development sometimes must wait for a new generation for full acceptance. Even so, it is evident that organized medicine has begun to accept the new specialty of Emergency Medicine, and there is widespread agreement that specialty content can be defined.

Physicians who have completed three years of postgraduate training are now entering clinical practice in increasing numbers. Both these newly trained residents and those younger practitioners who have made Emergency Medicine their primary career choice have begun to have a substantial impact on the field. These physicians have developed valuable skills and are expanding the diagnostic, monitoring, and therapeutic capabilities of medical practice in Emergency Departments. Those whose inclinations are toward research already are studying some heretofore unexplored areas. The impact of this first-line of trained emergency physicians on community hospitals has been encouraging and, although there has been insufficient time for comparative evaluation, it is apparent that the array of skills they bring will result in improved services to patients.

Although the basic skills and the most effective means to educate physician trainees require further study, much uniformity in the residency programs has resulted through review by the American College of Emergency Physicians. Moreover, the presence of four distinct career paths for those who complete the postgraduate programs are becoming clear. These are:

(a) Emergency group practice in urban or suburban hospitals

(b) Administrative positions in large groups or systems

(c) Faculty/teaching positions in medical school sections or departments

(d) Further fellowship training in critical care to become full-time staff in critical care units.

Of the four paths, the area of greatest need and general preference is (a), Group Practice. However, it is of great importance that many of the residents completing training return to university centers to become the core faculty of new postgraduate programs. Researchers are urgently needed as well. In this regard, a nationally funded research center in emergency care would be a giant step forward.

Emergency Medicine is unique because of its important nonclinical aspects, which are also being clarified. The Emergency Physician must provide the necessary knowledge and leadership for:

(1) The Emergency Response System. This includes transport and communication as well as the over-all organization of the Emergency Medical System and the direction of mobile ICU ambulances and EMT training.

(2) The administrative management of the Emergency Department, including the direction and training of nurses and paraprofessionals as well as the business aspects of the department and its interaction with government agencies.

EMERGENCY PHYSICIAN'S ROLE IN SYSTEMS DEVELOPMENT

For at least the past decade, physicians pioneering in emergency and critical care medicine have stressed that nationwide implementation of treatment guidelines could save money. It costs, for example, about 1 million dollars to maintain a patient for life who has sustained brain injury after cardiac arrest because of substandard or delayed initiation of proper care.

Even as recently as 1973, the shockingly poor state of most components of the EMS System were summarized in the documents that supported the EMS Systems Act. Among the deficiencies found were:

(a) About one-half of the nation's ambulances were operated by undertakers; one-quarter by volunteers.

(b) Almost no ambulance vehicles were adequately designed to permit life-support measures.

(c) Most Emergency Departments had no 24-hour coverage (Safar, 1976).

Spurred by the leaders in America, particularly those who visited other countries and saw how our nation was lagging behind some others in the effectiveness of EMS, recommendations were made. These were principally:

(1) Recognition of the emergency and first-aid by bystanders.

(2) EMS response systems—development of call numbers and training of the public.

(3) On-scene treatment by ambulance personnel.

(4) Transport with continued life support.

(5) Receiving patients and continuing intensive treatment in the Emergency Department to allow either stabilization or maintenance and rapid transfer to the critical care unit.

The role of the Emergency Department is crucial and emergency physicians are the obvious medical force to assist in EMS development, not only through providing training, but also by some physicians' assuming the helm of such systems. To rely on nonmedical administrators for a comprehensive understanding of an EMS system without emergency physician consultation and suitable direction is illogical and practically unsound. In fact, in some regions, emergency physicians clearly have spearheaded EMS development and have served as consultants in other areas.

More than in any other medical field, contact with the public, with paraprofessionals, and with legislators is required. Administrative abilities are being developed by some of the postgraduate education programs, and, although the emergency physician must first be a skillful clinician, the administrative role is vital for the development of adequate EMS systems. Those emergency physicians who further specialize in administration of emergency medical systems are in the position of understanding the roles and responsibilities at each level of personnel and can exert quality control.

Impartial medical experts must also work to develop regional centers so that patients with specific problems will have the greatest chance of a favorable outcome: e.g., spinal cord injury centers, trauma centers, etc.

Concomitant with the training of more Emergency Medicine specialists should be the development of special research and education centers in emergency and critical care medicine to attract the best minds to devote their efforts to improving the care of the critically ill or injured patient.

Although much of Emergency Medicine is, in Lewis Thomas' framework, "half-way technology," i.e., methods of postponing death or treating existent conditions, it is one area in which the cost-to-benefit ratio is potentially lowest, since a relatively small amount of well-placed effort can result in salvaging a productive life: e.g., defibrillating a heart in a younger person, treating shock from blood loss, etc. Thus, whereas the so-called "high technology" (embodying protection, prevention, and basic understanding of disease and cure) is certainly most desirable, Emergency Medicine offers potential benefits of "halfway technology" beyond those of other medical areas, and thus should receive a proportionately larger share of Federal funds in the future.

CONCLUSIONS

Emergency Medicine is developing as a specialty because of evolutionary changes in American medicine and profound changes in our society. There has been no great leap in scientific understanding or technologic development, but changes have reached a sufficiently high level so that the Emergency Department can offer special advantages for sick and injured patients. What has become evident is a great need for physicians to perform suitable tests and procedures that will facilitate rapid diagnosis and improve on-the-spot treatment. Those in the field are working to develop new tests and to stimulate clinical research that will increase diagnostic accuracy. Suitable standards, long overdue, are being developed now with care and sophistication.

More years must pass before Emergency Medicine can become a separate department in most medical schools. Political struggles are just beginning. There will be opposition, some of it based on valid reasoning. For example, board certification procedures must be established, and we must have enough well-trained emergency physicians to make up a core faculty. Others will object because of self-interest and territoriality, and simple inertia will, in some instances, slow the trend.

But, when emergency physicians demonstrate that they can improve patient care, and as valuable research material is produced, the place of the specialty will become secure. There is no stopping an idea whose time has come.

References

Barnoon, S., and Wolfe, H.: Measuring the Effectiveness of Medical Decisions. Springfield, Ill., Charles C Thomas, 1972.

Barry, R., Shortliffe, E., and Wetstone, H.: Hospital emergency departments: case study predicts load variation patterns. Hospitals 34:34, 1960.

Boyd, D., and Flashner, B.: The Critically Injured Patient: Concept and the Illinois Statewide Plan for Trauma Centers. Illinois Department of Public Health,

Division of Emergency Medical Services, May 1972, p. 67.

DeHoff, J. B.: Emergency departments: multi-purpose medical centers. Maryland Med. J. 21:2, 55–57, 1972.

Dickson, J.: Automation in Clinical Laboratories, Proceedings of Institute of Electrical and Electronics Engineers. 57:1974, 1969.

Gibson, G.: Guidelines for research and evaluation of emergency medical services. Health Services Reports 89:2, 99, 1974.

Ginsberg, A. S., and Ofensend, F. L.: An application of decision theory to a medical diagnosis-treatment problem. IEEE Transactions on Systems Science and Cybernetics, 4:3, Sept. 1968.

Gorry, G. A., et al.: Decision analysis as the basis for computer-aided management of acute renal failure. Am. J. Med. 55:473, 1973.

Gorry, G. A., and Barnett, G. O.: Sequential diagnosis by computer. J.A.M.A. 205:849, 1968.

Graves, H. B.: Interview-emergency medicine progress. J. Am. Coll. Emerg. Physicians 5:1, 55, 1976.

Gross, P. F.: Development and Implementation of Health Care Technology: The U.S. Experience. Inquiry, IX:2, 34–45, 1970.

Hanlon, J. J.: Emergency Medical Care as a Comprehensive System. Health Services Reports 88:579, 1973.

Harrison, T. R.: The most distressing symptom. J.A.M.A. 198:1, 170, 1966.

Haviland, J. W.: Why so long? Accreditation or recognition for emergency medicine. J. Am. Coll. Emerg. Physicians 5:2, 133, 1976.

Huntley, H. C.: National Status of Emergency Health Services. Proceedings of the 2nd National Conference on Emergency Health Services, Dec. 2–4, 1971. Publication No. DEHS-16, Washington, D.C., U.S. Government Printing Office, 1966.

Ingelfinger, F. J.: Decision in medicine. N. Engl. J. Med. 293:5, 254, 1975.

Jelliffe, R. W.: Quantitative aspects of clinical judgment. Am. J. Med. 55:4, 431, 1973.

Katz, M. A.: A probability graph describing the predictive value of a highly sensitive diagnosis test. Med. Intelligence 291:21, 1115, 1974.

Kosasa, T. S., et al.: Use of a radioimmunoassay specific for HCG in Dx of early ectopic pregnancy. Obstet. Gynecol. 42:868, 1973.

Lee, S., Solon, J., and Sheps, C.: How new patterns of medical care affect the emergency unit. Mod. Hosp. 94:97, 1960.

Lusted, L. B.: Decision-making studies in patient management. N. Engl. J. Med. 284:416, 1971.

McNeil, B. J., Keeler, E., and Adelstein, S. J.: Primer on certain elements of medical decision-making. N. Engl. J. Med. 293:5, 211, 1975.

Mills, J. D.: Emergency medicine: a developing specialty. J. Am. Coll. Emerg. Physicians. 2:2, 113–115, 1973.

National Academy of Sciences – National Research Council: Accidental Death and Disability: The Neglected Disease of Modern Society. Washington, D.C., 1966.

Paulker, S. G., and Kassirer, J. P.: Therapeutic decision making: a cost-benefit analysis. N. Engl. J. Med. 293:5, 229, 1975.

Powers, D. L., and Mandell, G. L.: Intraleukocytic bacteria in endocarditis patients. J.A.M.A. 227:3, 312, 1974.

Proliferation of certification in medical specialities: productive or counterproductive? Sounding Board 294:9, 497, 1976.

Raiffa, H.: Decision Analysis: Introductory lectures on choices under uncertainty. Reading. Mass., Addison-Wesley Publishing Company, 1968, p. 240.

Rasmussen, H.: Medical education—revolution or reaction. Pharos 38:2, 53, 1975.

Rockwell, M., et al.: Shock III—a computer system as an aid in the management of critically ill patients. Communication of Association for Computing Machinery. 9:355, 1966.

Rosenfield, L. S., et al.: Regional Emergency Medical Services in North Carolina: Monitoring and Evaluation. University Program in Health Services Evaluation, University of North Carolina at Chapel Hill, 1974.

Safar, P.: Testimony before the U.S. Senate Health Subcommittee, Jan. 23, 1976.

Satin, D. G., and Duhl, F. J.: Help?: The hospital emergency unit as community physician. Med. Care X:3, 248, 1972.

Schwartz, W. B., Gorry, G. A., and Kassirer, J. P.: Decision analysis and clinical judgment. Am. J. Med. 55:459, 1973.

Siegel, J. H., and Strom, B. L.: An Automated Consultation System to Aid the Physician in the Care of the Desperately Sick Patient. In Stacy, R. W., and Waxman, B. D. (eds.): Computers in Biomedical Re-search. New York, and London, Academic Press, 1972.

Siegel, J. H., et al.: A computer-based clinical assessment, research, and education system to facilitate continuing education in the care of the critically ill patient. Surgery 68:238, 1970.

Siegel, J. H., and Strom, B. L.: The computer as a "living textbook" applied to the care of the critically injured patient. J. Trauma 12:739–753, 1972.

Southwick, A. F.: The Hospital as an institution—expanding responsibilities change its relationship with the staff physician. California Western Law Review 9:429, 1973.

Spiro, H. M.: My kingdom for a camera—some comments on medical technology. N. Engl. J. Med. 291:20, 1070, 1974.

Straus, R.: Departments and disciplines: stasis and change. Science 182:895, 1973.

Walker, L. L.: Inpatient and emergency department utilization: the effect of distance, social class, age, sex and marital status. J. Am. Coll. Emerg. Physicians 5:2, 105, 1976.

Williamain, T. R.: The Status of Performance Measures for Emergency Medical Services. Technical Report, TR-06-74, Operations Research Center, M.I.T., Cambridge, Mass., 1974.

Part I

PATHOPHYSIOLOGY OF VITAL ORGAN SYSTEMS FAILURE

OVERVIEW OF PART I

Staff physicians and physician trainees working in Emergency Departments are confronted with the broadest spectrum of problems seen anywhere in the health care system. These range from minor complaints or injuries, which could be handled by the primary or family physician, to critical illnesses or injuries with multiple organ failure, which should be managed by a team of specialists coordinated by a physician with special competence in critical care medicine. Although at this time in the U.S. only about 2 to 5 per cent of patients coming to hospital Emergency Departments are critically ill or injured, Emergency Department personnel should be knowledgeable about the pathophysiology and therapy of acute life-threatening conditions for at least two reasons:

1. Emergency Department physicians will be seeing an ever-increasing number of critically ill or injured patients as regionalized centralization of special care decreases the number of Emergency Departments. Furthermore, the proportion of critically ill patients will increase as patients with minor complaints are seen more consistently by primary or family physicians outside the Emergency Department.

2. The Emergency Department physician is the pivotal figure in determining the effectiveness of the entire Emergency Medical Services System.* Through his command of paramedics attending patients before they reach the hospital, through the care he and his staff render the patient in the Emergency Department, and through his influence on the organization and standards of the entire

___

Part I is dedicated to the memory of Dr. Herbert Shubin, a pioneering clinical investigator on vital organ systems failure.

*The Emergency Medical Services System consists of: (1) Recognition of the emergency and aid by bystanders. (2) Initiation of the Emergency Medical Services response system. (3) Rescue, extrication, and treatment at the scene by members of the System. (4) Transportation with life support. (5) Treatment in the most appropriate Emergency Department. (6) Treatment in the operating room. (7) Treatment in the intensive care unit. (8) Organization and communication for (1)–(7). (9) Planning, education, and evaluation for (1)–(8). (10) Research. (From Safar, P.: Public Health Aspects of Critical Care Medicine and Anesthesiology, Chapter 4. Philadelphia, F. A. Davis Co., 1974; and Club of Mainz Recommendations. J. Am. Coll. Emergency Physicians *4/1*:60, 1975.)

system, the Emergency Department physician significantly affects the quality of care accorded critically ill patients.

Part I of this book treats the fundamentals of multiple vital organ systems failure, with the object of adding to the basic concepts in physiology, pathology, and therapeutics acquired in medical school some newer emergency care-oriented information. Relevance of this information to life support measures is stressed, since, in a book for clinicians, reviews of pathophysiologic mechanisms cannot and should not be viewed entirely separate from therapeutics. It is hoped that Part I will stimulate emergency and critical care physicians to re-orient their patient care attitudes and habits from "management by rounding and prescription"—the common practice in managing patients hospitalized for noncritical illness—to "management by titration." The latter requires personal, continuous monitoring of vital organ systems' function and titrating therapeutic interventions from moment to moment according to clinical observations, changes of measured variables, and the physician's knowledge of the pathophysiologic mechanisms involved. All this is done in an attempt to restore optimal homeostasis through correction of deranged physiologic variables.

Titrated life support measures should commence upon recognition of the emergency in the pre-hospital phases of care, and should be continued until pharmacologic, surgical, or divine intervention corrects the underlying disorder—or until the patient dies or is considered hopeless. Practical experience with such titrated management is best acquired through supervised life support practice in physiology and resuscitation laboratories, operating room anesthesia and intensive care units.

Chapter 2 summarizes the events occurring in acute, potentially lethal conditions, since such events best illustrate the dynamics of acute multiple organ failure and its reversal. Chapters 3–7 deal with newer concepts on the failure of the respiratory, circulatory, central nervous, and renal systems, as well as with the metabolic and endocrine response to trauma. These chapters focus on subacute (not immediately lethal) deteriorations, and stress the fact that uncompensated single organ system failure almost invariably leads to multiple organ system failure and, if not reversed, to death.

These pages provide a deeper understanding of the mechanisms involved in often reversible dying processes and should thereby promote recognition of the need for early and continuing resuscitative efforts — at the scene, during transportation, in the Emergency Department, and, in selected cases, during early transfer to special care centers. We hope that such understanding will lead to improvements in initial care of the critically ill and injured so that the need for subsequent advanced, expensive intensive care — all too often incapable of influencing processes gone beyond reversibility — can be minimized.

Acknowledgments: Dr. Nancy Caroline added valuable ideas in the writing and edited Chapters 2 and 5, and Ms. Vicki Shidel assisted with the preparation of the manuscripts of Part I.

Chapter 2

THE MECHANISMS OF DYING AND THEIR REVERSAL

Peter Safar

INTRODUCTION

This chapter summarizes what we know of the general pathophysiologic events which occur during dying and resuscitation. There remain, however, many unanswered questions in this field, owing to a paucity of studies on dying processes in man — whether the death be precipitate and unexpected or slow and expected ("natural"). Controlled *clinical* data have, for obvious reasons, been difficult if not impossible to obtain, and controlled *animal* studies can be applied only in limited respects to man. Further, some dying processes are still poorly understood and resuscitation techniques still unproved because of the great variety of animal models used by different investigators — models which do not, in many instances, adequately simulate actual clinical events.* However, as we shall discuss later, some valuable information has been gained from laboratory experiments, starting with the pioneering work of Swann in the U.S. (1949) and Negovskii's group in Moscow (1962) in the 1940s, up to 1974/75 when this chapter was written.

The late Claude Beck of Cleveland, whose vision not only resulted in the first successful internal defibrillation of the human heart in 1947, but also in the concept of "the heart too good to die" (most primary cardiac deaths are reversible!) stated in his introduction to Negovskii's book on resuscitation (1962):

...our attitudes must be revolutionized because the experiment is far beyond the clinician.

---

*A. Gurvich, 1974; Lind, 1975.

This revolution would be facilitated if we had in this country an institute for the study of the Environment of Death. One such institute (comparable to our many cancer institutes) would focus attention on the prevention of death, the reversal of death and the complex biological problems of the dying process. There is scarcely any more pressing medical problem. Strange, indeed, that America needs this nudge from Russia — and fortunate that we have had it.

In the U.S., the development of resuscitation techniques and emergency cardiac care systems began to flourish during the 1960s and 1970s, and many "hearts too good to die" have been salvaged as a consequence (Beck, 1960). However, an institute for the study of dying and resuscitation still does not exist. The issue of the 1970's has become "brains too good to die." Therefore, specialists from various disciplines should now be drawn together for the study of acute dying processes and their reversal, with emphasis on the target organ of resuscitation: the human brain.

The viability of the brain defines human life. In the absence of therapeutic intervention, the terminal stages of life, in both rapid and protracted dying, are followed by biologic *panorganic death*, i.e., irreversible over-all tissue destruction (Fig. 1). This is a slow process, ranging from an estimated 10 minutes required for some brain cells to die, to about 20 to 30 minutes for the cardiac muscle to cease electric activity, to hours or days for epidermal cells to cease replication. In view of this variable longevity of different body tissues, *brain death* (Chapter 5) (Grenvik, 1974) has recently been designated as the most meaningful indicator of death in a human sense. By contrast to brain death, *clinical death* occurs immediately upon car-

STAGES AND REVERSIBILITY OF DYING

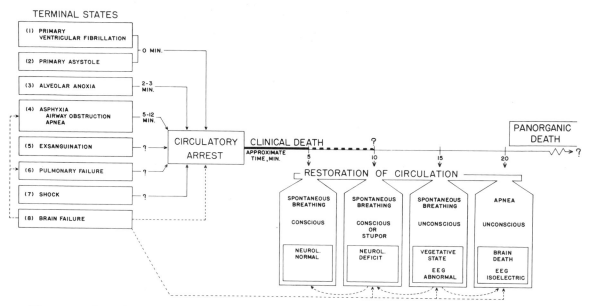

Figure 1. Flow chart illustrating diagrammatically the development of circulatory arrest from eight basic variations of terminal states; clinical death with reversible brain failure, with its presently undefinable duration; and the various possible outcomes.

diac arrest and is defined as "the period of respiratory, circulatory, and brain arrest during which initiation of resuscitation can lead to recovery with pre-arrest central nervous system (CNS) function" (Negovskii, 1962; Safar, 1974a).

Until recently, patient and animal data indicated that cessation of circulation longer than about five minutes resulted in irreversible neurohistologic changes and neurologic deficit (Gurvitch; Stephenson, 1974). However, the temporal limits of clinical death are no longer so certain.

Recent investigations in our laboratory have shown that special, immediate postresuscitative therapy aimed at transiently depressing cerebral metabolism (i.e., barbiturate loading) or promoting the cerebral reperfusion with blood, can result in complete neurologic recovery of monkeys after 16 minutes of total brain ischemia, and of dogs after 12 minutes of ventricular fibrillation (Safar; Bleyaert, 1975). Both insults, without such special post-ischemic therapy, result in permanent severe neurologic deficit, coma, or death as assessed by the termination of the study one week after the insult. In the above studies, periods of clinical

death are preceded by adequate arterial oxygen transport. Other studies, however, have indicated that, if preceded by low oxygen transport—as in asphyxia, anemic hypoxia (carbon monoxide poisoning), or shock states—and not followed by newer methods of postresuscitative therapy, clinical death of *less* than five minutes may result in irreversible neurologic damage. Under such circumstances, the brain may sometimes be irreversibly damaged even before cessation of circulation.

When the circulation is restarted soon after the end of the period of clinical death, the result is recovery of spontaneous breathing and consciousness or stupor, with some residual neurologic deficit (Fig. 1). Little animal or human data are available concerning the integrity of the higher, more subtle activities of the human brain after resuscitation. There have been few, if any, attempts to measure impairment of learned knowledge, loss of skills, or derangement of emotions resulting from ischemic-anoxic insults in patients who have apparently achieved full neurologic recovery (Bengtsson, 1969; Barber, 1970).

If restoration of circulation is delayed

further beyond the limits of clinical death (exactly how long is not known), resuscitation results in return of spontaneous breathing, but continued coma with an abnormal electroencephalogram (EEG),* i.e., the *vegetative state* (coma prolongé); and if delayed even longer, the result is persistent apnea and coma with an isoelectric EEG, namely *brain death* (coma depassé) (Fig. 1). In brain death, the entire brain is irreversibly functionally silenced, but spinal cord reflexes may continue (Grenvik, 1974). When there is no restoration of circulation, the result is biologic or panorganic death. While brain death is by definition irreversible, the vegetative state may secondarily lead either to brain death or sometimes to awakening, with variable defects persisting.

Although resuscitation attempts are almost always indicated in the acute situation, subsequent intensive care should be terminated when brain damage becomes certain and there appears to be no chance that human life with mentation can be restored on the basis of available knowledge (Safar, 1963). Where cardiopulmonary resuscitation (CPR) attempts inside or outside the hospital have succeeded in restoring some cerebral oxygenation within about four minutes of arrest, and adequate spontaneous circulation is accomplished within minutes thereafter, one-half to two-thirds of patients so treated recovered completely, with CNS function judged equivalent to that in the pre-arrest state (Safar, 1974b). Most of the remaining patients died before leaving the hospital from complications secondary to coma or from their underlying diseases. Among the long-term survivors of all CPR attempts, including the delayed attempts, about 20 per cent seem to have permanent major neurologic deficit (Lund, 1973; Bell, 1974; Schaffer, 1975). These survivors with unremitting neurologic damage represent a great burden to their families, society at large, and, if the patient has recovered to the point of recognition of his own defects, to himself as well.

Dying in the terminal stages of incurable disease is not cardiac arrest. We define *cardiac arrest* as "the clinical picture of sudden cessation of circulation in a person who was not expected to die at that time" (Safar, 1963). Cardiac arrest is clinically diagnosed when at least the following four conditions coexist: (1) unconsciousness; (2) apnea or gasping respirations; (3) pulselessness in large arteries (carotid, femoral); and (4) deathlike appearance.

Cardiac arrest may be primary, as in sudden, complete cessation of cardiac pumping action, or secondary, as initiated rapidly or more slowly by non-cardiac causes (Fig. 1).

Examples of *primary* cardiac arrest include VF (common) or asystole (less common) in patients with ischemic heart disease and in VF from electric shock (Fig. 1, conditions 1 and 2). Such sudden primary cessation of circulation in well-oxygenated persons results in unconsciousness within about 10 seconds and an isoelectric EEG in about 30 seconds; agonal gasping may continue for 30 to 60 seconds; and apnea and maximal pupillary dilatation begin at about 60 seconds.

Examples of *rapid secondary* cardiac arrest include: alveolar anoxia (e.g., inhalation of oxygen-free gas; fulminating pulmonary edema); asphyxia (airway obstruction, apnea); and exsanguination (Fig. 1, conditions 3–5). Examples of *slow secondary* cardiac arrest are severe hypoxemia, as in subacute pulmonary edema or consolidation (Chapter 3), various shock states (Chapter 4), and intracranial pathology (Chapter 5) (Fig. 1, conditions 6–8), any of which may stop the circulation within minutes, hours, or days.

In this chapter we shall first describe the pathophysiologic changes occurring during the terminal state and resuscitation as observed in one example, exsanguination. Then we shall comment briefly on the fundamentals of a variety of dying mechanisms. Finally, a selection of specific lethal conditions will be summarized (Fig. 1). Although the basic steps of CPR (Airway, Breathing, Circulation) are applicable in most cases of sudden death (Safar, 1968), definitive therapeutic measures (CPR step D) inevitably differ with the different mechanisms of terminal states.

THE TERMINAL STATE

The "terminal state" begins with decompensation of the organism's defenses from derangement of vital organ systems.

---

*An alphabetical list of abbreviations and terms and their definitions is given at the end of this chapter (p. 47).

The pathophysiologic pattern and duration of the terminal state vary to some extent with the initiating cause of dying (Fig. 1). In exsanguination cardiac arrest, for instance, the terminal state includes the following:

(1) *Sequential losses,* first of rational mentation, then of consciousness, airway, breathing, and circulation.

(2) *Terminal apnea,* when profound hypotension or pulselessness supervene.

(3) *Agonal state,* i.e., the period during which, following the onset of pulselessness (cessation of circulation) and the brief period of terminal apnea, gasping respirations and sometimes also low arterial pressure pulsations return (Negovskii, 1962).

(4) *Clinical death,* namely coma, apnea, no gasping, no pulse (no blood flow), but CNS failure still reversible.

The mobilization of compensatory mechanisms, for instance protection of the cerebral cortex by maximal vasodilatation, will depend on the rapidity of arrest. Whereas in acute respiratory insufficiency or shock states, tissue deprivation of oxygen and substrate usually progresses sufficiently slowly for compensatory mechanisms to come into play, rapid exsanguination and other precipitate causes of cardiac arrest do not permit these mechanisms to develop. We will use the observations on exsanguination cardiac arrest in dogs made by Negovskii's group (1962, 1974) and by our group (Kirimli, 1965, 1969, 1970) as prototypes to describe the general pattern and mechanisms of sudden death and its reversal. When reference is made to other causes of dying and other species, it will be so stated.

DYING

In awake dogs under opiate or barbiturate sedation, exsanguination through a femoral artery cannula induces hyperventilation, arterial hypotension, tachycardia, and agitation within the first one to two minutes, owing to the well-known protective reflexes of the carotid and aortic pressor- and chemoreceptors and to discharges from many regions of the brain. From Minutes 5 to 8, the heart rate begins to decrease, the electrocardiogram (EKG) shows signs of myocardial ischemia, and the animal begins to grow somnolent. During Minutes 8 to 15, the animal continues to breathe regularly, but at a slower rate, the heart rate decreases further (due to increased vagal tone), and the mean systemic arterial pressure (SAP) falls to 20 to 30 torr when about one-half of the blood volume has been lost. Such rapid hemorrhage results in an acute decrease in hematocrit caused by a decrease in intravascular pressure and subsequent transfer of extravascular fluid into the vascular compartment.

At this point, sludging and segmentation become apparent in the retinal arteries, and the brain begins to fail: the animal is comatose, the cerebral arteriovenous oxygen difference is greatly increased, and brain metabolism begins to switch from the aerobic form to the more primitive anaerobic form (glycolysis) (Fig. 2).

Just before the onset of pulselessness, electrocortical silence and apnea start; although the arterial P_{O_2} is still normal, the arterial P_{CO_2} is low (from hyperventilation),

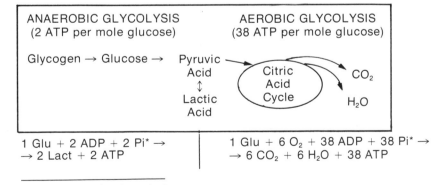

CELLULAR GLUCOSE METABOLISM

ANAEROBIC GLYCOLYSIS (2 ATP per mole glucose)	AEROBIC GLYCOLYSIS (38 ATP per mole glucose)
Glycogen → Glucose → Pyruvic Acid ↕ Lactic Acid	Citric Acid Cycle → CO_2 / H_2O
1 Glu + 2 ADP + 2 Pi* → → 2 Lact + 2 ATP	1 Glu + 6 O_2 + 38 ADP + 38 Pi* → → 6 CO_2 + 6 H_2O + 38 ATP

*Pi = Inorganic phosphate

Figure 2. Diagram of cellular energy metabolism for glucose.

and the blood-base deficit is only slight because terminal circulation is inadequate to wash out fixed acids accumulating in the ischemic-anoxic tissues. Circulation and bleeding stop when total blood loss is about one-half to two-thirds of estimated blood volume, with an SAP (aortic pressure) of about 15 torr without pulse waves. EKG complexes continue. Onset of pulselessness is accompanied by abolition of corneal and lid reflexes, by pupillary dilatation, and cessation of retinal capillary flow.

The rate at which hypotension, coma, and pulselessness develop depends on the speed of exsanguination, the anesthesia used, and several other factors. Usually, circulation stops in asystole. In about 5 per cent of the dogs, spontaneous ventricular fibrillation developed after about 4 to 5 minutes of pulselessness. A higher incidence of ventricular fibrillation occurred later, during resuscitative efforts, when the heart was massaged.

The agonal state which follows is of varying duration (two or more minutes) and is characterized by resumption of gasping respirations, which are a sign that the bulbar centers are still active. The agonal gasps are insufficient to ventilate the lungs, since inspiratory, expiratory, and auxiliary muscles contract simultaneously. In about 50 per cent of the animals, the mean SAP rises transiently to about 20 to 30 torr with good pulsations, which occasionally may be accompanied by a brief recovery of the EEG and consciousness. When these last flickers of life, which are inadequate for "self-resuscitation" cease, clinical death begins. EKG complexes continue for some time during clinical death at a diminishing rate (anoxic depression), first with sinus rhythm, later with nodal and ventricular rhythms, and finally (at the end of five minutes of clinical death) with bizarre biphasic or monophasic ventricular complexes.

During dying, cerebral cortical function fails first, while the phylogenetically older brain stem and medulla (respiratory and vasomotor centers) continue to function, although in a disorganized fashion.

When mean SAP decreases to about 30 torr or less, the EEG develops high amplitude sinusoidal delta waves and, with progressive ischemia-anoxia, a decrease in frequency and amplitude; finally, there is electrical silence. Electric discharges from the reticular formation are the last to cease.

Biochemical Events in the Brain. During dying, metabolic changes in all organs reflect depletion of oxygen and substrate and accumulation of metabolic end-products (Drewes; Siesjö, 1973). The brain's energy requirements must be met entirely by glucose metabolism (Fig. 2), whereas the heart and other vital organs can—at least in part—get energy also from metabolizing fat and proteins. Normally, at least 95 per cent of brain metabolism goes all the way to the high energy-producing aerobic form of glucose metabolism, which occurs primarily in mitochondria and which produces 38 moles of ATP per mole of glucose (or 690,000 calories). In contrast, oxygen deprivation results in partial or complete interruption of the glucose metabolism at the end of the anaerobic pathway, i.e., burning glycogen via glucose only to pyruvic and lactic acid. This results in an accumulation of lactic acid and an increase in the lactate–pyruvate ratio (Huckabee, 1958). This anaerobic metabolism produces only 2 moles of ATP per mole of glucose (or 54,000 calories) (Fig. 2).

Hypoxemia below a PaO_2 of 50 torr without circulatory arrest causes an increase in brain intra- and extracellular lactate, and below a PaO_2 of 35 torr, also a decrease in phosphocreatine. These and even more severe degrees of hypoxemia which reduce cerebral venous PO_2 to 10 torr (normally about 30 torr), however, will not be accompanied by a significant decrease in brain ATP, as long as there is no drastic decrease in SAP, because of compensatory cerebral vasodilatation and a sixfold increase in glucose metabolism during anoxia (Pasteur effect) (Siesjö, 1973). Thus, as long as there is *some* perfusion, a reduction in PaO_2 must be very severe to reduce total brain energy production and thus threaten neuronal survival.

Sudden circulatory arrest, in contrast, induces unconsciousness and a flat EEG immediately after the brain oxygen stores have become exhausted and aerobic brain metabolism ceases. Given *oxygen stores* (which are mainly in capillary hemoglobin) of about 0.26 μmole/gm. brain and a cerebral oxygen consumption of approximately 1.5 μmoles/gm. brain per minute, brain oxygen stores are depleted within less than 10 seconds of circulatory arrest. This equals the time to unconsciousness.

Brain glucose stores, based on an anaerobic glucose consumption of about

1.5 μmoles/gm. brain per minute will last only about four minutes for anaerobic energy metabolism (Nemoto, personal communication). As brain ATP and glucose are consumed, brain lactic acid, ADP, AMP, and inorganic phosphate accumulate. In about four to five minutes of clinical death, brain glycolysis and attendant lactic acid production cease. At five minutes of circulatory arrest, brain ATP has decreased to less than 25 per cent of normal (Michenfelder, 1970) and brain phosphocreatine to zero (Negovskii, 1974). In rats, brain ATP is zero after 15 minutes of circulatory arrest (Siesjö, 1973). It is encouraging to learn that there is this biochemical basis for the clinical period of circulatory arrest tolerated by the brain—i.e., four to five minutes.

In summary, cessation of aerobic glucose metabolism within seconds is followed by cessation of anaerobic glucose metabolism within minutes, beyond which point energy production and, therefore, cell membrane mitochrondrial and enzyme functions cease, and irreversible cellular changes begin. It seems unlikely that circulatory arrest of more than five minutes allows complete functional restoration of all neurons, unless new resuscitative measures are employed which have not yet been studied in terms of their metabolic effects.

RESUSCITATION

The pattern of recovery after arrest, starting with *restoration of circulation*, varies with different species, mechanisms of dying, experimental models, and resuscitative techniques. In normothermic unanesthetized dogs after exsanguination cardiac arrest, complete neurologic recovery is possible if clinical death lasted less than about five minutes. For resuscitation, Negovskii used rapid *arterial* reinfusion of the arterially shed, oxygenated, heparinized blood (which, under clinical circumstances, is not immediately available) with epinephrine added; intermittent positive pressure ventilation (IPPV) with air was also provided (1962). Cardiac compression is not necessary in this situation, since the arterial reinfusion perfuses the coronary arteries in a retrograde fashion, which restarts cardiac electrical activity immediately and spontaneous mechanical activity within seconds. Within one to two minutes, after 10 to 20 per cent of the shed blood has been reinfused,

spontaneous circulation with near-normal arterial perfusion pressure is re-established.

When volume is repleted through the *venous* route and circulation restored with external cardiac compression, spontaneous circulation returns, but not quite as rapidly as with arterial reperfusion; however, venous infusion is effective also with the use of readily available plasma substitutes (Ringer's solution, dextran) and bank blood, whereas these nonoxygenated, acidic solutions often fail to restore spontaneous circulation when given through the arterial route (Kirimli, 1965, 1969). Venous infusion plus CPR permits oxygenation of blood and blood substitutes on the way through the lungs. However, different blood substitutes vary in their effectiveness. The infusion of Ringer's solution alone, for example, in a volume two and one-half times that of the volume of blood shed, can restore circulation, but cannot sustain arterial pressure. With more salt solution tissue edema results. In contrast, colloid solutions infused in volumes equal to those of the blood shed enable survival in 100 per cent of animals. With either the arterial or venous technique, heart pumping action can easily be restored, even after circulatory arrest of up to about 10 minutes. The EKG recovers in mirror image sequence of its disappearance—namely, first with ventricular, then nodal, and finally, sinus rhythms. After four minutes of reperfusion, spontaneous *breathing* resumes, signalling respiratory center recovery. The first gasps appear to return earlier when ventilation is with air rather than 100 per cent oxygen. This does not imply that ventilation with air is to be preferred over that with oxygen; it may merely indicate that the hypoxic and acidotic stimuli are less profound when high oxygen concentrations are used. Spontaneous breathing returns first with agonal gasping, which is replaced by a pattern of periodic respirations (Cheyne-Stokes) with a higher than normal frequency, and then by normal respiratory patterns with interposed gasps, which progressively diminish until a fully normal breathing pattern is established.

The vasomotor center recovers at the same time breathing begins. Continuation of the more primitive gasping type respirations for over 20 minutes after the beginning of reperfusion is a poor prognostic sign in terms of cerebral recovery. Following return of the first gasps, corneal reflexes, EEG, and muscular tone recover in rapid sequence. At about five minutes of reperfusion, the pupils start constricting.

The *cerebral cortex* is more vulnerable than the brain stem to the effects of hypoperfusion, and therefore recovers more slowly. Although anesthesia and hypothermia induced before and maintained during circulatory arrest protect the cortex to some extent, in the normothermic unanesthetized animal the sequence of EEG recovery is not always the mirror image of the disappearance of electric impulses during dying, probably because of many small, scattered areas of underperfusion persisting in the brain during the postresuscitative period (Ames, 1968).

Usually EEG recovery first takes the form of sinusoidal oscillations (nine to 12 per second), forming spindles, which are synchronous with breathing movements. The brain stem provokes electrical cortical activity at a time when the cortex itself is inactive. The spindles have some prognostic significance: they occur after long periods of clinical death which results in permanent neurologic deficit; spindles are not, however, common after either very long periods of clinical death resulting in brain death or after short periods of clinical death (or newer postresuscitative therapy) resulting in complete CNS recovery. Spastic breathing and focal or generalized convulsions are poor prognostic signs but, if controlled, can be followed by near-normal CNS recovery.

At 24 hours after restoration of circulation, the EEG appears grossly normal, even when the animal is still uncoordinated. Nonetheless, subtle EEG abnormalities can be seen throughout the first week, and these EEG derangements often may be worsened by postresuscitative complications. Such secondary worsening of the cerebral status has been seen (*a*) on the second day in monkeys after 20 minutes of total cerebral ischemia (secondary silencing of the EEG with intracranial hypertension) (Bleyaert, 1973; Nemoto, 1975); and (*b*) on Days 5 to 7 postischemia in dogs after over five minutes of clinical death from exsanguination (Negovskii, 1974; Nemoto, 1977).

In man, with sluggish CNS recovery, subtle changes can be seen which are not obvious in animals. Slow awakening involves passage through stages of rigidity, mental stupor and sensory aphasia, and retarded inarticulate speech and disorientation in space and time. Impaired memory and peculiar behavior last for some time. Memory and intellect may be completely or partially restored. After two weeks, any further restoration of CNS function is very slow (Negovskii; A. Gurvitch, 1974).

Although the resistance of the brain to hypoxia has definite limits, these have not yet been precisely defined. Individual neuronal cells (as distinguished from mentation) can recover in terms of protein metabolism and electric activity following circulatory arrest of as long as 60 minutes in cats (Hossmann, 1973). In dogs, continuous EEG recovery with an amplitude greater than 25 to 50 μvolts within five minutes of the beginning of reperfusion is a favorable sign, whereas delay in EEG recovery beyond 30 minutes (in the absence of CNS depressant drugs) is an unfavorable one. Sustained reduction in cerebral oxygen consumption and cerebral blood flow (CBF) due to ischemic anoxia to 20 to 40 per cent of normal or less suggests permanent coma (Shalit, 1970; Snyder, 1975).

Post-ischemic-anoxic *neurohistologic* changes are the result of the initial ischemic-anoxic insult, plus postresuscitative changes (Chapter 5). Such neurohistologic alterations are spotty, probably because of regional variations of oxygen consumption–blood flow ratios, and can be correlated with neurologic deficit and physiologic changes (Brierley, 1971, 1973; Nemoto, 1975; Bakay, 1968). They can be seen as early as five minutes or more after circulatory arrest and are most evident when brain sampling is performed two to three days after reperfusion. Post-ischemic-anoxic neurohistologic changes range from reversible swelling and vacuolization of neuronal and glial cells (particularly astrocytes) to irreversible pyknosis of neuronal cells. At the end of the first week, most acute reversible changes have taken place, and histologic examination reveals mainly loss of neuronal cells, necrotic foci, and glial scars. Most vulnerable are the cerebral cortex (primarily the occipital cortex), and midbrain (J. Moossy, personal communication).

Cerebral blood flow after circulatory arrest of 10 to 15 minutes in the dog responds to reperfusion first with brief hyperemia and then with a decrease in flow to about 50 per cent of control levels or less, where it remains (Snyder, 1975). Regional CBF seems to be mismatched in relation to *metabolic needs,* which are high during reperfusion because of an oxygen debt. An interesting concept in this respect has been raised by our laboratory findings, which showed that postresuscitative brain damage after 16 minutes of brain ischemia in monkeys can be dramatically prevented or ameliorated by giving large doses of thiopental intravenously after reperfusion (Bleyaert, 1975; Nemoto, 1977). One may speculate that barbiturate improves the perfusion–metabolism relationship in underperfused, hypermetabolic areas of brain tissue by decreasing metabolism throughout the brain and reducing regional blood flow in healthy areas, and by "putting the brain at rest" during the crucial restoration phase of metabolism.

Spotty postischemic hypoperfusion ("no reflow" phenomenon), in spite of normal SAP and cardiac output, seems to be due to capillary pinching by swollen endothelial and glial cells, to blood sludging, and later perhaps also to vasospasm (Ames, 1968; Fischer, 1973; Hossmann, 1973). Postischemic hypoperfusion, which seems to occur also in other organs such as liver and kidney, sets up the vicious cycle of postresuscitation disease—that is, hypoperfusion-ischemic anoxia-edema-hypoperfusion, and resultant deterioration.

Clotting disturbances in the recuperative phase are poorly characterized. Hypercoagulability with spotty areas of intravascular coagulation does seem to attend cessation of circulation and is a by-product of activation of the sympathoadrenal system. During resuscitation, there seems to be an early period of hypocoagulability, then normal clotting starting at about one hour), followed by alternating episodes of hypo- and hypercoagulability throughout the recovery phase.

Metabolic changes during resuscitation have not been studied thoroughly. After five minutes of clinical death, it takes about two to three minutes of reperfusion before carbohydrate metabolism returns to aerobic pathways and brain ATP and PK levels are replenished. Brain organic acid levels continue to be elevated for more than 30 minutes after the beginning of reperfusion. Although there is hyperglycemia, glucose metabolism and transport into brain cells seem impaired (Snyder, 1975). Full recovery of brain metabolism to the aerobic form requires one to two hours, and complete normalization of carbohydrate and phosphorus metabolism in the brain takes about 72 hours. Elevated intracellular sodium levels and low intracellular potassium levels persist in the brain for a longer time (Negovskii, 1974).

During dying and the early phases of resuscitation, the nature of the metabolic changes depends greatly on the pattern of dying. For instance, in exsanguination or ventricular fibrillation, hyperventilation causes a low arterial PCO_2 and normal or elevated PO_2, whereas poor peripheral perfusion leads to lactic acidosis in the venous blood; asphyxia, in contrast, results in hypercarbia, hypoxemia, and lactacidemia, owing to the combined effects of hypoventilation and hypoperfusion prior to arrest.

Although during dying metabolic abnormalities vary with the mechanism of dying, during resuscitation these derangements seem to follow a similar pattern, irrespective of the initiating insult. There is a wash-out of CO_2 and inorganic acids from tissues, producing transient hypercarbia, which is quickly changed by spontaneous or artificial hyperventilation to hypocarbia. There is, as well, a prolonged rise in arterial lactate values (to five to ten times normal), resulting in a low arterial pH (about 7.0) and a concomitant reduction in cardiac output for several hours (Kampschulte, 1969). At four to five hours, arterial pH may increase above 7.4 from hyperventilation and I.V. bicarbonate, but normalization of cerebral spinal fluid (CSF) acidosis often lags significantly behind. CSF lactate levels of 10 to 20 times normal seem to define the critical limits of tolerance in terms of brain recovery (Siesjö, 1973). With further passage of time, arterial pH continues to rise, and at 24 hours one may also see metabolic alkalemia (arterial pH above 7.4 and increased base excess), the cause of which is unknown.

Postresuscitative hypoxemia on breathing air is common—particularly in subjects with pre-existing cardiopulmonary disease or after prolonged periods of arrest and resuscitation—and occurs as a result of ventilation–perfusion mismatching with shunting, primarily from pulmonary edema and contusion (external heart compressions) and atelectasis. Controlled ventilation with 50 to 100 per cent oxygen should therefore be continued long into the recovery period (Smith, 1968).

Hepatic and renal functions halt immediately upon cessation of circulation. The liver thus fails in its vital role of detoxification, and noxious metabolites no longer are cleared from the circulation. Such metabolites doubtless contribute to cerebral dysfunction, since exchange transfusion, plasmaphoresis, and liver perfusion employed during the resuscitative period have all been shown to increase somewhat the tolerance of the CNS to the ischemic-anoxic insult (Negovskii, 1974). The kidneys also cease functioning immediately upon arrest and show subtle changes in function for several weeks post-ischemia; anuria, however, is less likely to occur after total cessation of circulation of several minutes than following hypovolemic shock of one hour or more (Chapter 6).

The role of *endocrine function* in dying and resuscitation is controversial. Increased production of glucocorticoids and ACTH in the terminal state is believed to exert a protective effect. However, the value of steroid medication in the postischemic phase is not established (Chapter 5). Selye's concept of the adaptation syndrome (increased adrenal cortical function, increased lymphocytes, decreased eosinophils, gastrointestinal hemorrhage) is not, in the view of Negovskii, significant in rapid dying and resuscitation where viability of the brain dictates survival, and the endocrine system, particularly its sympathetic component, is already maximally strained, as evidenced by vasoconstriction (except for vessels to the brain and heart), hyperventilation, tachycardia, and mobilization of glycogen. Recent discovery of "brain hormones" makes neuroendocrinology a promising research area within resuscitology.

In summary, the *postresuscitative disease* includes widespread disturbances of microcirculation, derangement of metabolic and electrolyte relationships, accumulation of toxic wastes, translocation of fluids among body compartments—all of which combine to predispose vital organ systems to secondary failure. Some of these processes can be interrupted before such secondary failure supervenes. The pathophysiology of the terminal state and its recovery phase deserve more attention, as do the immediate postresuscitative life support requirements dictated thereby. We concur with Negovskii that, "It is important not only to revive, but also to survive" (1962).

FUNDAMENTAL MECHANISMS OF RAPID DYING AND RESUSCITATION

The patterns of dying and resuscitation summarized in this section, in the same sequence as that shown in Figure 1, illustrate the most common underlying mechanisms of a variety of lethal conditions encountered in emergency care (Safar, 1977).

VENTRICULAR FIBRILLATION

Ventricular fibrillation (VF) is "irregular continuous peristaltic quivering motion of the ventricles of the heart," which does not pump blood and which is associated with the characteristic EKG pattern of oscillations without intermittent ventricular complexes.

Primary VF, in the strictest sense, is that occurring from electric shock (see later) or in patients without premonitory signs and symptoms of myocardial infarction. Generally, however, the term "primary VF" is used whenever this type of cardiac arrest occurs suddenly without evidence of preceding cardiovascular or pulmonary failure, even in those with known ischemic heart disease. The majority of sudden deaths in patients with pre-existing myocardial ischemia seem to be caused by VF, and thus in most cases of witnessed cardiac arrest VF should be suspected as the cause. High concentration of beta adrenergic agents, either exogenously administered or endogenously released, also may trigger VF—particularly in the presence of sensitizing drugs such as cyclopropane or halothane. Catecholamine release secondary to an increase in $PaCO_2$ has also been blamed for triggering VF during anesthesia.

Secondary VF may occur spontaneously or may be provided by stimuli such as heart massage in the weakly beating or arrested heart with bizarre EKG complexes or asystole—for instance, in asphyxia, exsanguination, or other causes of rapid dying. Secondary VF is more likely to occur in the anoxic (acidotic) heart and in the presence of high catecholamine levels (Gerst, 1966). The larger and the more diseased the heart, the more likely it is to fibrillate.

Sudden VF in the conscious person produces unconsciousness within about 10 to 15 seconds (Rossen, 1943). Terminal gasping may continue for 20 to 30 seconds during VF, which may produce minimal arterial pulse waves (probably without significant blood flow) because of the intrathoracic pressure fluctuations of gasping. Irreversible brain damage occurs as rapidly as with asystole, namely, within about five to ten minutes in man.

VF can be proved as the cause of pulselessness only by EKG or by direct visualization of the heart. Inspection and palpation of the fibrillating heart reveal wormlike movements all over the myocardium. The fibrillating heart is at first pink, while the EKG shows strong, rhythmic sinusoidal patterns with high amplitude. Later, the quivering motions become weaker and the heart grows cyanotic, while the EKG shows arrhythmic, polymorphous patterns with low amplitude. In the unanesthetized dog, electrically-induced VF fades into cardiac electrical silence in about 10 to 20 minutes. After 10 to 15 minutes or more of VF in dogs, the EKG pattern is so weak and the heart so anoxic and acidotic that CPR attempts often fail to restore spontaneous circulation (Safar, 1975).

VF in man does not ordinarily terminate spontaneously, but in most instances can be terminated by electric defibrillation, giving way to effective cardiac contractions, provided the myocardium is adequately oxygenated when defibrillation is attempted. However, VF in man has been seen very occasionally to stop spontaneously (Harben, 1963), for instance in about 50 per cent of patients developing "runs" of VF from coronary hypoperfusion due to bradycardia in heart block (Adams-Stokes syndrome). Very rarely, also, have prolonged CPR efforts, including the administration of bicarbonate, led to spontaneous defibrillation. The likelihood of VF stopping spontaneously varies inversely to the size of the heart. Although in man, dogs, sheep, and goats, electrically-induced VF does not stop spontaneously, it does usually terminate spontaneously in small monkeys, puppies, rabbits, guinea pigs, rats, mice, and birds.

There is still some disagreement concerning the mechanism of VF. There are at least two theories: (1) VF occurs secondary to excitation from many newly developed heterotopic foci which are independent of each other. (2) VF arises due to a circus movement, most likely triggered by an ectopic focus, creating a wave of excitation with multiple re-entry of impulses circulating continuously into areas which recently depolarized. Support of the triggering role of ectopic foci derives from the fact that in ischemic heart disease frequent premature ventricular contractions (PVC's) or ventricular tachycardia (VT) with or without pulse usually precede VF. Support for the circus movement derives from the efficacy of electric defibrillation. PVC's, electric shock, or other stimuli are most likely to throw the heart into VF when they occur during late systole, specifically the vulnerable period of the EKG, i.e., the upstroke of the T wave.

The triggering foci seem prone to develop when there are regional perfusion differentials in the myocardium—the "checkered, pale/pink heart" (Beck, 1955, 1960). The resulting electric instability is worsened by exertion, which further exaggerates the oxygen differential among regions. *Autopsies conducted shortly after sudden death have shown that one-third of the patients did not have myocardial infarction or major coronary artery obstruction* (Adelson, 1961). These events can be explained by coronary spasm from emotion, reflexes, and other causes—a mechanism difficult to prove in man but highly probable in view of suggestive clinical cases (Hellstrom, 1973).

Defibrillation. Although myocardial depressant drugs such as lidocaine, procainamide, quinidine, and potassium have some place in the occasional patient with intractable or recurrent VF when given in sufficient doses to terminate VF during CPR, they may make restoration of effective spontaneous cardiac contractions difficult. Therefore, the most reliable method at present for defibrillating the ventricles and restoring effective spontaneous circulation, is electric shock, applied either directly to the heart or externally across the chest (Prevost, 1899; N. Gurvich, 1946; Beck, 1947; Kouwenhoven, 1954; Zoll, 1956).

The principle of electric cardiac defibrillation is that a strong, brief shock of alternating current or capacitor discharge direct current produces synchronized depolarization of all heart muscle fibers, thereby eliminating the uncoordinated ectopic foci or circus movements of electric activity and converting all electric activity into a single contraction. This massive synchronous depolarization is followed by a refractory period and, if the heart is adequately oxygenated at that time, through early application of countershock or effective CPR, by spontaneous sinus rhythm and cardiac contractions.

There is no evidence that a manual precordial thump produces a sufficiently strong electric impulse to the heart to have a defibrillating effect. Very occasionally, however, VT has been terminated by precordial thump.

The likelihood of success in stopping VF with electrical countershock and restoring spontaneous circulation depends on the degree of myocardial hypoxia and acidosis, the duration of fibrillation, the size of the heart, the degree of coronary disease, and other factors. When, following prolonged circulatory arrest, a previously healthy heart is difficult to defibrillate in spite of adequate reoxygenation, or repeatedly reverts to VF after defibrillation, we may speculate that spotty areas of myocardial underperfusion, similar to those seen in the brain, are responsible.

The physiologic requirements for electric defibrillation, modified after Wiggers (1940), are: (1) reoxygenation of the myocardium; (2) arterial pH normalization (acidosis weakens the myocardium and increases its resistance to catecholamines); (3) enough energy to arrest fibrillation throughout the myocardium; (4) not so much energy as to overwhelm the pacemaker needed to initiate coordinated contractions; (5) resumption of function of a single pacemaker, since multiple pacemakers may cause return to VF; (6) a heart muscle capable of contracting vigorously: weak, uncoordinated contractions are prone to revert to VF (Stephenson, 1974).

Some of the above requirements are met by CPR, plus the intravenous administration of bicarbonate and epinephrine (Stewart, 1964; Redding, 1968). The beta receptor (inotropic) effect of epinephrine can induce VF, but, when given during VF, epinephrine makes VF more vigorous and thus promotes response to countershock and resumption of strong contractions. The alpha receptor (vasoconstrictor) effect of epinephrine increases the artifically induced arterial pressure during heart compressions, and thus coronary perfusion and myocardial oxygenation. The greater importance of the latter mechanism is evident from the ability of primarily alpha adrenergic agents (e.g., norepinephrine, phenylephrine, methoxamine) also to enhance electric defibrillation and restoration of spontaneous circulation (Pearson, 1965).

ASYSTOLE

The electrocardiographic definition of asystole is "pulselessness with cardiac standstill and isoelectric EKG." When discussing asystole here, we include "electromechanical dissociation," namely, pulselessness and cardiac standstill (no blood flow), with the isoelectric EKG intermittently interrupted by normal or abnormal EKG complexes at regular or irregular intervals.

Primary asystole in the strictest sense would occur only with sudden overwhelming overdose of myocardial depressant drugs (e.g., intravenous potassium, barbiturate, or local anesthetic); in sustained high energy electric shock (systolic arrest), such as used to occur with electrocutions; and in patients with severe bradycardia (Adams–Stokes syndrome) from atrioventricular block, which is usually caused by focal ischemic lesions in the conduction system. In the last type of arrest, syncope may occur without chest pain or premonitory hypotension. Myocardial underperfusion from severe bradycardia may easily trigger VF.

More common is asystole *secondary* to increased vagal tone, particularly in patients with underlying heart disease. Vagotonia depresses the sinus node, then the atrioventricular node, and finally the atrioventricular conduction system, which may lead in the diseased heart to idioventricular rhythm (heart block) with bradycardia of 30 to 40 per minute. In the healthy heart, such vagotonia usually leads simply to "vagal escape."

Asystole may also develop in the wake of marked sinus bradycardia. Although sinus bradycardia is considered physiologic in athletes, sinus bradycardia with a ventricular rate of less than 40 to 50 per minute occurring in some healthy persons—or, more likely, in patients with pre-existing heart disease—can occasionally result in asystole. Predisposing factors include: hypercarbia; hypoxemia; hypothermia; hypothyroidism; drugs (e.g., beta receptor blockers, reserpine, morphine); vagal maneuvers (e.g., nausea and vomiting, oculocardiac reflex in eye surgery, pressor receptor reflex of carotid sinus massage); hyperpotassemia (e.g., severe burns); and obstructive jaundice. Secondary asystole furthermore is the typical end-point in exsanguination and asphyxia.

Vasovagal syncope occurring in persons with heart disease or resulting in unconsciousness and airway obstruction is another possible mechanism of secondary asystole. In healthy young people, an emotional insult may cause a sudden reduction in heart rate and arterial pressure, leading to syncope from cerebral underperfusion. The skin becomes cold and sweaty, breathing is shallow, and the pupils are narrow, then wider. The mechanism of vasovagal syncope is not clear; it probably is in part a result of pooling of blood into capacitance vessels. Positioning the person horizontally and raising his legs usually promptly reverses this emergency. If necessary, additional measures, if available, should include oxygen inhalation, I.V. fluids, and atropine. Pulselessness calls for CPR. In patients with myocardial infarction (particularly diaphragmatic wall infarcts) cardiac slowing for any reason decreases cardiac contractility, cardiac output, and coronary perfusion, and predisposes to asystolic arrest, as well as to PVC's, VT, and VF.

Treatment of asystole centers around CPR and abolition of the cause. The oxygenated heart with atrioventricular block and bradycardia or asystole responds to mechanical or electric stimulation with effective contractions. Thus, episodes of unconsciousness which are accompanied by severe bradycardia or pulselessness are best treated with "fist pacing," i.e., blows over the precordium, with each blow resulting in a contraction. External heart compressions serve the same purpose and in addition pump blood, which is particularly important in the event the heart has already become hypoxic. This manual pacing or heart compressions can tide the patient over until drugs are administered intravenously. In severe bradycardia, atropine should be tried first to prevent asystole. Atropine will not be effective, however, if the block is below the atrioventricular node, in the bundle of His, or beyond, or if the block results from structural damage to the conduction system. In such cases, isoproterenol will increase the heart rate, but must be given with caution, as it increases cardiac irritability and the tendency to develop VF. The definitive treatment of severe bradycardia is electric pacing. External pacing is painful and unreliable, and insertion of pacing wires directly into the heart through a transcutaneous intracardiac needle is effective, but hazardous and difficult. The optimal method is transvenous pacing (Procedures, p 00). Transvenous pacemaker insertion with EKG or fluoroscopic guidance requires time, which must be bridged by drugs and/or fist pacing. Sudden asystole developing in patients with Adams-Stokes syndrome who already have an implantable pacemaker is usually due to pacemaker failure.

ALVEOLAR ANOXIA

"Anoxia" means "no oxygen." "Hypoxia" means "less than normal oxygen" (usually referring to PO_2). "Alveolar anoxia" is rare, but an active Emergency Department will see occasional examples, namely cases secondary to inhalation of oxygen-free gas (e.g., laboratory, industrial, mining, or anesthetic accidents), or to rapid decompression (in a pressure chamber or in high altitude flying).

A sudden switch from breathing air or oxygen to breathing oxygen-free inert gas causes cerebral failure, followed rapidly by cessation of breathing movements and circulation. This pattern of dying is one of pure oxygen lack, as there is continued removal of CO_2 and other metabolites from anoxic tissues until oxygen lack stops the heart. The resulting neuronal failure, therefore, is associated with *less acidosis* than in asphyxia from airway obstruction or apnea. A sudden change to breathing oxygen-free inert gas in unanesthetized dogs results instantaneously in spontaneous hyperventilation, and within one minute in hypotension, bradycardia and pupillary dilatation. Within three minutes, cardiac arrest develops in systole. The dogs continue hyperventilating almost to the point of cardiac arrest (Swann, 1949). Clinical death after about five minutes is easily reversed with promptly initiated CPR.

Rapid decompression causes cerebral brain failure even more rapidly than does pure nitrogen breathing, since decompression does not require washing out of alveolar oxygen. In man, rapid decompression to an atmospheric pressure of 75 torr produces an arterial oxygen saturation of 15 per cent or less, and unconsciousness within 15 seconds (Luft, 1956). This is almost as rapid as in neck-cuff occlusion, which produces unconsciousness within four to ten seconds (Rossen, 1943). With decompression, in about five seconds (minimum circulation time from lungs to brain), there is amnesia and automatic behavior (staring, arrested position); then the eyes turn upward, consciousness is lost, and respirations cease; finally, posture fails at about 15 seconds, accompanied by a complete flattening of the EEG and exaggerated reflex actions (decerebration) (Luft, 1956). Immediately upon switching to atmospheric pressure, the pattern of clinical and EEG recovery is the mirror image of the preceding deterioration.

Comparative data on the recoverability of the human brain following alveolar anoxia as compared to ischemia or asphyxia are not available.

Less fulminating alveolar hypoxia is common, for instance in exposure to high altitude (Safar, 1964), or inhalation of gases with decreased oxygen concentration. Alveolar hypoxia kills by the same mechanism as hypoxemia from pulmonary disease (Chapter 3). A decrease of PaO_2 to about 60 torr or less induces hyperventilation through the peripheral chemoreceptor reflex. At a PaO_2 of 30 torr or less, cerebral vessels are maximally dilated and further decrease in PaO_2 will lead to cerebral anaerobiosis (Figure 2). In unacclimatized adults dying from hypoxemia, cardiac arrest may occur at a PaO_2 of 15 to 25 torr. In acclimatized adults (e.g., patients with acutely decompensated chronic obstructive lung disease, with polycythemia and increased base excess), we have occasionally seen pulse and some cortical function continue during resuscitation attempts at a time when blood gas determinations unexpectedly revealed PaO_2 values of 15 to 20 torr. Obviously, such severe degrees of hypoxemia cannot be tolerated long by heart and brain.

ASPHYXIA

"Hypoxemia" denotes reduced arterial Po_2 (PaO_2); "hypercarbia" (hypercapnia) increased arterial Pco_2 ($PaCO_2$); and "asphyxia" a combination of both. Hypoventilation is a reduction in alveolar ventilation (minute volume minus deadspace minute ventilation). This results, in the air-breathing animal or person, in a progressive increase in $PaCO_2$ and an inversely related decrease of PaO_2. The extremes of hypoventilation are complete airway obstruction and apnea (no breathing movements), and these comprise the two principal causes of asphyxia.

By far the most common cause of rapid dying from obstructive asphyxia is coma (irrespective of the cause), which may result in (a) upper airway soft tissue obstruction from malpositioning (flexion) of the head (Safar, 1959); or (b) airway obstruction by foreign matter (e.g., vomitus) (Chapters 3, 9 and 10).

Other causes of upper airway obstruction include trauma with soft tissue obstruction or inhalation of blood, inflammatory swelling of tissues (e.g., cellulitis of the floor of the mouth, croup, epiglottitis), and food bolus obstruction.

Foreign matter usually obstructs the airway only partially, but may trigger reflex laryngospasm which in turn completes the obstruction. The larynx may then relax only when the dying process reaches the stage of severe hypoxemia, which may be at a moment when breathing movements already have ceased. If started prior to cardiac arrest, skillfully applied positive pressure artificial ventilation usually can revive the patient, even if the foreign matter was not removed.

Moderate *partial* airway obstruction, as in bronchospasm, first stimulates increased respiratory efforts, which usually can maintain normal or even low $PaCO_2$ values for some time. Hypoxemia may occur early because of ventilation–perfusion mismatching and shunting. When the patient becomes exhausted or the obstruction worsens, asphyxia develops, with rapidly progressive hypoxemia and hypercarbia leading to secondary apnea and cardiac arrest.

The events accompanying *complete* airway obstruction in unanesthetized air-breathing dogs were studied by Swann (1949), our group (Redding, 1960, 1962), and Kristoffersen (1967). Although these investigators used slightly different models, we have reason to believe that the following is the approximate course of events, not only in dogs, but also in man (Figure 3): struggling and increased breathing efforts (with exaggerated intrathoracic pressure fluctuations causing intercostal and suprasternal retractions) are accompanied by a sympathetic discharge with arterial hypertension and tachycardia. Anesthesia, which mitigates the struggling and its attendant oxygen consumption, or clamping the airway at end-inspiration instead of end-expiration, which increases the alveolar oxygen reserve, retards, but does not prevent, this asphyxial process.

Unconsciousness starts at about two minutes after complete airway obstruction, when PaO_2 reaches 30 torr (arterial oxygen saturation 50 per cent) or less. Apnea occurs at 2 to 6 minutes, and pulselessness (asystole

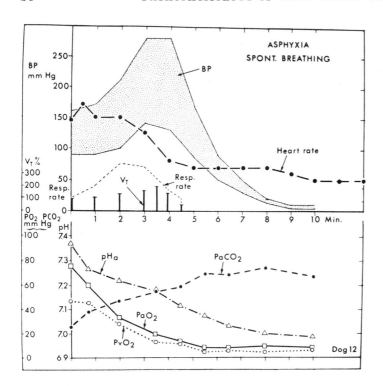

Figure 3. Pattern of deterioration of physiologic variables in mechanical asphyxiation, using a spontaneously breathing dog as a representative example (From Kristoffersen, M. B., et al.: Anesthesiology, 28:488, 1967).

in diastole) at 5 to 10 minutes. Hypoxia and acidosis (from accumulation of CO_2 and fixed acids) in blood and tissues combine as a cause of circulatory failure. When PaO_2 is 20 to 30 torr, pHa about 6.8 to 7.0, and $PaCO_2$ about 80 torr, the SAP falls to about 30 to 50 torr; further decreases in SAP below 30 torr lead to pupillary dilatation and the onset of an isoelectric EEG. Pulselessness occurs when the PaO_2 is about 10 torr or less, and pHa is 6.5 to 6.8.

The EKG develops nodal rhythm and, when hypotension occurs, bizarre ventricular complexes with gigantic T waves. At the time of pulselessness, the EKG shows asystole or electromechanical dissociation (i.e., some EKG complexes without pulse). Usually, toward the end of a five-minute period of clinical death, the EKG is flat.

When IPPV is started before the critical SAP is reached, resuscitation is prompt. When CPR is started within 2 to 5 minutes of cardiac arrest, recovery with an intact CNS is common. After 5 to 10 minutes of clinical death from asphyxia in animals, restoration of spontaneous circulation by CPR is still possible, although the severe acidemia requires administration of large amounts of both epinephrine and bicarbonate, since epinephrine's effect is blocked at such low

pH values; recovery of the brain in such circumstances is questionable. In some human cases of slow asphyxiation, as little as 1 to 2 minutes of arrest or even no circulatory arrest at all have resulted in permanent neurologic deficit, particularly when pre-existing illness or injury caused a decrease in arterial oxygen transport prior to the beginning of airway obstruction.

In asphyxial arrest, the medulla does not remain active as long, nor does electric cardiac activity persist as long as in exsanguination arrest, perhaps because the former is associated with more tissue acidosis. Also, brain recovery is less likely following asphyxial arrest than exsanguination arrest of equal duration, perhaps because, in the former case, stagnant blood in cerebral vessels hampers reperfusion.

Sudden apnea in an air-breathing patient or animal results in a similar itinerary toward asphyxial cardiac arrest, but events proceed at a somewhat slower pace than in airway obstruction, because in apnea less vigorous respiratory efforts and less profound struggling entail lower oxygen consumption during the terminal state. Sudden apnea may occur as a result of high energy electric shock, intravenous injection of a paralyzing dose of muscle relaxant (anesthesia), sudden severe increase in intracranial pressure with brain herniation, and large doses of anesthetics, narcotics, or hypnotics.

Hypercarbia without hypoxemia can be produced by inhalation of an oxygen-enriched atmosphere prior to hypoventilation or apnea. The rate of $PaCO_2$ rise in apnea is about 4 to 6 torr per minute. The rate of deoxygenation in apnea can be calculated from alveolar oxygen, functional residual capacity, and oxygen consumption. Preventilation with 50 per cent oxygen can maintain PaO_2 above normal values for at least five minutes of apnea in persons with healthy lungs. Preventilation with 100% oxygen and complete denitrogenation (Chapter 10) will, in animals or man with healthy lungs, initially produce a PaO_2 of over 600 torr and subsequently sustain the PaO_2 above 75 torr for over one-half hour, provided the oxygen-filled alveoli and airways remain connected to an oxygen reservoir without other gases (Roth, 1947). This process is called "apneic diffusion oxygenation" (Holmdahl, 1956) and is believed to work through the "hemoglobin–oxygen pump." Through continuous absorption of oxygen into the blood, this "pump" creates a negative pressure in the alveoli, which draws oxygen from the reservoir down into the lungs. The PaO_2 will decline below normal when alveolar oxygen is displaced by CO_2, and right-to-left shunting occurs from absorption atelectasis of oxygen-filled alveoli. Without administration of buffers, circulatory collapse begins when pHa falls to about 6.8, and cardiac arrest occurs when pHa decreases to about 6.5. In dogs, this may occur as late as after one and one-half hours of apnea, when the $PaCO_2$ has risen to about 340 torr but the PaO_2 is still above 80 torr (Kristoffersen, 1967).

Whereas alveolar anoxia without hypercarbia stops the heart in systole, hypercarbia alone (without hypoxemia), as well as asphyxia, produce acidemia, which stops the heart in diastole. Hypercarbia per se rarely kills; the dog, for example, can tolerate artificial ventilation with up to 70 per cent CO_2 (30 per cent oxygen) without circulatory embarrassment (Graham, 1960). But acidemia causes potassium loss from blood cells into plasma, which may produce dangerous arrhythmias in individuals with heart disease. Rapid lowering of $PaCO_2$ from extremely high levels can precipitate sudden VT or VF, presumably due to re-entry of potassium into cells, even in healthy individuals or animals.

Apneic diffusion oxygenation is a principle applied in prophylactic oxygen inhalation for patients whose respiratory movements or airway patency are at risk (e.g., convulsive states). A clinical example of hypercarbia without hypoxemia, at least in its initial stages, is the chronic obstructive lung disease patient inhaling an enriched oxygen mixture without assisted or stimulated breathing. Consequent normalization of PaO_2 through abolition of hypoxemia, which ordinarily provides the predominant respiratory drive in such patients, results in hypoventilation and possibly apnea. At that point, however, apneic oxygenation does *not* occur because these patients usually have not been breathing 100 per cent oxygen, but rather lower oxygen concentrations. Thus, at the moment of apnea, severe hypoxemia rapidly develops and asystolic arrest can occur. This problem is avoided, not by withholding oxygen, but by administering oxygen together with assisted or stimulated spontaneous ventilation.

In alveolar anoxia, asphyxia, and hypercarbia without hypoxemia, the depletion of oxygen stores progresses ten times more rapidly than the accumulation of lethal quantities of hydrogen ions (Kristoffersen, 1967). In dogs, the lethal values are about 10 torr for PaO_2 and 6.5 for pHa, irrespective of the rate of deoxygenation and accumulation of hydrogen ions.

A further example of asphyxia is that which develops in *neonates*. Every vaginal delivery is an asphyxial experience for the baby. Before, during, and/or sometimes after birth, a combination of respiratory asphyxia (hypoxemia and hypercarbia) and lactic acidosis from hypoperfusion develops. Asphyxia neonatorum can lead to brain damage and sometimes cardiac arrest. Predisposing factors include prematurity, postmaturity, prolonged labor, prolapsed cord, placental separation, placenta previa, uterine tetany (oxytocic drugs), general anesthesia and analgesia (narcotics), and traumatic delivery.

In newborn monkeys, experimental asphyxia results in a sequence of hyperventilation, primary apnea (during which external stimuli can still restart breathing), gasping, and secondary apnea (when stimuli are ineffective in eliciting respiration). Neurohistologic brain damage has been seen with four minutes or more of secondary apnea, even without cardiac arrest (Hook, 1974). This makes prolonged CPR efforts in pulseless neonates appear ill-advised.

EXSANGUINATION

This mechanism of dying was described earlier under "Terminal State" where it served as a model for understanding the detailed dying processes and the "postresuscitation disease."

PULMONARY FAILURE

Sudden death from airway obstruction or apnea was discussed under "asphyxia." Most critically ill or injured patients develop hypoxemia during air breathing because of ventilation–perfusion mismatching, including right-to-left shunting of unoxygenated blood through nonventilated alveoli. Common causes of shunt are atelectasis from airway obstruction and/or surfactant failure, alveolar edema, and pneumonic exudate. The degree and rapidity with which such hypoxemia develops vary considerably (Chapter 3).

Acute pulmonary disease usually stimulates spontaneous hyperventilation through hypoxemic stimulation of peripheral chemoreceptor reflexes and mechanical stimulation of pulmonary stretch receptor reflexes. Since as little as 20 per cent of lung tissue suffices to keep $PaCO_2$ within normal limits during spontaneous or artificial hyperventilation, we are dealing in acute pulmonary failure, usually with progressive hypoxemia, rather than hypercarbia, and indeed $PaCO_2$ values are often low. Sudden anoxic death is unusual but may occur, for example in acute pulmonary edema, aspiration, near-drowning, and in rare cases of fulminating hemorrhagic influenza pneumonitis. The dying pattern resembles more that of gradual alveolar anoxia than of asphyxia. Superimposed lactacidemia occurs when the circulation fails or sepsis is present. Hypercarbia occurs late, particularly when artificial ventilation is used.

Dying in the terminal stages of chronic lung disease can be a slow torture from moderate hypoxemia, which causes CNS excitement, if the patient is not permitted to slip into CO_2 narcosis. Sometimes it is complicating events rather than the underlying respiratory pathophysiology that irrevocably tip the patient toward death, as for instance alveolar rupture with tension pneumothorax and interstitial emphysema.

SHOCK

"Shock" is "the clinical picture of overall tissue perfusion inadequate to meet tissue needs." This definition encompasses inadequate transport of oxygen and substrate, as well as inadequate removal of metabolites. Shock, if not reversed in time, may lead to lethal multiple organ failure from the vicious cycle of hypoperfusion-tissue acidosis-cellular metabolic failure-capillary and cellular membrane failure-hypoperfusion. In slow dying from shock, vital organs may become irreversibly damaged by the time circulation ceases entirely.

Shock states have recently been reclassified by Weil and Shubin according to the following mechanisms (Chapter 4): (1) oligemia (decrease in circulating blood volume, for instance from external or internal loss of blood); (2) cardiac pump failure (cardiogenic shock); (3) total blood flow obstruction (e.g., pulmonary embolism, cardiac tamponade); and (4) altered blood flow distribution (e.g., septicemia, intoxication, sympathetic paralysis).

The main difference between acute dying as previously described, and dying in shock is *duration*, which depends on the underlying problem, the patient's general condition, therapeutic interventions, and other factors. In shock states, there usually is time for compensatory mechanisms to come into play. These may give short-term protection through cerebral and coronary vasodilatation and systemic vasoconstriction. In spite of these mechanisms, however, the brain may suffer permanent damage during shock (Kovach, 1961). Furthermore, shock states, owing to decreased coronary perfusion pressure, uneven myocardial oxygenation, acidosis, and other factors, predispose the heart to VF or asystole, which can be triggered by minor interventions, such as transportation or airway suctioning (hypoxemia).

BRAIN FAILURE

The mechanisms by which acute destruction of the brain (e.g., crushing head injury, gunshot wound, massive intracerebral hemorrhage) or a rapid increase in intracranial pressure without subarachnoid bleeding (e.g., epidural hemorrhage) may result in cardiac arrest are not well understood (Chapter 5). Hemorrhage into the cranial cavity does not produce oligemic shock, but rather results in coma and intracranial hypertension, which in some cases tends to raise the SAP concomitant with downward displacement of the brain. When the medulla herniates, tachycardia, hypotension, and apnea occur. In the absence of airway control and artificial ventilation, therefore, brain death usually kills via asphyxia. When the comatose, brain-dead patient receives respiratory and circulatory support by artificial ventilation, blood volume expansion and other measures, circulation can continue for many days, although vasomotor center failure usually results in arterial hypotension; only rarely does this advance to cardiac arrest. Brain damage can also kill by hypoxemia from neurogenic pulmonary edema, CNS-induced cardiac arrhythmias, infections, and other complications (Figure 1).

Regional or diffuse acute brain damage with coma in the presence of continued circulation may be followed by awakening, but with permanent neurologic damage; or in the vegetative state (active EEG, but stupor or coma); or brain death (permanently silent EEG) (Figure 1). The vegetative state can improve or worsen, whereas brain death will eventually lead to cardiac arrest and panorganic death, even when artificial ventilation is continued, because of abolition of all protective reflexes and complications.

SOME SPECIFIC MECHANISMS OF DYING AND RESUSCITATION

The following brief comments on some selected emergencies are intended to stimulate interest in the pathophysiologic mechanisms involved, since understanding of these mechanisms will facilitate appraisal of currently accepted therapeutic approaches and future innovations. Most of the emergencies described here, and the resuscitation requirements attendant upon them, are variations of one or more of the fundamental mechanisms discussed in the previous sections of this chapter. For in-depth reviews, the reader is referred to the literature quoted subsequently and to the other appropriate chapters of this book.

ELECTROCUTION

Accidental electrocution each year in the United States accounts for about 300 deaths from lightning (high energy, direct current, DC shock) and about 1000 deaths from household current (low energy, alternating current, AC shock). Cessation of circulation after high energy shock occurs over minutes and is due to apnea without ventricular fibrillation; in low energy shock circulation ceases instantaneously from ventricular fibrillation. The likelihood of electric current to produce VF depends on the intensity of the current, its frequency of oscillations, its path (whether or not the heart is included), and the duration of contact. DC current is more injurious than AC current of the same voltage, as DC produces electrolytic tissue damage and burns. AC current of several thousand volts, by contrast, is used in physiotherapy machines without hurting human nerves or even contracting muscle because of the high frequency of oscillations (e.g., 0.5 million cycles per second).

Chances of recovery are best when neither brain nor heart lies directly in the path of the current.

Lightning may produce an estimated energy of millions of volts and over 20,000 amperes. Usually, only stray currents hit people or animals; and for every person killed by lightning, there are at least three who sustain a nonlethal exposure to current. Many persons struck by lightning are merely stunned and may transiently have difficulty moving, hearing, or feeling. Some suffer burns, primarily at the entry and exit points of the often erratic paths traveled by lightning currents.

If lightning current passes through brain and heart, the following sequence seems to occur: the victim suddenly loses consciousness (electronarcosis) and becomes apneic, probably because of instantaneous cessation of brain metabolism; at the same time, the heart is thrown into a sustained contraction. Soon after termination of the electric shock, the contracted heart relaxes and resumes spontaneous contractions with sinus rhythm, while the respiratory center remains paralyzed—perhaps for days (!). Thus, the heart goes into secondary asystole (not ventricular fibrillation) from asphyxia, due to apnea, unless artificial ventilation is started before the onset of cardiac arrest (Kouwenhoven, 1930).

Usually, the brain arrest is reversible. Very high energy currents, however, can burn and destroy brain tissue permanently. On the other hand, some victims of lightning stroke have survived more than four minutes of clinical death with complete CNS recovery, which may be because the cessation of metabolic activity in brain cells is so instantaneous that the onset of degenerative processes is delayed (Taussig, 1969).

In 1960, we resuscitated a 10-year-old boy who was struck by lightning while riding a bicycle. He was found unconscious and apneic; however, he apparently had a pulse. Ambulance personnel failed to administer artificial ventilation during transport to Baltimore City Hospital. About 22 minutes after having been struck, he arrived at the Emergency Department in cardiac arrest and his circulation was immediately restarted with open chest cardiac resuscitation. He remained comatose at first, but following treatment with hypothermia, intravenous urea and artificial ventilation he awoke on the sixth day after the accident and recovered completely. This course of events would have been impossible with 22 minutes of ventricular fibrillation (Ravitch, 1961).

Household current (100 to 120 volts, 50 to 60 cycles per second) when traversing the human heart from hand to foot, usually results in VF. Very rarely, if at all, household current may go directly through the head, producing respiratory paralysis without VF. Many unrecognized accidental electrocutions occur in hospitalized patients with even lower currents (maximum permissible current, 10 microamperes through the heart) because of improperly grounded apparatus connected to patients having catheter or wire leads going directly into the heart. In patients with heart disease, low voltage currents may cause arrhythmias without cardiac arrest, which in turn can trigger VF later on.

Household current seems to produce no long-range deleterious effect on the myocardium. External burns, frequently seen in lightning and high voltage power line accidents, are absent in most cases of household current accidents. The noxious effects of household current depend to a significant extent on resistances encountered, which in turn determine the amperage going through the heart itself. The resistance of an adult person's thorax is about 70 to 100 ohms and varies with the type of skin contact. Dry skin offers resistance of several thousand ohms. Inside the body, bone tissue and air-filled lungs offer high resistance.

Animal and human data suggest the following "dose-response" of man to a 60-cycle AC current applied from hand to foot (Kouwenhoven, 1930; Hooker, 1933): with less than 0.01 ampere, the person will merely feel a "funny" sensation; with 0.01 ampere, he will freeze to the circuit; between 0.1 and 1 ampere, the likelihood of inducing VF and sudden death is greatest; and with more than 1 ampere, the current is strong enough to throw the heart into a contraction (unless it hits by chance during the "vulnerable period" represented by the upswing of the T wave of the EKG, which may cause VF). Thus, more than 1 ampere may defibrillate; the original AC external defibrillator, which discharges 500 volts at 5 amperes, probably gets 1.5 to 2 amperes through the heart. High voltage line accidents result in either VF or the pattern described for lightning, depending on the amount of current traversing heart and brain.

NEAR-DROWNING

About 7000 deaths from drowning occur annually in the United States. Resuscitative efforts have apparently saved many persons who were removed from the water cyanotic, unconscious, and apneic — some even pulseless. Neither accounts by rescuers nor postmortem examinations, however, yield conclusive information on the pathophysiologic changes which take place during submersion. Therefore, we have to rely for this information primarily on controlled animal experiments.

When unanesthetized dogs were completely submerged, they struggled, held their breaths, swallowed, vomited, and finally made terminal gasps with inhalation of water; death ensued within 3 to 5 minutes (Swann, 1949; Redding, 1961a). An estimated 10 per cent of human near-drowning victims removed from the water, by contrast, show no evidence that they inhaled water. They most likely suffered asphyxia from laryngospasm and/or reflex apnea. Laryngospasm due to submersion seems to be more prolonged and pronounced in man than in animals. Members of any species removed from the water with a pulse, and before anoxic relaxation of the larynx and agonal gasps occur, are easily resuscitated with IPPV/exhaled air or air, since the lungs are normal (Redding, 1960a). If water is inhaled, the picture becomes more complicated.

Inhaled *fresh water* rapidly passes into the circulation, so that a subject removed prior to circulatory arrest may have dry lungs (Revensdorf, 1902). The result of fresh water aspiration is not only hypoxemia, hypercarbia, and acidemia, but also hypervolemia, hemodilution (with reduced serum electrolyte values), hemolysis, and hyperpotassemia (from acidemia and hemolysis) (Swann, 1949, 1962; Karpovich, 1933; Redding, 1961a,b).

We simulated in unanesthetized dogs events in human near-drowning, by first clamping the tracheal tube ("laryngospasm") until apnea occurred, and after 30 seconds of apnea, flooding the lungs with water for 30 seconds. Subsequently, we drained the water for 30 seconds and started resuscitation. All dogs with fresh water flooding developed VF within less than three minutes after the start of IPPV/air (Redding, 1961b). At the moment of VF, the dogs had inhaled and absorbed about 40 ml./kg. of water (50 per cent of blood volume). With CPR, IPPV/100 per cent oxygen, epinephrine, and electric countershock, most dogs could be fully resuscitated. It appears that VF is primarily the result of anoxia and hypervolemia, not of the moderate hyperpotassemia and hemolysis to which it was attributed in the past. It is not certain whether human near-drowning victims with fresh water in the lungs also usually develop VF. Chlorinated water (customary swimming pool concentration) causes about the same pattern of dying as does fresh water (Modell, 1969).

Inhalation of *sea water* (which is hypertonic, 3 to 5 per cent salt), leads in the same dog model to transudation of water from the circulation into the alveoli and of electrolytes from the alveoli into the circulation, resulting in hypovolemia (about 30 per cent decrease in blood volume) and hemoconcentration (increases in serum sodium, magnesium, potassium, and chloride). It also produces damage to the capillary-alveolar membrane, resulting in plasma protein loss into the alveoli and fulminating, foaming pulmonary edema with hypoxemia, which is proportional to the quantity of sea water inhaled. Hypoxemia, bradycardia, and oligemic hypotension lead to asystole within hours. Following prolonged IPPV/100 per cent oxygen and plasma volume normalization, all dogs survived (Redding, 1960b). About twice as much sea water is needed to kill dogs as fresh water. Sea water is worse

for the lungs; fresh water is worse for the heart.

In human near-drowning victims with evidence of fresh or sea water inhalation who are rescued before cardiac arrest, electrolyte disturbances are minimal or absent one-half to one hour after removal from the water. Apparently, the organism can rapidly correct the electrolyte changes and clear the free plasma hemoglobin (Modell, 1968, 1969).

The limiting factors in human near-drowning cases are: (1) the severe and prolonged hypoxemia from the damage any type of water causes in the lungs; and (2) anoxic-ischemic brain damage.

As little as 2 ml./kg. of any type of water can produce hypoxemia, bronchospasm and pulmonary vasospasm. Larger amounts of fresh or brackish water inhaled cause primarily alveolar atelectasis from surfactant loss; whereas sea water produces pulmonary edema in addition. Additional regurgitation and aspiration of gastric contents, which is not uncommon, complicates the pulmonary pathologic changes. It is astounding, however, that in survivors of near-drowning, even after many days of severe hypoxemia from pulmonary edema and consolidation, sophisticated respiratory care, including prolonged CPPV/oxygen, pHa normalization, and other life support measures, has resulted not only in complete recovery of the patient, but also in normal pulmonary function values assessed at long-term follow-up (Butt, 1970; Hasan, 1971; Modell, 1968).

When cardiac arrest occurs during submersion, after rescue or during resuscitation, the principal factor limiting survival is brain damage. Prevention of brain damage calls for immediate special postresuscitative therapy (Chapter 5). Absence of early awakening is no reason to give up, particularly if drowning occurred in cold water, which protects the brain. This is illustrated by the survival with normal CNS of a five-year-old boy after documented 40 minutes of submersion in ice cold fresh water; his pulmonary edema was controlled by respiratory care, and he regained consciousness within about two days (Siebke, 1975).

Scuba divers can drown secondarily to complications from increased pressure, which may cause coma and loss of reflexes. This is described elsewhere in this book (Chapter 39G). These hyperbaric injuries can be due to (*a*) nitrogen narcosis (which may occur below 200 feet depth when breathing air); (b) nitrogen bubbles released into all tissues, including the brain, during rapid ascent after nitrogen loading at a depth of over 30 feet (decompression sickness—"bends"); or (c) cerebral air embolism. Decompression sickness can be avoided by slow ascent according to decompression tables. Systemic arterial air embolism, fortunately rare, is the most threatening potentially lethal complication, as it cannot always be avoided, even with sound diving practices. This accident can be caused by rapid ascent of just a few feet resulting in expansion of trapped gas in the lungs (trapped because of breath holding, emphysema, asthma, or other causes), and alveolar rupture. This may lead to entry of air into the pulmonary veins, causing cerebral and/or coronary air embolism and sudden death (see later, "Pulmonary Embolism").

TENSION PNEUMOTHORAX

An opening into the pleural space, either through the chest wall or through the lung, results in pneumothorax. When the opening is persistent and pressure in the pleural space becomes atmospheric throughout the respiratory cycle, the ipsilateral lung collapses. People or animals with previously healthy lungs and heart will merely become hypoxemic from the resulting 40 to 50 per cent of blood flow shunted through nonventilated alveoli. They will not die suddenly. If, however, the opening operates as a one-way valve, for instance in lung contusion or rupture of alveolar blebs, positive pressure breathing or coughing can force increments of gas into the pleural space where the gas cannot escape, and a tension pneumothorax develops. Alveoli may also rupture into the pulmonary interstitial spaces, resulting in mediastinal and subcutaneous emphysema (noticed in the form of crepitation about the neck) and subserosal blebs, which can rupture secondarily into the pleural space.

Tension pneumothorax can occur, for example, in newborn infants (even without positive pressure ventilation) and following blunt chest injury (with or without rib fracture). Predisposing factors include positive pressure ventilation and coughing in the presence of valvelike bronchial obstruction, as in asthma and emphysema. This may lead to overdistention of alveoli and surface alveolar rupture.

Tension pneumothorax should be suspected when there is progressive difficulty in ventilating the lungs, progressive inability of the lungs to deflate passively, progressive deterioration of the circulation (decrease in venous return, arterial hypotension, tachycardia), mediastinal shift (evidenced by tracheal shift or changes noted on percussion), and progressive distention of the abdomen. The latter is due to inversion of the diaphragm from a distended pleural space, and may also be due to pneumoperitoneum from air dissecting through diaphragmatic openings and breaking through the thin serosal membranes. Circulatory arrest seems to be the combined result of severe hypoxemia (from total compression atelectasis of the ipsilateral lung and partial compression of the contralateral lung) and compression and kinking of bronchi and major vessels. The asphyxial component seems to be more important than the shock component in this dying process. In some cases, cardiac tamponade from the interstitial mediastinal emphysema also may contribute to mortality.

When a pneumothorax is suspected in a person who still has a pulse, the diagnosis should be quickly confirmed by needle puncture and the pneumothorax drained by large bore tube (Chapter 10). When, in the presence of pulselessness, quick tube drainage without interruption of external heart compressions proves difficult, open chest cardiac resuscitation is indicated (Chapter 9).

CARDIAC TAMPONADE

Cardiac tamponade produces a type of obstructive shock (Chapter 4), and should be suspected under circumstances which may disrupt the integrity of the heart wall. These circumstances include stab wound, intracardiac needle injection, cardiac surgery or open chest heart compressions followed by closure of the pericardium, cardiac perforation by stiff intravascular catheter, and perforation of an infarcted portion of the ventricular wall. The patient with developing cardiac tamponade shows signs of compromised cardiac output, elevated venous pressure, venous pulsations, and pulsus paradoxus (the SAP during deep spontaneous inhalations decreases precipitately). There may be substernal pain. If time permits, a roentgenogram of the chest will show a widened heart shadow.

With cardiac tamponade, the SAP, pulse pressure, and cardiac output decline while the venous pressure and heart rate increase. Death in asystole or VF is due to progressive inability of the heart to fill during diastole. The rapidity of dying depends on the underlying status of the heart and on the rapidity with which blood accumulates in the pericardium.

Treatment includes pericardial needle aspiration, preferably under EKG monitoring; aspiration may have to be repeated and perhaps followed by the surgical creation of a pleural-pericardial window. In pulselessness, suspicion of cardiac tamponade is an indication for open chest cardiac resuscitation, with opening and drainage of the pericardial sac and direct surgical control of the bleeding site.

PULMONARY EMBOLISM

Pulmonary embolism may also produce a type of obstructive shock (Chapter 4). The potentially lethal obstruction may be caused by embolized thrombi, gas, fat, tissue, or amniotic fluid; some of these agents may cause sudden massive main pulmonary artery obstruction; others may produce showers of small obstructive matter, clogging many small vessels.

Acute pulmonary thromboembolism may be the most common cause of death in hospitals, particularly among old and chronically ill patients (Sasahara, 1967). Extensive clinical and laboratory research has dealt with humoral and nervous factors which may affect pulmonary vessels and bronchi remote from the embolic obstruction. Recent appraisal of available data, however, suggests that the overriding factor determining the degree of shock and likelihood of sudden death from pulmonary thromboembolism is the proportion of the total cross-sectional area of the pulmonary arterial tree blocked by thrombus. In patients with previously healthy lungs and heart, more than about 50 per cent of the vascular tree must be obstructed to produce shock. Sudden cardiac arrest from pulmonary thromboembolism usually is caused by a large thrombus blocking the pulmonary artery bifurcation. Under such circumstances, CPR may be only occasionally and partially effective (Stephenson, 1974). In patients with cardiopulmonary disease, a smaller proportion of the pulmonary vasculature suddenly blocked may cause shock or cardiac arrest. In this circumstance, cardiac arrest may be due to a variety of associated insults to an already diseased myocardium.

In shock or cardiac arrest from pulmonary thromboembolism, there is no pulmonary infarction — thus no hemoptysis. Pulmonary infarction is more likely to occur when a pulmonary end-artery becomes blocked in a patient with left heart failure and pulmonary congestion. The uncongested lung parenchyma, by contrast, can survive pulmonary artery obstruction without developing infarction because of uncompromised bronchial artery blood supply.

Single or multiple small emboli entering one or both lungs to the extent of 50 per cent obstruction of the vascular bed result in arterial hypotension, tachycardia, venous hypertension, diffuse pulmonary artery spasm and bronchospasm. Chest roentgenography in such cases reveals areas with reduced pulmonary vascularity. A lung scan and arterial PaO_2 measurement permit a rapid screen for suspected emboli, since a normal lung and normal oxygen tension virtually rule out significant embolization. If the lung scan is positive and time permits, a pulmonary angiogram confirms the diagnosis.

Acute pulmonary thromboembolism which does not lead instantaneously to cardiac arrest increases not only physiologic deadspace (ventilated lung areas which are unperfused), but also increases right-to-left shunting of venous blood (perfused but unventilated lung areas), the cause of hypoxemia and a high alveolar-arterial PO_2 gradient (Chapter 3). Although the exact mechanism of hypoxemia in pulmonary embolism is not clearly understood, it is related at least in part to complex ventilation-perfusion disturbances, including those induced by patchy bronchoconstriction and by pulmonary edema in the hyperemic portion of the pulmonary vascular bed.

Management of the patient with pulmonary thromboembolism is aimed at prevention of recurrent embolization and support of vital functions during the critical few days required for natural thrombolysis and recanalization of obstructed vessels. Embolectomy has been associated with very poor results. Heparinization primarily prevents secondary thrombus formation. In shock, management should include IPPV–CPPV/ 100 per cent oxygen, maintenance of arterial perfusion pressure by vasopressor, use of bronchodilator and pulmonary vasodilators (the best pulmonary vasodilator is 100 per cent oxygen), and perhaps, as well, more definitive measures including: (a) intravenous infusion of a thrombolytic agent such as urokinase or streptokinase (urokinase study, 1973); or (b) emergency partial cardiopulmonary bypass with venoarterial pumping to ameliorate right heart overload and improve arterial flow.

Gas embolism is suspected when a predisposed patient suddenly develops tachypnea, hypotension, tachycardia and venous hypertension. The diagnosis is further supported by the typical "mill wheel murmur" heard over the precordium. Conditions which may lead to lethal *right heart* gas embolism include craniotomy in the sitting position (the negative intrathoracic and venous pressures suck air into open veins), pressure transfusion from bottles pressurized with air, vaginal gas insufflation, and therapeutic pneumoperitoneum. Prevention is the best cure. In neurosurgical operations where the patient is in the sitting position, the anesthesiologist anticipates gas embolization by auditing heart sounds with a Doppler monitor and esophageal stethoscope and placing a right atrial catheter for aspiration of the gas if needed.

Fatal right heart gas embolism is caused by obstruction of the right atrium and pulmonary outflow tract. The degree of reduction of cardiac output and the likelihood of developing cardiac arrest depend on the volume and solubility of the gas, the position of the patient, and the condition of the heart. In man, probably over 300 ml. of air must enter the venous system in order to cause sudden cardiac arrest. In dogs, 50 to 100 ml. of air intravenously often causes VF.

Treatment of right heart gas embolism includes: (a) administration of 100 per cent oxygen by IPPV; (b) positioning of the patient left-side-down and head down in order to favor exit of foam within the right heart from the pulmonary outflow tract; (c) use of vasopressor as needed; and (d) when cardiac arrest develops, opening the chest to perform open chest heart resuscitation, including needle aspiration of the right ventricle.

Left heart gas embolism involves entry of gas into the systemic arterial circulation—either through the pulmonary veins (e.g., lung rupture), or from a pump or air bubbles entrapped in the left side of the heart during open heart surgery. Systemic gas embolism of as little as 1 ml. can lead to cardiac arrest through obstruction of coronary arteries and to severe neurologic deficit, including coma, from cerebral embolization. Coronary embolization may be ameliorated through cardiac massage, which can force bubbles from the arterial to the venous side of the circulation. Cerebral embolism should be treated promptly by measures to ameliorate brain ischemia (Chapter 5). Prophylaxis and therapy should include denitrogenation of lungs and blood with 100 per cent oxygen inhalation in order to increase the rate of air bubble reabsorption. Hyperbaric oxygenation seems a sound and effective approach, but secondary thrombosis in vessels obstructed by gas may limit its effectiveness.

Fat embolism rarely causes sudden death. Lipemia is common in shock and trauma, owing to: (a) liberation of catecholamines and other substances which promote lipid mobilization; (b) direct entry into veins of fat from broken bones and other traumatized fat tissue. The "pulmonary fat embolism syndrome" (the clinical picture of pulmonary edema and consolidation with bronchospasm) may be followed by evidence of systemic fat embolization (cerebral, cutaneous, coronary) (Peltier, 1974). Fat embolism is more likely to occur when a prolonged period of hypoperfusion or manipulation of large bone fractures preceded. The often severe, sometimes lethal progressive pulmonary consolidation (acute respiratory distress) which ensues (Chapter 3) is due to pulmonary capillary obstruction by fat globules and secondary thrombi and hemorrhagic destruction of lung tissue by fatty acids (Herndon, 1971). Aggressive respiratory support, including CPPV–oxygen and steroids, should be augmented by measures such as I.V. dextran-40 and heparin. Some of these measures require further evaluation.[*]

Bone marrow emboli are the result of multiple fractures such as frequently occur during external cardiac compression. They are not in themselves lethal and are usually either asymptomatic or overshadowed by the underlying problem (cardiac arrest, multiple trauma).

Amniotic fluid embolism can kill rapidly through mechanisms not yet clearly under-

---

[*]See Fat Embolism, pp. 94 and 786.

stood. The incidence of death ascribed on the basis of clinical and postmortem findings to promote amniotic fluid embolism is about one in 8000 deliveries. Multiparous women are affected more commonly than the primipara. Experimental amniotic fluid embolism in animals causes systemic vasodilatation, attendant systemic arterial hypotension, and venous hypertension (Reis, 1969). The pulmonary bed is vasoconstricted and there is hypoxemia with a greatly increased alveolar-arterial oxygen gradient (the picture of pulmonary edema and consolidation, i.e., shock lung). A consumptive coagulopathy with hypofibrinogenemia also may be present.

One should suspect pulmonary amniotic fluid embolism when, in patients with placenta accreta, cesarean section, uterine rupture, retention of the products of conception, or premature separation of the placenta, sudden collapse occurs during or after labor and delivery. This is particularly true when collapse is associated with dyspnea, cyanosis, and shock. Therapy includes aggressive respiratory care (Chapters 3 and 10), SAP support by vasopressor, pulmonary broncho- and vasodilatation, and measures directed against intravascular coagulation.

TEMPERATURE EMERGENCIES

Man is homoiothermic through a delicate mechanism which maintains core body temperature near 37°C. (98°F.). The hypothalamic temperature regulating center controls the required balance of heat production (primarily from muscular work and hepatic metabolism) and heat retention or elimination (primarily through cutaneous vasoconstriction and vasodilatation, sweating and pulmonary ventilation). Specific diseases, injuries, and drugs can overstress or derange the temperature-regulating mechanism, leading rapidly to lethal hypothermia or hyperthermia.

Hypothermia. By reducing oxygen consumption, hypothermia protects vital organs during apnea and circulatory arrest, and for this reason hypothermia is sometimes used therapeutically in circumstances where delivery of oxygen and substrate to tissue is impaired (Chapter 5). However, hypothermia can itself cause cardiac arrest in man when the heart temperature reaches about 22 to 28°C. (70 to 82°F.). Healthy, unmedicated man exposed to low environmental temperatures without protection,

fights the cold with cutaneous vasoconstriction, shivering, and catecholamine release, which result in a transient increase in oxygen consumption, heart rate, SAP, and cardiac irritability. With persisting exposure, the defense mechanism finally becomes overwhelmed and the core body temperature decreases. When core temperature falls to 30 to 35°C. (86 to 95°F.), a further decrease in temperature usually will be unopposed by shivering and vasoconstriction. CNS depressant and vasodilating drugs (including alcohol) and muscle relaxants (used in anesthesia) foster a more rapid downward drift in core temperature in a cold environment, as they inhibit initial defense mechanisms of hypermetabolism and diversion of circulation away from the periphery. The decline in body temperature is accompanied by a decline in total and cerebral oxygen consumption, cardiac output, cerebral blood flow, microcirculation (hence, there is increased blood sludging and viscosity), SAP, heart rate, respiratory minute volume, and electrical activity of the brain. Oxygen consumption falls to about 50 per cent of normal at a core temperature of 30°C. (86°F.) and 15 per cent of normal at 20°C. (68°F.), at which point the EEG is isoelectric. Body temperatures in man below about 22 to 28°C. (70 to 82°F.) cannot be reached safely without artificial circulation, since the human heart stops in asystole or VF in that temperature range. Restoration of spontaneous circulation, including defibrillation, may be difficult unless the heart temperature is rapidly increased during cardiac compressions, which may require thoracotomy and direct rewarming of the heart or partial extracorporeal circulation with a heat exchanger.

In progressive reduction of heart temperature (from external cooling or rapid infusion, for example, of cold blood), the contractions of the cooled heart become weaker, and discharges from ectopic foci increase. Coronary perfusion is reduced because of retarded systole, particularly when diastole is further shortened by tachycardia. Diminished coronary perfusion, in turn, predisposes to focal coronary ischemia and VF, particularly in patients with underlying ischemic heart disease. Other factors which promote VF in the hypothermic patient include acidemia, alkalemia, changes in the calcium/potassium ratio, mechanical stimuli (external heart compressions), electric stimuli (pacing), sympathetic stimuli, catecholamine release, and certain drugs (Stephenson, 1974). The hibernating animal's heart does not fibrillate, probably because it has no adrenergic fibers (Nielsen, 1969).

While hypothermia thus carries considerable hazard to the myocardium, at the same time it offers a certain degree of protection to the brain (Chapter 5), partially through preservation of cerebral enzyme function. The peculiar combination of cardiac vulnerability and brain protection is illustrated by a recent case of our ambulance series: an inebriated patient was found with a core temperature of 25°C. (77°F.), unconscious, but still breathing spontaneously and with a palpable pulse. Upon being moved into the ambulance, he developed VF. Multiple defibrillation attempts at the scene failed. CPR during transportation and in the hospital had to be continued intermittently for seven hours before uninterrupted spontaneous circulation finally was restored. He made a complete recovery with prearrest CNS status. Another example is the patient described under "Drowning"—a child who survived submersion of 40 minutes in ice water with complete CNS recovery. Also, during rewarming VF may occur, triggered by shivering with increased oxygen consumption and uncontrolled acidemia or other factors. To prevent this, rewarming should be slow, with control of shivering by drugs and blood gas and pH normalization.

Hyperthermia. Emergencies arising from extremes of heat vary from benign electrolyte imbalances to rapidly lethal derangements of multiple organ systems, and may reflect both normal (albeit exaggerated) and defective responses to increased temperature.

Heat cramps, usually most marked in the muscles of the legs and abdomen, are a relatively benign sequela to electrolyte loss through sweating. They are easily corrected by administration of sodium chloride and cause no permanent disability.

Heat exhaustion is essentially a form of hypovolemic shock caused by the body's exaggerated response to high environmental temperatures; massive fluid loss through sweating leads to peripheral vasomotor collapse. The patient has a pale, cold, clammy skin, wide pupils, arterial hypotension, tachycardia, and a decreased core temperature. Nausea and vomiting frequently accompany this syndrome and further exacerbate hypovolemia. Emergency treatment is aimed at restoring vascular volume and consists of providing a cool environment, positioning the patient supine with legs raised, and infusing isotonic saline.

Heat stroke (heat pyrexia) represents a failure of the mechanism of heat regulation through sweating. The patient's skin is flushed and dry, and cardiac output, SAP, heart rate, minute volume of breathing, and core temperature are all increased. The cerebral cortex can suffer irreversible heat damage, especially at temperatures of about 41°C. (106°F.) or above. The insult to the brain depends on the duration and degree of hyperthermia, as well as on the adequacy of arterial oxygen transport. Thermal damage involving the brain stem results in apnea prior to cardiac arrest. Just before pulselessness ensues, the skin becomes gray and cyanotic. Treatment consists of rapid cooling; ventilation with oxygen; intensive therapy for shock, respiratory failure, and brain failure; and CPR where appropriate. Cooling should be carried to the point of normothermia or hypothermia by external means, cold intravenous and rectal fluids, and perhaps extracorporeal circulation with heat exchanger.

Malignant hyperpyrexia is a very rare, sudden, unexpected, and fulminating increase in metabolism and body temperature that occurs during induction or maintenance of anesthesia with a variety of agents. It happens in apparently healthy individuals because of a familial error in skeletal muscle metabolism. This anesthesia-related complication can result within minutes in lethally high body temperatures, mixed acidemia, cell membrane and capillary failure, and intravascular coagulation, followed by brain destruction. Immediate recognition and resuscitation, including rapid cooling, pHa normalization, and I.V. procainamide, may result in complete recovery.

ACUTE ANEMIA

Slowly developing chronic anemia with normal or elevated blood volume, even to severe reductions in blood hemoglobin content (e.g., 3 gm. per cent), is compatible with life and work. *Chronic* anemia merely predisposes to other lethal insults. An *acute* decrease in blood hemoglobin concentration of life-threatening proportions without a decrease in blood volume is rare. It may, for example, occur during the treatment of massive hemorrhage with plasma or plasma substitutes without blood or red cell infusion.

Our experiments with rapid normovolemic hemodilution in dogs (withdrawal of 10 ml./kg. body weight of blood and replacement with the same volume of dextran every 10 minutes) demonstrated four sequential phases of response (Takaori, 1967):

(1) Complete compensation of arterial oxygen transport through increase in cardiac output (largely due to decreased blood viscosity) and an increase in the coefficient of oxygen extraction (arteriovenous oxygen content difference/arterial oxygen content) was observed until the hemoglobin values had decreased to approximately 5.5 gm. per cent. Oxygen consumption remained unchanged, and there was no lactacidemia.

(2) Partial compensation occurred when the hemoglobin levels fell to between 5.5 and 4 gm. per cent; oxygen consumption began to decline, although cardiac output reached its maximal compensatory increase.

(3) Reversible decompensation occurred after about 10 blood replacements or 100 minutes, when the hemoglobin had fallen to about 3 to 4 gm. per cent; at this point, cardiac output declined from its maximal compensatory increase, arterial pressure and heart rate decreased, right ventricular end-diastolic pressure increased (heart failure), venous oxygen values decreased sharply, and blood lactate values and base deficit increased. Animals could still survive this degree of hemodilution without requiring hemoglobin-containing solutions.

(4) Irreversible decompensation occurred when the hemoglobin dropped below approximately 3 gm. per cent (10 per cent hematocrit) breathing air (or below about 2 gm. per cent hemoglobin with 100 per cent oxygen breathing). This stage was characterized by a dramatic decrease in cardiac output, oxygen consumption, and venous oxygen values. The lowest hemoglobin values measured before cardiac arrest were 1.5 to 2 gm. per cent. Asystole occurred at an arterial oxygen content of about 2 to 3 volumes per cent.

Patients with oligemia or cardiopulmonary disease may decompensate earlier because of an inability to increase cardiac output and/or because of a reduced PaO_2. Monitoring patients with normovolemic hemodilution should include assessments of central or mixed venous PO_2 (even better, mixed cerebral venous PO_2). When mixed venous PO_2 reaches about 30 to 35 torr, or cerebral venous PO_2 reaches 20 torr or less, metabolism in vital organs can be assumed to become anaerobic, and there is consequently a need for increasing the arterial oxygen-carrying capacity by infusion of blood or red blood cells.

CARBON MONOXIDE POISONING

Carbon monoxide (CO), an inert odorless gas, is probably not a cellular poison per se, but, by virtue of its affinity for hemoglobin, produces acute normovolemic anemic hypoxia. Hemoglobin binds CO about 200 to 300 times more readily than it binds oxygen; the carboxyhemoglobin produced is subsequently not available for oxygen transport.

The uptake of CO depends on the inhaled concentration, duration of exposure, ventilation volumes, and state of metabolism at the time of exposure (Forbes, 1962; Tomashevsky, 1961). A person doing light work who is exposed to as little as 0.2 per cent CO inhaled, will form CO hemoglobin at a rate of 1 per cent per minute. If he is doing heavy work, this rate will be 2.4 per cent per minute, and within about 45 minutes CO will saturate 76 per cent of his hemoglobin—a lethal concentration.

CO poisoning may occur with exposure to products of combustion in closed spaces, automobile exhaust, or CO-containing gases used in industry. Environments commonly hazardous in this regard include tunnels during rush hour (automotive exhaust may contain over 10 per cent CO), mines, poorly ventilated rooms with blocked chimneys and some household gases (not in the U.S.).

Humans breathing low concentrations of CO develop a sequence of headache, vertigo, yawning, dimmed vision, tachycardia, and vomiting. Higher concentrations or longer exposure result in coma, twitching, collapse, pupillary dilatation, Cheyne-Stokes respirations, apnea, and cardiac arrest (asystole). The skin is warm; a cherry red color of the skin, while pathognomonic of CO poisoning, is seen only rarely.

The pathophysiology of acute CO poisoning has been studied in conscious dogs inhaling 1 per cent CO. These animals reach 80 per cent CO hemoglobin saturation almost instantaneously, and death is sudden (Swann, 1949). There is no increase in respiratory drive, since the peripheral chemoreceptors are sensitive to a decrease in arterial oxygen tension (PaO_2), not oxygen content, and PaO_2 in CO poisoning is normal. The sequence of events in these animals is loss of consciousness, rapidly followed by hypotension, convulsions, apnea from cerebral hypoxia, and cardiac arrest in asystole. If, prior to cardiac arrest, IPPV with 100 per cent oxygen is begun, the animal survives and resumes spontaneous breathing, but he may have permanent cerebral damage. Dogs inhaling lower concentrations of CO in air (0.17 to 0.25 per cent) develop cardiac arrest in four to seven hours.[*] Resuscitation of cardiac function and spontaneous breathing is easily achieved, but the animals die in coma within days thereafter. Thus, irreversible cerebral damage apparently occurs before cardiac arrest, particularly when there was a prolonged antecedent period of arterial hypotension. The latter seems to be a more crucial parameter in determining the outcome of the brain than the per cent of CO hemoglobin and duration of exposure.

The organism tolerates better a reduction of hemoglobin by normovolemic hemodilution with colloid plasma substitutes, as described earlier, than the same degree of reduction by blockage of hemoglobin with CO. This may be because CO, in addition to usurping oxygen's place on the hemoglobin molecule, also shifts the oxyhemoglobin dissociation curve to the left, rendering release of oxygen at the tissue level less efficient. Certain respiratory enzymes similarly have greater affinity for CO than for oxygen. The question whether CO also damages the brain directly has not been resolved. Neurohistologically, there are not only the well-described areas of necrosis in the globus pallidus, but also nonspecific hypoxic changes in white and gray matter, particularly in the cortex, as well as cerebral edema, as in ischemic-anoxic encephalopathy of other types (Chapter 5).

Treatment includes IPPV/100 per cent oxygen and CPR where indicated. CO_2 inhalation has not proved valuable; hyperbaric oxygenation has, but is rarely available early enough to influence the outcome. As early as possible after exposure, deliberate hypothermia or other measures known to ameliorate

postanoxic brain damage (e.g., barbiturates) should be undertaken (Chapter 5).

HYPOGLYCEMIA

The CNS depends on glucose and oxygen for energy metabolism. Fat and proteins are unable to substitute fully for glucose. Whereas oxygen deprivation is the cause of sudden death very frequently, glucose deprivation is rare and kills more slowly (Sussman, 1967). Hypoglycemia often results in brain failure without cardiac arrest.

Hypoglycemia occurs in overdose of insulin (less likely in overdose by oral hypoglycemic drugs), or islet cell tumor of the pancreas. Alcohol, salicylates and some other drugs, as well as the increased glycogen turnover in neonates, are factors predisposing to hypoglycemia. The symptomatology and outcome depend on the degree and speed of reduction in blood sugar, the underlying disease, and other factors.

A decrease of blood sugar levels to about 30 to 50 mg. per cent results in hunger, yawning, irritability, sweating, hyperventilation, tachycardia, and arterial hypertension — most a response to the released epinephrine. A rapid reduction in blood sugar to 30 mg. per cent or less produces exhaustion of glucose and glycogen stores, which results in coma, convulsions, wide pupils, pale skin, hypoventilation, bradycardia and hypotension (insulin shock) — and cardiac arrest in asystole, if the blood sugar drops further and remains below 30 mg. per cent over one to two hours. Beyond that time and degree of hypoglycemia, CNS recovery may be with neurologic deficit.

Neurohistologically, the damage caused by hypoglycemic brain failure is almost indistinguishable from that caused by ischemic-anoxia, namely, diffuse cortical neuronal cell degeneration and myelin degeneration of central and peripheral nerves.

Since hypoglycemia may be a factor in any emergency associated with shock, convulsions, and cardiac arrest, and since glucose transport and brain glucose stores are reduced in ischemic-anoxia, *administration of 30 to 50 per cent glucose during resuscitation — irrespective of the underlying problem — seems indicated.* Hypertonic glucose may help ameliorate intracellular edema because of its osmotherapeutic effects and put

---

[*]Soboleva, 1957, as quoted in Negovskii, 1962.

potassium back into cells in brain, heart, and elsewhere. To accomplish the latter, a combination of hypertonic glucose, potassium, and insulin I.V. has been recommended for critically ill patients with myocardial infarction (Sodi-Pallares, 1968). The heart is more resistant to hypoglycemia than to hypoxemia, since it also lives on substrates other than glucose. How long the human brain can tolerate perfusion with glucose-free but normally oxygenated blood without suffering permanent neuronal loss has not been defined to our knowledge. The period is definitely much longer than that of clinical death in oxygen deprivation states. For glucose stores and metabolism, see "Terminal State" above.

DRUGS AND OTHER POISONS

Sudden death from poisons, some of which we have adapted for therapeutic use, is as old as mankind. The mechanism of dying, where understood, depends on the mechanism of the given drug's action. Often, poisons kill by nonspecific means, e.g., by inducing coma, hypotension, or bronchospasm, all of which are readily controllable by standard resuscitation and life support measures. Reviews of drugs and other poisons are given elsewhere in this book and in other textbooks (Goodman, 1970; Arena, 1974). Here are only a few examples:

Any drug which depresses consciousness and induces coma may cause sudden death from hypoxemia due to upper airway soft tissue obstruction (malpositioning of the head, foreign matter inhalation), hypoventilation, and apnea (Chapter 3). The lethal potential of depressant drugs, particularly barbiturates, is not dose-related, since a variety of contributing factors may influence mortality. For example, the minimal blood concentration of a hypnotic or narcotic drug required to induce coma without apnea may result in asphyxia and irreversible brain damage, if the person happens to have a pillow under his head and his neck remains flexed during loss of consciousness and if resuscitation and life support are started late. In contrast, much higher blood concentrations of these drugs (30 × or more) may be survived without residual damage if the person's position favors an open airway and spontaneous breathing, or if artificial ventilation, oxygenation and circulatory support are begun early (Clemmeson, 1961).

Barbiturates and many other anesthetics, when given in doses much larger than those causing coma and vasodilatation, may also depress myocardial contractility and produce cardiac arrest—particularly in the presence of hypovolemia or cardiac disease. Other hypnotics such as glutethimide (Doriden) cause, in addition, capillary and pulmonary membrane damage, arterial hypotension, and pupillary dilatation. These toxic manifestations do not obviate complete CNS recovery, provided support of arterial oxygenation and circulation is started early.

Narcotics (e.g., heroin), injected intravascularly, may cause fulminating pulmonary edema through mechanisms that are not well understood. Talcs and other adulterants contaminating illicitly used narcotics may, further, produce pneumonitis and vascular damage. Cardiac arrest in narcotic overdose usually is secondary to airway obstruction and apnea, as with other depressants.

Drugs such as local anesthetics first produce stimulation (e.g., convulsions), followed by cardiovascular collapse and apnea. Other drugs may kill through their specific pharmacologic effects. For example, anticholinesterases (nerve gases, some insecticides, poisonous mushrooms) may kill through the muscarinic actions of acetylcholine, which affect smooth muscles, heart, and glands, leading to hypersalivation, vomiting, defecation, bronchospasm, bronchorrhea, obstructive asphyxia, arterial hypotension, bradycardia, and asystole; further, the nicotinic actions of anticholinesterases on ganglia and skeletal muscles, first stimulation then depression, result in synaptic block, paralysis, and apnea. *Atropine* reverses the muscarinic effects, while IPPV supports life until the nicotinic effects subside.

Salicylates stimulate spontaneous hyperventilation (hypocarbia, respiratory alkalemia), which is followed by metabolic acidemia, circulatory collapse, coma, convulsions, and asphyxial death—unless artificial ventilation, intravenous bicarbonate, and other life support measures interrupt the sequence.

Overdose with sympathomimetics of the alpha-adrenergic stimulating type (e.g., norepinephrine, phenylephrine, methoxamine) produces arterial hypertension with the possibility of cerebral hemorrhage and pulmonary edema. Their prolonged use results in renal ischemia and failure. Sympathomimetics of the beta-adrenergic stimulating variety elicit tachycardia, VT, and VF, particularly when the heart is sensitized by certain anesthetics such as cyclopropane or halothane. Sympathomimetics with both alpha and beta properties (e.g., epinephrine) will produce a mixed picture.

Poisons which have traditionally been popular for suicide or murder include arsenic and cyanide. The exact mechanism by which arsenic, a cellular poison, causes death is unknown, but the terminal event in arsenic poisonings appears related to defibrillation-resistant VT and VF. Coma and convulsions may also contribute to mortality. Cyanide, the most rapidly lethal poison, inhibits the cytochrome oxidase system for cellular oxygen utilization, producing cellular anoxia. Cyanide poisoning can result almost simultaneously in cerebral silence, apnea, and asystole without hypoxemia or hypercarbia (unless dying is slow). The reversibility of coma and cardiac arrest from cyanide poisoning and the dose-time relationship have not been studied, to our knowledge. Specific antidotes to cyanide are amyl nitrite or sodium nitrite, which produce ferric iron, displacing cyanide from cytochrome oxidase, and sodium thiosulfate, which converts cyanide to nontoxic thiocyanide.

ANAPHYLAXIS*

Anaphylaxis may be viewed as a manifestation of the immune system gone berserk in which antibodies, elaborated in response to a previous exposure to antigen — usually a foreign protein — reappear in full force upon re-exposure to the antigen and trigger a potentially lethal process. The antigens most often incriminated in this immune catastrophe include insect poisons, vaccine proteins, antitoxic sera (especially those derived from heterologous sources), and drugs (e.g., penicillin). However, virtually any antigen or haptene may elicit an anaphylactic response in the specifically sensitized individual.

The mechanism of anaphylactic shock is complex. Briefly, the following events seem to occur: The antigen–antibody complex adsorbs to cells (primarily mast cells) which liberate histamine and probably also serotonin, slow-reacting substance (SRS), acetylcholine, kinins, and other vasoactive materi-

*See also pp. 309–310.

als. These are smooth muscle and membrane poisons, and their most significant target organs are the airway, lungs, and vascular bed. Development of pharyngeal and laryngeal edema, bronchospasm, and edema of the bronchial mucosa is instantaneous and leads rapidly to asphyxia. The peripheral vascular bed reacts with vasodilatation, capillary leakage, and shock. There is suggestive evidence that the chemical mediators of anaphylaxis may also exert direct effects on the myocardium, and may, together with hypoxemia, be a factor in the development of EKG changes and cardiac arrest (Booth, 1974).

Management of suspected anaphylactic shock should include intravenous epinephrine 0.2 to 0.5 mg./70 kg.; IPPV/oxygen, CPR, and intravenous fluids as needed. When the antigen has been introduced by injection in an extremity (as in insect stings or injection of medication), a tourniquet may be applied proximal to the injection site to delay absorption of the antigen. I.V. steroids are also indicated, although their effects will not be significant for several hours. Antihistamines are unlikely to be of value, since they cannot reverse the action of histamine already liberated and are entirely ineffective against the many other chemical mediators (serotonin, kinins) involved in anaphylaxis.

SEVERE MULTIPLE TRAUMA

Multiple trauma, particularly that involving head or chest injury, can lead to sudden death by a variety of mechanisms including: asphyxia from complete airway obstruction by soft tissues (malpositioning of the head), or blood, or vomitus — secondary to coma per se; asphyxia from apnea due either to the primary impact or secondary to intracranial hemorrhage with intracranial hypertension; internal or external exsanguinating hemorrhage from injury of great vessels; obstructive shock from cardiac tamponade secondary to myocardial rupture; VF or asystole from cardiac contusion; tension pneumothorax from lung laceration and positive pressure breathing; asphyxia from tracheal or bronchial rupture with pneumothorax, interstitial emphysema, or atelectasis; crushing chest injury with severe flailing, resulting in inadequate lung expansion and hypoxemic arrest. Combinations of several of these and other mechanisms make the management of multiple injury patients in terminal states one of the greatest challenges of emergency and critical care medicine.

MISCELLANEOUS CAUSES OF RAPID DYING

In addition to the general and specific mechanisms of sudden death summarized in the previous sections, it appears justified to add a few "mixed" thoughts on this subject.

One-third of *sudden deaths* in previously healthy *adults* seem to be the direct result of alcohol intoxication (Kuller, 1970), which kills by asphyxia (upper airway soft tissue obstruction from coma, regurgitation and aspiration); arterial hypotension from vasodilatation and myocardial depression, as well as accidental hypothermia are additional factors leading to morbidity and mortality in the alcohol intoxicated patient. Sudden cardiac deaths are the second most common mode of acute exitus, and have been described in an earlier section of this chapter.

Sudden deaths of apparently healthy unattended *infants* (crib deaths) are common, accounting for an estimated 10,000 to 25,000 infant deaths per year in the United States (Beckwith, 1967; Strimer, 1969). Autopsies on these infants usually are unrevealing. The mechanism(s) of death are unknown; the most plausible current hypothesis is that occurrence of upper airway soft tissue obstruction from malpositioning of head and jaw in infants rendered stuporous, comatose, or "sluggish" by a variety of acute disease states, leads to asphyxial death. Increased airway resistance from laryngotracheobronchitis may be a predisposing factor in some cases.

Generalized *convulsions* can cause asphyxia from pharyngo-laryngospasm and apnea. The cumulative effects of convulsions with associated hypoxemia may contribute to the mental deterioration of epileptics observed over time. Neurons suffer not only from the hypoxemia secondary to impaired oxygenation during convulsions, but also from the hypoxic acidosis induced by the increased metabolic (electric) activity of neurons themselves. Thus, management of generalized convulsions requires IPPV/oxygen (if necessary with the aid of a muscle relaxant) and, as soon as possible thereafter, a CNS depressant (e.g., diazepam, thiopental, phenobarbital, diphenylhydantoin) to minimize the electric discharges from the brain.

In addition to precipitating respiratory deaths, seizure disorders may lead to death from cardiac causes. Temporal lobe seizures, for example, can stimulate a variety of cardiac arrhythmias, among them VT and VF, although the mechanism is unclear.

Electroconvulsive therapy can cause asphyxia from airway obstruction and apnea, as the result of the deliberately induced convulsions, the postictal coma, or the use of anesthetics and relaxants.

Electrolyte disturbances can be the primary cause of cardiac arrest (Stephenson, 1974). A normal serum sodium level is required to maintain cardiac excitability and contractility. Disturbances of the calcium/potassium ratio can cause asystole or VF. Calcium increases myocardial contractility and, if present in excessive concentration, stops the heart in systole. Potassium, on the other hand, depresses myocardial contractility and stops the heart in diastole or VF. Not only the absolute values of each electrolyte but also their ratios are important; the normal calcium/potassium ratio is about 1 to 1.5. Hyperpotassemia occurring in patients with extensive burns, because of tissue breakdown, may be worsened by succinylcholine (used as a relaxant in anesthesia), as that agent causes muscle contractions and further release of potassium. The resultant rise in serum potassium may precipitate cardiac arrest. Paralyzed, degenerated muscle tissue (as in paraplegics) also seems prone to liberate potassium under the influence of succinylcholine. Magnesium, which may be absorbed in high concentration during aspiration of sea water, can stop the heart in diastole. An abnormal increase in sodium and other osmotically active substances such as glucose and urea can result in hyperosmolality. This, however, is rarely acutely lethal, but may cause gradual brain damage (Chapter 5).

Acid-base disturbances, as reflected in abnormal blood pH values (which often do not reflect the acid-base milieu in tissues), have been, in part, discussed before. Usually well compensated arterial pH abnormalities lie between 7.2 and 7.6. In man, such extremes as 6.9 or less or 7.8 or more can result rapidly in shock states or cardiac arrest — extreme acidemia in circulatory collapse and cardiac standstill, extreme alkalemia in VT and VF.

One must keep in mind the possibility of paradoxic phenomena. For example: (1)

During dying and its reversal, alkalemia may coexist at times with tissue acidosis (e.g., bicarbonate infusion raises pHa, causing a shift to the left of the oxygen-hemoglobin dissociation curve which may reduce oxygen release at the tissue level; this adds to the shock-induced tissue acidity for which bicarbonate was administered). (2) In patients with high CO_2 and bicarbonate (e.g., emphysema), rapid lowering of $PaCO_2$ by artificial hyperventilation may lead to coma with cerebral anoxia due to cerebral vasospasm from high CSF pH (Chapter 5). (3) Increased hydrogen ion concentration from low oxygen and/or high CO_2 in the extracellular fluid of the brain causes vasodilatation and, in the lungs, causes vasoconstriction. (4) Hypercarbia per se in the fit person causes little circulatory disturbance, probably because it releases norepinephrine from nerve endings, which results in systemic vasoconstriction and some inotropic effect on the heart; this is offset in the healthy person by the direct effect of hypercarbia, one of vasodilatation and myocardial depression (Nahas, 1957; Brobeck, 1973).

Sometimes, sudden death is caused by members of the medical profession rather than by Nature's arbitrary chances. *Iatrogenic insults* leading to sudden death include those occurring during surgery, e.g., from anesthesia or uncontrollable hemorrhage. The mechanisms of sudden death with anesthesia as the primary factor are, in order of decreasing frequency: mechanical asphyxiation, overdose with myocardial depression, and vasodilatation hypotension (e.g., spinal or epidural anesthesia). The incidence of anesthesia-related deaths ranges from 1:500 anesthesias among patients in poor physical status to 1:10,000 among patients in good physical status (Phillips, 1974). There are as well iatrogenic sudden deaths associated with diagnostic procedures, such as cardiac catheterization (e.g., cardiac perforation, acute ischemia and VF), and roentgen studies (e.g., hypersensitivity to contrast agents, airway obstruction, and hypotension due to postural changes or the dark environment).

WHY RESUSCITATE? A PHILOSOPHIC APPRAISAL

In the foregoing discussion we have dealt at length with the pathophysiologic aspects of acute dying and its reversal. It is necessary, however, to step back for a moment from technical details and consider some philosophic implications inherent in reanimation. Specifically, is resuscitation worth the effort? Can it be justified—socially, morally, economically? Is it supportive of human evolution on this earth, or is it merely a quixotic, antievolutionary undertaking of arrogant homo sapiens?

Few would argue that resuscitation applied without judgment and compassion is morally and economically acceptable. The debilitated elderly patient, the terminal cancer patient in intractable pain, the severely brain-injured patient without prospect of human mentation—their dying should be permitted to proceed without the imposition of costly and, in these instances, dehumanizing life support technology. But what of those whose dying occurs from potentially reversible conditions imposed by the arbitrary mischances of Nature, before they have had time to live "full lives"? Is their reanimation defensible, or do we also tamper here with the sanctified laws of Nature?

Certainly, so long as the evolution of life is viewed as a statistical matter, and species-oriented, resuscitation of a few individual humans assumes trivial significance. Indeed, proponents of a laissez-faire stance on dying could with some justification assert that resuscitation, by promoting survival of the unfit, exerts an untoward effect on human evolution. Those who argue thus for resuscitative nihilism must, however, to be consistent, condemn the endeavors of Medicine in any form. For all of human disease and misery must then be viewed as part of Nature's selective process, and medical intervention of any kind be seen as ill-advised tampering with evolution. But the human brain—considered by its owners to be the peak of evolution destined to "build this earth" (Teilhard de Chardin)—and Medicine, which is a creation of the human brain, have declared that even a single human life is of inestimable value. The ethic of natural selection must of necessity be alien and repugnant to man, especially to man as physician. Medicine represents an imposition of human values on a random universe: an assertion that compassion, reason, and decency constitute a higher ethic than chance. Thus, the increasing change from a species-oriented toward an individuum-oriented society makes resuscitation evolutionarily positive. Those who fear that resuscitation of a handful of "unfit" will exert a negative impact on evolution of the species, might better concern themselves with the eradication of war, violent crime, and man-made disasters which destroy primarily the young and fit.

Science and medicine, products of the cultural evolution of man, have influenced and should continue to influence human values. Research on the mechanisms of dying and its reversibility—so far less advanced than research on the beginnings of human life—should be fostered, not only for medical and public health reasons, but also for the acquisition of new knowledge per se. Science, art, and humanism (with medicine being a mix of the three) are prime examples of increasing consciousness on this earth, and must therefore be considered evolutionarily positive. Bertrand Russell said, "For man only the examined life is worth living." I want to add that only the examined death is worth fighting or accepting.

But quite aside from evolutionary considerations, resuscitation implies a commitment on the side of Life. To devote one's energies to the restoration of lives cut short before fulfillment is to declare that life is intrinsically valuable—that it is worth living. And while the therapeutic impact of resuscitation may affect only a few, the moral impact of this endeavor and the commitment it represents may have a much broader influence in a world where life has too often been regarded as cheap.

Those of us who choose to pursue the study of dying and its reversal must constantly bear in mind the over-all goal of our efforts, namely, the restoration not only of circulatory and respiratory functions, but of human mentation as well. Those who return from the shores of Lethe should be enabled to re-enter the community of the living in a manner approaching the ancient ideal: "Mens sana in corpore sano" (Juvenal).

ABBREVIATIONS AND DEFINITIONS

Abbreviations and Terms	*Definitions*
AC	Alternating current
Acidemia	Arterial pH less than 7.35
Acidosis	Reduced pH (tissues)
ACTH	Adrenocorticotropic hormone
ADP	Adenosine diphosphate
Alkalemia	Arterial pH over 7.45
Alkalosis	Increased pH (tissues)
AMP	Adenosine monophosphate
Anoxia	No oxygen
Apnea	No breathing movements
Arterial Oxygen Transport	Cardiac output (resting adult about 5 liters/min.) times arterial oxygen content (normally about 20 ml./100 ml.)
Asphyxia	Hypoxemia plus hypercarbia
Asystole	Cessation of circulation with heart in standstill and EKG flat
ATP	Adenosine triphosphate
BE	Blood base excess. Normal value 0 ± 3 mEq./liter
°C.	Centigrade (degrees Celsius)
CBF	Cerebral blood flow (see Chapter 5)
CNS	Central nervous system
CO	Carbon monoxide
CPPV	Continuous positive pressure (controlled) ventilation (IPPV + PEEP, positive end-expiratory pressure) (Chapter 10)
CPR	Cardiopulmonary resuscitation. Basic life support: ABC (airway, breathing, circulation); advanced life support: D (definitive therapy, including drugs, defibrillation, and postresuscitative therapy)
CVP	Central venous pressure
DC	Direct current
EEG	Electroencephalogram
EKG	Electrocardiogram
°F.	Degrees Fahrenheit
gm.	Gram(s)

Hypercarbia	Arterial P_{CO_2} over 45 torr
Hyperventilation	Increased alveolar ventilation, resulting in a Pa_{CO_2} of less than 35 torr
Hypocarbia	Arterial P_{CO_2} less than 35 torr
Hypoventilation	Decreased alveolar ventilation, resulting in a Pa_{CO_2} of over 45 torr
Hypoxemia	Arterial P_{O_2} less than 75 torr
Hypoxia	Reduced oxygen (tissues)
IPPB	Intermittent positive pressure (assisted) breathing
IPPV	Intermittent positive pressure (controlled) ventilation
I.V.	Intravenous
kg.	Kilogram(s)
M	Molar, i.e., molecular weight in grams per liter
mEq	Milliequivalent(s); i.e., millimole(s) per liter
mg.	Milligram(s)
ml.	Milliliter(s)
mM	Millimole(s) per liter; i.e., milliequivalents per liter
O_2	Oxygen
Pa_{CO_2}	Arterial carbon dioxide tension (pressure). Normal value: 35 to 45 torr
Pa_{O_2}	Arterial oxygen tension (pressure). Normal values: 75 to 100 torr when breathing air; 550 to 650 torr when breathing 100 per cent oxygen
pHa	Arterial pH (negative logarithm of hydrogen ion concentration) Normal value: 7.35–7.45
PVC	Premature ventricular contraction (ventricular extrasystole)
SAP	Systemic arterial pressure. Normal value: 90 to 100 torr, mean
torr	Unit of pressure equal to 1 mm. Hg (named for Torricelli)
VF	Ventricular fibrillation
VT	Ventricular tachycardia

Selected Books and Reviews

Arena, J. M.: Poisoning. Springfield, Charles C Thomas, 1974.

Brierley, J. B., and Meldrum, B. S. (eds.): Brain Hypoxia. Philadelphia, J. B. Lippincott Co., 1971.

Brobeck, J. R. (ed.): Best & Taylor's Physiological Basis of Medical Practice. 9th Ed. Baltimore, The Williams & Wilkins Company, 1973.

Elam, J. O.: Respiratory and Circulatory Resuscitation. In Handbook of Physiology. Respiration, Vol. II, Chapter 50, pp. 1265–1312. American Physiologic Society, 1965.

Goodman, L. S., and Gillman, A. (eds.): The Pharmacological Basis of Therapeutics. 4th Ed., New York, The Macmillan Co., 1970.

Ingvar, D. H.: The pathophysiology of cerebral anoxia. Acta Anaes. Scand. Suppl. 29:47, 1968.

Plum, F. (ed.): Symposium of the threshold and mechanisms of anoxic ischemic brain injury. Arch. Neurol. 29:359, 1973.

Safar, P.: Cardiopulmonary-Cerebral Resuscitation. Philadelphia, W. B. Saunders Co., in press.)

Safar, P., et al.: Emergency and Critical Care Medicine—Local Implementation of National Recommendations. In Safar, P. (ed.): Public Health Aspects of Critical Care Medicine and Anesthesiology. Philadelphia, F. A. Davis Co., 1974(b).

Safar, P. (ed.): Advances in Cardiopulmonary Resuscitation. The Wolf Creek Conference. New York, Springer Verlag, 1977.

Stephenson, H. E.: Cardiac Arrest and Resuscitation. 4th Ed. St. Louis: C. V. Mosby Co., 1974.

References

Adelson, L., and Hoffman, W.: Sudden death from coronary artery disease. A statistical study, Cuyahoga County Coroner's Office, Cleveland. J.A.M.A., 176:129, 1961.

Ames, A., III, et al.: Cerebral ischemia. II. The noreflow phenomenon. Am. J. Pathol., 52:437, 1968.

Bakay, L., and Lee, J. C.: The effect of acute hypoxia and hypercapnia on the ultrastructure of the central nervous system. Brain, 91:697, 1968.

Barber, R. E., et al.: A prospective study in patients with irreversible brain damage. N. Engl. J. Med., 283:1478, 1970.

Beck, C. S., and Leighninger, D. S.: Death after a clean bill of health. J.A.M.A., 174:133, 1960.

Beck, C. S., and Leighninger, D. S.: Scientific basis for the surgical treatment of coronary artery disease. J.A.M.A., 159:1264, 1955.

Beck, C. S., Pritchard, H., and Feil, S. H.: Ventricular fibrillation of long duration abolished by electric shock. J.A.M.A., 135:985, 1947.

Beckwith, B. M., et al.: The sudden death syndrome of infancy. Hosp. Pract., 2:42, 1967.

Bell, J. A., and Hodgson, H. J. F.: Coma after cardiac arrest. Brain, 97:361, 1974.

Bengtsson, M., et al.: A psychiatric-psychological investigation of patients who had survived circulatory arrest. Acta Psychiatr. Scand., 45:327, 1969.

Bleyaert, A., et al.: A method for total brain ischemia (TBI) without circulatory arrest in the Rhesus monkey. The Physiologist, 16:267, 1973.

Bleyaert, A. L., et al.: Amelioration of postischemic encephalopathy by sodium thiopental after 16 minutes of global brain ischemia in monkeys. The Physiologist, *18*:145, 1975.

Booth, B. H., et al.: Electrocardiographic changes during human anaphylaxis. J.A.M.A., *26*:627, 1970.

Brierley, J. B., Meldrum, B. S., and Brown, A. W.: The threshold and neuropathology of cerebral anoxic-ischemic cell damage. Arch. Neurol., *29*:367, 1973.

Butt, M. P., et al.: Pulmonary function after resuscitation from near-drowning. Anesthesiology, *32*:275, 1970.

Clemmeson, C., and Nilsson, E.: Therapeutic trends in the treatment of barbiturate poisoning. Clin. Pharmacol. Ther., *2*:220, 1961.

Drewes, L. R., Gilboe, D. D., and Betz, A. L.: Metabolic alterations in brain anoxic anoxia and subsequent recovery. Arch. Neurol., *29*:385, 1973.

Fischer, E. G.: Impaired perfusion following cerebrovascular stasis. Arch. Neurol., *29*:361, 1973.

Forbes, W. H.: Carbon monoxide. *In* Whittenberger, J. L. (ed.): Artificial Respiration. New York, Hoeber, Harper and Row, 1962.

Cerst, P. H., Fleming, W. H., and Malm, J. R.: Increased susceptibility of the heart to ventricular fibrillation during metabolic acidosis. Circ. Res., *19*:63, 1966.

Graham, G. R., Hill, D. W., and Nunn, J. F.: The effect of high concentrations of carbon dioxide on the circulation and respiration. Anaesthetist, *9*:70, 1960.

Grenvik, A.: Brain death and vegetative state. Symposium on Brain Resuscitation. Crit. Care Med. 1978 (in press).

Gurvich, N. L., and Yuniev, S. G.: Restoration of a regular rhythm in the mammalian fibrillating heart. Am. Rev. Sov. Med., *3*:236, 1946.

Gurvitch, A. M.: Determination of the depth and reversibility of post-anoxic coma in animals. Resuscitation, *3*:1, 1974.

Harben, K., MacKenzie, I. L., and Ledingham, I. M.: Spontaneous reversion of ventricular fibrillation. Lancet, *2*:1140, 1963.

Hasan, S., et al.: Near drowning in humans. A report of 36 patients. Chest, *59*:191, 1971.

Hellstrom, H. R.: Vasospasm in ischemic heart disease—a hypothesis. Perspect. Biol. Med., *16*:427, 1973.

Herndon, J. H., Riseborough, E. J., and Fischer, J. E.: Fat embolism: a review of current concepts. J. Trauma, *11*:673, 1971.

Holmdahl, M. D.: Pulmonary uptake of oxygen, acid-base metabolism, and circulation during prolonged apnoea. Acta Chir. Scand., Suppl., *212*, 1956.

Hook, R., and Davis, C. D.: Resuscitation of the New Born Infant. *In* Stephenson, H. E. (ed.): Cardiac Arrest and Resuscitation. St. Louis: C. V. Mosby Co., 1974.

Hooker, D. R., Kouwenhoven, W. B., and Langworthy, O. R.: Effect of alternating electrical currents on the heart. Am. J. Physiol., *103*:444, 1933.

Hossmann, K. A., and Kleihues, P.: Reversibility of ischemic brain damage. Arch. Neurol., *29*:375, 1973.

Huckabee, W. E.: Relationships of pyruvate and lactate during anaerobic metabolism. I. Effects of infusion of pyruvate or glucose and of hyperventilation. J. Clin. Invest., *37*:244, 1958.

Ingvar, D. H.: The pathophysiology of cerebral anoxia. Acta Anaes. Scand., Suppl. *29*:47, 1968.

Kampschulte, S., Morikawa, S., and Safar, P.: Recovery from anoxic encephalopathy following cardiac arrest. Fed. Proc., *28*:522, 1969.

Kampschulte, S., Smith, J., and Safar, P.: Oxygen transport after cardiopulmonary resuscitation. Anaes. Resuscit., *30*:95, 1969.

Karpovich, P. V.: Water in the lungs of drowned animals. A.M.A. Arch. Pathol., *15*:828, 1933.

Kirimli, B., Kampschulte, S., and Safar, P.: Resuscitation from cardiac arrest due to exsanguination. Surg. Gynecol. Obstet., *129*:89, 1969.

Kirimli, B., Kampschulte, S., and Safar, P.: Pattern of dying from exsanguinating hemorrhage in dogs. J. Trauma, *10*:393, 1970.

Kirimli, B., and Safar, P.: Arterial versus venous transfusion in cardiac arrest from exsanguination. Anesth. Analg., *44*:6, 1965.

Kouwenhoven, W., and Langworthy, O. R.: Effects of electric shock. Trans. Am. Inst. Elec. Engnr., *49*:381, 1930.

Kouwenhoven, W. B., and Milner, W. R.: Treatment of ventricular fibrillation using a capacitor discharge. J. Appl. Physiol., *7*:253, 1954.

Kovach, A. G. B., and Sandor, P.: Cerebral blood flow and brain function during hypotension and shock. Am. Rev. Physiol. *38*:571, 1976.

Kristoffersen, M. B., Rattenborg, C. C., and Holaday, D. A.: Asphyxial death: the roles of acute anoxia, hypercarbia and acidosis. Anesthesiology, *28*:488, 1967.

Kuller, L. K.: Preventive care to reduce sudden heart deaths. Mod. Med., *38*:169, 1970.

Liberthson, R. R., et al.: Prehospital ventricular fibrillation. N. Engl. J. Med., *291*:7, 1974.

Lind, B., Kampschulte, S., and Safar, P.: I. A review of total brain ischaemia models in dogs and original experiments on clamping the aorta. II. Total brain ischaemia in dogs: Cerebral physiologic and metabolic changes after 15 minutes of circulatory arrest. Resuscitation *4*:19(I) and 97(II), 1975.

Luft, U. C., and Noell, W. K.: Manifestations of brief instantaneous anoxia in man. J. Appl. Physiol., *8*:444, 1956.

Lund, I., and Skulberg, A.: Resuscitation of cardiac arrest by doctor-manned ambulances in Oslo. American Heart Association/National Research Council CPR/ECC Conference Proceedings, May, 1973, Washington, D.C., Dallas: Am. Heart Assoc., 1975.

Michenfelder, J. D., and Theye, R. A.: The effects of anesthesia and hypothermia on canine cerebral ATP and lactate during anoxia produced by decapitation. Anesthesiology, *33*:430, 1970.

Modell, J. H.: The Pathophysiology and Treatment of Drowning and Near-drowning. Springfield, Ill., Charles C Thomas, 1971.

Modell, J. H., and Davis, J. H.: Electrolyte changes in human drowning victims. Anesthesiology, *30*:414, 1969.

Nahas, G. G., and Cavert, H. M.: Cardiac depressant effect of CO_2 and its reversal. Am. J. Physiol., *190*:483, 1957.

Negovskii, V. A.: Introduction: Reanimatology—The Science of Resuscitation. *In* Stephenson, H. E.: Cardiac Arrest and Resuscitation. 4th Ed. St. Louis, C. V. Mosby Co., 1974.

Negovskii, V. A.: Resuscitation and Artificial Hypothermia. Consultant's Bureau, New York, 1962.

Nemoto, E.: Postischemic amelioration of brain damage In: Proceedings, 3rd Koelner Symposium on cerebral and coronary vascular disorders. June 1976. Heidelberg: Springer Verlag, 1977 (K. Zulch, ed.).

Nielsen, K. C., and Owman, C.: Control of spontaneous ventricular fibrillation during induced hypothermia in cats by acute cardiac sympathectomy. Acta Physiol. Scand., *76*:73, 1969.

Pearson, J. W., and Redding, J. S.: Influence of peripheral vascular tone on cardiac resuscitation. Anesth. Analg., *44*:746, 1965.

Peltier, L. F., et al.: Fat embolism. Arch. Surg., *109*:12, 1974.

Phillips, O. C., and Capizzi, L. S.: Anesthesia Mortality. *In* Safar, P (ed.): Public Health Aspects of Critical Care Medicine and Anesthesiology. Philadelphia, F. A. Davis Co., 1974.

Prevost, J. L., and Batelli, F.: On some effects of electrical discharges on the hearts of mammals. Ct. R. Acad. Sci. (Paris), *129*:1267, 1899.

Ravitch, M., et al.: Lightning stroke. Recovery following cardiac massage and prolonged artificial respiration. N. Engl. J. Med., *264*:36, 1961.

Redding, J., et al.: Resuscitation from drowning. J.A.M.A., *178*:1136, 1961(a).

Redding, J. S., and Pearson, J. W.: Resuscitation from asphyxia. J.A.M.A., *182*:283, 1962.

Redding, J., and Pearson, J. W.: Resuscitation from ventricular fibrillation. J.A.M.A., *203*:93, 1968.

Redding, J., Voigt, G. C., and Safar, P.: Drowning treated with intermittent positive pressure breathing. J. Appl. Physiol., *15*:849, 1960(a).

Redding, J., Voigt, C., and Safar, P.: Treatment of sea water aspiration. J. Appl. Physiol., *15*:1113, 1960(b).

Reis, R. L., et al.: Hemodynamic effects of amniotic fluid embolism. Surg. Gynecol. Obstet., *129*:45, 1969.

Revenstorf: Über den Wert der Kryoskopie zur Diagnose des Todes durch Ertrinken. Muenchner Med. Wschr., *2*:1880, 1902.

Rossen, R., Kabat, H., and Anderson, J. P.: Acute arrest of cerebral circulation in man. Arch. Neurol. Psychiatr., *50*:510, 1943.

Roth, L. W., Whitehead, R. W., and Draper, W. B.: Studies on diffusion respiration. II. Survival of the dog following a prolonged period of respiratory arrest. Anesthesiology, 8:294, 1947.

Safar, P.: Resuscitation: Controversial Aspects. Chairman of International Symposium (Vienna). New York, Springer, 1963.

Safar, P.: Über Philosophie, Geschichte und Zukunft der Wiederbelebung (Philosophy, history and future of reanimation). Anaesthesist, *23*:507, 1974(a).

Safar, P., et al.: Intensive care unit and the anesthesiologist. South. Med. J., *54*:8, 1961.

Safar, P., Escarraga, L. A., and Chang, F.: Upper airway obstruction in the unconscious patient. J. Appl. Physiol., *14*:760, 1959.

Safar, P., Stezoski, W., and Nemoto, E. M.: Amelioration of brain damage following 12 minutes of cardiac arrest in dogs. Arch. Neurol. *33*:91, 1976.

Safar, P., and Tenicela, R.: High altitude physiology in relation to anesthesia and inhalation therapy. Anesthesiology, *25*:515, 1964.

Sasahara, A. A., et al.: Clinical and physiologic studies in pulmonary thromboembolism. Am. J. Cardiol., *20*:10, 1967.

Schaffer, W. A., and Cobb, L. A.: Recurrent ventricular fibrillation and modes of death in survivors of out-of-hospital ventricular fibrillation. N. Engl. J. Med., *293*:259, 1975.

Shalit, M. N., et al.: The blood flow and oxygen consumption of the dying brain. Neurology, *20*:740, 1970.

Siebke, H., et al.: Survival after 40 minutes submersion without cerebral sequelae. Lancet, *1*:1275, 1975.

Siesjö, B. K., Carlsson, C., Hägerdal, M., and Nardström, C. H.: Brain metabolism in the critically ill. Crit. Care Med. *4*:283, 1976.

Smith, J., et al.: Need for oxygen enrichment in myocardial infarction, shock, and following cardiac arrest. Acta Anaesth. Scand., Suppl. *29*:127, 1968.

Snyder, J. V., et al.: Global ischemia in dogs: intracranial pressures, brain blood flow and metabolism. Stroke, *6*:21, 1975.

Sodi-Pallares, D., et al.: Polarizing solution in myocardial infarction. Am. J. Cardiol., *21*:275, 1968.

Stewart, J. S.: Management of cardiac arrest with special reference to metabolic acidosis. Br. Med. J., *1*:476, 1964.

Strimer, R., et al.: Epidemiologic features of 1,134 sudden, unexpected infant deaths. J.A.M.A., *209*:1493, 1969.

Sussman, K. E.: Acute problems, hypoglycemia. *In* Williams, P. H. (ed.): Diabetes. New York, Hoeber, Harper & Row, 1967.

Swann, H. G.: Resuscitation in semi-drowning. *In* Whittenberger, J. F. (ed.): Artificial Respiration. New York, Hoeber, Harper and Row, 1962.

Swann, H. G., and Brucer, M.: The cardiorespiratory and biochemical events during rapid anoxic death. I-VII, Tex. Rep. Biol. Med., *7*:511, 1949.

Takaori, M., and Safar, P.: Treatment of massive hemorrhage with colloid and crystalloid solutions. J.A.M.A., *199*:297, 1967.

Taussig, H. B.: "Death" from lightning and the possibility of living again. Am. Sci., *57*:306, 1969.

Tomashefski, J. F., and Billings, C. E., Jr.: Carbon monoxide poisoning—the physiologic basis for treatment. Ohio State Med., J., *57*:149, 1961.

Urokinase Pulmonary Embolism Trial: A National Cooperative Study. Circulation, *47* (Suppl. 2): 50, 1973.

Wiggers, C. J.: The physiological bases for cardiac resuscitation from ventricular fibrillation. Method for serial defibrillation. Am. Heart J., *20*:413, 1940.

Zoll, P. M., et al.: Termination of ventricular fibrillation in man by externally applied electric counter shock. N. Engl. J. Med., *254*:727, 1956.

Chapter 3

ACUTE RESPIRATORY INSUFFICIENCY*

Peter Safar,
and Nancy Caroline

INTRODUCTION

Acute respiratory insufficiency (ARI) and associated acid-base (AB) derangements are often the initiating events that decisively trigger a chain reaction of pathophysiologic misadventures in the critically ill and injured. Still under-appreciated and under-diagnosed, respiratory insufficiency takes its toll in a variety of clinical settings — its significance too often recognized only after the patient cannot be saved.

Those who record the destinies of patients may diagnose by retrospect. Those who care for patients, especially critically ill patients, do not have that luxury. Clinicians must be sensitized to suspect ARI in the appropriate clinical settings, to recognize its frequently subtle early signs, and to take action before more blatant and irretrievable manifestations of respiratory insufficiency supervene. The purpose of this chapter is to stimulate, in those who care for the critically ill and injured, a heightened awareness of ARI and its presentations.

This is a chapter on *applied* respiratory pathophysiology; we take for granted that the reader has a grasp of basic anatomy, respiratory physiology and pathology, and that he has read (or will read) Chapters 2, 9 and 10 of this book. Furthermore, the emphasis in this chapter is on *acute* events, and we will not dwell here on the morphology of chronic processes. Rather, in the pages that follow,

we hope to provide a framework for thinking and learning about the various ways in which the respiratory system may be menaced. Through examination of several disparate pathophysiologic processes, we shall try to derive more general concepts of how the respiratory mechanism fails.

We begin, in the latter section of this introduction, with some general definitions. Detailed definitions of physiologic variables — including their symbols, abbreviations and normal values — are provided in the Glossary at the end of this chapter.† In subsequent sections, we consider acid-base derangements, disturbances of ventilation and oxygenation, and pulmonary clearing and defenses. The final section of this chapter provides a discussion of selected pathophysiologic conditions, presented as prototypes for more general mechanisms of ARI.

The priorities and views presented in this chapter, reflect the authors' clinical and research experiences in resuscitation and respiratory care since the 1950s — at Baltimore City Hospitals and at the University Health Center of Pittsburgh; their and their associates' teaching of respiratory pathophysiology and therapy to medical students and house staff; and their associates; experiences with concepts and techniques in respiratory intensive care. We do not pretend to have all the answers. Indeed, we will be well satisfied with Chapters 2, 3, 9 and 10 if

*Acknowledgments: Dr. Ake Grenvik made valuable suggestions concerning content, and edited this chapter. Drs. George Schwartz and Michael Loughhead contributed material and thoughts. Patricia Sands, M.P.H., edited this chapter. Vicki Shidel and Katharine Leslie prepared the manuscript.

†For glossary, see pp. 99–103. In the absence of international agreements on terminology, abbreviations and symbols, we have used those introduced or accepted by the Department of Anesthesiology/Critical Care Medicine of the University of Pittsburgh. Most conform to those of the American Physiologic Society and the American College of Chest Physicians (Chest 67:583, 1975).

51

they provoke the reader to search for better answers than we can presently provide.

Definitions

Respiratory insufficiency may be defined as the "inability of the lungs to arterialize fully the blood flowing through them" (E. Robin). Normal arterialization of blood entails the achievement of an arterial PO_2 (PaO_2) of 75 to 100 mm. Hg (torr) (the lower values in elderly persons) during breathing of air and an arterial PCO_2 ($PaCO_2$) of 35 to 45 torr. The American College of Chest Physicians defines "pulmonary insufficiency" as "the altered function of the lungs which produces clinical symptoms, usually including dyspnea." Thus, respiratory insufficiency is also present when there is an increase in airway resistance (airway obstruction) sufficiently severe to cause dyspnea, even if PaO_2 and $PaCO_2$ values are still normal.

Acute respiratory insufficiency (ARI), also called *acute respiratory failure* (ARF), is respiratory insufficiency occurring rapidly and to a degree that causes malfunction of vital organs. For example, coma of any cause is considered under the heading of "acute respiratory insufficiency" because it results in hypopharyngeal obstruction by the base of the tongue when the head is not tilted backward, and it represents a threat to airway patency because of upper airway areflexia. Moreover, coma usually interferes with respiratory control mechanisms. "Acute ventilatory failure" is synonymous with hypercarbia, i.e., an increased $PaCO_2$. "Pulmonary failure" indicates incapacitating disease of the pulmonary parenchyma, such as pulmonary edema-consolidation (adult respiratory distress syndrome). Notably, many of the above terms are used without precision or careful definition in the general literature.

Chronic respiratory insufficiency is chronic hypoxemia or hypercarbia due to a disorder of the respiratory system. The specific duration of the condition and the degrees of PaO_2 reduction or $PaCO_2$ increase required for this category have not been well established.

Hypoxemia is a PaO_2 lower than 75 torr. *Hypercarbia* is a $PaCO_2$ higher than 45 torr. *Hypocarbia* is a $PaCO_2$ lower than 35 torr. *Asphyxia* is a combination of hypoxemia and hypercarbia, usually caused by hypoventilation when breathing air. *Hypoxia* is oxygen deprivation at the tissue level, which may be the result of hypoxemia, reduced blood flow, anemia, or impaired tissue oxygen utilization (see later). *Alkalemia* is an arterial pH (pHa) of over 7.45, and *acidemia* a pHa of less than 7.35. The terms *alkalosis* and *acidosis* should be used only when also stating the site of the pH abnormality. The metabolic component of the acid base derangement may be expressed clinically in changes of *total buffer base*, i.e., base excess (BE) or base deficit (BD) in milliequivalents per liter (mEq./L.) from a normal of zero.

Most mechanical abnormalities of pulmonary function can be grouped into restrictive patterns, obstructive patterns, or small airway dysfunction. Restrictive patterns are signified by a reduction of vital capacity (VC) not explainable by airway obstruction. Obstructive patterns cause a slowing of air flow during forced ventilatory maneuvers. "Small airway dysfunction" is a term which should be used when abnormalities of new function test values are found, such as closing volume, frequency dependent compliance, or flow-volume curves.

Airway obstruction is any increase in airway resistance that causes dyspnea (in the conscious patient), noisy breathing, intercostal and suprasternal retraction, or blood gas abnormalities. Airway obstruction may be partial or complete, high or low. High (upper) airway obstruction is a narrowing of the air passages at the level of the larynx or above.

Airway obstruction stimulates breathing movements reflexly. If the obstruction is only partial and not severe or prolonged, it may initially be accompanied by normal blood gas values. However, if allowed to continue, airway obstruction may subsequently result in sudden exhaustion with hypoventilation, decreased PaO_2, increased $PaCO_2$, stupor, coma, complete airway obstruction, secondary apnea, and cardiac arrest. Sudden complete airway obstruction results in asphyxia and asystole within five to 12 minutes (see Chapter 2).

Recognition of Acute Respiratory Insufficiency

Hypoxemia and hypercarbia are laboratory diagnoses, established on the basis of arterial blood gas determinations; however, their presence should be suspected when certain circumstances or clinical signs exist, and blood gas confirmation should be sought (Table 1). Failure to suspect early ARI often permits progression of the disorder to a less salvageable stage.

In the conscious patient, *hypoxemia* should be suspected when there is restlessness, tachycardia, tachypnea, sweating, or cyanosis. Arterial blood PO_2 values are used to confirm the suspicion. Absence of cyanosis is no proof of adequate oxygenation, since anemia or cutaneous vasodilatation may permit a pink color in spite of hypoxemia. On the other hand, cyanosis may be present when there is a normal PaO_2 — for example, in polycythemia, or when there is slow blood flow, which causes increased oxygen extraction at the capillary level and dark blood in the venules. This produces bluish color of the skin and mucous membranes, locally or

TABLE 1 *Recognition of Acute Respiratory Insufficiency*

CONDITION (DEFINITION, PROOF)	SUSPICION
A CONSCIOUS PATIENT	
1. Hypoxemia (PaO_2<75 torr/FIO_2 0.21)	Restlessness, tachycardia, tachypnea, sweating, cyanosis at the tongue. Acute lung disease
2. Hypercarbia ($PaCO_2$>45 torr)	Somnolence. Very shallow and/or slow breathing (i.e., severe hypoventilation)
3. Asphyxia ($PaCO_2$>45 torr + PaO_2<75 torr)	Combination of (1) and (2) above. Shallow and/or slow breathing of air. Airway obstruction, see (A4)
4. Partial airway obstruction during spontaneous breathing (increased airway resistance). PaO_2 normal or ↓; $PaCO_2$ normal or ↑.	Noisy breathing. Inspiratory retraction of intercostal and/or suprasternal areas. Dyspnea
Complete airway obstruction (leads to coma from asphyxia within 1–3 minutes).	No air flow felt or heard at mouth and nose
5. Increased work of breathing (increased airway resistance, decreased lung/chest compliance, increased ventilatory requirement)	Dyspnea. Labored breathing. (May lead to sudden exhaustion and asphyxia)
B. UNCONSCIOUS PATIENT	
1. Hypoxemia	Coma of any cause. Airway obstruction
2. Hypercarbia } (See A)	
3. Asphyxia	Very shallow and/or slow breathing (breathing volumes unreliable; check arterial blood gases with 100% O_2 test!)
4. Partial airway obstruction (a) During spontaneous breathing movements	Noisy breathing (snoring, crowing, gurgling, wheezing). Inspiratory retraction of intercostal and/or suprasternal areas
(b) During apnea	Recognized only during artificial positive pressure ventilation attempts: noisy air flow, increased resistance to inflation, slowed exhalation
5. Complete airway obstruction (a) During spontaneous breathing	Movements of chest or abdomen, but no air flow felt or heard at mouth or nose Inspiratory retraction of intercostal and/or suprasternal areas
(b) During apnea	Recognized only during artificial positive pressure ventilation attempts: complete resistance to inflation, no chest deflation, gastric insufflation, excessive gas leaks

ACUTE RESPIRATORY INSUFFICIENCY, PARTICULARLY HYPOXEMIA, IS ONE OF THE MOST UNDER-DIAGNOSED DERANGEMENTS IN CRITICALLY ILL OR INJURED PATIENTS.

regionally. In individuals with melanotic skin, the blue versus pink color of the capillary blood is best differentiated at the tongue. Cyanosis of the nail beds and lips often is unreliable in assessing these individuals.

In the conscious person, *hypercarbia* should be suspected when he becomes somnolent. Heart rate and arterial pressure may not change with hypercarbia, as often the central circulatory effects of hypercarbic acidemia (sympathetic stimulation) are offset by its peripheral effects (vasodilatation and cardiac depression). When there are signs of airway obstruction or very shallow or slow breathing movements in the air-breathing person, asphyxia (hypercarbia plus hypoxemia) should be suspected.

In contrast to hypoxemia and hypercarbia, airway obstruction *is* largely a clinical diagnosis. Signs of airway obstruction and modalities of treatment vary according to whether spontaneous breathing movements are present or absent, whether obstruction is partial or complete, and whether the patient is conscious or unconscious.

In the spontaneously breathing person, conscious or unconscious, *partial airway obstruction* is recognized when there is noisy air flow, such as snoring (usually soft tissue hypopharyngeal obstruction by the tongue when the neck is flexed); crowing or stridor (usually laryngospasm); gurgling (usually foreign matter in the upper air passages); or wheezing (usually bronchial narrowing, as in asthma or emphysema). *Complete airway obstruction* is recognized when there is no air flow felt or heard at mouth or nose. In partial *or* complete obstruction, there may also be retraction of the neck and chest with each inspiratory effort, particularly retraction of the intercostal spaces and the suprasternal area.

In the *apneic patient*, partial or complete airway obstruction can be recognized only during artificial positive pressure ventilation attempts. There is increased resistance to inflation. In *partial obstruction*, air flow may be noisy or slowed during inflation or exhalation. In *complete obstruction*, there is complete resistance to inflation attempts. In this case, gas may follow the path of least resistance into the stomach.

The treatment of airway obstruction in the *conscious* person depends on its cause. Emergency airway control in the *unconscious* person should follow a rapid sequence of action in stepwise fashion, with diagnosis and treatment going hand-in-hand as described in Chapter 9: (1) Tilt head backward. (2) Try to inflate the lungs with positive pressure after each step, as this may ameliorate or overcome the obstruction. (3) Clear mouth and pharynx manually, if necessary. (4) Perform the triple airway maneuver (backward tilt of the head, forward displacement of the mandible, plus opening of the mouth). (5) Suction upper airway, if necessary. (6) Insert oro- or nasopharyngeal tube. (7) Insert the esophageal obturator airway in the prehospital setting in an unconscious apneic patient (as alternative to tracheal intubation). (8) Intubate the trachea. (9) If tracheal intubation is impossible, consider alternatives, such as cricothyroid membrane puncture, or translaryngeal oxygen jet insufflation. Tracheotomy is a long-term airway control measure, to be performed if at all possible under controlled conditions in the well oxygenated, well ventilated patient.

ACID-BASE DERANGEMENTS

Vital organ function depends on a near-normal acid-base milieu. This milieu can be evaluated only approximately by monitoring blood acid-base changes, for these reveal extracellular fluid (ECF) changes and only partially reflect the intracellular acid-base abnormalities that influence organ function. Nonetheless, measurement of acid-base parameters in the arterial blood remains the most practical and readily available means of gauging over-all body acid-base status.

A review of some fundamental concepts is useful here. Acids are hydrogen ion (H^+) donors, and bases are hydrogen ion acceptors. An acid in solution dissociates with formation of a hydrogen ion; the degree of dissociation determines the amount of free H^+, which in turn determines the actual acidity. The H^+ concentration $[H^+]$ is customarily expressed in the form of its negative logarithm, namely, the pH. Thus, the actual H^+ concentration for a pH of 7.4 is 40 nano equivalents (nEq.)/ L.; for a pH of 7.0, 100 nEq./L; and for a pH of 7.8, 16 nEq./L. Thus, the pH scale is nonlinear. A certain increase in $[H^+]$ is better tolerated than the same degree of decrease.

Even under normal conditions of primarily aerobic metabolism, the body produces an excess of acid which must be neutralized or eliminated in order to maintain the internal environment at a near constant pH. Normally the body produces two forms of acid: volatile carbonic acid (H_2CO_3, about 20,000 mEq. produced every 24 hours) and fixed, nonvolatile organic acids (50 to 70 mEq. produced every 24 hours). To deal with this acid load, the body employs three principal mechanisms: buffering; pulmonary excretion; and renal excretion.

The most rapidly acting of these defense mechanisms is the *buffer system* in the extracellular fluid, which acts within seconds; intracellular buffering occurs within hours. The *respiratory mechanism*, through which excess carbonic acid is excreted in the form of CO_2, works within minutes, whereas the *renal mechanism*, which accounts for excretion of bicarbonate and fixed acids (40 per cent titratable acids, 60 per cent ammonia) requires hours to days. Clearly, any dysfunctions of the lungs or kidneys thus imply potential disruption of acid-base equilibrium.

The most important buffering mechanism is the $NaHCO_3/H_2CO_3$ system. At a normal pH of 7.4, the ratio of sodium bicarbonate to carbonic acid is normally 20:1. H^+ reacts with bicarbonate to form water and CO_2:

$$H^+ + HCO_3^- \rightleftharpoons H_2CO_3 \rightleftharpoons H_2O + CO_2$$

The pH-bicarbonate-CO_2 relationship, then, is expressed by the Henderson-Hasselbalch equation:

$$pH = pK + \log\frac{HCO_3^-}{H_2CO_3}$$

$$7.4 = 6.1 + \log\frac{20}{1}$$

(K is the dissociation constant of carbonic acid)

One *measures* blood pH and PCO_2 and *calculates* the plasma bicarbonate from these values, using any of the commonly used nomograms representing the Henderson-Hasselbalch equation, such as the Siggaard-Andersen nomogram (Chapter 10). As a very rough guide, in pure respiratory changes, for each 10 torr rise or fall in $PaCO_2$, pHa changes in the opposite direction by about 0.08, and bicarbonate increases or decreases parallel with PCO_2 by about 1 to 2 mEq./L. (Fig. 1; see also Chapter 10).

While bicarbonate constitutes about 53 per cent of the total blood buffer base, hemoglobin represents about 35 per cent, protein 7 per cent, and phosphate 5 per cent. The total blood buffer base amounts to about 48 mEq./L. A deviation from this normal value

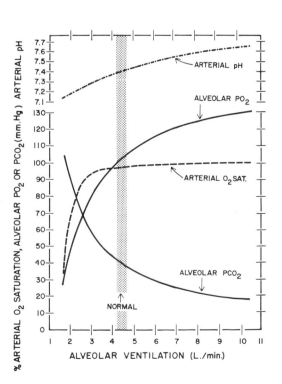

Figure 1. Blood gas changes (vertical axis) during progressive hypoventilation with air (horizontal axis, read from right to left), FIO_2 0.21 (air): As alveolar ventilation decreases, arterial (which in normal lungs equals alveolar) PO_2 decreases, and arterial (which equals alveolar) PCO_2 increases. Arterial O_2Hb saturation is maintained above 90 per cent until alveolar ventilation decreases to 50 per cent of normal or less, because of the S-shape of the O_2Hb dissociation curve (see Fig. 2). With a rise in $PaCO_2$, pHa decreases, and bicarbonate rises. A reduction in $PaCO_2$ (hyperventilation) results in an increase in pH and a decrease in bicarbonate (see text). During hyperventilation with air, PaO_2 cannot increase over about 130 torr. With FIO_2 0.5–1.0 (not shown), PaO_2 remains high (above this scale) during hypoventilation to apnea. $PaCO_2$ increases in apnea about 5 torr per minute. (These values are for a resting oxygen consumption of 250 ml./70 kg. body weight per minute.) (From Comroe, J. H., Jr.: The Lung, 2nd ed., Chicago, Yearbook Medical Publishers, 1962.)

is called "base excess" or "base deficit," which normally is zero; and its deviation is expressed as $\pm$ mEq./L. The calculated *blood base excess* (or deficit), which includes bicarbonate and hemoglobin, as calculated from the Siggaard–Andersen nomogram (Chapter 10), expresses the *metabolic component* of the acid-base derangement. The $Paco_2$ indicates the *respiratory component*. Determinations of total CO_2 are less meaningful. Although standard bicarbonate and base excesses are based in part on assumptions, *measurements of arterial Pco_2, pH, and hemoglobin, and calculation of bicarbonate and base excess, are the keystones for acid-base therapy* (Chapter 10).

In describing *blood* acid-base abnormalities, we prefer the terms "acidemia" and "alkalemia" to "acidosis" and "alkalosis," since a pH change in one direction in the blood may be accompanied by a pH change in the opposite direction in some tissues. For example, there may be severe tissue acidosis in shock, while the blood pH is normal or elevated due to compensatory hyperventilation, bicarbonate administration, or both.

It is generally agreed that pHa changes between 7.2 and 7.6 do not in themselves demand therapeutic intervention, but rather an effort should be made to correct the underlying disorder (e.g., shock, hyperventilation). Beyond these limits, however, or when there seems to be vital organ system malfunction associated with even a lesser pHa derangement per se, direct manipulation of pHa is justified. An acidemia of 6.9 or less pHa results in asystole, and an alkalemia of 7.8 or higher pHa induces lethal tachyarrhythmias.

Respiratory Alkalemia

Alveolar hyperventilation results immediately in hypocarbia, followed within minutes by a decrease in plasma $[H^+]$, $[HCO_3^-]$ and $[K^+]$. Chronic hyperventilation provokes renal response in which H^+ excretion is decreased while sodium loss is increased (without potassium loss). As H^+ leaves cells, K^+ enters them, causing a relative deficit of K^+ in ECF. These changes tend to bring pHa back toward normal.

Strictly speaking, respiratory alkalemia refers to a *primary* deficit in hydrogen ions. When there is accumulation of fixed acids

(see later), the organism tries to compensate with hyperventilation. This should be called "base deficit," and "respiratory alkalemia" only if the pHa is increased above normal. Chronic respiratory alkalemia is rarely dangerous, but acute respiratory alkalemia can cause life-threatening arrhythmias in patients with cardiac disease. Respiratory alkalemia may be caused by respiratory stimulation from brain injury, hepatic failure, fever, mechanical hyperventilation, and acute hypoxemia of any cause. Spontaneous hyperventilation may result in tetany. For unknown reasons, this is rarely seen with artificial (passive) hyperventilation. Extreme passive hyperventilation, however, may result in a decrease in cardiac output and a decrease in tissue oxygenation because of a leftward shift of the HbO_2 dissociation curve.

Except for the patient with decompensated chronic obstructive lung disease, in whom rapid mechanical hyperventilation can cause cerebral alkalosis and ischemia (see later), hyperventilation with a moderate increase in pHa to not more than about 7.6 is rarely dangerous and does not require specific therapy. $Paco_2$ values below 25 torr should be avoided, as they may cause excessive cerebral vasoconstriction, increased oxygen consumption, and reduction in cardiac output. If large mechanical ventilation volumes are required for oxygenation, increase in inhaled CO_2 with a CO_2 mixer attached to the O_2/air mixer of the ventilator and increasing mechanical deadspace are convenient ways to normalize $Paco_2$, and thus pHa. When a patient with metabolic or brain disease hyperventilates himself to a $Paco_2$ below 20 torr or seems to exhaust himself, CNS depressant agents or even muscle relaxants may be required to permit control of ventilation volumes and pHa.

Respiratory Acidemia

Respiratory acidemia results from overall alveolar hypoventilation, i.e., a minute volume of ventilation inadequate to remove CO_2 at the rate it is produced. Hypoventilation results in an immediate increase in $Paco_2$ (hypercarbia) followed by a decrease in pHa. Accumulated CO_2 enters the red cells, where it becomes H_2CO_3, dissociating into bicarbonate ions (which move into plasma) and hydrogen ions (bound by hemoglobin). At the same time, chloride shifts into the red cells and potassium moves out of the red cells to maintain electrical neutrality. These are not very effective buffer mechanisms. Thus, acutely, for each 10 torr rise in $PaCO_2$, pHa decreases by about 0.08 and bicarbonate increases by about 1 mEq./L. CO_2 narcosis sets in when the $PaCO_2$ reaches 80 to 100 torr. The narcosis is reversible if the brain was not previously damaged. If progressive hypercarbia leads to cardiac arrest, it is not through the CO_2 rise per se, but through associated hypoxemia or a decrease in pHa to 6.9 to 6.5. To normalize pHa in the presence of hypercarbia, renal compensation, in the form of increased bicarbonate reabsorption, is mobilized within hours and reaches maximal efficacy within about one week. However, the renal compensatory mechanism is not an unmixed blessing, for sodium and water retention accompanying bicarbonate reabsorption may contribute to tissue edema.

Although many central and peripheral factors can produce over-all alveolar hypoventilation and respiratory acidemia, the most common cause of hypercarbia is COPD. Total ventilation volumes are inadequate because of increased alveolar deadspace. In addition, there is "parasitic ventilation" (J. B. West), that is, some alveoli plunder alveolar gas from others rather than fresh gas. Hypercapnic patients breathing air are always hypoxemic as well. It is this hypoxemia, not the hypercarbia, which may result in irreversible vital organ damage. When diuretics are given to patients with COPD, metabolic alkalemia from chloride and potassium loss may be superimposed on the chronic respiratory acidemia. Treatment of respiratory acidosis is hyperventilation to normalize pHa.

Metabolic Acidemia

Metabolic acidemia represents an increase in circulating H^+ concentration in the form of fixed acids rather than increased H_2CO_3. The fixed acids consume buffer base, resulting in a base deficit. Furthermore, the increased concentration of fixed acids leads to a decrease in blood pH unless compensatory hyperventilation, stimulated by the acidemia, produces a commensurate decline in $PaCO_2$.

Causes of metabolic acidemia include ingestion of excess H^+ (e.g., salicylic acid), accumulation of ketoacids (e.g., beta-hydroxybutyric acid, acetoacetic acid) in diabetes, alcohol intoxication or starvation; accumulation in ischemic-anoxic tissues of lactic acid (e.g., shock, heart failure, severe hypoxemia), which is concomitantly or subsequently washed out into the circulation; lactacidemia secondary to alcohol ingestion, phenformin idiosyncrasy, and of unknown etiology; renal failure with decreased excretion of H^+ (primarily ammonia) and loss of bicarbonate; and loss of alkali in diarrhea or intestinal fistulas.

Treatment of metabolic acidemia should be directed primarily at the underlying condition. Only when the pHa decreases below approximately 7.2 is it usually necessary to take steps to increase pHa per se toward normal—by hyperventilation, administration of buffer base (e.g., bicarbonate, tris buffer), or both. It is not entirely clear at what level of base deficit intervention is required. A reasonable clinical compromise is first to let moderate spontaneous or artificial hyperventilation normalize pHa, while attempts are made to treat the underlying disorder. Excessive hyperventilation should be avoided, as it causes a decrease in cardiac output and cerebral blood flow. If modest hyperventilation cannot maintain pHa above 7.2, or if, in spite of a pHa of 7.2 to 7.4, there is evidence of vital organ malfunction, we tend to correct the base deficit using the following formula: The mEq. of bicarbonate required to bring base deficit to zero equals the base deficit in mEq./L. times $\frac{1}{5}$ of body weight (which approximates the ECF in liters).

$$\text{mEq. } HCO_3^- \text{ required} = BD \times \frac{BW}{5}$$

For example, with a base deficit of 20 mEq./L. in a 60-kg. adult, $20 \times 60/5$ (i.e., 240) mEq. of $NaHCO_3$ given intravenously (best in a 1 mEq./ml. solution) usually will bring the base deficit to zero, at least transiently. Bicarbonate infusion should be slow to minimize red blood cell damage and hyperosmolality. Caution also should be exercised to correct hypokalemia, if present, before administering a bicarbonate load. In existing hyperventilation, overbreathing should be slowed down after the initial CO_2 load from bicarbonate has been exhaled, lest an overshoot of pHa occur.

A word on the choice of buffering agents is warranted. Since bicarbonate is transiently a CO_2 donor and tris-buffer (THAM) is not (THAM also enters cells more readily), buffering in respiratory acidemia, mixed acidemia (e.g., status asthmaticus), or cerebral edema (e.g., postcardiac arrest) might be more logically accomplished with THAM; whereas buffering in pure metabolic acidemia may be done with either bicarbonate or THAM. Use of THAM is associated with some difficulties, such as the unavailability of a readily prepared concentrated solution, the production of apnea, and hypoglycemia.

Metabolic Alkalemia

Metabolic alkalemia is an increase of buffer base, particularly bicarbonate, in extracellular fluid. It occurs, when, in COPD, CO_2 retention stimulates H^+ secretion and bicarbonate reabsorption. Other causes include potassium depletion in hypopotassemia (H^+ enters cells, resulting in extracellular alkalosis); hypochloremia (which promotes H^+ secretion and bicarbonate reabsorption); and reduction in extracellular fluid volume from diuretics. Primary metabolic alkalemia with low serum sodium and chloride is seen in loss of H^+ via gastric juice, use of diuretics, or hyperventilation in COPD with chronic hypercarbia. Primary metabolic alkalemia with high urine and serum chloride is seen in primary aldosteronism, Cushing's syndrome, potassium depletion, bicarbonate infusion, and chronic alkali ingestion (ulcer patients). Spontaneous compensation with hypoventilation is unpredictable and undesirable, particularly without oxygen breathing. Treatment should be directed at the cause, and pHa increase above 7.6 avoided. Treatment includes KCl administration according to specific formulas (Chapter 10). Normalization of pHa without hypoventilation is possible with I.V. ammonium chloride or L-arginine monohydrochloride.

DISTURBANCES OF VENTILATION

In order to understand disturbances of ventilation, one must be familiar with the concepts of alveolar ventilation, CO_2 transport, control of breathing, and ventilatory mechanics. (For definitions, see the Glossary, and for clinical examples, see the final section of this chapter.)

Alveolar Ventilation

The $PaCO_2$ represents a summation of over-all adequacy of alveolar ventilation to meet metabolic demands. *Alveolar ventilation* equals minute volume (sum of tidal volumes/minute), minus deadspace ventilation/minute ("wasted ventilation"):

$$\text{Alv. Ventil.} = \text{Min. Vol.} - (\text{DS} \times \text{R})$$
$$\dot{V}_A = \dot{V}_E - (V_D \times f)$$
$$\text{Example: } \dot{V}_A = 8 \text{ L.} - (150 \text{ ml.} \times 20) = 5 \text{ L.}$$

Anatomic *deadspace* (approximately 2 ml./kg. body weight) is the gas volume, from mouth and nose to terminal bronchioles, that does not participate in the gas exchange with the blood. Alveolar deadspace is the volume of gas in alveoli that are ventilated but not perfused (Figure 3, A); this is an abnormal entity. Total deadspace, also called "physiologic deadspace" (actually a misnomer because it is in part "pathologic"), is anatomic deadspace plus alveolar deadspace. Under conditions of respiratory care, one must also consider mechanical deadspace beyond the patient's natural airway, e.g., exhaled gas contained in tubings and valves and reinhaled.

Increased alveolar deadspace is one extreme of the potpourri of changes called "ventilation/perfusion mismatching" (the other extreme is shunting), which exists in some lung units in essentially all types of lung disease and critical illness or injury, even without primary lung disease. For example, in oligemic shock, the uppermost portions of the lungs are hypoperfused or nonperfused; and in COPD, poorly perfused units, particularly bullous emphysema, represent deadspace. This increase in the alveolar deadspace calls for increased tidal volumes in order to maintain normal $PaCO_2$.

The deadspace/tidal volume ratio (V_D/V_T) normally is about 0.3. When ventilation volumes required to maintain normal $PaCO_2$ are larger than estimated and there is no reason for assuming increased metabolism, increased V_D/V_T should be suspected. Quantitation is possible by measuring alveolar CO_2 concentration (F_ACO_2), assuming it equals end-tidal CO_2 ($F_{ET}CO_2$) and mixed exhaled CO_2 ($F_{\bar{E}}CO_2$); and solving the *Bohr equation:*

$$\frac{V_D}{V_T} = \frac{F_ACO_2 - F_{\bar{E}}CO_2}{F_ACO_2},$$

or the simpler modification (Enghoff):

$$\frac{V_D}{V_T} = \frac{PaCO_2 - P_{\bar{E}}CO_2}{PaCO_2}.$$

With a normal ventilation/perfusion ratio of 1, approximately 1 liter of alveolar ventilation is required for every liter of cardiac output. Attempts to determine the adequacy of alveolar ventilation (and thus $PaCO_2$) from minute volume nomograms (predicted from age, sex, height and weight), have proved unreliable—more so for patients with sick lungs than for those with healthy ones—because metabolic rate and alveolar deadspace vary unpredictably. Only obvious severe hypoventilation (e.g., a minute volume of 4 liters or less in the average adult, or all tidal volumes not larger than estimated deadspace volume) justifies the clinical assumption of hypercarbia (hypoventilation) without confirming $PaCO_2$ measurement. If in doubt, one obviously must ventilate artificially.

Regional hypoventilation of one or more lung units is readily compensated by relative hyperventilation of other lung units. Thus, theoretically at least, up to about 80 per cent of perfused lung tissue could be without ventilation, and hyperventilation of the remaining 20 per cent would enable maintenance of a normal $PaCO_2$. In clinical reality, however, this is not possible, because such an 80 per cent shunt would concomitantly produce a degree of hypoxemia incompatible with life. The efficiency of oxygen absorption simply cannot keep pace with that of CO_2 elimination because of the greater diffusibility of CO_2 (20 times that of oxygen), the smaller veno-arterial PCO_2 difference (5 torr), and the linearity of the CO_2 dissociation curve.

Over-all reduction in alveolar ventilation during *air* breathing always results not only in increased $PaCO_2$, but also in decreased PaO_2 (Figure 1). When the hypoventilating patient is breathing *oxygen,* however, hypercarbia may develop without hypoxemia. Thus, prophylactic oxygen inhalation is indicated in conditions such as coma, which may result unexpectedly in hypoventilation. Notably, if the lungs are filled with 100 per cent oxygen and connected via a leak-free system to a reservoir filled with 100 per cent oxygen, the patient may remain apneic without becoming hypoxemic for up to 30 minutes. This is possible because the blood passing through the alveoli picks up oxygen and thereby slightly reduces alveolar pressure, which draws more oxygen into the alveoli (*apneic diffusion oxygenation*). During apnea, CO_2, lacking a comparable transport mechanism and thus unable to diffuse outward, accumulates at a rate of about 5 torr/minute. The limiting factor, then, with such a nitrogen-free system, is not hypoxemia nor hypercarbia itself, but rather the hypercarbia-induced acidemia, which, when severe, can cause arrhythmias and cardiac arrest.

Over-all hypoventilation in *clinical practice* is likely to occur during and following anesthesia (e.g., use of neuromuscular blocking agents), in obstructive airway disease (COPD, chronic bronchitis), and in CNS (respiratory center) depression by drugs. Less common causes include muscular weakness (myasthenia gravis, polyneuritis), trauma, chest wall deformities, and pulmonary fibrosis. Hypoventilation can be the result of restrictive lung or chest wall abnormalities (evident from reduced total VC), or obstructed airways (reduced timed VC, reduced MEFR), or both (Chapter 10).

Barbiturates, particularly when combined with alcohol, diazepam (Valium), opiates, phenothiazines, and other depressant drugs tend to decrease the response to elevated $PaCO_2$ in doses which per se are insufficient to cause hypoventilation without a CO_2 challenge. A rare accident of nature is "Ondine's curse," named after the mean mythical nymph who took her lover's ability to breathe without thinking about breathing; this sleep-induced, potentially lethal hypoventilation is due to respiratory center damage of often unknown etiology, sometimes misdiagnosed as "heart attack" or "stroke." A rare cause of hypoventilation due to increased work of breathing leading to fatigue is decreased chest wall compliance (see later) from obesity, i.e., the "Pickwickian syndrome." This causes even worse hypoxemia than that expected from hypoventilation, owing to alveolar collapse from an elevated diaphragm.

Acute pulmonary parenchymatous diseases (e.g., pneumonia, pulmonary edema), on the other hand, usually decrease lung compliance and, in turn, vital capacity; only when very severe do they reduce tidal volumes. Even in those circumstances, compensatory increases in respiratory frequency (tachypnea) tend to offset tidal volume reductions (provided tidal volumes are larger than deadspace), so that the result is hypoxemia with a normal or low $PaCO_2$.

Carbon Dioxide Transport

Metabolism produces a PCO_2 in the tissues of over 50 torr, which drives CO_2 down a diffusion gradient into plasma and erythrocytes, passing through tissue capillaries. When the blood leaves the capillaries, its PCO_2 has increased from about 40 torr on the arterial side to about 45 torr on the venous side, with a corresponding increase in CO_2 content from about 45 ml./100 ml. blood on the arterial side to about 50 ml./100 ml. blood on the venous side. The veno-arterial pH difference is minimal because reduced hemoglobin is a better buffer than oxyhemoglobin, and therefore any tendency toward pH decrease on the venous side is offset by more efficient buffering. CO_2 is transported to the lungs primarily in the form of bicarbonate (90 per cent); the remainder is found in combination with protein as carbamino compounds primarily carbamino Hb (5 per cent), and in simple solution (5 per cent). Of the CO_2 released into the alveoli (arteriovenous difference), 60 per cent is in the form of bicarbonate, 30 per cent comes from carbamino compounds (primarily Hb), and 10 per cent from dissolved CO_2. With a CO_2 solubility coefficient of 6 ml./100 ml./100 torr, about 3 ml. of CO_2 is in physical solution in 100 ml. of venous blood with a PO_2 of 50 torr (Henry's Law: the amount of gas dissolved in a liquid is proportional to its partial pressure). Since reduced Hb binds more CO_2 than oxyhemoglobin, oxygen unloading in tissues facilitates CO_2 loading, and the reverse occurs in the lungs. CO_2 diffuses readily from plasma via the capillary wall into the alveolus with a negligible arterio-alveolar PCO_2 gradient $P(a-A)CO_2$. CO_2 elimination is cata-

lyzed by the enzyme carbonic anhydrase in the red blood cells, from where CO_2 diffuses in exchange for chloride ions (the chloride shift).

Control of Breathing

The volumes, frequencies, rhythms, and patterns of spontaneous breathing are controlled by impulses from the respiratory center, which lead to contractions of the diaphragm and the external intercostal muscles. Auxiliary inspiratory muscles are activated only when the diaphragm and intercostals do not meet the demand the CNS "senses." The diaphragm is the primary muscle producing inspirations at rest and is innervated by the phrenic nerve (which originates from 3.–5. cervical segments of the spinal cord). Exhalations are usually passive, due to the elastic recoil of lungs and chest. Forced exhalations ("bucking," coughing) are promoted by contractions of the internal intercostal muscles and the abdominal wall, which must be considered as a functional part of the chest wall. A normal maximal inhalation (VC) is produced by contraction of the diaphragm (about 50 per cent of the force) plus contraction of the intercostal and auxiliary muscles (the other 50 per cent). With normal lungs under basal conditions, loss of function of either the diaphragm or intercostals does not reduce tidal volume and frequency, and thus CO_2 elimination, although it does reduce VC.

The respiratory center is a neuronal switchboard located immediately beneath the floor of the fourth cerebral ventricle. The activity of the respiratory center cells reflects the net result of many stimuli: (1) the PCO_2, pH, and temperature of the blood perfusing the respiratory center (hypercarbia, acidemia, and hyperthermia stimulating breathing movements); (2) the acidity of the CSF (normal CSF pH is 7.3) (increases in acidity stimulate the central medullary chemoreceptor cells located at the anterior surface of the medulla, which send messages to the respiratory center cells); (3) a reduction in PaO_2 (probably to 50 torr or less) or pHa (probably to 7.3 or less), stimulating the peripheral chemoreceptors (carotid and aortic bodies), which send impulses via the ninth and tenth cranial nerves to the respiratory center; (4) stimulation of the bronchopulmonary stretch receptors (Hering–Breuer reflexes), which through stimuli via the tenth cranial nerves normally terminate lung inflations and deflations. These reflexes cause tachypnea and decreased VC when there is increased airway resistance, tracheobronchial irritation, atelectasis, pneumonia, pneumothorax, or accumulation of pleural fluid; (5) arterial hypotension stimulating, and arterial hypertension suppressing, respiratory impulses via baroreceptor (carotid sinus) reflexes carried along via the ninth cranial nerves; (6) stimuli from the entire periphery, particularly muscles, joints, and skin, stimulating breathing or causing breath-holding; (7) impulses from the cerebral cortex (e.g., voluntary impulses, senses, emotions) modifying the otherwise semiautomatic respiratory cycles. All these afferent impulses combined influence the respiratory center output.

From the length and variety of the above list, it is readily apparent that a whole host of factors may engender ventilatory embarrassment by disturbing respiratory control mechanisms. To enumerate but a few examples:

¶Spontaneous *hyperventilation* is common in patients with arterial hypotension, acidemia, CSF acidosis (e.g., head injury), anxiety, or hysteria.

¶Voluntary hyperventilation with air immediately prior to breath-holding and diving, which has been tried to enable longer submersion, may permit the development of hypoxemia to the point of coma, while the $PaCO_2$ remains below the threshold required to stimulate air hunger and a need to surface.

¶In compensated COPD, the hypoxemic drive to breathe transcends the usual hypercarbic drive, because of compensatory changes in the CSF where pH is normalized by elevation of bicarbonate. Administration of high concentrations of inspired oxygen to patients who have switched their allegiance to a hypoxemic drive may result in hypoventilation.

¶Spontaneous *hypoventilation* is common in patients with drug-induced CNS depression (from barbiturates, narcotics), greatly increased intracranial pressure, increased work of breathing (obesity, markedly increased airway resistance), or deafferentation (e. g., high spinal block).

¶Control of artificial ventilation in the patient who is "fighting the ventilator" is usually facilitated by decreasing respiratory drive factors, e.g., by increasing PaO_2, decreasing $PaCO_2$, normalizing pH, reversing shock, etc.

Ventilatory Mechanics

Breathing volumes and patterns and static lung volumes are influenced not only by nervous impulses to the respiratory muscles, but also by the mechanical characteristics of the lungs and chest wall. The forces which must be overcome in order to move gas in and out of the lungs—by the patient's respiratory muscles, the operator's hand on the resuscitator bag, or the mechanical ventilator—are essentially the following three: (1) elastic resistance of lungs and thorax (i.e., elastance), the reciprocal of compliance (i.e., distensibility); (2) airway resistance (the reciprocal of airway conductance); and (3) tissue viscous resistance. While compliance is expressed as volume change per unit pressure under static conditions (when no air is moving), airway and tissue viscous resistances are expressed in terms of pressure change per unit flow (in liters per second or liters per minute). Tissue viscous resistance is negligible.

LUNG VOLUMES (Chapter 10)

These can be determined and monitored with a standard spirometer or ventilation meter. Clinically important volumes and flow variables include vital capacity (VC), maximum expiratory flow rate (MEFR), functional residual capacity (FRC), and inspiratory capacity (IC) (see Glossary). VC and MEFR can be measured only in the conscious, cooperative patient. Normal VC (inspiratory reserve volume plus tidal volume plus expiratory reserve volume) and MEFR can be predicted from nomograms based on age, height, sex, and weight. VC measured during forced coached rapid exhalation in the conscious person is called "forced expiratory volume" (FEV). Any changes that limit lung expansion reduce VC and FEV. Thus, reduction in *total* FEV indicates *restrictive* lung/thorax changes. If the proportion of the total FEV exhaled within the first second is less than about 80 per cent of the total FEV (timed FEV 1 sec.), however, airway *obstruction* is present. Likewise, reduced MEFR indicates partial obstruction of medium and large airways. Periodic MEFR measurements are useful to monitor bronchodilator therapy.

The *functional residual capacity* (FRC), or the volume of gas left in the lungs at the end of normal exhalation (i.e., resting volume), is reduced when alveoli are collapsed or fluid-filled. This usually results in increased right-to-left shunting of non-oxygenated blood, and thus a lower than expected PaO_2 (FIO_2 1.0), and decreased lung compliance. FRC is also decreased when the diaphragm is pushed upward, as in obesity or ascites; it is increased when the diaphragm is low or when there is air trapping, as in emphysema or asthma.

The inspiratory capacity (IC), i.e., tidal volume plus inspiratory reserve volume (also called "sighing volume") is significant because without periodic sighing (normally occurring about every 10 to 15 minutes or more often (even during sleep), "miliary atelectasis" would develop, with progressive hypoxemia from resultant shunting and decreased compliance. Such atelectasis, furthermore, enhances the likelihood of secondary infection (pneumonia). Sighing sufficient to keep the alveoli open (either spontaneously or by coached or passive periodic lung inflations) requires inspired volumes of about 15 ml./kg. body weight (about 1 liter in a 70-kg. adult) or more, at least every 15 to 30 minutes.

COMPLIANCE

Lung elastance is the result of the retractile forces of the elastic fibers in the pulmonary stroma, vessels and bronchi (about one-half of elastic recoil force), and *surface tension* at the alveolar liquid/gas interface (the other half). The pressure inside a soap bubble (alveolus) on a tube (airway) is inversely proportional to the radius (Laplace's Law):

$$Pressure = \frac{4 \times surface\ tension}{radius}$$

The surface tension of saline solution would be 70 dynes/cm.², a force sufficient to collapse alveoli and empty small alveoli into larger ones. However, Nature provided us with a special surface tension-reducing lipoprotein called "surfactant" (a phospholipid, dipalmitoyl lecithin), which lines the alveoli and reduces surface tension of lung extract below that of saline, namely to 5–40 dynes/cm.², varying with the radius. This "lung soap" is produced by round alveolar Type II lining cells, which contain surfactant inclusion bodies. Alveolar stabilization is accomplished by the actions of surfactant as well as by the structural interdependence of alveoli. The efficacy of alveolar stabilization is enhanced by the fact that surfactant molecules are compacted (surface tension further reduced) when alveoli become smaller during exhalation. Any insult to the lung tissue tends to stiffen it by impairing the surfactant mechanism. Furthermore, direct damage to the surfactant layer or to the alveolar Type II cells which produce it increases surface tension, thereby promoting alveolar collapse, increasing hypoxemia from shunting, and decreasing lung compliance.

Compliance (C) is measured and expressed as "lung volume change per unit airway pressure change when no air is moving":

$$C = \frac{\Delta V}{\Delta P} \text{ (static), in ml./cm. } H_2O$$

When assessing lungs-plus-thorax compliance in the apneic patient, the pressure used is alveolar pressure (which equals airway pressure under static conditions) minus atmospheric pressure. For lung compliance alone, measured either under apnea or during spontaneous breathing, the pressure is alveolar (airway) pressure minus intrapleural pressure.

Measurements of lung compliance alone in spontaneously breathing patients is technically difficult and therefore considered "semi-research," as it requires use of a body box or continuous intrapleural pressure monitoring (with intrapleural catheter or esophageal balloon) simultaneously with volume and flow measurements (pneumotachogram).

Lung-chest compliance is easier to measure, i.e., as volume change per airway pressure change. (Under static conditions, airway pressure equals alveolar pressure.) Ideally, inflations have to be sustained for several seconds, until flow ceases. In conscious, healthy, breath-holding adults, lung-chest compliance is about 100 ml./cm. H$_2$O pressure; whereas it is about 50 ml./cm. H$_2$O in anesthetized, curarized, apneic adults. The apparently greater compliance in the conscious person is due to an inability to abolish voluntarily all inspiratory muscle tone. The latter volume would be about double for the same lung volume range if one were to measure lung compliance alone.

Chest wall compliance is decreased with abdominal wall contraction (straining, coughing, bucking); postural changes (prone, lateral, head-down positions); or increased weight on the chest wall (obesity). *Lung compliance* is *decreased* with most lung diseases, owing to a reduction in FRC (e.g., complete airway obstruction; alveolar collapse, compression or fluid filling) or a true increase in elastic recoil force (i.e., "specific compliance," FRC corrected compliance). To follow changes in lung compliance by measurement of lung-thorax compliance, one must keep the thoracic components constant by, for instance, voluntary or drug-induced relaxation of the abdominal and other respiratory muscles, and by making measurements in the same body position.

COPD is associated with *increased* specific *lung compliance* because of reduced elastic recoil. Difficulty in ventilating the emphysematous patient is due instead to increased airway resistance and air trapping, leading to overdistention of lungs and chest and ventilation at the top of the compliance curve, where higher pressures are required for the same volume changes.

Since static compliance measurements interfere with ventilation and oxygenation, lung-thorax compliance changes are clinically estimated in apneic critically ill or injured patients on mechanical ventilation by monitoring the airway pressure change under near-static conditions (i.e., end-inflation pressure minus end-expiratory pressure), with known volumes of inflations. This "clinical compliance," "effective compliance," or "dynamic compliance" thus includes a component of airway conductance; i.e., the values are reduced also when there is partial airway obstruction. Lung-thorax compliance measurements in some adults with respiratory distress syndrome during mechanical ventilation have been as low as 8 to 10 ml./cm. H$_2$O, still with the possibility of improvement and complete recovery.

AIRWAY RESISTANCE

Airway resistance is expressed as pressure gradient (in cm. H$_2$O) per flow (in L./min. or L./sec.). Gas flow through the respiratory tree is in part laminar, which depends primarily on the gas viscosity; and in part turbulent, which depends, among other things, on the gas density. The resistance to laminar flow through tubes depends on the length of the tubing, the number of patent airways, the cross-sectional area of the airways, and their stability *(Poiseuille's law)*:

$$R \text{ (resistance)} = \frac{8 \times \text{viscosity} \times \text{length}}{\pi \times r^4}$$

Thus, a very small decrease in airway caliber (r = radius) results in a large increase in airway resistance. No "law" exists for turbulent flow. In toto, airway resistance normally, during quiet breathing, should not exceed 2.5 cm. H$_2$O/30 liters per minute (or 500 ml./sec.) flow.

Airway resistance increases as the patient exhales, and most small airways are closed at the bottom of VC; on the other hand, airway resistance decreases as lung volume increases. Airway resistance measurements are complicated and usually are reserved for laboratory tests of the conscious patient, as they require the use of the body box, an interruptor technique, or the esophageal balloon for intrathoracic pressure recording. Clinically, increased airway resistance is recognized from auscultatory changes (wheezing, stridor), increased resistance to positive pressure inflation attempts, and/or increased time required for passive exhalation. Furthermore, in the conscious cooperative patient, FEV$_1$, MEFR, and MVV measurements can detect over-all increase in airway resistance.

Normally, small bronchi begin closing at 10 per cent of the VC above residual volume (called "closing capacity"). In old age, the closing volume is higher, i.e., 10 to 40 per cent above RV; and in COPD and asthma patients, some airways may start closing considerably above FRC. Measurement of closing volume during an expiratory VC is a more sensitive technique to use for early recognition of asthma and COPD than timed FEV and MEFR (Chapter 10).

Mechanisms of increased upper airway

resistance are discussed in Chapter 9. Increased lower airway resistance may be caused by foreign bodies, tumors, bronchial spasm, edema, congestion, and/or secretions (e.g., asthma); bronchial collapse (COPD); and kinking, torsion, or compression of the air passages (e.g., from tension pneumothorax).

The greatest narrowing of the airway in the normal person is usually at the level of the medium-sized bronchi. The elastic retractile force of the lungs which stretches the bronchi open is reduced with age and lost altogether in emphysema. This causes intrapulmonary airways not held open by cartilaginous support to collapse passively or even to be compressed when the pressure in the surrounding alveoli is higher than in the bronchial lumen, as during forced exhalation. This results in a "check-valve" mechanism, i.e., expiratory obstruction, causing air trapping. Maintaining intraluminal pressure positive by expiratory retardation, as with pursed lip breathing, reduces air trapping.

DISTURBANCES OF OXYGENATION

Hypercarbia alone may impair organ function, but usually in a reversible fashion unless there is associated brain injury. In contrast, "hypoxemia not only stops the motor, but also wrecks the machinery" (J. B. S. Haldane).

Asphyxia, a combination of hypoxemia and hypercarbia, usually results from airway obstruction or depression of respiratory movements while breathing air. Asphyxia progresses most rapidly when, during air breathing, the airway suddenly becomes completely obstructed (e.g., choking on food) or breathing movements cease (apnea). Complete sudden airway obstruction in lightly anesthetized air-breathing dogs results in a decrease of PaO_2 to less than 20 torr within five minutes, and cardiac arrest at a PaO_2 of about 10 torr or pHa of 6.5 (see Chapter 2). Asphyxia associated with complete airway obstruction leads more rapidly to cardiac arrest when breathing movements continue than it does during induced apnea, since the former usually is associated with a higher oxygen consumption because of struggling and catecholamine release.

Hypoxemia (PaO_2 less than 75 torr) may be caused by any one or a combination of the following: (1) reduced FIO_2 (e.g., anesthetic accident, inert gas displacing air) or reduced PIO_2 (e.g., high altitude); (2) increase of alveolar CO_2 from hypoventilation while breathing air; and (3) ventilation/perfusion mismatching (particularly its extreme, right-to-left shunting of blood through nonventilated alveoli), the cause of hypoxemia in most specific lung diseases and almost all nonspecific lung changes of critically ill or injured patients. Hypoxemia due to conditions (1) and (3) stimulates breathing movements because of stimulation of the peripheral chemoreceptors, which results in normal or low $PaCO_2$.

While a rise in $PaCO_2$ is the only reliable proof of inadequacy of alveolar ventilation (breathing volumes), a decrease in PaO_2 during breathing of air (hypoxemia) in the absence of hypercarbia or a PaO_2 lower than expected during breathing of 100 per cent oxygen (i.e., an increased alveolar-arterial PO_2 gradient) is an indication of right-to-left shunting of blood.

In normal man with mild to moderate hypoxemia, irreversible organ changes usually are forestalled by compensatory vasodilation and an increase in blood flow to vital organs. However, when the PaO_2 falls to about 30 torr or less, compensatory mechanisms are generally exhausted, as for instance, in the case of cerebral vasodilation from hypoxemia. Thus, more important for the organism at large than PaO_2 is total arterial oxygen transport and its distribution to various organ systems. Total *arterial oxygen transport* equals arterial oxygen content times cardiac output:

$$\text{Art. } O_2 \text{ Tr.} = \text{Art. } O_2 \text{ Content} \times \text{C.O.}$$
$$\overset{\circ}{C}aO_2 = CaO_2 \times \overset{\circ}{Q}_T$$

Example:
1 L. O_2/min. = 0.2 L./100 ml. × 5 L./min.

Blood oxygen content depends on hemoglobin (Hb) concentration and the percentage oxygen saturation of Hb, which in turn depends on PO_2. When oxygen diffuses from a normal alveolus into plasma, it exerts there a partial pressure about equal to that in the alveolus, with only a minimal alveolar-arterial PO_2 gradient [$P(A - a)O_2$; or $D(A - a)O_2$]. Ninety-eight per cent of arterial oxygen is carried in red blood cells, where each molecule of Hb (molecular weight approximately 65,000) has the capacity to combine with four molecules of oxygen to form O_2Hb. The minimal amount of oxygen carried in physical solution in blood is determined by the coefficient of solubility of oxygen in plasma (0.0031), which permits only 0.3 ml. of oxygen to be dissolved in 100 ml. of blood at a PO_2 of 100 torr (Henry's Law). However, the amount of dissolved oxygen may become significant when the PaO_2 is increased from 100 torr to 600 torr by 100 per cent oxygen inhalation (in healthy lungs), which raises the oxygen content in solution from 0.3 to 1.5 ml./100 ml. blood—a significant amount in the case of severe anemia or reduced blood flow. A higher than normal PaO_2 per se may also improve oxygen delivery from the arterial side of capillaries to mitochondria in the presence of tissue edema, e.g., cerebral edema.

The relationship between blood PO_2 and oxygen saturation of Hb (and thus blood oxygen content) is not linear, but S-shaped, in the form of the O_2Hb *dissociation curve* (Fig. 2). The curve is obtained by equilibrating blood at 37° C. with gas at a PCO_2 of 40 torr and at PO_2 values ranging from zero to 150 torr, at which point full saturation is reached. The oxygen saturation does not vary with changes in blood Hb concentration. When fully saturated with oxygen, 1 gm. of Hb holds 1.34 to 1.39 ml. of oxygen. A normal arterial PO_2 of 100 torr gives an O_2Hb saturation of 97 per cent. Assuming a normal Hb content of 15 gm./100 ml. blood, the oxygen-carrying capacity of blood, and thus the

arterial oxygen content, is approximately 20 ml./100 ml. blood. The oxygen-carrying capacity is reduced in reduced Hb concentration (anemia), abnormal hemoglobin (e.g., methemoglobin), or when the Hb is blocked by a substance which has an even greater affinity to it than oxygen (e.g., carbon monoxide).

In critically ill or injured patients, it is wise to adjust therapy so that PaO_2 is maintained at no less than 60 torr, the knee of the curve, above which a large further increase in PO_2 has little effect on oxygen content, but below which even a small decrease in PO_2 reduces oxygen content drastically. Thus, above 60 torr, a modest decrease in alveolar PO_2 does not immediately jeopardize arterial oxygen content (Fig. 1).

Many factors influence the position of the S-shaped curve (Fig. 2) and thus oxygen binding and release. The position of the curve at a pH of 7.4 and 37° C. is defined by the value "P-50," namely, the PO_2 at which Hb is 50 per cent saturated. The normal P-50 is 27 torr. A shift of the curve to the right (increased P-50) means that a greater PO_2 is required for a given percentage saturation, i.e., the affinity of Hb to oxygen is decreased. This is beneficial to tissues, as it fosters release of oxygen from Hb at the lower PO_2 values of the venous side of the capillary. A shift to the left (decreased P-50) means a relatively higher saturation for a given PO_2; this might be considered advantageous, but in reality this increased affinity

Figure 2. Normal Oxygen-Hemoglobin Dissociation Curve. Horizontal axis = PO_2; vertical axis = O_2 saturation.

Note clinically important PO_2 values: (1) Keep PaO_2 in critically ill patients above 60 torr, the knee of the curve, below which deoxygenation is abrupt. (2) Normal mixed venous PO_2 is about 40 torr. (3) Normal P-50 is 27 torr. (4) PaO_2 20 is lethal; $P\bar{v}O_2$ 20 means danger. On the right, arteriovenous oxygen extraction (about 5 ml./100 ml. blood). This oxygen availability is decreased with shift of curve to the left due to decreased temperature (T), increased pH, or decreased 2,3-DPG.

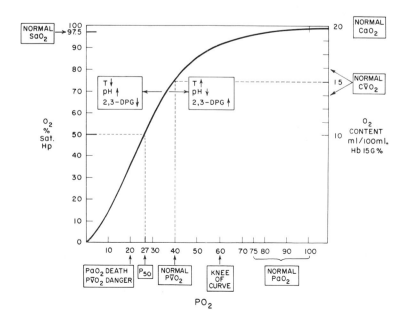

of Hb to oxygen is detrimental to delivery of oxygen to the tissues.

Thus, P-50 varies directly with the erythrocyte content of high energy phosphates (2,3-diphosphoglycerate; i.e., 2,3-DPG), which bind to Hb and decrease its affinity for oxygen. In chronic hypoxia with a reduction in tissue Po_2, as occurs in natives of high altitudes and in patients with COPD or congenital cyanotic heart disease, Nature increases the DPG level by influencing glycolysis within the cell; hemoglobin oxygen affinity is thereby decreased and the organism is better adapted to tolerate low Po_2 states. In contrast, P-50 is decreased, because of decreased DPG, in cases of massive bank blood infusion (stored ACD blood loses DPG), abnormal hemoglobin, intravenous alimentation, and other blood-traumatizing events. In these instances, the affinity of hemoglobin for oxygen rises, and tissue oxygenation suffers commensurately.

Independent of DPG content, falls in pH (e.g., at the tissue level due to the metabolic production of CO_2 and fixed acids) shift the Hb dissociation curve to the right (Bohr effect), while pH increases (e.g., in alkalemia from excessive controlled hyperventilation or bicarbonate administration) shift the curve to the left. Accordingly, hypercarbia causes a shift to the right by decreasing pH (CO_2 in addition forms carbamino Hb, which decreases oxygen affinity), and hypocarbia shifts the curve to the left by increasing pH. Thus, both hypercarbia and acidemia mitigate toward greater oxygen release in the tissues. Finally, an increase in temperature shifts the curve to the right, thus favoring tissue oxygenation during exercise or fever; whereas hypothermia shifts the curve to the left.

We have said that more important than Pao_2 is arterial oxygen transport. The normal total arterial oxygen transport in a resting 70-kg. adult is about 1 liter oxygen per minute. We may go one step further and consider the relationship of transport to oxygen consumption (need, demand). This relationship is stated by the Fick formula and by the oxygen utilization coefficient. The *Fick formula* expresses the relationship between cardiac output and oxygen consumption, as follows:

$$\mathring{Q}_T = \frac{\mathring{V}o_2}{C(a-v)O_2}, \text{ or } \mathring{V}o_2 = \mathring{Q}_T \times C(a-v)O_2$$

The *oxygen utilization coefficient* (O_2UC) is as follows:

$$O_2UC = \frac{\mathring{V}o_2}{Cao_2} = \frac{\mathring{Q}_T \times C(a-\bar{v})O_2}{\mathring{Q}_T \times Cao_2} =$$

$$\frac{C(a-\bar{v})O_2}{Cao_2}$$

Example: $0.25 = \dfrac{250 \text{ ml.}}{1000 \text{ ml.}} = \dfrac{5 \text{ vol. \%}}{20 \text{ vol. \%}}$

Oxygen utilization is normally about 25 per cent of total arterial oxygen transport. When the supply decreases in relation to demand, the O_2UC increases, which can be an ominous sign in critical illness or injury. An exception is systemic shunting (e.g., sepsis) or histotoxic anoxia, which reduces the O_2UC and also oxygen consumption as the condition worsens.

Normally, under basal conditions, the brain receives about 13 per cent of the total body blood flow and consumes 20 per cent of the total oxygen used by the organism; the corresponding approximate values for the heart are 4 per cent of blood flow and 11 per cent of oxygen consumption, the kidneys 19 per cent of blood flow and 7 per cent of oxygen consumption, the splanchnic bed 24 per cent of blood flow and 25 per cent of oxygen consumption, the skeletal muscles 21 per cent of blood flow and 30 per cent of oxygen consumption, and for skin only 9 per cent of blood flow and 2 per cent of oxygen consumption.

Whenever total arterial oxygen transport is reduced, whether by a decrease in arterial oxygen content, blood flow, or both, below the tissue needs, tissue hypoxia develops. The conditions of *tissue hypoxia* (in contrast to hypoxemia, which refers only to a reduced Pao_2) are classified according to their etiologies (Table 2). In the presence of tissue hypoxia or whenever the transport of oxygen does not keep up with organ needs, cellular metabolism switches from aerobic glycolysis (producing 38 moles ATP net energy per mole glucose) to the less efficient anaerobic glycolysis (producing only 2 moles ATP per mole glucose), with attendant production of fixed acids, particularly lactic acid (Chapter 2).

TABLE 2 *Classification of Hypoxias (Inadequate Supply of O_2 to Tissues)*

TYPE	PRIMARY DISTURBANCE(S)	EXAMPLES
(1) Atmospheric hypoxia (results in 3 below)	Reduced inhaled PO_2 Reduced inhaled O_2 concentration	High altitude, decompression Anesthesia accident, confined space, inert gas displacing air
(2) Alveolar hypoxia (results in 3 below)	Reduced PO_2 in alveolar gas	Hypoventilation (reduced alveolar ventilation) with normal or abnormal lungs
(3) Arterial hypoxia (hypoxic hypoxia)	Decreased arterial PO_2 (hypoxemia)	Right-to-left shunting of blood through non-ventilated alveoli or cardiovascular shunts. Ventilation/perfusion mismatching without shunting. Alveolar-capillary diffusion impairment (decreased surface area, increased membrane thickness).
(4) Anemic hypoxia	Decreased arterial O_2 content Decreased arterial O_2 carrying capacity	Anemia. Carbon monoxide poisoning. Methemoglobinemia.
(5) Stagnant hypoxia (circulatory hypoxia)	Reduced tissue blood flow, general or local	Shock states, vasoconstriction, local stasis, intravascular coagulation, etc.
(6) Tissue hypoxia; histotoxic hypoxia	Various	Impaired release of O_2 from Hb (shift of Hb dissociation curve to left) Impaired O_2 diffusion (e.g., tissue edema) Increased tissue demand (e.g., hyperthermia) Poisoning (e.g., cyanide, which blocks O_2 use by cytochrome oxidase, as in nitroprusside overdose)

Ventilation/Perfusion Mismatching and Shunting

Most critically ill or injured patients are hypoxemic (PaO_2 75 torr or less) during air breathing, because of variable mismatching of ventilation and perfusion in different regions of the lung (Fig. 3). This mismatching ranges from one extreme of the spectrum, in which alveoli are ventilated but not perfused at all (increased alveolar deadspace) to the other extreme, the one most difficult to treat, namely, lung units that are perfused but not ventilated at all (pulmonary right-to-left shunting; venous admixture). Between these extremes are intermediate situations of mismatching, for example, areas with relatively more ventilation than perfusion (gravitational effect on the pulmonary apices, especially in oligemia or shock) and areas with relatively more perfusion than ventilation (dependent portions of the lung, partial airway obstruction, pulmonary congestion).

Nature has given us various mechanisms to normalize ventilation/perfusion relationships, which ideally should be 1:1. These mechanisms include intrapulmonary pressure effects and the ability of the pulmonary arterioles to constrict in the presence of low PO_2 and/or low pH (the opposite of the reaction of brain arterioles, which dilate with low pH). A decrease in alveolar PO_2 below 70 torr (e.g., high altitude exposure, COPD) causes hypoxic vasoconstriction in the lungs and increased pulmonary vascular resistance; whereas a decrease in mixed venous PO_2 (common in extreme exercise) does not produce vasoconstriction. Increased alveolar PCO_2 produces pulmonary vasospasm and bronchodilation, whereas low alveolar PCO_2 produces pulmonary vasospasm and bronchospasm. Pulmonary vasoconstriction in the fetus seems to be due to a combination of antenatal lung collapse and low pH. The subsequent pulmonary vasodilation after birth is the result of lung expansion and oxygenation (i.e., pH normalization).

Pulmonary vascular diameter is also locally controlled by gravity (i.e., blood volume) and the degree of alveolar distention. The latter is dependent on transpulmonary (alveolar–pleural) pressure gradients. Dur-

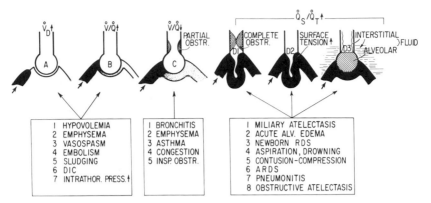

Figure 3. *Ventilation-Perfusion Mismatching.* Mechanism of Hypoxemia in Critical Illness or Injury during Breathing of Air.

Variable combinations of the following co-exist: (*A*) alveoli ventilated but not perfused (i.e., alveolar deadspace); (*B*) alveoli more ventilated than perfused; (*C*) alveoli perfused more than ventilated; (*D*) alveoli perfused but not ventilated at all (right-to-left shunting; "venous admixture").

(*A*) does not produce hypoxemia unless during breathing of air ventilation is not increased to compensate for increase in deadspace and $PaCO_2$ is increased. (*B*) in itself also does not produce hypoxemia. (*C*) is the most common cause of hypoxemia; it is readily correctable by oxygen inhalation. (*D*) hypoxemia due to shunting cannot be corrected by oxygen inhalation alone, but may yield in part to a continuous increase in airway pressure plus increased FIO_2 which may recruit and stabilize collapsed or fluid-filled alveoli. The 100 per cent oxygen test (see text and Chapter 10) permits differentiation between (*C*) and (*D*).

Clinical examples are listed below. Those under (*D*) are listed in the order of likelihood of improvement by positive pressure; e.g., (*D2*) from increased surface tension as in newborn respiratory distress syndrome, or (*D3*) from acute pulmonary edema, permit alveolar reexpansion with positive pressure more likely than (*D1*) from complete airway obstruction (absorption atelectasis) or (*D3*) from pneumonia.

ing spontaneous breathing, the deeper and more forceful the inhalation, the greater is the pressure gradient produced, and the more vasodilation at the capillary level occurs. Further, negative intrapleural pressure promotes venous return to the right heart, thereby tending to increase cardiac output. During positive pressure ventilation of healthy lungs, optimal pulmonary capillary diameter and perfusion can be expected during intermediate degrees of alveolar distension. Both alveolar collapse and alveolar overdistention produce an increase in pulmonary vascular resistance and a shift of blood from the capillaries to the major vessels. In stiff, acutely diseased lungs, positive pressure ventilation by "recruiting" alveoli sometimes may even decrease pulmonary vascular resistance and not reduce cardiac output, since the noncompliant lung in a sense "buffers" transmission of the increased airway pressure to the venae cavae.

Surfactant production and function are impaired by pulmonary hypoperfusion, as may occur in atelectasis as well as overdistention of alveoli. Surfactant production is also reduced by alveolar collapse itself. Thus, in acutely diseased or injured lungs, a slight continuous increase in airway pressure and ventilatory movements are beneficial for both pulmonary blood flow and surfactant production and function.

Impaired diffusion of oxygen or CO_2 between alveoli and blood has clinical significance only in terminal conditions of severe lung disease, e.g., far advanced ARDS with loss of most alveoli and capillaries. Diffusion capacity of the lungs is measured by the carbon monoxide single breath or steady state test (Chapter 10). Diffusion of gases in a liquid is slower than in a gas. Nevertheless, diffusion of oxygen from alveolar spaces into blood normally takes only 0.3 seconds, while capillary transit time is longer (0.75 seconds at rest, 0.4 seconds during exercise). CO_2 transfer is even faster because of its higher solubility and the carbonic anhydrase activity in the erythrocytes. The *diffusion* of oxygen or CO_2 is proportional to the area (A), multiplied by the diffusion constant (D) and the partial pressure gradient (P) of the gas, and divided by the tissue thickness (l = length):

$$\dot{V}O_2 \text{ or } \dot{V}CO_2 \propto \frac{A \times D \times (P_1 - P_2)}{l}$$

The *diffusion constant* (D) is proportional to the solubility (S) of the gas in water (0.3 ml./100 ml. per 100 torr for oxygen; 6 ml./100 ml. per 100 torr for CO_2), divided by the square root of the molecular weight of the gas.

$$D \propto \frac{S}{\sqrt{MW}}$$

The term "alveolar-capillary block" has been used to describe hypoxemia seen in the presence of normal alveolar ventilation. Theoretically, diffusing capacity of the lungs for oxygen may be decreased because of increased alveolar membrane thickness, decreased capillary suface area, or decreased capillary blood volume. However, probably only severe fibrosis or inflammation may represent a true block to the diffusion of oxygen when blood flow is greatly increased by exercise, and then only when the patient is breathing air. Hypoxemia with an FIO_2 of 1.0 almost never can be attributed to diffusion block. Even a decrease in PaO_2 during exercise while breathing oxygen should not be attributed a priori to diffusion impairment, since hypoxemia from shunting may also worsen with exercise.

Alveolar-Arterial PO_2 Gradient and 100 Per Cent Oxygen Test

Normally, the alveolar-arterial PO_2 gradient ($P(A-a)O_2$ or $D(A-a)O_2$ during breathing of air is negligible; less than 9 torr; in the aged, up to 10 to 20 torr. This minimal gradient is due to ventilation/perfusion mismatching, including right-to-left shunting (venous admixture) of not more than 5 per cent of cardiac output (of anatomic shunts from the Thebesian veins entering the left ventricle and from bronchial veins, and reduced ventilation:perfusion ratios in dependent lung areas). With an FIO_2 of 1.0, the normal gradient becomes more pronounced, but should be less than 150 torr.

Alveolar PO_2 with FIO_2 at 1.0, the 100 per cent oxygen test, is calculated as follows:

$$PAO_2 = PB - PaCO_2 - 47$$

(47 torr is PH_2O at 100% relative humidity and 37° C.)

The $P(A-a)O_2$, then, is calculated as follows:

$$P(A-a)O_2 = (PB - PaCO_2 - 47) - PaO_2$$

A person breathing 100 per cent oxygen for at least ten minutes, the time required for replacing all nitrogen with oxygen (up to 20 minutes is required for sick lungs), would increase his PaO_2 to at least 500 torr; i.e., would show a $P(A-a)O_2$ of 173 torr, namely, 760 minus 40 (PCO_2) minus 47 (PH_2O) minus 500. However, since the calculation of the $P(A-a)O_2$ is cumbersome, it has become clinically customary to follow the relative changes in PaO_2 with FIO_2 1.0 as an indication of venous admixture in the lungs. However, PaO_2 also depends on oxygen consumption and cardiac output (Figure 4). For the quantitation of right-to-left shunt in terms of percent of cardiac output shunted through non-ventilated alveoli ($\dot{Q}_S/\dot{Q}_T$), solving the shunt equation is necessary. This requires determination of mixed venous (pulmonary artery) and arterial oxygen content, not readily available in emergency situations. The *shunt equation* with FIO_2 1.0 is as follows:

$$\frac{\dot{Q}_S}{\dot{Q}_T} = \frac{Cc'O_2 - CaO_2}{Cc'O_2 - C\bar{v}O_2}$$

(where $Cc'O_2$ is pulmonary end-capillary O_2 content, CaO_2 is arterial O_2 content, $C\bar{v}O_2$ mixed venous O_2 content, $\dot{Q}_S$ is shunted blood flow, and $\dot{Q}_T$ is cardiac output).

Capillary oxygen content is calculated as:

$$Cc'O_2 = (1.34 \times Hb \text{ cont. } (O_2 Hb \text{ Sat.}) + P_AO_2 (0.0031)$$

The determination of capillary oxygen content during less than 100 per cent oxygen breathing is more complicated, since the expected O_2 saturation of Hb is difficult to estimate. Therefore, shunt measurement is more easily accomplished during 100 per cent oxygen breathing, which gives 100 per cent oxygen saturation in most patients. However, use of 100 per cent oxygen introduces some inaccuracy in the direction of over-reading quantitation and estimation from $D(A-a)O_2$ of the shunt; this error, usually not of clinical significance, is introduced because 100 per cent oxygen causes vasodilation in the hypoxic (shunted) lung areas and also some degree of absorption atelectasis.

More important and practical than quantitating the shunt are serial determinations of PaO_2 (FIO_2 1.0); i.e., *100 per cent oxygen tests*. The relationship between decrease in PaO_2 and increase in shunt is not linear. With an arteriovenous O_2 content difference of 6 ml./100 ml., a decrease in PaO_2 (FIO_2 1.0) from a normal value of 500 torr or more to 100 torr would be produced by an increase in shunt fraction to about 22 per cent. A PaO_2 (FIO_2 1.0) of 40 torr would indicate a shunt of 50 per cent, which usually can be survived only with continuous positive pressure ventilation. A *complete 100 per cent oxygen test* consists of PaO_2 determinations during *three conditions*.

Step (1): During spontaneous breathing of air (FIO_2 0.21). This first step should be omitted if the patient's condition calls for immediate oxygen inhalation.

Step (2): During spontaneous breathing and FIO_2 1.0 at atmospheric pressure. This must be done by a leak-free non-rebreathing system with mask, mouthpiece, or tracheal tube.

Step (3): During some form of positive pressure ventilation, preferably controlled ventilation with IPPV or CPPV and FIO_2 1.0.

If the reduced PaO_2 (FIO_2 0.21) (Step 1) is increased to 400–500 torr during Step 2, the predominant problem is ventilation/perfusion mismatching without shunting. FIO_2 of 1.0 produces an alveolar PO_2, even in underventilated alveoli, of about 600 torr. If the PaO_2 with an FIO_2 of 1.0 (Step 2) is lower than 500 torr, increased shunting exists. If the PaO_2 (FIO_2 1.0) during breathing at atmospheric pressure is significantly increased by positive pressure ventilation (change from Step 2 to Step 3), it indicates that positive pressure ventilation may be therapeutically useful. In many pathologic conditions, increased airway pressure recruits alveoli or thins alveolar fluid, and thereby increases FRC, oxygen diffusion, and PaO_2. Examples include acute pulmonary edema and miliary atelectasis from lack of sighing and surfactant, with increased surface tension (Figure 3). Positive pressure with an FIO_2 of 1.0 will increase PaO_2 less dramatically in pulmonary compression, contusion, and consolidation; and least in obstructive atelectasis or pneumonitis. If the PaO_2

remains the same when going from Step 2 to Step 3, one may assume that the shunt is not reversible with positive pressure ventilation at low levels, and may require high PEEP (Chapter 10). Finally, a decrease in PaO_2 with positive pressure (FIO_2 1.0) could result from increased pulmonary vascular resistance in open lung areas (with concomitant increase in shunt), or from reduction in cardiac output secondary to elevated intrathoracic pressure.

The 100 per cent oxygen test gives earlier and more sensitive information of the degree of pulmonary consolidation than do physical examination or roentgenograms, and thus it is a particularly valuable tool for determining *when* positive pressure ventilation should be started in progressive pulmonary deterioration, such as that following chest injury, pulmonary edema, or pneumonia, In the critically ill or injured patient, the 100 per cent O_2 test and resuscitation can be accomplished simultaneously by reoxygenating the patient using a self-refilling bag-valve-mask unit with 100 per cent oxygen reservoir (e.g., Laerdal unit).

Monitoring PaO_2 (FIO_2 1.0) periodically and minimizing the $P(A-a)O_2$ are important in gauging and treating the pulmonary status. However, more important to the organism as a whole are the *interactions* be-

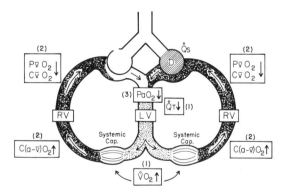

Figure 4. Hypoxemia-cardiac output-oxygen consumption relationships. Diagrammatic illustration of mechanisms by which, in patients with increased (but unchanged) right-to-left shunting ($\dot{Q}s/\dot{Q}T$) a decrease in cardiac output (*1*) or an increase in oxygen consumption (*1*) results in a decrease in oxygen values in venous blood (*2*) and thereby a decrease in PaO_2 (*3*) (i.e., worsening of hypoxemia). The more hypoxic the blood shunted through nonventilated alveoli, the greater the degree of venous admixture. In normal lungs without shunt, a decrease in cardiac output or an increase in oxygen consumption does not produce hypoxemia (see text).

tween changes in PaO_2, *cardiac output*, and *oxygen consumption* (Figure 4). When there is a significant increase in shunt fraction, the already hypoxemic patient will suffer a further decrease in PaO_2 if his cardiac output falls, as in shock. By the same token, an increase in oxygen consumption (e.g., fever, convulsions) may decrease PaO_2, even if FIO_2 and $\dot{Q}s/\dot{Q}_T$ remain constant. This is due to the fact that a decrease in venous oxygen values will qualitatively worsen the effects of venous admixture. A decrease in cardiac output and/or increase in oxygen consumption leads to an increase in the arteriovenous O_2 content difference. Without any shunt, such a decrease in venous oxygen values should not decrease arterial PO_2, since oxygenation of blood going through the intact alveoli is rapid and efficient. In the severely hypoxemic patient, one may attempt to manipulate PaO_2 by improving cardiac output (e.g., by volume expansion, inotropic agents, or arrhythmia control), and/or depressing metabolism (e.g., by sedation, analgesia, curarization, or hypothermia)—even if FIO_2 and shunt fractions cannot be changed.

PULMONARY CLEARING AND DEFENSES

The mechanisms keeping our 300 million alveoli open and their surface area of 50 to 100 m² clean are among the most miraculous accomplishments of Nature. Air breathing creatures, including man, require highly efficient and delicately balanced clearing and defense mechanisms against environmental and endogenous contaminants. Inhalation of air with variable temperature and humidity, and inhalation of variable concentrations of particulate and molecular air pollutants and microbes are conditions of life on Earth. In addition, enormous amounts of cellular residues and their breakdown products within the lungs have to be eliminated.

The functions of the lungs, besides arterialization of blood and provision of a blood reservoir, include such less appreciated roles as filtration of blood; production of surfactant, mucopolysaccharides, proteolytic enzymes, vasoactive substances, heparin (produced by mast cells), and immunoglobulins; and inactivation of serotonin, kinins, and other injurious endogenous and exogenous substances, particles, and microorganisms. All this is part of complex pulmonary defenses which, when excessive, in themselves become the source of morphologic and functional changes and disease.

Airway Defenses

Upper airway defense mechanisms from the mouth and nose to the glottis include closure of the larynx during swallowing, breath holding, reflex laryngospasm, filtration, warming and humidification of air, and movement by the ciliated nasal epithelium of a mucous carpet with trapped foreign particles toward the pharynx. Defense mechanisms in the tracheobronchial tree include primarily the ciliary escalator system of the tracheobronchial mucosa, coughing, and warming and humidification of inhaled air by the mucosa. Particles transported by the nasal and tracheobronchial ciliary activity have been observed to move at a normal rate of approximately 0.5 cm./minute. All these defense mechanisms may be depressed by drugs or disease.

The hairs at the nares filter only gross foreign material. The slitlike nasal passages, lined by highly vascular mucous membranes with ciliated epithelium, provide not only conditioning of inspired air to body temperature and 100 per cent relative humidity (44 mg. H_2O/L. gas at 37° C.), but also effective filtration of inhaled particles and absorption of foreign gases. These mechanisms are almost unaffected by even extreme changes of relative humidity and temperature of the inhaled air. The nose also absorbs watersoluble gases such as SO_2, and clears dust and common pollutants injurious to the lungs.

The mucous carpet lining the tracheobronchial tree and clearing it of inhaled particles is transported upwards by the ciliated epithelium toward the oropharynx, from which point the cleared material is swallowed. Infection and other disease can reduce the effectiveness of the nasal and pulmonary defenses. The most common breakdown of the nasal defense mechanism is created by tracheal intubation or tracheotomy, which "decapitates the patient's respiratory tract" (Proctor). Therefore, whenever the nasal air passage is bypassed, inhaled gases must be warmed and humidifed, or if not warmed, at least supersaturated with water droplets (mist) (Chapter 10).

Breathing through a slitlike mouth also humidifies and warms the gas but not as effectively as does nose breathing. Furthermore, breathing through a wide open mouth, as in exercise, bypasses the protective mechanisms. When therapeutic aerosols are inhaled, most drain out in nose and partially open mouth, but about 50 per cent reach the small bronchi when inhaled via wide open mouth, tracheal tube, or tracheostomy tube. Normally, the trachea and large bronchi are poor air conditioners. Farther down, good clearance takes place in the smallest bronchi, which have a large surface area and slow flow; they also have greater reactivity in terms of smooth muscle spasm, edema, and congestion.

The tracheobronchial mucus is produced primarily by goblet cells, which normally end at the 15th generation bronchi. Cilia exist farther down to the terminal bronchioles, but are sparse in the smallest air passages between the 15th and 30th generation bronchi. In lung diseases such as asthma and bronchitis, goblet cells can be found beyond that level, even in areas where cilia are scarce, either normally as in the smallest bronchi or pathologically where islands of ciliated epithelium have been replaced by squamous metaplasia from chronic infection. This impairs the ability to clear the thick mucus present in these conditions.

Alveolar Defenses

Alveolar defenses are difficult to study because of the inaccessibility of the smallest bronchi and alveoli. Their external *enemies* include changes in humidity, temperature and P_{O_2}; microbes; and pollutants that escape upper airway clearing. Their internal sanitation problems include, under normal conditions, about 8 gm. of alveolar lining cells and 12 gm. of surfactant "sloughed" and replaced each day (Clements). Alveolar *defenses* include primarily the following: (1) the alveolar surfactant film, which is suctioned upward by the ciliary escalator with which it is contiguous, a process promoted by intermittent lung inflations; (2) phagocytes (macrophages) from blood monocytes, which swallow endogenous and exogenous

particles, and are probably also cleared upward via the surfactant-ciliary escalator system, carried off via lymphatics into the blood (whence they can be cleared into the gastrointestinal lumen), or left in the lung tissue. Macrophages, if damaged by some types of dust (e.g., silica) or if provoked into releasing enzymes, can cause tissue damage such as silicosis-fibrosis. (3) The proliferative ability of alveolar lining cells Type II, the round granular cells which produce surfactant and which also produce the flat Type I cells. (4) The inflammatory reactions of the tracheobronchial and pulmonary tissues.

The Lungs' Reaction to Injury

In general, the bronchopulmonary apparatus reacts to a large number of specific exogenous and endogenous insults in a relatively small number of nonspecific ways. Endothelial and alveolar lining cells are most vulnerable. Mechanical, chemical, metabolic, infectious, hydrostatic, or neoplastic insults may result in any or several of the following responses:

(1) Loss or inactivation of surfactant, or cessation of its production (surfactant has a half-life of about 12 hours), resulting in increased alveolar surface tension and alveolar collapse.

(2) Capillary plugging with aggregates of red and white blood cells, thrombocytes or fat, causing pulmonary parenchymal ischemia with secondary (disseminated intravascular) coagulation and clot lysis.

(3) Capillary endothelial cell swelling and subsequent leakage; depending on the pore sizes in capillary walls, water, crystalloids, globulins, albumin, fibrinogen, and blood cells may breach the capillary wall and diffuse into pulmonary parenchyma. Such molecules and cells seep first into the interstitial spaces around small vessels and bronchi (the histologic picture of which is called "cuffing"); subsequently edema fluid accumulates between endothelial and epithelial cells, lifting them off their basement membranes; and, finally, edema fluid floods the alveoli. In cases of pulmonary edema-consolidation, the pathologist sees completely fluid-filled and empty alveoli side by side; for, because of the peculiar permeability and pressure relationships within the pulmonary parenchyma, alveoli either fill

completely or not at all. When alveolar edema containing fibrinogen is thinned out and dried by ventilation, hyaline membranes form. In adult respiratory distress syndrome (ARDS) the main factor causing this inspissated type of edema is capillary membrane damage. In infant respiratory distress syndrome (IRDS), on the other hand, the initiating factor is increased alveolar surface tension from lack of surfactant (due to prematurity, asphyxia, acidosis, and other factors). Increased surface tension promotes transudate, which mixes with cell debris and amniotic fluid to form the "membranes."

(4) Tissue hypoxia (probably ECF acidosis) and certain endogenous poisons (e.g., serotonin) cause pulmonary arteriolar spasm. Whether pulmonary venules in man can contract as they do in certain animals is controversial.

(5) The intrapulmonary airways react to endogenous and exogenous insults with bronchospasm, mucosal edema and congestion, slowing of the ciliary escalator system, and increased production of mucopurulent secretions.

(6) Nonspecific inflammatory responses. Some viruses and bacteria cause morphologically more specific inflammatory reactions, including specific cell types and inclusion bodies (e.g., tuberculosis, fungal infections) (Chapter 53).

The *end results* of these processes are also usually nonspecific. If the pulmonary parenchyma is the primary site of the insult, alveolar lining cell proliferation, interstitial edema and exudate provoke proliferation of interstitial fibroblasts with resulting fibrosis within one to two weeks and the likelihood of permanent stiffening of the lungs. However, as long as the capillary and alveolar basement membranes and some alveolar lining cells remain intact, regeneration of endothelial and alveolar lining cells can result in lung healing and functional recovery, which is often surprisingly complete, even after apparent hepatization of lung tissue. If the *pleural space* is the primary site of the insult, blood or inflammatory exudate, if not drained promptly, can become organized and form thick pleural scars; connective tissue thereby grows into the pulmonary parenchyma, causing potentially irreversible, severe respiratory insufficiency (chronic restrictive pulmonary disease,

CRPD). Finally, if the *airways* are the focus of injury, reactions there, when protracted, may also not revert to normal. Sloughing of ciliated epithelium may be followed by squamous metaplasia, resulting in impaired bronchial clearing and severe bronchial inflammation; tracheobronchial wall damage with chondromalacia may then ensue.

Pulmonary oxygen toxicity, an iatrogenic insult to lungs, provides an example of the lungs' nonspecific polymorphic response to a specific insult. Pulmonary capillaries and alveoli are acclimatized to inhaled air with a PaO_2 of about 100 torr. Substantially higher FIO_2, which may be required to sustain life, carries potential danger to lung tissue thus acclimatized. At an FIO_2 between 0.21 and 0.6, if there is pulmonary damage at all, it is mild and reversible. Patients on mechanical ventilation have received 40–60 per cent oxygen for months to years without permanent harm to lungs or other vital organs. However, uninterrupted breathing of an FIO_2 of 1.0 at one atmosphere is a very different matter. By six to 12 hours, tracheobronchial irritation and pulmonary congestion become manifest. These changes are probably reversible up to about 48 hours. If exposure to FIO_2 of 1.0 is longer than two to three days, however, irreversible pulmonary edema and consolidation can follow. The end-point is hemorrhagic pulmonary necrosis, red hepatization, and death from anoxia. Positive pressure artificial ventilation neither enhances nor diminishes this injury, but can keep the patient alive longer. Pulmonary oxygen toxicity is related to PIO_2 and time — not to FIO_2. Severe hypoxemia from shunting (which is usually the indication for high FIO_2) ameliorates and postpones the pulmonary oxygen toxicity, but does not abolish it. Breathing oxygen under hyperbaric conditions leads to damage earlier, and breathing 100 per cent oxygen at a reduced atmospheric pressure (as in space craft) is as safe as breathing air.

Microscopically in pulmonary oxygen toxicity, there is an exudative phase (congestion, interstitial and alveolar edema, hemorrhage, hyaline membranes) and a proliferative phase (fibroplasia, hyperplasia of alveolar lining cells, thickening of alveolar walls). The healed lung has fewer alveoli and capillaries. Pulmonary oxygen toxicity is entirely preventable by limiting the time of exposure to an FIO_2 of 1.0 and reducing the

FIO$_2$ to 0.6 or less as soon as feasible. With-holding oxygen inhalation from hypoxemic patients for fear of creating pulmonary oxygen damage is unwarranted. ("The brain softens before the lung hardens."—A. Sladen.)

EXAMPLES OF PATHOPHYSIOLOGIC MECHANISMS CAUSING ACUTE RESPIRATORY INSUFFICIENCY (ARI)

Introduction

In this final section, we shall briefly examine a variety of pathophysiologic entities illustrating aspects of acute respiratory insufficiency (ARI). Some of these entities are common, whereas others are rarely encountered in clinical practice. All, however, provide insight into aspects of ARI and resuscitation therefrom. Clinical entities will be reviewed here according to the categories shown in Fig. 5. A more detailed description of etiologies, diagnoses, and therapies for each can be found elsewhere in this book.

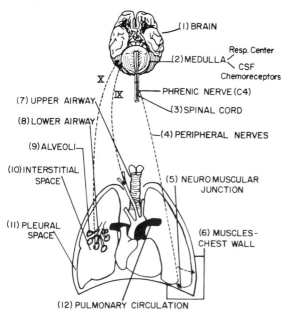

Figure 5. The twelve principal sites of the initiating mechanisms of acute respiratory insufficiency (hypoxemia, hypercarbia, airway obstruction, increased work of breathing) (see text).

As pictured in Fig. 5, the pathophysiologic entities relevant to ARI fall into the following general categories:

(1) Acute pathophysiologic changes anywhere in the *brain* can influence the respiratory center to alter normal respiratory impulses, reflexes, and muscle tone.

(2) *Medullary* (respiratory) *center* depression by drugs or other insults, particularly ischemia from increased intracranial pressure, may cause hypoventilation. On the other hand, bloody or acid CSF can result in hyperventilation by stimulation of CSF medullary chemoreceptors.

(3) Lesions of the *spinal cord*—for instance, high spine injury or disease—can cause hypoventilation and apnea when the injury extends to the outflow tracts of the phrenic nerves at the level of C3 to C5. Lesions anywhere in brain and spinal cord from a variety of inflammatory processes, such as multiple sclerosis (probably an autoimmune disease), may cause ARI.

(4) Interruption of *peripheral nerves* supplying the respiratory muscles (e.g., polyneuritis) and spastic peripheral neuropathy like tetanus are rare causes of hypoventilation.

(5) Blockade at the *neuromuscular junctions* of the respiratory muscles is the most common potential cause of hypoventilation in surgical patients who receive anesthesia with depolarizing (e.g., succinylcholine) or nondepolarizing (e.g., curare) muscle relaxants. Myasthenia gravis, nerve gases, insecticides, botulism, and many antibiotics (particularly aminoglycosides) are rare examples of ARI caused by similar mechanisms.

(6) Disorders of the *chest wall* or its muscles can cause ventilation/perfusion mismatching, hypoventilation, atelectasis with shunting, and hypoxemia. These disorders include upward displacement of the diaphragm (e.g., abdominal distention) and paradoxic motion of the paralyzed diaphragm.

(7) *Upper airway obstruction* by the tongue (prevalent in coma), vomitus, water (near-drowning), blood, laryngospasm, inflammatory processes (e.g., croup), or tumors is a common cause of ARI.

(8) *Lower airway obstruction* is the most common cause of chronic respiratory insufficiency, e.g., asthma, bronchitis, and emphysema.

(9) *Collapsed or fluid-filled alveoli* are

the most common cause of hypoxemia from shunting, usually without hypercarbia (e.g., miliary atelectasis, acute pulmonary edema, pneumonia, inhalation of toxic substances).

(10) *Changes in interstitial tissue spaces* of the lungs, which precede (as in pulmonary edema) or follow (as in pneumonitis) alveolar changes may lead to interstitial fibrosis, i.e., restrictive lung disease with decreased compliance.

(11) Changes of the *pleural space* (e.g., pneumothorax, tension pneumothorax, pleural exudate, hemothorax, bronchopleural fistula, diaphragmatic hernia) can acutely cause hypoxemia or asphyxia and, when permitted to persist, lead to pulmonary fibrosis.

(12) Generalized and localized changes in the *pulmonary vasculature* are caused by numerous insults; many lead to pulmonary hypoperfusion, increased deadspace, shunting, and obstructive shock (e.g., pulmonary thromboembolism, fat embolism).

The above mechanisms result in identifiable patterns of arterial blood gas and acid-base abnormalities, some of which are summarized in Table 3. Although etiologies and mechanisms of these conditions vary, therapy of most should follow the general principles of modern resuscitation (Chapter 9) and respiratory care (Chapter 10), titrated according to the pathophysiologic derangement. Because of the many secondary complications associated with ARI, patients requiring long-term mechanical ventilation should, where possible, be transferred to regional critical care (intensive care) centers staffed and equipped for sophisticated respiratory care. Life support during transfer by mobile ICU may require sophisticated measures including CPPV (Chapter 10).

Cerebral Disorders (Fig. 5, Site 7)

(1) Coma

Various types of insults may cause confusion, delirium, stupor, and coma (Chapter 5). Any type of coma tends to produce ARI through airway obstruction, depression of airway and respiratory reflexes, and respiratory center depression. Causes of airway obstruction in coma include obstruction by hypopharyngeal soft tissue when the head is not tilted backward, inability to clear secretions, laryngospasm, regurgitation and aspiration of gastrointestinal contents, and—in upper airway injuries—bleeding or anatomic

TABLE 3   *Examples of Arterial Blood Gas and Acid Base Abnormalities in Critically Ill Patients*

	Condition	(N) Normal	Asthma Attack	Status Asthmaticus	Compensated COPD	Decompensated COPD	Pulmonary Edema	ARDS	Miliary Post-op. Atelectasis	Brain Injury with Coma	Vomiting from Pyloric Stenosis
Pulmonary Status (100% O₂ Test) — PaO₂ (torr)	SB PB FIO₂ 0.21	75–100	(↓)	↓↓	↓↓	↓↓	↓↓↓	↓↓↓	↓↓↓	↓↓	N
	SB PB FIO₂ 1.0	>500	N	↓	N	(↓)	↓↓	↓↓↓	↓↓	(↓)	N
	CV, AR Pos Pres FIO₂ 1.0	>500	N	↓	N	(↓)	(↓)	↓↓	N	N	N
O₂ Transport	Hb, gm.%	13–15	(N)	(N)	↑	↑	(N)	(N)	(N)	(N)	(N)
Ventilation	PaCO₂ torr	35–45	N (↓)	↑↑	↑	↑↑↑	(↓)N	(↓)N	(↓)N	↓↓	(↓)
Acid-Base Status	pHa	7.35–7.45	N (↑)	↓↓	N	↓	(↑)N	(↑)N	N	↑	↑
	HCO₃ mEq./L.	22–26	N	(↓)	↑	↑↑	N	N	N	↓	↑↑
	BE mEq./L.	0 ± 3	N	↓	↑	↑↑	N(↓)	N(↑↓)	N	N	↑↑

deformation. Further, in most coma states, respiratory movements are depressed, resulting during air breathing in hypercarbia plus hypoxemia, although some mechanisms causing coma may stimulate breathing, as, for instance, in brain injury, renal failure, diabetic coma, hepatic coma, and salicylate intoxication. From whatever cause, however, prolonged partial airway obstruction or respiratory depression may result in miliary atelectasis and accumulation of tracheobronchial secretions with secondary infection.

Hypnotic drug intoxication is one of the more common causes of prolonged coma. In most instances, complete recovery from coma of this type, without brain damage, can be achieved if airway control, oxygenation, ventilation, and circulatory support are started before hypoxic brain damage has occurred and are continued until the drug effect has worn off. In animals with straight, unobstructed airways, the lethal dose of an hypnotic or narcotic drug equals the apneic dose. In man, however, there is no predictable lethal dose. A dose sufficient to produce coma but insufficient to produce apnea may kill readily because the kinked human upper airway tends to obstruct when the neck is flexed or in the midposition. In contrast, many times an apneic dose can be survived without brain damage if artificial ventilation is instituted early. When coma is due to opiate overdose, specific opiate antagonists (naloxone) should supplement general life support measures. Nonspecific antidotes, however, particularly those with side-effects (e.g., analeptics for barbiturate poisoning), should be avoided; such nonspecific drugs may cause unnecessary lethal complications (e.g., convulsions, prolonged depression) where basic life support alone, when started in time, enables survival without residuals.

(2) Convulsive states

A wide variety of disease states may produce seizures, with or without morphologic changes in the brain. Such epileptogenic states include meningitis, encephalitis, uremia, post-ischemic-anoxic encephalopathy (e.g., after cardiac arrest, alveolar anoxia, CO poisoning), intoxication with convulsant drugs or heavy metals, sepsis, hepatic coma, intracranial tumor, and — most common — idiopathic epilepsy. All these effect a global type of encephalopathy, of which seizures represent a nonspecific manifestation. In *focal* ischemia or hemorrhage (stroke), generalized convulsions are rare.

Convulsive states produce respiratory insufficiency primarily by discoordination of upper airway reflexes and spasm of the respiratory muscles. The resulting tissue hypoxia may be accelerated by the hypermetabolism of muscle contractions. Trismus associated with seizures may preclude effective mouth-to-mouth ventilation and require mouth-to-nose ventilation instead. If in addition muscle spasms interfere with airway control and ventilation, a short-acting muscle relaxant (succinylcholine) is indicated initially, but only in the hands of personnel trained in anesthesiology. All patients in coma or convulsions should receive glucose intravenously.

Long-term resuscitation in convulsive states (Chapter 10) should include suppression of neuronal hyperactivity, which in itself can cause neuronal damage — using a short-acting barbiturate (e.g., thiopental or pentobarbital) or diazepam (Valium) — and attempts to correct the cause of convulsions. After stabilization, long-term anticonvulsant therapy with a long-acting barbiturate (phenobarbital) or diphenylhydantoin (Dilantin) or both should be considered. In the hospitalized conscious patient considered at risk of episodic convulsions, prophylactic inhalation of oxygen will buy time for therapeutic action should airway obstruction or apnea occur suddenly.

Medullary Depression by Increasing Intracranial Pressure (Fig. 5, Site 2)

Acute medullary drug depression or subsequent medullary damage can cause hypoventilation and apnea (Chapter 5). Furthermore, when there is intracranial hypertension, airway obstruction may occur from coma itself. While supratentorial intracranial hypertension tends to produce hyperventilation, medullary herniation causes apnea.

Cerebral hypoxia or intracranial hypertension can produce a neurogenic form of pulmonary edema, the mechanism of which is not clear. Neurogenic factors are presumed to play a role since denervated animal lung is protected. Systemic arterial hypertension and pulmonary venospasm caused by the CNS lesion have been implicated as possible pathophysiologic factors in neurogenic pulmonary edema, but conclusive evidence for the etiology of this phenomenon is still lacking.

Spinal Cord Injury (Fig. 5, Site 3)

If the cervical spinal cord becomes "transected" *below* C4, diaphragmatic breathing can maintain minute volume and $PaCO_2$ at normal levels even though VC is reduced to about one-half. However, this reduction in "sighing volume," together with immobilization in one position, may result in miliary atelectasis and hypostasis, leading to progressive hypoxemia, decreased compliance, and possibly secondary pneumonia. Furthermore, diaphragmatic breathing with chest retraction can, in itself, cause hypoxemia from ventilation/perfusion mismatching.

When a cervical lesion is higher in the spinal cord and *includes* C4, asphyxia from hypoventilation may rapidly ensue unless artificial ventilation is begun immediately. In addition, high cervical (percutaneous or operative) cordotomy for intractable pain can occasionally, when the lesion extends beyond the lateral spinothalamic tract, result in sleep-induced apnea, perhaps because the lesion produces damage to the cervical extension of the reticular formation or deafferentation with diminished stimuli to the respiratory center from the periphery.

Peripheral Nerve Disorders (Fig. 5, Site 4)

(1) POLYNEURITIS

Now that an effective vaccine has rendered poliomyelitis a clinical rarity, the most common syndrome causing ventilatory insufficiency from peripheral nerve paralysis is polyneuritis of the Landry-Guillain-Barré type. After mild respiratory or gastrointestinal symptoms, the patient becomes weak, and within a few days may be fully paralyzed. Sensory symptoms are rare, but any motor fibers may be involved and, occasionally, some autonomic fibers as well, which may cause circulatory disturbances. Higher centers usually are not affected, and these patients remain conscious unless they are permitted to asphyxiate or are given CNS-depressant drugs. Attempts to isolate an etiologic virus have failed so far, and some investigators believe that the disease may be the result of an autoimmune reaction affecting primarily peripheral nerves; the presence of perineural lymphocytic infiltrates followed by demyelinization of nerve fibers is suggestive of an immunologic phenomenon. However, despite these morphologic changes, most patients recover completely or with only mild residual deficit after variable periods (weeks to months) on mechanical ventilation. The utility of steroid therapy in shortening or mitigating the course of this disorder is still unproved.

The possibility of respiratory paralysis occurring within hours after the onset of symptoms in Landry-Guillain-Barré syndrome makes it mandatory in cases of suspicion to monitor the inspiratory capacity (IC). Reduction in IC to about 15 ml./kg. BW calls for tracheal intubation and mechanical artificial ventilation, followed by tracheotomy in prolonged paralysis.

(2) TETANUS

Tetanus, a major killer until World War II, should be an historical curiosity only, because of the effectiveness of active mass immunization and modern wound care. However, it remains a common disease in underdeveloped countries, not least among newborn babies. When the anaerobic bacillus, *Clostridium tetani*, penetrates deeply into tissues, the low PO_2 of necrotic materials enables its spores to germinate. With clostridial proliferation, tetanus exotoxin enters the CNS through retrograde spread along the perineurium of peripheral nerves and also via lymphatics and the blood stream. Muscular rigidity starts with spasms of the jaw muscles ("lockjaw") and pharyngeal muscles, and later involves respiratory muscles; thus asphyxia may occur through airway obstruction and/or ventilatory movement arrest. These spasms may be initiated or exaggerated by various external stimuli.

In mild and moderate cases, with only trismus and rigidity but without ventilatory impairment, observation in a stimulus-free, dark room with respiratory resuscitation facilities on hand, suffices. In severe cases, with upper airway spasms or IC reduced to

15 ml./kg. body weight or less, the patient should be preoxygenated, anesthetized, curarized, his trachea intubated, and prolonged mechanical ventilation begun. With modern long-term airway care and support of ventilation, oxygenation, and circulation, patients have survived this dramatic illness with complete recovery of the CNS and muscle function after many weeks of partial curarization and sedation. As soon as the diagnosis is made, human tetanus immune globulin (antitoxin) should be given; active immunization (toxoid) should also be undertaken, since the disease does not leave a reliable immunity.

Blockade of Neuromuscular Junctions
(Fig. 5, Site 5)

(1) MYASTHENIA GRAVIS

This disease of unknown etiology is incurable, but symptomatically controllable. An abnormal function of the neuromuscular endplates produces a curare-like (nondepolarizing) type of weakness and paralysis of muscles, usually starting with muscles of the eye, face, larynx, and pharynx. Later it involves the muscles of respiration as well. Muscle weakness can be monitored by periodic tests of IC, inspiratory force, grip strength, and response to electric stimulation of peripheral nerves. The weakness can be reversed by curare antagonists, i.e., anticholinesterase drugs, either for diagnosis (e.g., edrophonium) or for treatment (e.g., neostigmine).

The pathogenetic mechanism of myasthenia gravis is unknown, but there is suggestive evidence that antibodies inhibit the action of acetylcholine. Histologic examination reveals early lymphocytic infiltration between muscle fibers and around small blood vessels, and sometimes also in other organs; degeneration of the neuromuscular endplates; and later replacement of paralyzed muscles by fat and fibrous tissue. About 10 per cent of these patients have a thymoma. Thymectomy, however, is followed by a cure in fewer than one-half of these cases.

Mild cases need treatment with anticholinesterase drugs only during episodes of intensified paralysis. The muscarinic side-effects of neostigmine (i.e., hypotension, bradycardia, bronchospasm, salivation, gastrointestinal cramps) can be blocked by atropine, which, however, is not always required. Mestinon (pyridostigmine) is longer acting than neostigmine and produces fewer muscarinic side-effects. In resistant cases, long-term artificial ventilation and steroid therapy may induce remission. ARI in patients on anticholinesterase therapy can be the result of either myasthenic crisis (resistance to anticholinesterase drugs) or cholinergic crisis (muscarinic and nicotinic effect, i.e., paralysis from overdose with anticholinesterase drug). Irrespective of which type of crisis is suspected, if the IC is less than 15 ml./kg. body weight and there is inability to clear bronchial secretions, it seems wise to discontinue all drug therapy temporarily, intubate the trachea, and resume mechanical ventilation with individualized advanced respiratory care. After improvement of the pulmonary status, maintenance drug therapy can be resumed and readjusted to a more effective dose after the neuromuscular junctions have been put "at rest."

(2) ANTICHOLINESTERASE POISONING

Insecticides and nerve gases of the organophosphate type (e.g., Parathion, Malathion, TEPP, HETP, OMPA) or of the carbamate type (Dimetal, Matacil), which are inhaled, ingested, or absorbed through the skin, may produce ARI. These agents act by inhibiting cholinesterase activity, which results in accumulation of acetylcholine in the CNS (leading to convulsions, coma, and apnea), the autonomic ganglia, the parasympathetic nerve endings (causing miosis, tenesmus, bronchorrhea, bronchospasm, bradycardia, and hypotension), and finally at the motor nerve endings (causing fasciculations followed by paralysis). The muscarinic effects of cholinesterase inhibitors, at the parasympathetic nerve endings, usually can be reversed by very large (titrated) doses of atropine. Oximes (e.g., pralixomine) have been tried as cholinesterase reactivators, but require considerable time to restore plasma cholinesterase levels; their use should not supplant that of atropine. The combination of bronchial obstruction, respiratory muscle paralysis, and circulatory depression makes the treatment of insecticide or nerve gas poisoning victims challenging, particularly since complete reversal of the condition is possible if hypoxemia is prevented.

(3) BOTULISM

Ingestion of improperly canned or uncooked food containing toxin elaborated by *Clostridium botulinum* may produce potentially lethal, progressive, descending, bulbar and skeletal muscle paralysis. The botulinus exotoxin is produced under anaerobic conditions, most commonly in home-canned vegetables, smoked meats, and vacuum-packed fish. It acts by blocking release of acetylcholine from nerve endings, thereby preventing neuromuscular transmission in cholinergic fibers. The toxin can be destroyed by boiling for 20 minutes. Symptoms of poisoning usually begin with cranial nerve palsies as manifested by diplopia and loss of accommodation; other symptoms include dry mouth, dysphagia, and sometimes nausea and vomiting. Muscular weakness is marked, and respiratory paralysis may occur very rapidly. The temperature usually is normal and the sensorium clear. However, asphyxia may lead to unconsciousness. If endotracheal intubation and artificial ventilation are instituted before hypoxic damage has occurred, recovery is complete. Adjunctive therapy includes administration of trivalent botulinus antitoxin. Guanidine hydrochloride, which presumably binds the toxin, has also been used, although its benefit is still unproved.

Disorders of Muscles and Chest Wall
(Fig. 5, Site 6)

(1) MYOTONIA

Congenital myotonia (Thomsen's disease) is an hereditary disorder characterized by hyperexcitability and hypertrophy of muscles, which also tend to relax slowly. This disease and many other rare muscle spasm and muscle stiffness syndromes interfere with voluntary action, but only occasionally compromise ventilation. It is incurable, but symptomatic improvement of congenital myotonia may be obtained by quinine or procaine amide.

(2) SCLERODERMA (PROGRESSIVE SYSTEMIC SCLEROSIS)

This disease of unknown etiology, with onset later in life, is characterized by progressive interstitial fibrosis of many organ systems. The skin shows epidermal atrophy, and the gastrointestinal tract develops muscularis atrophy and mucosal ulcerations. Glomerulosclerotic changes may be seen in the kidney; fibrotic changes in the myocardium may lead to conduction defects. Subcutaneous and submucosal tissues become fibrotic and hypertrophied. Pulmonary involvement is characterized by pulmonary interstitial fibrosis, thickening of alveolar membranes and breakdown of alveolar septa leading to bullous emphysema (restrictive plus obstructive lung disease). Hypoxemia develops slowly, however; muscular hypertrophy of pulmonary arterioles also may be seen. Rare are restriction of chest movements from skin changes and aspiration pneumonia from esophageal malfunction.

(3) KYPHOSCOLIOSIS

This chest deformity may be idiopathic, congenital, or the result of bone or neuromuscular disorders (e.g., poliomyelitis). The chest wall is deformed and stiffened and the lungs distorted and partially compressed. The resulting ventilation/perfusion mismatching leads to chronic hypoxemia which, in turn, causes pulmonary vasospasm and finally a fixed increase in pulmonary vascular resistance with cor pulmonale. All lung volumes and VC are decreased and obstructive lung disease may occasionally occur later in life from airway distortion and compression. Patients with kyphoscoliosis are more prone to atelectasis and pneumonia, which may result in hypercarbia in addition to hypoxemia.

Pectus excavatum (funnel chest), a congenital deformity of the anterior chest wall, is primarily a cosmetic problem, as it usually is not associated with any abnormalities in pulmonary function values.

(4) FLAIL CHEST

If the integrity of the chest wall is disrupted by trauma or disease, the unstable segment may be paradoxically sucked in with inspiratory movements, while the rest of the chest wall moves normally outward. Such "flailing" usually is caused by trauma (including external heart compressions) but occasionally by chest wall resection (thoracoplasty) or multiple pathologic rib fractures. Automobile accidents are the most common cause of flail chest. Lateral flailing is seen with multiple rib fractures; anterior flailing may result from costochondral separations and sternal fractures, as occur from steering wheel trauma. Flailing with posterior rib fractures is rare. The presence of flail chest should alert the physician to search for a variety of other injuries, for blunt chest injury may result in (besides flail chest) any one or a combination of the following: multiple rib fractures, pneumothorax, tension pneumothorax, interstitial emphysema, lung contusion with or without lung lacerations, tracheal or bronchial rupture, hemothorax, mediastinal hemorrhage, pericardial hemorrhage and tamponade, cardiac contusion, etc.

In the past, it was assumed that lateral flailing causes "pendel air," i.e., downward movement of the diaphragm drawing gas from the lung on the flail side and into the lung on the normally expanding side. However pendel air—if it exists—is a minor factor in producing ARI, since $PaCO_2$ rise is rare and, indeed, concomitant tachypnea often leads to mild hypocarbia. Rather, ARI occurs due to progressive shunting. The unstable chest wall prevents development of negative intrathoracic pressure required for deep lung expansion, thus favoring progressive atelectasis (decreased FRC). Development of ARDS results in progressive hypoxemia and increasing $P(A-a)O_2$ (FIO_2 1.0). This ARDS is the result of a combination of many factors: lack of periodic deep breaths; inability to cough, resulting in secretional obstruction; lung contusion; hypoperfusion from shock; trauma; as well as other pathogenetic factors of ARDS that are still not well understood. The lung may, in addition, rupture on the surface (causing pneumothorax) or into the interstitial space (causing mediastinal and subcutaneous emphysema). Tension pneumothorax occurs when a valvelike pulmonary leak is exposed to increased airway pressure (e.g., coughing, positive pressure ventilation).

Because they are at risk of hypoxemia from so many mechanisms, all patients with chest injury should breathe 50 to 100 per cent oxygen at atmospheric pressure during transport to the hospital. When attended by ambulance personnel unable to recognize and treat pneumothorax, positive pressure ventilation should be avoided, since this measure may provoke pneumothorax and thus requires pleural drainage standby. For interhospital transport, prophylactic pleural drainage may be considered.

Treatment of chest injuries in the hospital has advanced considerably over the past two decades. Previous management using tracheotomy with spontaneous breathing and external surgical stabilization was accompanied by high mortality. The breakthrough in the salvage of patients with crushing chest injury came with the introduction in the 1950s of intermittent or continuous positive pressure controlled hyperventilation (IPPV CPPV) via tracheotomy (T. Moerch). This both stabilizes the chest wall internally and raises PaO_2 in the presence of ARDS. Controlled ventilation should be continued for at least one week to enable fibrous stabilization of the chest wall. Older patients may require more prolonged periods of controlled ventilation. Active diaphragmatic contractions, as in assisted breathing or intermittent mandatory ventilation, should be avoided in cases of severe flailing.

In *moderate* flailing, less than one week of tracheal intubation and IMV plus PEEP may suffice (Chapter 10). Only *mild* degrees of flailing should be treated "expectantly" with spontaneous breathing and pain control (e.g., multiple intercostal blocks or catheter epidural analgesia) to enable otherwise painful sighing and coughing.

Subcutaneous or mediastinal emphysema accompanying flail chest is rarely a problem in itself. Several hours of 100 per cent oxygen breathing at atmospheric pressure for denitrogenation will permit more rapid reabsorption of interstitial air, thus giving leaks a chance to seal. If, however, the interstitial emphysema persists, a bronchial or tracheal tear should be suspected, and bronchoscopy and/or bronchography will be required to determine the necessity for surgical repair.

Airway Obstruction (Fig. 5, Site 7)

The causes, mechanisms, and management of *upper* airway obstruction are discussed under Coma (above) and in Chapter 9. Aspiration and near-drowning will serve here as prototypes for *lower* airway obstruction with pulmonary injury.

(1) ASPIRATION

With good care, aspiration should not occur: attention to positioning the patient and intubating the airway in comatose patients should minimize the incidence of this complication. Nevertheless, regurgitation or vomiting followed by inhalation of gastrointestinal contents has been the most common cause of morbidity and mortality associated with general anesthesia, coma, or other conditions that impair upper airway protective reflexes. When neglected, aspiration still causes unnecessary deaths and crippling. With immediate recognition and modern respiratory care, however, aspiration has become potentially a completely reversible complication.

The extent and reversibility of the lung lesion and the clinical picture (bronchospasm, pulmonary edema, atelectasis) following aspiration depend on acidity and volume aspirated, host defenses, and therapy. Massive aspiration of solid or semisolid material can cause acute asphyxial cardiac arrest. Inhalation of even small amounts of liquid material causes bronchospasm, pulmonary vasospasm, surfactant failure, and leakage of blood components into the alveoli. Hypoxemia occurs from both shunting and ventilation-perfusion mismatching. In addition, there is often tachycardia, fever, and hypotension.

Aspiration of acid gastric juice (the pH of which can be as low as 1.0) causes bronchial epithelial and alveolar damage. Profound hypoxemia and regional or total pulmonary consolidation and necrosis may follow if treatment is not undertaken. Gastric juice of pH over 3.0 is relatively benign. Inhaling duodenal or intestinal material (as is common in ileus) causes less chemical damage but more obstructive atelectasis and bacterial contamination, resulting in pneumonitis and, sometimes, abscess formation.

Emergency management in symptomatic aspiration consists of tracheal intubation (if necessary under brief succinylcholine paralysis followed by coughing to help clearing); tracheobronchial suctioning via curved tip catheter (for selective insertion into right and left bronchus) and using a sputum trap for inspection, pH determination, and bacteriologic examination of the suctioned material; in the case of semisolid aspirate, tracheobronchial irrigation with 3- to 5-ml. increments of isotonic saline solution; in suspicion of solid matter aspirate, clearing under vision with rigid ventilating bronchoscope; and optimized CPPV (FIO_2 1.0 to 0.6). Prophylactic broad spectrum antibiotics started immediately should be readjusted according to sputum culture reports; prophylactic antibiotics may not be required if the aspirate is of very low pH. Bronchodilator therapy is necessary if wheezing is a prominant feature. In spite of controversial experimental results, therapeutic doses of steroid probably should be started immediately upon suspicion of aspiration and discontinued when the lung lesion is improving—based on the fact that short-term steroid therapy may ameliorate the asthmatic reaction of the human lungs without being harmful in itself.

(2) NEAR-DROWNING

ARI in near-drowning may occur by a variety of mechanisms. Reflex laryngospasm and bronchospasm, induced by water in the hypopharynx and larynx (even without entry of water into the tracheobronchial tree) can, by themselves, lead to asphyxia and coma. If, however, resuscitation is started before flooding of the lungs occurs and before cardiac arrest, recovery is quick and complete. Even if water enters the alveoli, the resulting hemodilution from fresh water inhalation or hemoconcentration from sea water inhalation is not an insuperable obstacle to resuscitation. However, in these instances, the pulmonary lesion does cause acute hypoxemia, which calls for 100 per cent O_2 administration as soon as possible. With prompt and modern respiratory care, the lesion usually is entirely reversible (Chapt. 2).

Inhaled *fresh water*, although absorbed, tends to produce severe shunting from surfactant failure and atelectasis; therefore, optimized CPPV (FIO_2 1.0–0.6) is indicated until the $P(A-a)O_2$ normalizes (usually in 24 to 48 hours). Hypertonic *sea water* produces shunt from pulmonary edema and capillary-alveolar membrane damage, similarly requiring prolonged $CPPV/O_2$. Also, in salt water aspiration plasma loss by transudation must be replaced. Near-drowning in either fresh or salt water frequently is complicated by additional inhalation (during drowning or resuscitation) of gastric contents, which may produce further damage. Furthermore, even small amounts of any type of water inhaled cause bronchospasm, bronchial edema, and pulmonary vasospasm. Although steroid therapy does not seem to improve the outcome in dogs, we consider it indicated in human near-drowning victims whose clinical picture resembles that of an asthmatic response and in those who become comatose because of anoxic brain damage. In the last analysis, it is the degree of hypoxic brain damage that determines the outcome; even some near-drowning victims with cardiac arrest have been completely resuscitated.

Chronic Nonspecific Intrapulmonary Airway Obstruction (Fig. 5, Site 8)

Chronic obstructive pulmonary (lung) disease [COPD, COLD] is not really a single disease or syndrome. We suggest the term "chronic nonspecific intrapulmonary airway obstruction" for the triad of asthma, chronic bronchitis and emphysema. These three conditions can be present clinically and morphologically in any given patient either separately or in variable combinations. Physicians diagnose one to the exclusion of the others usually merely on the basis of clinical impression. All three conditions, however, have multiple causes and unknown etiologies and pathogeneses and are not mutually exclusive. They overlap clinically also with bronchiectasis, pneumoconiosis, and mucoviscidosis (cystic fibrosis). The total VC (FEV total) may or may not be reduced. Asthma, chronic bronchitis and emphysema, however, have in common reduced timed FEV, MEFR, FEV/VC ratio, and MVV, all of which indicate closure of medium-sized airways. Even early in the development of asthma and emphysema, though, when the above values may still be normal, one can already recognize small airway closure from an increase in closing volume or decrease in frequency-dependent compliance.

By definition, "asthma" is increased reactivity of the airways with episodic overall bronchospasm as one of its principal features. "Chronic bronchitis" is productive cough with excessive sputum production, with or without infection, over about three months per year for over three years. "Emphysema" is loss of pulmonary elasticity

with progressive loss of support and thus collapse of small airways (check-valve obstruction) and distended, rarified alveoli. Chronic bronchitis can have a bronchospastic (asthmatic) component; and both chronic asthma and bronchitis can lead to emphysema.

(1) ASTHMA

The word "asthma" derives from the Greek word meaning "panting," and orginally referred to any disorder causing dyspnea, wheezing, and cough. In common usage today, however, asthma specifically implies "episodic or continuous bronchial obstruction caused by a variable combination of allergic, infectious, emotional and environmental factors."

Bronchospasm plus variable degrees of mucosal edema-congestion and obstructing mucus combine to produce bronchial obstruction. There is also eosinophilia of blood and sputum, mucosal infiltration with eosinophils and mononuclear cells, hypertrophy of bronchial muscles, and hyperplasia of mucous glands and goblet cells. When excessive mucus production is dominant, chronic bronchitis may supervene. Sympathetic nervous system tone in the lungs seems decreased episodically, for instance during sleep. Between attacks, blood gas and pH values usually are normal. During brief and mild to moderate attacks, there is usually only slight hypoxemia during air breathing (from ventilation/perfusion mismatching without shunting) and normal or low $PaCO_2$, as mild partial airway obstruction at first reflexly stimulates breathing movements. Prolonged severe bronchial obstruction, however, may become intractable and the patient's respiratory drive in relation to the obstruction becomes exhausted; when this occurs, he develops status asthmaticus.

Status asthmaticus has been defined as "epinephrine-resistant diffuse wheezing with signs of asphyxia" and represents a failure of basic asthma therapy. Until recently, it has killed about 5000 persons in this country per year through interaction and progression of *hypoxemia* (shunting from spasm and atelectasis, the latter caused by inspissated secretions) and *mixed acidemia* (hypercarbia, lactacidemia from tissue hypoxia and catecholamine overdose, ketoaci-

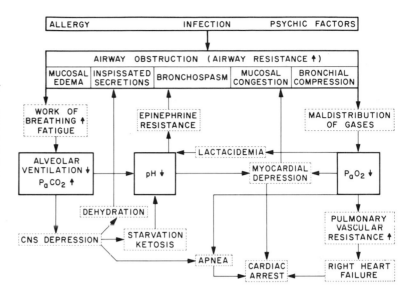

Figure 6. *Pathophysiology of status asthmaticus.*

Vicious cycles and progression of asphyxiation. Hypoxemia and acidemia (respiratory plus metabolic) are the focal derangements leading to death, and thus are the focal points for therapeutic intervention.

(From Safar, P.: J.A.M.A. *208:* 1008, 1969.)

dosis from starvation and dehydration) (Fig. 6). Further, alveoli overdistended due to air trapping may rupture into the pleural or interstitial spaces during spontaneous or positive pressure ventilation.

Therapy of chronic asthma should include prevention and treatment of allergic, infectious, emotional, and environmental factors (particularly air pollution). Symptomatic treatment relies heavily on sympathomimetic amine bronchodilators (e.g., metaproterenol by aerosol, ephedrine by mouth), aminophylline, steroid, and bronchial clearing (Table 4).

Sympathomimetic bronchodilator aerosols seem to act in part topically and in part via absorption into the blood stream. Beta receptor stimulators (e.g., isoproterenol) relax circumferential bronchial smooth muscles. Sometimes alpha receptor stimulation (e.g., phenylephrine) is needed, in addition, to provide mucosal vasoconstriction and decongestion. Epinephrine, the most potent bronchodilator, is both a beta and alpha receptor stimulator. Isoproterenol (Isuprel) is a pure beta stimulator and is widely used in aerosols. Because it stimulates at both beta-1 (pulmonary) and beta-2 (cardiac) receptor sites, however, isoproterenol may cause considerable tachycardia. Agents acting primarily at beta-2 sites, such as metaproterenol, provide a proportionally greater therapeutic effect in the lungs with fewer undesirable cardiac effects (Table 4).

Sympathomimetic amines seem to work by converting ATP to cyclic AMP, while the *xanthines* (e.g., aminophylline) inhibit breakdown of cyclic AMP. Thus both, through different mechanisms, cause accumulation of cyclic AMP in the tracheobronchial smooth muscles; and can be used together for augmented effect. Increased cyclic AMP binds calcium and thereby promotes smooth muscle relaxation through stabilization of cell membranes. In addition, cyclic AMP seems to impede antigen-antibody mediated release of histamine from mast cells and leukocytes. Histamine and other mediators produce smooth muscle spasm, increased capillary permeability, and slowing of mucociliary transport. Parasympathetic stimuli, by contrast, cause accumulation of cyclic GMP (guanosine 3,5 phosphate). Their action can be blocked by the vagolytic agent atropine which, however, is not favored for use in asthma, as it thickens bronchial secretions; but in selected cases, atropine can prolong the actions of catecholamines. Antihistamines given orally or parenterally sometimes worsen asthma, probably because of their drying effect. Antihistamine aerosols have not been evaluated.

Steroids are indicated when the response to bronchodilators is unsatisfactory. Steroids reduce inflammation (particularly mucosal edema), sensitize receptors to sympathetic agonists and, through an unknown mechanism, reduce mucus production and plugging. Adrenal cortical insufficiency from chronic steroid medication can be avoided by alternate day, low dose steroid medication (increased during exacerbation) or use

TABLE 4 Effects of Drugs on Bronchopulmonary System

DRUG	COMMON ROUTES OF ADMINISTRATION	DESIRABLE EFFECTS	UNDESIRABLE EFFECTS
SYMPATHOMIMETIC AMINES		Enhance production of cyclic AMP	
epinephrine (Adrenalin, Vaponefrin, Micronefrin)	aerosol sc, (I.V. infusion)	Alpha + beta receptor stimulation. Relieves bronchospasm. Decongests mucosa. Increases cardiac output.	Tachyarrhythmias. Hypertension. Potent. Short action.
ephedrine	oral, (aerosol)	Same as epinephrine, but longer acting. Releases norepinephrine in tissues.	Tachyarrhythmias. CNS stimulation. (Hypertension.) Tachyphylaxis.
isoproterenol (Isuprel, Aludrin)	aerosol (I.V. infusion)	Beta 1 + 2 receptor stimulation. Relieves bronchospasm. Pulmonary vasodilation. Increases mucociliary clearing.	Tachyarrhythmias. Systemic vasodilation (hypotension). CNS stimulation. (Bronchospastic metabolites.)
isoetharine (Dilabrom, Bronkosol)	aerosol, (oral)	Beta 2 receptor stimulation. Relieves bronchospasm. Pulmonary vasodilation. Increases mucociliary clearing.	(Tachycardia.)
metaproterenol (Alupent)			
salbutamol (Ventolin)			
terbutaline (Bricanyl)			
carbuterol			
phenylephrine (Neo-Synephrine)	aerosol, (oral) (in combination with other drugs)	Alpha receptor stimulator. Decongests mucosa. Prolongs action of isoproterenol.	Hypertension (bradycardia).
METHYL XANTHINES			
aminophylline (Theophylline ethylene diamine)	oral, rectal, (I.V. infusion)	Inhibits breakdown of cyclic AMP. Relieves bronchospasm. Increases mucociliary clearing. Cardiac stimulant. Diuretic. Pulmonary vasodilator.	Tachyarrhythmias. Hypotension. CNS stimulation.
MISCELLANEOUS DRUGS			
atropine	sc, oral, (aerosol)	Vagolytic. Relieves bronchospasm.	Tachyarrhythmias. Drying of mucosa. Decreases mucus velocity.
antihistamines	oral, sc, I.V.	(Antiallergic)	CNS depression. Drying of mucosa. Decreases mucus velocity.
corticosteroids hydrocortisone prednisolone dexamethasone	oral, I.V.	Sensit. of sympathetic agonists. Decongests mucosal edema. (Relieves bronchospasm.) Reduces mucus plugging. Normalizes eosinophilia.	Adrenocortical atrophy (with long-term use). Onset of action delayed.
beclomethasone (Vanceril) triamcinoline	aerosol	Same as above.	Minimal systemic absorption. Oral candidiasis.

Table continued on opposite page.

TABLE 4 *Effects of Drugs on Bronchopulmonary System* (Continued)

DRUG	COMMON ROUTES OF ADMINISTRATION	DESIRABLE EFFECTS	UNDESIRABLE EFFECTS
acetylcysteine (Mucomyst)	aerosol, bronchial instillation	Softens mucus by breaking S-S bonds of mucopolysaccharides.	Bronchospasm. Spreading secretions. Use with bronchodilator.
streptokinase	aerosol, bronchial instillation	Softens pus by lysing proteins	Bronchospasm. Spreading secretions.
disodium cromoglycate (Cromolyn, Intal)	dust inhalation	Blocks histamine release from mast cells. Long-term therapy. Reduction of wheezes. Facilitates weaning from steroid.	Bronchospasm. Slow onset, long-term action only as steroid substitute. Use with bronchodilator.

Abbreviations:
sc = subcutaneous
I.V. = intravenous

of topically acting, poorly absorbed steroids e.g., beclomethasone, i.e., Vanceril).

Disodium cromoglycate (Cromolyn, Intal) has been recently introduced as a possible alternative to steroids. It is not a bronchodilator, but blocks histamine release from mast cells. When given on a regular basis by dust inhalation (it is not soluble), disodium cromoglycate may be useful prophylactically in allergic asthma and may permit weaning from steroids in young asthmatics. It has no place in emergency and critical care.

IPPB therapy sessions have been overrated as a mode of bronchial clearing. Their effectiveness has not been demonstrated, and some aerosols inhaled during IPPB may in fact increase airway resistance. For this reason sputum-softening acetylcysteine (Mucomyst) and ultrasonic mist, when needed, should be given with a bronchodilator, as they may provoke bronchospasm.

Status asthmaticus. The diagnosis is made if two doses of epinephrine (at least 20 minutes apart) each 0.01 mg./kg. body weight (0.5 mg. in adults) given subcutaneously do not improve the obstruction. *Therapy of status asthmaticus* requires the use of sophisticated measures by an experienced team. Priorities for therapy: (1) oxygenation with IPPB by mask, or IPPV (FIO_2 1.0) via tracheal tube if indicated (with "titrated" expiratory retardation); (2) bronchodilation with pHa normalization; (3) additional measures.

The bronchodilator effect of catecholamines is decreased by acidosis; pHa normalization restores this effect and may thereby obviate the need for tracheal intubation and

mechanical ventilation. Normalization of pHa is possible with bicarbonate (1–2 mEq./kg., followed by titrated doses according to pHa) or THAM, and bronchodilator titration by vein (e.g., aminophylline, 4 mg./kg./6 hours) and aerosol (e.g., epinephrine by titration). In intractable bronchospasm, intravenous titration of epinephrine or isoproterenol by infusion *or* general anesthesia (e.g., halothane) may be required. In all cases of status asthmaticus, EKG and blood pressure monitoring are mandatory, as the combination of hypoxemia, acidemia and bronchodilator can cause life-threatening dysrhythmias and cardiac arrest.

Hydrocortisone, 5 mg./kg. (or dexamethasone 0.2 mg./kg., or methylprednisolone 1 mg./kg.) should be given I.V. immediately, even though the effect of steroid begins only after several hours. Steroid doses should be repeated every six hours so long as there is severe wheezing. A broad spectrum antibiotic should be started and readjusted according to sputum smear and culture results. Circulatory support is essential because hypovolemia (plasma loss) and reduction in cardiac output from increased intrathoracic pressure are common. Thus *hydration is essential*, e.g., with 5 per cent dextrose in 0.25 per cent NaCl (plus potassium, 2 mEq./100 ml.); over 24 hours, 100 ml./kg. in infants, 50 ml./kg. in small children, and 20 ml./kg. in adults. Additionally about 50 ml./kg. should be given for rehydration. Colloid may also be indicated. Curarization, sedation, tracheal intubation and controlled ventilation are indicated when the patient cannot clear secretions spontaneously or becomes comatose (Chapter 10).

(2) CHRONIC BRONCHITIS

The typical bronchitic patient has, in the mucosa of the tracheobronchial tree, an increased number of mucous glands and goblet cells, edema, and inflammatory infiltrates. In many areas, furthermore, ciliated epithelium is replaced by squamous metaplasia, resulting in an impairment of clearing. Clearing of the periphery by cough is further impeded by inflammatory softening of the bronchial walls; additional bronchial compression from without is enhanced by secondary emphysematic airway collapse and alveolar distention. Early in chronic bronchitis, chest roentgenograms, lung volumes, and diffusion capacity are normal. The PaO_2 (FIO_2 0.21) is reduced, however, because of ventilation/perfusion mismatching without significant shunting. With time, the chronic hypoxemia can provoke polycythemia, increased pulmonary vascular resistance, and right heart failure. Further, as the disease progresses and the work of breathing increases, chronic hypercarbia may also ensue. These morphologic and laboratory derangements are reflected in the clinical picture of the chronic bronchitic. The classic "blue bloater" is plethoric (polycythemia) and cyanotic (hypoxemia), chronically coughing voluminous quantities of sputum (mucous gland hyperplasia). Jugular venous distention, hepatomegaly, and peripheral edema signal accompanying right heart failure. Treatment is symptomatic (Chapter 10) with special emphasis on prevention and long-term antibiotic treatment of infection. Mechanical clearing of the tracheobronchial tree should not rely on IPPB therapy sessions alone, which have been over-valued and over-used, but rather on an individualized combination of mist and bronchodilator aerosol inhalation (with IPPB only if its value is proved by MEFR tests), chest physiotherapy, and a change in habits (e.g., cessation of smoking). Periodic short-term tracheal intubation with suctioning may be useful in patients unable otherwise to clear secretions.

(3) EMPHYSEMA

Emphysema is diagnosed when the chest roentgenogram shows overinflated lungs (e.g., flat diaphragms) and pulmonary function studies reveal increased TLC and RV and decreased timed FEV and MEFR. Greatly increased alveolar deadspace and "parasitic ventilation" between lung units result in chronic hypoxemia with compensatory polycythemia and chronic hypercarbia, with compensatory rise in bicarbonate, and usually normal or only slightly reduced pHa. In uncomplicated emphysema, the hypoxemia is the result of ventilation/perfusion mismatching without shunting, and thus is readily corrected by FIO_2 0.3–0.6. There may or may not be asthmatic or bronchitic symptoms.

The classic "pure" emphysematous patient, or "pink puffer," is asthenic and only mildly dyspneic at rest. Hypoxemia is modest early in the course, hence the designation as "pink." Similarly, hypercarbia is a late finding, and cor pulmonale is less frequent than in the "pure" chronic bronchitic.

The predominant pathogenesis of emphysema is loss of elastic fiber traction on small airways, leading to collapse of these airways and a consequent valvelike respiratory obstruction; overdistention and gradual rarification of alveoli follow. Rapid exhalation increases closing volume and compresses the entire tracheobronchial tree, which results in trapping of secretions. The previous distinction between panlobular emphysema (diffuse distention of all alveoli) and centrilobular emphysema (dilation of respiratory bronchioles and alveolar ducts only) is not useful, since both can exist in the same patient.

The etiology of emphysema is not known. Among the factors thought to contribute to its development are: deficiency of alpha-1 anti-trypsin (causing "autodigestion" of connective tissue); hypoperfusion of bronchial arteries; destruction of elastic fibers by chemical air pollutants; and alveolar overdistention from obstruction by asthma or bronchitis. Smoking, occupational hazards, infections, and genetic variables have all been linked to the development of emphysema.

Basic therapy of compensated emphysema is symptomatic. It includes control of asthmatic and bronchitic symptoms (see above); teaching the patient slow (pursed lip) exhalations to "splint" bronchi; supporting upward movement of the diaphragm manually, with posture or adjuncts; and chest physiotherapy. While treatment sessions with IPPB-mist-bronchodilator or ultrasonic mist help individual patients, these measures do not seem to alter the course of the disease statistically. Ambulatory low flow oxygen inhalation helps to improve exercise tolerance.

Acute decompensation of chronic emphysema and/or bronchitis usually is due to respiratory infection, sedatives (e.g., alcohol, hypnotics), left heart failure (with superimposed pulmonary edema), or pulmonary thromboemboli. With decompensation, the $PaCO_2$ rises further, causing somnolence (CO_2 narcosis), and pHa decreases. Hypoxemia is intensified and, without resuscitation, can be the cause of cardiac arrest. The PaO_2 will decrease further due to shunting from secretional obstruction, atelectasis or pneumonia or left heart failure (perhaps with pulmonary thromboemboli) with pulmonary edema, calling for FIO_2 1.0–0.6 with positive pressure. The latter measure will be more effective in increasing PaO_2 in pulmonary edema than in pneumonia.

Do not withhold *oxygen* from the COPD patient who needs it! It is true that respiratory movements in many patients with COPD are controlled more by the hypoxemic peripheral chemoreceptor drive than by increase in $PaCO_2$, and that raising PaO_2 to about 80 torr or more tends to depress spontaneous breathing movements in these patients. These changes, in the *unattended* patient who inhales oxygen, have occasionally led to hypoventilation, further CO_2 rise, coma, airway obstruction, apnea, and asphyxial cardiac arrest. However, this does not mean FIO_2 must be limited in decompensated COPD with worsening hypoxemia; to the contrary, this situation calls for an FIO_2 as high as needed to bring PaO_2 to 60–80 torr. The conscious patient should concomitantly be stimulated to breathe by coaching or careful intravenous titration of an analeptic drug (e.g., doxapram). Even FIO_2 1.0 is justified when needed if mechanical ventilation is used. The stuporous or comatose patient should have his trachea intubated, the tracheobronchial tree suctioned, mechanical ventilation with FIO_2 control used with individualized adjustment (Chapter 10) to oxygenate rapidly and normalize $PaCO_2$ slowly. Weaning with IPPB or IMV should be started as early as possible. These patients may be difficult to wean because of increased work of breathing, large deadspace, and poor respiratory drive. Additional measures include antimicrobial therapy, correction of sodium and chloride depletion, and diuresis (in heart failure).

$PaCO_2$ reduction to the patient's habitual level should proceed *gradually*, not permitting pHa to rise above 7.45. Rapid reduction of $PaCO_2$ in emphysematics and in an animal model has resulted in secondary coma and convulsions; these manifestations are related to cerebral alkalosis with cerebral vasoconstriction and anoxia, since CO_2 passes the blood-brain barrier rapidly, but bicarbonate ions pass it only slowly. Thus bicarbonate in brain cells and cerebral arteriolar smooth muscles remains high. When this cerebral alkalosis syndrome occurs, the brain can be quickly reacidified with acetazolamide (Diamox) 0.5 gram I.V.

Decompensated COPD is often attended by *decompensated cor pulmonale*. In the emphysematic patient, there is a fixed increase in pulmonary vascular resistance due to a reduced cross-sectional area of the pulmonary vascular bed. This increase in PVR imposes an increased afterload on the right ventricle, leading over a period of time to the right ventricular hypertrophy of cor pulmonale. When, in addition, a further increase in PVR is superimposed—as occurs by pulmonary arteriolar spasm in the presence of hypoxia and acidosis—acute decompensation with right ventricular failure may supervene. Such decompensation is signalled by jugular venous distention, hepatomegaly and peripheral edema. Signs of left heart failure, if previously present, may at the same time be ameliorated, because of decreased output to the left heart from the failing right ventricle.

The treatment of choice for decompensated cor pulmonale is oxygen, along with measures to normalize $PaCO_2$ and pHa. Digitalis is of little if any benefit in the right ventricular failure of cor pulmonale, and indeed may be dangerously arrhythmogenic, especially in the presence of hypoxemia and acidosis.

It should be pointed out that the most common cause of right heart failure—in emphysematous patients as well as in the general patient population—is not cor pulmonale but rather left heart failure. The etiologic distinction is a significant one, since right heart failure secondary to left heart failure *is* likely to benefit from digitalis. Clinical signs of pulmonary edema as well as roentgenologic and EKG signs of left ventricular enlargement should alert the physician to the possiblity of a primary myocardial disorder.

Acute Alveolar Disorders (Fig. 5, Site 9)

(1) PULMONARY EDEMA AND CONSOLIDATION

A delicate balance among pressures, permeabilities, and lymphatic drainage protects us against drowning in our own plasma. This balance can be described in mathematical terms by the *modified Starling equation:*

Fluid movement across capillary walls =

$$K \times [(P_c - P_{if}) + (\pi_{if} - \pi_c)]$$

(to this, lymphatic drainage should be added)

where K is the filtration coefficient (depending on surface area and membrane permeability), P is hydrostatic pressure, π is colloid osmotic (oncotic) pressure, "c" is in capillaries and "if" is in interstitial fluid.

Although the equation is somewhat oversimplified in that it assumes an inert capillary membrane, it does identify the four most significant parameters in determining fluid movement across capillary walls, namely: (1) membrane permeability; (2) the hydrostatic pressure gradient from capillaries into interstitial spaces and alveoli; (3) the colloid osmotic gradient from interstitial spaces into capillaries; and (4) lymphatic drainage.

When the balance among these parameters is disturbed, molecular and cellular species of various sizes may leak from the pulmonary capillaries. Under normal circumstances, electrolytes and plasma proteins diffuse with variable efficiency through the capillary wall, but are rapidly cleared back into the vascular system by the lymphatics. Leakage of significant amounts of larger molecules, such as albumin and fibrinogen, or of blood cells is distinctly abnormal, however. When such leakage is copious or prolonged, pulmonary edema and consolidation can ensue.

Acute or protracted pulmonary edema may be suspected when there is dyspnea, tachypnea, rales, expectoration of white or pink foam, decreased vital capacity, hypoxemia, and increased $P(A-a)O_2$. The diagnostic problem, however, does not end with affixing a label of pulmonary edema to the patient. Appropriate management depends critically upon accurate identification of the pathogenetic mechanism underlying the pulmonary edema; and in this phase of diagnosis it is useful to return to the four parameters of the modified Starling equation.

Factor (1), increased membrane permeability, is predominant in shock lung (ARDS), aspiration, inhalation of noxious fumes, endotoxin, various poisonings, and pulmonary fat embolism. An increased hydrostatic pressure gradient, factor (2), predominates whenever left atrial pressure, and thus pulmonary capillary pressure increase, e.g., in mitral stenosis or, more commonly, left ventricular failure from coronary ischemia or hypertension. Factor (3), reduced blood colloid osmotic pressure, rarely by itself causes pulmonary edema, but may facilitate its development. Thus, in the presence of serum albumin levels (which are primarily responsible for plasma colloid osmotic pressure) below about 2.5 gm. per cent (normal value 5 gm. per cent) a modest rise in left atrial pressure (factor 2) or moderate degrees of membrane damage (factor 1) may cause pulmonary edema. Factor (4), impaired lymphatic drainage, may also be an adjunctive factor, particularly in fibrotic and emphysematic lungs, which seem to be pulmonary edema-prone because of reduced lymphatics, and in high CVP.

Acute pulmonary edema starts in the interstitial spaces of the lungs, with accumulation of edema fluid around vessels and bronchi ("cuffing"). Alveoli are flooded secondarily, in a scattered, all-or-none fashion. Interstitial edema may cause wheezes and ventilation/perfusion mismatching, while alveolar edema produces rales and shunting. Even before edema is recognizable on auscultation or roentgenogram, however, an increased $P(A-a)O_2$ (FIO_2 1.0) is demonstrable. Thus the 100 per cent oxygen test is the simplest clinical tool presently available to follow changes in shunt fraction and to guide therapy. Only when fluid leaves the alveoli and enters the bronchi and is churned up into foam can one hear rhonchi and encounter expectoration of foam.

Acute pulmonary edema kills by hypoxemia. Thus the first priority of *treatment* is to improve oxygenation. Immediate increase in PaO_2 is usually possible with 100 per cent oxygen administered by some form of continuous positive airway pressure. While IPPB (assisted breathing) does not reliably increase PaO_2, probably because tachypnea does not enable oxygen distribution, SB-CPAP or, even better, CPPV usually does (Chapter 10). The simplest positive pressure treatment is spontaneous breathing with CPAP by mask. Unnecessary tracheal intubation, an arrhythmogenic procedure, should be avoided in cardiogenic pulmonary edema. However, if the patient is stuporous or comatose or cannot cough up the edema fluid, or if PaO_2 cannot be kept above 60 torr with spontaneous breathing of 100 per cent O_2 by CPAP, or if CO_2 rises, tracheal intubation and controlled mechanical ventilation with CPPV (IPPV plus PEEP)—facilitated if necessary by curarization—and 100 per cent O_2 is indicated. In pulmonary edema, positive airway pressure raises PaO_2, not by increasing the alveolar-capillary pressure gradient (since the capillaries are also exposed to the positive pressure), but most likely by expanding FRC; fluid-filled alveoli are "recruited" and edema fluid is thinned out, thereby facilitating oxygen diffusion into blood.

Acute pulmonary edema, particularly of the cardiogenic type, benefits from a reduction in venous return. This is best accomplished by the measure which also increases PaO_2, namely an increase in airway pressure; the resultant increase in intrathoracic pressure is transmitted to the venae cavae, thereby reducing over-all venous return. Morphine titrated intravenously to cause vasodilation (particularly of capacitance vessels) also facilitates the reduction of venous return; morphine is of additional value because it relieves the anxiety and slows the tachypnea associated with acute pulmonary edema. In left heart failure, the patient should be rapidly digitalized. The choice of further therapy depends on the mechanism and cause, and may include use of a vasodilator more potent than morphine (e.g., Arfonad, nitroprusside, chlorpromazine, spinal anesthesia); phlebotomy; postural adjustment (sitting position); rapid diuresis with I.V. furosemide to reduce blood volume; possible peritoneal dialysis (in the presence of uremia); bronchodilation with aminophylline, which also increases sodium and water excretion, promotes systemic and pulmonary vasodilation, and enhances cardiac contractility; arrhythmia control; and normalization of pHa, $PaCO_2$, base deficit, and oncotic pressure. The use of rotating tourniquets, although traditionally advocated in pulmonary edema, is of no clinically proved benefit, and indeed may produce deleterious degrees of tissue acidosis and increased afterload. Finally, the underlying cause of the pulmonary edema should be sought and treated.

Therapy of acute pulmonary edema should be guided by careful monitoring of arterial blood gases and vital signs. Furthermore, periodic measurements of pulmonary artery wedge pressure as well as on-line determinations of cardiac output may help greatly in the physiologic management of intractable pulmonary edema. Experimental noninvasive methods (e.g., chest impedence, inert gas methods) for the early recognition of increased pulmonary water appear promising.

Progressive pulmonary consolidation (shock lung, ARDS) is a form of subacute, protracted pulmonary edema. It occurs when the integrity of the pulmonary capillary-alveolar membrane is disrupted by a combination of multiple, usually noninfectious insults. The patient with shock, trauma or sepsis develops a progressive decrease in PaO_2 (FIO_2 1.0) below that expected, i.e., a progressive increase in $P(A-a)O_2$ (FIO_2 1.0), together with a progressive decrease in compliance. Cardiac arrest can supervene when PaO_2 decreases below 30 torr in spite of modern therapy. The pathophysiology of the acute, subacute, and healing phases of pulmonary edema and consolidation is described elsewhere in this chapter.

Since the 1960s, when ARDS was first recognized as a treatable clinical entity, this author has considered the lesion to be the pulmonary counterpart of acute tubular necrosis (ATN) in the kidney, in the sense that both ARDS and ATN derive from cell damage due to the coexistence of multiple injurious factors and are potentially reversible. Principal among these factors are shock (hypoperfusion of the lungs), trauma, and sepsis. Notably, oligemic shock alone, if reversed early by adequate fluid resuscitation, causes an increased alveolar deadspace but not pulmonary shunting. When trauma or sepsis is superimposed, however, the outlook is very different. These insults produce capillary damage through release of amines, peptides, endotoxins, or other bacterial products. Furthermore, hypoperfusion is aggravated by capillary plugging with aggregates of erythrocytes, thrombocytes, and leukocytes. The latter, when attached to the capillary wall, release lysosomal enzymes, which augment the membrane damage. At the same time, catecholamines, generated in response to stress, cause thrombocyte aggregation and peptide release. Additional factors, which may in themselves or combined with shock, trauma, or sepsis cause ARDS, include: aspiration, lung contusion, fat embolization, uremia, pulmonary oxygen toxicity, bank blood embolization (particularly with use of large pore blood filters), overinfusion with salt solutions (by decreasing colloid osmotic pressure), overinfusion with colloid solutions (by increasing pulmonary capillary pressure), and pulmonary infection. Rare causes of ARDS include numerous lung toxins, such as antineoplastic drugs (e.g., adriamycin, bleomycin); turpentine (excreted through the lungs); and paraquat (a weed killer which is taken up by the lungs and may result in pulmonary edema after a lucid period).

Prevention of ARDS in susceptible individuals requires preventing or promptly reversing hypoperfusion with appropriate I.V. solutions, maintaining urine flow over 25 ml./hour, draining pus where present, using aseptic catheter and airway care techniques (patients in shock are infection-prone), providing gastric drainage, and optimizing cardiac, respiratory, and blood variables.

Early recognition and reversal of ARDS are enhanced by continuous monitoring and optimizing of arterial pressure, CVP, PAP (PAWP), EKG, urine flow, temperature, and lung-chest compliance (in patients on mechanical ventilation); and frequent monitoring of PaO_2 (FIO_2 1.0, i.e., 100 per cent O_2 test) fluid intake/output, serum and urine osmolality, serum electrolytes, protein and colloid osmotic pressure, hematologic values, body weight, sputum contamination, and chest roentgenograms.

Modern treatment of established ARDS includes intratracheal mechanical controlled ventilation with optimized CPPV (IPPV + PEEP) and FIO_2 control; measures to increase cardiac output (including normalization of $PaCO_2$); diuresis; if necessary, hemodialysis; and therapeutic doses of steroid. Types and volumes of intravenous fluids must be wisely chosen. A test bolus of 5 per cent albumin, 200 ml., may result in an increased PaO_2 if reduced colloid osmotic pressure was a causative factor in the pulmonary edema. If, on the other hand, increased membrane permeability had a significant role, a test bolus of albumin may leak out of the pulmonary capillaries, and the PaO_2 worsen as a consequence.

In hypoxemia intractable in spite of all the above measures, long-term extracorporeal membrane oxygenation may be considered. The technique, however, is still experimental and, to date, the mortality from heparin-induced intracranial bleeding has been high.

Another disorder in this group is the *infant respiratory distress syndrome (IRDS)*. Surfactant production reaches a peak between the twenty-eighth and thirtieth week of fetal life. In the amniotic fluid, a lecithin: sphingomyelin ratio of less than 1.5 is often associated with severe IRDS, 1.5 to 2.0 with mild to moderate IRDS, and over 2.0 with the absence of IRDS. IRDS becomes apparent in the neonate following a brief normal period and can be correlated with the degree of prematurity; perinatal asphyxia, shock and acidosis; cesarian section; and maternal diabetes. The surfactant deficit is related in part to the asphyxial pulmonary vasoconstriction. Acidosis inhibits the production of lecithin from choline, which requires a pH of 7.4 for enzyme function of this pathway.

For prevention, at least in the experimental model, steroid administered to pregnant animals has induced fetal surfactant production. The severity of IRDS is decreased by maintaining pHa near normal with bicarbonate. Continuous positive pressure spontaneous (and in severe cases, artificial) breathing with controlled FIO_2 (Chapter 10) and prompt treatment of acidosis and shock have drastically reduced mortality from IRDS.

(2) PNEUMONIA

Infection and accompanying inflammation at the alveolar level may be caused by numerous viruses, bacteria, fungi and parasites. Pneumonias complicate many illnesses and in the preantibiotic era they figured as a major killer, especially among the very young and very old. Even today, pneumonias of various types exact an unjustifiably high mortality—a mortality which could, we believe, be decreased by modern respiratory intensive care as it is now being applied to ARDS.

The most common type of pneumonia is that produced by the *Pneumococcus* and is usually lobar in distribution. In the aged, however, pneumococcal pneumonia may occur as patchy bronchopneumonia, which in turn can cause obstructive atelectasis of various lung areas. In a large proportion of the population, pneumococci are normal inhabitants of the upper respiratory tract. Infection probably occurs by auto-innoculation in a compromised host, and there is little risk of cross-infection. Thus, the pneumococcus may establish a beachhead in situations where defense mechanisms are diminished, as, for instance, after aspiration, pulmonary edema, viral infection, inhalation of irritant gases, or lung contusion. In the early stages of infection, pneumococci are protected from phagocytosis by their polysaccharide capsules, and they multiply readily in alveoli. The bacterial proliferation provokes an outpouring of protein-containing fluid, which provides a hospitable culture medium for the microorganisms and facilitates their spread to contiguous regions of lung. Meanwhile, the body's defenses are geared up, and polymorphonuclear leukocytes begin to migrate into the alveolar spaces. This leukocyte mobilization may be delayed, however, by alcohol, anesthesia, or steroid.

As this drama is unfolding in the alveoli, the patient manifests a sudden rigor, often pleuritic pain, and soon thereafter coughs up rusty sputum. He becomes hypoxemic from shunting due to fluid-filled alveoli. There is leukocytosis and, in one-fourth of the patients, a positive blood culture. If the pneumonia is untreated, fever, pleuritic pain, and cough continue for about one week; the recovery period, beginning at this time, is heralded by diaphoresis and sudden defervescence ("crisis"). Over the ensuing two to three weeks, debris is cleared upward and via the lymphatics, and the pulmonary lesion is completely resolved. In patients with compromised defenses, however, death may occur from hypoxemia due to shunting and/or

sepsis with distributive-type shock; or there may be delayed resolution with fibrosis.

With modern antibiotics and respiratory therapy the disease process is shortened and most patients survive. Even the compromised host can be saved through use of bactericidal agents such as penicillin, which do not depend upon intact host defenses for their effectiveness. Treatment is more difficult when complications occur, such as development of abscesses (rare) or spread of the infection to the pleural space (empyema) or extrapulmonary sites (metastatic infections).

Staphylococcus pneumonia is less uniform than pneumococcal pneumonia in its manifestations, and afflicts primarily infants and debilitated adults. Distributive-type shock is common, and recovery is often delayed by empyema and abscess formation. Pneumonia from the gram-negative bacterium *Klebsiella* (Friedlander bacillus), may cause aggressive necrotizing pneumonitis and cavitation, with pulmonary scar formation following in its wake. Alcoholics are more susceptible, as are patients with diabetes and COPD. The gram-negative rod, *Hemophilus influenzae*, produces primary pneumonia chiefly in children. In adults, hemophilus pneumonia usually is secondary to a viral infection such as influenza. In susceptible individuals the hemophilus organisms may produce a purulent infection of larynx, trachea, bronchi, and alveoli, with the picture of bronchiolitis in children. Complications such as otitis and meningitis are not infrequent. Associated epiglottitis may cause death from acute upper airway obstruction.

Influenza virus pneumonia has menaced the lives of large numbers of patients ever since the pandemics of 1889 and 1918, in which an estimated 20 to 40 million people died. Such epidemics or pandemics seem to recur about every ten years. Their prevention through immunization is hampered by rapid antigenic shifts, enabling the virus to elude type-specific antibodies. Furthermore, viral infections are not amenable to antibiotic therapy. During the influenza virus pandemic of 1968, some nonimmunized people suffered viral invasion of the entire tracheobronchial tree in one to two days, causing necrosis of the ciliated epithelium and alveolar-septal edema, disruption and intra-alveolar hemorrhage. Although viremia and invasion of other vital organs was seen, death invariably was due to a syndrome of pulmonary edema-consolidation from the virus alone or from superinfection with staphylococcus, hemolytic streptococcus, or other bacteria.

At the onset of influenza virus pneumonia, there is leukopenia for two to four days. Untreated, the primary viral pneumonia or secondary bacterial pneumonia may have a fulminating course with fatal outcome. However, early recognition of ARDS (100 per cent oxygen test) and sophisticated life support (see ARDS above) with optimized CPPV/O$_2$ can "turn the tide" in patients moribund from this basically reversible disease. Unfortunately patients are often permitted to die from such pneumonias without advanced critical care being given a chance. In forthcoming influenza epidemics, therefore, physicians should recognize pulmonary consolidation early and transfer such patients to advanced respiratory intensive care centers.

(3) INHALATION OF NOXIOUS FUMES

Although death from smoke inhalation is usually due to "anemic anoxia" from carbon monoxide poisoning (Chapter 2), the smoke of burning objects may also contain irritant gases and vapors that produce primary pulmonary damage. Furthermore, some gases when combined with water become corrosive acids or alkali, as in the case of sulfur dioxide (sulfuric acid), nitrogen oxide (nitric acid), ammonia (ammonium hydroxide), or phosgene. These substances and others can cause chemical burns of the upper airway and tracheobronchial tree, and can sometimes produce alveolar damage with pulmonary edema as well. Acute anoxic death is avoided by treatments similar to those given to patients with pulmonary edema-consolidation and/or status asthmaticus. Steroids seem useful. The mainstay of therapy is optimized CPPV with oxygen. When there is sloughing of the tracheobronchial tree, careful frequent extraction of the debris by bronchoscope may be life-saving.

Interstitial Pulmonary Fibrosis
(Fig. 5, Site 10)

Diffuse infiltration of the lung parenchyma can be caused by numerous different types of infectious agents including bacteria, viruses, fungi, and parasites, as well as by dust, fumes, and various diseases (neoplasm, sarcoidosis, histiocytosis, uremia, unresolved pulmonary edema, fat emboli, oxygen toxicity, radiation, heat, blast injury, hemosiderosis, farmer's lung, alveolar proteinosis, rare collagen diseases, and rare congenital and familial diseases). Also, pleural scars from pleuritis may grow into the lungs, causing interstitial fibrosis.

Although most lung infections occur from bronchial spread and are thus usually focal, insults to the lungs from the hematogenous route may cause diffuse lesions with variable chest x-ray changes. These lesions result in exertional dyspnea and increased pulmonary vascular resistance. Hypoxemia occurs from ventilation/perfusion mismatching (without significant shunting); and VC, RV, FRC, and compliance are all decreased. Nonetheless PaCO$_2$ is usually low because of tachypnea stimulated by hypoxemia and pulmonary receptors. Chronic interstitial fibrosis calls for specific drug therapy according to the underlying disorder, including steroids in selected cases. Prognosis depends on the underlying disorder.

Emergencies Involving the Pleural Space
(Fig. 5, Site 11)

Air enters the pleural and interstitial spaces as a common complication of various types of acute lung disease. Patients on mechanical ventilation are more susceptible to pneumothorax (Chapter 2), especially when subjected to positive end-expiratory pressure (PEEP). Tension pneumothorax develops when there is a valvelike lung leak and airway pressure increased by coughing or positive pressure ventilation.

The normal intrapleural pressure of about -3 (exhalation) to -8 (inhalation) cm H$_2$O becomes less negative, or even positive, in emphysema or when the pleural space fills with gas or fluid. The latter collapses the underlying lung and causes hypoxemia from shunting. Greatly increased positive intrapleural pressure (tension pneumothorax) in addition causes kinking and compression of the tracheobronchial tree and large veins. These pathophysiologic changes are reflected in the clinical signs of tension pneumothorax: tympanism; distant breath sounds; tracheal and mediastinal shift; and progressive airway obstruction, circulatory deterioration, hypoxemia, and distention of chest (with impaired exhalation) and abdomen (inverted diaphragm). When air is not under pressure, its absorption from the pleural space and elsewhere in the body can be hastened by 100 per cent O_2 breathing, which denitrogenates the lungs, blood, and gas pockets. However, tension pneumothorax requires prompt decompressive therapy; diagnostic needle puncture to confirm the presence of air under pressure should be followed by large-bore pleural drainage in the second or third intercostal space anteriorly in the midclavicular line.

Spontaneous pneumothorax occurs (and recurs) most commonly in seemingly healthy young males with apparently healthy lungs, most likely due to rupture of blebs. If the volume of intrapleural air is minimal, observation is sufficient. When the volume of air is sufficient to cause symptoms or compromise cardiorespiratory function, pleural drainage is required. Recurrence can be prevented by surgery to create adhesion of the parietal to the visceral pleura.

Fluid in the pleural space can be either transudate or exudate. Transudates occur when mechanical factors influencing formation or resorption of pleural fluid are disturbed, for example when there is a decrease in plasma oncotic pressure or in systemic or pulmonary hydrostatic pressure (congestive heart failure, cirrhosis, nephrosis). *Transudates* are characterized by a pleural fluid-to-serum protein ratio of less than 0.5, a pleural fluid LDH less than 200 I.U., and a pleural fluid-to-serum LDH ratio less than 0.6. *Exudates*, on the other hand, show the reverse characteristics and occur in the wake of inflammation or other disease of the pleural surface (tuberculosis, pneumonia with effusion, malignancy, pancreatitis, etc.)

Exudates containing large numbers of leukocytes are referred to as *empyema* and may be seen in various types of bacterial pneumonias, subdiaphragmatic abscesses, peritonitis, lung cancer, perforated esophagus, mediastinitis, and other infections. Unresolved or undrained infected fluid or blood in the pleural space results in chronic adhesive pleuritis, which in turn can produce secondary infiltration and fibrosis of the lungs. Thus the lung may or may not expand with surgical decortication.

Treatment of pleural fluid accumulation is by chest tube drainage, preferably through a lower intercostal space in the midaxillary line. The presence of bronchopleural fistula will complicate drainage and may require strong pleural suction with high flow rates to keep the lung expanded. Acute infected empyema may benefit from continuous intrapleural irrigation with antibiotics. In chronic empyema, open drainage and thoracoplasty for closure of the cavity may be required.

Diaphragmatic herniations, depending on size and acuteness, can produce intestinal obstruction and hypoxemia from lung compression. Although ARI is unlikely to be the result of the common hiatal hernia, it is common in congenital hernia (through foramen of Morgagni or Bochdalek) or blunt trauma resulting in usually central diaphragmatic rupture. These may require resuscitation with thoracotomy and emergency surgical repair.

Pulmonary Hypoperfusion
(Fig. 5, Site *12*)

(1) PULMONARY THROMBOEMBOLISM (PTE)

Probably about 8000 persons die each year in the U.S.A. with PTE as the principal cause. Variable combinations of vascular stasis, hypercoagulability, and intimal changes probably are responsible for PTE seen in 25 to 60 per cent of autopsies; however, only 10 to 30 per cent of these cases are diagnosed before death. Small pulmonary emboli may produce neither shock (because of the adaptability of the remaining vascular tree) nor infarct (because of bronchial artery collateral circulation). PTE is also underdiagnosed because the fibrinolytic system initiates clot lysis within one to two days, and resolution is complete within about one to two weeks; further clot resolution may continue in the immediate postmortem period. This natural process of resolution provides impetus for resuscitation efforts. For if the patient can be tided over the acute phase of PTE, there is a good likelihood that pulmonary vascular patency will be restored in the meanwhile. Even clots which are organized before embolizing and do not dissolve by lysis may become organized in the pulmonary vessels, with shrinkage and recanalization.

In a previously healthy person, 50 per cent or more of the total pulmonary arterial cross-sectional area must be blocked to produce increased pulmonary artery pressure, tachycardia, right heart failure, and reduction in cardiac output (obstructive shock). Although this mechanical factor is the most important one in man, additional reflex and humoral components (e.g., serotonin released from platelets that coat fresh emboli), causing vaso- and bronchoconstriction throughout both lungs, have been identified as significant pathogenetic factors in work with experimental animals. Pulmonary infarction is rare because the lung is supplied with oxygen from the pulmonary and bronchial arteries as well as from the airways. Probably more than one of these routes must be defective (as in left heart failure) to enable infarction.

One should *suspect* acute PTE when there are predisposing factors and when there is a sudden onset of dyspnea, tachypnea, wheezing, chest pain, and tachycardia. Auscultation may reveal a right ventricular gallop, systolic murmur, or widely split second heart sound. EKG changes (tall P wave, right shift of QRS axis), increased CVP and pulmonary artery pressure, and perhaps hypotension and reduced cardiac output are also sometimes associated. The chest roentgenogram may be normal or may show regional translucency or disappearance of a vessel shadow. When infarction follows PTE, there may be fever and, subsequently, roentgenographic evidence of infiltrates and hemorrhagic pleural fluid.

Acute PTE is associated with acute arterial blood gas derangements. Deadspace is increased with alveolar (end tidal) CO_2 lower than arterial CO_2. Bronchoconstriction from regional hypocarbia mitigates the increase in deadspace, however. Surfactant failure due to hypoperfusion starts in two to three hours and can produce atelectasis in one to two days. Thus, in addition to increased deadspace, there is hypoxemia with increased $P(A-a)O_2$ (FIO_2 1.0). The mechanism of this shunt effect is not clear, although several hypotheses have been entertained, e.g., too rapid passage of cardiac output through unoccluded capillaries; development of subclinical pulmonary edema around unobstructed, overloaded capillaries; opening of normally closed intrapulmonary shunt vessels; and recanalization of shunt vessels. Further, shock (with low cardiac output), if present, decreases venous oxygen values and thereby worsens the hypoxemia from shunting.

One should try to *prove* PTE by photoscanning or angiography. The former uses I.V. macroaggregated albumin labeled with iodine-131 or technetium-99m; or xenon-133 I.V. (with breath holding). Capillaries behind embolized vessels fail to fill and thus are not visualized. Although many lung disorders can cause scanning defects, emboli will not simultaneously produce ventilation defects, which can be demonstrated by xenon-133 inhalation. Pulmonary angiography is more specific than scanning, showing cut-off, decreased filling or filling defects of affected pulmonary arteries.

Modern *treatment* includes titrated heparinization, which prevents secondary thrombosis both at the site of origin and in the lungs. Heparin also enhances fibrinolysis in fresh thrombi and may inhibit serotonin release by inhibiting platelet breakdown. PTE with shock and hypoxemia calls for intratracheal mechanical ventilation with optimized $CPPV/O_2$ (oxygen is the best pulmonary vasodilator); support of coronary and cerebral perfusion pressure with vasopressors; digitalization in patients with heart failure; and perhaps cautious use of broncho- and vasodilator drugs (e.g., chlorpromazine, isoproterenol, papaverine, atropine). PTE with shock and cardiac arrest is a challenge for titrated resuscitation. Experimental use of thrombolytic agents (e.g., plasmin, streptokinase, urokinase) or long-term assisted circulation (partial extracorporeal venoarterial pumping via membrane oxygenator) has occasionally turned the tide in moribund patients. Surgical thromboembolectomy should be discouraged as it carries a 50 per cent mortality and, theoretically at least, should not be necessary, since PTE is spontaneously reversible if life is maintained for at least one week. Vena cava ligation, clipping, or insertion of an "umbrella" is used to reduce the likelihood of recurrent emboli. Ligation is indicated when multiple septic emboli originate from the pelvis.

(2) FAT EMBOLISM*

Blood obtained from a normal subject after a meal normally contains aggregates of

---

*See also pp. 38 and 786.

triglycerides, which are of no pathologic significance. Larger aggregates, causing significant injury, however, can be produced by mechanical factors (fat entering veins in fractures of bones containing fatty marrow and in trauma to other fatty tissues) and humoral factors; the latter are mediated in massive trauma and shock through platelet aggregates, catecholamines, and release of noxious substances. Scattered and transient plugging of pulmonary capillaries without symptoms probably occurs frequently in trauma; but particularly when there has been a period of hypoperfusion (shock), this plugging can become symptomatic (fat embolism syndrome). The "dose" of fat embolization also increases when large bone fractures are manipulated. Thus, key factors in the prevention of fat embolism syndrome are prevention or immediate treatment of hypoperfusion (primarily by maintaining high circulating blood volume) and immobilization of fractures.

Circulating fat globules produce an ARDS-like picture of ARI through immediate capillary plugging plus subsequent release of fatty acids; there is resultant endothelial damage, hemorrhagic pneumonitis, and further pulmonary ischemia from secondary thrombosis (disseminated intravascular coagulation) at sites obstructed by fat.

In severe and prolonged pulmonary fat embolism syndrome, fat can lodge also in capillaries of the brain (producing stupor, coma, hyperthermia), the kidneys (producing lipuria, hematuria), the retinal vessels (producing blindness), and the skin (producing petechial hemorrhages). Such manifestations of systemic fat embolization are usually preceded by the pulmonary syndrome and probably are the result of fat globules passing through the pulmonary circulation via shunt vessels or capillaries and chemically induced aggregation of fat in the systemic vessels.

After trauma, there is a variable period of relatively normal pulmonary status prior to the development of the pulmonary syndrome. The clinical picture of this syndrome includes dyspnea, tachypnea, tachycardia, wheezes, and sometimes fever. Arterial blood gases reveal an increase in $P(A-a)O_2$ (FIO_2 1.0), while chest x-rays show "snow storm appearance." The platelet count falls. Lipemia, lipuria, elevated serum lipase, fat in CSF and fat in sputum occur, although these can all be present without the syndrome. $PaCO_2$ on spontaneous breathing is normal or low. Many of these signs and symptoms are not pathognomonic and could be present with ARDS or aspiration, which are also common in traumatized victims; however the CNS symptoms and cutaneous and retinal petechiae should elicit suspicion of fat embolization.

Therapy includes optimized $CPPV/O_2$, heparinization, steroid (doses as in status asthmaticus), and other supportive measures. Blood volume expansion with dextran-40, I.V. alcohol for lipolysis and Trasylol (for disseminated intravascular coagulation) have been tried with variable results. The outcome following the pulmonary syndrome is good, but residual retinopathy and neurologic deficit have been seen in patients who survive.

COMMENT

Throughout the world, advanced research in respiratory physiology, pathology, and therapy has proceeded at an accelerated pace during the past 25 years. Corresponding advances in clinical practice, however, have lagged seriously and needlessly behind. It is not simply a matter of technology. By and large, we *have* the hardware we need to provide sophisticated life support, although much improvement is still possible. The problem, rather, is a much more fundamental one—the failure of many health professionals to suspect and recognize acute respiratory insufficiency early enough to take appropriate action.

ARI is legion, and its early manifestations are subtle. In this chapter, we have attempted to sensitize the reader to this stealthy killer as well as to the multiple derangements of other organ systems that may follow in its wake. We have tried also to demonstrate that ARI is not simply an isolated disruption of pulmonary function. In many, if not all, cases, the pulmonary dysfunction of ARI is reparable, and it is the failure of other organ systems, attendant upon ARI, which ultimately kills. Thus, once pulmonary injury has done its mischief, life support measures must be directed not only at reversing the pulmonary lesion but also at maintaining other vital organs until the lungs can heal. Therapy represents a compromise among the demands of multiple organs, with unabashed favoritism to the brain. Life support under these circumstances thus aims at optimizing, not necessarily normalizing, the functions of each organ system.

References*

Books and Reviews

American Physiologic Society: Handbook of Physiology. Section 3, Volumes I & II, Respiration. Washington, D.C., American Physiological Society, 1964.
Bates, D. V., Macklem, T. T., and Christie, R. V.: Respiratory Function in Disease: An Introduction to the Integrated Study of the Lung, 2d ed. Philadelphia, W. B. Saunders Co., 1971.
Bendixen, H. H., et al.: Respiratory Care. St. Louis, C. V. Mosby Co., 1965.
Brain, J. D., Proctor, D. F., and Reid, L.: Respiratory Defense Mechanisms. In Lenfant, C. (ed.): Lung Biology in Health and Disease. New York, M. Dekker, 1974.
Brecher, G. A.: Venous Return. New York, Grune & Stratton, 1956.
Campbell, E. J. M.: The management of acute respiratory failure in chronic bronchitis and emphysema. Am. Rev. Resp. Dis. 96:626, 1967.
Campbell, E. J. M., Agostoni, E., and Davis, J. N.: The Respiratory Muscles: Mechanics and Neural Control. Philadelphia, W. B. Saunders Co., 1970.
Casarett, L. J.: Toxicology: the respiratory tract. Ann. Rev. Pharmacol. 11:425, 1971.
Cherniak, R. M., et al.: Respiration in Health and Disease, 2d ed. Philadelphia, W. B. Saunders Co., 1972.
Clements, J. A.: Pulmonary surfactant. Am. Rev. Resp. Dis. 101:984, 1970.
Comroe, J. H., Jr., et al.: The Lung: Clinical Physiology and Pulmonary Function Tests, 2d ed. Chicago, Year Book Medical Publishers, Inc., 1962.
Davenport, H. W.: The ABC of Acid-Base Chemistry. Chicago, University of Chicago Press, 1969.
Farrell, P. M., and Avery, M. E.: Hyaline membrane disease. Am. Rev. Resp. Dis. 111:657, 1975.
Fishman, A. P.: Pulmonary edema. The water-exchanging function of the lung. Circulation 46:390, 1972.
Goodman, L. S., and Gillman, A. (eds.): The Pharmacological Basis of Therapeutics, 5th ed. New York, Macmillan Co., 1975.
Harrison, T. R. (past ed.), and Wintrobe, M. M. (ed.): Principles of Internal Medicine, 7th ed. New York, McGraw-Hill Book Co., 1974.
Hayek, H. von: The Human Lung (Anatomy). Translated by Krahl, V. E. New York, Hafner, 1960.
Hedley-Whyte, J., and Winter, P. M.: Oxygen therapy. Clin. Pharmacol. Ther. 8:696, 1967.
Henderson, L. J.: Blood, A Study in General Physiology. New Haven, Yale University Press, 1928.

Herndon, J. H., Riseborough, E. J., and Fischer, J. D.: Fat embolism: a review of current concepts. J. Trauma 11:673, 1971.
Liebow, A. A., and Carrington, C. B.: The eosinophilic pneumonias. Medicine (Baltimore) 48:151, 1969.
Mead, J.: Mechanical properties of lungs. Physiol. Rev. 41:281, 1961.
Moore, F. D., et al.: Post-traumatic Pulmonary Insufficiency. Philadelphia, W. B. Saunders Co., 1969.
Moser, K. M., and Stein, M. S. (eds.): Advances in Cardiopulmonary Diseases—Pulmonary Thromboembolism. Chicago, Year Book Medical Publishers, Inc., 1973.
National Academy of Sciences/National Research Council: Pulmonary effects of non-thoracic trauma. Proceedings of a conference conducted by the Committee on Trauma, Division of Medical Sciences. J. Trauma 8:621, 1968.
Nunn, J. F.: Applied Respiratory Physiology with Special Reference to Anesthesia. New York, Appleton-Century-Crofts, 1969.
Peltier, L. F., et al.: A panel by correspondence. Fat embolism. Arch. Surg. 109:12, 1974.
Pontoppidan, H., Geffin, B., and Lowenstein, E.: Acute Respiratory Failure in the Adult. New England Journal of Medicine Progress Series. Boston, Little, Brown and Co., 1973.
Plum, F., and Posner, J. B.: The Diagnosis of Stupor and Coma, 2d ed. Philadelphia, F. A. Davis Co., 1972.
Robin, E. D., Cross, C. E., and Zelis, R.: Pulmonary edema. N. Engl. J. Med. (part I) 288/5:239, 1973; (part II) 288/6:292, 1973.
Safar, P., (ed.): Advances in Cardiopulmonary Resuscitation. The Wolf Creek Conference. New York, Springer Verlag, 1977.
Safar, P. (ed.): Respiratory Therapy. Philadelphia, F. A. Davis Co., 1965.
Safar, P.: Management of Ventilatory Failure—Steps of Emergency Airway Control. In Weil, M (ed.). Critical Care Medicine, New York, Harper & Row, 1976.
Safar, P., and Tenicela, R.: High altitude physiology in relation to anesthesia and inhalation therapy. Anesthesiology 25:515, 1964.
Slonim, N. B., and Hamilton, L. H.: Respiratory Physiology, 2d ed. St. Louis, C. V. Mosby Co., 1971.
Spencer, H.: Pathology of the Lung, 2nd ed. Oxford, Pergamon Press, 1968.
Staub, N. C.: The pathophysiology of pulmonary edema. Hum. Pathol. 1:419, 1970.
Sykes, M. K., McNicol, M. W., and Campbell, E. J. M.: Respiratory Failure. Blackwell Scientific Publications. Philadelphia, F. A. Davis Co., 1969.
Weibel, E. R.: Morphometry of the Human Lung. New York, Academic Press, 1963.
West, J. W.: Respiratory Physiology—The Essentials. Baltimore, Williams & Wilkins Co., 1975.

Papers

Anthonisen, N. R., et al.: Airway closure as a function of age. Resp. Physiol. 8:58, 1969.
Astrup, P.: A new approach to acid-base metabolism. Clin. Chem. 7:1, 1961.
Barach, A. L., Martin, J., and Eckman, M.: Positive pressure respiration and its application to the treatment of acute pulmonary edema. Ann. Intern. Med. 12:754, 1938.
Barber, R. E., Lee, J., and Hamilton, W. K.: Oxygen toxicity in man: a prospective study in patients with irre-

---

*Because of the great number of relevant publications on respiratory physiology and pathology, no quotes were made in the text and only selected books and papers are listed here.

versible brain damage. N. Engl. J. Med. 283:1478, 1970.

Bates, D. V.: Medical progress: chronic bronchitis and emphysema. N. Engl. J. Med. 278:546, 1968.

Beecher, H. K., Bennett, H. S., and Bassett, B. L.: Circulatory effects of increased pressure in the airway. Anesthesiology 4:612, 1943.

Behnke, A. R., et al.: The effect of oxygen on man at pressures of from 1 to 4 atmospheres. Am. J. Physiol. 110:565, 1935.

Bendixen, H. H., Hedley-Whyte, J., and Laver, M. B.: Impaired oxygenation in surgical patients during general anesthesia with controlled ventilation: a concept of atelectasis. N. Engl. J. Med. 269:991, 1963.

Bergofsky, E. H., Turino, G. M., and Fishman, A. P.: Cardiorespiratory failure in kyphoscoliosis. Medicine 38:263, 1959.

Bjork, V. O., and Engstroem, C. G.: The treatment of ventilatory insufficiency after pulmonary resection with tracheostomy and prolonged artificial respiration. J. Thorac. Surg. 30:356, 1955.

Breivik, H., et al.: Normalizing low arterial CO_2 tension during mechanical ventilation. Chest 63:525, 1973.

Burger, E. J., Jr., and Macklem, P.: Airway closure: demonstration by breathing 100% O_2 at low lung volumes and by N_2 washout. J. Appl. Physiol. 25:139, 1968.

Campbell, E. J. M.: A method of controlled oxygen administration which reduces the risk of carbon-dioxide retention. Lancet 2:12, 1960.

Cheng, T. O., Godfrey, M. P., and Shepard, R. H.: Pulmonary resistance and state of inflation of lungs in normal subjects and in patients with airway obstruction. J. Appl. Physiol. 14:727, 1959.

Cherniack, R. M.: Respiratory effects of obesity. Can. Med. Assoc. J. 80:613, 1959.

Cherniack, R. M., and Snidal, D. P.: The effect of obstruction to breathing on the ventilatory response to CO_2. J. Clin. Invest. 35:1286, 1956.

Chinard, F. P., and Enns, T.: Transcapillary pulmonary exchange of water in the dog. Am. J. Physiol. 178:197, 1954.

Clark, L. C.: Monitor and control of blood and tissue oxygen tensions. Trans. Am. Soc. Artif. Intern. Organs 2:41, 1956.

Clements, J. A.: Surface phenomena in relation to pulmonary function (6th Bowditch lecture). Physiologist 5:11, 1962.

Clemmesen, C., and Nilsson, E.: Therapeutic trends in the treatment of barbiturate poisoning. Clin. Pharmacol. Ther. 2:220, 1961.

Comroe, J. H., et al.: Oxygen toxicity: the effect of inhalation of high concentrations of oxygen for 24 hours on normal men at sea level and at a simulated altitude of 18,000 feet. J.A.M.A. 128:710, 1945.

Coryllos, P. N., and Birnbaum, G. L.: Studies in pulmonary gas absorption in bronchial obstruction. Am. J. Med. Sci. 183:317, 1932.

Cournand, A., et al.: Physiological studies of the effects of intermittent positive pressure breathing on cardiac output in man. Am. J. Physiol. 152:162, 1948.

Donald, D. W., and Christie, R. V.: The respiratory response to carbon dioxide and anoxia in emphysema. Clin. Sci. 8:33, 1949.

Draper, W. B., and Whitehead, R. W.: The phenomenon of diffusion respiration. Anesth. Analg. 28:307, 1949.

Eckenhoff, J. E., and Dam, W.: The treatment of barbiturate poisoning with or without analeptics. Am. J. Med. 20:6, 1956.

Egbert, L. D., and Bendixen, H. H.: Effect of morphine on breathing pattern. J.A.M.A. 188:113, 1964.

Egbert, L. D., Laver, M. B., and Bendixen, H. H.: Intermittent deep breaths and compliance during anesthesia in man. Anesthesiology 24:57, 1963.

Emerson, H.: Artificial respiration in the treatment of edema of the lungs. A suggestion based on animal experimentation. Arch. Intern. Med. 3:368, 1909.

Fenn, W. O.: Mechanics of respiration. Am. J. Med. 10:77, 1951.

Frumin, M. J., Epstein, R. M., and Cohen, G.: Apneic oxygenation in man. Anesthesiology 20:789, 1959.

Greenfield, L. J., Ebert, P. A., and Benson, D. W.: Effect of positive pressure ventilation on surface tension properties of lung extracts. Anesthesiology 25:312, 1964.

Gregory, G. A., et al.: Treatment of idiopathic respiratory distress syndrome with continuous positive airway pressure. N. Engl. J. Med. 284/24:1333, 1971.

Grenvik, A.: Respiratory, circulatory, and metabolic effects of respirator treatment: a clinical study in postoperative thoracic surgical patients. Acta Anaesth. Scand. (suppl.) 19:1, 1966.

Guyton, A. C., and Lindsey, A. W.: Effect of elevated left atrial pressure and decreased plasma protein concentration on the development of pulmonary edema. Circulation 7:649, 1959.

Hamilton, W. (ed.): Symposium on Intensive Care. National Research Council. Anesthesiology 25:192, 1964.

Hamilton, W. K., et al.: Postoperative respiratory complications: a comparison of arterial gas tensions, radiographs and physical examination. Anesthesiology 25:607, 1964.

Holmdahl, M. D.: Pulmonary uptake of oxygen, acid-base metabolism, and circulation during prolonged apnoea. Acta Chir. Scand. (supple.)212, 1956.

Huckabee, W. E.: Relationships of pyruvate and lactate during anaerobic metabolism. I. Effects of infusion of pyruvate or glucose and of hyperventilation. J. Clin. Invest. 37:244, 1958.

Ibsen, B.: The anaesthetist's viewpoint on treatment of respiratory complications in poliomyelitis during the epidemic in Copenhagen, 1952. Proc. R. Soc. Med. 47:72, 1954.

Jenkins, M. T., and Luhn, N. R.: Active management of tetanus. Anesthesiology 23:690, 1962.

Kampschulte, S., Marcy, J., and Safar, P.: Simplified physiologic management of status asthmaticus in children. Crit. Care Med. 1:69, 1973.

Klein, R. L., Safar, P., and Grenvik, A.: Respiratory care in blunt chest injury—retrospective review of 43 cases. American Society of Anesthesiologists Meeting Abstracts, New York, October, 1970, p. 145.

Lassen, H. C. A.: Preliminary report on the 1952 epidemic of poliomyelitis in Copenhagen. With special reference to the treatment of acute respiratory insufficiency. Lancet 1:37, 1953.

Leifer, K. N., and Wittig, H. J.: The beta-2 sympathomimetic aerosols in the treatment of asthma. Ann. Allergy 35:69, 1975.

Lenfant, C.: Measurement of ventilation/perfusion distribution with alveolar–arterial differences. J. Appl. Physiol. 18:1090, 1963.

Macklem, P. T., et al.: Chronic obstructive disease of small airways. Ann. Intern. Med. 74:167, 1971.

Mead, J., and Collier, C.: Relation of volume history of lungs to respiratory mechanics in anesthetized dogs. J. Appl. Physiol. 14:669, 1959.

Messer, J. W., Peters, G., and Bennett, W. A.: Causes of death and pathologic findings in 304 cases of bronchial asthma. Dis. Chest 38:616, 1960.

Mithoefer, J. C., Runser, R. H., and Karetzky, M. S.: The use of sodium bicarbonate in the treatment of acute bronchial asthma. N. Engl. J. Med. 272:1200, 1975.

Modell, J.: Pathophysiology and treatment of drowning. Proceedings of the Second International Symposium on Resuscitation. Acta Anaesth. Scand. (suppl. 29:263, 1968.

Moerch, E. T., Avery, E. E., and Benson, D. W.: Hyperventilation in the treatment of crushing injuries of the chest. Surg. Forum 6:270, 1956.

Morissette, M., Weil, M. H., and Shubin, H.: Reduction in colloid osmotic pressure associated with fetal progression of cardiopulmonary failure. Crit. Care Med. 3:115, 1975.

Nims, R. G., Conner, E. H., and Comroe, J. H.: The compliance of the human thorax in anesthetized patients. J. Clin. Invest. 34:744, 1955.

Pautler, S., et al.: Pulmonary oxygen toxicity at one ATA. Acta Anaesth. Scand. (suppl.)24:51, 1966.

Petty, T. L., and Ashbaugh, D. G.: The adult respiratory distress syndrome. Chest 60:233, 1971.

Prys-Roberts, C., Kelman, G. R., and Greenbaum, R.: The influence of circulatory factors on arterial oxygenation during anesthesia in man. Anaesthesia 22:257, 1967.

Rahn, H., et al.: The pressure-volume diagram of the thorax and lung. Am. J. Physiol. 146:161, 1946.

Redding, J., et al.: Resuscitation from drowning. J.A.M.A. 178:1136, 1961.

Riley, R. L., Cournand, A., and Donald, K. W.: Analysis of factors affecting partial pressures of oxygen and carbon dioxide in gas and blood of lungs. Theory: J. Appl. Physiol. 4:77, 1951; Methods: J. Appl. Physiol. 4:102, 1951.

Robin, E. R., et al.: Capillary leak syndrome with pulmonary edema. Arch. Intern. Med. 130:66, 1972.

Rosenow, E. C.: Drug-induced pulmonary disease. Ann. Intern. Med. 77:977, 1972.

Rotheram, E. B., Safar, P., and Robin, E. D.: CNS disorder during mechanical ventilation in chronic pulmonary disease. J.A.M.A. 189:993, 1964.

Sackner, M. A., Epstein, S., and Wanner, A.: Effect of beta-adrenergic antagonists aerosolized by Freon propellant on tracheal mucous velocity and cardiac output. Chest 69:593, 1976.

Safar, P., and Escarraga, L. A.: Compliance in apneic anesthetized adults. Anesthesiology 20:283, 1959.

Safar, P., Escarraga, L. A., and Chang, F.: Upper airway obstruction in the unconscious patient. J. Appl. Physiol. 14:760, 1959.

Safar, P., et al.: Cuffed tracheotomy tube vs. tank respirator for prolonged artificial ventilation. Arch. Phys. Med. Rehabil. 43:487, 1962.

Safar, P., Grenvik, A., and Smith, J.: Progressive pulmonary consolidation: review of cases and pathogenesis. J. Trauma 12:955, 1972.

Safar, P.: Recognition and management of airway obstruction. J.A.M.A. 208:1008, 1969.

Safar, P., Nemoto, E., and Severinghaus, J.: Pathogenesis of CNS disorder during artificial hyperventilation in compensated hypercarbia in dogs. Crit. Care Med. 1:5, 1973.

Said, S. I., et al.: Pulmonary gas exchange during induction of pulmonary edema in anesthetized dogs. J. Appl. Physiol. 19:403, 1964.

Sasahara, A. A.: Therapy for pulmonary embolism. J.A.M.A. 229:1795, 1974.

Severinghaus, J. W.: Blood Gas Concentrations. In Handbook of Physiology, American Physiological Society, Section 3, Vol. II, Washington, D.C., 1964, p. 1475.

Severinghaus, J. W.: Electrodes for blood and gas P_{CO_2}, P_{O_2} and pH. Acta Anaesth. Scand. (suppl.) 11:207, 1962.

Severinghaus, J. W.: Oxyhemoglobin dissociation curve corrections for temperature and pH variation in human blood. J. Appl. Physiol. 12:485, 1958.

Severinghaus, J. W., and Bradley, A. F.: Electrode for blood P_{O_2} and P_{CO_2} determinations. J. Appl. Physiol. 13:515, 1958.

Siggard-Andersen, O.: Blood acid-base alignment nomogram. Scales for pH, P_{CO_2}, base excess of whole blood of different hemoglobin concentrations, plasma bicarbonate and plasma total CO_2. Scand. J. Clin. Lab. Invest. 15:211, 1963.

Smith, J. D., et al.: Positive pressure ventilation and control of inspired oxygen concentration in pulmonary edema and consolidation. American Society of Anesthesiologists Meeting, Abstract 83, San Francisco, October, 1969.

Smith, J. D., Grenvik, A., and Safar, P.: Fatal influenza pneumonitis. Crit. Care Med. 1:123, 1973.

Urokinase Pulmonary Embolism Trial: A National Cooperative Study. Circulation 47(suppl. 2):70, 1973.

Winter, P. M., et al.: Modification of hyperbaric oxygen toxicity by experimental venous admixture. J. Appl. Physiol. 23:954, 1967.

GLOSSARY

Physiologic Variables

SYMBOL/ ABBREVIATION	VARIABLE	APPROX. NORMAL VALUES (70-KG. RESTING ADULT)
(A) *Oxygenation*		
BP (or AP)	Barometric pressure (Atmosph. press.)	760 torr (760 mm. Hg) at sea level
FIO_2	Fraction (concentration) of inhaled oxygen	0.21 (air), 1.0 (100% O_2)
PIO_2	Partial pressure of inhaled oxygen°	150 torr (FIO_2 0.21, BP 760 torr)
PAO_2	Partial pressure of alveolar oxygen°	100 torr (FIO_2 0.21, BP 760 torr)
PaO_2	Arterial blood oxygen tension (pressure)	75–100 torr (FIO_2 0.21) 500–600 torr (FIO_2 1.0)
Hb	Hemoglobin content	13–15 gm./100 ml. blood
Hct	Hematocrit	35–45%
SaO_2	Saturation of arterial (blood) Hb with oxygen	>95% (PaO_2 >80 torr)
CaO_2	Content of oxygen in arterial blood°	20 ml./100 ml. blood (with Hb 15 gm %)
P-50	Blood PO_2 at SO_2 50%, signifying the position of the HbO_2 dissociation curve (Hb-O_2 affinity)	27 torr
PcO_2	Capillary oxygen tension	100–40 torr
$P\bar{v}O_2$	Mixed venous PO_2	40–45 torr
$C\bar{v}O_2$	Mixed venous oxygen content	15 ml/100 ml. blood
$C(a-\bar{v})O_2$	Arteriovenous oxygen content difference	5 ml./100 ml. blood
Q	Volume of blood	
$\dot{Q}$	Volume flow of blood per unit of time	
$\dot{Q}_T$	Total flow of blood = cardiac output°	5 liters/min.
$\dot{C}aO_2$	Arterial oxygen transport ($\dot{Q}_T \times CaO_2$)	1000 ml. O_2/min.
$\dot{V}O_2$	Oxygen consumption per minute (STPD) = $\dot{Q}_T(Ca-\bar{v}O_2)$	250 ml./min.
O_2UC	Oxygen utilization coefficient° $\dot{V}O_2/\dot{C}aO_2$	0.25
VCO_2	CO_2 production per minute (STPD)	200 ml./min.
RQ	Respiratory exchange ratio (respiratory quotient), i.e., $\dot{V}CO_2/\dot{V}O_2$	0.8
V/Q	Pulmonary ventilation: perfusion ratio	Overall approx. 1 (regional variations)
$\dot{Q}s/\dot{Q}T$	Proportion of cardiac output shunted through nonventilated alveoli (or otherwise from right to left side of heart)°	<5%
$P(A-a)O_2$	Alveolar-arterial oxygen tension difference°	Near zero
DCO	Diffusion capacity for carbon monoxide (pulmonary function test)	25 ml./min./torr
La	Arterial blood lactate concentration	1 μ Mole/ml. = 9 mg.%
ECF	Extracellular fluid	20% of BW in liters
ICF	Intracellular fluid	50% of BW in liters
(B) *Ventilation*		
$PaCO_2$	Partial pressure of arterial CO_2	35–45 torr
$PACO_2$	Partial pressure of alveolar CO_2	Same as $PaCO_2$
$PETCO_2$	Partial pressure of end-tidal CO_2	Same as $PaCO_2$
$P\bar{v}CO_2$	Partial pressure of mixed venous CO_2	45–50 torr
VT	Tidal volume	500 ml. (7 ml./kg. BW)
f	Frequency (rate) of breathing	12–20/min.

°For calculations and explanation, see text.

SYMBOL/ ABBREVIATION	VARIABLE	APPROX. NORMAL VALUES (70-KG. RESTING ADULT)
$\dot{V}_E$	Minute volume ($V_T \times f$) = exhaled volume per min. (BTPS)	8 liters/min.
V_D	"Physiologic" (total) deadspace (BTPS), i.e., anatomic deadspace (V_{DAN}) plus alveolar deadspace (V_{DA}); also called "wasted ventilation"	2 ml./kg. BW (V_{DAN}) near zero (V_{DA})
V_D/V_T	Deadspace/tidal volume ratio	0.3
$\dot{V}$	Gas flow per unit time	
$\dot{V}_A$	Minute alveolar ventilation (BTPS) = $\dot{V}_E - (V_D \times f)$	5 liters/min.

(C) *Abnormalities*

Asphyxia	Hypoxemia plus hypercarbia	
Hypoxemia	Reduced arterial P_{O_2}	$Pa_{O_2} < 75$ torr
Hypoxia	Reduced oxygenation (of tissues)	
Cyanosis	Bluish discoloration of mucous membranes and/or skin due to excessive amount of reduced Hb	
Hypercarbia (Hypercapnia)	Increased arterial P_{CO_2}	$Pa_{CO_2} > 45$ torr
Hypoventilation	Reduced alveolar ventilation (from decrease of V_T or f)	$Pa_{CO_2} > 45$ torr
Hypocarbia (Hypocapnia)	Reduced arterial P_{CO_2}	$Pa_{CO_2} < 35$ torr
Hyperventilation	Increased alveolar ventilation (from increased V_T or f)	$Pa_{CO_2} < 35$ torr
Tachypnea	Increased respiratory frequency	
Bradypnea	Decreased respiratory frequency	
Hyperpnea	Increased respiratory frequency and volume	
Dyspnea	Subjective sensation of difficult or labored breathing	
ARDS	Adult respiratory distress syndrome (i.e., shock lung, progressive pulmonary consolidation)	
COPD (COLD)	Chronic obstructive pulmonary (lung) disease; i.e., emphysema and/or chronic bronchitis	
CRPD (CRLD)	Chronic restrictive pulmonary (lung) disease; i.e., fibrosis	
ARI (ARF)	Acute respiratory insufficiency; acute respiratory failure (see text)	
DIC	Disseminated intravascular coagulation	

(D) *Lung Volumes*

TLC	Total lung capacity (lung volume; i.e., $RV + ERV + V_T + IRV$)	6 liters
RV	Residual volume (volume of air left in lungs after maximal exhalation)	1 liter
ERV	Expiratory reserve volume (maximal volume of air exhaled from end-expiratory level; i.e., from FRC)	1.5 liters
IRV	Inspiratory reserve volume (maximal volume of air inhaled from the end-inspiratory level; i.e., from $FRC + V_T$)	3 liters
FRC	Functional residual capacity (volume of air in lungs and deadspace at end point of normal exhalation; i.e., $RV + ERV$)	2.5 liters
IC	Inspiratory capacity (maximal volume of air inhaled from FRC; i.e., $V_T + IRV$). Also called "sighing volume."	3.5 liters

Symbol/ Abbreviation	Variable	Approx. Normal Values (70-kg. resting adult)
VC	Vital capacity (maximal volume of air exhaled from point of maximal inhalation; i.e., ERV + V_T + IRV)	5 liters
IVC	Inspiratory vital capacity (maximal volume of air inhaled from point of maximal exhalation)	5 liters
FEV (FVC)	Forced expiratory volume (forced vital capacity) (expiratory VC performed with forced effort). Reduction in FEV, VC or IVC reflects restrictive disease.	Total FEV = >80% of predicted FEV (FVC). For predicted values see nomogram, Chapter 10.
FEVt	Forced expiratory volume (timed), specify seconds; e.g., FEV_1 is proportion of FEV exhaled during first second. Reduction in FEV_1, MEFR, or $\dot{V}max$ reflects obstructive disease.	FEV 1 sec. = >80% and FEV 3 sec. = >95% of patient's total FEV
MEFR (PEFR)	Maximal (peak) expiratory flow rate. The highest forced expiratory flow measured with a peak flow meter.	>500 liters/min. For predicted values see nomogram, Chapter 10
CV	Closing volume; i.e., % of expir. VC above RV, where, during exhalation, intrapulmonary airways begin to close. (At RV, most terminal bronchioles are closed.)	Ranging from 10% of VC in the young to 40% of VC in the aged
CC	Closing capacity; i.e. closing volume plus RV	
$\dot{V}max$	Maximal forced expiratory flow rate, related to % of total lung volume remaining when measurement is made	
MVV (MBC)	Maximal voluntary ventilation (maximal breathing capacity); the volume of air exhaled in a specified period of time during repetitive maximal respiratory efforts.	Rarely used

(E) *Mechanics*

C	Compliance (distensibility). Static volume change per unit pressure change ($\Delta V/\Delta P$), of lungs (C_L) or thorax (C_T) or both (C_{LT})	C of lungs plus thorax = 50–100 ml./cm. H_2O (apnea, anesthesia)
E	Elastance; elastic resistance. Reciprocal of compliance; i.e., static pressure change per unit volume change.	
Cdyn	Dynamic compliance; compliance measured at zero gas flow during active breathing.	Lower than C in apnea (includes some airway resistance)
C/Vl	Compliance related to lung volume; i.e., specific compliance.	
Gaw	Airway conductance; gas flow (in liters/ min) per unit of pressure change (in cm. H_2O).	
Raw	Airway resistance; reciprocal of airway conductance; i.e., pressure change (alveoli-mouth pressure) per flow (liters/min.)	0.6–2.4 cm. H_2O/30 liters per minute (i.e., 500 ml./sec.)
Ppl	Intrapleural pressure	
Paw	Pressure in the airway	
W	Mechanical work of breathing	

SYMBOL/ ABBREVIATION	VARIABLE	APPROX. NORMAL VALUES (70-KG. RESTING ADULT)
(F) *Acid-Base Status*		
$[H]^+$	Hydrogen ion concentration.	
pH	Negative logarithm of hydrogen ion concentration	
pHa	Arterial pH.	7.35–7.45
art. $[HCO_3^-]$	Bicarbonate ion concentration in arterial blood.	22–26 mEq./L.
BE	Base excess; i.e., deviation from normal of total buffer base.°	0 ± 3 mEq./L.
SBic	Standard bicarbonate, i.e., bicarbonate conc. with P_{CO_2} corrected to 40 torr.	
Acidemia	Above normal hydrogen ion concentration in arterial blood.	pH = <7.35
Alkalemia	Less than normal hydrogen ion concentration in arterial blood.	pH = >7.45
Hypobasemia	Low blood bicarbonate level.	$[HCO_3^-] = < 22$ mEq./L.
Hyperbasemia	High blood bicarbonate level.	$[HCO_3^-] = > 26$ mEq./L.
Acidosis } Alkalosis }	Referring to the body-at-large. May or may not be accompanied by acidemia or alkalemia. Indicate site (e.g., tissue acidosis) and whether respiratory or nonrespiratory.	
(G) *Circulation*		
$\overline{SAP} = MAP$	Mean systemic arterial pressure	90 torr (120/75 torr)
$\overline{CVP}$	Mean central venous pressure	3–10 torr
$\overline{PAP}$	Mean pulmonary artery pressure	15 (25/10) torr; range 14–17 torr
PAWP, PAOP	Pulmonary artery wedge (occlusive) pressure°	10 torr; range 6–12 torr
COP (π)	Plasma colloid osmotic (oncotic) pressure	25 torr
SVR	Systemic vascular resistance; i.e., TPR (total peripheral resistance) = $$\frac{(\overline{SAP} - \overline{CVP}) \times 60 \times 1.332}{\mathring{Q}_T}$$	700–1400 dynes sec. cm^{-5}
PVR	Pulmonary vascular resistance = $$\frac{(\overline{PAP} - \overline{LAP}) \times 60 \times 1.332}{\mathring{Q}_T}$$	75–150 dynes sec. cm^{-5}
BW	Body weight	
BV (Q)	Blood volume	8–10% of BW in liters
ECF	Extracellular fluid volume; i.e., plasma volume (5% of BW) plus interstitial fluid volume.	20–30% of BW in liters
ICF	Intracellular fluid volume	50% of BW in liters
$\mathring{Q}_T$	Cardiac output	5 liters per min.
(H) *Miscellaneous*		
STPD	Standard temperature (0°C.) and pressure (760 torr), dry.	
BTPS	Body temperature (37° C.) and pressure saturated with water vapor (47 torr)	
ATPS	Ambient temperature and pressure saturated with water vapor	
P_{H_2O}	Water vapor pressure	At full saturation and 37°C., 47 torr

---

°For calculations and explanation, see text.

Symbol/ Abbreviation	Variable	Approx. Normal Values (70-kg. resting adult)
SB, BP	Spontaneous breathing at atmospheric (barometric) pressure.	
SB, CPAP (EPAP)	Spont. breathing with continuous (expiratory) positive airway pressure.	
IPPV	Intermittent positive pressure (controlled) ventilation. (Artificial ventilation)	
IPPB	Intermittent positive pressure (assisted) breathing. (artificial ventilation)	
PEEP	Positive end-expiratory pressure.	
CPPV	Continuous positive pressure (controlled) ventilation; i.e., IPPV plus PEEP.	
IMV	Intermittent mandatory ventilation; i.e., SB, BP (or CPAP) plus IPPV	

Chapter 4

CARDIOVASCULAR SYSTEM FAILURE

Herbert Shubin,* Max Harry Weil,
Richard W. Carlson, and Uri Freund

Circulatory competence is maintained by an integrated functioning of the primary components of the cardiovascular system (Fig. 1), including: (1) the heart serving as a pump; (2) the arterial tree, as the resistance bed, which serves as the conduit to deliver blood to the capillaries through which metabolites are exchanged; (3) the low pressure veins as the return system, which also serves as the capacitance bed; and (4) the fluid within the heart and blood vessels. Cardiovascular system failure reflects malfunction of one or more of these primary components.

Studies forming the basis for this chapter were supported by United States Public Health Service Research Grants HL-05570 from the National Heart, Lung, and Blood Institute; GM-16462 from the National Institute of General Medical Sciences; RO1 HS 01474 from Health Resources Administration; the Parker B. Francis Foundation; and the Cardiopulmonary Research Foundation.

*Manuscript was submitted June 26, 1975; Dr. Shubin died unexpectedly on June 29, 1975.

HEART

The strength of myocardial contraction, as pointed out by Starling, is related to the length of the cardiac muscle fibers. When the diastolic volume is increased so that the muscle fibers are elongated, the subsequent stroke volume will increase. This holds until a critical diastolic volume is reached. When this volume is exceeded the stroke volume and cardiac output decrease and the pulmonary capillary pressure increases. These are features of cardiac decompensation and heart failure. During exercise, sympathetic stimulation, or treatment with certain vasoactive drugs the relationships between stroke volume, diastolic pressure, and muscle length change. Myocardial failure is characterized by a ventricular function curve in which increases in stroke volume are

For abbreviations, definitions, and normal values, see Chapter 3.

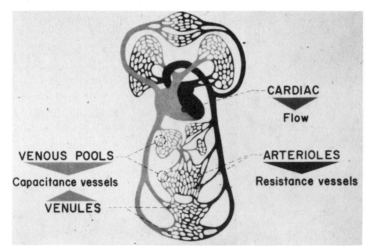

Figure 1. Primary components of the cardiovascular system which form the basis for hemodynamic functions. The capillary (exchange) vessels and intravascular volume are not separately labeled.

CARDIAC Flow

ARTERIOLES
Resistance vessels

VENOUS POOLS
Capacitance vessels

VENULES

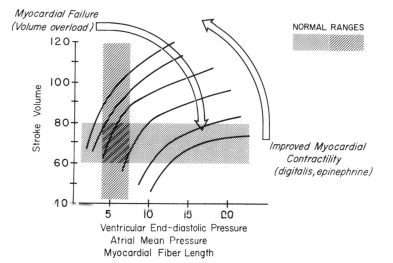

Figure 2. A series of ventricular function curves. Increases in myocardial competence are indicated by shifts to the left and decreases by shifts to the right.

achieved at high end-diastolic pressure levels (Fig. 2). Digitalis and beta adrenergic drugs improve myocardial contractility. Their actions are best explained in terms of a shift in the ventricular function curve to the left; greater stroke work is achieved at a lower ventricular end-diastolic pressure.

The cardiac output, when standardized for body surface area, is referred to as the cardiac index (CI). The normal values of CI range from 2.5 to 4.5 liters/min./m². Cardiac output and peripheral blood flow increase with elevation in body temperature. A decrease in cardiac output occurs with hypothermia, and this is directly related to a concurrent decrease in oxygen uptake and myocardial function.

ARTERIES

Changes in the diameter and tone of vessels are controlled primarily by neurohumoral reflexes. In cardiogenic shock, for example, there is an increase in arterial tone. This is regarded as a compensatory mechanism to maintain the arterial perfusion pressure when cardiac output is reduced. The increase in arterial resistance is similar to that which follows administration of vasopressor drugs. The term "peripheral resistance" is used to quantify the relationship between the cardiac output and the peripheral vessels. This term, although widely used, must be viewed with reservations. Some regional blood vessels may constrict while others dilate. The value of the calcu-

lated total peripheral resistance,* however, fails to indicate the relative contributions of individual circuits. Nevertheless, the concept is useful in the differentiation of the shock syndromes.

VEINS

There is a considerable difference in the functions of the high- and low-pressure systems. In the arteries, a large change in pressure is required to increase the volume of blood carried in these vessels. The resistance of the arteries to stretch is about 140 times greater than that of the veins. In the veins, however, small increments in pressure cause a large increase in the volume of fluid contained in these thin-walled vessels. The arterial system regulates the pressure and distribution of blood flow by local and generalized changes in peripheral resistance. The return of blood to the heart is maintained by alterations in the capacity of the venous system.

BLOOD VOLUME

The red cells normally comprise about 45 per cent of the total blood volume and

---

*Total peripheral resistance (TPR) represents the ratio of mean arterial pressure (MAP) and total systemic blood flow. When expressed in dynes sec. cm.⁻⁵

$$TPR = \frac{MAP \text{ in mm. Hg} \times 80}{\text{cardiac output in L./min.}}$$

plasma the other 55 per cent. The total blood volume usually ranges from 65 to 75 ml./kg. About 70 per cent of the total blood volume is normally contained in the low-pressure venous system, with another 15 per cent each in the arteries and in the capillaries. Nearly 20 per cent of the blood is contained in the splanchnic bed and liver and about 25 per cent in the thoracic vena cava, heart, pulmonary circuit, and the thoracic aorta.

The plasma contains many solutes and colloids, including about 7 gm./100 ml. of protein. The concentrations of plasma proteins are regulated within a narrow range. These proteins, and in particular albumin, are responsible for plasma colloid osmotic pressure, which in turn affects the relationship of fluid between the intravascular and extravascular compartments. As the colloid osmotic pressure rises, and if other factors remain constant, fluid leaves the tissue spaces and is drawn into the intravascular compartment.

The interstitial fluid and plasma have similar electrolyte concentrations. The distinctive and important difference between the composition of these fluids, however, is the presence of approximately 7 gm./100 ml. of proteins in the plasma and of less than one-half this concentration of protein in the interstitial fluid. The plasma albumin exerts an osmotic pressure which serves to hold fluid in the intravascular compartment. An alteration in either the concentration of plasma proteins or the permeability of the capillaries may account for a rapid shift of fluid between the plasma and the extravascular spaces. Damage to the capillaries by burns, foreign proteins, or bacterial toxins increases capillary permeability and results in rapid leakage of proteins from the plasma.

The critical functional reserves differ from one organ to another. A patient will survive with only approximately 15 per cent of normal liver function, 25 per cent of renal function, 35 per cent of red cell mass, and 45 per cent of lung tissue. Plasma volume provides the least reserve: a loss of more than 30 per cent of the initial volume is critical. For this reason, fluid replacement becomes a major consideration early in the course of treatment of a critically ill patient. In contrast to the plasma volume, there is an almost threefold reserve of red blood cells, provided the reduction in red cell mass occurs over a period of days.

HEMODYNAMIC MEASUREMENTS

ARTERIAL PRESSURE

When direct measurements of blood flow at the bedside are not generally available, clinicians rely on indirect evidence of adequate perfusion of the skin, brain, kidney, and heart. Arterial pressure often is looked upon as an indirect indicator of systemic blood flow. The clinical measurement of arterial blood pressure with a sphygmomanometer, however, may be quite misleading in a patient in shock, for in the presence of vasoconstriction the "cuff blood pressure" may be less than that obtained from direct intra-arterial measurements. For this reason, and for the purpose of facilitating the repeated sampling of arterial blood for gas analyses, an intra-arterial catheter is routinely inserted into the patient with acute circulatory failure (see Chapter 9).

CENTRAL VENOUS PRESSURE (CVP)*

For the past decade, central venous catheterization has been widely used in the assessment and management of the critically ill patient. Central venous catheterization provides a means for obtaining: (1) measurements of central venous pressure; (2) blood samples for laboratory analyses; (3) blood for phlebotomy; (4) recordings of atrial electrograms; (5) a route for the administration of drugs; and (6) a route for the administration of fluids, including hyperosmolar fluids for parenteral alimentation, which would cause thrombosis if given via peripheral vein.

Blood volume deficit may be an obvious cause of shock in patients who present with gross evidence of blood or fluid loss or with documented fluid deprivation. Less apparent are losses after blunt trauma or tissue infarction. In patients in whom a volume deficit is suspected, measurements of CVP provide a practical bedside guide for fluid repletion. The CVP, of itself, does not indicate hypovolemia. It may even be increased to levels exceeding 10 cm. H_2O after marked blood or fluid loss, particularly in older patients with limited cardiac reserve. This paradoxic elevation in CVP with reduction in blood volume may be attributable to

---

*See procedure, p. 351, for insertion technique.

a concomitant decrease in the venous return to the heart. This accounts not only for a decrease in cardiac output and arterial pressure but also for a critical reduction in the blood flow to the coronary arteries. If the blood flow to the coronary arteries is diminished, myocardial contractility is likely to be reduced and ventricular end-diastolic volume and CVP increased. During volume repletion, cardiac output, arterial pressure, and coronary blood flow may be restored to more normal values and CVP returned to normal levels. The level of CVP thus does not reflect the vascular volume per se; rather, it indicates the relationship between the volume of blood which enters the heart and the effectiveness with which the heart ejects that volume.

Although individual measurements of CVP are not reliable indicators of blood volume, serial measurements of CVP nevertheless may be very helpful in the treatment of patients with blood volume deficits. When such patients are challenged with fluid, serial measurements of CVP serve as a dynamic indicator of the competence of the right ventricle to accept and expel the blood returned to it. A question arises as to whether changes in CVP during volume loading reflect pressure changes in the left atrium (LA). In studies by Hanashiro and Weil in dogs during intravenous volume loading, such a relationship was demonstrated. The changes in CVP, although parallel to those in the left atrium, were of smaller magnitude.

PULMONARY ARTERY PRESSURE*

Despite the many other advantages of the central venous catheter, there now is little doubt that measurements of the pulmonary artery pressure, and particularly the pulmonary artery wedge pressure, provide a more precise indication of left ventricular function than do measurements of CVP. The development of a flow-directed balloon-tipped catheter has greatly facilitated the passage of the catheter into the pulmonary artery. The catheter is inserted into a peripheral vein and advanced into the superior or inferior vena cava. The balloon at the tip is then inflated with air and the catheter

*See procedure p. 285, for insertion of balloon catheter.

is advanced through the right atrium and ventricle into the pulmonary artery. Since the value of pulmonary artery wedge pressure closely approximates the left ventricular end-diastolic pressure, it serves as a measure of the preload, and thus helps to delineate the position of the left ventricle with respect to its Starling curve. If there is evidence of perfusion failure (e.g., elevated lactate values, low cardiac output) and the pulmonary artery wedge pressure is not elevated or is in a borderline range (12 to 20 torr), patients may be subjected to a fluid challenge. Conversely, when the pulmonary artery wedge pressure or left ventricular end-diastolic pressure exceeds 20 torr, myocardial failure should be suspected and treatment with diuretic drugs may be warranted. Recently, however, it has been demonstrated by members of our unit that in some patients the pulmonary artery wedge pressure may be normal in the presence of clinical and radiographic signs of pulmonary edema. This may be related in part to a decrease in plasma colloid osmotic pressure or to changes in capillary permeability. Conversely, a fluid challenge may be undertaken, with care, in patients in shock and in whom the wedge pressure exceeds 20 torr, since volume deficits may in themselves decrease coronary blood flow and thereby engenders left ventricular failure.

BLOOD VOLUME

During the course of acute blood loss or in the immediate period following blood loss, measurements of hemoglobin and hematocrit are often misleading—particularly when there has not been enough time for volume compensation by hemodilution. Measurements of blood volume by radioisotopic methods may be helpful under these circumstances, provided that rigorous techniques are used, including multiple sampling over a period of at least 45 minutes to assure complete mixing of the indicator. The measurement of red cell mass and plasma volume by radioactive techniques, while very valuable in assessing patients in shock, may not be available routinely in some institutions because of limitations in instrumentation and technicians on an around-the-clock basis. Under those circumstances, performance of a fluid challenge, while monitoring pulmonary artery or central venous pressure, provides an alternative means of assessing blood volume.

CARDIAC OUTPUT AND ARTERIAL OXYGEN TRANSPORT

The cardiac output is not an entirely dependable measure of tissue perfusion. Under some circumstances, the cardiac output may be normal, but the amount of blood delivered to tissues may be considerably reduced. In patients with hepatic cirrhosis, for example, the cardiac output may be high because of large arteriovenous shunts. Even in patients in whom the total blood flow is normal, the effective flow to vital tissues may be inadequate because there is shunting away from the capillary beds in which the critical exchange occurs. Tissue anoxia with accumulation of lactic acid is characteristic of shock under such circumstances, even when cardiac output is normal or elevated.

Measuring Cardiac Output. Indocyanine green dye is commonly used as an indicator for the measurement of cardiac output. After intravenous injection the dye is bound to plasma albumin and rapidly taken up by the liver cells. Indocyanine green is nontoxic and is rapidly and exclusively removed from the circulation by the liver. The amount of protein-bound dye carried to the liver per unit time is a fuction of hepatic blood flow. The rate of its removal reflects the functional competence of the liver cells. The rate of disappearance from the plasma after injection is measured, and the plasma half-life of indocyanine green is calculated. In patients who are in shock, liver perfusion is decreased or locally altered by shunts and sludging of cellular aggregates.

Repeated measurements of the half-life of indocyanine green are clinically useful. For evaluation of the severity and progression of shock, changes in the half-life of indocyanine green are indicative of changes in visceral perfusion. Measurements on critically ill patients have demonstrated that the delay in the clearance of indocyanine green dye is correlated with the reduction in cardiac output and increase in blood lactate. This simple liver function test, therefore, is of practical value not only for the rapid identification of hepatic insufficiency but also for objective assessment of the perfusion deficit of patients in shock.

The extent to which the reduction in cardiac output is a critical determinant of survival is dependent on the concurrent reduction in oxygen availability. Thus, in addition to systemic blood flow, factors which must be taken into account include pulmonary gas exchange, circulating hemoglobin, and the affinity of the hemoglobin for oxygen. Blood carries oxygen in physical solution and in chemical combination as oxyhemoglobin. In both instances the amount of oxygen is dependent on the oxygen tension to which the blood is exposed. At an arterial oxygen tension of 100 torr, the volume of dissolved oxygen in 100 ml. of blood is only 0.30 ml. One gram of hemoglobin can combine chemically with 1.39 ml. of oxygen (STPD). If 100 ml. of blood contains 15.0 gm. of hemoglobin it can combine with 20.8 ml. of oxygen. The amount of oxygen which combines with the hemoglobin is dependent on the partial pressure of oxygen in the blood; it is not linearly related to the oxygen tension, but is described by the S-shaped oxygen hemoglobin equilibrium curve (Chapter 3).

The affinity of the hemoglobin for oxygen is quantitatively assessed by the P_{50}, which is the oxygen tension at which 50 per cent of the hemoglobin is saturated with oxygen, at pH 7.4 and 37°C. The value of the P_{50} identifies the position of the oxygen hemoglobin equilibrium curve. Normally the P_{50} value is 26.6 torr. Increases in the P_{50} indicate a rightward shift of the oxyhemoglobin equilibrium curve and, therefore, a decrease in the affinity of hemoglobin for oxygen. This favors oxygen unloading, thus increasing oxygen delivery to tissues. Decreases in the P_{50} indicate a leftward shift of the oxygen hemoglobin equilibrium curve, with increased affinity of hemoglobin for oxygen and therefore decreased oxygen release in the capillaries.

Patients may compensate for a reduction in cardiac output by increased tissue extraction of oxygen. In studies in our unit on patients with acute myocardial infarction and shock, the extraction of oxygen was increased, as demonstrated by a difference in the oxygen content of arterial and venous blood which exceeded 6 volumes per cent. This compares to normal values which range from 3.5 to 4.5 vol per cent.

SHOCK*

Shock may be regarded as a hemodynamic defect of such severity that delivery of oxygen is not adequate to meet the metabolic needs of the tissues. A number of biochemical disturbances follow ischemic injury to tissues. These include the liberation of lysosomal enzymes, histamine, serotonin, and kallikrein; alterations in blood clotting; reduction in reticuloendothelial activity; and the release of protein breakdown products, especially uric acid, urea, and creatinine. Acidemia due to an excess of these acids, as well as lactic and pyruvic acid, fatty acids, ketones, and amino acids, ensues. Signs of diffuse injury appear, including increases in serum transaminase and lactic dehydrogenase. Indocyanine green clearance by the liver is impaired, reflecting a decrease in hepatocellular function. Of the numerous metabolic parameters that are repetitively measured under experimental and clinical conditions, the arterial blood lactate content (normal value 1.3 mM/l) serves as the best single indicator of the severity of shock. The increase in arterial blood lactate is an indirect measure of oxygen deprviation. Lactacidemia may be suspected when there is a base deficit (see Chapter 3), but other acids, for example those increased in renal failure or diabetic coma, also cause a base deficit. Experimentally, reduction in oxygen consumption during shock is predictively related to survival, since the extensiveness of cellular dysfunction and ischemic injury quantitatively reflect the oxygen debt.

The labeling of shock as "irreversible" has been a source of controversy. This designation might most appropriately be regarded as a statistical expression, indicating the likelihood of a fatal outcome in an experimental animal. The use of the term in the clinical sense has been strongly refuted in recent years. The concept is valid only in the experimental laboratory in which a well defined experimental technique is used to produce shock with a statistically predictable mortality. Clinically, what seemed "irreversible" in the past might well be reversible now with our improved understanding of the pathophysiology of the shock state and the more specifically targeted treatment procedures available today.

*See also Chapter 31 for treatment.

CLASSIFICATION OF SHOCK STATES

Until recent years, shock was classified on an etiologic basis. We referred to: (1) shock due to blood loss (hypovolemic shock); (2) cardiogenic shock (pump failure); (3) bacterial shock (bacteremia); (4) acute hypersensitivity reactions (anaphylactic shock); (5) neurogenic shock (barbiturate and narcotic overdose, transection of the spinal cord); (6) shock associated with obstruction to blood flow (pulmonary embolization, dissecting aneurysm); and (7) endocrine shock (myxedema, pheochromocytoma, adrenocortical insufficiency). Although the terminal pathophysiologic changes in these conditions are similar, they represent the end stages of the disease processes and do not necessarily illuminate the options for therapy.

On the basis of additional information, gathered primarily from studies on patients, we have proposed a modification of our earlier classification (Table 1). We *now* refer to: (1) "hypovolemic shock" as the condition in which the volume contained within the intravascular compartment is inadequate for tissue perfusion; (2) "cardiogenic shock" as the condition in which the cardiac pump is impaired to the extent that it cannot adequately circulate available volume; (3) "obstructive shock" as the condition in which there is obstruction in the great veins, the heart, the pulmonary arteries, or the aorta, to a degree which physically impedes the main stream of blood flow. These three categories are comparable to those in our earlier classification. In our new classification, we have introduced a term which designates changes in the distribution of blood volume. We have brought together into this category, bacteremia, hypersensitivity, and neurogenic types of shock and have termed this (4) "distributive shock." Each of these conditions represents a distributive defect due to a major defect in arterial resistance or venous capacitance or both of these. In distributive shock, in contrast to the other three categories, the defect is primarily in the small arteries and veins that make up the resistance and capacitance portions of the circuit. In this new classification we have deleted one of the previous categories—endocrine shock. Adrenocortical insufficiency, myxedema coma, pheochromocytoma, and other endocrine crises which may be com-

TABLE 1   *Classification of Shock*

Type of Shock	*Associated Features*
I. *Hypovolemic*	
A. Exogenous	Blood loss due to hemorrhage
	Plasma loss due to burn, inflammation
	Electrolyte loss due to diarrhea, dehydration
B. Endogenous	Extravasation due to inflammation, trauma, anaphylaxis, pheochromocytoma, envenomation
II. *Cardiogenic*	Myocardial infarction
	Acute mitral insufficiency, ruptured ventricular septum
	Cardiac failure
	Arrhythmia
III. *Obstructive* (by anatomic site)	
A. Vena cava	Compression
B. Pericardium	Tamponade
C. Cardiac chambers	Ball-valve thrombus
D. Pulmonary circuit	Embolism
E. Aorta	Dissecting aneurysm
IV. *Distributive* (mechanisms of altered blood flow distribution not fully understood)	
A. *High or normal resistance* (increased venous capacitance; selective or general) Cardiac output normal or low	Bacillary shock (gram-negative enteric bacilli) Barbiturate intoxication Ganglionic blockade (after volume load)
B. *Low resistance*, vasodilatation, systemic arterio-venous shunts Normal or high cardiac output	Cervical spinal cord transsection Inflammation (g + pneumonia) Peritonitis Reactive hyperemia

plicated by shock have volume, cardiac or distributive defects, and often a combination of these.

Hypovolemic Shock.* The circulatory changes which occur in association with hemorrhage are determined by the rate, volume and duration of blood loss. With very rapid blood loss, such as occurs after rupture of a major artery, acute coronary insufficiency and myocardial failure may occur early. However, when the loss of blood extends over a period of days, the plasma volume expands and there may be no evidence of circulatory failure. The values of the hemoglobin and hematocrit are not of immediate help in estimating blood loss during acute bleeding. Red cells and plasma are lost together, consequently the hemoglobin and hematocrit do not change acutely. Subsequently, when the extracellular fluid and protein reserves augment the plasma volume, dilution of the hemoglobin and hematocrit are noted.

When external bleeding is followed by shock there is a clear-cut indication for blood replacement. The blood loss may be estimated and the volume replaced. In circumstances where the site of hemorrhage is concealed, however, the cause of shock is

*See also p 553 for evaluation and clinical management.

obscure and the need for transfusion may not be apparent. The physician is challenged to recognize the hidden hemorrhage, detect its site and cause, and estimate the volume of blood lost. Important conditions in the differential diagnosis are hemorrhagic pancreatitis, bowel infarction or strangulation, cardiac tamponade, bleeding from arteriosclerotic or post-traumatic aneurysm of the aorta, and bleeding associated with fractures. Another setting in which concealed hemorrhage occurs is after surgery, with bleeding from a vascular pedicle or dislodgment of a ligature. Less frequently, capillary oozing after extensive surgical procedures causes an insidious form of shock due to blood loss.

In some instances, such as bowel obstruction or peritonitis, large volumes of fluid may accumulate in the lumen of the bowel or in the peritoneal cavity. The loss of intravascular fluid into this so-called "third space" may be of sufficient degree to result in hypovolemia and perfusion failure.

Cardiogenic Shock. Loss of contracting myocardial muscle mass due either to ischemia or infarction is the most common cause of cardiogenic shock. Acute mitral insufficiency and ruptured ventricular septum also may cause cardiogenic shock. These conditions are difficult to distinguish on the basis of the physical examination, since both produce a harsh holosystolic murmur, often with a precordial thrill. Pulmonary artery catheterization provides a means of identifying these conditions. Acute mitral insufficiency is recognized by the presence of a giant "V wave" in the pulmonary capillary (wedge) pressure tracing. Rupture of the ventricular septum is detected by a step-up in oxygen saturation between the right atrium and right ventricle.

The degree of "backward failure" as assessed both clinically and by chest x-ray usually is related to the degree of elevation of pulmonary capillary wedge pressure. In the presence of a normal colloid osmotic pressure, signs of pulmonary congestion appear when the pulmonary capillary pressure exceeds 18 torr, are slight to moderate between 18 and 25 torr, moderate to marked between 25 to 30 torr, and florid above 30 torr. The earliest x-ray changes associated with an increase in pulmonary artery wedge pressure are redistribution of flow to the upper lobes of the lung. If the pulmonary capillary pressure is increased further, there is a loss of fluid from the pulmonary capillaries to the perivascular and interstitial tissues. This leads to diminished clarity of the borders of medium-sized pulmonary vessels and the appearance of perihilar haze. When the pressure continues to increase, the fluid moves into the perialveolar spaces and radiolucent grapelike clusters appear. As the pulmonary capillary pressure increases further, the clusters coalesce and there is the characteristic x-ray appearance of acute pulmonary edema.

The severity of "forward failure" correlates with the degree of reduction in the cardiac index. Normally the cardiac index ranges between 2.5 and 4.5 liters/min./m.^{2}. Between 2.0 and 2.2 liters/min./m.^{2}, the signs and symptoms of forward failure begin to appear. In most patients in cardiogenic shock the cardiac index is less than 2.0 and at times as low as 1.0 liters/min./m.^{2}.

Obstructive Shock. The major causes of obstructive shock are listed in Table 1. *Pericardial tamponade* is a classic example. The etiology of pericardial tamponade is as varied as that of pericardial effusion. While it occurs most often in association with inflammatory disease, traumatic causes are increasing in frequency. Traumatic tamponade may result from chest injury, from bullet or stab wounds, or from iatrogenic causes, such as diagnostic cardiac catheterization or following cardiac surgery. Since the blood often is clotted, aspiration may yield no blood even in the presence of severe tamponade. If there has been associated blood loss, tamponade may involve as little as 200 ml. of blood, because hemodynamic mechanisms of compensation are limited.

Pericardial tamponade interferes with the diastolic filling of the heart. This results in decreased cardiac output, hypotension, and, if unchecked, clinical signs of shock with fatal progression. Because of the limitation in pericardial compliance, the increase in fluid produces an increasing pressure in the pericardial sac, and the diastolic expansion of the ventricles is impaired. The rapid increase in the ventricular diastolic pressure results in a reduction of the atrioventricular gradient, premature closure of the atrioventricular valves, inadequate filling of the ventricles, reduction of the stroke volume and cardiac output, and hypotension. The autonomic nervous system responds by increasing the release of endogenous catecholamines. This results in tachycardia, increased myocardial stimulation, increased stroke volume at a given end-diastolic pressure, arterial and venous constriction, with an increase in arterial pressure and a shift of blood to the central veins. As the tamponade increases a point is reached at which the venoatrial gradient cannot be restored and the ventricles are unable to fill with blood.

The presence of pulsus paradoxus is most reliably confirmed by direct arterial pressure measurements, since the Korotkoff's sounds on which the indirect (cuff) measurements are based often are not dependable. Since the severity of pulsus paradoxus is a function of the pulse pressure, this criterion fails when the pulse pressure is reduced to levels of less than 20 torr.

The conventional chest x-ray usually demonstrates cardiomegaly with clear lung fields. Confirmation of pericardial effusion is achieved by x-ray contrast studies, echocardiography, or pericardiocentesis (see procedure, p. 327).

Acute pulmonary embolism is another classic cause of obstructive shock. When an embolus or emboli obstruct more than 60 to 70 per cent of the pulmonary vasculature, there is an acute elevation in the pulmonary artery pressure. The wedged pulmonary artery pressure remains normal, unless there is associated left ventricular failure. The increased pressure load may cause dilatation and failure of the right ventricle. This is reflected by an increase in the right ventricular end-diastolic filling pressure and an increase in the right atrial and central venous pressures. The increased pulmonary arterial and right ventricular diastolic pressures are reflected by a loud pulmonic second sound, parasternal heave, diastolic gallop, and distended neck veins. Other physical signs include tachypnea, tachycardia, and often cyanosis and hypotension. Supporting findings include the presence of an enlarged right ventricle and pulmonary artery segment on chest x-ray and electrocardiographic signs of acute strain of the right ventricle, with right axis deviation, a $S_1Q_3T_3$ pattern, or right bundle branch block. The arterial blood gases characteristically show a reduction in both oxygen and carbon dioxide tensions.

When massive pulmonary embolism is the cause of shock, the central venous pressure characteristically is increased to levels exceeding 15 cm. H_2O. In patients with prior left ventricular dysfunction, acute pulmo-nary embolism may lead to left ventricular failure, and this is reflected by an elevation in pulmonary artery wedge pressure.

The lung scan, especially perfusion and ventilation scanning, is an excellent screening test, particularly when the chest x-ray is normal. A normal scan excludes pulmonary embolism as the cause of acute circulatory failure. If the lung scan shows segmental perfusion defects that ventilate normally, the diagnosis of pulmonary embolism is clear. When the findings are equivocal, pulmonary angiography is indicated. In addition to securing the diagnosis, pulmonary angiography provides a basis for estimating the degree of pulmonary vascular obstruction.

Distributive Shock. We regard bacterial shock, the shock state following release of endotoxin or endotoxin-like materials, as a primary disorder of venous capacitance. Blood appears to be selectively sequestered in the veins. In contrast to the more generalized increase in venous capacitance which responds to a fluid load in shock states due to altered neuromotor control, e.g., barbiturate intoxication, ganglionic blockade, and transection of the spinal cord, the defect in sepsis does not appear to be reversed by infusion of large volumes of fluid.

The patient with *bacterial shock* due to *gram-negative* enteric bacteremia is likely to have a low arterial pressure and cardiac index and a high peripheral arterial resistance. The mean circulation time is increased, indicating that the velocity of blood flow is decreased. These features are characteristic of high or normal resistance distributive defects. In these circumstances, infusion of large volumes of fluid usually fails to restore hemodynamic balance, presumably due to ballooning of a selective portion of the venous capacitance bed with selective sequestration of blood.

In patients with *peritonitis* the hemodynamic defect is quite different. The decrease in arterial pressure is associated with a relative increase in cardiac index and a reduction in peripheral arterial resistance. Although the cardiac index is normal or increased, perfusion is critically reduced, and this is reflected by the high blood lactate. The mean circulation time, which is prolonged in patients in shock due to gram-negative bacteremia, is normal or short in patients with peritonitis. These findings are best explained by arteriovenous shunting; in the context of the new classification, they are categorized as a low-resistance type of distributive shock.

When shock occurs as a complication of *barbiturate intoxication,* it is often assumed that the circulatory failure is due to arterial vasodilatation. However, that is not the case. More frequently there is evidence of arterial vasoconstriction which serves to maintain the arterial pressure near normal levels despite the concurrent decrease in cardiac output. The reduction in cardiac output is rarely due to heart failure. The central venous pressure usually is decreased. The blood volume, and more specifically the plasma volume usually is reduced. The reduced effective blood volume reflects either an absolute decrease in plasma volume or an expansion of the capacity of the vascular bed so that the available blood volume is not adequate to fill it. In either instance, the return of blood to the heart is reduced and there is a consequent reduction in cardiac output and arterial pressure. The hemodynamic defect thus is related to an increase in vascular capacity without a concurrent increase in blood volume.

ACUTE PULMONARY EDEMA

Acute pulmonary edema is characterized by a sudden and relatively rapid transudation of fluid from the pulmonary capillaries into the alveoli. Failure of the left ventricle is the most common cause of acute pulmonary edema. Other cardiac causes are disorders of atrial and ventricular rhythm or mechanical interference with pulmonary venous drainage, such as occurs with mitral stenosis. However, acute pulmonary edema also may occur after a variety of noncardiac disturbances, such as inhalation of irritating gases, pulmonary embolism, intracranial hemorrhage and intravenous fluid overload, particularly with crystalloid solutions.

CARDIOGENIC PULMONARY EDEMA

The fundamental disorder in acute cardiogenic pulmonary edema is the inability of the left ventricle to serve as an effective pump, owing to an imbalance between the load imposed on the myocardium and the myocardial contractile strength. Such an imbalance is, in turn, related to a loss of or damage to myocardial contractile units. Clin-

ical examples of this type of defect are myocardial infarction and myocarditis. An increase in the work load on the heart due to arterial hypertension, valvular heart disease, or intravenous overinfusion of fluids also may account for such an imbalance. The left ventricle can eject only a portion of the volume that is delivered to it by the right ventricle. The left ventricular end-systolic volume and end-diastolic volume and the mean left atrial pressure all increase.

The increase in left ventricular end-diastolic and left atrial pressures is accompanied by an increase in the pulmonary blood volume and the pulmonary venous and capillary pressures. When the pulmonary capillary pressure increases, so that the gradient between the oncotic pressure and the pulmonary capillary (or wedge) pressure is less than 5 torr, transudation occurs from the pulmonary capillaries via the perivascular interstitial spaces to the alveolar spaces. An increase in capillary permeability also may contribute to the loss of fluid from the intravascular compartment.

The diminished stroke volume and the decelerated blood flow in the aorta lead to a reduction in aortic baroreceptor activity. Consequent to neurogenic reflexes involving the vasomotor center, sympathetic activity is increased, and this results in increased systemic venous tone. Blood in the systemic veins consequently is thrust centrally into the already engorged pulmonary blood vessels and the pulmonary congestion is intensified, leading to the development of an edematous lung, which has reduced compliance (reduced distensibility). Resistance to air flow in the bronchioles is increased and wheezing may occur. The fluid which accumulates in the alveoli diminishes surfactant, and there is collapse of some alveoli. As the pulmonary edema increases, pulmonary gas exchange is compromised and hypoxemia ensues.

The clinical manifestations of left ventricular failure include tachycardia and pulsus alternans. There may be a reduction in systolic pressure, and with the exception of patients with severe hypertension, a small pulse pressure is noted. The pulmonic component of the second heart sound is increased, and a diastolic gallop commonly is heard. The pulmonary congestion is manifested by cough and dyspnea. The frothy, blood-tinged sputum, fine rales, and, with more severe pulmonary edema, the moist bubbling rales and wheezes are due to fluid in the larger bronchi. When the impairment of pulmonary gas exchange becomes more marked, cyanosis appears. In patients with right ventricular congestive heart failure, signs of generalized venous hypertension are distended neck veins, hepatomegaly, hepatojugular reflux, and peripheral edema. The venous pressure, especially the central venous pressure, is elevated.

NONCARDIOGENIC PULMONARY EDEMA

Pulmonary edema is a frequent complication in critically ill patients. The development of pulmonary edema most often is attributed to either "hemodynamic" changes, e.g., elevation of the left ventricular filling pressure, or increased capillary permeability. The level of the left ventricular filling pressure, however, does not always correlate with radiographic signs of pulmonary edema. Guyton and Lindsey demonstrated in dogs that pulmonary edema occurred at left atrial pressure levels of 24 torr when the albumin concentration in the plasma was normal. After the albumin concentration was reduced to about 50 per cent of the control values, pulmonary edema appeared when left atrial pressure was increased to only 12 torr.

Reliable measurements of plasma colloid osmotic pressure, using methods recently developed in our laboratory, are now feasible for clinical purposes. Measurements of the pulmonary artery wedge pressure also are routinely obtainable with the use of the Swan–Ganz flow-directed pulmonary artery catheter. It is now possible, therefore, to assess simultaneous changes in the hydrostatic and colloid osmotic pressure in patients.

An increase in hydrostatic pressure is generally regarded as the main cause of pulmonary edema after acute myocardial infarction. However, increases in left ventricular filling pressure do not always account for the presence of pulmonary edema. Reduction of colloid osmotic pressure, regardless of the cause, could by itself facilitate transudation of fluid into the pulmonary interstitium and alveoli even at normal left ventricular filling pressures. In a number of patients in our unit who developed acute pulmonary edema after acute myocardial infarction, the pulmo-

nary artery wedge pressure averaged only 15 torr. However, when both the plasma colloid osmotic pressure and pulmonary wedge pressure were taken into account by computing the oncotic–hydrostatic gradient, a more sensitive index for separating patients with and without pulmonary edema emerged. All patients with pulmonary edema had a gradient of less than 9 torr.

Intravenous administration of large volumes of crystalloid solutions in critically ill patients may result in pulmonary edema in the absence of pulmonary venous hypertension. Measurements of left ventricular filling pressure, therefore, may fail to alert the physician to the development of this complication, for in many of these patients the left ventricular filling pressure may be normal. Since a reduction in colloid osmotic pressure may be a contributing factor, measurement of the plasma colloid osmotic pressure and calculation of the gradient between the colloid osmotic pressure and the left ventricular filling pressure may prove helpful in alerting the physician to the patient receiving large volumes of crystalloids who is at risk of developing pulmonary edema.

References

Burch, G. E., and DePasquale, N. P.: Congestive heart failure—acute pulmonary edema. J.A.M.A. *208*:1895, 1969.

Forrester, J. S., and Swan, H. J. C.: Acute myocardial infarction: a physiological basis for therapy. Crit. Care Med. *2*:283, 1974.

Lewin, A. J., and Maxwell, M. H.: Acute renal failure: diagnostic and therapeutic criteria. Crit. Care Med. *2*:305, 1974.

Nishijima, H., Weil, M. H., Shubin, H., and Cavanilles, J. M.: Hemodynamic and metabolic studies on shock associated with gram-negative bacteremia. Medicine *52*:287, 1973.

Shubin, H., and Weil, M. H.: Routine Central Venous Catheterization for Management of Critically Ill Patients. *In* Ingelfinger, F. J., et al. (eds.): Controversy in Internal Medicine. Philadelphia, W. B. Saunders Co., 1974, pp. 177–184.

Shubin, H., and Weil, M. H.: Shock associated with barbiturate intoxication. J.A.M.A. *215*:265, 1971.

Shubin, H., Weil, M. H., Nishijima, H.: Bacterial Shock. *In* Weil, M. H., and Shubin, H. (eds.): Critical Care Medicine Handbook. New York, John N. Kolen, Inc., 1974. pp. 189–185.

Shubin, H., Nishijima, H., Weil, M. H.: Clinical Features in Shock Associated with Gram-Negative Bacteremia. *In* Urbascheck, B., Urbascheck, R., and Neter, E. (eds.): Gram-Negative Bacteria Infections and Mode of Endotoxin Actions—Pathophysiological, Immunological, and Clinical Aspects. New York, Springer Verlag, 1974.

Stein, L., et al.: Pulmonary edema during fluid infusion in the absence of heart failure. J.A.M.A. 229:65, 1974.

Stein, L., Shubin, H., and Weil, M. H.: Recognition and management of pericardial tamponade. J.A.M.A. 225:503, 1973.

Weil, M. H., et al.: Routine plasma colloid osmotic pressure measurements. Crit. Care Med. 3:229, 1974.

Weil, M. H., and Shubin, H. (eds.): Critical Care Medicine Handbook. New York, J. N. Kolen, Inc., 1974.

Weil, M. H., and Shubin, H.: Diagnosis and Treatment of Shock. Baltimore, The Williams and Wilkins, Co., 1967.

Weil, M. H., and Shubin, H.: Proposed Reclassification of Shock States with Special Reference to Distributive Defects. In Hinshaw, L. N., and Cox, B. B. (eds.): The Fundamental Mechanisms of Shock. New York and London, Plenum Press, 1972, pp. 13–23.

Weiss, M. H.: Head trauma and spinal cord injuries: diagnostic and therapeutic criteria. Crit. Care Med. 2:311, 1974.

Chapter 5

PATHOPHYSIOLOGY OF ACUTE CENTRAL NERVOUS SYSTEM FAILURE*

Peter Safar

INTRODUCTION

A comprehensive discussion of the pathophysiology of acute central nervous system failure would require a separate book. Therefore, this chapter will focus merely on a few aspects of acute total brain failure which are important for providing short-term brain homeostasis in emergency and critical care medicine. It will comment only very briefly on failure of the spinal cord. It will *not* review neuroanatomy, neurophysiology, or neuropathology, nor concern itself with the mechanics of head injury or the mechanisms by which certain drugs produce CNS failure, as these areas are covered elsewhere.

Preservation of brain function should be the pivotal concern in the management of critically ill or injured patients, for the status of the brain will determine the quality of life subsequent to recovery. The brain reacts to acute focal or total anoxic-ischemic, traumatic, inflammatory, metabolic, hemorrhagic, or neoplastic insults with (*a*) depressed neuronal function (coma); (*b*) metabolic disturbances (tissue acidosis); (*c*) edema; and (*d*) blood flow disturbances (depressed CBF autoregulation and CO_2 reactivity). This leads to a vicious cycle of brain failure, which at first is in part reversible and later may become irreversible (Fig. 1). Also, a wide variety of insults to other organ systems may ultimately jeopardize cerebral function. Some of these secondary (postresuscitative) changes can be ameliorated or prevented with the use of "titrated therapy," which, by restoring cerebral homeostasis, may enhance the chance for neuronal recovery (Safar, 1970–75).

With this chapter and Chapter 2, the author intends to promote the brain as the target organ of resuscitation and life support (emergency and critical care), since failure of any vital organ other than the brain (Chapters 3, 4, 6, 7), if not rapidly reversed, leads to multiple organ system failure, which ultimately includes the brain (Chapters 2 and 5). Therefore, all physicians involved in emergency and critical care, not only neurosurgeons and neuroanesthesiologists, should understand the pathophysiologic concepts of acute brain deterioration, and be able to provide life support measures aimed at creating intracranial homeostasis. The above concepts of secondary changes following the insult and therapeutic possibilities also hold true for the spinal cord.

*Adapted from—Safar, P.: Brain Homeostasis in Critical Care, lectures since 1970. Including Critical Care Medicine Symposia, University of Pittsburgh, 1970–1976; and the American Society of Anesthesiologists' Refresher Course, 1973.

Acknowledgments: Drs. E. Nemoto, J. Snyder, and J. Mickell made valuable suggestions. Dr. M. Albin contributed to the section on spinal cord injury. Dr. N. Caroline edited this chapter.

For an explanation of terms and abbreviations in this chapter, see p. 146.

116

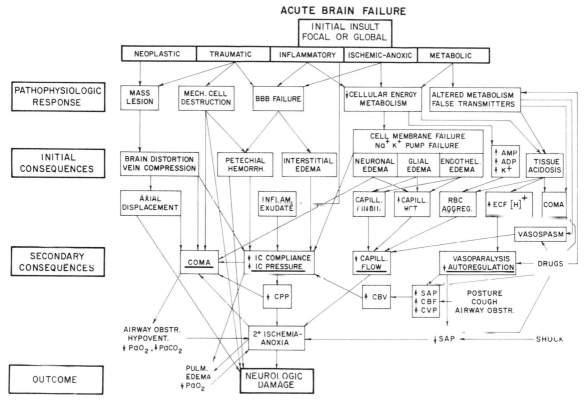

Figure 1. Progression from brain insult to neurologic damage as outcome, with vicious cycles. The pathophysiologic changes lead to vasoparalysis (loss of autoregulation), capillary blood flow reduction, mismatching of flow with metabolic needs, coma and ICP rise, as the key factors in deterioration. The key cycles are ischemia—edema and acidosis—CBV rise—ICP rise—etc. The factors not boxed can be therapeutically influenced most readily. For abbreviations see glossary, p. 146. Not illustrated is extracerebral organ failure, caused by the initial insult or the resulting coma and neurologic damage, which in turn may augment cerebral edema and ischemia. (Illustration by Safer and Nemoto, 1975.)

I THE BRAIN

Pathophysiology and Monitoring

VULNERABILITY AND DEATH OF THE BRAIN

The human brain, with its 10 billion neurons, 100 billion glial cells, and 500 trillion synapses, makes up only about 2 per cent of the body weight, but accounts for about 20 per cent of the total body oxygen consumption and requires 15 per cent of the cardiac output. The brain is the most vulnerable organ for several reasons, including its high energy and blood flow requirements mentioned above, its dependency primarily on aerobic glucose metabolism, the probable

importance of brain protein synthesis for learning and memory, and the limitation imposed by a rigid cranium on the brain's latitude for swelling when injured.

Sudden total cessation of cerebral circulation results in unconsciousness within 10 seconds (the time when brain oxygen stores are depleted); a flat electroencephalogram (EEG) within about 20 to 30 seconds; dilated, fixed pupils within about 60 seconds; and irreversible neuronal damage within about five minutes (using conventionally applied therapeutic measures after the start of reperfusion). Anaerobic glucose metabolism, which produces only two moles of ATP per mole of glucose (in contrast to aerobic metabolism, producing 38 moles of ATP per mole of glucose), is inadequate to sustain consciousness, and cannot sustain the integrity of neuronal cells for more than a few minutes (Siesjö, 1973; Nilsson, 1975). When brain ATP is decreased to 20 per cent or less of normal levels, which happens within about five minutes of circulatory arrest (Michenfelder, 1970), glucose stores are depleted and lactic acid production and accumulation cease. This coincides with the duration of circulatory arrest required to produce irreversible neuronal damage, according to concepts espoused until 1975. Recent work indicates that this critical duration of ischemia may be longer with novel postischemic therapy (Safar, 1976; Bleyaert, 1975; Nemoto, 1977).

When there is no restoration of circulation, the result is biologic, or panorganic, death. Restoration of arterial oxygen transport to the brain after this critical period of *"clinical death"* results in recovery with deficits of variable degrees. There may be return of breathing and consciousness, but transient or permanent intellectual, psychologic, or neurologic deficits, whose morphologic and physiologic bases have not been thoroughly studied. More prolonged ischemic-anoxic insults may result in the "vegetative state" or "coma prolongé." Finally, the initial insult or secondary deterioration after initial partial recovery following resuscitation may culminate in persistent apnea and coma with cerebral cortical silence—namely "brain death" or "coma depassé" (Chapter 2, Figure 1).

Brain death determination and certification should be carried out according to strict rules (Grenvik, 1974; Harp, 1974). Clinical criteria (including apnea, dilated fixed pupils, no spontaneous movements, and deteriorating circulation) are as important as an isoelectric EEG. The agreed-upon minimal time of EEG silence required for brain death certification varies and is not based on scientific data. A recent multi-institutional study revealed that the usual brain death certification criteria, including EEG silence for two hours or more, was never associated with recovery of consciousness. The author's institution uses two hours of EEG silence, in addition to the clinical criteria (Table I) (Wecht, 1969; Grenvik, 1978). Although "irreversible" stupor or coma *without brain death* cannot be proved at this time in the individual patient with 100% certainty, orderly discontinuance of seemingly senseless life support in such hopeless cases was introduced by our group and proved feasible (Loughhead, 1976).

INTRACRANIAL CONTENTS

The cranium is a closed box (Monro-Kelly doctrine), the total volume of which is almost constant. Its contents are essentially noncompressible, and consist of brain water (65 per cent), brain solids (25 per cent), CSF (7 per cent), and capillary blood (3 per cent) (Rosomoff, 1963)—excluding large vessel volume. Total intracranial blood volume, i.e., the blood in capillaries, arteries, and veins (including the venous sinuses), constitutes about 10 per cent of total intracranial volume. Small volume changes result in large intracranial pressure (ICP) changes.

Cerebral neurons are protected by the following: (1) glial cells, a syncytium which transfers nutrients and waste products between blood and neurons and acts as a potassium "sink"; (2) the blood/brain barrier (BBB), i.e., capillaries with unusually tight cell junctions; (3) the blood/cerebrospinal fluid (CSF) barrier, i.e., the choroid plexus; and (4) extracellular fluid (ECF, about 10 to 20 per cent of brain volume), which bathes brain cells and is contiguous with CSF.

Hypercarbia and hypoxemia, which increase CBF, as well as increased venous pressure and increased arterial pressure, all increase intracranial blood volume and in turn, increase ICP. Some of these alterations may also result in cerebral edema, particularly if they are prolonged and the integrity of the BBB is disturbed.

CEREBROSPINAL FLUID

CSF (Table 2) is formed at a rate of about 0.5 ml. per minute, about 70 per cent by the choroid plexus and 30 per cent via brain ECF, and is absorbed mainly through the arachnoid villi. Normal CSF is low in protein and has electrolyte concentrations similar to those in plasma. However plasma electrolyte *changes* are reflected only slowly in the CSF. And, although CSF in the cerebral ventricles and supracortical, supratentorial space equilibrates with cisternal CSF within minutes, equilibration with lumbar CSF occurs only after one to two hours of a change in composition.

CSF plays both mechanical and chemical roles. In its mechanical function, CSF protects the brain and spinal cord within a rigid enclosure and adapts its volume, within limits, to changes of intracranial blood volume and brain volume. The chemi-

TABLE 1 Guidelines for Diagnosis of Brain Death*

Two clinical examinations must be performed;
the second no sooner than two hours after the first.

	Date of Exam:	_____	_____
	Time of Exam:	_____	_____

A. Absence of induced hypothermia and absence of central nervous system depressant drugs. Body temperature should be recorded:

		(yes, no)	(yes, no)
1. Body Temperature:			
2. Ethanol level:	_____	_____
3. Toxicology screen:	_____	_____

B. Generalized flaccidity, no spontaneous movements, and no evidence of postural activity or shivering (all in the absence of muscle relaxants): _____ _____

C. Cranial Nerve Reflexes and Responses
   1. Pupils dilated and light-fixed: _____ _____

   2. Absent corneal reflexes: _____ _____

   3. Unresponsiveness to intensely painful stimuli, e.g., supraorbital pressure: _____ _____

   4. Absent response to upper and lower airway stimulation (e.g., pharyngeal and endotracheal suctioning): _____ _____

   5. Absent ocular response to head turning (no ocular movement): _____ _____

   6. Absent ocular response to irrigation of the ears with 10 to 20 ml. of ice water (no ocular movement): _____ _____

D. Isoelectric electroencephalogram recorded in part at full gain
   Date and time of tracings must be recorded: _____ _____

E. Absence of spontaneous breathing movements for 3 minutes (in absence of hypocarbia and muscle relaxants). $PaCO_2$: _____ _____

F. Comments:

CERTIFICATION

Having considered the above findings, we hereby certify the death of:

_____

Date: _____   Time: _____

Physicians' Signatures: _____   _____

Names Printed: _____ M.D. _____ M.D.

This document should be signed by two licensed physicians, who must not be the physicians of a proposed organ recipient.

*A. Grenvik, 1971; revised May 1977, Pittsburgh, Pa.

TABLE 2   Composition of CSF in Man:
Normal Values

	PLASMA (or arterial blood)	CSF
pH	7.4	7.3
$Paco_2$, torr	35–45	>45
Pao_2, torr ($FIO_2 = 0.21$)	75–100	<75
Bicarbonate, mEq./liter	23–26 (art.)	22–25
Lactate, μmoles/ml.	0.5–1.0 (art.) ⎱ cf.* 9.0	⎰ 1.5–2.0
mg./100 ml.	4.5–9.0 (art.) ⎰	⎱ 14–18
Cell count		0.5/mm.[3]
Total osmolality, mEq./liter	280–295	280–295
Sodium, mEq./liter	135–145	142–147
Potassium, mEq./liter	3.5–5.0	2.8–3.1
Magnesium, mEq./liter	1.5–2.5	2.23
Calcium, mEq./liter	2.1–2.6	2.28
Chloride, mEq./liter	100–106	120–130
Bromide, mEq./liter	-0-	0.9
Inorg. phosph., mEq./liter	1.0–1.5	1.0
Protein, mg./100 ml.	6000–8000	15–45
Albumin, mg./100 ml.	4000–5000	12–36
Globulins, mg./100 ml.	2000–3000	3–9
Glucose, μmoles/ml.	3.9–5.6 ⎱ cf. 0.05551	⎰ 2.8–4.2
mg./100 ml.	70–100 ⎰	⎱ 50–75
Amino nitrogen, μmoles/ml.	2.1–3.9	0.8
Bilirubin, total μmoles/liter	<12.0 ⎱ cf. 17.1	-0-
mg./100 ml.	<0.7 ⎰	-0-
Phospholipids, μmoles/ml.	2.9–5.2 ⎱ cf. 0.3229	⎰ 0.11
mg./100 ml.	9–16 ⎰	⎱ 0.35
Glutamic oxalacetic transam., (GOT), μM/hr./ml.	1.00	0.66
Lactic dehydrogenase (LDH), mU./ml.	60–120	60–120

*cf = correction factor.

cal function of the CSF is mediated principally through changes in acid-base balance. CSF pH is normally 7.3 at a $Paco_2$ of 40 torr, and is more finely regulated than blood pH owing to a system of balances among blood and CSF CO_2, brain CO_2 production, CSF bicarbonate concentration, and CSF lactate, the latter normally slightly higher than arterial lactate. Changes in arterial pH will be reflected in the CSF at a rate dependent on whether the arterial changes are respiratory or metabolic in origin. CO_2 crosses the BBB readily, but charged ions such as hydrogen or bicarbonate cross only slowly. Therefore, hypocarbia rapidly increases and hypercarbia rapidly decreases brain and CSF pH, whereas in metabolic alkalemia or acidemia (with controlled $Paco_2$ levels), CSF pH is maintained near normal over a wide range of blood pH values for some time.

In acute systemic acid-base disturbances, it is the brain pH — reflected in the CSF pH — rather than arterial pH, that determines the level of consciousness (Posner, 1965). *CSF sampling* provides a valuable means of assessing cerebral acid-base balance which, for the reasons mentioned above, is not always accurately reflected in arterial samples. CSF samples for pH and Pco_2 must be entirely bubble-free and cleared of deadspace, since even a small loss of CO_2 into a bubble or by diffusion through plastic catheters can cause a measured Pco_2 lower and pH higher than actual values. Use of a low-deadspace connecting catheter with mobile stopcock and a glass syringe facilitates accurate CSF sampling. For calculation of CSF bicarbonate from pH and Pco_2 (Henderson-Hasselbalch equation), the Severinghaus slide rule is recommended (Severinghaus, 1966). CSF Po_2 values, unless extremely low, are of little value in guiding therapy.

CSF pH significantly influences both respiration and cerebral blood flow. In its respiratory actions, low CSF pH stimulates the medullary surface chemoreceptors and thereby increases respiratory efforts. A decrease in CSF pH may thus be the principal cause of hyperventilation in patients with brain injury. The effects of CSF pH on cerebral blood flow are believed to occur through relaxation of cerebral arterioles when the smooth muscle of the arteriolar walls is bathed in an ECF of high hydrogen ion concentration (Cotev, 1969). In addition, CSF Po_2 and Pco_2 values, normally in a range between those of arterial and cerebral venous values, tend to decrease and increase respectively in areas surrounding ischemic lesions (Gordon, 1971); thus local hypoxia and hypercarbia further lower the pH in ischemic areas, thereby contributing to arteriolar dilatation and CBF augmentation.

Lactate, the end-product of anaerobic metabolism, is increased in CSF following brain hypoxia, ischemia, or trauma. The presence of blood in the subarachnoid space also results in vasospasm and CSF lactic acidosis. In brain ischemia or injury, there appears to be a correlation between CSF lactate concentration and prognosis—with lactate values over about 15 micromoles/ml. (over 10 times normal) being rarely associated with recovery of consciousness (Siesjö, 1976). The diagnostic and prognostic values of CSF enzyme elevations, however, and of cytologic examinations for sloughed cells have not yet been established.

CEREBRAL EDEMA

Data on brain edema, primarily gained from studies of histologic changes, brain impedance, and wet:dry weight ratios, are confusing, as the results vary with different experimental techniques. Abnormal imbibition of water by the brain may increase intracellular or extracellular fluid, or both. Cerebral edema following head trauma, for example, seems to be both intra- and extracellular, as there is injury to the BBB. Following ischemia or anoxia (e.g., cardiac arrest), on the other hand, accumulation of excess fluid in the brain seems to be primarily intracellular; cessation of brain perfusion appears to result immediately in a shift of sodium and water from the extracellular into the intracellular space (vanHarrevelt, 1956; Lind, 1975) because of failure of the cell membrane so-

dium pump, increase in brain tissue osmolality due to breakdown of molecules (Bandaranayake, 1975), and other factors. The BBB withstands ischemia better than brain cell membranes and mitochondria. About 45–60 minutes of circulatory arrest is required to produce BBB breakdown and interstitial edema and hemorrhage.

Reperfusion after moderate periods of ischemia rapidly reverses intracellular edema; however, after prolonged insults edema persists or worsens following reperfusion. Furthermore, swelling of glial, neuronal, and endothelial cells may pinch capillaries. This, in addition to intravascular sludging of blood cells, may impair reperfusion ("no-reflow phenomenon") (Fig. 1). Even focal ischemic or other types of brain lesions are surrounded by a "trouble zone" of edema.

In the injured (acidotic) brain, cerebral edema may be triggered or worsened by the combination of impaired CBF autoregulation (from injury or anesthesia—discussed subsequently), and arterial hypertension and hypercarbia, which increase CBF, CBV, and ICP—harmless in the normal brain, but edema-producing in the damaged brain. Cer-

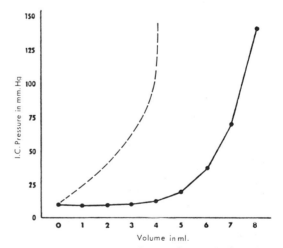

Figure 2. Intracranial compliance (volume/pressure) test; i.e., "acceptance" by intracranial space of additional volume increments without intracranial pressure rise due to displacement of CSF (solid curve). E.g. in the monkey, extradural balloon inflation with 1 ml./hour at first does not increase ICP, and at about 5 ml. a sharp rise in ICP begins, with 1 ml. capable of raising ICP above arterial pressure. In spite of normal resting ICP, this test may reveal reduced compliance in case of intracranial pathology, e.g., brain edema (interrupted curve). (Modified from Langfitt, T. W., et al. *In* Coveness, W. F. and Walker, A. E., (eds.) Head Injury: Conference Proceedings, Philadelphia, J. P. Lippincott Company, 1966.)

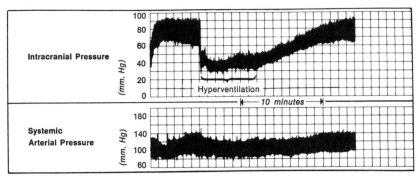

Figure 3. Simultaneously monitored ICP and SAP. Clinically unrecognized ICP rise—acutely reversed by controlled hyperventilation. (From Pizzi, F. J., et al., Am. Family Physician, November, 1974, p. 163.)

ebral edema first increases the pressure within brain tissue without increasing ICP, as the swelling brain first displaces CSF and blood. As intracranial compliance (displaceable CSF volume) decreases (Fig. 2), even slight arterial or venous hypertension (e.g., coughing, straining, hypercarbia) can increase ICP greatly (Fig. 3).

Cerebral electric impedance to a weak, high frequency test current is a promising, but still experimental, non- or semi-invasive method for *monitoring* shifts of extracellular fluid (a good conductor) into the intracellular space (a poor conductor). There are unidentified errors from current spread outside the brain, and from brain or blood displacing CSF. Techniques, apparatus, and interpretations have yet to be worked out. In general, intracellular edema increases brain impedance (van Harrevelt, 1956).

Cerebral edema cannot be proved clinically, but is suspected when signs of intracranial hypertension occur (see below).

INTRACRANIAL PRESSURE
(Lundberg, 1960, 1974; Langfitt, 1973)

Physiologic Considerations. Intracranial pressure (ICP) is controlled by many factors: distensibility, volume, and pressures of arteries and veins; venous outflow rate; rate of formation and absorption of CSF; and osmotic gradients between CSF, brain, and plasma. In the presence of space-occupying lesions (e.g., tumor, abscess, bleeding), increased CSF absorption and compression of intracranial veins first provide a temporary spatial compensation for ICP rise (intracranial compli-

ance, Fig. 2). Supratentorial mass lesions can expand acutely, either in the form of hemorrhage or through the vicious cycle of edema (or hemorrhage)–ICP rise–ischemia–edema, etc. When CSF is displaced, brain distortion blocks the CSF pathways or bridging veins, or arachnoid villi become compressed, the system decompensates, and ICP rises unchecked (Fig. 3).

With the patient in the horizontal position, normal ICP and lumbar CSF pressure are 0 to 15 cm. H_2O (0 to 11 torr); more than 20 cm. H_2O lumbar CSF pressure with the patient in the horizontal position is abnormal. In the sitting position, ICP is negative and lumbar CSF pressure is about 50 cm. H_2O. Pressure should be measured before fluid displacement, either with a water manometer or with a strain gauge. Lumbar subarachnoid puncture or catheterization is hazardous in patients with signs of a tentorial pressure cone, as it may provoke brain herniation; however, it is not absolutely contraindicated in the presence of papilledema, provided a thin needle is used and rapid CSF drainage is avoided (Langfitt, 1973). Lumbar puncture or catheterization probably is safe in patients with diffuse brain pathology without suspected ICP rise.

Intracranial hypertension cannot be recognized reliably clinically without direct measurement of ICP. Even serious increases in ICP may escape clinical detection. In various types of brain failure, particularly in children, baseline ICP may be normal but high ICP pressure waves occur suddenly and unexpectedly (Fig. 3).

Increased ICP damages the brain primarily (but not exclusively) by decreasing *cerebral perfusion pressure* (CPP) (Schutz, 1973). CPP is mean systemic arterial pressure ($\overline{SAP}$) minus mean ICP or jugular vein pressure, whichever is higher. Increased ICP in the "healthy" brain elicits compensatory vasodilatation; in spite of this, however, when CPP is reduced from a normal value of about 80 torr to about 50 torr or less, CBF declines. One should make an effort to treat an ICP over about 15 torr, and a CPP decrease to below about 50 torr in the "injured" brain. Direct pressure on the brain, for instance in neurosurgery by retractors, over venous pressure (20 torr or more), produces hemorrhagic cerebral necrosis—particularly in the presence of arterial hypotension (Albin, personal communication). When ICP equals $\overline{SAP}$, CBF is zero and brain death occurs. Consciousness occasionally seen in spite of a CPP of 0–10 torr may be due to higher systolic pressure waves.

A sustained increase in ICP to values greater than 50 torr is sometimes associated with decreased consciousness, even without a decrease in CPP, more likely in the presence of mass lesions which cause brain distortion, than with diffuse evenly distributed ICP rise (Langfitt, 1973). A key factor in the vicious cycle of ICP rise seems to be compression of the small veins of the arachnoid villi draining into the sinuses. When baseline ICP is elevated to over 20 torr, ICP waves, probably caused by cerebral blood volume variations, are seen unexpectedly (Lundberg, 1960). These plateau waves of 50 to 100 torr may last five to 20 minutes, and occasionally hours, and are terminated spontaneously or by therapy. There seems to be some correlation between duration and degree of ICP rise and outcome in terms of mortality and morbidity in patients suffering from head injury or metabolic failure (Mickell, 1976).

Usually, ventricular and cisternal ICP and lumbar CSF pressures change in the same direction and to the same degree. However, localized brain lesions may cause *ICP pressure gradients* between these compartments. Tissue pressure (e.g., pressure in the cortex underlying a subdural hematoma) may be higher than mean supratentorial ICP. Cranial extradural pressure may exceed ICP, for instance in extradural hematoma, because of the dura's elasticity. Localized or diffuse brain injury, with or without hemorrhage, may result in a vicious cycle of edema/hypoperfusion/impaired venous drainage/edema, which, after displacement of CSF, increases ICP. A mass lesion (but not intracranial fluid injection) may cause tentorial brain herniation with compression of the brain stem and, finally, medullary herniation, both resulting in ICP differences between supra- and infratentorial and lumbar CSF spaces (Fig. 4).

ICP Monitoring. Direct measurement of ICP is indicated in patients with coma commonly associated with ICP increases, such as following head injury (Lundberg, 1960; Johnston, 1970; Moody, 1971; Langfitt, 1973), in certain types of metabolic brain failure (Cook, 1975), and in selected patients with coma of unknown etiology. Monitored ICP rise is used to guide titrated measures for ICP reduction (e.g., CSF drainage, hyperventilation, osmotherapy, barbiturate, hypothermia—see later), and to signal termination of measures which may increase ICP (e.g., SAP rise, tracheal suctioning, CPPV).

Direct continuous intraventricular pressure monitoring has become feasible and safe (Langfitt, 1973; Lundberg, 1960). Much experience has been gained with insertion of an *intraventricular catheter* through a drill

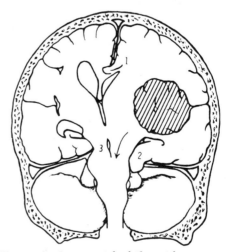

Figure 4. Intracranial shifts with supratentorial lesions:

(1) Herniation of the cingulate gyrus under the falx.

(2) Herniation of the temporal lobe into the tentorial notch.

(3) Downward displacement of the brain stem through the tentorial notch. (From Plum, F., and Posner, J. B.: The Diagnosis of Stupor and Coma, Philadelphia, F. A. Davis Co., 1972; as modified from Blackwood, W., et al., An Atlas of Neuropathology, Edinburgh, Livingstone Publishing, 1949.)

hole in the skull into the anterior horn of the lateral ventricle of the nondominant hemisphere (Lundberg, 1960). Such a catheter permits ICP monitoring, clinical analysis of the CSF, and therapeutic CSF removal for decreasing ICP, either by intermittent withdrawal or continuous drainage. Limitations are failure to catheterize the ventricle in cerebral edema with compressed or distorted ventricles, and an infection rate of about 2 per cent.

In the presence of normal ICP, a space-occupying intracranial lesion can be detected by the *intracranial compliance test* (Fig. 2). Normally, rapid intraventricular injection of 0.1 to 1.0 ml. of isotonic saline will not result in a sustained rise of monitored ICP, while in the presence of edema or a space-occupying lesion, this measure will cause a sustained ICP rise. This test must be performed with caution, via a freely draining catheter, and using saline without preservative.

In the supracortical subarachnoid space or the epidural space, fluid-filled soft catheters, micro-straingauges and *hollow skull screws* are used for ICP monitoring. The hollow fluid-filled screw (Vries, 1973) is inserted through a drill hole in the skull and a small opening made through the dura into the supracortical subarachnoid space. The hollow screw has become a popular means of monitoring ICP, but it does not permit CSF drainage and sampling.

SAP or CPP should be monitored together with ICP (Fig. 3) (Pizzi, 1974). Both arterial pressure and ICP strain gauges should be zeroed at heart level and all pressures recorded in mm. Hg (torr). The ventricular catheter or skull screw may be connected via a small-deadspace tubing to a stopcock and miniature strain gauge incorporated into the head dressing, which obviates artifacts from postural changes (Shapiro, 1975).

The Clinical Picture. Increased ICP should be suspected when there is headache, nausea, vomiting, and depression of consciousness (lethargy, drowsiness, stupor, coma). Chronically elevated ICP produces radiologic changes of the skull (e.g., thinning of sella turcica, shift of intracranial structures), and papilledema. Papilledema usually develops slowly, after about two days of increased ICP, and persists after normalization of ICP.

Neurologic deterioration from increased ICP may be rapid in intracranial hemorrhage, and slow in subdural hematoma or tumor. An increase in ICP does not invariably cause the "Cushing reflex," i.e., systemic arterial hypertension and bradycardia (Plum, 1972). The Cushing reflex is more common with posterior fossa lesions or rapidly expanding supratentorial lesions (e.g., epidural hemorrhage), and seems more useful in monitoring children than adults. Isolated global cerebral ischemic anoxia in monkeys may produce arterial hypertension, even when ICP remains normal (Nemoto, 1975).

Expanding *supratentorial mass lesions* (Fig. 4) cause sequential changes in breathing, circulation, and eye signs as the diencephalon, midbrain, pons, and finally the medulla, progressively fail. The clinician must try to recognize and reverse an ICP rise before the diencephalic changes (Cheyne-Stokes breathing, drowsiness, localizing signs such as contralateral hemiplegia and homolateral stiffening, and pupillary constriction) lead to compression and displacement of the midbrain (Plum, 1972). The latter is suspected when there are hyperventilation, nondilating fixed pupils of mid-size, and disappearing ciliospinal reflex, plus absence of oculovestibular reflex (caloric test) and loss of oculocephalic reflex (doll's eye phenomenon). The doll's eye test may be dangerous in patients with head injury because of frequent concomitant neck injury. Therefore, the oculovestibular test is preferred (20 to 100 ml. iced saline flushed into the ear canal, which normally gives conjugate deviation of the eyes toward the side of the cold stimulus).

Accompanying motor derangements may be reflected in *decorticate rigidity*, i.e., flexion of arms, wrists, and fingers; and extension, internal rotation, and plantar flexion of the lower extremity, due to interruption of the corticospinal pathways, provoked by vigorous external stimuli. This progresses to *decerebrate rigidity* from midbrain transsection (opisthotonos; arms extended, adducted and pronated; legs extended with plantar flexion; accompanied by shivering and hyperpnea). Hypothalamic damage may result in hyperthermia. Finally, tentorial herniation due to supratentorial ICP rise causes *axial displacement*, either symmetrically or, with unilateral lesions, by herniation of the brain across the falx and one side of the tentorium. This axial displacement results in the pontine and medullary changes of hypoventilation (with sighs or gasps), tachycardia, progressive arterial hypotension, maximally dilated pupils, and finally apnea. A unilaterally dilating pupil is the principal early sign when the uncus is herniated over the edge of the tentorium, compressing the third nerve. This can result in immediate midbrain transsection because of direct compression. All this is accompanied by a progressive decrease in consciousness from drowsiness to stupor to coma.

Subtentorial lesions can also increase ICP and cause herniation, both downward through the foramen occipitale magnum and upward through the tentorium. Such lesions, when they involve the reticular formation, cause coma. Those not involving the reticular formation may produce the peculiar clinical picture of an awake patient who is tetraplegic, apneic, and aphasic. Subtentorial lesions (e.g., tumor) can produce a noncommunicating hydrocephalus. While CSF shunting procedures can save cortical function, they are no substitute for definitive surgery to alleviate the pressure on the brain stem exerted by the subtentorial mass (Shapiro, 1975). Patients with subtentorial lesions must be watched for respiratory and circulatory disturbances. Even when conscious, their protective upper airway reflexes may be obtunded.

A special condition causing coma from increased ICP is *hydrocephalus*. In communicating hydrocephalus, deterioration is usually slow. Mass lesions and herniation through tentorium or foramen occipitale magnum causing obstructive hydrocephalus may result in rapid deterioration, which calls for an operation to shunt CSF.

Pseudotumor cerebri, i.e., signs of chronic ICP rise with papilledema, without mass lesion or hydrocephalus, is cerebral edema of unknown etiology. Operation may be indicated for saving vision.

It should be noted that not all intracranial pathology is associated with elevated ICP. For example, coma following shock, cardiac arrest, hypoxemia, or hypoglycemia may have as morphologic bases focal areas of cerebral hypoperfusion, edema, locally increased tissue pressure (without over-all ICP rise), and neuronal cell damage (Lind, 1975; Snyder, 1975; Nemoto, 1975). After very severe ischemic-anoxic insults, ICP seems to increase when secondary brain death develops (Nemoto, 1975).

CEREBRAL ELECTRIC ACTIVITY

In general, high CO_2, tissue acidosis, acidemia, *severe* hypoxemia, and ischemia all exert a depressant effect; whereas *mild* hypoxemia, tissue alkalosis, and alkalemia exert a stimulating effect on the electrical activity of cerebral cortical neurons measured by EEG. In epileptics, focal or general *seizures* may or may not be triggered by focal lesions such as brain scars. Death during convulsions usually is due to asphyxia from respiratory muscle spasm and airway obstruction. However, artificial ventilation, if necessary facilitated by a muscle relaxant, will not suffice to prevent long-term brain damage. The electric overactivity of neurons per se can stop protein synthesis and cause cerebral acidosis and permanent brain damage. Therefore, depression of the EEG manifestations of convulsions is indicated, for instance with the use of diazepam (Valium) or thiopental, followed by long-term depressants such as phenobarbital or diphenylhydantoin (Dilantin).

The vast information gained from animal experiments with invasive studies of the electric activity of most brain regions and even of single neurons is contrasted by a paucity of information on critically ill patients because of the limitations of and artifacts associated with noninvasive EEG monitoring. Clinically, cerebral electric activity monitored through surface electrodes reflects primarily (but not exclusively) the electrocorticogram. In the assessment of critically ill patients, the EEG is widely used to determine brain death (isoelectric EEG) and to detect convulsions in curarized patients. Less well developed is EEG monitoring in critically ill or injured patients without electrocortical silence. Multiple EEG tracings can be analyzed by computer for average voltage and frequency, enabling assessment of the depth of CNS depression, perhaps more reliably than is possible from clinical signs, (Bergamasco, 1968; Prior, 1971; Stockard, 1974).

Monitoring of average cortical-evoked EEG potentials (Larson, 1973), recorded via scalp electrodes and elicited by somatosensory, auditory, and/or visual stimuli, can enable early detection of deterioration and thus allow early surgical or pharmacologic intervention. The equipment needed is expensive and includes an averaging computer with memory. Unilateral lesions (hematoma, stroke) cause a decrease in the amplitude of evoked potentials on the affected side, while the latency remains unchanged. Demyelinization or compression of pathways increases the latency and makes the normally polyphasic-evoked wave form monophasic. Unconsciousness, for instance in head injury, is associated with decreased amplitude, even in the absence of mass lesions. Recovery is associated with improved amplitude of evoked potentials.

CEREBRAL BLOOD FLOW AND METABOLISM

CBF is normally about 50 ml./100 g. brain per minute (Table 3; Fig. 5). CBF decreases when cerebrovascular resistance increases. Cerebrovascular resistance (CVR) is CPP divided by CBF. Lassen and associates (personal communication.) discovered ischemia thresholds for regional CBF reduction (in baboons): (1) impairment of neuronal function occurs with CBF reduction to 20 ml./100 g. per minute; (2) cessation of neuronal function at 15; and (3) cell death at 10.

Regional CBF is normally matched with tissue demands by the arteriolar dilating effect of the brain ECF (CSF) hydrogen ion concentration (primarily from lactic acid and CO_2). The effect of the sympathetic and parasympathetic nervous systems and their transmitters on CBF in man seems minimal or absent (Lassen, 1974). Thus, CBF in *shock* is primarily CPP and $PaCO_2$ dependent; CNS symptoms occur when the compensating cerebral vasodilation reaches a maximum; irreversible neuronal damage may occur with SAP less than about 30 torr for over about 15 min. (Stone, 1965; Kovach, 1976; Safar, 1977; Slater, 1973).

CBF decreases during hypocarbia (lev-

TABLE 3   Cerebral Variables

VARIABLES	ABBREVIATION	APPROXIMATE NORMAL VALUES		CONVERSION FACTOR
		(a) RECOMMENDED UNITS	(b) TRADITIONAL UNITS	(a) TO (b)
Cerebral Blood Flow	CBF	0.50 ml./g. brain per min.	50 ml./100 g. per min.	×100
Cerebrovascular Resistance CPP/CBF	CVR	200 torr/ml. per g. per min.	2.0 torr/ml. per 100 g. per min.	÷100
Cerebral arteriovenous O_2 content difference	cer(a−v)O_2	3.0 μmoles/ml. blood	6.7 ml./100 ml.=vol.%	×2.24
Cerebral arteriovenous glucose difference	cer(a−v)G	0.5 μmole/ml. blood	9.0 mg./100 ml.=mg.%	×18.0 (MW gluc. 180)
Cerebral arteriovenous lactate difference	cer(a−v)L	−0.05 μmole/ml. blood	−0.45 mg./100 ml.=mg.%	×9.0 (MW lact. 90)
Cerebral metabolic rate for oxygen (O_2 consumption): CBF × cer(a−v)O_2	CMRO$_2$	1.5 μmoles/g. per min.	3.36 ml/100 g. per min.	×2.24
Cerebral metabolic rate for glucose. (gluc. consumption): CBF × cer (a−v)G	CMRG	0.25 μmole/g. per min.	4.5 mg./100 g. per min.	×18.0
Cerebral metabolic rate for lactate (−production + consumption), CBF × cer(a−v)L	CMRL	−0.023 μmole/g. per min.	−0.21 mg/100 g. per min.	×9.0
Mixed cerebral venous PO_2	P$\overline{c}$vO_2	35–45 torr		
Intracranial pressure	ICP	<20 torr		×1.3
Cerebral perfusion pressure°	CPP	>80 torr	<26 cm. H_2O	

°Systemic arterial pressure minus jugular vein pressure or ICP, whichever is higher.

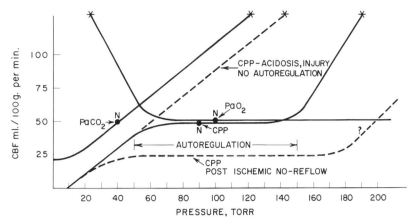

Figure 5. CBF changes due to changes in CPP (SAP minus ICP), PaCO₂, and PaO₂ in normal brain (N) (solid lines); and CBF changes due to changes in CPP in damaged brain (*interrupted line*). The latter is a variable combination of arteriolar vasoparalysis (loss of autoregulation) and capillary pinching and sludging ("false autoregulation" with fixed reduced CBF). (Illustration by Safar and Nemoto, 1975.)

eling off at about 50 per cent of normal with a $PaCO_2$ of 15 to 20 torr) and increases during hypercarbia (normally levels off at about 200 per cent of normal at a $PaCO_2$ of 80 to 100 torr) (Fig. 5). After one to two days of hypercarbia or hypocarbia, however, CBF returns toward normal levels owing to normalization of CSF pH (Severinghaus, 1965; Lassen, 1974).

CBF normally remains unchanged when CPP ranges between 50 and 150 torr (autoregulation), but CBF decreases with a decrease in CPP to below about 50 torr and increases with a rise in CPP to above 150 torr (Fig. 5). In hypertensive patients, the lower knee of this curve is at a higher pressure. Hypoxemia, ischemia, subarachnoid hemorrhage, trauma, and volatile anesthetics diminish or abolish this CBF autoregulation and, to a lesser extent, the changes in CBF due to changes in $PaCO_2$ as well. Thus, CBF may be drastically reduced with hypotension in such cases (Schneider, 1963). Changes in CBF give parallel changes in CBV. In the traumatized brain, any measure which increases CBF or SAP can cause a dangerous, not easily reversible ICP rise because of loss of autoregulation and decreased intracranial compliance.

Hypoxemia increases CBF only at a PaO_2 of 50 torr or less, giving maximal vasodilatation at about 20 to 30 torr PaO_2 (Fig. 5). Hyperoxia (PaO_2 500 torr) decreases CBF only about 10 per cent.

The autoregulation with SAP changes may be overwhelmed in hypertensive patients in whom an acute severe $\overline{SAP}$ rise may result in a breakdown of the BBB, resulting in cerebral edema and hemorrhages, i.e., hypertensive encephalopathy (Johansson, 1974).

In damaged acidotic brain tissue, there is vasoparalysis. If such acidotic foci are surrounded by normal brain, hypercarbia will "steal" blood flow from the vasoparalyzed areas and hypocarbia will produce a "reverse steal" effect, and thus improve regional CBF distribution (Soloway, 1968; Lassen, 1974).

Recent research data suggest that it is spotty, multiple, focal, microcirculatory changes rather than the over-all degree of CBF reduction which largely determine the amount of damage to neurons in post-ischemic-anoxic states (Ames, 1968; Fischer, 1973; Lind, 1975; Snyder, 1975). Later there may be vasospasm in addition (Kovach, (1976). This does not conflict with the concept of "selective vulnerability" (Brierley, 1976). Notably, total brain ischemia from normovolemic arrest (ventricular fibrillation, asphyxial asystole) seems to result in greater vascular changes and greater neurologic deficit than the same period of total brain ischemia with brain vessels empty (e.g., exsanguination cardiac arrest, intracranial hypertension) (Chapter 2) (Farmati, 1968; Hossman, 1973). This observation could be explained by greater impairment of reflow after blood has been stagnant in capillaries, which seems to occur in all organs after cardiac arrest and also during the resuscitative phase from shock states without cardiac arrest (Kovach, 1961, 1976; Vranova, 1968).

Monitoring of CBF utilizing brain saturation or desaturation curves of an inert gas (Kety, 1950) is still predominantly a research technique. CBF can be measured by experts in operating rooms and ICUs with the use of expensive equipment, including a portable gamma camera, computer and surface probes (single probe for hemispheric CBF; multiple probes for regional CBF) (Lassen, 1974; Sveindottir, 1975), and techniques such as intracarotid, venous, or inhaled administration of radioactive Xenon. CBF determination by the inhalation method is possible within 10 minutes with computerized mathematical corrections of "smeared" clearance curves and extracranial components (Obrist, 1975).

Cerebral angiography (used to evaluate vessel diameter and vessel displacement by space-occupying lesions) or brain scanning do not give information on CBF, since tracer transit time is influenced also by CBV. In brain death from intracranial hypertension, angiography showing nonfilling of intracranial arteries indicates a CBF of zero.

CBF monitoring gives more relevant information if combined with the use of a *superior jugular bulb catheter* to obtain arterial and mixed cerebral venous contents of oxygen, glucose, and lactate (Cohen, 1967; Mostert, 1970). When arterial blood hemoglobin is fully saturated with oxygen (PaO_2 over 100 torr) and cerebral oxygen consumption is constant, a decrease in CBF results in a decrease in mixed cerebral venous PO_2 ($P\overline{cv}O_2$), and mixed cerebral venous oxygen content ($C\overline{cv}O_2$); i.e., an increase in cerebral arteriovenous oxygen content difference. Conversely, an increase in CBF causes an increase in $P\overline{cv}O_2$. These estimates of changes in CBF from changes in cerebral venous oxygen content or tension or from arteriovenous oxygen content difference are called "CBF equivalent." They reflect overall CBF changes only when cerebral oxygen consumption does not change. Localized reduction in CBF as in a "stroke" may not decrease $P\overline{cv}O_2$, cerebral venous oxygen content difference, or total CBF values.

The above limitations make clinical CBF measurements in the Emergency Department or ICU difficult. Moreover, the usefulness of the information gained from total CBF monitoring in guiding therapeutic intervention is limited at present. *Hemispheric or regional CBF values may not change when there are multiple areas of focal hypoperfusion, as is common after ischemic-anoxic, metabolic, or infectious brain insults, unless these areas are extensive.* Also, CBF determinations are discontinuous, and ICP waves, often occurring suddenly and unexpectedly, may be missed.

The cerebral metabolic rates for oxygen ($CMRO_2$, cerebral oxygen consumption) for glucose (CMRG, glucose uptake), and for lactate (CMRL, lactate production) are calculated from CBF multiplied by cerebral arteriovenous gradients of oxygen, glucose, and lactate, respectively (Table 3). $CMRO_2$ is remarkably constant during consciousness, about 3.5 ml./100 g. per minute; $CMRO_2$ increases during convulsions, in hyperthermia, or with epinephrine, and decreases during anesthesia, coma, severe hypercarbia or hypothermia. Changes in $CMRO_2$, particularly persistently low levels (decreases to less than 2 ml./100 g. per minute), may have prognostic value in determining the irreversibility of coma in the absence of depressant drugs or hypothermia (Shalit, 1970; Tabbador, 1972; Bruce, 1973).

Superior jugular bulb catheterization (performed percutaneously via catheter inserted into the internal jugular vein in the neck, or with fluoroscopic guidance from an arm vein) permits monitoring of mixed cerebrovenous blood oxygen, glucose, lactate, and jugular vein pressure. A decrease of $P\overline{cv}O_2$ from the normal value of 30 to 40 torr to about 10 to 27 torr suggests anaerobic metabolism somewhere in the brain and can serve as a warning that there is need for therapy aimed at increasing CBF. A normal $P\overline{cv}O_2$, however, does not rule out focal areas of hypoperfusion.

Knowing cerebral arteriovenous oxygen, glucose, and lactate gradients theoretically permits estimation of the degree of brain anaerobiosis without the need for CBF measurement by the oxygen-glucose index (OGI) and the lactate-glucose index (LGI) (Cohen, 1967):

$$OGI = \frac{(a\text{-}v)\,O_2}{6\,x\,(a\text{-}v)\,G} \times 100 \quad \bigg| \quad LGI = \frac{(a\text{-}v)\,L}{2\,x\,(a\text{-}v)\,G} \times 100$$
$$\text{in molar values}$$

Normally, the brain burns only about 5 per cent of glucose to lactate (LGI) and 95 per cent to oxygen (OGI). OGI and LGI should add up to 100 per cent. The accuracy, and thus the clinical value of OGI/LGI determinations, however, is limited by difficult analytical methods and small concentration gradients.

SOME SPECIFIC PATHOPHYSIOLOGIC ENTITIES

Focal Cerebral Ischemia (Stroke). This results in a necrotic focus which is surrounded by a "trouble zone" of edema, impaired CO_2 reactivity, and impaired autoregulation (vasoparalysis). This "trouble zone" may be surrounded by normal brain tissue, with normal vascular reactivity. A decrease in the size of experimental infarcts has been accomplished by immediate postischemic hyperventilation (Soloway, 1968); hypothermia (Rosomoff, 1957); or barbiturate loading (Smith, 1974). Although ICP is rarely increased in ischemic stroke, the reduced regional CBF could be increased in some patients by CSF drainage (Reivich, personal communication). Cerebral angiograms may be normal after focal ischemia with neurologic deficit, probably due to clot lysis (Lassen, 1974, 1975). Hemorrhage into the necrotic tissue may produce a red infarct.

In patients with intermittent ischemic attacks from extracranial artery disease, CBF studies during carotid surgery confirm the ischemic threshold values mentioned above under "CBF" (Boysen, 1974). Volatile anesthetics offer no protection in focal brain ischemia (Hoff, 1975); while steroids (Patten, 1972; Bauer, 1973), arterial hypertension (Farhat, 1967; Wise, 1972), heparinization, hemodilution using dextran 40 (Gilroy, 1969), and osmotherapy (Meyer, 1971) may, provided they are started within 1–2 hours of onset of symptoms. Some patients develop symptoms of focal brain ischemia in conjunction with hypotensive episodes, e.g., myocardial infarction, postural hypotension, Valsalva maneuver. Since the early 1960s, we have proposed the exploration of the effect of a resuscitative approach on acute stroke, namely, immediate application of some of the above measures by physicians at the scene, continued in the hospital. *Such an approach may serve to preserve vital brain tissue.*

Cerebral arterial embolization may cause focal neurologic deficit (e.g., from bubbles, thrombi) or, if diffuse (e.g., from fat), convulsions and coma. Cerebral fat embolism syndrome usually follows pulmonary fat embolism syndrome. Autopsy reveals fat in pulmonary capillaries with perivascular hemorrhages. Gas and fat emboli can cause secondary thrombosis. Cerebral air embolism, the second most common cause of death in scuba diving (the first is drowning), is relatively unexplored.

Total Brain Ischemia. In animals, histopathologic neuronal changes and death of some neurons in scattered brain areas can be seen after as little as seven minutes of total circulatory arrest. With reperfusion following cell damage from the ischemic-anoxic insult, (Brierley, 1976) there secondary damage from edema, scattered areas of hypoperfusion, and probably other poorly understood factors (Fig. 6) (Moossy, *In* Nemoto, 1975). In acute experiments on cats and monkeys, some brain cells have been seen to recover after as long as 60 minutes of ischemia, at least in terms of electric discharges and protein synthesis (Hossmann, 1973). Although this is not a sign of recovery of even primitive cerebral function (Wolin, 1972), it shows that cerebral neurons are less vulnerable than previously assumed. Reperfusion of brain capillaries after an ischemic-anoxic insult is impaired at first due to capillary pinching from tissue cell edema and plugging from cell aggregates (Ames, 1968; Fischer, 1973); and later perhaps from other factors such as vasospasm (Hossmann, 1973). The acute secondary post-ischemic changes last probably not longer than about seven days (Chapter 2). The damage from total brain ischemia seems to be worse with postischemic arterial hypotension and less with normo- or mild hypertension (Miller, 1970; Myers, 1973); and also less following ischemia produced by ICP rise or exsanguination (bloodless brain) than by normovolemic circulatory arrest (e.g. primary cardiac arrest) (Hossmann, 1973; Schutz, 1973).

In the past, little research has been done on total brain ischemia and therapy *after* the insult. Results are confusing because of variability of species, models, and postischemic care (Gurvitch, 1974). Studies on total brain ischemia in our department began in 1970 with the development of animal

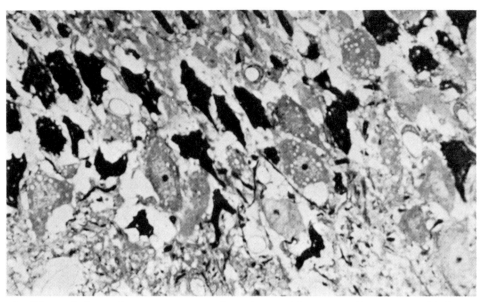

Figure 6. Histopathologic changes in neurons of rats (pyramidal neurons of hippocampus) following ischemic anoxic insult and a one-hour survival. Microvacuolation, "loosening" of neuropil, and other changes. Stained with toluidine blue. Magn. 750×. From: Brown, A. W. and Brierley, T. B., Chapter 6 in Brain Hypoxia; Brierley, T. B. and Meldrum, B. S. (eds.). Clinics in Developmental Medicine 39/40; Spastics International Med. Publ., London: Heinemann, 1971. pg. 49–60.

models (Lind, 1975; Nemoto, 1977). In dogs, after 15 minutes of total circulatory arrest, reperfusion resulted in brief transient CBF increase, followed by a sustained decrease of total CBF to about 50 per cent of control and impaired metabolism; there was no sustained increase in ICP (Lind, 1975; Snyder, 1975). In dogs after 12 minutes of ventricular fibrillation and resuscitation, reflow-promoting measures (combination of arterial hypertension, hemodilution, heparinization, and carotid artery flush with dextran-40) resulted in great amelioration or prevention of neurologic deficit (Safar, 1976). These four therapeutic modalities are now being tested separately in monkeys before clinical use.

A total brain ischemia model in primates was developed which includes post-ischemic intensive care for seven days, and permits neurologic, physiologic, and histologic studies (Nemoto, 1977). After 20 minutes of isolated total brain ischemia, there was persistent coma, and after transient partial improvement, delayed intracranial hypertension and brain death about the second day. After 16 minutes of isolated total brain ischemia, there was survival with severe perm-

anent neurologic deficit. At autopsy, there were scattered microscopic areas of cell death and edema throughout the brain, particularly in areas in which there is normally high metabolism and blood flow; e.g., the occipital cortex (Moossy, *In* Nemoto, 1977).

Many therapeutic modalities are being tested by this model. Barbiturate loading with thiopental in large doses, started as early as possible after reperfusion (but not later than 1–2 hours postischemia), resulted in amelioration of brain damage (Bleyaert, 1975, Nemoto, 1977). See p. 137, "Barbiturate loading."

Intracranial Hemorrhage. Intracranial hemorrhages range from petechial (as in brain contusion or hypertensive encephalopathy, fat embolism, or encephalitis) to massive arterial subarachnoid or intracranial hemorrhage (as in hemorrhagic stroke, ruptured aneurysm, or arteriovenous malformation).

The most rapid rise of ICP to arterial pressure level, although usually transient, occurs in subarachnoid hemorrhage from *rupture* of an *intracranial aneurysm*. In such a situation, the CPP should be kept between about 60 and 80 torr if possible; increasing CPP above 80 torr with ICP reduction and $\overline{SAP}$ rise may provoke rebleeding. Keeping $\overline{SAP}$ very low will reduce hemorrhage, but if prolonged, may enhance brain infarction, which occurs in such patients and is probably the result of vasospasm from bleeding or (postoperatively) from aneurysm clipping. Most authorities advise against craniotomy in the acute bleeding phase and favor interim neck vessel ligation. Since subacute subarachnoid hemorrhage can cause obstructive hydrocephalus, CSF drainage by ventriculotomy before operation may be indicated (Shapiro, 1975).

Although small amounts of blood are absorbed when the bleeding stops, intracranial hemorrhage damages the brain permanently, not only by increasing ICP, but also through direct injury, bleeding into brain tissue, and the toxic effect of blood break-down products in the subarachnoid and ventricular spaces. Some of these break-down products cause vasoconstriction, further reducing blood flow.

Head injury may cause subdural hematoma (usually from torn bridging veins), which may become symptomatic slowly, even after clinically lucid periods; and/or epidural hematoma (usually from a torn meningeal artery or its branches) which usually becomes symptomatic rapidly.

Cerebral Trauma and Space-Occupying Lesions. The results of these insults have been described previously, and are summarized in Fig. 1. The BBB seems tougher than neuronal and glial cell membranes. Therefore, breakdown of the BBB is more predominant in cerebral mechanical injury and in permanent focal ischemia than in temporary global ischemia. In trauma, petechial cerebral hemorrhages, space-occupying hemorrhages (contusion; intracerebral, sub- and epidural hemorrhages) may be worsened by arterial hypertension. The progression of changes with several vicious cycles occurring following cerebral injury and leading to partial or total permanent brain failure depend on the factors listed in Fig. 1, and other, still poorly understood, mechanisms, such as the release of vasoactive substances causing secondary focal vasospasm—after the period of reactive hyperemia. The mechanism by which expanding mass lesions (e.g., hematoma, tumor) may lead to coma and death were described under "ICP" above. Prolonged controlled hyperventilation increases survival rates, but does

not unequivocally decrease neurologic damage (Gordon, 1971).

Metabolic Brain Failure. The most common metabolic brain failure, ischemic anoxia, was mentioned above. The exact pathophysiologic bases for coma in liver failure (e.g., hepatic coma, Reye's syndrome) (Reye, 1963), renal failure (uremia), diabetic coma, and various intoxications are poorly understood. So far, advanced monitoring of cerebral physiologic variables has not been common in such patients, and autopsy results often merely show diffuse brain swelling. The clinical pictures of various types of metabolic brain failure are well described in textbooks (Plum, 1972). Some types of metabolic encephalopathy are associated with increased muscle tone (paratonia), multifocal myoclonic jerks or asterixis (flapping tremor).

Structural changes in hepatic encephalopathy, for instance, have usually been seen only in very chronic cases. In acute metabolic brain failure, CSF lactate and pH values, as well as CBF, $CMRO_2$, and ICP, may be normal at a time when the patient is unconscious. In hepatic coma, therapy should include efforts to decrease blood ammonia (e.g., by sterilizing the gut), but CSF and blood ammonia levels cannot be correlated well with coma and survival. Disturbances of glucose metabolism in the Krebs cycle and the accumulation of false neurotransmitters have been demonstrated. Brain pH may be high with increased excitability of neurons. Therapeutic trials with 1-dopa are promising.

Metabolic coma may be reversible if intracranial homeostasis is maintained and the etiologic factors eliminated. For example in *Reye's syndrome*—a rare acute reversible liver failure with often lethal brain failure in children of all ages—ICP monitoring and normalization seems to enhance recovery (Cook, 1975; Kindt, 1975). The etiology of Reye's syndrome is unknown, but according to the literature and local experience, we consider a combination of viral infection with an exogenous toxin possible. While trials with total body washout, exchange transfusion, amino acid infusions, blood dialysis and hypothermia gave no convincing results (DeVivo, 1976), osmotherapy and barbiturate loading increased survival (Marshall, 1978).

Osmotic Brain Failure. In acute *hyperosmolar* states (e.g., hyperglycemia, diabetes insipidus, hypernatremia, hyperalimentation, dehydration, use of glucocorticoids, mannitol, glycerol), coma may develop when serum osmolality increases from a normal value of 290 to about 340 milliosmols per liter or higher (Macaulay, 1961; Mattar, 1973). In some osmolar states such as infant hypernatremia and hyperosmolality from concentrated feeding formulas, petechial brain hemorrhages have been observed (Luttrell, 1959).

In acute *hypo-osmolar* states with serum osmolality reduced acutely to less than 250 milliosmols per liter (e.g., water intoxication), cerebral edema, convulsions, and coma may occur. Treatment of coma due to such extreme up- or downward changes in serum osmolality include pharmacologic control of convulsions, general life support measures, correction of the cause, and corrective fluid therapy: 0.45 per cent sodium chloride I.V. in hyperosmolality; 3 per cent sodium chloride, sodium bicarbonate, potassium, glucose, and a diuretic in water intoxication.

Extracranial Organ Failure Due to Brain Failure. All vital organ systems are under the influence of the CNS (Brown, 1972). Examples include impairment of sensory and motor function in coma resulting in upper airway soft tissue obstruction, hypoventilation, or apnea; hypothalamic-pituitary injury resulting in diabetes insipidus and/or hyperthermia; autonomic cardiovascular changes; hypermetabolism and catabolism (nitrogen loss) in head-injured, hyperventilating, hyperactive, comatose patients; increased gastric acidity with peptic ulceration; and pulmonary failure.

Neurogenic pulmonary edema may interfere with the maintenance of high PaO_2. The mechanisms underlying this type of pulmonary edema are not fully understood (Luisada, 1967; Bean, 1969). It has been seen in patients within one to two hours of an acute ICP rise (Shapiro, 1975). Hypotheses include cerebral hypoxia affecting lung innervation (Moss, 1974); and (alveolar) hypoxia causing pulmonary artery hypertension (from vasospasm) and leakage, resulting in interstitial-alveolar edema (Severinghaus). Sometimes acute pulmonary edema in coma is preceded or accompanied by a severe increase in systemic peripheral vascular resistance which may or may not be triggered by ICP rise. In these situations, control of arterial hypertension may reverse the pulmonary edema. In primates with isolated global brain ischemia, the development of pulmonary edema immediately upon reperfusion of the brain could be counteracted by preventing the resulting arterial hypertension with vasodilators or anesthesia (Nemoto, 1977). Secondary CNS deterioration following ischemic-anoxic insults with signs of increased ICP and brain death are often accompanied by decreasing PaO_2 values. Because of the frequency of pulmonary edema in patients with brain failure, serial PaO_2-100 per cent oxygen tests and advanced respiratory intensive care are required. (Chapters 3 and 10).

Patient Management

CLINICAL OBSERVATIONS

In coma, general life support, clinical observation, brain monitoring, and definitive therapy are interdependent, and must be carried out concomitantly. Clinical evaluation of patients with brain failure should focus on the change in the state of consciousness (lethargy, disorientation, delirium, stupor, coma), as determined by responses to verbal, tactile, and painful stimuli; respiratory patterns; cranial nerve functions; and, when they can be assessed, sensory and motor functions (Plum, 1972; Weiss, 1974). Furthermore, periodic examination of the eye grounds is indicated to assess perfusion defects and hemorrhage-edema (papilledema). The pupils should not be dilated artificially to avoid masking this sign for monitoring.

The most common causes of coma are supratentorial mass, ischemic-anoxic insults, lesions of the reticular formation, metabolic depression, electrolyte imbalances, and poisons (including drugs). Cerebral edema is *suspected* when there is headache, nausea, vomiting, decrease of consciousness, pupillary dilatation, convulsions, or papilledema (which develops slowly). Cerebral edema cannot be *proved* clinically. The changes accompanying rostrocaudal compression, axial displacement or unilateral herniation of the temporal lobe include unconsciousness, unilateral or bilateral pupillary dilatation, hyperventilation or hypoventilation, hyper- or hypotension, and brady- or tachycardia. Such changes must be detected immediately, since prompt surgical intervention—preceded by angiographic examination if time permits — may be required. This applies particularly to epidural hemorrhage and acute (sometimes delayed) subdural hemorrhage which, when properly managed, should not result in permanent neurologic deficit. Flow sheets are recommended to record continuous or frequent periodic neurologic observations (Bouzarth, 1968; Teasdale, 1974). Echoencephalography permits recognition of midline shifts without having to move the patient to the x-ray department (Brown, 1968). Computerized x-ray tomography brain scanning is a promising new noninvasive method suitable for the detection of intracranial ventricle size, blood clots, infarcts, tumors, and midline shifts (Ambrose, 1974). Patient observers must keep in mind that cerebral edema often becomes maximal 24 to 48 hours after ischemic-anoxic or traumatic (including operative) insults.

GENERAL MEASURES

In comatose patients, extracranial changes and general life support measures, particularly respiratory care measures, can greatly influence intracranial dynamics (Michenfelder, 1969; Safar, 1970–75; Shapiro, 1975). *Minimally, general monitoring requires arterial, central venous, and bladder catheters.* CVP line insertion should be without air leaks in order to prevent air embolism, "bucking" (sustained increase in airway pressure) should be avoided, as it can cause a dangerous rise in ICP. Variables to be monitored and optimized (not necessarily normalized) include arterial and central venous pressures; EKG, urine volume; arterial PO_2, PCO_2, pH and base excess; blood glucose and hematocrit; and serum electrolytes, albumin, oncotic pressure, and osmolality. Of paramount importance is avoidance or immediate correction of conditions which increase ICP, such as hypercarbia and hypoxemia, and avoidance of arterial hypotension. General therapeutic measures should begin as soon as possible after recognition of the emergency, and should include the following:

Airway Control. Personnel involved in the care of critically ill patients must be experienced and skillful with rapid intubation. Safe, rapid intubation is difficult particularly in restless comatose patients at risk of aspiration, and may require complete paralysis with succinylcholine (Stept, 1970). This should be done by the most experienced person available. $PaCO_2$ rises about 5 torr per minute in apnea! Coughing and straining (bucking) should be minimized, as these complications increase CVP, ICP, and SAP, produce hypoxemia and promote intracranial bleeding. Long-acting relaxants, narcotics, and anticonvulsants should be postponed until initial neurologic examination has been carried out, as they may obscure neurologic signs. In each case, the need for pulmonary cleaning and the jeopardy to the airway from aspiration must be weighed against the possibility of ICP rise from reflexes, hypercarbia, hypoxemia, and SAP rise (Fig. 1). ICP and CBF responses to airway control measures are unpredictable; therefore, these measures must be individualized. Once ICP rises, it may be impossible to normalize it. Manipulation of the head must be with caution in suspected cervical cord injury (common concomitant of head injury with coma) and in subtentorial lesions. Anteflexion and lateral rotation of the head may worsen the injury; maximal backward tilt of the head should be avoided, but moderate backward tilt with forward displacement of the mandible (triple airway maneuver) and intubation with the head held in the midposition, are recommended (Chapter 9).

Blood Gas and Acid-Base Balance. Adequate cerebral oxygenation is critical to maintenance of neurologic integrity and thus even brief periods of hypoxemia must not occur. *Arterial PO_2 should be maintained above 100 torr* to allow a margin of safety and thereby protect against hypoxemic episodes during convulsions, hypoventilation, or apnea. An adequate PaO_2 is best achieved by administration over several hours of 60 to 100 per cent oxygen, decreasing to 60 per cent or below, if possible, after no longer than 12 to 24 hours, to prevent pulmonary oxygen toxicity. If PaO_2 cannot be maintained above 100 torr with 60 per cent oxygen (e.g., in pneumonitis, aspiration syndrome, pulmonary edema), some form of continuous positive pressure breathing (e.g., CPPV) is indicated. This should be adjusted to enable optimal oxygenation without undue increase in cerebral venous pressure. Extreme elevation of the head has been used to counteract the ICP-raising effect of CPPV (Shapiro, 1975). The use of hyperbaric oxygenation in various acute cerebral states needs reappraisal (Ingvar, 1964). PaO_2 control and early detection of pulmonary edema may be by periodic 100 per cent oxygen tests which demonstrate pulmonary shunting earlier than clinical signs or roentgenograms. In neurogenic pulmonary edema (with aspiration, fat embolism, left heart failure, and other causes ruled out), general anesthesia and, in intractable ICP rise, operative decompression may be required to reverse the increased alveolar-arterial PO_2 gradient. In patients with pulmonary edema and stiff lungs, the needed CPPV fortunately causes a lesser increase in CVP and ICP than in patients with normal lungs. In persistent pulmonary edema, an indwelling pulmonary artery catheter for pulmonary artery and wedge pressure determinations may be helpful in guiding therapy.

Artificial ventilation is often needed, since even slight hypercarbia threatens cerebral homeostasis. Controlled ventilation with IPPV is preferred. PNPV, in an attempt to decrease mean intrathoracic pressure and thus jugular vein pressure and ICP, may be tried in the absence of an increased alveolar-arterial PO_2 gradient, but should be discontinued if it produces wheezes or signs of pulmonary edema. IPPV correctly performed in patients with healthy lungs, and CPPV in patients with sick lungs (recently modified through IMV which interferes less with spontaneous breathing efforts) do not in themselves produce dangerous increases in ICP. For details, see Chapters 3 and 10.

HYPERVENTILATION.   Most patients with acute brain failure hyperventilate spontaneously, mainly because of moderately increased ICP or CSF lactacidosis. Moderate *controlled hyperventilation* is indicated when the patient does not hyperventilate himself, or when he exhausts himself from doing so. Whether by spontaneous or artificial respirations, $PaCO_2$ should be kept at 25 to 35 torr. Hypocarbia decreases ICP (Fig. 3) (Lundberg, 1960; Zervas, 1972; Langfitt, 1973), normalizes CSF pH in CSF acidosis, and may improve intracerebral CBF distribution through the "reverse-steal" effect (see "CBF"). $PaCO_2$ values below 20 to 25 torr, however, are not recommended over a long term, as extreme degrees of hypocarbia may produce vasoconstriction in collateral circulatory channels. Also, pHa values over 7.6 should be avoided if possible. Guidance of ventilation volumes by CSF pH may have merit. Muscle relaxants can augment the

ICP-reducing effect of controlled hyperventilation; perhaps because of decreasing intrathoracic pressure, thereby decreasing CVP and CBV. Hypocarbia will lose its ICP-reducing effect with time, as CSF pH and CBF normalize after several days (Severinghaus, 1965). Hypocarbia decreases ICP by decreasing CBF and therapy CBV (Rosomoff, 1963).

Gordon (1971) reported a slight decrease in mortality after head injury with prolonged controlled hyperventilation, but this therapy did not significantly decrease neurologic deficit in the survivors. In another clinical study of patients with stroke, there was no obvious benefit from prolonged controlled hyperventilation.

Whereas comatose patients should be moderately hyperventilated following ischemic-anoxic or traumatic insults, those comatose due to chronic hypercarbia with decompensation of *chronic obstructive lung disease* should be oxygenated rapidly, but their increased $PaCO_2$ should be normalized gradually. Vigorous controlled hyperventilation in these patients to a "normal" $PaCO_2$ (40 torr) has resulted in transient awakening, followed by alkalotic brain failure and death (Rotheram, 1964). In these patients, PCO_2 and bicarbonate concentrations are high in blood and brain. Passive controlled hyperventilation results in CO_2 elimination without bicarbonate elimination from the brain, resulting in brain and blood alkalosis, cerebral vasoconstriction, and left shift of the hemoglobin/oxygen dissociation curve, both resulting in cerebral hypoxia (Safar, 1973). Should coma or convulsions occur in the presence of a high arterial and CSF pH, acetazolamide (Diamox) 0.5 g. I.V. is indicated, as this carbonic anhydrase inhibitor can acidify the brain rapidly (Severinghaus).

Control of Circulation.   Mean systemic arterial pressure ($\overline{SAP}$) should be maintained between about 80 and 120 torr in previously normotensive patients (higher in the hypertensive); but kept slightly higher following brain ischemia and slightly lower than normal following head trauma or in suspected intracranial hemorrhage. SAP can be raised by volume expansion and short-term infusion of a vasopressor and lowered by a vasodilator such as nitroprusside or trimethaphan (Arfonad). Increasing CPP briefly with vasopressor after circulatory arrest and CPR may improve the cerebral microcirculation, but sustained severe hypertension and hypotension may augment brain damage (Safar, 1976; Hossmann, 1973; Bleyaert, 1977). *However, when the ICP is found to be elevated, measures to lower it should have priority over those aimed at increasing SAP*, since the elevated SAP may itself increase ICP further, and since, as well, ICP rise over about 40 to 50 torr, even with maintained CPP, can depress consciousness. Raising SAP is contraindicated in brain lesions with vascular damage (head injury) as it may increase bleeding, edema, and ICP (Langfitt, 1973). Actually, arterial hypotension seems to reduce cerebral edema in experimental brain contusion (Klatzo, 1967). In focal ischemia (stroke), therapeutic hypertension is controversial, as it may produce bleeding into the infarct.

Total cardiac output and blood volume are of less importance to the brain than to extracranial organs which participate in compensatory vasoconstriction in shock (splanchnic and renal vessels); nonetheless, these variables should also be maintained at optimal levels. Cardiac arrhythmias, which may disturb cerebral circulation, should be monitored, recognized, and controlled.

Control of Posture. Attention to the patient's position is a matter of some importance. The head-down (Trendelenburg) position should be avoided, as it increases arterial, venous, and intracranial pressures. The supine position is preferred over sitting, as the latter may produce postural hypotension and cerebral hypoperfusion. Flexion or torsion of the neck should be avoided, as it may cause neck vein compression.

Control of Blood Variables. Hematocrit should be kept between 30 and 40 per cent, lower when deliberate hemodilution is sought. In experimental animals, normovolemic *hemodilution* during or immediately following reperfusion after an ischemic-anoxic insult, in addition to other measures, ameliorates or prevents brain damage, particularly if SAP is maintained normal or high (Cyrus, 1962; Fischer, 1972; Safar, 1976; Nemoto, 1975). Reduction in hematocrit, and thus viscosity, not the type of plasma substitute used, seems crucial for capillary flow promotion (Gregersen, 1963). However, this approach has not yet been tested clinically. Likewise, heparinization, which may promote reperfusion after an ischemic-anoxic insult (Stullken, 1976; Safar, 1976), needs further study before clinical trials are undertaken: Heparinization is contraindicated following trauma or other insults associated with damage to the BBB. Serum electrolyte concentration should be normalized, oncotic pressure maintained near normal, and albumin maintained above about 2.5 g. per cent.

Fluid Balance and Alimentation. Dehydration, as well as administration of salt-free dextrose 5 per cent in water, should be avoided. Since glucose transport across the BBB may be impaired, dextrose administration is advised. Thus, continuous infusion of 5–10% dextrose in 0.25–0.5% sodium chloride, with potassium added as needed, should be started as soon as possible (about 30 to 50 ml./kg./24 hr. in adults and children; 100 ml./kg./24 hr. in infants). Additional fluid may be necessary to correct for increased diuresis from diabetes insipidus, osmotherapy, or other causes. In contrast, trauma may activate the renin-angiotension-aldosterone system (sodium retention), and stimulate antidiuretic hormone release (water retention), which calls for adjustment of fluid therapy accordingly.

Except in the case of brain death, patients with head injury usually have high caloric requirements (3000 to 5000 cal./24 hr./70 kg.) and considerable catabolism (Bryan-Brown, 1973; Haider, 1975). This calls for early institution of parenteral alimentation and a switch to gastric feeding as soon as the bowel is active. Administration of antacids via gastric tube may prevent or ameliorate peptic ulcerations and prevent severe acid-induced aspiration pneumonitis should accidental reflux and aspiration occur, which is possible even in the presence of a cuffed tracheal tube. Monitoring should include daily measurements of body weight.

Control of Body Temperature. Hyperthermia, irrespective of the cause, calls for rapid normalization of body temperature (e.g., with drugs and external cooling). Hyperthermia increases cerebral metabolism and edema (Clasen, 1974), increases signs of brain injury, and seems to add permanent neurologic damage at core temperatures over about 41° C. (105° F.). Hypothermia is better tolerated than hyperthermia, and, under some circumstances, a moderate degree of hypothermia may be desirable as a means of decreasing cerebral metabolic rate (see later).

Control of Convulsions. Prompt control of seizures is essential to minimize cerebral oxygen and metabolic demands. Seizure control is accomplished initially by the use of a muscle relaxant, which will facilitate ventilation and oxygenation, but which may be discontinued intermittently to permit periodic neurologic assessment. Cerebral electric hyperactivity, however, also should be suppressed, using diazepam (Valium) or thiopental for short-term management, and for long-term management, pentobarbital, phenobarbital or diphenylhydantoin (Dilantin).

SPECIAL BRAIN THERAPY

Special brain monitoring, such as monitoring of ICP, CPP, CSF chemistry, and EEG, is indicated in most patients with potentially reversible coma from causes that may increase ICP (see above). Monitoring of cerebral venous blood oxygen, CBF, CMR, and cerebral electric impedance are still considered semiexperimental. Acute severe ICP rise with incipient herniation calls for immediate action: controlled hyperventilation, mannitol 1 to 2 g./kg. I.V., diuretic (furosemide) and—if operation is anticipated—neuromuscular blockade and barbiturate to gain time for surgical decompression and definitive therapy.

Osmotherapy. This is the most popular treatment for suspected cerebral edema. It reduces brain size during craniotomies and usually (but not always) can ameliorate or entirely reverse elevated intracranial pressure in various types of brain failure. Osmotherapy may increase CBF even when over-all ICP is not increased (Langfitt, 1973), perhaps by decongesting swollen cells that pinch capillaries. For reversal of acute increases of ICP, osmotherapy should be used in combination with CSF drainage and hyperventilation.

Osmotherapeutic solutions raise serum osmolality and thereby draw water from the intracellular and interstitial compartments into the vascular compartment (Javid, 1958). However, this mechanism provides only a symptomatic reduction of edema, as osmotherapeutics remove water (not sodium) from brain cells temporarily, do not restore membrane intergrity, and fail to shrink edematous brain in areas with damaged BBB (Pappius, 1967). The reduction in cerebral edema and ICP is followed by rebound brain swelling when the osmotic agent equilibrates back into cells. This rebound is most marked with urea (because of its low molecular weight (60), less following mannitol,

and least following glycerol (Tourtellotte, 1972; Newkirk, 1972; DeSousa, 1975). The latter does not pass the BBB, and is almost entirely metabolized. A mild osmotherapeutic effect is produced also by hypertonic glucose, dextrans, and albumin. The rapidly acting intravenous diuretic furosemide reduces experimental traumatic cerebral edema (Clasen, 1974). Ethacrynic acid given before mannitol seems to enhance the ICP-reducing effect (Wilkinson, 1971). Furosemide and acetazolamide (Diamox) (Huttenlocher, 1965) by different mechanisms reduce CSF production and may decrease ICP in hydrocephalus, but only transiently.

Vigorous osmotherapy, by shrinking the brain, can augment intracranial bleeding (Gjerris, 1974) or provoke subdural bleeding by tearing bridging veins (Luttrell, 1959; Marshall, 1962).

Commonly used intravenous osmotherapeutic techniques include: *Mannitol* 0.5 to 1.0 g./kg. body weight once, followed by 0.3 g./kg./hr. for continuous I.V. infusion. *Glycerol* has been tried in many different forms by gastric tube and I.V. One formula combines osmotherapy, hydration, and supply of calories, i.e., 5 per cent dextrose, 0.5 per cent saline, 10 per cent glycerol; infusion of this solution I.V. at a rate of about 1g./kg. of glycerol every two hours (0.5 g./kg. in the first 30 minutes, followed by 0.5 g./kg. over the next 90 minutes). This method provides intermittent bolus effects (Mickell).

Ideally, osmotherapy should be titrated by adjusting infusion rates according to monitored ICP. If osmotherapy is considered essential, glycerol is probably safer than other agents. However, all osmotherapeutic agents complicate fluid balance and can produce excessive degrees of hyperosmolality. Glycerol, furthermore, may produce hemolysis. Thus, "blind" administration of osmotherapeutic agents is discouraged. Serum osmolality should be monitored during osmotherapy; for although osmolality usually increases only from 290 to not more than 310 mOsm/liter, at times it may rise to dangerous levels—i.e., above 340 mOsm/liter, unless care is taken to assess osmolar changes.

Hypothermia. Hypothermia decreases cerebral oxygen consumption (about 15 per cent per degree temperature decrease), CBF, cardiac output, and heart rate. Furthermore, hypothermia decreases the brain's inflammatory response to injury, diminishes edema formation, and may as well protect enzyme activity (Rosomoff, 1957; Kramer, 1968). Experimentally, hypothermia results in smaller focal ischemic or focal traumatic brain lesions, more so when cooling is induced before than after the insult (Rosomoff, 1957; 1960). Prolonged controlled hypothermia following total brain ischemia-anoxia has not yet been satisfactorily evaluated in terms of neurologic outcome and histopathologic changes. Recent experiments with focal ischemia in monkeys suggest that post-insult cooling may worsen the outcome (Michenfelder, 1977).

Therapeutic hypothermia is a hazardous and complex technique that requires an experienced intensive care team, including an anesthesiologist. Cooling to 30° C. itself does not mask neurologic warning signs. Uncontrolled hypothermia with unchecked shivering and vasoconstriction, however, increases ICP and oxygen consumption and is arrhythmogenic, particularly in aged patients and in those with cardiac disease. Usually, at about 25 to 28° C. cardiac (esophageal) temperature, asystole or ventricular fibrillation develops. Hypothermia increases blood viscosity and depresses defense mechanisms against infections.

Usually, hypothermia is produced by surface cooling; poikilothermia (vasodilatation and hypothalamic depression) and inhibition of shivering are produced by drugs. At present, in the young, previously healthy patient with acute traumatic, inflammatory, or ischemic-anoxic brain damage, and perhaps even with metabolic brain damage and deep, persistent coma, induction of hypothermia (the earlier the better) may be justified, particularly in cases of intractable intracranial hypertension. The ICP-reducing effect of hypothermia is augmented by barbiturate (Shapiro, 1974).

Although the complexity and hazards and uncertain benefits derived from hypothermia have resulted in its disappearance as a usual therapy, re-evaluation with improved animal models for ischemic-anoxic and traumatic brain damage and clinical trials with modern intensive care seems warranted.

Barbiturate loading. Short-acting barbiturates decrease cerebral oxygen consumption, CBF, and ICP, and, when given before the insult, increase the brain's tolerance of ischemic-anoxia (Wechsler, 1953; Wilhjelm, 1965; Secher, 1968; Yatsu, 1972). In experimental animals with *focal* brain ischemia (middle cerebral artery ligation), or focal cold injury ("contusion") barbiturates

have reduced infarct size and edema when given before and (less clearly established) after the insult (Smith, 1974, 1976, 1977; Hoff, 1975). In patients with head injury, thiopental or pentobarbital, particularly when combined with hypothermia, have been effective in rapidly controlling intractable intracranial hypertension in traumatic and metabolic coma (Shapiro, 1973; Marshall, 1978).

In our laboratory, large doses of thiopental given to monkeys (90 mg./kg. I.V.), immediately *after total* brain ischemia of 16 minutes and reperfusion, dramatically prevented or ameliorated postischemic brain damage (Bleyaert, 1975; Nemoto, 1977). Starting thiopental with 30–60 min. delay or giving a smaller dose was less effective. Normotension was maintained with vasopressor and plasma volume expansion. The mechanism of this ameliorating action of barbiturate has not yet been clarified. One may speculate that the barbiturate has a beneficial effect on intracranial blood flow distribution by sustaining autoregulation while it reduces ICP, and by decreasing neuronal metabolism at a time when spotty hypermetabolism coexists with underperfusion. Also barbiturates can "scavenge" free radicals which are developed in anoxic tissue and tend to "burn up" lipid cell membranes (Siesjö, 1976). Reducing $CMRO_2$ is not the whole explanation. Various barbiturates give brain protection (pre-treatment) or resuscitation (post-treatment). Optimal durations of therapy and dosages are not known. Low (anticonvulsive) and medium (metabolism depressant) doses are less likely to produce myocardial depression than massive doses perhaps needed for membrane stabilizing effect.

Patients comatose 5–10 min. after cardiac arrest of over 5 min. duration might benefit from cautious, expertly performed barbiturate therapy. Initiating uncontrolled clinical trials with the Pittsburgh protocol of 1975 (Safar, 1977) showed that a massive dose of thiopental (30 mg./kg.) by careful titrated infusion with arterial pressure support is feasible even immediately after myocardial infarction cardiac arrest (Breivik). Current protocols and results of prospective (randomized) collaborative trials are available from the author (Safar, 1977). The "ultimate" brain resuscitation method will not be barbiturate alone, but a combination of drugs and measures resulting from ongoing research by several groups.

Steroids. The use of steroid therapy for

treatment of suspected cerebral edema is popular, but its value has not yet been proved (Rovit, 1968; Pappius, 1969; Bartko, 1972; Ransohoff, 1972; Reulen, 1972; Bauer, 1973). Steroids must not be relied upon to normalize acutely increased ICP. Therapeutic doses of steroids seem to activate the sodium-potassium pump, enabling a reduction in intracellular sodium concentration (and water volume) and an increase in intracellular potassium; these changes in turn result in membrane hyperpolarization and an increase in the electric shock seizure threshold. In addition, steroids may stabilize lysosomal membranes, preventing release of lytic enzymes, and stabilize mitochondria and capillary walls.

Since the only life-threatening complication associated with short-term steroid medication, stress ulceration of the gastrointestinal tract, has not been proved to be the result of steroid medication itself, a reasonable compromise in patients with suspected cerebral edema is the administration (as early as possible) of pharmacologic doses of dexamethasone (0.2 mg./kg.) or methylprednisolone (1 mg./kg.) every six hours until there is an improvement in the state of consciousness, but not longer than three to four days. If the membrane stabilizing effect of steroid action is true, larger doses would be indicated (e.g., 5 times the above single dose as "priming dose," then continue as above).

Cranial decompression. Wide surgical decompression has been effective in a few cases for diffuse cerebral edema with severely increased ICP following traumatic, metabolic, or other type of brain injury, when the patient approached brain death (Kerr, 1968). Salvage has been reported when surgical intervention was carried out within about 30 minutes after the onset of apnea and dilating pupils.

Anesthesia. In acutely brain damaged comatose patients, anesthetic management should include the above principles of general life support (Michenfelder, 1969; Shapiro, 1975). In coma from brain failure requiring operation, general anesthetics may be needed for brain homeostasis but not for decreasing pain perception. Immobilization with a muscle relaxant and controlled ventilation with oxygen are favored. Anesthesia and concomitant life support for patients

with acute brain failure should ideally be under the direction of an anesthesiologist experienced with neuroanesthesia. Airway control and respiratory care measures as well as anesthetics and other drugs used for the anesthetic management influence brain homeostasis considerably. All volatile anesthetics cause a dose-dependent increase in CBF, CBV, and ICP, and a decrease in $CMRO_2$ — harmless for the normal brain, but potentially harmful to the injured brain. There is blockage of CBF autoregulation produced by some anesthetics, particularly halothane. This can be reversed partially by hyperventilation. Spontaneous breathing of halothane should be avoided. Once ICP rise occurs under anesthesia, the damage is difficult to reverse. Among the volatile agents, N_2O is least harmful to the brain. Intravenous anesthetics, however, (thiobarbiturates, narcotics and neuroleptic drugs) tend to support CBF autoregulation, improve regional CBF/metabolic balance, and decrease ICP. Barbiturates also prevent or ameliorate postischemic-anoxic brain damage. The I.V. anesthetic ketamine, however, increases cerebral metabolism, CBF, CBV, and ICP, and should be avoided in patients with damaged brains. Halothane, methoxyflurane, trichloroethylene, ethrane, ether, and cyclopropane tend to increase ICP by increasing CBF and CBV, particularly in the presence of decreased intracranial compliance (space-occupying lesions) or arterial hypertension. Volatile anesthetics block autoregulation and decrease cerebral metabolism, but do not protect against or ameliorate postischemic brain damage.

Among relaxants, pancuronium may be preferred over d-tubocurarine, since the latter can produce histamine release, which may increase ICP (Shapiro, 1975). Relaxation per se decreases ICP. Some anesthetics and other CNS depressants such as reserpine (Clasen, 1974) may ameliorate the reaction of the brain to injury by depleting serotonin, which seems to cause cerebral edema (Osterholm, 1969).

In summary, halothane depresses and barbiturates preserve autoregulation and brain homeostasis. The anesthesiologist has means to control ICP and CPP, primarily by hyperventilation, SAP control, and an intelligent choice and titration of drugs.

II THE SPINAL CORD*

The following are merely a few summarizing comments on spinal cord injury. Since space in this section does not permit a separate chapter on spinal cord failure, the reader is referred to Chapter 38 and to the review papers on the subject listed in the References for this chapter.

Acute spinal cord injury is the most common type of spinal cord failure the emergency physician encounters. An estimated 11,000 new acute spinal cord injury cases occur in the U.S. yearly, 4,000 of these rendering the patient quadriplegic and the remaining 7,000 patients becoming paraplegic. The overwhelming majority of these injuries result from vehicular, sports, and industrial accidents and occur mainly in young people between 18 and 25 years of age (Bosch, 1971; Bucy, 1973; Botterell, 1975). Although hard statistical data are not available, it is suspected that paraplegia or tetraplegia, which otherwise might have been preventable, often results from inappropriate maneuvers during rescue and transportation, during diagnostic procedures in the Emergency Department, and in transporting the patient within the hospital environment. The need for immediate immobilization with head-neck-chest alignment (head in midposition) in trauma which is followed immediately by weakness or paresthesias in arms or legs or complaints of pain in the neck area, is now usually appreciated by most health care personnel. Much less appreciated is the fact that spinal cord injuries are often associated with head trauma (Tribe, 1963; Jacobson, 1970; Botterell, 1975), and the combination of these two entities often is lethal. *The primary adage in handling all comatose trauma victims is to suspect they have cord injury until proved otherwise.* Equally important is to realize that early respiratory failure is the primary cause of death among traumatic quadriplegics (Tribe, 1963; Jacobson, 1970; Botterell, 1975), and that improper immobilization, retrieval and handling can easily convert an incomplete lesion to a complete one.

The physician who trains paramedics, whose actions at the scene are crucial in determining the outcome of spinal cord injury

victims, and the physician who sees the patient first on arrival in the hospital must understand some pathophysiologic concepts in order to appreciate the opportunity he has to prevent these most tragic and costly outcomes encountered in traumatology.

Prior to the early 1960s, clinically complete lesions were considered irreversible from inception, and research efforts were more rehabilitation-oriented than concerned with mechanisms of injury and early treatment.

The experimental work of Albin, White, and co-workers in the early 1960s demonstrated the dynamic temporal characteristic of the expanding spinal cord injury; developed an animal impact-injury model for studying sequential physiopathology and evaluating therapy; suggested the use of localized hypothermia to limit lesion expansion and lessen edema; and in general stimulated research into the pathology and treatment of acute cord injuries (Albin, 1968; White, 1970; Wagner, 1972; Bucy, 1973; Osterholm, 1974). Application of new treatment modalities developed under laboratory conditions becomes difficult to evaluate in the human, however, because of lack of controls.

The spinal column may be flexed, extended, compressed, and/or rotated. The mobile cervical spine is particularly vulnerable. Although the spinal cord may be injured primarily when bony deformity results from the impact, cervical cord damage has been seen even without fracture dislocation, particularly in patients with pre-existing spondylosis. The spinal cord adapts to protruding bone by "plastic deformation." The arterial blood supply of the spinal cord normally is not as abundant as that of the brain. In addition, cord blood supply may be limited by impairment of major vertebral blood supply in injury.

The changes that occur within minutes of an injury and the speed with which they progress can be correlated with the severity of trauma (Hung, 1975). Albin and associates showed that the amount of energy required to produce paralysis is large (6.0×10^4 g. cm.) if applied externally over the spine of an experimental animal, while as little as 4.0×10^2 g. cm. of impact injury delivered to the exposed cord with intact dura will produce an irreversible lesion (work in progress). This indicates the energy absorption capacity of the anatomic structures in-

---

*Dr. Maurice Albin supplied valuable suggestions and references.

terposed between spinal cord and skin. It must also be emphasized how rapid impact injury can occur, since maximal cord deformation develops in about 6.0 milliseconds in irreversible experimental trauma (Hung, 1975).

The sequence of events that follow injury are trauma, hemorrhage, ischemia, edema, and repair. With the exception of immediate spinal cord transsection from severe fracture dislocation, these post-traumatic events will determine in part whether the lesion will be complete or incomplete, or whether a transient or permanent paralysis will occur.

In general, somatosensory cortically evoked responses are changed immediately after trauma, even when the cord may appear to be histologically normal, and within minutes small perivascular hemorrhages are seen, more preponderant in gray matter. These hemorrhages coalesce, and within a few hours ischemic changes in the gray matter can be seen. After about one hour of injury, an increase in injury site tissue norepinephrine has been reported (Osterholm, 1974), which has not been verified by other investigators (Hedeman; Ducker; Albin, 1974). Direct experimental observation and analysis have shown immediate reduction in blood flow of cord vessels following impact trauma, a decrease in tissue O_2 tension, and a vicious cycle of focal hemorrhage, edema, and hypoperfusion (Ducker, 1969, 1971; Wagner, 1971; Kelly, 1972).

The edema in experimental spinal cord injury seems to be maximal within three to six hours after impact. This is followed by progressive hemorrhagic necrosis, which, at least in part, is due to secondary post-traumatic impairment of the microcirculation. Sometimes, acute central softening of the spinal cord has been seen, possibly due to anterior spinal artery insufficiency following trauma.

While immobilization is sustained, the spine of the traumatized subject should be examined by x-ray, and the consultant neurosurgeon should decide on lumbar puncture and/or myelography or other diagnostic procedures. He may take scalp EEG recordings (and computerized analysis of the record) from the sensory cortex during peripheral stimulation (cortical evoked potentials).

Since some novel experimental therapeutic approaches, such as hypothermia, and others involving surgical exposure of the cord, may ameliorate the neurologic deficit from spinal cord injury if applied as early as possible, all patients with spinal cord injury should be taken immediately to the nearest spinal cord injury center.

Clinically, recent research has revealed as crucial the immediate and sustained immobilization with head-neck-chest alignment; cervical traction in unstable cervical fractures; cardiopulmonary life support; and, in selected cases, operative procedures to provide stability in an unstable column, to decompress a "trapped" cord and to provide a field for open selective hypothermic perfusion.

Therapeutically, several modalities have been evaluated both in animals and man. These have included localized spinal cord hypothermia (White, 1970), hyperosmotic agents (Joyner, 1963), steroids (Ducker, 1969), alpha-episilonaminocaproic acid (Goodkin, 1969), normothermic perfusion (Tator, 1973; Thienprasit, 1975), and catecholamine blockers such as alpha-methyl tyrosine (Osterholm, 1974). Of these, localized hypothermia has been with us the longest, and has been shown by many investigators to have a significant therapeutic effect in tightly controlled animal experiments. Unfortunately, the clinical data relating to its use are meager, although some investigators have applied this method clinically with promising results (Yashon, 1971; Gildenberg, 1972; Meacham, 1973). If applied early, localized hypothermia has been shown to reduce spinal cord edema, decrease the inflammatory responses, and arrest the expanding lesion (Albin; White, 1969).

It can be assumed, however, that some of the other measures listed above under "Head Injury" may also become rationale for use in spinal cord injury after evaluation in the animal model.

CONCLUDING COMMENT

Physicians involved in the care of critically ill patients should familiarize themselves with the pathophysiology of acute brain failure and newer therapeutic approaches to restoration of intracranial homeostasis. The breakthroughs in respiratory resuscitation in the 1950s and in cardiovascular resuscitation in the 1960s are being followed by breakthroughs in resuscitation of the arrested brain in the 1970s (Safar, 1970–1978). We are now witnessing the orderly progression of control and reversal of rising

ICP by CSF drainage, hyperventilation, osmotherapy, barbiturate, and hypothermia (Lundberg, 1960; Langfitt, 1973; Shapiro, 1975). At the same time, the previously sacrosanct five-minute limit of clinical death is being challenged by experimental studies in which dramatic amelioration or prevention of postischemic brain failure has been achieved after 12 to 16 minutes of cessation of circulation using therapy promoting reflow (Safar, 1975) or barbiturate loading (Bleyaert, 1975; Nemoto, 1977). Other recent studies have shown chemical and electrical recovery of some neurons in cats after 60 minutes of circulatory arrest (Hossmann, 1971; 1973). Neuronal salvage by a rapid resuscitative approach has been documented for spinal cord injury (Albin, 1968) and should be explored for focal brain ischemia (stroke). Microneurosurgery has minimized iatrogenic brain injury and has led to the discovery of previously obscure disease mechanisms and of new, surgically correctible lesions (Jannetta, 1975). Brain researchers are increasingly pursuing unanswered questions that are therapeutically relevant (Plum, 1973; Safar, 1976, 1977, 1978).

In the Emergency Department, operating room, and ICU, the acutely injured brain can now be accorded scientific monitoring and titrated therapy such as that given to other vital organ systems aimed at restoring homeostasis, in order to prevent or ameliorate permanent neurologic, intellectual, or psychologic deficits. Neuroanesthesia has advanced from witchcraft to a clinical science. On the basis of such findings and developments, the pessimism of the past concerning the salvability of the "black box" (CNS) is yielding to optimism. Laboratory researchers and clinicians should communicate and collaborate in order speedily to close the gap between what is known and what is applied. Much remains to be learned in this fascinating field of resuscitation of "the brain too good to die."

References

I The Brain

Reviews

Albin, M. (ed.): Anesthetic management of the patient with head injury. Neuroanesthesia, International Anesthesia Clinics 15:297, 1977.
Alexander, E.: Medical management of closed head injuries. Clin. Neurosurg. 19:240, 1971.

Alexander, S. C., and Lassen, N. A.: Effects of anesthesia on cerebral blood flow. Refresher Course Synopsis 227, 1975. American Society of Anesthesiologists, Chicago.
Brierley, J. B.: Cerebral Hypoxia. In Blackwood, W., and Corsellis, J. A. N. (eds.): Greenfield's Neuropathology, London, Arnold, 1976. pp. 43–85.
Brock, M., and Dietz, H.: Intracranial Pressure—Experimental and Clinical Aspects. New York, Springer Verlag, 1972.
Cohen, P.: The metabolic function of oxygen and biochemical lesion of hypoxia. Anesthesiology 37:148, 1972.
Davson, H.: Physiology of CSF. Boston, Little, Brown and Co., 1967.
Grenvik, A.: Brain death certification and discontinuance of life support in vegetative state. Crit. Care Med. May 1978.
Harp, J. R.: Criteria for the determination of death. Anesthesiology 40:391, 1974.
Klatzo, I., and Seitelberger, F. (eds.): Proceedings of the Symposium on Brain Edema. New York, Springer Verlag, 1967.
Kovach, A. G. B., and Sandor, P.: Cerebral blood flow and brain function during hypotension and shock. Ann. Rev. Physiol. 38:571, 1976.
Langfitt, T. W.: Increased Intracranial Pressure. In Youmans, J. R. (ed.): Neurologic Surgery, Vol I, Chapter 18. Philadelphia, W. B. Saunders Co., 1973.
Lassen, N. A.: Control of the cerebral circulation in health and disease. Circ. Res. 34:749, 1974.
Michenfelder, J. D., Gronert, G. A., and Rehder, K.: Neuroanesthesia. Anesthesiology 30:65, 1969.
Moss, I. R., Wald, A., and Ransohoff, J.: Respiratory functions and chemical regulation of ventilation in head injury. Ann. Rev. Resp. Dis. 109:205, 1974.
Pizzi, F. J., et al.: A protocol for the management of head trauma. American Family Physician 10:163, 1974.
Plum, F., and Posner, J. B.: The Diagnosis of Stupor and Coma, 2nd ed. Philadelphia, F. A. Davis Co., 1972.
Plum, F. (ed.): Symposium on the threshold and mechanisms of anoxic-ischemic brain injury. Arch. Neurol. 29:359, 1973.
Safar, P. (ed.): Brain resuscitation. Symposium Issue. Crit. Care Med. May 1978.
Safar, P. (ed.): *Advances in Cardiopulmonary Resuscitation.* (Wolf Creek Conference Proceedings, Oct. 1975). New York, Springer Verlag, 1977. Chapters 27–30.
Safar, P., and Nemoto, E.: Brain resuscitation in cardiac arrest and shock. In Proceedings, International Symposium on Shock. Utrecht, Netherlands, Springer Verlag, 1977.
Siesjö, B. K. et al.: Brain metabolism in the critically ill. SCCM Annual Lecture, May 1976. Critical Care Medicine 4:283, 1976.
Shapiro, H. M.: Intracranial hypertension. Therapeutic and anesthetic considerations. Anesthesiology 43:445, 1975.
Trubuhovich, R. V. (ed.): Management of intracranial catastrophes. Internat. Anesthesia Clinics, 1978.

SELECTED REFERENCES

Albin, M. S., et al.: Brain retraction pressure during intracranial procedures. Surg. Forum 26:499, 1975.
Ambrose, J.: Computerized x-ray scanning of the brain, J. Neurosurg. 40:679, 1974.

Ames, A., III, et al.: Cerebral ischemia. II. The no-reflow phenomenon. Am. J. Pathol. 52:437, 1968.

Bandaranayake, M. N., and Nemoto, E. M.: Rat brain osmolality during ischemic anoxia. Physiologist 18:128, 1975.

Bartko, D., et al.: Effect of Dexamethasone on the Early Edema Following Occlusion of the Middle Cerebral Artery in Cats. In Steroids and Brain Edema. New York, Springer Verlag, 1972.

Bauer, R. B., and Tellez, H.: Dexamethasone as treatment in cerebrovascular disease. 2. A controlled study in acute cerebral infarction. Stroke 4:547, 1973.

Bean, J. W., and Beckman, D. L.: Centrogenic pulmonary pathology in mechanical head injury. J. Appl. Physiol. 27:807, 1969.

Bergamasco, B., et al.: EEG sleep patterns as a prognostic criterion in post-traumatic coma. Electroenceph. Clin. Neurophysiol. 24:374, 1968.

Bleyaert, A. L., et al.: Amelioration of postischemic encephalopathy by sodium thiopental after 16 minutes of global brain ischemia in monkeys. Physiologist 18:145, 1975; Acta Neurol. Scand. (Suppl. 64) 56:144, 1977.

Bleyaert, A. L., et al.: Augmentation of postischemic brain damage by repetitive hypertension. Anesthesiology (to be submitted, 1978).

Bouzarth, W. F.: Neurosurgical watch sheet for craniocerebral trauma. J. Trauma 8:29, 1968.

Boysen, G., Fieschi, C., and Lassen, N. A.: On the critical lower level of cerebral blood flow in man. Circulation 49:1023, 1974.

Brierley, J. B., Meldrum, B. S., and Brown, A. W.: The threshold and neuropathology of cerebral "anoxic-ischemic" cell change. Arch. Neurol. 29:367, 1973.

Brown, R. E.: Analysis of echoencephalograms. Neurology (Minneap.) 18:237, 1968.

Brown, R. S., and Shoemaker, W. C.: Sequential hemodynamic changes in patients with head injury: evidence for an early hemodynamic defect. Ann. Surg. 177:187, 1972.

Bruce, D. A., et al.: Regional cerebral blood flow, intracranial pressure, and brain metabolism in comatose patients. J. Neurosurg. 38:131, 1973.

Bryan-Brown, C. W., et al.: Cerebral edema unresponsive to conventional therapy in neurosurgical patients with unsuspected nutritional failure. Crit. Care Med. 1:125, 1973.

Clasen, R. A., Pandolfi, S., and Laing, I.: Experimental study of fever in cerebral edema. J. Neurosurg. 41:576, 1974.

Clasen, R. A., Pandolfi, S., and Casey, D.: Furosemide and pentobarbital in cryogenic cerebral injury and edema. Neurology (Minneap.) 24:642, 1974.

Clasen, R. A., Pandolfi, S., and Casey, D.: Reserpine in experimental cerebral edema: further observations. Neurology (Minneap.) 24:594, 1974.

Cohen, P. J., et al.: Effects of hypoxia and normocarbia on cerebral blood flow and metabolism in conscious man. J. Appl. Physiol. 23:183, 1967.

Cook, D. R., et al.: Resuscitation of the brain in metabolic failure. Experience with Reye's syndrome. In Total Parenteral Alimentation. (Rome, Italy, 1975 Congress). New York, American Elsevier Publ. Co., 1976.

Cotev, S., and Severinghaus, J. W.: Role of cerebrospinal fluid in the management of respiratory problems. Anesth. Analg. 48:42, 1969.

Cyrus, A., et al.: Effect of low molecular weight dextran in cerebral infarction. Marquette Med. Rev. 4:180, 1962.

DeVivo, D. C., and Keating, J. T.: Reye's syndrome. Adv. Ped. 22:175, 1976.

DeSouza, S. W., Dobbing, J., and Adlard, B. P. F.: Glycerol in treatment of cerebral oedema. Lancet 1:835, 1975.

Farhat, S., and Schneider, R.: Observations on the effect of systemic blood pressure on intracranial circulation in patients with cerebrovascular insufficiency. J. Neurosurg. 27:441, 1967.

Farmati, O., et al.: Retinal observations in dying and resuscitation. Anesthesiology 29:189, 1968.

Fischer, E. G.: Impaired perfusion following cerebrovascular stasis. Arch. Neurol. 29:361, 1973.

Fischer, E. G., and Ames, A., III: Studies on mechanisms of impairment of cerebral circulation following ischemia: effect of hemodilution and perfusion pressure. Stroke 3:538, 1972.

Gilroy, J., Barnhart, N., and Meyer, J.: Treatment of acute stroke with dextran 40. J.A.M.A. 210:293, 1969.

Gjerris, F., and Schmidt, K.: Chronic subdural hematoma: surgery or mannitol treatment. J. Neurosurg. 40:639, 1974.

Gordon, E.: Controlled respiration in the management of patients with traumatic brain injuries. Acta Anaesth. Scand. 15:193, 1971.

Gordon, E.: The acid-base balance and oxygen tension of the cerebrospinal fluid and their implications for the treatment of patients with brain lesions. Acta Anaesth. Scand. (Suppl.) 39:7, 1971.

Gregersen, M. I., et al.: Blood viscosity at low shear rates. Effects of low and high molecular dextrans. Biorheology 1:247, 1963.

Gurvitch, A. M.: Determination of the depth and reversibility of postanoxic coma in animals. Resuscitation 3:1, 1974.

Haider, W., et al.: Metabolic changes in the course of severe acute brain damage. Europ. J. Int. Care Med. 1:19, 1975.

Harvard Medical School Ad Hoc Committee to Examine the Definition of Brain Death: A definition of irreversible coma. J.A.M.A. 205:337, 1968.

Hoff, J. T., et al.: Barbiturate protection from cerebral infarction in primates. Stroke 6:28, 1975.

Hossmann, K. A.: Cortical steady potential, impedance and excitability changes during and after total ischemia of cat brain. Exper. Neurol. 32:163, 1971.

Hossmann K. A., and Kleihues, P.: Reversibility of ischemic brain damage. Arch. Neurol. 29:375, 1973.

Hossmann, K. A., Lechtape-Gruter, H., and Hossman, V.: The role of cerebral blood flow for the recovery of the brain after prolonged ischemia. Z. Neurol. 204:281, 1973.

Huttenlocher, P. R.: Treatment of hydrocephalus with acetazolamide. Results in 15 cases. J. Ped. 66:1023, 1965.

Ingvar, D. H., and Lassen, N. A.: Focal cerebral ischemia treated with hyperbaric oxygen. Nord. Med. 72:1352, 1974.

Jannetta, P. J.: Observations on the etiology of trigeminal neuralgia, hemifacial spasm, acoustic nerve dysfunction and glossopharyngeal neuralgia. Definitive microsurgical treatment and results in 117 patients. Neurochirurgia, in press, 1977.

Javid, M.: Urea—new use of an old agent. Reduction of intracranial and intra-ocular pressure. Surg. Clin. North Am. 38:907, 1958.

Johansson, B., Strandgaard, S., and Lassen, N. A.: On the pathogenesis of hypertensive encephalopathy. The hypertensive "breakthrough" of autoregulation of cerebral blood flow with forced vasodilatation, flow increase, and blood brain barrier damage. Circ. Res. 34 (suppl. 1) *1*:167, 1974.

Johnston, I. H., Johnston, J. A., and Jennett, B.: Intracranial pressure changes following head injury. Lancet 2:433, 1970.

Kerr, F. W. L.: Radical decompression and dural grafting in severe cerebral edema. Mayo Clin. Proc. *43*:852, 1968.

Kety, S. S.: Circulation and metabolism of the human brain in health and disease. Am. J. Med. 8:205, 1950.

Kindt, G. W., et al.: Intracranial pressure in Reye's syndrome. J.A.M.A. *231*:822, 1975.

Kramer, R. S., et al.: The effect of profound hypothermia on preservation of cerebral ATP content during circ. arrest. J. Thorac. Cardiovasc. Surg. 56:699, 1968.

Kovach, A. G. B.. Importance of nervous and metabolic changes in the development of irreversibility in experimental shock. Discussion of paper by Levenson. Fed. Proc. 20/2 (part 3):122, 1961.

Larson, S. J., et al.: Non-invasive evaluation of head trauma patients. Surgery *74*:34, 1973.

Lind, B., et al.: A review of total brain ischemia models in dogs and original experiments on clamping the aorta. Resuscitation (Brit.) 4:19, 1975.

Lind, B., Snyder, J., and Safar, P.: Total brain ischemia in dogs. Cerebral physiologic and metabolic changes after 15 minutes of circulatory arrest. Resuscitation 4:97, 1975.

Loughhead, M., et al.: ICU patient categorization. Crit. Care Med. *4*:108, 1976.

Luisada, A. A.: Mechanism of neurogenic pulmonary edema. Am. J. Cardiol. *20*:66, 1967.

Lundberg, N.: Continuous recording and control of ventricular fluid pressure in neurosurgical practice. Acta Psychiat. Neurol. Scand. 36:Suppl. 149, 1960.

Luttrell, C. N., Finberg, L., and Drawdy, L. P.: Hemorrhagic encephalopathy induced by hypernatremia. II. Experimental observations on hyperosmolarity in cats. A.M.A. Arch. Neurol. *1*:153, 1959.

Macaulay, D., and Watson, M.: Hypernatraemia in infants as a cause of brain damage. Arch. Dis. Child. *36*:543, 1961.

Marshall, L. F., et al.: Pentobarbital therapy for intracranial hypertension in metabolic coma. Crit. Care Med. Jan. 1978.

Marshall, S., and Hinman, F., Jr.: Subdural hematoma following an administration of urea for diagnosis of hypertension. J.A.M.A. *182*:813, 1962.

Mattar, J. A., Weil, M. H., and Shubin, H.: A study of the hyperosmolal state in critically ill patients. Crit. Care Med. *1*:293, 1973.

Meyer, J. S., et al.: Treatment with glycerol of cerebral edema due to acute infarction. Lancet 2:993, 1971.

Michenfelder, J. D., and Theye, R. A.: The effects of anesthesia and hypothermia on canine cerebral ATP and lactate during anoxia produced by decapitation. Anesthesiology 33:430, 1970.

Michenfelder, J. D.: Failure of prolonged hypocapnia, hypothermia or hypertension to favorably alter acute stroke in primates. Stroke 8:87, 1977.

Mickell, J. J., et al.: Intracranial pressure monitoring in Reye–Johnson syndrome. Crit. Care Med. *4*:1, 1976.

Mickell, J. J., et al.: ICP monitoring and normalization therapy in children. Pediatrics 58:606, 1977.

Miller, J. R., and Myers, R. E.: Neurological effects of systemic circulatory arrest in the monkey. Neurology *20*:715, 1970.

Moody, R. A., and Mullan, S.: Head injury monitoring: a preliminary report. J. Trauma *11*:458, 1971.

Moss, G.: The role of the central nervous system in shock: the centroneurogenic etiology of the respiratory distress syndrome. Crit. Care Med. 2:131, 1974.

Mostert, J. W., Kenny, G. M., and Murphy, G. P.: Safe placement of central venous catheter into internal jugular veins. Arch. Surg. *101*:431, 1970.

Myers, R. E.: Two classes of dysergic brain abnormality and their conditions of occurrence. Arch. Neurol. 29:394, 1973.

Nemoto, E. M., et al.: Postischemic encephalopathy (PIAE): a long-term monkey model for therapy evaluation. (a) Fed. Proc. *34*:384, 1975 (abst. #933). (b) Stroke 8:558, 1977.

Nemoto, E. M., Erdmann, W., and Strong, E.: Regional brain Po₂ after 16 minutes global cerebral ischemia in monkeys. Crit. Care Med. 4/2:129, 1976.

Nemoto, E. M., et al.: Global ischemia in dogs: cerebrovascular CO₂ reactivity and autoregulation. Stroke 6:425, 1975.

Nemoto, E. M., et al.: Amelioration of post-ischemic-anoxic brain damage by thiopental. *In* Safar, P. (ed.): Advances in CPR. (Wolf Creek Conference Proceedings, Oct. 1975.) New York, Springer Verlag, 1977.

Newkirk, T. A. Tourtellotte, W. W., and Reinglass, J. L.: Prolonged control of increased intracranial pressure with glycerin. Arch. Neurol. 27:95, 1972.

Nilsson, B., Norberg, K., and Siesjö, B. K.. Biochemical events in cerebral ischemia. Br. J. Anaesth. 47:751, 1975.

Obrist, W. D., et al.: Regional cerebral blood flow estimated by ¹³³Xenon inhalation. Stroke 6:245, 1975.

Osterholm, J., et al.: Experimental effects of free serotonin on the brain and its relation to brain injury. J. Neurosurg. *31*:408, 1969.

Pappius, H. M.: Biochemical Studies on Experimental Brain Edema. *In* Klatz, I. and Seitelberger, F. (eds.): Brain Edema. New York, Springer Verlag, 1967.

Pappius, H. M., and McCann, W. P.: Effects of steroids on cerebral edema in cats. Arch. Neurol. 20:207, 1969.

Patten, B. M., et al.: Double blind study of the effects of dexamethasone on acute stroke. Neurology (Minneap.) 22:377, 1972.

Posner, J. B., Swanson, A. G., and Plum, F.: Acid-base balance in cerebrospinal fluid. Arch. Neurol. *12*:479, 1965.

Prior, P. F., et al.: Monitoring cerebral function: clinical experience with new device for continuous recording of electrical activity of brain. Br. Med. J. 2:736, 1971.

Ransohoff, J.: The Effects of Steroids on Brain Edema in Man. *In* Reulen, H. J.: Steroids and Brain Edema. New York, Springer Verlag, 1972.

Reulen, H. J.: Steroids and Brain Edema. New York, Springer Verlag, 1972.

Reye, R. D. K., Morgan, G., and Baral, J.: Encephalopathy and fatty degeneration of the viscera: a disease entity in childhood. Lancet 2:749, 1963.

Rosomoff, H. L.: Hypothermia and cerebral vascular lesions. II. Experimental middle cerebral artery interruption followed by induction of hypothermia. A.M.A. Arch. Neurol. Psychiatr. 78:454, 1957.

Rosomoff, H. L., et al.: Experimental brain injury and delayed hypothermia. Surg. Gynecol. Obstet. *110*:27, 1960.

Rosomoff, H. L., and Zubibe, F. P.: Distribution of intracranial contents in experimental edema. Arch. Neurol. 9:26, 1963.

Rotheram, E. B., Safar, P., and Robin, E. D.: CNS disorder during mechanical ventilation in chronic pulmonary disease. J.A.M.A. *189*:993, 1964.

Rovit, R. L., and Hagan, R.: Steroids and cerebral edema: the effect of glucocorticoids on abnormal capillary permeability following cerebral injury in cats. J. Neuropathol. Exper. Neurol. 27:277, 1968.

Safar, P.: Maintenance of brain homeostasis in critical care. Proceedings of Annual Symposia on Critical Care Medicine, Univ. of Pittsburgh, May, 1975.

Safar, P., Nemoto, E. M., and Severinghaus, J. W.: Pathogenesis of central nervous system disorder during artificial hyperventilation in compensated hypercarbia in dogs. Crit. Care Med. *1*:5, 1973.

Safar, P., Stezoski, W., and Nemoto, E. M.: Amelioration of brain damage following 12 minutes of cardiac arrest in dogs. Fed. Proc. *34*:384, 1975; Arch. Neurol., 33:91, 1976.

Safar. P.: Cardiopulmonary-cerebral resuscitation (CPCR). *In* Advances in CPR. (Wolf Creek Conference Proceedings, Oct. 1975.) New York, Springer Verlag, 1977.

Schneider, M.: Circulation, Blood Flow, Oxygen Diffusion and Metabolism. Part I. Critical Blood Pressure in the Cerebral Circulation. *In* Schade, J., and McMenemey, W. (eds.): Selective Vulnerability of the Brain in Hypoxemia. Philadelphia, F. A. Davis Co., 1963.

Schutz, H., et al.: Brain mitochondrial function after ischemia and hypoxia. I. Ischemia induced by increased intracranial pressure. II. Normotensive systemic hypoxemia. Arch. Neurol. 29:408, 1973.

Secher, O., and Wilhjelm, B.: The protective action of anesthetics against hypoxia. Canad. Anaes. Soc. J. *15*:423, 1968.

Severinghaus, J. W.: Role of cerebrospinal fluid pH in normalization of cerebral blood flow in chronic hypocapnia. Acta Neurol. Scand. (Suppl.) *14*:116, 1965.

Severinghaus, J. W.: Blood gas calculator. J. Appl. Physiol. *21*:1108, 1966.

Shalit, M. N., et al.: The blood flow and oxygen consumption of the dying brain. Neurology 20:740, 1970.

Shapiro, H. M., et al.: Rapid intraoperative reduction of intracranial pressure with thiopentone. Br. J. Anaes. 45:1057, 1973.

Shapiro, H. M., Wyte, S. R., and Loeser, J.: Barbiturate augmented hypothermia for reduction of persistent intracranial hypertension. J. Neurosurg. *40*:90, 1974.

Siesjö, B. K., and Ljunggren, B.: Cerebral energy reserves after prolonged hypoxia and ischemia. Arch. Neurol. 29:400, 1973.

Slater, G. I., et al.: Sequential changes in distribution of cardiac output in hemorrhagic shock. Surgery 73:714, 1973.

Smith, A. L., et al.: Barbiturate protection in acute focal cer. ischemia. Stroke 5:1, 1974; Anesthesiology 47: 285, 1977.

Smith, A. L., and Margue, J. J.: Anesthetics and cerebral edema. Anesthesiology 5:64, 1976.

Snyder, J. V., et al.: Global ischemia in dogs: intracranial pressures, brain blood flow and metabolism. Stroke 6:21, 1975.

Soloway, M., et al.: The effect of hyperventilation on subsequent cerebral infarction. Anesthesiology 29:975, 1968.

Stept, W., and Safar, P.: Rapid induction–intubation for prevention of gastric content aspiration. Anesth. Analg. 49:633, 1970.

Stockard, J. J., et al.: Hypotension induced changes in cerebral function during cardiac surgery. Stroke 5:730, 1974.

Stone, H. H., et al.: The Effect of Acute Hemorrhagic Shock on Cerebral Circulation and Metabolism of Man. *In* Shock and Hypotension. New York, Grune & Stratton, 1965.

Stullken, E. H., and Sokoll, M.D.: The effects of heparin on recovery from ischemic brain injuries in cats. Anesth. Anat. Analg. 55:683, 1976.

Sveinsdottir, E., and Lassen, N. A.: A 254-Detector System for Measuring Regional Cerebral Blood Flow. *In* Langfitt, McHenry, Reivich & Wollman (eds.): Cerebral Circulation and Metabolism. New York, Springer Verlag, 1975.

Tabaddor, K.: Prognostic value of cerebral blood flow and cerebral metabolic rate of oxygen in acute head trauma. J. Trauma *12*:1053, 1972.

Teasdale, G., and Jennett, B.: Assessment of coma and impaired consciousness. Lancet, pg. 81, July 13, 1974.

Tourtellotte, W. W., Reinglass, J. L., and Newkirk, T. A.: Cerebral dehydration action of glycerol. I. Historical aspects with emphasis on the toxicity and intravenous administration. Clin. Pharmacol. Therap. *13*:159, 1972.

vanHarrevelt, A., and Ochs, S.: Cerebral impedance changes after circulatory arrest. Am. J. Physiol. *187*:180, 1956.

Vranova, Z., Keszler, H., and Vrana, M.: Oxygen tension in the cerebral cortex of dogs in haemorrhagic shock and its changes after oxygen therapy. Acta Anaesth. Scand. *12*:171, 1968.

Vries, J. K., Becker, D. P., and Young, H. F.: A subarachnoid screw for monitoring intracranial pressure. J. Neurosurg. 39:416, 1973.

Wechsler, R. L., Dripps, R. D., and Kety, S. S.: Blood flow and oxygen consumption of the human brain during anesthesia produced by thiopental. Anesthesiology *12*:308, 1953.

Wecht, C. H.: Determination of death. Bull. Allegheny Co. Med. Soc. 58:29, 1969.

Weiss, M. H.: Head trauma and spinal cord injuries: diagnostic and therapeutic criteria. Crit. Care Med. 2:311, 1974.

Wilhjelm, B. J., and Arnfred, I.: Protective action of some anaesthetics against anoxia. Acta Pharmacol. Toxicol. 22:93, 1965.

Wilkinson, H. A., Wepsic, J. G., and Austen, G.: Diuretic synergy in the treatment of acute experimental cerebral edema. J. Neurosurg. 34:203, 1971.

Wise, G., Sutter, R., and Burkholder, J.: The treatment of brain ischemia with vasopressor drugs. Stroke 3:135, 1972.

Wolin, L. R., and Massopust, L. C., Jr.: Behavioral effects of arrest of cerebral circulation in the Rhesus monkey. Exp. Neurol. 34:323, 1972.

Yatsu, F. M., et al.: Experimental brain ischemia: protection from irreversible damage with a rapid-acting barbiturate (methohexital). Stroke 3:726, 1972.

Zervas, N. T., and Hedley-Whyte, J.: Successful treatment of cerebral herniation in five patients. N. Engl. J. Med. *286*:1075, 1972.

II The Spinal Cord

Albin, M. S., and Bunegin, L.: Catecholamine synthesis rates in traumatized spinal cord. Anat. Rec. *178*:296, 1974.

Albin, M. S., et al.: Study of functional recovery produced by delayed localized cooling after spinal cord injury in primates. J. Neurosurg. 29:113, 1968.

Albin, M. S., et al.: Effects of localized cooling on spinal cord trauma. J. Trauma 9:1000, 1969.

Bosch, A., Stauffer, E. S., and Nickel, V. L.: Incomplete traumatic quadruplegia. J.A.M.A. 216:473, 1971.

Botterell, E. H., et al.: A model for the future care of acute spinal cord injuries. Ann. Royal Coll. Physicians Surgeons Can., 193, 1975.

Bucy, P. C.: Edgar A. Kahn Lecture—Spinal cord injury. Univ. Mich. Med. Center J. 39:71-77, 1973.

Ducker, T. B., and Assenmacher, D. R.: The microvascular response to experimental spinal cord trauma. Surg. Forum 20:428, 1969.

Ducker, T. B., and Hamit, H. F.: Experimental treatments of acute spinal cord injury. J. Neurosurg. 30:693, 1969.

Ducker, T. B., and Lucas, J.: Recovery from Spinal Cord Injury. In Seeman, P., Brown, G. M. (eds.): Frontiers in Neurology and Neuroscience Research, 1st Inter. Symp. of Neuroscience Inst., Univ. of Toronto. pp. 142-154, 1974.

Ducker, T. B., and Perot, P. L., Jr.: Spinal cord oxygen and blood flow in trauma. Surg. Forum 22:413, 1971.

Gildenberg, P. L., Dohn, D. F., and Henoch, M.: Local hypothermia in the treatment of spinal cord injuries. Cleveland Clinic Quarterly 39/3:109, 1972.

Goodkin, R. V., et al.: A survey of the management of experimental spinal cord trauma. Proc. 17th Spinal Cord Injury Conf., pp. 12-16, Sept. 1969.

Hedeman, L. S., Shellenberger, M. K., and Gordon, J. H.: Studies in experimental spinal cord trauma. I. Alterations in catecholamine levels. J. Neurosurg. 40:37, 1974.

Hung, T. K., et al.: Biomechanical responses to open experimental spinal cord injury. Surgical Neurol. 4:271, 1975.

Jacobson, S. A., and Bors, E.: Spinal cord injury in Vietnamese combat. Paraplegia 7/4:263, 1970.

Joyner, J., and Freeman, L. W.: Urea and spinal cord trauma. Neurology 13:69, 1963.

Kelly, D. L., Jr., et al.: Effects of hyperbaric oxygenation and tissue oxygen studies in experimental paraplegia. J. Neurosurg. 36:425, 1972.

Meacham, W. F., and McPherson, W. F.: Local hypothermia in the treatment of acute injuries of the spinal cord. South. Med. J. 66:95, 1973.

Osterholm, J. L.: The pathophysiological response to spinal cord injury. The current status of related research. J. Neurosurg. 40:3, 1974.

Tator, C. H., and Deecke, L.: Value of normothermic perfusion, hypothermic perfusion and durotomy in the treatment of experimental acute spinal cord trauma. J. Neurosurg. 39:52, 1973.

Thienprasit, P., et al.: Effect of delayed local cooling on experimental spinal cord injury. J. Neurosurg. 42:150, 1975.

Tribe, C. R.: Causes of death in the early and late stages of paraplegia. Paraplegia 1/1:19, 1963.

Wagner, F. C., Jr., and Bucy, P. C.: Recent research on spinal cord injury (editorial). Arch. Neurol. 27:465, 1972.

Wagner, F. C., Dohrmann, G. J., and Bucy, P. C.: Histopathology of transitory traumatic paraplegia in the monkey. J. Neurosurg. 35:272, 1971.

White, R. J., and Albin, M. S.: Spine and Spinal Cord Injury. In Gurdjian, et al. (eds.): Impact Injury and Crash Protection, Springfield, Ill., Charles C Thomas, pp. 63–85, 1970.

White, R. J., et al.: Spinal cord injury sequential morphology and hypothermia stabilization. Surg. Forum 20:432, 1969.

Yashon, D., Albin, M. S., and Demian, Y. K.: The technique of localized spinal cord hypothermia in the human. Proc. 17th Spinal Cord Inj. Conf. of Veterans Administration, 1971, p. 58.

GLOSSARY[*]

ATP	adenosine triphosphate
BBB	blood/brain barrier
CBF	cerebral blood flow
CBV	cerebral blood volume
$C\overline{cv}O_2$	mixed cerebral venous oxygen content, ml./100 ml.
CMRG	cerebral metabolic rate for glucose
CMRL	cerebral metabolic rate for lactate
$CMRO_2$	cerebral metabolic rate for oxygen
CNS	central nervous system
CPP	cerebral perfusion pressure, torr; ($\overline{SAP}$ minus $\overline{ICP}$)
CPPV	continuous positive pressure (controlled) ventilation, (IPPV plus positive end-expiratory pressure, PEEP)
CSF	cerebrospinal fluid
CVP	central venous pressure, torr
CVR	cerebrovascular resistance (i.e., CPP/CBF)
ECF	extracellular fluid
EEG	electroencephalogram (-graph)
EKG	electrocardiogram (-kardiogram) (-graph)
ICF	intracellular fluid
ICP	intracranial pressure, torr
IMV	intermittent mandatory ventilation (spontaneous breathing at atmospheric or positive pressure with rate controlled IPPV or CPPV superimposed)
IPPV	intermittent positive pressure (controlled) ventilation
IVP	intraventricular pressure (ICP)
F_IO_2	inhaled oxygen concentration
FIO_2	inhaled oxygen concentration
mEq./l.	milliequivalents per liter (or mEq./L.)
$Paco_2$	arterial carbon dioxide pressure, torr
Pao_2	arterial oxygen pressure, torr
$P\overline{cv}o_2$	mixed cerebral venous oxygen pressure, torr
PNPV	positive negative pressure (controlled) ventilation
$\overline{SAP}$	mean systemic arterial pressure, torr
torr	unit of pressure equal to 1 mm. Hg (named for Torricelli)

---

[*]Also see Tables 1 and 2.

Chapter 6

RENAL FAILURE AND FLUID-ELECTROLYTE IMBALANCE

Robert E. Binda

INTRODUCTION

This chapter will discuss the pathophysiology of acute fluid and electrolyte disturbances and required fluid therapy in emergency situations of patients with varying degrees of renal dysfunction. Under these conditions, fluid balance must become a more exacting endeavor since the kidneys are no longer capable of compensating for fluid and electrolyte changes as they do in the normal person. Since renal failure kills slowly and since the management of patients in Emergency Departments is brief, it was decided to focus in this chapter on facts that might help prevent further damage in the renal failure patient. This chapter will not attempt a comprehensive discussion of the pathophysiology of acute or chronic renal failure.

We will first review normal renal function and the body's ability to regulate fluid and electrolytes in the face of severe insults.

NORMAL RENAL FUNCTION

This section will be a brief review of how the kidney functions to effect salt and water homeostasis. It should establish a framework for the discussion of fluid balance in an emergency situation occurring in a patient with renal disease. Readers wishing a more detailed discussion of normal renal function can find this in several reference texts (Guyton, 1976; Strauss, 1971; Harvey, 1974).

Although the control of the body's fluid environment is the result of all nephrons working in concert, the regulatory role of the kidney can best be viewed by seeing how an individual nephron functions under a variety of conditions.

The basic function of a nephron is to clear the plasma of unwanted substances. These include some of the end-products of metabolism—for example, uric acid, urea, and creatinine—and excesses of many non-metabolic substances, such as sodium, potassium, and hydrogen ions. At the same time, the kidney conserves quantities of these same electrolytes and water in order to maintain the body's osmolality in a range essential for reasonable cellular function. Individual nephrons accomplish this task by filtering a large proportion of the plasma (approximately one-fifth) into the nephron's tubules, where unwanted substances fail to be reabsorbed.

The rate at which plasma is filtered into the nephron, the glomerular filtration rate (GFR), varies from 2 to 200 ml./min. in the adult (averaging 2 ml./kg./min.). Ninety-nine per cent of this fluid is reabsorbed during its course through the nephron. The GFR controls urine volume and, indirectly, plasma volume. Reduced plasma volumes produce vasoconstriction of the efferent arteriole of the glomerulus, which leads to a reduced GFR. Such diminished urine production will correct mild plasma volume deficits.

The nephron is also able to regulate the plasma osmolality. Water can be reabsorbed from the glomerular filtrate under the influence of the posterior pituitary's antidiuretic hormone (ADH). The free water (absence of

147

solutes) that is reabsorbed serves to reduce the osmolality of plasma while increasing that of urine. The normal range of osmolality found in the nephron's collecting duct is between 70 and 1200 mosm/L. depending on the presence (1200 mosm./L.) or absence (70 mosm./L.) of ADH. Plasma osmolality changes less than urine osmolality, because the smaller volume of urine is affected to a greater degree by a given change in free water clearance than is the larger plasma volume.

Regulation of sodium reabsorption by the kidney serves to maintain a functional quantity of this cation within certain body fluids and has a significant effect on the osmolality and the quantity of plasma and interstitial volumes. The kidney can limit the amount of sodium excreted to 0.5 to 1.0 mEq./L. of urine, thus allowing the patient to function with practically no sodium intake. On the other hand, sodium loading in a patient or experimental animal results in brisk excretion of sodium in the urine, provided the subject is neither sodium-depleted nor under the influence of aldosterone (as a result of hypovolemia, previously-forced diuresis, or dysfunction of the glomerulosa layer of the adrenal cortex) (DeWardener, 1961; Cortney, 1965; Johnston, 1966).

Finally, potassium, hydrogen ions, chloride, and bicarbonate are also subject to renal regulation. Since chloride and bicarbonate are the major anions reaching the renal tubules, their uptake and elimination follows that of the cation sodium to preserve electrical neutrality. As a corollary, a deficiency of either chloride or bicarbonate will lead to increased reabsorption of the other anion.

Potassium is almost completely reabsorbed in the proximal tubule, only about 20 per cent of the filtered potassium reaching the end of the proximal tubule. This proximal reabsorption of potassium is tied with sodium reabsorption in the same section of the nephron, and therefore is independent of both dietary intake and the potassium balance of the patient. In the potassium-depleted patient additional potassium is reabsorbed in the distal tubule, so that only 1 per cent of the filtered potassium is excreted in the urine. In the hyperkalemic patient, potassium is secreted into the tubule fluid by the distal segments of the nephron.

This distal secretion of potassium is tied with excretion of hydrogen ions. A deficiency of either of these cations leads to excretion of the other, often leading to depletion exemplified by the hypokalemia associated with metabolic alkalemia.

EFFECTS OF RENAL FAILURE

Renal disease is the result of a reduction in the number of functioning nephrons. Man is born with about 20 million nephrons, and it has been stated that one can survive, although with some difficulty, if only 20,000 function. The remaining nephrons, however, must increase their work load. If, for example, the number of functioning nephrons were reduced to 50 per cent of normal, the remaining nephrons would have to handle twice the solute load of a normal nephron. This added solute load then prevents the urine from being concentrated to its maximum of 1200 mosm./L. In this situation, therefore, the maximum response to dehydration would be a urine osmolality of 600 mosm./L. instead of the normal 1200 mosm./L., and the patient with this degree of renal dysfunction would be limited in his ability to tolerate fluid deprivation. In addition, as a result of this reduction in the number of functioning nephrons, there is also a diminished ability to excrete a water load. Renal disease, therefore, leaves the patient with little reserve, and dehydration or overhydration may develop rapidly. Therefore, great care must be exercised in establishing a fluid balance in these patients.

Until now, we have concentrated on the function of the individual nephron. Since renal disease puts an excessive load of fluid and solutes on individual nephrons, the range of function of each nephron begins to be reduced.

Here it is appropriate to discuss the role of the renal system, as a whole, in the regulation of fluid and electrolyte status of a patient with renal dysfunction. The body loses water by two means.

(1) Through evaporation from skin and lungs and elimination within the feces (the volume eliminated through the GI tract in the absence of diarrhea is small, in the range of only about 150 ml./day). The total magnitude of these so-called insensible losses varies with the environmental temperature and humidity, but usually is around 300 ml./m²/day in the hospital environment, or about 10 ml./kg./day.

TABLE 1 Water Losses in a Hospital Environment

	NORMAL	RENAL DISEASE
Insensible Water Loss	300 l/m²/day or 10 ml./kg./day	Same as normal
Urinary Water Loss	10–25 ml./kg./day	0–50 ml./kg./day
Total	20–35 ml./kg./day	10–50 ml./kg./day

(2) In the form of urine. The usual loss via the kidney is 0.5 to 1.0 ml./kg./hour, or 10–12 ml./kg./day as a minimum value and 20–25 ml./kg./day as an average. Therefore, the minimum amount of fluid lost in a hospitalized patient would be about 10 ml./kg./day (in the absence of any urine production), and the maximum losses would depend on the volume of water eliminated by all routes combined, particularly by the kidneys. The polyuria of renal failure can be as much as 4 liters/day (approximately 50 ml./kg./day), while the urine production by normal kidneys is dependent on and varies with the fluid intake.

Table 1 summarizes the wide range of water losses that may exist in patients with renal disease. It is important, therefore, in assessing the water requirements of the patient to know his urinary losses, since his requirement may not be different from, and actually may exceed, that of patients without renal dysfunction. It also is important, when assessing water requirements, to remember that a patient ingesting a normal diet will accumulate about 750 ml. (10 ml./kg./day) from metabolism.

With regard to the handling of sodium, the patient with renal disease does vary significantly from the normal patient. With a GFR of 120 ml./min. (2 ml./kg./min.) there normally is reabsorbtion of all but approximately 1 per cent of the filtered sodium. The doubling of the sodium intake results only in an increase of this sodium extraction from the filtered load to about 2 per cent to maintain sodium balance. A normal person can triple his intake of sodium from approximately 150 mEq. to 400 mEq. without going into positive sodium balance by increasing the extraction rate up to about 15 per cent.

The patient with a decreased GFR secondary to loss of nephrons does not have a compensatory urinary excretion of sodium in the face of sodium loads. If the GFR is reduced from 120 to 10 ml./min., the extraction rate required to maintain sodium balance with an intake of 150 mEq. Na⁺ per day increases from 1 per cent to 10 per cent, and if this person's sodium intake were doubled, the required increase in extraction rate (20 per cent) would exceed his kidney's capabilities to eliminate sodium, and he would enter into positive sodium balance. Therefore, the patient with significant renal impairment may tolerate only about 300 mEq. of sodium per day without developing positive sodium balance and fluid retention.

Among the many molecular species that the *acute* renal failure patient is unable to excrete, postassium proved to be the most life-threatening. Hyperpotassemia should be suspected when there are bradycardia, hypotension, and typical EKG changes (high T wave, widened QRS complex). The occurrence of cardiac arrest (asystole or ventricular fibrillation) could not be correlated with specific serum potassium values, since tissue and serum K^+/Ca^+ concentration ratios vary with electrolyte shifts ongoing in acute critical illness or injury. Nevertheless, acute increases in serum K values to about 7 mEq/L. (normal value 3.5 to 5.5 mEq/L.) should not be left untreated. Treatment includes intravenous calcium and attempts to normalize serum potassium with intravenous glucose, plus insulin (1 unit regular insulin per 2 g. glucose), K-exalate enemas, peritoneal dialysis, and hemodialysis—in this approximate order of complexity.

Hemodynamic characteristics of the *chronic* renal failure patient usually include a high cardiac output with increased blood volume and interstitial volume, the tissue edema being the result of sodium and water retention as well as proteinuria and hypoproteinema.

Having reviewed the kidney's ability to regulate a patient's fluid and electrolyte balance, we can now outline an approach to the renal patient who presents to the Emergency Department with an alteration in his fluid and electrolyte status. Evaluation of this patient should include an assessment of his renal function, determination of the nature and degree of his fluid and electrolyte disorder, rational choice of an appropriate replacement fluid, and, finally, monitoring techniques to be employed in assessing the progress of therapy.

ASSESSMENT OF RENAL FUNCTION

Laboratory methods utilized to assess renal function often fail to detect any abnormalities until more than 60 per cent of this function is lost. Fortunately, up to this stage of impairment there are few overt problems of electrolyte and water balance. In spite of this limitation, in the emergency situation the tests listed below often are the only means available for delineating the renal status of the patient requiring fluid therapy. We will discuss the most commonly used tests and their shortcomings.

Blood Urea Nitrogen

The BUN blood level is dependent on renal function, nitrogen metabolism, and the state of hydration of the patient. Abnormal production of urea is often responsible for the alterations in BUN values clinically encountered. Urea is produced in the liver from amino acids, some of which come from the GI tract and others from the body's protein catabolism. Therefore, generalized reduction in liver function may result in a fall in the serum urea level (since amino acids are not converted to urea), and an increased delivery of amino acids to the liver secondary to GI bleeding will elevate the BUN.

In addition to the effect on the BUN of a variable synthesis of urea, the reliability of the urea nitrogen as a measure of the GFR is reduced because urea is not excreted simply as a function of the glomerular filtration as is inulin, but approximately 20 to 30 per cent of the filtered urea can be reabsorbed in the distal tubules and collecting ducts under the influence of ADH (Goldstein, 1969). As the number of functioning nephrons is reduced, the BUN becomes a better measure of the GFR.

Therefore, although the BUN can be utilized like the inulin clearance as a measure of the GFR, a dehydrated patient, or one with a GI hemorrhage, may have normal renal function and an elevated BUN level.

Creatinine and Creatinine Clearance

Creatinine is produced from phosphocreatine liberated with muscle contractions. Serum creatinine and endogenous creatinine clearance are more reliable than the use of an isolated measurement of the BUN. The difficulty with the serum creatinine is that creatinine is secreted as well as filtered, and with increasing serum levels of creatinine there is a compensatory increase in tubular secretion. Therefore, the serum creatinine reflects variable tubule function rather than GFR (Kim, 1969). In addition, although the creatinine clearance value should provide a reasonable measure of renal function, the above-mentioned difficulty with the serum creatinine, and errors in collection of a 24-hour urine sample, limit its usefulness. Twenty-three per cent of patients with a moderate decrease in their GFR were found to have a normal endogenous creatinine clearance (Price, 1972; Kim, 1969).

Urine Osmolality

The osmolality of the urine must be quite variable, in order to maintain normal serum osmolality. As the number of functioning nephrons begins to diminish, the ability to vary the urine osmolality also diminishes. Early in the course of renal disease, there is a loss of concentrating ability due to an osmotic diuresis that exists in the functional nephrons; as the GFR continues to decline, the urine osmolality begins to approach that of the plasma. Therefore, the elevated BUN found in dehydration can be separated from the elevated BUN associated with significantly compromised renal function, because, in dehydration, urine osmolality is often above 400 mosm./L., whereas in renal failure it is 250 to 350 mosm./L.

Urinary Sodium

Another test of renal function is the measurement of urinary sodium. A 24-hour measurement is best; however, spot checks of urine sodium can be used clinically as a guide to diagnosis and therapy while awaiting a 24-hour determination. As mentioned previously, urinary sodium excretion depends on sodium intake, but, with normal or restricted sodium diets, urine concentrations should remain below 20 mEq./L. The patient who has lost a significant number of nephrons and, as a result, his sodium-retaining capabilities, will generally have values of urinary sodium above 20 mEq/L. in spite of normal sodium intake.

ASSESSMENT OF FLUID AND ELECTROLYTE ALTERATIONS

The patient with renal disease can be subjected to the same alterations in fluid and electrolyte balance as a normal patient, and with the same consequences. For this discussion, we will consider fluid and electrolyte imbalances as falling into one of two categories: (1) absolute fluid and/or electrolyte changes in which either water and/or salt is gained or lost from the body; (2) distributional changes in which fluid and electrolyte changes occur within the body, resulting in a shift from one fluid compartment to another.

Absolute Imbalances

Here, fluid and electrolytes are either lost from or gained by the body. The volume of these changes can be measured either directly by collecting the losses and recording the gains, or indirectly by noting change in body weight. The composition of the fluids can be directly measured or estimated from knowledge of the fluid content (see Table 2).

Treatment of these absolute derangements in fluid balance in the renal patient should follow the same principles as in the normal person, keeping in mind the limited tolerance of renal patients for excess or insufficient fluid replacements. The safest approach is an accurate measurement of the

volume lost or gained and determination of the electrolyte content. In the absence of this capability, estimates made by noting weight changes and estimates of fluid composition are important substitutes required for therapy.

Distributional Imbalances

The management of these types of problems is more involved because they do not result in external fluid loss, and therefore the magnitude and composition of these losses are not readily measurable. As a result of this complexity and the surrounding controversy over therapy, more time will be devoted to the discussion of the management of these types of problems (see also Chapters 4 and 7).

Tissue trauma and ischemia-anoxia, as in hemorrhagic shock, with subsequent replenishment of blood volume by infusion of shed blood, are followed by a state of reduction in plasma volume and interstitial fluid volume. Although this loss of interstitial fluid into a "third space" has been demonstrated experimentally and clinically, there is continuing controversy about where this fluid goes. Possibilities include edema of traumatized tissue as well as shift of fluid from the extracellular into the intracellular spaces, due to hypoxic cell membrane failure. Distributional changes result in variation in volume and composition of the interstitial fluid as the result of changes occurring at the capillary level in response to trauma, hypoxia, or severe infection. The result of significant shifts in interstitial fluid volume and composition may be an impairment of transport between the intravascular and extracellular spaces. This would then impair nutrition of cells and elimination of waste-products, both of which will alter cell function and possibly tissue survival.

The magnitude and composition of these distributional changes is a subject for controversy arising from various interpretations of the events that occur in response to insults to the capillaries. The classic description of fluid movement across the capillaries was by Starling (1896), who hypothesized that there was no net gain or loss of fluid across the capillary bed. Recently, people have begun to question the validity of Starling's hypothesis (Intaglietta, 1973 and 1974), since in order to study the factors operative

TABLE 2   Solute Composition of Body Fluids°

FLUID	Na	K	CL	PROTEIN GM. %
		MEQ/L		
Gastric	20–80	5–20	100–150	
Pancreatic	120–140	5–15	90–120	
Sm. Intestine	100–140	5–15	90–130	
Bile	120–140	5–15	80–120	
Ileostomy	45–135	3–15	20–115	
Diarrhea	10–90	10–80	10–110	
Sweat:				
Normal	10–30	3–10	10–35	
Cystic Fibrosis	50–130	5–25	50–110	
Burns	140	5	110	3–5

°From Harriet Lane Handbook, Children's Medical and Surgical Center, The Johns Hopkins Hospital, Baltimore, Maryland 21205.

in the capillaries and tissues an artifical situation is created that interferes with and alters the very parameters being measured.

The simplified equation describing *Starling's hypothesis* is as follows:

$$Jw = K \times S \times [(Pc - Pi) + (\pi i - \pi c)]$$

where the net flow of water (Jw) across the capillary is related to capillary hydraulic conductivity (K), surface area (S), and the sum of the hydrostatic pressure difference between capillary (Pc) and tissue interstitial space (Pi) and the osmotic pressure difference between tissue interstitial space (πi) and capillary (πc).

Any stress that results in a decrease in capillary blood flow decreases capillary hydrostatic pressure, which favors reabsorption of interstitial fluid to maintain blood volume. In the absence of replacement of this volume, survival of tissues—and even the patient—has been thought to be compromised (Carrico, 1976). The composition of this interstitial fluid shift is approximated by the electrolyte content of the so-called balanced salt solutions. This has led many to advocate the use of these types of fluids for the treatment of conditions resulting in distributional fluid shifts. In dogs subjected to oligemic shock of a duration and severity sufficient to cause death in spite of reinfusion of all blood shed, approximately 50 ml./kg. body weight of fluid was lost into this "third-space" (Carrico, 1976). These volumes, when first replaced and subsequently mobilized from the "third space," could have significant consequences for the patient with renal impairment who may have difficulty in handling large quantities of fluid and sodium.

It should, however, be evident that the renal patient would get into trouble only with excessive intravascular volumes. He develops problems sooner than a normal person because his cardiovascular system is already compromised as a result of his renal disease. He has a greater intravascular volume to begin with, because of his decreased GFR. In addition, he has greater cardiac output because of chronic anemia (Neff, 1971). Both these factors put significant strain on his myocardial function, which then may deteriorate in the face of further volume stress resulting from intravascular volume overload during resuscitation. This is often evidenced by pulmonary edema or acute right heart failure, both of which may be difficult to treat in the patient with significantly compromised renal function, since the removal of this excess fluid is limited by the functional state of the kidneys. Having accepted a lesser ability to tolerate an overload of the intravascular space as the differentiating factor in the management of patients with compromised renal function, it then is apparent that careful assessment and continuous monitoring of intravascular volume is an essential part of fluid therapy in renal disease.

It should be recalled that the interstitial volume is in equilibrium with the intravascular volume. (Even though some investigators have questioned the validity of Starling's hypothesis, as mentioned above, they do not dispute this equilibrium.) Therefore, if there is a "third space" deficit, intravascular volumes will not remain elevated until this deficit is corrected. The patient with kidney disease not only can tolerate, but may well require the same magnitude of salt and water replacement as a normal individual as long as the losses are similar. The end-point of therapy should then be either when the clinical status of the patient stabilizes, or when evidence of an increased intravascular volume persists for a reasonable time.

In summary, the patient with renal disease may present to the Emergency Department with an alteration in either the intravascular or the interstitial volume, or both.

TABLE 3

| | BLOOD VOLUME | | |
	INCREASED	UNCHANGED	DECREASED
INTERSTITIAL VOLUME Increased (Edema)	Circulatory Overload	Mild Overload (Peripheral Edema)	Capillary Leak Syndrome (Sepsis, Peritonitis)
Decreased		Compensated Hypovolemia	Uncompensated Hypovolemic Shock

Some of these conditions are listed in Table 3. The magnitude and composition of these losses can either be directly measured or estimated from data similar to those found in Table 2. When one is dealing with a patient whose fluid and electrolyte disturbance is the result of changes at the capillary level, estimates of this volume can be made and should guide therapy. The important aspect is monitoring the intravascular volume by some method, and reassessing the patient's condition as it changes during significant changes in his intravascular volume. Again, one may accept as an end-point in therapy either replacement of the estimated losses with sustained improvement of the patient's condition, or a protracted increase in the intravascular volume before the estimated volume of fluid required has been administered.

We will now discuss the choice of fluids that can be used in fluid and electrolyte therapy for patients with renal dysfunction.

REPLACEMENT FLUIDS

The choice of fluid should be influenced by the deficit one is trying to correct, whether intravascular, interstitial, or both. We will discuss each of these deficits and the advantages and disadvantages of the three types of fluids used in fluid replacement.

At the outset, let us point out that a deficit in the *intravascular volume* rarely exists by itself, with the exception of the so-called "capillary leak syndromes" mentioned in Table 3. The body tends to maintain this volume at all costs because of its important influence on the cardiac output. As mentioned above, interstitial fluid can be absorbed at the capillary level in an attempt to maintain the intravascular volume. Much of what will be said about the various fluids will be based on this concept.

Without forgetting this bias, the existing intravascular deficit still needs to be treated, and many solutions are advocated.

Blood

This may be in the form of packed RBCs or whole blood. This component of therapy is important, because patients with significant renal disease have chronic anemia,

which the body tries to compensate for by an increase in cardiac output. Further reduction in the circulating red cell mass, as would occur with blood loss, may exceed the ability of the cardiovascular system to compensate, and the result will be a reduction in oxygen delivery to the cells. When significant intravascular volume losses result in significant reductions in the hematocrit, transfusions are required. In healthy dogs, acute normovolemic hemodilution, as would occur with concurrent treatment of hemorrhage by colloid plasma substitutes (such as dextrans or hydroxyethyl starch), without red blood cells, results in reversible (slight) decompensation of cardiac output (which had increased to compensate for the anemia) at hematocrit levels between 10 and 25 per cent, and an irreversible decompensation at hematocrit values below 10 per cent (Takaori, 1968). Neff found the cardiac index to be above 5 L./m.²/min. when the hematocrit was below 23 per cent (1971). Limits of tolerance of acute anemia can be monitored by detecting an increase in blood lactate values and a decrease in mixed venous (central venous) oxygen values (Chapter 2).

Although maintenance of the hematocrit is important, the administration of blood is not without significant risks. There is a reported incidence of hepatitis occurring in 1.4 per cent of one-unit transfusions from volunteer donors, and 3 per cent of two-unit transfusions (Allen, 1972). With donor screening programs, the incidence of hepatitis can be reduced to two-thirds, but not eliminated. In addition, the use of blood transfusions in potential renal allograft recipients may sensitize them and hasten rejection of a donor kidney at a later date. Some investigators have recently questioned the validity of this concept (Festenstein, 1976). These risks must be weighed against the risk of the development of worsening anemia, and should not, when indicated, militate against transfusion. One must keep in mind, however, that any attempts to normalize hematocrit long-range in uremic anemia are futile, since impaired erythropoesis continues and the erythrocytes infused for the emergency eventually break down.

Albumin Solutions

These are effective intravascular volume expanders where the deficit is limited to this space. As pointed out above, an isolated reduction in intravascular volume rarely occurs, and, under circumstances in which changes have occurred in the interstitial volume of the patient, the use of albumin-containing solutions above may be associated with complications.

The popularity of albumin-containing solutions is based on the assumption that albumin remains in the intravascular space for extended periods, where it preserves the capillary osmotic pressure that, according to Starling's hypothesis, is important in preventing fluid from leaking into the interstitial space and preserving the intravascular volume. If this were indeed the case, intravascular deficits could be treated with the hepatitis-free human serum albumin, and interstitial deficits could be treated with appropriate fluids.

Unfortunately, there are several loopholes in these assumptions. As already stated, several investigators question Starling's hypothesis that albumin remains exclusively in the intravascular space. It appears that albumin leaks from the venular end of the capillary into the interstitial spaces of tissues. The interstitial and intravascular spaces are in equilibrium, and the interstitial spaces communicate with the intravascular space via the lymphatics. Total lymph flow rate is about 0.1 per cent of cardiac output a day. Protein that has left the intravascular space can thus be returned by the lymphatic route. The rate of protein exchanged is about 5 per cent per hour in normal adults (Parving, 1973-B); i.e., 5 per cent of the body's albumin leaves and re-enters the intravascular space each hour. The corresponding figure in normal infants is 18 per cent per hour (Parving, 1973-A). If exogenous albumin is administered, these turnover rates can increase up to threefold (Rossing, 1972).

The fact that 60 per cent of the body's albumin is actually extravascular, combined with the turnover rates of albumin as stated, gives the body an ability to maintain a stable serum albumin concentration under a variety of conditions. This albumin mobilization explains why, for each 10 per cent of intravascular volume lost, there is a decrease of only 2 per cent of the serum albumin concentration. Therefore, a loss of 50 per cent of the intravascular volume would result in only a 10 per cent decrease in the serum albumin concentration; this cannot be de-

tected accurately by the clinical methods presently available. The hypoproteinemia (hypoalbuminemia) of certain chronic illnesses (e.g., renal failure, hepatic failure) can be corrected only transiently with albumin infusion, since the underlying problems of protein loss (e.g., proteinuria in renal failure) or failure of albumin synthesis continue.

What are the clinical implications of these facts about the dynamics of albumin? In the first place, if the body can compensate for losses of albumin, the need to replace it obviously is reduced, especially if replacement is not without risk. The risk is related to the resulting increased escape of protein associated with the administration of exogenous albumin. Marty (1974) has alluded to some of the consequences of the increased interstitial albumin concentration that results from this increased turnover rate of infused albumin. Increased interstitial concentrations of protein will reduce lymphatic flow, and may exacerbate, not ameliorate, accumulations of interstitial fluid. Second, by increasing the concentration of albumin in the interstitial space of the liver, the endogenous hepatic production of albumin is reduced (Rothschild, 1969). Finally, an important consideration in dealing with patients with renal disease is that tubule reabsorption of sodium and water can be decreased as much as 20 per cent when the protein content of the renal interstitial fluid is increased. This may explain the greater renal dysfunction associated with albumin versus crystalloid fluid resuscitation from shock of various etiologies (Moncrief, 1973; Carey, 1971).

Another argument against the indiscriminate use of protein-containing solutions is the expense that this form of therapy involves (Skillman, 1976), but costs should not be a primary consideration when albumin may be life-saving. Weil's group has shown that in critically ill or injured patients without renal failure, particularly those with pulmonary failure, normalizing colloid osmotic pressure (normal values 22–29 torr) with albumin infusion can be life-saving, even if the effect of albumin is transient (Stein, 1975; Morissette, 1975). Also, there is a revival of the concept that not all colloid solutions have an equal effect on the microcirculation; dextran 40, for example, has a beneficial effect on capillary blood flow beyond the hemodilution itself, since it seems to reduce blood cell sedimentation rate and aggregation, and coats thrombocytes; its use results in a more effective increase in plasma volume, blood flow, and oxygen consumption in various shock states than either the same amounts of albumin or two to four times the volumes of crystalloid solutions (Shoemaker, 1976).

Crystalloid Solutions

These are solutions composed of water and electrolytes with or without supplemental dextrose (dextrose, 5 per cent in water without salt, should not be used).

The chief value of these solutions is their similarity to interstitial fluid, and therefore their ability to replace losses from this compartment. This discussion will be concerned with those solutions whose electrolyte concentrations approximate those of the interstitial space, namely, sodium in the range of 120 to 150 mEq./L. and potassium of 3 to 15 mEq./L.

Use of crystalloid solutions is advantageous since the composition is essentially the same as that of fluid lost from the interstitial spaces, and they are without the problems associated with blood and albumin. They are economic and, if given with adequate monitoring in large enough volumes to compensate for leakage into the interstitial space and for concomitant urine loss, can be used effectively to replace intravascular volume and sustain it for limited periods. Eventually, endogenously produced or externally-administered colloid is necessary, however, to sustain blood volume.

These fluids, however, have some theoretic and practical disadvantages of which the clinician should be aware. The commercially available preparations of Hartman's solution or lactated Ringer's solution contain small amounts of potassium. This is of little consequence to the patient with normal renal function, but it may be a significant problem to the patient with severe renal dysfunction. Therefore, when severe renal disease is present or when adequacy of renal function is in doubt, it is best to avoid this type of solution. Second, there is still concern expressed in the literature that the use of large quantities of crystalloid solutions may increase the incidence of pulmonary edema. Moss (1973) has shown, however, that, at least in the case of hemorrhagic

shock, changes of pulmonary edema were present before any resuscitative measures were instituted, and that the pulmonary edema that frequently complicated shock was not the result of saline infusions.

The still ongoing controversy between those favoring colloid solutions and those preferring crystalloid solutions in shock and trauma can be reconciled by interpretation of experimental and clinical data and physiologic reasoning: most *moderate* losses of plasma volume and interstitial fluid volume into the still undefined "third space" can be corrected with isotonic salt solution only — in the renal failure patient, isotonic sodium chloride. Long-term maintenance of normovolemia after *severe* blood loss, however, may require colloid in addition to crystalloid solutions, since the disadvantages of albumin are greater in the renal failure patient. As in the modern treatment of severe burns, it seems that a titrated "artistic" mix of various types of intravenous solution is the most reasonable approach for the critically ill or injured patient. This mix should include crystalloid, colloid (albumin and/or dextran 40 for specific indications) and erythrocytes to maintain hematocrit at 25 to 35 per cent. Clinical methods are needed to determine the altered permeability of capillary walls that would influence the choice of crystalloid versus colloid solutions; e.g., the use of albumin would be more logical if most of it did not leak from the intravascular space. Research is needed to determine the advantages and disadvantages of an overfilled as opposed to a dry interstitial space to the function of vital organs.

MONITORING DURING FLUID THERAPY

This aspect of care cannot be overstressed. Adequate monitoring is the cornerstone for the prevention of overload of the intravascular space, for which these renal patients have little tolerance. The two major systems requiring monitoring are the renal and cardiovascular.

Monitoring of the Renal System

When dealing with disease affecting any organ system, an assessment of the severity of that disease and the response of the organ system to stress is essential for the management of the patient. The same is true when the patient has varying degrees of renal dysfunction.

Earlier, we discussed various tests available to help the clinician to determine the degree of renal dysfunction present in a patient. Serial repetition of these measurements allows for monitoring of progress or improvement in the process being treated.

Information on the quantity and quality of urine the patient produces (normally 0.5 to 1.0 ml./kg. per hour of urine) is essential for the clinician. Access to urine flow may be necessary more often than just when and if the patient voids. Therefore, catheterization of the bladder is important in moderate-to-severe fluid disturbances. Renal failure with mild electrolyte and fluid disturbances can often be managed without an indwelling urinary catheter, which introduces an infection hazard.

Monitoring the Cardiovascular System

Since these patients have a limited tolerance of circulatory overload, we have advocated monitoring in order to prevent this complication.

Measurement of blood pressure, heart rate, urine flow, and central venous pressure may suffice in mild-to-moderate fluid derangements; however, with severe disturbances, intra-arterial blood pressure, pulmonary artery wedge pressure, red cell mass (chromium-tagged red cell method), and plasma volume (radioactive iodinated serum albumin method) may be of benefit when large quantities of fluids are to be administered.

Ancillary Measurements

Every patient's response to injury and therapy is different to some degree, and other measurements may need to be made.

The status of the respiratory system may be affected early in either the fluid imbalance or therapy, and serial determination of arterial blood gases will warn of the development of interstitial and alveolar pulmonary edema far in advance of any x-ray changes (Chapter 3). At the same time, the patient's acid-base status may reflect the adequacy of cardiac output. When doubt still exists, direct determination and serial moni-

toring of cardiac output can often be helpful in therapeutic endeavors.

In addition to the measurement of serum and urine osmolality, the monitoring of colloid oncotic pressure may influence care, although "normal" values for humans at bedrest range from 26 to 47 cm. H_2O (Parving, 1973).

CLINICAL APPLICATIONS

Using Table 3 for a framework, we can now apply some of these principles to the management of patients in the Emergency Department.

The important goal of initial therapy is to achieve an adequate intravascular volume, since insufficient volume limits cardiac output, and excessive volume may exceed the tolerance of an already over-stressed circulatory system. The assessment of intravascular volume in the Emergency Department needs to be a clinical one based on the vital signs and monitoring techniques that are readily available.

Excessive intravascular volume may be removed through the judicious use of diuretics, careful phlebotomy, and/or dialysis (time permitting).

Intravascular hypovolemia will respond to almost any type of fluid. The choice should be the clinician's, based on his experience and (it is hoped) influenced by the limitations of albumin solutions and the risk of potassium-containing solutions. Normal saline and packed red cells are associated with the least theoretic controversy. The volume of fluid required, of course, must be determined by titrated therapy. Aliquots of 20 ml./kg. to 30 ml./kg./hr. are reasonable estimates, but greater or lesser volumes may be required, and the physician should be guided by the patient's response and not by a preconceived estimate of the required amount of fluid.

Once the patient's intravascular volume has been temporarily stabilized, attention can be turned to the correction of interstitial volume disturbances. Here again, since the intravascular and interstitial spaces are in equilibrium, correction of the former with crystalloid will also correct the latter, and therapy can continue until the intravascular space begins to stabilize, reflecting a stabilization of the interstitial space. As with the intravascular volume, estimates of losses should be kept in perspective and therapy should actually be based on the patient's response.

SUMMARY

We have advocated here a titrated approach based on monitoring and a clinical impression of the patient's response to aliquots of fluid.

The patient in the Emergency Department should have his intravascular volume assessed and continually monitored while aliquots of crystalloid and packed red cells (when indicated by hematocrit changes) are administered, until a sustained stabilization of the vital signs and appearance of the patient is achieved. If, during the course of this approach, another vital organ system begins to fail, such as the pulmonary or cardiovascular, support of these systems is essential while fluid therapy is re-evaluated.

The management of fluid and electrolyte imbalances in patients with renal disease can be approached in a manner not too dissimilar from that employed in those with normal renal function. The frequent and accurate monitoring of intravascular volumes and renal function is an essential aspect of this approach to treatment.

References

Allen, J. G.: The case for the single transfusion. N. Engl. J. Med. 287:984, 1972.

Baue, A. E., et al.: Hemodynamic and metabolic effects of Ringer's lactate solution in hemorrhagic shock. Ann. Surg. 166:29, 1967.

Bennett, E. J., et al.: Fluid requirements for neonatal anesthesia and operation. Anesthesiology 32:343, 1970.

Carey, L. C., et al.: Hemorrhagic shock. Curr. Probl. Surg. January, 1971, pp. 3–48.

Carrico, E. J., et al.: Fluid resuscitation following injury. Rationale for the use of balanced salt solutions. Crit. Care Med. 4:46, 1976.

Cortney, M. A., et al.: Renal tubular transport of H_2O, solute, and PAH in rats loaded with isotonic saline. Am. J. Physiol. 209:199, 1965.

DeWardener, H. H., et al.: Studies on the efferent mechanism of the sodium diuresis which follows the administration of intravenous saline in the dog. Clin. Sci. 21:249, 1961.

Festenstein, H., et al.: Influence of HLA matching and blood transfusion on outcome of 502 London transplant group renal graft recipients. Lancet 1:24:157, 1976.

Giutierrez, V., et al.: Relationship of hypoproteinemia and prolonged mechanical ventilation to the development of pulmonary insufficiency in shock. Ann. Surg. 71:385, 1970.

Goldstein, M. H., et al.: Effect of urine flow rate on urea reabsorption in man: urea as a "tubular marker." J. Appl. Physiol. 26:594, 1969.

Guyton, A.: Textbook of Medical Physiology. Philadelphia, W. B. Saunders Co., 1976.

Harvey, R. J.: The Kidneys and the Internal Environment. New York, John Wiley & Sons, 1974.

Intaglietta, M., and Rosell, S.: Isovolumetric capillary pressure during rest and sympathetic nerve activity in canine subcutaneous adipose tissue. Acta Physiol. Scand. 87:532, 1973.

Intaglietta, M., and Zweifach, B. W.: Microcirculatory Basis of Fluid Exchange: Advances in Biological and Medical Physics. In Laurence, J. T., et al. (eds.). Vol. 15. Chicago, Year Book Medical Publishers, Inc., 1974.

James, P. M. et al.: Tolerance to long and short term lactate infusion in men with little penalties subjected to hemorrhagic shock. Surg. Forum 20:543, 1969.

Johnston, C. I., and Davis, J. O.: Evidence from cross-circulation studies for a humoral mechanism in the natriuresis of saline loading. Proc. Soc. Exp. Biol. Med. 121:508, 1966.

Kim, K. E., et al.: Creatinine clearance in renal disease. Br. Med. J. 4:11, 1969.

Marty, A. T.: Hyperoncotic albumin therapy. Surg. Gynecol. Obstet. 139:105, 1974.

Moncrief, J. A.: Burns. N. Engl. J. Med. 288:444, 1973.

Morissette, M., Weil, M. H., and Shubin, H.: Reduction in colloid osmotic pressure associated with fatal progression of cardiopulmonary failure. Crit. Care Med. 3:115, 1975.

Moss, G. S., et al.: The effect of saline solution resuscitation on pulmonary sodium and water distribution. Surg. Gynecol. Obstet. 136:934, 1973.

Neff, M. S., et al.: Hemodynamics of uremic anemia. Circulation 43:876, 1971.

Parving, H. H., et al.: Simultaneous determination of plasma volume and transcapillary escape rate in ^{131}I-labelled albumin and T-1824 in the newborn. Acta Paediatr. Scan. 62:248, 1973-A.

Parving, H. H., and Gyntelberg, F.: Transcapillary escape rate of albumin and plasma volume in essential hypertension. Circ. Res. 32:643, 1973-B.

Price, M.: Comparison of creatinine clearance to inulin clearance in the determination of the GFR. J. Urol. 107:339, 1972.

Rossing, N., et al.: Plasma Protein Catabolism in the Capillary Wall? Protides of the Biological Fluids. In Peeters, H. (ed.). New York, Pergamon Press, Inc., 1972, pp. 437–441.

Rothschild, M. A., et al.: Serum albumin. Am. J. Dig. Dis. 14:711, 1969.

Shoemaker, W. C.: Comparison of the relative effectiveness of whole blood transfusion and various types of fluid therapy in resuscitation. Crit. Care Med. 4/2:71, 1976.

Skillman, J. J., et al.: Peritonitis and respiratory failure after abdominal operations. Ann. Surg. 170:122, 1969.

Skillman, J. J.: The role of albumin and oncotically active fluids in shock. Crit. Care Med. 4:55, 1976.

Starling, E. E.: On the absorption of fluids from the connective tissue spaces. J. Physiol. 19:312, 1896.

Stein, L., et al.: Pulmonary edema during volume infusion. Circulation 52:483, 1975.

Strauss, M. B., and Welt, L. G.: Diseases of the Kidney. Boston, Little, Brown, & Co., 1971.

Takaori, M., and Safar, P.: Treatment of massive hemorrhage with colloid and crystalloid solutions. J.A.M.A. 199/5:297, 1967.

Chapter 7

GENERAL BODY RESPONSE TO TRAUMA

Donald S. Gann

The over-all response of the body to injury is the product of myriad changes in autonomic and endocrine functions. Despite the apparent complexity, however, this response can be viewed as a highly coordinated part of a sequence of reactions designed to preserve and restore the perfusion of tissues and the volume of blood. This chapter will examine the so-called metabolic response to injury as a part of the system mediating regulation of blood volume, and will examine the neurohumoral mediators of the metabolic response in terms of that regulation.

THE METABOLIC RESPONSE TO INJURY AND BLOOD LOSS

Before proceeding, it would be well to examine the pattern of response we are seeking to explain. The earliest and one of the most prominent features of the response to injury is hyperglycemia, described over 100 years ago by Claude Bernard. Together with this, there is an increase in circulating free fatty acids and in the turnover rate of amino acids. The latter commonly is accompanied by an increase in the plasma concentration of potassium. Depending on the severity of injury, there may also be an increase in circulating lactate and a systemic acidosis. Hemodilution follows, with a fall in the hematocrit and often in the plasma concentration of sodium.

Prominent changes in renal function also form part of the response to injury. Principal among these is the retention of salt and water, together with a somewhat less prominent increase in excretion of potassium and hydrogen ions. It is important to note at the

outset that these changes can prevent further loss of body fluids, but in the absence of an increased intake they cannot lead to a net positive balance of sodium or of water.

REGULATION AND CONTROL

At times it is useful to distinguish between the concept of regulation and that of control. By *regulation* is meant a special kind of control in which the range of a particular variable is held constant within very narrow limits. In contrast, in *control* the values of output variables may vary widely. Negative feedback, through which features of an output variable affect the response of the system, is a prominent feature of all regulating systems and of many other control systems as well. In addition to limiting the magnitude of a response, negative feedback also in general accelerates the response of a system. This response may also be affected by a less commonly known feature of control, feedforward, in which through a parallel path a feature of a stimulus may alter the gain or temporal features of a response. In this context, gain is meant to imply the ratio of a change in response to a change in stimulus. Thus, in a regulating system, such a change is minimized.

The circulating blood volume is one of the most tightly regulated variables in the body. Any perturbation of blood volume leads to immediate and far-ranging changes that act to offset this disturbance and to restore the blood volume to its initial value. Blood pressure tends to be less well regulated, but is still held within narrow limits. In contrast, certain features of body composition, including concentrations of circulat-

158

ing glucose and other small molecules and secretion rates of a variety of hormones, are well controlled but vary widely over a broad range. Indeed, it is the wide range of operation of these control subsystems that permits the tight regulation of a function such as blood volume.

THE NEUROENDOCRINE RESPONSE TO INJURY

As pointed out almost 40 years ago by Blalock, the most prominent characteristic of trauma is a loss of circulating body fluids. This loss is the result not only of hemorrhage per se, but also of a shift of fluids into the so-called "third space," a region of fluid collection and edema that is the direct result of injury. Pain is also a prominent feature of trauma that, depending on the circumstances and level of consciousness, is commonly accompanied by anxiety, fear, and anger. As illustrated in Figure 1, hemorrhage and the associated loss of extracellular fluid volume impair the general functions of the cardiovascular system. This system, however, operates to provide a general inhibitory control over a variety of autonomic and endocrine functions. Some of these endocrine functions are controlled directly by the central nervous system; others through autonomic peripheral control. A loss of circulating volume thus decreases the cardiovascular inhibition of neural control and results in a general increase in a variety of functions of the sympathetic nervous system and of the endocrine glands. A few prominent exceptions to this will be discussed subsequently. At the same time pain and, if present, anxiety, fear, and anger, are prominent feedforward features of this response that bring the neuroendocrine response into action before changes in circulating blood volume have been sufficient to activate them.

As discussed below, the concerted effect of the neuroendocrine response is to restore the initial state of the cardiovascular system, initially through increases in myocardial contractility and heart rate as well as in peripheral resistance, and subsequently through the shift of fluids into the vascular system. Thus, the system operates over-all to regulate certain cardiovascular functions and to offset the effect of volume loss. It does this both through a negative feedback system which senses the effects of loss of volume and operates to correct them, and through a feedforward mechanism which operates to anticipate the occurrence of volume loss.

BLOOD VOLUME RESTITUTION

The acute loss of blood volume sets in motion a set of mechanisms that operate first, to restore and maintain hemodynamic stability, i.e., arterial perfusion pressure; second, to restore a portion of the volume lost by transcapillary refilling from the interstitial fluid; third, to restore the remainder of the volume lost, as well as albumin which has also been lost by a shift of fluid from the intracellular to the interstitial volume, with concomitant increase in lymphatic return of preformed albumin and increase in lymphatic flow and in transcapillary refilling; fourth, to add newly synthesized albumin to the circulation to restore intravascular and extravascular stores; and fifth, to replenish the lost red cell mass. In addition, two auxiliary mechanisms are brought into action: through one, the renal excretion of sodium and water is decreased to prevent additional losses of volume; through the other, thirst and the appetite for salt are increased to stimulate ingestion of added water and salt.

The various phases involved in restitution of blood volume after hemorrhage occur

Figure 1. The neuroendocrine response to injury, general view. For details, see text. Abbreviations: ECF, extracellular fluid; CVS, cardiovascular system; CNS, central nervous system; SNS, sympathetic nervous system; +, stimulation; −, inhibition.

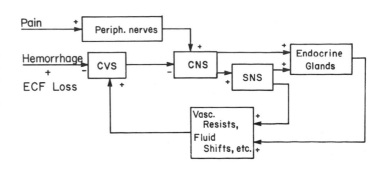

in the sequence indicated above, not all at once. The reflexes involved in hemodynamic stabilization occur in a matter of seconds to minutes. The initial phase of transcapillary refilling is completed in two to six hours, but the remaining restitution of fluid and of protein occurs over the next 18 to 24 hours. Newly synthesized protein is added to the circulation from 24 to 72 hours, and the synthesis of red cells is complete at only two to four weeks. Furthermore, this sequence is important not only because the organism might not survive to a later step if the earlier steps do not occur, but also because the early steps actually play a role in setting the later ones in motion. For example, precapillary vasoconstriction, which is a major component of the phase of hemodynamic stabilization, leads to a fall in capillary pressure. This decrease in capillary hydrostatic pressure is the principal force leading to an increase in transcapillary filling of fluid.

The phase of *hemodynamic stabilization* is set in motion in response to a change in activity of stretch receptors located in the arteries and in the atria. These receptors normally respond to mean arterial pressure, to the rate of change of arterial pressure, to atrial filling volume, and to the rate of change of that volume. A loss of circulating blood volume is sensed first in the low pressure portions of the circulation by the atrial receptors, and later by the arterial receptors. These receptors project to the central nervous system, where their activity leads to tonic inhibition of the vasomotor centers, which in turn mediate a variety of autonomic functions. When this inhibition is released secondary to the loss of volume, sympathetic nervous activity is stimulated and parasympathetic nervous activity is inhibited, with a resultant increase in myocardial force, heart rate, arteriolar constriction, and to some extent venular constriction. These changes operate to maintain perfusion pressure generally and to maintain flow itself to critical vascular beds, including the brain and myocardium. However, they do so by limiting perfusion of other vascular beds, including particularly the splanchnic region. This hypoperfusion of "less critical" beds leads to progressive tissue anoxemia and acidosis. If the loss of blood has been of sufficient magnitude, the ensuing prolonged vasoconstriction ultimately will prove fatal to the organism as the acids, kinins, prostaglandins,

and perhaps other toxic substances formed in these tissues are washed back into the general circulation.

This physiologic pattern for the restitution of blood volume may be impaired by major loss of volume with shock and reduced peripheral perfusion. The toxic substances (e.g., acids, kinins, and prostaglandins) formed during hypoperfusion may increase the permeability of capillaries, and thus lead to further leakage of fluid from the circulation. Further, with prolonged anoxia, the sodium pump may fail, leading to the sequestration of additional fluid within cells.

The *subsequent phases* which operate to restore lost volume also operate to relieve the intense sympathetic stimulation that underlies the phase of hemodynamic stabilization at the expense of limited perfusion of so-called "less critical" vascular beds. However, as noted above, the later phases are slower in their operation, so that if the initial loss of blood has been severe, or if the initial injury is profound enough to involve major translocations of functional extracellular fluid, vigorous fluid therapy is necessary if the harmful effects of the sympathetic component of the response are to be avoided. The effectiveness of such therapy lies not only in obviating the need for other phases of the response, but also in increasing pressures and volumes in the critical vascular beds containing the dominant receptors so that the initial reflex is turned off. Thus, what can be viewed in general terms as a baroreceptor reflex is the dominant organizing principle of the phase of hemodynamic stabilization and of the response to therapy. As will be seen below, this reflex also plays a central organizing role in the mediation of most of the other phases of the response to loss of volume.

Details of the Neuroendocrine Response to Loss of Volume

The various phases of restitution of blood volume after loss of blood volume are set in motion initially by losses in the rate of filling and in the amount of filling in the atria, augmented by subsequent decreases in arterial pulse and mean pressures. The details of the subsequent neuroendocrine reaction and of the principal effects of the components of this reaction on the restitution of blood volume are illustrated in Figure 2. In-

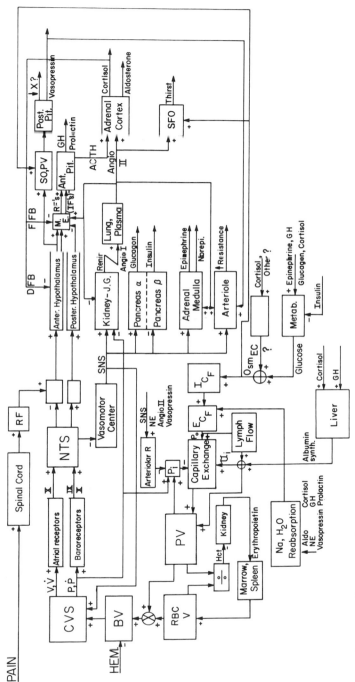

Figure 2. The neuroendocrine response to injury, detailed view. For details, see text. Abbreviations: RF, reticular formation; CVS, cardiovascular system; V, atrial filling volume; V̇, rate of atrial filling; P, arterial mean pressure; Ṗ, arterial pulse pressure; NTS, nucleus tractus solitarius; BV, blood volume; RBCV, red blood cell volume; PV, plasma volume; P_i, capillary hydrostatic pressure; π_i, capillary oncotic pressure; P_o, interstitial hydrostatic pressure; ECF, extracellular fluid volume; ICF, intracellular fluid volume; Hct, hematocrit; OSM_{EC}, extracellular osmolality; DFB, delayed feedback; FFB, fast feedback; ME, median eminence; RF's, releasing factors; IF's, inhibitory factors; SO, supraoptic nucleus; PV, paraventricular nucleus; GH, growth hormone; Angio, angiotensin II; JG, juxtaglomerular; SFO, subfornical organ; +, stimulation; −, inhibition.

formation is conveyed to the nucleus tractus solitarius and its surrounding areas in the medulla through the ninth and tenth cranial nerves. This nucleus not only sends inhibitory information to the vasomotor centers, but also projects through the midbrain reticular formation to the anterior and posterior hypothalamus. The activity of the reticular formation is also enhanced through pain sensations that reach the brain stem through spinal pathways and act in a feedforward manner as suggested above. As volume is lost and the inhibition of the vasomotor centers is decreased, sympathetic activity increases, as indicated previously.

Sympathetic stimulation, combined with a decrease of arterial pressure, stimulates the juxtaglomerular apparatus of the *kidney* to release the enzyme, renin, which results in the conversion of angiotensinogen to angiotensin I in the plasma. Most of the angiotensin I is converted in the lung to angiotensin II, but a small portion is also converted in the plasma itself. As will be shown subsequently, angiotensin II plays a central role in a feedforward manner, increasing the gain of many of the other components of the reflex. Sympathetic stimulation also acts on the *pancreatic* alpha cells to increase the rate of secretion of glucagon, and on the pancreatic beta cells to inhibit the secretion of insulin. These sympathetic effects are further augmented by reciprocal decreases in *parasympathetic* activity, since parasympathetic innervation normally acts to inhibit secretion of glucagon and to stimulate secretion of insulin. *Sympathetic* activity also leads to increased secretion of norepinephrine and epinephrine by the adrenal medulla. The epinephrine–norepinephrine ratio is determined by the availability of the adrenal cortical hormone, cortisol, which induces the enzyme N-methyltransferase in the adrenal medulla.

PITUITARY STIMULATION

The anterior hypothalamic projection from the solitary tract projects in part to supraoptic and paraventricular nuclei of the *hypothalamus,* where biosynthesis of vasopressin takes place. The vasopressin is transported to the *posterior pituitary,* and its release is thus augmented by loss of blood volume. The synthesis and release of vasopressin are also enhanced by increases in plasma osmolality, as indicated below. Furthermore, there is recent evidence to suggest that a factor (labeled "X" in Figure 2) which may play the role of a natriuretic hormone may be present in the posterior pituitary, and that its release may be inhibited by loss of volume. Both anterior and posterior hypothalamus also project to the hypothalamic median eminence. Although all details are not clear, it appears that a variety of anterior hypothalamic nuclei are responsible for the synthesis and transport to the median eminence of the various hypothalamic releasing factors. Projections from the posterior hypothalamus appear to act on the median eminence to inhibit the release of these releasing factors. In addition, for some anterior pituitary hormones, there are inhibitory factors which are also stored in the median eminence. In response to loss of blood volume, changes in the release of these factors ensue, which in turn change their rate of presentation via the hypophyseal portal vessels to the anterior pituitary gland.

The net effect is increased secretion of at least three anterior pituitary hormones: ACTH, growth hormone, and prolactin. The secretion rates of other pituitary hormones also may change, but have not been well studied.

ADRENAL CORTEX

If hemodynamic stabilization has taken place, the increased ACTH release from the anterior pituitary will be presented to the adrenal cortex and will result in increased secretion of cortisol and, to some extent, of aldosterone. The secretion of aldosterone is also stimulated primarily by angiotensin II, formed as described above. As the concentration of cortisol rises in plasma, there is an inhibition of the release of corticotropin releasing factor from the median eminence, which is critically dependent on the rate of rise of concentration of cortisol and which is termed "rate-sensitive" or "fast" feedback. Furthermore, after the peripheral concentration of cortisol has stabilized at an increased level for approximately one hour, the synthesis of corticotropin releasing factor is inhibited through a mechanism termed "proportional" or "delayed" feedback. There is some evidence that cortisol acts in a similar manner to inhibit the secretions of vasopressin and of growth hormone.

EFFECTS OF ANGIOTENSIN II

There is another internal feedback mechanism whereby angiotensin II acts on the juxtaglomerular apparatus to inhibit the release of renin. There may be additional negative feedback loops in this portion of the system, but they have not been well defined. Angiotensin II also acts on the median eminence to release corticotropin releasing factor. Finally, there is evidence that angiotensin II acts on the subfornical organ and/or in the lateral hypothalamus to increase thirst, which is also augmented by the so-called "intracellular mechanism" through changes in plasma osmolality.

Details of Restitution of Blood Volume

The effects of the neuroendocrine changes described above are illustrated in diagrammatic form in the lower and left sections of Figure 2. Sympathetic activity, circulating norepinephrine, angiotensin II, and vasopressin all increase arteriolar resistance. The latter two agents are particularly effective in the splanchnic bed. An increase in arteriolar resistance leads to a decrease in capillary hydrostatic pressure. The greater this pressure, the greater the propensity of fluid to move out of the capillary, so that a decrease in the pressure leads to an increase in *transcapillary filling*. As this filling takes place, however, the interstitial fluid pressure and capillary oncotic pressure fall, decreasing the rate of transcapillary filling. This decrease can be offset only by restoration of interstitial fluid through a shift of fluid from the cells to the interstitium. Such a shift, however, can occur only down an osmotic gradient.

An appropriate osmotic gradient occurs very rapidly following hemorrhage and other stresses, and may be sustained for two to six hours. Not all the components of the solute which account for this increase in osmolality have been defined, but glucose plays a minor role if the rate of hemorrhage is relatively small, and a major role if it is relatively large. The extracellular concentration of glucose is increased through the action of a number of the endocrine components of the neuroendocrine response, particularly including epinephrine and glucagon (which increase the rate of glycolysis) and growth hormone and cortisol (which act to decrease the rate of glucose entry into cells and thus to produce a transient diabetic state). Cortisol and glucagon also enhance gluconeogenesis, adding to the increase in circulating glucose concentration. Furthermore, since the secretion of insulin falls, the entry of glucose into cells is further impeded, with a still greater increase in extracellular concentration of glucose. For reference, an increase in glucose concentration of 18 mg./100 ml. is equivalent to an increase in solute concentration of one milliosmole/kg. H_2O.

INCREASE IN NONGLUCOSE SOLUTE

The nonglucose elements responsible for the increased concentration of solute have not been completely identified. However, it appears that changes in concentrations of amino acids and of free fatty acids, and, if the volume loss is sufficiently large, of lactate, may account for at least a portion of this solute. The concentration of free amino acids in the extracellular fluid will be increased through the antianabolic actions of cortisol and of glucagon, which impede the entry of amino acids into cells and thus lead to the net catabolic effect that is a major component of the metabolic response to injury. As nitrogen is lost from cells, potassium and water also move out of cells to maintain electrical neutrality and osmotic equilibrium, thus accounting for the increase in potassium in the extracellular fluid and for a portion of the fluid shift. The increase in free fatty acids results from the concerted actions of epinephrine, glucagon, ACTH, cortisol, and growth hormone, all of which act to induce lipolysis. The increase in nonglucose solute which follows volume loss has been shown to depend critically on an increase in rate of secretion of cortisol. However, it does not occur if cortisol concentration is increased but there is no concomitant stress. As indicated above, the increase in plasma osmolality may stimulate both thirst and the secretion of vasopressin, but from the point of view of restitution of blood volume its principal effect is to mediate the shift of fluid from the intracellular to the interstitial compartment.

Thus, the principal features of the metabolic response to injury all participate in this *shift of fluids*. As interstitial pressure increases, not only is capillary exchange facilitated but the rate of flow through the lymphatics is increased. Because the extracellular compartment is relatively rich in protein, the albumin store in this compartment is returned to the circulation through the increase in the lymphatic flow. This results in an increase in intravascular oncotic pressure which further facilitates transcapillary refilling and which also acts to prevent further loss of fluid from the capillaries. If the restoration of lost protein does not occur in this manner, the initial phase of transcapillary refilling and the accompanying decrease in arteriolar resistance will result in a fall of plasma oncotic pressure and a subsequent loss of fluid which has been reabsorbed during the first phase. Later, as a result of the actions of growth hormone and of cortisol, the synthesis of new albumin is stimulated and this albumin is added to the circulation to increase oncotic pressure, as well as to the interstitium.

RENAL EFFECTS

Renal excretion of salt and water is limited. Initially this may occur through a fall in glomerular filtration rate resulting directly from loss of blood volume and pressure. However, filtration rate is usually restored rapidly during the phase of cardiovascular stabilization unless volume loss is very large, since sympathetic stimulation leads to constriction of the efferent arteriole, which restores filtration pressure and rate. As this happens, however, and fluid is filtered from the glomeruli, the oncotic pressure of the peritubular capillary increases, leading to increased proximal tubule reabsorption of salt and water. This increase may be further facilitated through the action of circulating norepinephrine and through the decreased synthesis of intrarenal kinins, which may result directly, or from changes in the circulating level of the posterior pituitary natriuretic hormone described above. There is also some evidence that both growth hormone and prolactin may act to increase proximal reabsorption of salt and water. In the distal tubule, reabsorption of water occurs down an osmotic gradient in response to vasopressin. Also in the distal tubule, aldosterone leads to a reabsorption of sodium chloride together with water. In the late distal tubule and collecting duct, aldosterone facilitates sodium–potassium and sodium–hydrogen exchange, resulting in further reabsorption of sodium. As discussed earlier, this increased reabsorption serves only to limit further losses of fluid, but may contribute to additions to the extracellular fluid and plasma volumes if ingestion is increased through the stimulation of thirst, or if fluid therapy is undertaken.

As the plasma volume is restored, blood volume returns toward normal. However, during this process the concentration of *red cells* in the blood is reduced through hemodilution, and the hematocrit falls. This fall in hematocrit appears to signal the kidney to secrete erythropoetin, a hormone which stimulates red cell synthesis in the bone marrow and spleen. This stimulus leads gradually, over a two- to four-week period, to restoration of the volume of red blood cells. As this late contribution to blood volume occurs, intracellular stores of fluid are replenished, and the remaining excess fluid is lost through renal excretion as a result of reversal of the mechanisms described previously.

SUMMARY

According to the view outlined above, the principal effects of trauma are to reduce the blood volume both through hemorrhage and through shifts of extracellular fluid into the traumatized area. This volume loss stimulates the afferent limb of a generalized baroreceptor reflex, which leads to a reflex increase in sympathetic activity as well as to increased secretion of various hormones from the pituitary gland. This effect on the sympathetic nervous system not only leads to cardiovascular stabilization, but also to changes in the rates of secretion of other hormones. The combined autonomic and endocrine effects lead to restitution and retention of plasma volume, which may be supported or augmented by renal conservation of salt and water and by increased ingestion. Finally, as a result of hemodilution, red cell synthesis and restoration is stimulated. This set of reflexes can be viewed as an exquisite case of physiologic regulation effected through a variety of internal mechanisms for physiologic control. The process is accelerated and supported by certain feedforward processes stimulated by pain, anxiety, fear, and anger. It is important to note, however, that the time courses vary widely for different aspects of the process, and that various components are important to different degrees quantitatively. Finally, it is likely that our understanding of the details of the process will change as a result of further investigation in the near future, but that the general pattern will remain. Thus, the metabolic and hormonal responses to trauma can be viewed as by-products of a process organized fundamentally to restore and maintain the blood volume.

References

Abbot, W. E., Krieger, H., Babb, L. I., Levey, S., and Holden, W. D.: Metabolic alterations in surgical patients. I. The effect of altering the electrolytic, carbohydrate and amino acid intake. Ann. Surg. *138*:434, 1953.

Blalock, A.: Principles of Surgical Care: Shock and Other Problems. St. Louis, C. V. Mosby Company, 1940.

Cope, O., and Litwin, S. B.: Contribution of lymphatic system to replenishment of plasma volume following hemorrhage. Ann. Surg. *156*:655, 1962.

Cryer, G. L., and Gann, D. S.: Right atrial receptors mediate the adrenocortical response to small hemorrhage. Am. J. Physiol. *227*:325, 1974.

Dallman, M. F., and Jones, M. T.: Corticosteroid Feedback Control of Stress-Induced ACTH Secretion. *In* Brodish, A., and Redgate, E. S. (eds.): Brain–Pituitary–Adrenal Interrelationships. Basel, Karger, 1973, p. 176 (International Symposium.)

Deaux, E., and Kakolewski, J. W.: Emotionally induced increases in effective osmotic pressure and subsequent thirst. Science *169*:1226, 1970.

Gann, D. S.: Parameters of the stimulus initiating the adrenocortical response to hemorrhage. Ann. N.Y. Acad. Sci. *156*:740, 1969.

Gann, D. S., and Cryer, G. L.: Models of adrenal cortical control. Adv. Biomed. Engnr. *2*:1, 1972.

Gann, D. S., and Cryer, G. L.: Feedback Control of ACTH Secretion by Cortisol. *In* Brodish, A., and Redgate, E. S. (eds.): Brain–Pituitary–Adrenal Interrelationships. Basel, Karger, 1973, p. 197.

Gann, D. S., and Pirkle, J. C., Jr.: Role of cortisol in the restitution of blood volume after hemorrhage. Am. J. Surg. *130*:565, 1975.

Gann, D. S., and Robinson, H. B., Jr.: Salt, Water, and Vitamins in Nutrition in Surgical Patients. *In* Ballinger, W. F., Collins, J. A., Drucker, W. R., Dudrick, S. J. and Zeppa, R. (eds.): Pre- and Postoperative Care Committee, American College of Surgeons. Philadelphia, W. B. Saunders Company, 1975, p. 73.

Grizzle, W. E., Dallman, M. F., Schramm, L. P., and Gann, D. S.: Inhibitory and facilitatory hypothalamic areas mediating ACTH release in the cat. Endocrinology *95*:1450, 1974.

Grizzle, W. E., Johnson, R. N., Schramm, L. P., and Gann, D. S.: Hypothalamic cells in an area mediating ACTH release respond to right atrial stretch. Am. J. Physiol. *228*:1039, 1975.

Haddy, F. J., Scott, J. B., and Molnar, J. I.: Mechanism of volume replacement and vascular constriction after hemorrhage. Am. J. Physiol. *208*:619, 1965.

Järhult, J.: Osmotic fluid transfer from tissue to blood during hemorrhagic hypotension. Acta Physiol. Scand. *89*:213, 1973.

Leung, K., and Munck, A.: Peripheral actions of glucocorticoids. Annu. Rev. Physiol. *37*:245, 1975.

Martini, L., and Ganong, W. F.: Neuroendocrinology. New York, Academic Press, 1967.

Meyer, V., and Knobil, E.: Growth hormone secretion in the unanesthetized Rhesus monkey in response to noxious stimuli. Endocrinology *80*:163, 1967.

Moore, F. D., and Ball, M. R.: Metabolic Response to Surgery. Springfield, Charles C Thomas, 1952.

Pirkle, J. C., Jr., and Gann, D. S.: Restitution of blood volume after hemorrhage: Mathematical description. Am. J. Physiol. *228*:821, 1975.

Skillman, J. J., Awwad, H. K., and Moore, F. D.: Plasma protein kinetics of the early transcapillary refill after hemorrhage. Surg. Gynecol. Obstet. *125*:983, 1967.

Starling, E. H.: On the absorption of fluids from the connective tissue spaces. J. Physiol. (Lond.) *19*:312, 1896.

Chapter 8

IMMUNOLOGIC ALTERATIONS IN ACUTE ILLNESS AND INJURY

S. C. Bansal and Y. K. Chitkara

INTRODUCTION AND BASIC CONCEPTS OF IMMUNE RESPONSE

Understanding the possible alterations in immunologic response both pre-existent or caused by acute illness or injury offers the emergency physician an important indicator which may be vital in directing subsequent therapy.

The host defense against a substance which is foreign to the body may be nonspecific or specific (Table 1). The nonspecific host response is not influenced by prior exposure to the foreign substance but is genetically determined. Specificity, memory, and the ability to recognize foreignness are the three cardinal features of the specific immune response. A substance that is able to evoke an immune response and react specifically with induced sensitized cells or antibodies is termed an *antigen.* Pre-existing disease states may involve alterations in immunologic capabilities, and acute disease processes can change the responses. Immunologic deficiencies occur with the poorly nourished, in infancy and old age, in alcoholics, and after burns, shock states, surgical trauma, and anesthesia.

NONSPECIFIC IMMUNITY

INFLAMMATORY RESPONSE

The development of inflammatory response is an important means of resistance to foreign invasion. The inflammatory response leads to elaboration of phagocytic cells (macrophage and polymorphonuclear leukocytes) and a host of other humoral factors that contribute to the elimination of foreign substances.

Acknowledgment: This work was supported by Alma Dea Morani Funds and PHS Grant Nos. A1-12074 and CA-16909-01.

TABLE 1   *Biologic Responses of Host Defense System*

NONSPECIFIC – INNATE IMMUNITY (PHAGOCYTIC CELL AND HUMORAL FACTORS)	SPECIFIC – ADAPTIVE IMMUNITY (LYMPHOCYTES, MACROPHAGES AND PLASMA CELLS)
Inflammatory Reaction Chemotaxis Phagocytosis Intracellular killing	Cell-mediated Immunity Delayed hypersensitivity reaction Homograft reaction
Antimicrobial Substances Lysozyme Interferon Complement Opsonin, etc.	Humoral Immunity Immunoglobulin formation (IgM, IgG, IgA, IgE, IgD)

CELLULAR RESPONSE IN NONSPECIFIC IMMUNITY—PHAGOCYTIC CELLS

The ability of cells to ingest particulate matter, from antigen-antibody complexes to living cells, is called phagocytosis. Several mechanisms enhance this system such as opsonic, natural, and specific antibodies. On the other hand, some factors such as uremia and shock decrease phagocytic activity.

The neutrophil microbicidal (phagocytosis) activity is impaired also in thermal and surgical trauma, malnutrition, iron deficiency anemia, infection, prematurity, and malignancy. These defects are transient but they correlate with the severity of the underlying disease process. With better understanding of the neutrophil function, it is likely that the use of antibiotics in infection will change.

There are two main categories of phagocytic cells, those that migrate (polymorphonuclear leukocytes and mononuclear cells) and those that are fixed in tissue (mononuclear macrophages). The process of phagocytosis is shown schematically in Figure 1. Many humoral factors (lysozyme, phagocytin, etc.) also contribute to the over-all capabilities of the phagocytes. It appears that a number of antimicrobial systems are present in phagocytes. However, the predominant activity of one system might depend on many factors, including the type of organism and the metabolic status of the phagocyte.

SOME HUMORAL FACTORS IN NONSPECIFIC IMMUNITY

Natural antibodies are present throughout the human organism. They react with substances with which the host had no previous contact. *Lysozyme* is found in tears, sweat, and neutrophils, but little is present in plasma, which has only a poor protective effect. *Properdin*, originally described as a

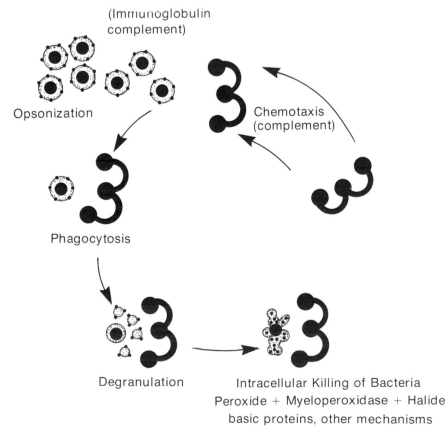

(Immunoglobulin complement)

Opsonization

Chemotaxis (complement)

Phagocytosis

Degranulation

Intracellular Killing of Bacteria
Peroxide + Myeloperoxidase + Halide
basic proteins, other mechanisms

Figure 1. Schematic representation of phagocytosis. (Reproduced with permission from monograph, Staphyloccocal Disease, published by The Upjohn Company 1974.)

naturally occurring euglobulin, has a broad spectrum of antibacterial activity and most likely activates a complement system. *Interferon* is a virus-neutralizing protein provided by a wide variety of mammalian cells when stimulated by virus and many other agents. The precise nature of interferon is not certain, but it holds a potential in future antiviral therapy. *Complement* may be considered as a group of nonspecific serum components belonging mostly to the α and β globulin class of proteins. The clinical implications of the complement system are of diagnostic and prognostic significance in immune complex diseases. Several diseases are marked by complement abnormalities, such as acute and chronic glomerulonephritis, systemic lupus erythematosus, lymphopenic agammaglobulinemia, and certain types of serum sickness.

INFLUENCES ON NONSPECIFIC IMMUNITY

The nonspecific immune response can be influenced by a variety of genetic and constitutional variables. Some diseases that decrease nonspecific immunity are diabetes, burns, cancer, uremia, shock, infection, radiation toxicity, and alcohol intoxication.

SPECIFIC OR ADAPTIVE IMMUNITY

In contrast to nonspecfiic immunity, acquired immunity is an adaptive response to an antigenic stimulus which results in the development of immunologic memory, sensitized cells, and synthesis of specifically reacting antibody molecules. Phylogenetic studies show that immune processes of adaptive immunity are present only in those animal species endowed by evolution with a thymus and an organized lymphoid structure. Ontogenetic studies demonstrate that the time of the first manifestation of these processes coincides with the time of the first appearance of circulating lymphocytes and the formation of organized lymphoid structure. Therefore, adaptive immunity could be expected to be diminished in premature infants. Adaptive immune response may be mediated by lymphocytes (cell-mediated immunity) or by circulating antibodies (humoral immunity).

CELL-MEDIATED IMMUNITY

Two functionally distinct populations of lymphocytes are recognized. Morphologically, under a light microscope these two populations of cells are indistinguishable. One cellular compartment is dependent for its development on thymus (called 'T' cells) and affects the cell-mediated immune responses of delayed hypersensitivity and homograft rejection. The second distinct population of lymphocytes, called 'B' cells, is not thymus-dependent and responds to antigenic stimulation by antibody production.

DELAYED HYPERSENSITIVITY

Intradermal injection of an antigen (e.g., tuberculin) in a sensitized subject results in the appearance in 24 to 48 hours of a skin reaction characterized by an area of erythema and induration at the site of injection. Histologically, the reaction site shows an accumulation of mononuclear cells. In sharp contrast to an antibody-mediated reaction, the delayed type of hypersensitivity reaction can be transferred to an unsensitized subject by sensitized lymphocytes only. Delayed hypersensitivity, which is principally mediated by T lymphocytes, provides protection against a number of bacterial, fungal, and viral agents.

THE HOMOGRAFT REACTION

This is an immune response that falls into the group of cell-mediated reactions. The specific immune response can be divided into three compartments which merge into each other but still are sufficiently defined to merit distinction for understanding (Fig. 2). The afferent arc of the immune response is concerned with sensitization which occurs as a result of contact of lymphocytes with the antigen. The antigen can be released by the graft or taken up by the lymphocytes when passing through the graft. The central arc is concerned with expansion by proliferation of the activated lymphocytes and possibly by recruitment of noncommitted cells by factors released from the activated lymphocytes. At present, the most vulnerable part of the immune response is the central proliferative phase. Most drugs used at present for immunosuppression act upon the proliferative phase to reduce the immune attack on the graft. The efferent or ef-

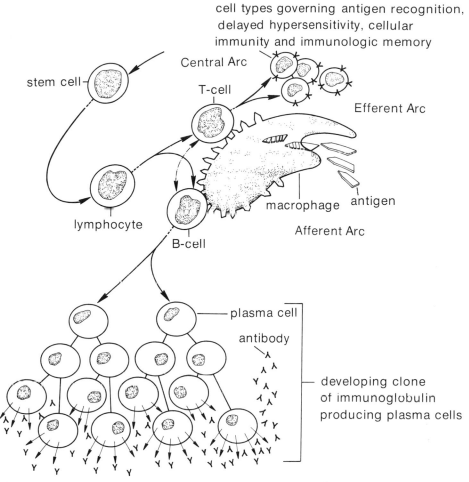

Figure 2. How an antigen is "processed."

Precursor stem cells in the bone marrow develop into lymphocytes that differentiate into B-cells and T-cells. When an antigen enters the body it encounters a macrophage and is "processed." The macrophage (with the processed antigen) interacts with (1) T-cells that differentiate into cells controlling immunologic memory and subsequent antigen recognition and (2) B-cells that differentiate and proliferate into clones of antibody producing plasma cells. (Reproduced with permission from monograph, Immunoglobulin Abnormality Detection, published by Millipore Corporation, 1973.)

fector arc is concerned with disposing the grafted tissue containing alien (non-self) antigens. The lymphocytes involved in this reaction are mainly the T cells.

HUMORAL IMMUNITY

Following an immunogenic stimulus, circulating antibody molecules are produced by the plasma cells formed as a result of differentiation of specific B lymphocytes (Fig. 2). All antibodies are gamma globulins in nature and are termed immunoglobulins. There are five major classes of immunoglobulins: IgG, IgM, IgA, IgD, and IgE.

IgG comprises 70 to 75 per cent of circulating antibodies and is probably the most important in man. Antibodies to pyogenic bacteria, viruses, hemagglutinins and incomplete hemolysins belong to the IgG class. It is actively transported across the placental barrier and therefore constitutes the entire specific humoral defense in the neonate. IgG is formed late in the primary immune response and probably has a regulatory effect on synthesis of IgM.

IgM is a large molecular weight protein and consists of five subunits. Antibodies in the IgM class appear first during the primary response. Lipopolysaccharide antigens typified by O antigens of gram-negative bacteria stimulate synthesis of the IgM class of immunoglobulins. Cold agglutinins, Wassermann antibodies, rheumatoid factor, and heterophil antibodies characteristically belong to this class.

IgA provides antibody activity in the external secretions of the body. A secretory piece of glycoprotein secreted by the epithelial cells is attached to the IgA molecule, as a result of which the latter is protected from the proteolytic activity in the secretions.

IgE is a minor component of serum gamma globulins. These antibodies sensitize human skin and leukocytes; the sensitized leukocytes release histamine and a slow releasing substance (SRS-A) on antigenic challenge. Some patients with allergies (e.g., asthma) or parasitic diseases have higher than normal IgE levels.

The role of *IgD* is poorly defined. There have been recent reports of antinuclear factors being identified in this class of immunoglobulins.

DISORDERS OF
IMMUNOGLOBULIN SYNTHESIS

These disorders may result in qualitative and/or quantitative alterations in serum immunoglobulins. A diffuse increase in all immunoglobulins may occur in many chronic diseases and is called *polyclonal gammopathy.* A decrease in one or more of the immunoglobulins (hypogammaglobulinemia) is usually congenital, but rarely may be acquired. Neoplasia of plasma cells and lymphocytes leads to the production of clones of such cells which retain their function and synthesize one type of immunoglobulins. Such disorders, called monoclonal gammopathies, are characterized by the presence in serum of homogenous immunoglobulins which appear on electrophoresis as "spikes" or M components. The presence of M component in an otherwise healthy individual may suggest an underlying plasma cell myeloma.

FACTORS THAT INFLUENCE
IMMUNE RESPONSE

For a long time there has been a general impression that the immune response may be influenced by a number of factors, e.g.,

age, nutrition, alcohol, hormones and drugs, etc. But there is a general lack of information with respect to their mechanisms. Regardless, these modifiers frequently are present in patients presenting with acute diseases and should be given weight in therapeutic management.

NUTRITION

Clinical and epidemiologic data suggest that protein calorie malnutrition predisposes to increased susceptibility to infection. The infection can lead to malnutrition by inducing a negative nitrogen balance and thus set up a vicious cycle.

In malnourished children, there is reduction of cortical thickness associated with a variable degree of depletion of the cortical lymphoid cells in the thymus. Partial atrophy of lymph nodes has also been reported (Awdeh et al., 1972). Delayed skin hypersensitivity to tuberculin, candida antigen, diphtheria toxoid, and dinitrochlorobenzene is impaired in severely malnourished children. Lymphocyte transformation in vitro using tetanus toxoid, streptolysin O, and nonspecific mitogen is depressed (Grace et al., 1973; Jose et al., 1970).

One or more of the serum immunoglobulins may be elevated in undernourished children (Chandra, 1972). The rate of synthesis of IgG has been found to be increased in children with kwashiorkor (Cohen and Hansen, 1962). However, humoral response to antigenic stimulus is impaired in malnourished individuals (Awdeh, 1972). The role of concomitant infections and exposure to various antigenic stimuli in particular geographic areas must be taken into consideration when correlating immunoglobulin levels and nutritional status.

It should be emphasized that although there is depression of immune response in malnutrition, the relationship between nutrition and the host defense is complex. Many other factors, including the onset and duration of malnutrition, concurrent infection, and other associated disorders, influence the immune response adversely.

AGE

The effects of aging on immune responses and the role of immune phenomena in the aging process have been studied extensively in animals, but there is a general paucity of information in man. There is an age-related decline in the immunocompetent cells. The decreased immunocompetence may be due to decreased proliferation of T and B lymphoid cells, defective cellular interactions, and/or an inappropriate T and B cell ratio (Heidrick and Makinodan, 1973).

Available data in man suggest that cell-mediated immune functions go awry with age. Another in vitro parameter of cell-mediated immunity, the phytohemagglutinin-induced lymphocyte blastogenic response is usually less than that observed in younger people.

Serum immunoglobulins belonging to IgA, IgG, and IgM have been found to be unrelated to age. As the isoimmune response declines, the incidence of autoantibodies has been consistently demonstrated to be high in healthy elderly people. In addition, diseases of old age such as amyloidosis, cancer, polyarteritis, and diabetes are associated with decreased immune response.

Some workers have correlated mortality in old people with failure of the cellular immune response; increased mortality has been reported in those who become anergic to dinitrochlorobenzene. Increased susceptibility to microbial invasion or emergence and/or proliferation of neoplastic clones have been considered as possible factors in contributing to such an increased mortality.

INFANCY

The immune response in infancy, particularly in premature infants, is often inadequate, resulting in increased risk of infection even from organisms usually considered normal flora. The cord blood contains antibodies which belong to the IgG class and have been transferred from the mother across the placental barrier. The IgG concentrations decrease rapidly after birth to a low level at three to six months of age, with subsequent increase to normal adult levels at the age of 10 to 14 years. Serum levels of IgA and IgM are negligible in infants. Increased levels of IgM in cord blood are highly suggestive of intrauterine infections such as syphilis, cytomegalovirus infection, or toxoplasmosis.

EFFECTS OF ALCOHOL

Alcoholic liver disease is associated with increased susceptibility to infection. A decrease in both relative proportions and absolute numbers of peripheral blood T cells has been observed in patients with alcoholic cirrhosis (Bernstein et al., 1974). Phytohemagglutinin-induced lymphocyte response has been shown to be depressed in liver damage due to alcohol (Hsu and Leevy, 1971). In addition, a majority of patients with alcoholic cirrhosis have been found anergic to dinitrochlorobenzene in a delayed skin hypersensitivity test (Berenyi et al., 1974). Serum immunoglobulins are usually elevated, especially IgM and IgG, and the absolute number of B cells is increased.

Few studies of immunologic parameters in alcohol ingestion without cirrhosis have been done. Serum IgA has been reported to increase following heavy drinking; the rise is, however, transient (Varsomis et al., 1974).

There is an obvious need to study the cumulative effects of drinking alcohol and to determine whether the immunologic aberrations observed in alcoholic liver disease precede or follow the development of hepatic pathology and complicating infectious diseases.

Alcohol ingestion affects the nonspecific immunity as well. This is demonstrated by depressed leukocyte chemotaxis, impaired mobilization of leukocytes, and depressed serum complement levels (Brayton et al., 1970). How these changes relate to particular susceptibilities (e.g., Klebsiella pneumonia) is not known.

IMMUNOLOGIC ALTERATIONS IN ACUTE CLINICAL CONDITIONS

Many acute conditions encountered in clinical practice are associated with abnormalities of the immune system. It is becoming increasingly clear that defects of immune response may significantly alter the clinical picture and prognosis in these disease states.

BURNS

The immunologic effects of thermal injury are complex. In spite of the advances made in the management of metabolic aspects of burn trauma, local wound care, and local and systemic antibiotics, the mortality in major burns continues to be high. This has led many workers to look into alterations in host defense mechanisms brought on by cutaneous burns.

There is a fall in all classes of immunoglobulins beginning two days after burns, followed by a gradual return to normal levels by 14 to 15 days postburn (Artruson et al., 1969). The mechanisms and functional significance of the decreased immunoglobulins are not known. Complement levels are decreased (Farrell, 1973). Moreover, primary and secondary antibody responses after antigenic stimulation have been found to be decreased (Alexander and Moncrief, 1966).

Several parameters indicate generalized suppression of cell mediated immunity. For example, skin graft rejection is delayed in proportion to the severity of burn trauma (Polk, 1968). Burn patients with involvement of 30 per cent or more body area show decreased reactivity to most tests of delayed hypersensitivity (Casson et al., 1966). An immediate and sustained fall in absolute T cells and depressed reactivity of lymphocytes in mixed lymphocyte culture also have been observed following thermal trauma (Sakai et al., 1974). Burn injury has profound inhibitory effects on granulocyte formation and function (Alexander, 1972). In order to boost the patient's immune defenses against potential bacterial contaminants of burn wounds, immunotherapy in the form of vaccination against *Pseudomonas aeruginosa* and other gram-negative organisms has been tried on a limited scale.

SHOCK

It has been suggested that the reticuloendothelial system (RES) is depressed in shock (Alexander, 1972). A reticuloendothelial depressing substance has been demonstrated in the plasma of dogs subject to hemorrhagic shock (Blattberg et al., 1972). However, stimulation of the RES has had variable effects on resistance to shock caused by endotoxin. In fact, most of the RES stimulants lead to increased mortality in experimental endotoxic shock. It is apparent that there is no simple relationship between enhanced phagocytic activity and the capacity to withstand endotoxic shock. It appears paradoxic that substances that induce increased phagocytic activity and resistance to challenge with virulent bacteria should cause increased susceptibility to one of the bacterial constituents, endotoxin. Since the increased susceptibility to endotoxic shock can be re-

versed by corticosteroids, it is likely that factors other than RES may be concerned in resistance to endotoxin challenge. It is speculated that although nonspecific stimulants cause proliferation of reticuloendothelial cells, the integrity and stability of lysosomal membranes essential for detoxifying endotoxin may be reduced by such stimulants (Lemperle, 1966).

SURGICAL TRAUMA AND ANESTHESIA

Several investigations suggest that the host immune response is depressed in the postoperative period. Postoperative depression of the lymphocyte response to phytohemagglutinin has been observed (Riddle and Berenbaum, 1967). Ether anesthesia may be associated with greater depression of B cell population to blastogenesis as compared to halothane (Jupert et al., 1973). Cyclopropane anesthesia has been considered to be more depressive than nitrous oxide in its effect on T and B cells. Therefore anesthesia should be chosen with at least these factors in mind.

There is an increased incidence of tumor "takes" in experimental animals if sarcoma cells are injected during the immediate postoperative period. Changes in serum immunoglobulins following surgical trauma have also been reported (Cohnen, 1972). Serum immunoglobulin concentrations were determined in 34 patients undergoing various surgical procedures under ether anesthesia. On the basis of duration of anesthesia, the patients were divided into two groups, the first group of 15 patients who were anesthetized for less than two and one half hours and the second group of 19 patients who required anesthesia for periods longer than two and one half hours but less than seven hours. No significant alterations of serum IgG, IgM, and IgA levels were observed in the first group. In the second group, a significant drop of IgG levels on the first and third postoperative days and an attempt at recovery on the seventh day were observed. A rise of serum IgM concentrations occurred during the period from the third to the seventh postoperative days; the increase was, however, not statistically significant. Serum IgA concentrations remained more or less unchanged (Table 2). It was concluded that changes in serum immunoglobulins could be related to the severity and extent of surgical trauma and/or duration of

TABLE 2   *Serum Immunoglobulins Before and After Surgery*

DURATION OF ANESTHESIA		1 – 2½ HOURS				2½ – 7 HOURS			
TIME IN DAYS AFTER SURGERY		0	1	3	7	0	1	3	7
IgG	Mean	1156	1101	1136	1153	1335	1088	934	1139
	S.D.	241	293	258	223	276	238	277	267
	P	–	N.S.°	N.S.	N.S.		0.01	0.01	0.05
IgM	Mean	101	106	116	114	110	109	117	120
	S.D.	32	30	39	40	22	23	39	32
	P	–	N.S.	N.S.	N.S.	–	N.S.	N.S.	N.S.
IgA	Mean	201	220	217	216	220	207	222	211
	S.D.	34	39	45	36	40	47	32	51
	P	–	N.S.	N.S.	N.S.	–	N.S.	N.S.	N.S.

°N.S. = Not Significant.
Serum immunoglobulin levels on days 1, 3 and 7 were compared to concentrations on day 0.

exposure to anesthesia. It is possible that defects in the immune system might contribute to the development of surgical infections.

Neutrophil killing capacity and phagocytosis have been reported to be considerably impaired after surgery (Donovan, 1967).

SPECIFIC PATIENT PROBLEMS

Some patients with chronic disease processes characterized by compromised host defense may present with acute clinical conditions. The management of such patients will be greatly facilitated by recognizing the patient as having a defective host defense mechanism and defining the extent and likely duration of such a derangement. The urgency of the situation and the need for more sophisticated diagnostic studies must be assessed in each case at the initiation of therapy.

CANCER

The tumor-bearing host does indeed possess sensitized lymphocytes capable of destroying the particular tumor cells, and it is now generally recognized that the host is capable of mounting an immune response to his tumor. Therefore, interest has now shifted to the understanding of the failure of the immune system to eradicate tumors.

The apparent contradiction between the presence of cytotoxic lymphocytes in vitro and the progressive tumor growth indicated the importance of factors that interfere with cell-mediated immunity both in vitro and in vivo (Hellstrom, 1974). Such factors have been detected in the sera of tumor-bearing individuals. It can be shown that sera containing such blocking factors are able to inhibit partially or completely the lymphocyte cytotoxicity against the tumor in question and promote their growth in vivo.

The importance to the tumor host of his immune response also emerges from experiments in which a normally lethal dose of Rous sarcoma was given to experimental animals. Stimulation of host defense mechanisms caused complete regression of tumor cells in 44 per cent of the animals as compared to 75 per cent mortality in controls (Bliznakov, 1968).

The neoplasms are common at the extremes of age. During these periods, i.e., early and old age, the host is immunodeficient because of immunologic immaturity and decay, respectively. There is also evidence that immunosuppressed (e.g., renal transplant recipients) and immunodeficient hosts show an increased incidence of malignant disease (Penn, 1970).

Inasmuch as the malignancy arises in an immunodeficient host more frequently, the tumor itself causes the depression of immune response in the host of origin. Patients with malignant disease are prone to get various infections more frequently and with increased severity.

IMMUNE DEFICIENCY DISEASES

The immune deficiency diseases may be either primary or acquired in association with certain other disorders. Primary diseases of the immune system include a number of rare syndromes characterized by deficiency of T cells or B cells or both. DiGeorge's syndrome is the classic example in which there is failure of development of thymus, resulting in predominantly deficient cell-mediated immunity. Bruton's type of agammaglobulinemia is marked by a deficiency of B cells and therefore a weakened humoral defense mechanism. Combined cellular and humoral deficiency diseases are more common and include the Swiss type of agammaglobulinemia, Wiskott-Aldrich syndrome, and ataxia telangiectasia. Primary immunodeficiency is seen mainly in children.

Secondary disorders of the immune system are important because they are seen more commonly in clinical practice. In patients with Hodgkin's disease, cell-mediated immunity is defective; the defect is explained by abnormalities of T cells. There is increased susceptibility to tuberculous, fungal, and viral infections. Sarcoidosis and chronic uremic states are also associated with impaired cellular immune response. In monoclonal gammopathies there is proliferation of one clone of antibody-producing cells which results in defective production of useful specific antibodies.

Patients with immune deficiency diseases present with recurrent infections. A history of repeated low grade infections or unusual reactions to vaccine, as progressive vaccinia, should make one suspicious of an underlying cellular immune defect. Recurrent infections caused by bacteria of high virulence, e.g., *Diplococcus pneumoniae* and *Haemophilus influenzae,* may suggest an abnormality of the humoral component of the immune system.

RENAL TRANSPLANT AND IMMUNOSUPPRESSIVE THERAPY

From the stage of tentative experiment in the early 1950s, the kidney transplant is passing to the stage of routine therapeutics. Some 17,936 patients have received 19,907 renal grafts and approximately 8000 of these patients are alive with functioning grafted kidneys (Bergan, 1975).

The sequence of events that follows a

TABLE 3   *Major Complications in a Renal Homograft Recipient (Related to Immunosuppressive Therapy)*

1. *Wound*
   Delayed healing
   Disruption
   Infection
2. *Hematologic*
   Leukopenia
   Chronic anemia
3. *Infective*
   Bacterial
   Viral
   Fungus
4. *Miscellaneous*
   Transplant lung
   Unexplained fever
   Hepatic dysfunction
   Pancreatitis
   Gastrointestinal bleeding
   Bone and joint (aseptic necrosis)
   Thromboembolic
   Eye complications
   Malignant tumors
   Urologic, cystitis
   Glomerulonephritis

homotransplantation has been discussed above. Until now we have been able to detect rejection only when the damage has been done. It is at present necessary to suppress continuously the host's immune response, which is achieved by nonspecific immune suppression, such as antimetabolites, steroids, and antithymocyte globulin. The recipient who receives nonspecific immunosuppression is vulnerable to several complications (Table 3).

Until this problem of organ rejection is solved by specific suppression of immune response, one will have to face the complications of nonspecific immunosuppressive therapy. Immunosuppressive drugs are not only being given to patients receiving organ transplants but also to those with autoimmune disease and cancer.

Such immunosuppressive assault has not only introduced a host of new problems but can modify the presentation of symptoms of established disease process owing to altered body immune defense (Simmons et al., 1972). Such new problems and altered clinical pictures will appear at the door of practicing emergency physicians more frequently. A thorough understanding of the host defense system will be required to manage these patients.

References

Alexander, E. L., and Wetzel, B.: Human lymphocytes: similarity of B and T cell surface morphology. Science 188:732, 1975.

Alexander, J. W.: Host defense mechanisms against infection. Surg. Clin. N. Amer. 52:1367, 1972.

Alexander, J. W., and Good, R. A.: Immunobiology for the Surgeon. Philadelphia, W. B. Saunders Co., 1970.

Alexander, J. W., Hegg, M., and Altemeier, W. A.: Neutrophil function in selected surgical disorders. Ann. Surg. 168:447, 1968.

Alexander, J. W., and Moncrief, J. A.: Alterations of the immune response following severe thermal injury. Arch. Surg. 93:75, 1966.

Allison, A. C.: Immunological Tolerance. In Bach, F. H. and Good, R. A. (eds.): Clinical Immunobiology. New York, Academic Press, 1972.

Artruson, G., Högman, C. F., and Johnsson, S. G. O.: Changes in immunoglobulin levels in severely burned patients. Lancet 1:546, 1969.

Awdeh, Z. L., et al.: A survey of nutritional-immunological interactions. Bull. W.H.O. 46:537, 1972.

Axelsson, U., and Hallen, J.: A population study of monoclonal gammopathy: Follow up after 5½ years on 64 subjects detected by electrophoresis of 6995 sera. Acta Med. Scand. 191:111, 1972.

Bansal, S. C., and Sjögren, H. O.: Antitumor immune response and its manipulation in a tumor-bearing host. Israel J. Med. Sci. 10:939, 1974.

Berenyi, M. R., Straus, B., and Cruz, D.: In vitro and in vivo studies of cellular immunity in alcoholic cirrhosis. Am. J. Dig. Dis. 19:199, 1974.

Bergan, J. J.: A review of human solid organ transplantation. Bull. Am. Coll. Surg. 60:24, 1975.

Bernstein, I. M., et al.: Reduction in circulating T lymphocytes in alcoholic liver disease. Lancet 2:488, 1974.

Blattberg, B., et al.: Purification of a reticuloendothelial system–depressing substance produced in shock. J. Reticuloendothel. Soc. 12:371, 1972.

Bliznakov, E. G.: Effect of reticuloendothelial system stimulation on resistance to Rous sarcoma infection in chickens. Int. J. Cancer 3:336, 1968.

Bode, F. R., Pare, J. A. P., and Fraser, R. G.: Pulmonary diseases in the compromised host. Medicine 53:255, 1974.

Bradley, J.: Immunoglobulins. J. Med. Genet. 11:80, 1974.

Brayton, R. G., et al.: Effect of alcohol and various diseases on leukocyte mobilization, phagocytosis and intracellular bacterial killing. N. Engl. J. Med. 282:123, 1970.

Casson, P. R., Solowey, H. C., and Converse, J. M.: Delayed hypersensitivity status of burned patients. Surg. Forum 17:268, 1966.

Chandra, R. K.: Immunocompetence in undernutrition. J. Pediatr. 81:1194, 1972.

Chandra, R. K.: Reduced bactericidal capacity of polymorphs in iron-deficiency anemia. Arch. Dis. Child. 48:861, 1973.

Coen, R., Grush, O., and Kander, E.: Studies of bactericidal activity and metabolism of the leukocyte in full-term infants. J. Pediatr. 75:400, 1969.

Cohen, S., and Hansen, J. D. L.: Metabolism of albumin and gammaglobulin in kwashiorkor. Clin. Sci. 23:351, 1962.

Cohnen, G.: Changes in serum immunoglobulins after surgical trauma. J. Trauma 12:249, 1972.

Donovan, D. J.: Effect of surgery on reticuloendothelial function. Arch. Surg. 94:247, 1967.

Farrell, M. F., Day, N. K., and Tskradlius, V.: Study of lymphocyte depletion and serum complement perturbations following acute burn trauma. Surgery 73:697, 1973.

Gewurz, H.: The Immunologic Role of Complement. In Good, R. A., and Fisher, D. W. (eds.): Immunobiology. Stamford, Conn., Sinauer Associates, Inc., 1971.

Good, R. A.: Disorders of the Immune System. In Good, R. A., and Fisher, D. W. (eds.): Immunobiology. Stamford, Conn., Sinauer Associates Inc., 1971.

Grace, H. J., Armstrong, D., and Smythe, P. M.: Reduced lymphocyte transformation in protein calorie malnutrition. S. Afr. Med. J. 46:402, 1972.

Heidrick, M. L., and Makinodan, T.: Presence of impairment of humoral immunity in non-adherent spleen cells of old mice. J. Immunol. 111:1502, 1973.

Hellström, I., and Hellström, K. E.: Lymphocyte-mediated cytotoxicity and blocking serum activity in tumor antigen. Adv. Immunol. 18:209, 1974.

Hsu, C. C. S., and Leevy, C.: Inhibition of P.H.A.–stimulated lymphocyte transformation by plasma from patients with advanced alcoholic cirrhosis. Clin. Exp. Immunol. 8:749, 1971.

Jerne, N. K.: The immune system. Scientific American 229:52, 1973.

Jose, D. G., Welch, J. S., and Doherty, R. L.: Humoral and cellular immune responses to streptococci, influenza and other antigens in Australian aboriginal school children. Austr. Pediatr. J. 6:192, 1970.

Jubert, A. V., Lee, E. T., Hersh, E. M., McBride, C. M.: Effects of surgery, anesthesia and intraoperative blood loss on immunocompetence. J. Surg. Res. 15:399, 1973.

Klebanoff, S. J.: Antimicrobial mechanisms in neutrophilic polymorphonuclear leukocytes. Sem. Hematol. 12:117, 1975.

Lemperle, G.: Effect of R.E.S. stimulation on endotoxic shock in mice. Proc. Soc. Exp. Biol. Med. 122:1012, 1966.

LoGrippo, G. A., Anselm, K., and Hayashi, H.: Serum immunoglobulins and five serum proteins in extrahepatic obstructive jaundice and alcoholic cirrhosis. Am. J. Gastroenterol. 56:357, 1971.

Meakins, J. L.: Host defense mechanisms: evaluation and roles of acquired defects and immunotherapy. Canad. J. Surg., May 1975, pp. 259–268.

Morton, D. L.: Cancer immunotherapy: an overview. Sem. Oncol. 1:297, 1974.

Nakamura, N. H.: Immunopathology: Clinical Laboratory Concepts and Methods. Boston, Little, Brown & Co., 1974.

Penn, I.: Malignant tumors in organ transplant recipients. Recent Results Cancer Res. 35:1, 1970.

Polk, H. C., Jr.: Prolongation of xenograft survival in patients with pseudomonas sepsis: a clarification. Surg. Forum 19:514, 1968.

Prehn, R. T., and Main, J. M.: Immunity to methylcholanthrene-induced sarcomas. J. Nat. Cancer Inst. 18:769, 1957.

Quie, P. G.: Pathology of bactericidal power of neutrophils. Sem. Hematol. 12:143, 1975.

Riddle, P. R., and Berenbaum, M. C.: Post-operative depression of the lymphocyte response to phytohaemagglutinin. Lancet 1:746, 1967.

Roberts-Thomson, I. C., et al.: Ageing, immune response and mortality. Lancet 2:368, 1974.

Rosner, F., et al.: Leukocyte function in patients with leukemia. Cancer 25:835, 1970.

Sakai, H., et al.: Mixed lymphocyte culture reaction in patients with acute thermal burns. J. Trauma 14:53, 1974.

Sbarra, A. J., and Karnovsky, M. L.: The biochemical basis of phagocytosis. II. Incorporation of C^{14}-labelled building blocks into lipid, protein and glycogen of leukocytes during phagocytosis. J. Biol. Chem. 235:2224, 1960.

Selvaraj, R. J., and Bhat, K. S.: Metabolic and bactericidal activities of leukocytes in protein-calorie malnutrition. Am. J. Clin. Nutr. 25:166, 1972.

Simmons, R. L., Kjellstrand, C. M., and Najarian, J. S.: Technique, complications and results. In Najarian, J. S., and Simmons, R. L. (eds.): Transplantation. Philadelphia, Lea & Febiger, 1972.

Sjögren, H. O.: Transplantation methods as a tool for detection of tumor specific antigen. Progr. Exp. Tumor Res. 6:289, 1965.

Sjögren, H. O., et al.: Suggestive evidence that the "blocking antibodies" of tumor-bearing individuals may be antigen-antibody complexes. Proc. Nat. Acad. Sci. U.S.A. 68:1372, 197

Taylor, G.: Immunology in Medical Practice. London, W. B. Saunders Co., Ltd., 1975.

Varsamis, J., et al.: Heavy drinking and IgA increase. Lancet 1:1291, 1974.

Waldorf, D. S., Willkens, R. F., and Decker, J. L.: Impaired delayed hypersensitivity in an ageing population. J.A.M.A. 203:111, 1968.

Yata, J., Tsukimoto, I., and Tachibana, T.: Human lymphocyte subpopulations. Human thymus-lymphoid tissue (HTL) antigen-positive lymphocytes forming rosettes with sheep erythrocytes and HTL antigen negative lymphocytes interacting with antigen-antibody-complement complexes. Clin. Exp. Immunol. 14:319, 1973.

Part II

FUNDAMENTAL PROCEDURES AND TECHNIQUES

Chapter 9

CARDIOPULMONARY– CEREBRAL RESUSCITATION INCLUDING EMERGENCY AIRWAY CONTROL

Peter Safar

INTRODUCTION

HISTORY

There were no immediately applicable effective emergency resuscitation techniques available before the 1950s. Modern respiratory resuscitation was pioneered in the 1950s, modern circulatory resuscitation in the 1960s, and therapeutically promising research on brain resuscitation began in 1970.

Cardiopulmonary resuscitation (CPR) evolved from the following: proof that ventilation with the operator's exhaled air is physiologically sound (Elam, 1954); proof of the ventilatory superiority of exhaled air ventilation (without equipment) over the manual chest-pressure arm-lift maneuvers (Safar, 1958 a, b; 1959); studies on the role of upper airway soft-tissue obstruction and the need for backward tilt of the head, forward displacement of the mandible, and opening of the mouth in unconscious patients (Safar, 1958a, 1959a; Morikawa, 1961a); proof of the ventilatory superiority of exhaled air ventilation in children (Gordon, 1958); rediscovery and development of external cardiac compression (Kouwenhoven, 1960); demonstration of the need to combine positive pressure ventilation with external cardiac compression (Safar, 1961); internal electric defibrillation of the heart in patients (Beck, 1947); the concept of "the heart too good to die" (Beck, 1960); external electric defibrillation of the heart in patients (Zoll, 1956); electric cardiac pacing (Zoll, 1956a); proof of the feasibility of teaching CPR not only to medical personnel but also to the lay public (Safar, 1958a; Elam 1961a; Lind, 1961; Winchell, 1966A; Berkebile, 1973A; Safar, 1974Aa); proof that lay people in the field will perform mouth-to-mouth breathing (Elam, 1961; Lind, 1963) and CPR (AHA, 1974A; Lund, 1976); production of realistic training aids by Laerdal since 1960; and agreements on details of techniques and

This chapter is in part adapted from:

(1) Safar, P.: *(a)* World Federation of Societies of Anesthesiologists. CPR Manual, 1968 (out of print); *(b)* Chapter 3 in Respiratory Therapy, Philadelphia, F. A. Davis, 1965 (out of print); *(c)* Advances in CPR, New York: Springer-Verlag, 1977; and *(d)* Chapter on Emergency Airway Control, Ventilation and Oxygenation, *In* Critical Care Medicine (Weil, M. H., ed.) Boston, Little, Brown & Co., 1975.

(2) American Heart Association/National Research Council; CPR Standards of 1973 (J A.M.A. Suppl., Feb. 1974).

Acknowledgments: Su Serafin and Vicki Shidel typed the manuscript.

A table of abbreviations used in this chapter and their definitions may be found on p. 101.

teaching methods through national committees (NAS, 1966A; AHA, 1974A) and international symposia (Poulsen, 1961; Lund, 1968).

The development of modern CPR is based on ideas conceived or accidentally discovered many years ago, which had been dormant until the 1950s because of lack of appreciation of their importance or lack of vision, communication, acceptance, develop-ment, promotion, or teaching. This applies to intermittent and continuous positive pressure artificial ventilation (IPPV, CPPV) (Vesalius, 1543); mouth-to-mouth breathing (Tossach, 1771); jaw-thrust (Esmarch, 1878; Heiberg, 1874); open chest cardiac resuscitation (Boehm, 1878; Schiff, 1882); internal defibrillation (Prevost, 1899; Wiggers, 1940); tracheal intubation (Kuhn, 1911); and exter-

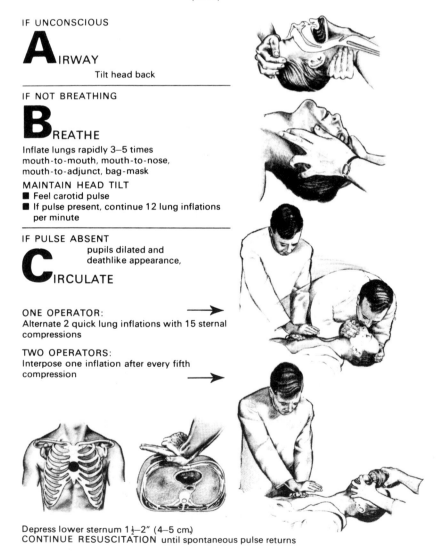

CARDIOPULMONARY-CEREBRAL RESUSCITATION
(CPCR)
PHASE I
EMERGENCY OXYGENATION BASIC LIFE SUPPORT
(BLS)

IF UNCONSCIOUS

AIRWAY
          Tilt head back

IF NOT BREATHING

BREATHE
Inflate lungs rapidly 3–5 times
mouth-to-mouth, mouth-to-nose,
mouth-to-adjunct, bag-mask
MAINTAIN HEAD TILT
■ Feel carotid pulse
■ If pulse present, continue 12 lung inflations
  per minute

IF PULSE ABSENT
          pupils dilated and
          deathlike appearance,
CIRCULATE

ONE OPERATOR:
Alternate 2 quick lung inflations with 15 sternal
compressions

TWO OPERATORS:
Interpose one inflation after every fifth
compression

Depress lower sternum 1½–2″ (4–5 cm.)
CONTINUE RESUSCITATION until spontaneous pulse returns

Figure 1 Phases and steps of cardiopulmonary–cerebral resuscitation. Phase I–Emergency oxygenation.

nal CPR (Maass, 1892) with external defibrillation by AC (Zoll, 1956, 1973) and DC (Gurvitch, 1946).

PHASES AND STEPS OF CPR

We have divided CPR for teaching and learning into *three phases* and *nine steps* which are easily memorized by using the letters of the alphabet from (A) through (I) (Fig. 1, Tables 1 and 2).

Phase I is for emergency oxygenation (basic life support, *BLS*). It consists of Steps (A) Airway control, (B) Breathing support, i.e., emergency artificial ventilation and oxygenation of the lungs; and (C) Circulation support, i.e., recognition of pulselessness and establishment of artificial circulation by heart compressions.

Phase II is for restarting spontaneous circulation (advanced life support, *ALS*). It is for restoring near-normal arterial oxygen transport (i.e., arterial oxygen content times blood flow). It consists of Steps (D) Drugs and fluids via venous life-line; (E) Electrocardioscopy (cardiography); and (F) Fibrillation treatment, usually by electric countershock.

Phase III is for *postresuscitative life support (PLS)*. It consists of Steps (G) Gauging, i.e., determining and treating the cause of demise and the patient's salvability; (H)

CARDIOPULMONARY-CEREBRAL RESUSCITATION

(CPCR)

PHASE II

ESTABLISHMENT OF NORMAL ARTERIAL OXYGEN TRANSPORT

(RESTART SPONTANEOUS CIRCULATION)

ADVANCED LIFE SUPPORT

(ALS)

DO NOT INTERRUPT CARDIAC COMPRESSIONS AND LUNG VENTILATION
INTUBATE TRACHEA WHEN POSSIBLE

DRUGS AND FLUIDS, I.V. LIFELINE
EPINEPHRINE:
0.5–1.0 mg. I.V. repeat larger dose as necessary

SODIUM BICARBONATE:
1 mEq/kg. I.V.
Repeat dose every 10 minutes until pulse returns.
Monitor and normalize arterial pH.

I.V. FLUIDS as indicated

E.K. G. Ventricular fibrillation? Asystole? Bizarre complexes?

FIBRILLATION TREATMENT
EXTERNAL DEFIBRILLATION:
D.C. 100–400 W/sec.
Repeat shock as necessary
LIDOCAINE
1–2 mg/kg. I.V. if necessary

IF ASYSTOLE,
repeat step **D**—calcium and vasopressors as needed
CONTINUE RESUSCITATION until good pulse
is maintained

D.C. 100–400 W/sec

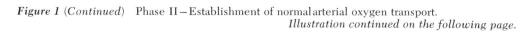

Figure 1 (Continued) Phase II—Establishment of normal arterial oxygen transport.
Illustration continued on the following page.

CARDIOPULMONARY-CEREBRAL RESUSCITATION

(CPCR)

PHASE III

POST-RESUSCITATIVE LIFE SUPPORT

(PLS)

GAUGING

Determine and treat cause of demise

Determine salvageability

HUMAN MENTATION-- **C**EREBRAL RESUSCITATION

Support perfusion pressure, oxygenation, ventilation

If arrest > 5 min., coma > 5 min. after reperfusion

---clinical trials (e.g., thiopental)

INTENSIVE CARE

$PaCO_2$ 25-35	Art., CV, (PA) catheters
PaO_2>100	Temp. Control, EKG
pHa 7.3-7.6	(Curarization)

ICP (osmotherapy, hypothermia)

Suppress convulsions

Steroid, Dextrose 5-10%, electrol., IV. Fluids, alimentation

Hct., plasma COP, serum osm.

Outcome

Figure 1 (*Continued*)   Phase III—Postresuscitative life support.

Human mentation—to be restored (it is hoped) by additional brain resuscitation; and (I) Intensive care (long-term life support).

Since the introduction of CPR this author has used the term "basic life support" for Steps A, B, and C and "advanced life support" for Steps D through I, irrespective of the use of equipment. The American Heart Association (AHA) recently decided to use the term "basic life support" for Phase I, Steps A, B, and C without the use of equipment; and the term "advanced life support" for steps A, B, and C with the use of equipment plus Phases II and III (Steps D through I) (AHA, 1974A). We are now proposing the terms *BLS* (Phase I), *ALS* (Phase II) and *PLS* (Phase III) (Fig. 1) because of the greater emphasis which postresuscitative pathophysiologic changes and life support deserve (Chapters 2 and 5).

"Decision trees" of basic and advanced life support have been proposed (AHA, 1974A; Shoemaker, 1976). Our extensive experience with CPR teaching and practice indicates that trying to memorize such decision trees confuses and complicates basically simple and logical steps. Memorizing the sequence of Steps A through I as presented in this chapter and using common sense when deviations from this sequence are required seem to be practical and effective.

The sequence of actions in performing Phases I and II, which lead to the establishment of adequate spontaneous circulation, should be as rapid as possible, since artificial circulation by external or internal cardiac compressions produces only 10 to 40 per cent of cardiac output or carotid blood flow (Redding, 1961; Del Guercio, 1965).

TABLE 1 *Steps of Emergency Airway Control*
(Phase I, Step A of CPR)

		PERSONNEL TO BE TAUGHT					
STEPS		LAY PUBLIC	POLICE, FIREMAN, LIFE-GUARD	EMT, HOSPITAL TECH-NICIAN	GENERAL RN	ICU-ED RN, RESP. THER., PARA-MEDIC	MED. STUD., MD, DDS	ECCM MD
A-1	Backward tilt of the head (accident victim: gentle tilt, support horizontal stable straight position)	X	X	X	X	X	X	X
A-2	IPPV-CPPV (after each step) (e.g., mouth-mouth)	X	X	X	X	X	X	X
A-3	Manual clearing of mouth and throat (crossed-finger, tongue-jaw lift, or finger-behind-teeth maneuver for wiping, finger probe, extraction); back blows, abdominal thrusts	X	X	X	X	X	X	X
A-4	Triple airway maneuver (tilt head, open mouth, displace mandible forward) with and without mouth-mouth (mask)	(X)	X	X	X	X	X	X
	(Oxygen equip. for pocket mask)	—	(X)	X	X	X	X	X
A-5	Suction (oro- and nasopharyn-geal)	—	X	X	X	X	X	X
A-6	Pharyngeal tube insertion (oro- and nasopharyngeal)	—	X	X	X	X	X	X
A-7	Esophageal obturator airway insertion	—	—	—	—	X	—	X
A-8	Tracheal intubation (orotracheal); tracheobronchial suctioning	—	—	—	—	X	X	X
A-9	Alternatives for tracheal intubation (a) cricothyroid membrane puncture	—	—	—	—	(X)	X	X
	(b) translaryngeal O_2 jet insufflation	—	—	—	—	(X)	X	X
A-10	Tracheotomy, bronchoscopy Bronchodilation and clearing	—	—	—	—	—	—	X

TABLE 2   *Steps of Cardiopulmonary-Cerebral Resuscitation (CPCR)*

STEPS	LAY PUBLIC	POLICE, FIREMAN, LIFE-GUARD	EMT, HOSPITAL TECH-NICIAN	GENERAL RN	ICU-ED RN, RESP. THER., PARA-MEDIC	MED. STUD., MD, DDS	ECCM MD
PERSONNEL TO BE TAUGHT							
PHASE I: EMERGENCY OXYGENA-TION; BASIC LIFE SUPPORT (BLS)							
A. *Airway Control* (see Table 1)	X	X	X	X	X	X	X
B. *Breathing Support*							
Direct Mouth-to-Mouth (Nose)	X	X	X	X	X	X	X
Mouth-Adjunct (Pocket Mask) with triple airway maneuver	(X)	X	X	X	X	X	X
O₂ and suction equipment	—	X	X	X	X	X	X
Mouth-Mask O₂	—	X	X	X	X	X	X
Bag-Valve-Mask-O₂	—	—	(X)	X	X	X	X
O₂ Hand Triggered Ventilator	—	—	X	X	X	X	X
C. *Circulation Support*							
Feel Pulse	X	X	X	X	X	X	X
External Heart Compression (single operator)	X	X	X	X	X	X	X
(Two Operators)	—	X	X	X	X	X	X
Mechanical CPR	—	—	(X)	—	X	—	X
Open Chest Cardiac Resuscitation	—	—	—	—	—	(X)	X
PHASE II: RESTORATION SPON-TANEOUS CIRCULA-TION; ADVANCED LIFE SUPPORT (ALS)							
D. *Drugs and Fluids via I.V. Lifeline*	—	—	—	—	X	X	X
E. *Electrocardioscopy*	—	—	—	(X)	X	X	X
F. *Fibrillation Treatment*	—	—	—	—	X	X	X
PHASE III: IMMEDIATE POST-RESUSCITATIVE LIFE SUPPORT (PLS)							
G. *Gauging* (Determine Salvageability)	—	—	—	—	—	(X)	X
H. *Human Mentation–Cerebral Resuscitation*	—	—	—	—	—	—	X
I. *Intensive Care*	—	—	—	—	X	—	X

Phase III (Safar, 1977Aa, 1978A) deserves more attention and perfection than it has received in the past (AHA, 1974A) and should be continued at least as long as the patient is comatose or until his condition is considered hopeless. The content of this chapter is organized according to the above phases and steps. This chapter is for persons already familiar with the techniques, at least from having viewed a CPR training film.

PHASE I: EMERGENCY OXYGENATION

(A) Airway Control

CAUSES OF AIRWAY OBSTRUCTION

The most common cause of airway obstruction is hypopharyngeal obstruction by the base of the tongue in patients in coma

(Fig. 2) (Safar, 1958a, 1959a). This type of obstruction occurs when the relaxed tongue and neck muscles fail to lift the base of the tongue from the posterior pharyngeal wall, because the patient's head and neck are in the flexed or mid-position. Holding the head tilted backward is therefore the most important step in resuscitation, since it stretches the anterior neck structures and thereby lifts the base of the tongue from the posterior pharyngeal wall (Fig. 2). Sometimes additional forward displacement of the mandible is required to produce this stretch, particularly when nasal obstruction necessitates opening of the mouth, which reduces this stretch (triple airway maneuver, Step A-4) (Safar, 1959a; Morikawa, 1961a). In about one-third of unconcious patients the nasal passage is open during inhalation but obstructed during exhalation because of valve-like behavior of the soft palate; moreover, the nose may be blocked by congestion or mucus (Safar 1959b, 1965).

Hypopharyngeal obstruction by the base of the tongue is contingent upon head-jaw position and occurs regardless of whether the patient is prone or supine (Safar, 1958a, 1959a; Asmussen, 1959). Although gravity may aid in the drainage of liquid foreign matter, it does not relieve hypopharyngeal soft tissue obstruction.

Another cause of airway obstruction is the presence of foreign matter such as vomitus or blood, which the unconscious patient cannot eliminate by swallowing or coughing. Laryngospasm usually is caused by upper airway stimulation in the stuporous or lightly comatose patient. Lower airway obstruction may be the result of bronchospasm, bronchial secretions, mucosal edema, inhaled gastric contents, or foreign matter.

Airway obstruction may be complete or partial. Complete obstruction leads to asphyxia (hypoxemia plus hypercarbia), apnea, and cardiac arrest within five to 10 minutes (Chapters 2 and 3). Partial obstruction must also be promptly corrected, as it can result in hypoxic brain damage, cerebral or pulmonary edema or other complications, and may result in exhaustion, secondary apnea, and cardiac arrest.

RECOGNITION OF AIRWAY OBSTRUCTION

Complete airway obstruction is recognized by inability to *hear* or *feel* air flow at the mouth or nose and by *seeing* inspiratory retraction of supraclavicular and intercostal areas when there are spontaneous breathing movements. During apnea complete airway obstruction is recognized if, when attempting to ventilate the patient, it is not possible to inflate the lungs. *Partial* airway obstruction is recognized by noisy air flow, which may also be accompanied by retraction. Snoring suggests hypopharyngeal obstruction by the tongue; crowing, laryngospasm;

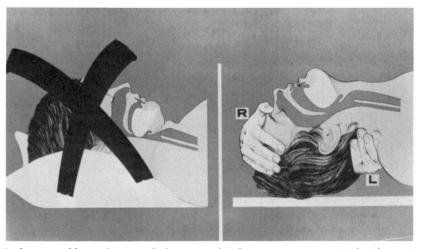

Figure 2 Mechanism of hypopharyngeal obstruction by the tongue in coma. *Left,* Obstruction with head in mid-position or flexed. *Right,* Backward tilt of the head stretches anterior neck structures and thereby lifts the base of the tongue off the posterior pharyngeal wall. R, Right hand; L, left hand. (From A. Laerdal, CPR Flip Charts.)

gurgling, the presence of foreign matter; and wheezing, bronchial obstruction.

Hypercarbia is suspected when there is somnolence and is confirmed by measurement of increased $PaCO_2$; hypoxemia is suspected when there is tachycardia, restlessness, sweating, or cyanosis and confirmed by measurement of decreased arterial Po_2 (Chapter 3). Absence of cyanosis does not rule out severe hypoxemia. During acute airway obstruction, attempts at clearing the airway and reoxygenation have priority over arterial blood gas determinations.

STEPS OF EMERGENCY AIRWAY CONTROL

Recognition of acute airway obstruction must go hand in hand with therapeutic action, step by step, considering training limitations and possible complications with the use of each step (Table 1). Upper airway control Steps A-1 through A-7 (Table 1) are meant primarily for the unconscious patient who requires progression from one step to the next within seconds if the obstruction is not controlled. Upper airway control Steps A-3, 5, and 8 (Table 1) are for the conscious as well as the unconscious patient.

Emergency airway control measures are being improved continuously. Still unproved measures are merely mentioned. The steps described here have withstood the test of time and therefore should be practiced to perfection on manikins and, when possible, also on unconscious (anesthetized) patients under the direction of an experienced anesthesiologist. Emergency oxygenation of the non-intubated patient is an art which no texts—only practice—can teach. Emergency airway control measures should be applied to the comatose patient in emergencies in the following sequence until the airway is successfully opened.

Step A-1: Backward Tilt of the Head. The unconscious patient in need of resuscitation should be positioned supine with his head tilted backward. He should be in the horizontal position, except for periods when clearing the airway is required, in which case a head-down tilt may promote gravity drainage of liquid foreign matter. The prone position should be avoided because it makes the face inaccessible, produces mechanical obstruction, and reduces thoracic compliance, The "stable side position" (NATO position) is recommended for the unat-

tended comatose patient to promote gravity drainage of liquid foreign matter from the mouth. This position consists of flexing the patient's lower leg and placing the lower arm behind his back, with the hand of the upper arm under his cheek; the head is tilted backward. We question the safety of it for accident cases, as it encourages abandonment of the patient and may aggravate a spinal injury and cause paralysis. In cases of coma following trauma, we prefer not the NATO position, but manual support of head-neck-chest in the supine horizontal straight aligned position by a helper. He must provide only *moderate* backward tilt and *no* lateral turning or flexing of the head. For clearing, the aligned patient may be turned.

Backward tilt of the head, forward displacement of the mandible, or both, prevent hypopharyngeal obstruction by the base of the tongue (Figs. 1–3). Either maneuver stretches the tissues between the larynx and mandible, and thereby lifts the base of the tongue from the posterior pharyngeal wall (Safar, 1958). Tilting the head backward is most easily accomplished by placing one hand under the patient's neck and the other at the patient's forehead. This usually results in opening the patient's mouth. If not, the hand under the neck may be moved to the chin to hold the mouth open (chin lift) (Guildner, 1976). Elevation of the shoulders facilitates head tilt. A pillow should never be placed under the head of an unconscious person, as it flexes his neck, causing hypopharyngeal obstruction.

Step A-2: Positive Pressure Inflation Attempts. Each airway control step should be followed as feasible by positive pressure inflation attempts, as they permit assessment of airway patency and may in part overcome

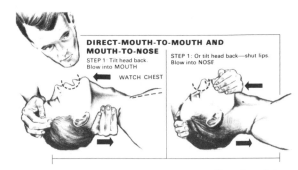

Figure 3 Step A-1, backward tilt of head, and Step A-2, positive pressure inflation with mouth-to-mouth (*left*) and mouth-to-nose (*right*) exhaled air inflation.

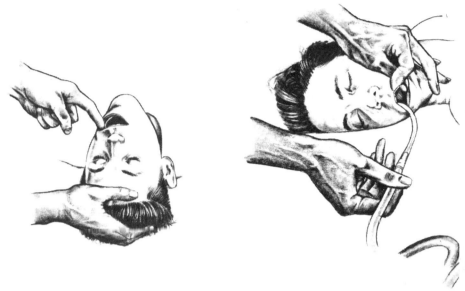

Figure 4   Forcing the mouth open for clearing or insertion of airway or laryngoscope. *Left,* Finger-behind-teeth maneuver for clenched jaw. Slide index finger between cheek and teeth, and wedge tip of index finger behind last molars. *Middle,* Crossed-finger maneuver for moderately relaxed jaw. In corner of mouth, press thumb against lower teeth and index finger, crossed over or under thumb, against upper teeth, and force mouth open. *Right,* Tongue-jaw lift maneuver (from Gordon, A. *In* Safar, 1977A) for fully relaxed jaw. Grasp and lift tongue and lower jaw with one hand, tilt head backward with other hand, if necessary grasp foreign body with two-finger tweezer maneuver.

the obstruction. Positive pressure inflation may be accomplished by IPPV, CPPV, IPPB, or IMV—using exhaled air ("rescue breathing," i.e., mouth-to-mouth, mouth-to-nose, mouth-to-adjunct) (Fig. 3); air (e.g., self-refilling bag-valve-mask unit); or oxygen (e.g., mouth-mask-oxygen, bag-mask-oxygen) (see Step B, below).

Emergency oxygenation attempts in the unconscious patient should start with backward tilt of the head and positive pressure inflation attempts (preferably with oxygen) with artistic (titrated) adaptation of inflation pressure, volume, rate, frequency, rhythm, and flow—according to airway-lung-chest resistances and gas leaks encountered. Positive pressure ventilation patterns with airway pressure curves are described and illustrated in Chapter 10. Depending upon whether the patient is apneic, controlled ventilation (IPPV, CPPV) or assisted (augmented) ventilation (IPPB, IMV) may be used, often alternating rapidly between these patterns, depending on need.

Recent trends have been to apply a slight amount of positive end-expiratory pressure (PEEP) (CPPV), for instance by not letting the patient fully exhale after the first few inflations of reoxygenation, to "recruit" collapsed or fluid-filled alveoli and thereby increase functional residual capacity (FRC). Positive pressure ventilation in the relaxed

patient without a tracheal tube tends to produce gastric insufflation with pharyngeal pressures exceeding 20 to 25 cm. H_2O (Ruben, 1961). Thus, when higher pressures are needed use of a tracheal tube is preferred.

Step A-3, Manual Clearing.   When positive pressure inflation attempts—in spite of backward tilt of the head—meet obstruction and you suspect foreign matter aspiration, force the mouth open and (in the absence of suction) sweep one or two fingers (perhaps covered with a piece of cloth) through mouth and pharynx. Clearing and drainage of liquid foreign matter is aided by turning the head to the side. However, in accident victims turning the head to the side or flexing it forward must be avoided since this may aggravate spinal cord injury. If head turning is necessary in accident victims, the entire patient should be turned, with an additional helper holding head, neck, and chest in alignment.

FORCING MOUTH OPEN.   The three maneuvers (Fig. 4) to be practiced on manikins and patients for forcing the mouth open are the "crossed-fingers maneuver" (for the moderately relaxed jaw) (Safar, 1957–61), the "tongue-jaw lift maneuver" (for the very relaxed jaw) (Gordon, in Safar, 1977A), and the "finger-behind-teeth maneuver" (for trismus) (Safar, 1957–61). These methods are useful for manual clearing, suctioning, and insertion of a pharyngeal tube or a laryngoscope blade.

For the *crossed-finger maneuver*, press your index finger against his upper teeth and your thumb (crossed over your index finger) against his lower teeth forcing his mouth open; insert your fingers in the far corner of his mouth to leave ample room for instrumentation.

For the *tongue-jaw lift maneuver* (in fully relaxed jaw only), insert your thumb into his mouth and throat, with the tip of your thumb lifting the base of his tongue while the other fingers grasp the mandible at the chin and lift anteriorly.

For the *finger-behind-teeth maneuver*, insert one index finger between the patient's cheek and teeth and wedge the tip of your index finger behind his last molar teeth. These maneuvers can be practiced on manikins, patients, and co-workers. Wipe liquid foreign matter with the index and middle fingers or suction; try to *extract* solid foreign matter from pharynx with hooked index finger or using index plus middle fingers like tweezers.

BLOWS AND THRUSTS. For cases of suspected foreign body obstruction with asphyxia (Haugen, 1963), visualization of mouth and pharynx with a laryngoscope (by trained personnel) or (in its absence) with a flashlight and tongue blade, is recommended by this author as the first, most direct and, potentially, most effective step. It permits inspection of the upper airway and extraction of the foreign body by fingers or by forceps or suction. Admittedly, this may be difficult while the patient is conscious. It is easy in the hands of physicians or paramedics trained with direct laryngoscopy after the patient has lost consciousness (Step A-8). If complete obstruction persists in spite of these measures, and if the necessary equipment is available, cricothyrotomy or translaryngeal oxygen jet insufflation may avert cardiac arrest (Step A-9).

The above direct approach should have priority over indirect methods such as back blows (Gordon, in Safar 1977A), and/or abdominal or chest thrusts (Heimlich, 1975, 1975a), which recently have been added to the CPR sequence with the consent of national organizations (NAS, 1976A; ARC, 1976A). These recommendations are based primarily on anecdotal evidence, particularly the abdominal thrust (Heimlich maneuver), which has been advertised because of

claims that patients with sudden complete foreign body obstruction will usually eject (or have ejected?) the foreign body when this maneuver is used. Physiologic evidence indicates that several sharp blows administered between the shoulder blades may dislodge a solid foreign object (Gordon, in Safar 1977A). In small children and infants, this may be accomplished by placing the child prone on one's hand or knee. Physiologic evidence indicates that manual abdominal thrusts (Heimlich, 1975) or chest thrusts (like EHC) (Guildner, 1976a), in curarized animals and man produce airway pressures (with upper airway closed) and air flows (with upper airway open) much lower than those produced by natural coughing (Gordon, in Safar 1977A; Guildner, 1976a). These thrusts may be even less effective in the choking patient who, after a coughing spell, may obstruct with a low lung volume. Complications of the Heimlich maneuver include gastric rupture (Visintine, 1975), injury to the liver and other organs, and the danger of provoking regurgitation. Chest thrust (EHC) may be safer.

The *National Research Council* (NRC) recommends the following sequence of action (NAS, 1976A):

Trained *lay persons* and emergency care personnel without equipment should treat the choking, *conscious* victim with a succession of (1) back blows (four in rapid succession); (2) manual thrusts (four in succession); and, if necessary, (3) repeat back blows and thrusts until they are effective or he becomes unconscious. Then proceed as below. If he suddenly collapses and becomes *unconscious*, proceed with (1) attempts to ventilate (Steps A and B of CPR); (2) if unable to ventilate, apply back blows; (3) manual thrusts; (4) finger probe; (5) ventilation attempts; and (6) continue this sequence until you can ventilate. Check for the pulse; if pulseless, start CPR.

The sequence recommended by the NAS/NRC for use by trained *emergency care personnel* is the same as for lay persons as long as the victim is *conscious*. If he becomes *unconscious*, (1) attempt to visualize the foreign body with laryngoscope or tongue blade and flashlight; (2) attempt to extract the foreign body with fingers or forceps (e.g., Kelly or Magill forceps); (3) if ineffective in relieving the obstruction or if the foreign body cannot be visualized, proceed with back blows, manual thrusts, finger probes, and ventilation attempts as recommended for lay persons; and (4) when all this fails, perform cricothyroid membrane puncture. There is no data to support the use of devices such as the "Choke Saver" or "Throat-E-Vac."

This author recommends a different approach for the victim suspected of having aspirated a foreign body, irrespective of whether he is still conscious or already comatose:

(1) Ask him to open his mouth (or force the mouth open with the crossed-finger, tongue-jaw lift, or finger-behind-teeth maneuver) and *probe* mouth and pharynx with your hooked finger or suction. Trained personnel with equipment should use laryngoscope and forceps (Magill forceps or Kelly clamp) for extraction under *vision*.

(2) Attempt to *ventilate* by mouth-to-mouth or other IPPV method, as it is often possible to deliver oxygen around the foreign body.

(3) If ventilation attempts meet complete obstruction, quickly and briefly turn him on his side (turn children prone) and administer several sharp back *blows*, followed by finger probe and ventilation attempts.

(4) If still obstructed keep him supine and administer several abdominal *thrusts* (Heimlich maneuver), again followed by finger probe and ventilation attempts.

(5) If you lack laryngoscope and forceps *continue* with the sequence—ventilation attempts, back blows, abdominal thrusts, finger probe, ventilation attempts—until you can get air into him.

(6) When you feel time has run out for repeating the sequence, use *cricothyrotomy* or translaryngeal oxygen jet insufflation (Step A-9) if you are trained in their use and have the equipment available.

These special measures for foreign body obstruction will fail when laryngospasm, laryngeal edema, or obstructing tumor cause the choking, which can mimic foreign body obstruction. It also must be stressed that most patients who suddenly collapse during meals do so because of ventricular fibrillation or asystole from ischemic heart disease; they require standard CPR measures. The special measures meant for treatment of foreign body obstruction are only applicable as initial steps when this condition is suspected, as in the case of a patient who is suddenly unable to speak or cough and/or may use the distress signal of choking (clutching his neck). He may rapidly become cyanotic and make exaggerated breathing ef-

forts while no air flow is felt or heard at mouth and nose. He may become unconscious within two minutes.

In witnessed foreign body aspiration with a patient conscious and *partially* obstructed (noisy breathing plus dyspnea), digital probing should be avoided, as it may worsen the obstruction; the patient should be taken rapidly to the nearest hospital Emergency Department, with oxygen inhalation en route.

The incidence of suffocation from an inhaled or ingested object is reported by national agencies to be about 3000 cases per year (few with autopsy proof of an inhaled foreign body). In contrast, there are about 600,000 acute deaths per year in the United States from ischemic heart disease (a fair number occurring at the dinner table) and over 100,000 from accidents (Safar, 1974A).

Step A-4: Triple Airway Maneuver. Backward tilt of the head alone fails to open the air passage in about 20 per cent of unconscious patients (Safar, 1959a) because of inadequate tongue lift caused by stretch of the anterior neck structures produced by head tilt alone; this calls for additional forward displacement of the mandible (Esmarch, 1878; Heiberg, 1874). In addition, closing the mouth with spontaneous or artificial breathing occurring through the nose reveals nasal obstruction in about one-third of unconscious patients (primarily expiratory obstruction through a valvelike behavior of the soft palate) (Safar, 1959b; Morikawa, 1961a; Safar, 1965). This calls for opening the mouth. When the mouth is opened, however, some stretch of the neck is lost, which can be regained by forward displacement of the mandible. An interesting additional observation is that forward displacement of the mandible by pulling on the extralaryngeal muscles can in part ameliorate "laryngospasm" (Fink, 1956). All these observations combined resulted in the introduction of the "triple airway maneuver" as the ideal manual method for producing supralaryngeal upper airway patency, i.e., the combination of: (*a*) backward tilt of the head; (*b*) opening of the mouth; (*c*) forward displacement of the mandible (Safar, 1957–61; 1975).

The triple airway maneuver is difficult to learn (Fig. 5). For the spontaneously breathing patient or for mouth-to-mask ventilation, position yourself at the patient's vertex. Grasp the ascending rami of his mandible in front of his earlobes, using fingers 2–5

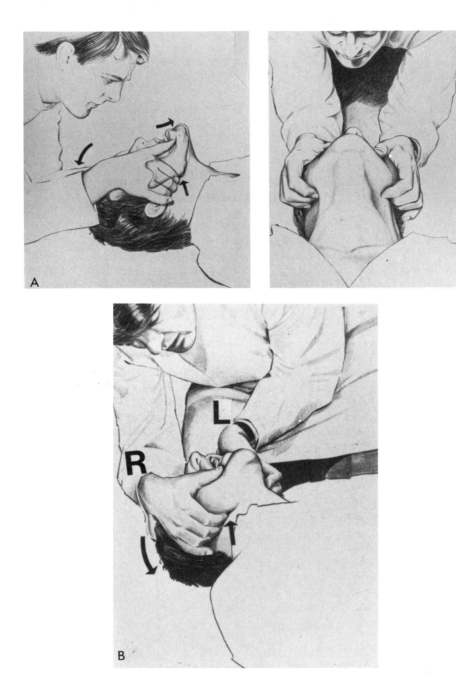

Figure 5 Step A-4, triple airway maneuver: tilt head backward, displace mandible forward, and open mouth. *A*, Triple airway maneuver, with operator at patient's vertex, for spontaneously breathing patient. Grasp ascending rami of mandible in front of earlobes and pull upward forcefully so that lower teeth move in front of upper teeth. Tilt head backward with pressure of the hand. Retract lower lip with thumbs. Do not grasp the horizontal ramus of the mandible, as this may close the mouth.

    B, Triple airway maneuver, as in *A*, but with operator at side of patient for direct mouth-to-mouth ventilation. Seal nose with cheek for mouth-to-mouth breathing; seal mouth with other cheek for mouth-to-nose breathing. R, Right hand; L, left hand. (From A. Laerdal, CPR Flip Charts.)

(or 2–4) of both hands and pull forcefully upward (forward). Retract his lower lip with your thumbs. (Do not grasp the horizontal ramus of his mandible as this may close his mouth.) Displace his mandible forward so forcefully that his lower teeth jut out in front of his upper teeth. This forceful thrust at the angles of the jaw is also an effective method for arousing the semiconscious patient. For direct *mouth-to-mouth* ventilation (Fig. 5B), position yourself at the side of his head, readjust your hands in a comfortable position (e.g., your elbows resting on the ground) and occlude his nose with your cheek when blowing. For mouth-to-nose ventilation occlude his mouth with your other cheek.

You can also perform the triple airway maneuver by displacing his mandible forward with your thumb in his mouth, but this may injure your thumb and hamper provision of a good seal between your mouth or a mask and his mouth. Thus, the jaw thrust with two hands in front of the earlobes is preferred.

In patients with suspected neck injury, in whom backward tilt of the head (as well as flexion and rotation) are contraindicated, the triple airway maneuver with *moderate* backward tilt of the head is the airway control method of choice, short of tracheal intubation and/or tracheotomy.

Practice the triple airway maneuver on manikins, patients, and co-workers.

Step A-5: Clearing by Suction. Suction has not been listed here together with manual clearing because it requires portable or stationary equipment; and because Steps A-1 through A-4 can be performed without equipment. For suctioning the mouth and pharynx, force the mouth open as described under Step A-3 (Fig. 4).

Suction equipment should be powerful enough to clear semisolid foreign matter from the pharynx. Ideally it should produce a negative pressure of at least 300 torr when the tube is occluded and air flow of at least 30 liters per minute when the tube is open (Rosen, 1960). No portable suction unit fulfills these specifications, although wall suction can be that forceful. The amount of suction should be controlled, particularly for use in children and for tracheobronchial suctioning. Suction devices, including yoke, collection bottle, water for rinsing, suction tube, etc. should be conveniently and practically situated.

Suction tips and catheters should be sterile. For suctioning of mouth and oro-pharynx the round multiple-hole pharyngeal (tonsil) rigid (metal or plastic) suction "tip" is recommended; for suctioning of the tracheobronchial tree and the nasopharynx, well lubricated soft curved-tipped catheters are recommended. They permit deliberate insertion into one or the other main stem bronchus. Straight catheters usually pass into the right main bronchus because of its lesser angle with the trachea (Kirimli, 1970). They should be used with a T or Y tube or lateral opening for on–off control. Suction equipment should include a suction trap which permits inspection and examination of the suctioned material. For tracheobronchial and nasal suctioning the catheter should be inserted without suction and withdrawn with intermittent suction. The diameter of the tracheobronchial suction catheter should leave ample room between suction catheter and wall of the tracheal tube through which it is inserted so that air can enter the lungs during suctioning.

Blind *nasotracheal suction* attempts in the non-intubated patient call for the sniffing position (raise occiput and tilt head backward), a well lubricated curved-tip catheter and topical anesthesia of the nasal passage. This technique is safe only in the conscious, cooperative patient, since in stupor or coma it may produce intractable laryngospasm, vomiting with aspiration, and asphyxial or reflex cardiac arrest.

Step A-6: Pharyngeal Intubation. Oropharyngeal and nasopharyngeal tubes, commonly known as "airways," hold the base of the tongue forward and obviate obstruction by lips, teeth, and nose (Fig. 6). Thus they usually are substituted for the jaw thrust and opening of the mouth in the triple airway maneuver, which is not easily maintained over long periods. Even with the pharyngeal tube in place, however, the patient's head must be held tilted backward because, with flexion of the neck, the tip of the tube becomes partially withdrawn and the base of the tongue is pressed against the posterior pharyngeal wall between the tip of the tube and the larynx entrance.

"Airways" should be inserted into comatose patients only to avoid laryngospasm or vomiting in persons with intact upper airway reflexes. Shortened airways, however, can be improvised to serve as mouth props in conscious or stuporous patients, as they do not stimulate the hypopharynx (Morikawa, 1961). We have used cut-off oropharyngeal airways for keeping the mouth

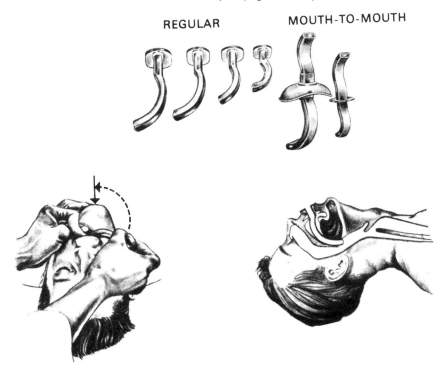

Oropharyngeal airways.

REGULAR   MOUTH-TO-MOUTH

Figure 6   Step A-6, oropharyngeal intubation. *Top*, Various sizes of regular Guedel-type airways and S-shaped mouth-to-mouth airways. *Left*, Insertion of oropharyngeal tube in moderately relaxed jaw. Force mouth open with crossed-finger maneuver and insert airway over tongue with the 180-degree rotation, without pushing the base of the tongue backward. *Right*, Correct position of appropriate size oropharyngeal airway.

open under the mask for stuporous patients requiring oxygenation and bronchodilator aerosol inhalation (which would rain out in the nasal passage). Forceful insertion of the pharyngeal tube must be avoided.

Oropharyngeal tubes of the Guedel type come in five sizes (large adult, adult, child, infant, newborn) and are made of rubber, plastic, or metal. For resuscitation, at least adult, child, and infant sizes should be on hand. For insertion, first force the mouth open with the crossed-finger tongue-jaw lift, or the finger-behind-teeth maneuver (Step A-3, Fig. 4). Then insert the tube *over* the tongue. This can be accomplished either by first inserting the tube into the mouth with the curve backward (convexity caudad) and then twisting it over the tongue 180° (Fig. 6) or without twisting with the aid of a tongue blade. Incorrect placement can push the tongue back into the pharynx and produce airway obstruction.

In patients with trismus, a *nasopharyngeal tube*, which is better tolerated by most patients, is preferred. It should be of very soft rubber or plastic and should be inserted parallel to the level of the palate until one

feels the "give" of the angle of the naso-pharyngeal air passage; then advance the tube until airflow is optimal. This should not be too deep, as it may cause laryngospasm or entry into the upper esophagus. Check air flow before securing. The double nasopha-ryngeal airway recommended by Elam pro-vides an even better air passage. In spite of the not uncommon complication of epistaxis, nasopharyngeal airways should be used more widely.

Step A-7: Esophageal Obturator Airway Insertion.   The esophageal obturator airway (EOA) (Don Michael, 1968; Gordon, in Safar, 1977A; Schofferman, 1976) was intro-duced for prevention of gastric regurgitation during positive pressure artificial ventilation in the hands of personnel not trained in or not permitted to perform tracheal intubation (Fig. 7). Its future role remains to be deter-mined.

The EOA is a large-bore tube of the size of a tracheal tube with a rounded closed tip to be inserted blindly through the mouth into the esophagus. An esophageal cuff is then inflated to prevent regurgitation and gastric insufflation. When mouth-to-tube or

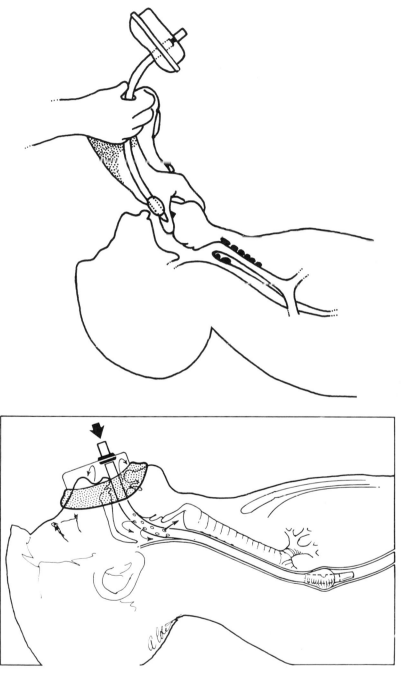

Figure 7 Step A-7, esophageal obturator airway (EOA) insertion (only for relaxed, apneic patient, as alternative to tracheal intubation). *Top*, Open mouth and elevate tongue with thumb. Insert EOA (a cuffed tube with tip closed) through the mouth into the esophagus. *Bottom*, Inflate the cuff. Apply the mask and ventilate via the holes in the tube at the hypopharyngeal level. Hold head tilted backward. (From AHA Advanced Life Support Slide Series, 1975; and Schofferman et al., Chest 69:67, 1976.)

bag-valve-tube ventilation is performed, air or oxygen is delivered through multiple openings at the hypopharyngeal level and through the larynx into the trachea. The EOA is to be used with a mask to seal oronasopharyngeal leaks. Various modifications to obviate these problems have been recommended (Elam, in Safar, 1977A). The device should be inserted only into relaxed comatose apneic patients. Most experience has been gained in cardiac arrest patients. Complications have occurred primarily in spontaneously breathing, not deeply comatose patients.

For insertion, hold the mandible with one hand, depressing the tongue with your thumb and blindly insert the EOA through the patient's mouth into the esophagus (Fig. 7). Then inflate the cuff according to instructions, apply the mask, hold the head tilted backward, and begin mouth-to-tube or bag-valve-tube ventilation.

When the patient is delivered to the Emergency Department with an EOA in place and is deeply comatose, intubate the trachea with a cuffed tube prior to removal of the EOA. Be prepared to suction regurgitated material which appears after removal of the EOA. When he is "light," leave the EOA in place until he is breathing spontaneously and conscious or at least has recovered protective upper airway reflexes, since removal of the EOA may be followed by massive regurgitation. Physicians and nurses working in Emergency Departments must be familiar with this device and the proper timing and techniques of extubation.

The use of the EOA is less desirable than tracheal intubation, but has evolved as an alternative to it. The potential *advantages* of the EOA are that no visualization of the larynx is required for its insertion and that it can be introduced more easily and quickly than a tracheal tube. It has been used in large series of cardiac arrest cases outside the hospital by paramedics. Potential *injury* with the EOA, however, has been reported, so its use should be restricted to adequately trained personnel (Johnson, 1976; Schofferman, 1976). The injuries encountered include esophageal rupture, asphyxia from inadvertent tracheal intubation (which seems to occur in almost 10 per cent of the cases but is of no consequence if immediately recognized), and provocation of laryngospasm, vomiting, and aspiration. The main *drawbacks* of use of the EOA are inabil-ity to control laryngospasm, inability to suction the tracheobronchial tree and inability to protect the lungs against aspiration of foreign matter or blood from the upper airway.

Step A-8: Tracheal Intubation. Tracheal intubation is *indicated* as the final step of emergency airway control in unconscious patients. It is warranted in most comatose patients unless they are so light that upper airway reflexes are intact, coma is expected to be brief in duration, and the patient is attended continuously by personnel experienced with airway control in the not intubated patient. Tracheal intubation is also indicated in the conscious patient with inadequate spontaneous clearing of the tracheobronchial tree; suspected aspiration, upper airway areflexia, or need for prolonged mechanical ventilation. After three to seven days a switch to tracheotomy should be considered—earlier in selected cases (Chapter 10). Improved tubes and cuffs have minimized laryngotracheal damage (Carroll, 1969, 1973; McGinnis, 1971; Hedden, 1969; Lindholm, 1969). In all these instances, tracheal tubes with proper use can isolate the airway, keep it patent, prevent aspiration, and facilitate ventilation and oxygenation.

Usually, airway control, ventilation, and oxygenation attempts without equipment or with simple adjuncts, should precede attempts at tracheal intubation. During CPR, however, lung inflations interposed between heart compressions require high pharyngeal pressures which may cause gastric insufflation. This interferes with adequate lung inflation and promotes regurgitation and aspiration. Therefore, during CPR, the trachea should be intubated as soon as possible without interrupting CPR for more than 15 seconds at a time. With use of a tracheal tube during CPR, lung inflations do not have to be interposed between chest compressions, which also can be performed at a higher rate.

Tracheal intubation may be performed through the *mouth* or through the *nose* (Gillespie, 1950; Applebaum, 1976A). Orotracheal intubation is preferable in an emergency situation, since it can be accomplished more rapidly and with less trauma than nasotracheal intubation.

EQUIPMENT FOR TRACHEAL INTUBATION. The equipment needed for laryngoscopy, upper airway foreign body extraction, and tracheal intubation (Fig. 8, Table 3)

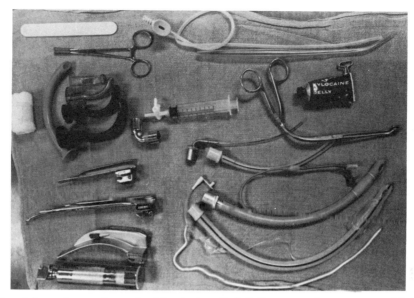

Figure 8 Step A-8, equipment for tracheal intubation. On left, from top to bottom, tongue blade, clamp for cuff, bite block, nasopharyngeal tube, oropharyngeal tubes, curved connector, laryngoscope handle with adult curved and straight blades and child straight blade. At right, from top to bottom, curved-tip tracheal suction catheter, pharyngeal rigid suction tip, lidocaine water-soluble jelly, Magill forceps, three-way stopcock and syringe for cuff inflation, assortment of tracheal tubes, stylette (see text).

must be in every prehospital life support station (AHA, 1974A), ambulance, emergency department, ICU, and other selected hospital locations. Details depend on individual preference. Immediate readiness is important. Most laryngoscopes have three sizes of detachable blades (adult, child, infant) on a battery handle. Laryngoscope blades may be straight or curved; anesthesiologists, critical care physicians, and emergency physicians should be able to intubate the trachea with both the straight and the curved blade. The straight blade is designed to pick up the epiglottis directly. The curved blade is designed to lift the epiglottis off the larynx indirectly, as its tip is placed just above the epiglottis at the base of the tongue, by pulling on the glosso-epiglottic frenulum. The curved blade does not touch the larynx itself and therefore probably produces less trauma and less reflex stimulation; it also permits more room for a view and for tube insertion.

Tracheal tubes should be available in various sizes ranging from an infant size of 12 French to a 38 French adult tube (Table 3). Most tubes supplied are too long and must be cut (Schellinger, 1964). The length of tube needed can be estimated by placing it alongside the patient's face and neck, with the bifurcation of the trachea being at the angle of Louis.

For adults and older children, tubes with large-volume low-pressure soft cuffs are recommended; for infants and small children, uncuffed tubes. Narrow small-volume high-pressure cuffs should *not* be used because they can cause necrosis of the tracheal mucosa. Overinflation of the cuff can be avoided by monitoring intracuff pressure (which in large soft cuffs equals airway and tracheal wall pressure) (Carroll, 1969) or by use of a pressure limiting balloon (McGinnis, 1971). The tubes should be made of nonirritating plastic. Those reinforced with coiled wire are less likely to kink or be compressed, but are more difficult to insert. All tubes must have standard 15-mm. male fittings.

A blunt-tipped metal or plastic malleable *stylet* makes the curvature of the tube controllable. It should be placed to avoid protrusion beyond the distal end of the tube. Use of a straight stylet, bent 45° at the distal fifth of its length and used with a curved laryngoscope blade facilitates intubation under difficult circumstances, even when only the rim of the epiglottis can be visualized.

TECHNIQUE OF ORO-TRACHEAL INTUBATION. Intubation techniques are best learned by observing and doing in the nonemergency setting. Equally important to in-

TABLE 3   Sizes of Tracheal Tubes, Laryngoscopes, and Bronchoscopes
(A) Tracheal Tubes

APPROXI-MATE AGE	WEIGHT (kg.)	OUTSIDE DIAMETER (mm.)	APPROX. INSIDE DIAMETER (mm.)	FRENCH SIZES	MAGILL SIZES	LENGTH OF TUBE (cm.)**	SUCTION CATHETERS (FRENCH SIZES)	TRACHE-OSTOMY TUBES (DIAMETERS LIKE TRACH. TUBES) APPROX. (mm.)
		14.0		42				
		13.3		40				
Adult male		13.0	9.0	39				
		12.7		38	10		14	60
F. (34–40)		12.3		37				
		12.0	8.0	36				
Adult female		11.7		35	9			
		11.3		34		20–24	12	60
(F. 32–36)		11.0		33				
		10.7	7.0	32	8	20–24		
13–14 yrs.		10.3		31	7		10	60
11–12 yrs.		10.0		30		19	10	
		9.7		29	6		10	
8–10 yrs.		9.3		28		18	10	
		9.0	6.0	27	5		10	55
6–7 yrs.		8.7		26		15	10	
		8.3		25	4		10	
4–5 yrs.	16–20	8.0	5.0	24		14	10	50
		7.7		23	3		8	
2–3 yrs.	11–15	7.3		22		13	8	
		7.0		21	2		8	
1–2 yrs.	9–11	6.7		20		12	8	
		6.3		19	1		8	
3–12 mo.	5–9	6.0	4.0	18		11	8	45
		5.7		17			6	
1–3 mo.	2.5–5	5.3		16	0	9	6	40
		5.0		15			6	
newborn	2–2.5	4.7		14		9	6	
(F. 12–14)		4.3		13	00		6	30
	1–2	4.0	3.0	12		8	6	

*For adults and large children, tubes with large-volume soft *cuffs* are recommended; for children under 8 years of age, uncuffed tubes.

**The lengths of orotracheal tubes given here are from J. Marcy (Children's Hospital of Pittsburgh) and are purposely very short, to be used with the adapter well within the mouth.

For length of *nasotracheal* tube, add 25 to 30 per cent of length of orotracheal tube.

sertion of the tube into the trachea are many ancillary steps before and after this act. The author recommends supervised practice to perfection of the following *sequence of action,* first on adult and infant intubation manikins, then on anesthetized patients (Figures 9 and 10):

Select, prepare, and check the equipment (do not depend on helpers). Select the appropriate size tracheal tube and a spare tube one size smaller. Lubricate the tracheal tube with a water soluble anesthetic jelly (e.g., lidocaine). Check the cuff by manipulation of cuff pilot tube-stopcock-syringe assembly, and deflate the cuff. Check the laryngoscope light. Have the patient in the supine position, with the occiput elevated and the head tilted backward (sniffing position) to bring laryngoscope blade and trachea into a straight line. Oxygenate the patient, preferably with 100 per cent O_2 for at least two minutes (e.g., with bag-valve-mask). Interrupt ventilation (in the apneic patient hold your breath and stop the intuba-

TABLE 3—Continued
(B) Laryngoscope Blades

SIZE	STRAIGHT BLADE		CURVED BLADE	
	LENGTH (mm.)	EXAMPLE	LENGTH (mm.)	EXAMPLE
Adult (large)	190	Flagg #4	158	Macintosh #4
Adult (medium)	160	Flagg #3	130	Macintosh #3
Child (2–9 yrs.)	133	Flagg #2	108	Macintosh #2
Child (3 mo.–2 yrs.)	115	Wis-Hipple #1-1/2	100	Macintosh #1
Infant (under 3 mo.)	102	Flagg #1		
Premature	75	Miller Premature		

(C) Rigid Tube Bronchoscopes
(use ventilation attachment)

AGE	INSIDE DIAMETER (mm.)	LENGTH (cm.)
Adult (large)	9	40
Adult (medium)	7	40
Child (5–8 yrs.)	5	30–33
Child (1–4 yrs.)	4	26
Infant (under 1 yr.)	3	26

tion effort when you become short of breath), and force his mouth open with your right hand, e.g., with crossed-finger maneuver. Grasp the laryngoscope handle firmly with the left hand, and insert the blade from the right corner of his mouth, pushing his tongue to the left so as not to obscure the view by the tongue bulging over the open side of the scope. Protect the lips from being injured between teeth and blade. Move the laryngoscope blade toward the sagittal plane and visualize his mouth, pharynx, uvula, and epiglottis while moving your right hand to the forehead or occiput for holding his head tilted backward.

Visualize the arytenoids and the midline (the most important landmarks) and finally the vocal cords (desirable but not essential), by lifting the epiglottis (directly with the straight blade or indirectly with the curved blade). Expose the larynx by pulling the laryngoscope handle upward (forward) at a right angle to the blade. Do not use the upper teeth as a fulcrum. (When using the curved laryngoscope blade, insertion too deep will push the epiglottis downward, whereas too superficial insertion will make the tongue bulge; with use of the straight blade, too deep an insertion into the esophagus will suspend the entire larynx.) These mistakes can be avoided by recognition of the arytenoid cartilages.

If necessary, ask your helper to push the larynx backward for better visualization. Ask him to retract the right corner of the mouth to gain space. Insert the tracheal tube (with your right hand) through the right corner of the patient's mouth while looking through the laryngoscope blade; twist the tube if necessary. Observe the tip of the tube and the cuff pass through the larynx and advance the tube so the cuff is placed just below the larynx. Ask your helper to hold the tube in place against the corner of the patient's mouth. Remove the stylet and connect the ventilation-oxygenation device (e.g., bag-valve/O_2 unit) and turn ventilation-oxygenation over to your helper. Remove the laryngoscope blade and insert a pharyngeal tube or bite block. During CPPV inflate the cuff (via three-way stopcock), but only to the point of abolishing audible leaks. Auscultate both lungs to rule out bronchial (usual right bronchial) intubation. Tape the tube securely to his face. Suction the tracheobronchial tree if necessary (in emergency cases through a suction trap for inspection and examination of the material removed). Establish nonkinking, nonslipping connections to the ventilation-oxygenation device. In deep coma or gastric distention insert a gastric tube (and an esophageal stethoscope for monitoring during anesthesia). Deliver O_2 via a heated humidifier or nebulizer and use atraumatic aseptic suctioning as needed (Chapter 10). During all these maneuvers do

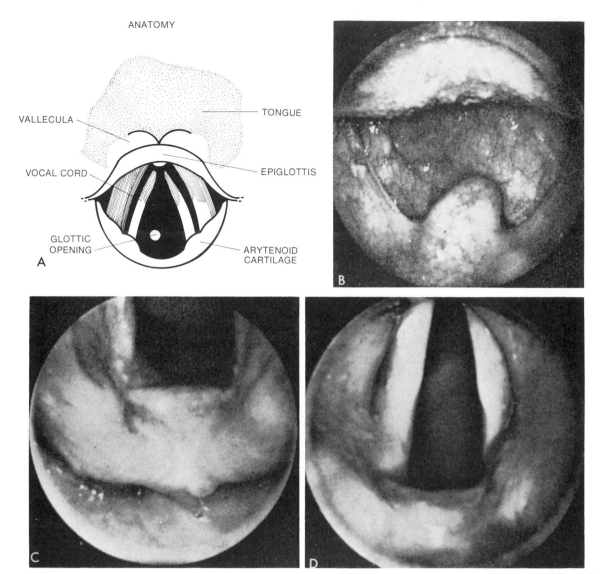

Figure 9 Step A-8, anatomic views for tracheal intubation. *A,* Diagram of anatomy of larynx entrance exposed by direct laryngoscopy. (From AHA Advanced Life Support Slide Series, 1976.)

B, First direct laryngoscopic view during tracheal intubation; exposure of epiglottis and uvula.

C, Second direct laryngoscopic view during tracheal intubation; exposure of arytenoids.

D, Third direct laryngoscopic view during tracheal intubation; exposure of glottis. The anterior commissure is not fully seen. The posterior commissure is below. (From Holinger, P. H., et al.: J. Thorac. Surg. *17*:178, 1948.)

not interrupt IPPV-CPPV/O$_2$ longer than about 30 to 60 seconds at a time (15 seconds during CPR).

The patient with a full stomach in need of general anesthesia or comatose from illness or injury may require *rapid ("crash") intubation* in the semi-sitting position (to combat regurgitation), after preoxygenation, rapid paralysis (by succinylcholine), and closure of the esophagus by pressure on the cricoid (Sellick, 1961; Snow, 1959; Stept,

1970A). The convulsing, asphyxiated patient with head injury is a challenging example. He should not be intubated without a muscle relaxant, since coughing and straining in the presence of brain contusion can cause additional cerebral edema and hemorrhage. Crash intubation is hazardous in the hands of the novice!

GASTRIC INTUBATION. In the conscious patient, gastric intubation is easy, as the patient assists by swallowing. In coma,

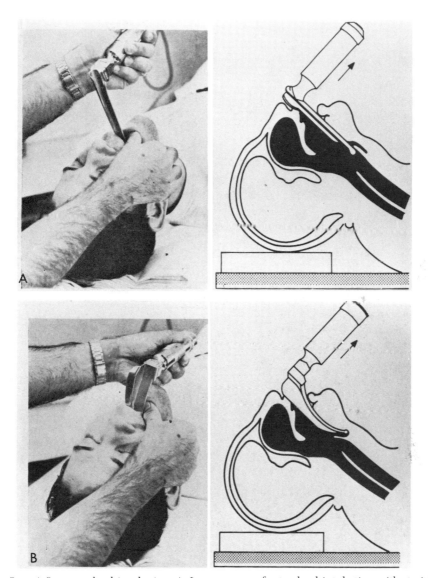

Figure 10 Step A-8, orotracheal intubation. *A,* Laryngoscopy for tracheal intubation with straight blade. *Left,* Insertion of scope; *right,* larynx exposed. Note elevated occiput with head tilted backward (sniffing position).

B, Laryngoscopy for tracheal intubation with curved blade. *Left,* Insertion of scope; *right,* larynx exposed. Note indirect elevation of epiglottis. (From Safar, P.: Respiratory Therapy. Philadelphia, F. A. Davis, 1965.)

particularly in CPR cases, after tracheal intubation, a nasogastric tube should be inserted. This may be difficult. In stupor and coma, gastric intubation before securing the airway with a cuffed tracheal tube is not advisable, since the gastric tube can provoke vomiting and passive regurgitation (as it inactivates the esophageal sphincters) and aspiration. This applies to insertion of both the small-bore Levine tube and the large-bore Ewald tube for gastric lavage. Ventilation-oxygenation and CPR should not be interrupted during gastric intubation. Insertion of a nasogastric tube in the relaxed comatose patient can be facilitated by use of ample (water soluble) lubricant. First, insert the well lubricated tube through the nose beyond the "give" of the nasopharyngeal angle; then pull the larynx forward from the outside (with the other hand) to open the upper esophageal sphincter, and finally advance the tube to engage into the upper esophagus and feed it into the stomach. If necessary an index finger is inserted into the hypopharynx for palpation, straightening, and bimanual advancement of the tube.

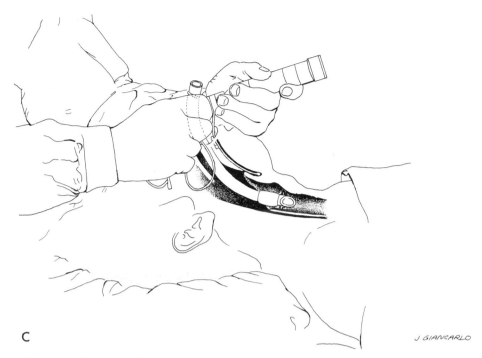

Figure 10 (*Continued*) C, While exposing larynx with curved blade, insertion of cuffed tube through right corner of mouth. (From Applebaum, E. L., and Bruce, D. L.: Tracheal Intubation, Philadelphia, W. B. Saunders Co., 1976.)

TECHNIQUE OF NASOTRACHEAL INTUBATION. Nasotracheal intubation is less predictable than orotracheal intubation, more time consuming, potentially more traumatic (epistaxis), and may introduce nasal bacteria into the trachea. It is not a suitable emergency airway control procedure for use in the asphyxiating patient. Nasotracheal intubation, however, may be required in cases of trismus, inability to tilt the head backward (suspected neck fracture), and similar circumstances when the patient is breathing spontaneously and is not asphyxiated.

For intubating through the nose, select the patient's most patent nasal passage by asking him to sniff. If he is conscious, apply a nasal vasoconstrictor, e.g., phenylephrine nasal spray, to widen the nasal air passage; and a nasal topical anesthetic, e.g., 4 per cent lidocaine in the form of drops or water soluble jelly. Cocaine 1 to 2 per cent also may be used in small amounts, as it is both a potent topical anesthetic and vasoconstrictor. Apply topical anesthesia to hypopharynx, larynx, and trachea as described below. Select a well lubricated, soft, smallbore nasotracheal tube (Table 3), cuffed for adults, and insert it through the more patent nostril parallel to the palate. Ideally the tube's bevel should face the nasal septum to avoid damaging the turbinates. Moderate backward tilt of the head and elevation of the occiput are desirable. The tube is advanced beyond the "give" of the nasopharyngeal angle. For blind nasotracheal intubation the tip of the tube is then maneuvered laterally by twisting and anteriorly or posteriorly by extending or flexing his head (not in suspected neck injury!). The tube is then advanced during inhalations, until coughing and air flow indicate entry into the larynx. If the patient's mouth can be opened, nasotracheal intubation can be facilitated by visualizing the larynx. In this case a Magill forceps or large Kelly clamp is used to direct the tube.

INTUBATING THE AWAKE PATIENT. Tracheal intubation of the conscious patient is difficult and thus requires skill, experience, and artistry. Topical anesthesia of the upper airway mucosa is provided by spraying a topical anesthetic (e.g., 4 per cent lidocaine) from a nebulizer, first onto the oropharyngeal mucosa, then under direct vision, with partially inserted laryngoscope blade, onto the hypopharynx and supraglottic laryngeal mucosa, avoiding stimulation of the gag reflex. The laryngotracheal mucosa is then sprayed with 2 to 3 ml. of 4 per cent lidocaine, either by instillation through the glottis using a cannula with multiple holes (e.g., Steiner cannula) or by translaryngeal injection through the cricothyroid membrane, using a thin (e.g., 22 gauge) needle. The procedure is facilitated by sedation and systemic analgesia using, for instance, titrated intravenous injections of small amounts of a narcotic (e.g., meperidine), with care taken not to abolish response to verbal command and with suction ready to cope with regurgitation. For intubation the laryngoscope blade and tracheal tube must be handled securely, gently applying pressure only when and where absolutely necessary. The operator's reassuring voice is an important adjunct.

DIFFICULT INTUBATION. Intubation attempts may fail when there is inadequate muscular relaxation, poor technique, or anatomic abnormality. Difficulty with intubation can be expected when the patient has taut neck tissues, a receding jaw, protruding teeth, inability to tilt the head backward, a narrow oral cavity, or a large tongue.

Patients difficult to intubate through mouth or nose with the regular technique described above should get the benefit of a try at intubation by the most skilled anesthesiologist immediately available. As a last resort, elective intubation in the spontaneously breathing, well oxygenated patient can be accomplished with the use of a flexible fiberoptic tracheoscope or bronchoscope (the latter being longer and having a suction channel). First, the tracheal tube to be used is inserted through the nose (preferable route) or mouth into the hypopharynx. Then a flexible fiberoptic tracheoscope, with a diameter considerably smaller than that of the tracheal tube (so that the patient can breathe around the scope), well lubricated, is inserted through the tube and directed under vision through the larynx into the trachea. Then the tracheal tube is slipped over the tracheoscope into the trachea and the tracheoscope is removed. For various other highly specialized intubation techniques to use in unusual circumstances, consult the anesthesia literature.

COMPLICATIONS OF TRACHEAL INTUBATION. Attempts at tracheal intubation can injure lips, tongue, teeth, pharynx, tonsils, and larynx. Nasotracheal intubation also can injure the adenoids and nasal mucosa and cause epistaxis. Accidental esophageal intubation is the most dangerous complication; it may be difficult to detect unless one carefully listens to breath sounds over chest and epigastrium. Other complications include tube obstruction by compression, kinking, secretions, biting, a bulging cuff, a too-narrow lumen, or obstructing adapters; accidental bronchial intubation (usually right main bronchus as it is in more direct line with the trachea than the left main stem bronchus); and tube dislodgment. Persistent coughing (bucking, chest wall spasm) calls for IPPV–CPPV with oxygen, and may require sedation, anesthesia, or even curarization to facilitate oxygenation and prevent asphyxia. In spite of these many possible complications, correct use of tracheal intubation has become the cornerstone of emergency resuscitation and long-term airway control in the critically ill patient.

EXTUBATION. The technique of extubation is hazardous, and its safety depends on special knowledge and skills. At the end of general anesthesia in the healthy person the tracheal tube is removed either under sufficient depth of anesthesia to obviate postextubation laryngospasm or when the patient has recovered upper airway reflexes and responds to command. Respiratory insufficiency (hypercarbia, large alveolar-arterial PO_2 gradient), acute acid base abnormalities and circulatory derangements should be ruled out prior to extubation. Ideally, the patient should be able to "sigh" himself upon command with an inspiratory capacity of at least 15 ml./kg. to avoid progressive atelectasis after extubation. Other signs of recovered muscle power include hand squeeze, raising the head, and no retraction during spontaneous breathing. The stomach should not be distended.

The technique of extubation starts with suctioning the mouth, oropharynx, and nasopharynx. The tracheobronchial tree is suctioned with a separate sterile curved-tip catheter. The lungs are filled with 100 per cent O_2. While positive pressure is applied into the trachea, the cuff is deflated, exsufflating secretions at the cuff into the pharynx, which should be suctioned by a helper. Then the tube is gently removed while positive pressure with 100 per cent oxygen is maintained in the trachea. Tracheal suction should not be continued during withdrawal of the tracheal tube, as this can empty the lungs and cause severe hypoxemia. After removal of the tube, oxygenation by mask is continued. Be prepared to treat postextubation laryngospasm with positive pressure oxygen, relaxation with succinylcholine and, if necessary, reintubation. In airway problems, extubation attempts should be accompanied with cricothyrotomy standby. Long-term complications following extubation may include aphonia, sore throat, and ulcers and granulomas of the larynx. For factors to be considered in the prevention and treatment of postextubation "croup," consult the anesthesia literature (Jordan, 1970).

Tracheal intubation in infants and small children. When intubating the trachea in infants and small children, the operator must keep in mind that the infant's larynx in relation to that of the adult is located higher, has a U-shaped epiglottis, and is funnel-shaped, with the narrowest diameter at the level of the cricoid ring. Selecting a tube with too large a diameter can cause croup with asphyxia following extubation from reactive narrowing at the cricoid level.

For intubation in infants, particularly in newborns, use of a straight pointed blade (e.g., Miller blade) is more satisfactory than the curved laryngoscope blade. Since the small dimensions of the infant make accidental bronchial intubation more likely, we recommend for newborn resuscitation a tapered "Cole" tube, which has a shoulder at the larynx entrance, thus preventing accidental bronchial intubation. For long-term use in infants, regular plastic tubes without shoulders are less injurious. Selecting the tube with the optimal diameter and length (Table 3), use of perfect atraumatic technique, and attention to details are important.

Step A-9: Alternatives to Tracheal Intubation. Cricothyroid membrane puncture (Proctor, 1965; Safar, 1967) and translaryngeal oxygen jet insufflation (Smith, 1974, 1975; Klain, 1976; Spoerel, 1971; Jacoby, 1956; Jacobs, 1972) are alternative final steps of last resort, when tracheal intubation is impossible in an asphyxiating patient and necessary tools are immediately available.

Cricothyroid membrane puncture (Fig. 11). This technique cannot be satisfactorily performed merely with a pen knife, since the opening must be kept patent and a standard connector to the tube in the cricothyroid space must permit connection of ventilation equipment. Blind, automatic cricothyrotomy techniques are hazardous and

therefore are to be discouraged. Cricothyroid membrane puncture cannulas should be adequate for spontaneous breathing of air, which in the adult is possible for over 30 minutes with a thin walled cannula of about 6-mm. outside diameter (in the large child with a cannula of about 3-mm. outside diameter). We have recommended the "cut-and-poke" cricothyrotomy technique using a curved cannula with a 15-mm. male adapter for connecting ventilation-oxygenation equipment (Safar, 1967). We now recommend a larger skin incision than in our original publication for better exposure of the cricothyroid space. The 6-mm. cannula also permits suctioning as well as spontaneous and artificial ventilation. Some of the air or oxygen delivered leaks through mouth and nose during positive pressure ventilation; this, however, can be minimized by closing mouth and nose by hand.

Translaryngeal oxygen jet insufflation (Fig. 12). This technique consists of insertion of a 12–16 gauge "extra-cath" needle through the cricothyroid membrane and insufflating oxygen intermittently from a high pressure source (20 to 50 psi) to overcome the resistance of connecting tube and stopcock (T-tube or valve). The chest must be carefully watched to prevent lung rupture, since the valve must be turned off the moment the chest rises. Also, the upper airway must be partially open for passive exhalation to avoid lung rupture. In complete obstruction a second large-bore tracheal needle, perhaps with intermittent suction, can be inserted to promote exhalations. Inflation starts with some air entrainment and ends with upward leakage through the larynx. The most life-threatening possible complication (which can be avoided with proper technique) is interstitial oxygen insufflation from lung rupture or from accidental insertion of the catheter into tissue spaces instead of into the tracheal lumen. Lung rupture has been avoided with the use of a specially designed fluidic ventilator triggered from a second pressure monitoring needle (Klain, 1976). Personnel taught cricothyroid membrane puncture should also be taught translaryngeal oxygen jet insufflation.

The jet insufflation technique seems to exsufflate upper airway secretions (Rock, 1976) and shows promise for long-term assisted or controlled ventilation. Recently, cycling rates of 100 to 200 per minute or

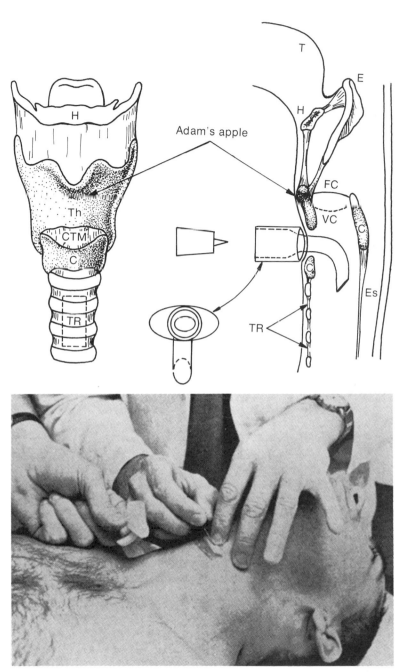

Figure 11 Step A-9, cricothyroid membrane puncture with curved cannula inserted by "cut-and-poke" technique. (From Safar, P., and Penninckx, J.: Anesthesiology 28:943, 1967.)

A, Anatomy with cannula in place. H, Hyoid cartilage; Th, thyroid cartilage; C, cricoid cartilage; TR, trachea; CTM, cricothyroid membrane; E, epiglottis; T, tongue; FC, false cords; VC, vocal cords; Es, esophagus. Curved cannula, 6 mm. outside diameter for adults (3 mm. for large children; use needle under vision for small children and infants); 15 mm. male adaptor for connecting ventilation equipment. Rubber stopper with pointed knife blade.

B, Techniques of cricothyrotomy with curved cannula. Grasp larynx with thumb and middle finger and identify cricothyroid membrane with index finger. Make adequate skin incision. Make stab incision through cricothyroid membrane. Poke blunt tip cannula through membrane into tracheal lumen (cannula available from Lanz Medical Products Company, Wilmerding, PA).

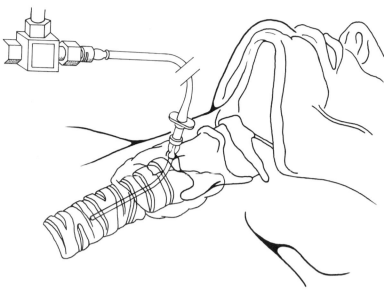

Figure 12 Step A-9, translaryngeal oxygen jet insufflation. Hold head tilted backward, hold larynx between thumb and middle finger and identify cricothyroid membrane with index finger. Insert 14–16 gauge extra-cath needle through cricothyroid space into tracheal lumen, pointing downward. Connect extension tube – stopcock or valve – high pressure tubing from 30–50 psi oxygen source. For lung inflation, turn valve or stopcock until chest moves; then turn off and let him exhale passively through mouth and nose. (From AHA Advanced Life Support Slide Series, 1975.)

more, using a fluidic jet ventilator, with tidal volumes smaller than estimated dead space (!) have been shown to maintain not only PaO_2 but also $PaCO_2$ normal values for hours. This new technique of *high frequency positive pressure jet ventilation* (HFPPJV) (Klain, 1977) may prove to be a breakthrough in assisted and controlled ventilation, for CPR and long-term use, as it is less injurious to the tracheal mucosa than the use of tracheal tubes, and it obviates the need for synchronizing the patient's breathing with that of artificial ventilation. The remaining principle disadvantage of the translaryngeal jet technique is inability to suction the tracheobronchial tree.

OTHER STEPS OF AIRWAY CONTROL

Tracheotomy (see Chap. 16) is an operation for long-term airway management. The skilled operator can perform tracheal intubation more rapidly than tracheotomy. Therefore, tracheotomy should be performed whenever possible in the oxygenated, well-ventilated patient – if necessary with a tracheal tube in place (Chapter 10).

Bronchoscopy is indicated for clearing the tracheobronchial tree in aspiration of solid foreign matter or obstruction by thick mucus or blood (Jackson, 1965; Muendich, 1953; Proctor, 1965; Safar, 1958). The technique of therapeutic and diagnostic bronchoscopy with the rigid tube bronchoscope or the flexible fiberoptic bronchoscope is beyond the scope of this chapter. For tracheobronchial clearing, however, the rigid tube bronchoscope is more effective than bronchoscopy with the fiberoptic flexible bronchoscope, which has only a narrow lumen for suctioning. Even bronchoscopy in the conscious critically ill person should be with oxygenation and assisted ventilation, which is made possible by use of the jet insufflation bronchoscope or ventilation bronchoscope (the scope functioning like a tracheal tube by virtue of a large-bore sidearm and window). The flexible fiberoptic bronchoscope has advantages for examination (Ikada, 1968). Lung rupture is possible during fiberoptic bronchoscopy via tracheal tube with IPPV–CPPV (Lindholm, 1974), as the scope within the tube impairs exhalation.

Bronchodilation and bronchial clearing are important in the management of status asthmaticus (Kampschulte, 1973), bronchitis with asphyxiation, in near-drowning and in aspiration (Chapters 3, 10). Lower airway control should include a combination of: (1) titrated positive pressure ventilation with oxygen—IPPV, CPPV, IPPB, IMV: (2) humidification to promote ciliary escalator clearing; (3) shrinkage of the decongested and edematous mucosa by sympathetic alpha-receptor stimulator aerosol or steroid; (4) bronchodilation by beta-2 receptor stimulator and aminophylline; and (5) arterial pH normalization (Chapters 3, 10). Special cases of subacute airway obstruction include laryngotracheobronchitis (which benefits from epinephrine aerosol administered to the upper airways with IPPV) (Adair, 1071, 1975); and tension pneumothorax (which can asphyxiate the patient by bronchial kinking and compression) (Chapters 3, 10). In massive aspiration of solid foreign matter, ventilation bronchoscopy can be a life-saving resuscitative measure.

B. Breathing Support—Emergency Artificial Ventilation

Most presently recommended methods of artificial ventilation (Chapter 10) depend on intermittent inflation of the lungs with positive pressure applied to the airway, i.e., controlled ventilation by IPPV or CPPV (i.e., IPPV with PEEP). Shallow spontaneous breaths may be augmented with intermittent positive pressure (assisted) breathing (IPPB) or with intermittent mandatory ventilation (IMV). All these methods may be performed with exhaled air, air, or oxygen. The forces opposing positive pressure lung inflation that must be overcome are essentially the elastic resistance of the lungs and thorax and airway resistance. Exhalation usually is passive.

DIRECT MOUTH-TO-MOUTH AND MOUTH-TO-NOSE VENTILATION

Research on emergency artificial ventilation without equipment in the 1950s (Safar, 1958a, 1959) proved the superiority of IPPV with exhaled air (by direct mouth-mouth, mouth-nose or mouth-adjunct) over the then-taught back-pressure and chest-pressure arm-lift maneuvers (Gordon, 1951); these in most instances fail to ventilate the lungs because of inadequate force of inflation and inability of the operator to control the patient's airway (Safar, 1958a). Exhaled air, which contains 16 to 18 per cent oxygen, was found to be an adequate resuscitative gas, provided the patient's lungs are normal and the operator uses about twice normal tidal volumes (Elam, 1954, 1958). This usually results in $PaCO_2$ values of 20 to 30 torr in the rescuer and 30 to 40 torr in the patient, and in PaO_2 values of over 75 torr (oxygen saturation over 90 per cent) in the patient with normal lungs. Emergency artificial ventilation should never be delayed by attempts to find and apply adjuncts; direct exhaled air ventilation is always readily available.

The recommended *technique* for direct exhaled air ventilation is as follows (Figure 3):

(1) If the patient is unconscious, tilt his head backward.

(2) If he is not breathing, inflate his lungs by blowing into his mouth.

(3) If this meets an obstruction, close his mouth and blow into his nose.

(4) If this is also unsuccessful, displace his mandible forward, retract his lower lip and blow into his mouth (triple airway maneuver, see Step A-4 above).

For *mouth-to-mouth* breathing, tilt the patient's head backward (which usually opens his mouth automatically); take a deep breath; seal your mouth around his mouth (mouth and nose in infants and small children) with a wide open circle; and blow forcefully into adults, gently into children (use only puffs for infants to avoid lung rupture). When blowing into his mouth, prevent air leakage through his nose either by pinching his nose with one hand, or by pressing your cheek against his nostrils while blowing. While blowing, watch his chest. When you see his chest rise, stop inflation, raise your head, turn your face to the side, and allow him to exhale passively. When his exhalation is finished, give him the next deep inflation. Volume is more important than rhythm.

Air can be blown into the *stomach*, particularly when the air passage is obstructed or the inflation pressure excessive (Safar, 1958a; Elam, 1960). Inflation of the stomach may make lung inflations more difficult and provoke vomiting. Therefore, if you see the patient's stomach bulging, press with your hand briefly over the epigastrium (between sternum and umbilicus). This will force air out of the stomach. Since this may also cause regurgitation, turn the patient's head and shoulder to one side and be prepared to clear his pharynx.

When his mouth is blocked, blow into his nose. For *mouth-to-nose* ventilation, however, close his mouth with your thumb; encircle his nose with your mouth (avoid pinching his nose with your lips); blow; and open his mouth during exhalation, as there may be expiratory nasal obstruction (Figure 3).

Always ensure adequate ventilation by *seeing* his chest rise and fall, *feeling* air moving from you into him, and *hearing and feeling* air escape during exhalations—and improvise accordingly. Direct exhaled air ventilation can be made more esthetic by blowing through a handkerchief placed over the patient's mouth and nose.

The start of ventilation-oxygenation fits into the entire CPR *sequence* as follows: after three to five rapid, deep lung inflations (without necessarily waiting for full exhalation to take place, which thus results in CPPV rather than IPPV), feel for the pulse. If the pulse is present, continue with one inflation every 5 seconds (about 12 inflations per minute). In children, a faster rate is desirable. If the pulse is absent, start external heart compressions (EHC) and proceed with CPR (Step C below).

In *children and infants,* exhaled air ventilation is performed with the same technique, except that in small children and infants the rescuer covers both the mouth *and* nose of the child with his mouth and uses small breaths with less volume to inflate the lungs at a more rapid rate, about once every 2 seconds. In newborn babies, the volume between your cheeks is adequate, i.e., ventilate with "puffs." Backward tilt of the head should not be exaggerated, since the infant's flexible hyperextended cervical spine may worsen the obstruction.

When you cannot ventilate him with head tilt alone, use the triple airway maneuver (Step A-4) and blow into mouth or nose, with the other orifice closed by your cheek pressed against it.

In victims of *trauma,* maximal backward tilt of the head should be avoided, and mouth-to-mouth breathing, if necessary, applied with the use of the triple airway maneuver (Step A-4), using only *moderate* backward tilt of the head. Also, flexion (chin on chest) and lateral turning of the head must be avoided.

In the *tracheotomized* patient or *laryngectomee,* perform direct mouth-to-

tracheostomy tube, or mouth-to-stoma inflations. Improvise control of leaks between tube and skin.

MOUTH-TO-ADJUNCT VENTILATION

Reports of the first exhaled air ventilation adjuncts published were of a mask (Elam, 1954) and the S-tube (Safar, 1957). They were recommended to make mouth-to-mouth ventilation more acceptable at a time when influential individuals and organizations objected to the introduction of mouth-to-mouth ventilation on esthetic grounds.

The S-tube, a double Guedel airway, overcomes the esthetic objection to direct mouth-to-mouth contact, keeps the mouth open, and assists in maintaining a patent airway. Like all pharyngeal tubes, however, it may induce laryngospasm and vomiting if inserted into the conscious or merely stuporous patient. Shortened S-tubes or mouth props may facilitate mouth-to-mouth inflation, but may cause problems with air leakage.

Subsequent events have shown that in emergencies people rarely hesitate to apply oral resuscitation directly and that adjuncts often are not immediately available. Therefore, the lay public should not be taught the use of S-tubes or other pharyngeal airways. In hospital and ambulance practice, however, the use of airway and ventilation adjuncts by trained personnel is indicated. The new Laerdal pocket mask (Figure 13) (Safar, 1974) is also appropriate for use by the lay public.

Mouth-to-Mask Oxygen (Figure 13). All types of trained personnel trying to ventilate manikins and patients seem to be more effective with the mouth-to-mask than with the bag-valve-mask technique. The latter leaves only one hand free for support of mask fit and head tilt (which closes the mouth under the mask), does not permit use of the triple airway maneuver during IPPV by one operator, and provides only 1 liter inflation volume—hardly enough to overcome leakage with poor mask fit. In contrast, using the Laerdal pocket (folding) mask with oxygen nipple delivers 50 to 100 per cent oxygen, provides 4 liters reserve volume (the rescuer's vital capacity) to overcome leakage, and keeps both hands free for mask fit and the triple airway maneuver (Safar, 1974, 1975). With the triple airway maneuver,

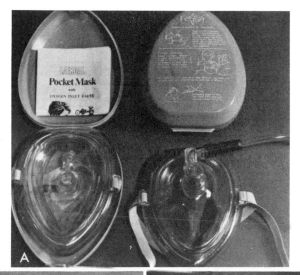

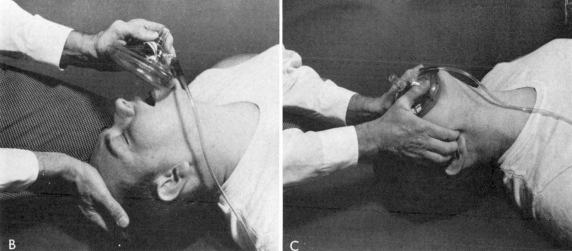

Figure 13 Triple airway maneuver, artificial ventilation and oxygen inhalation by mouth-to-pocket mask. *A*, Laerdal folding mask with 15 mm. male breathing port and oxygen insufflation nipple, inflated cushion, and head strap, pocket size and transparent.

B, In comatose patient, tilt head backward. Open mouth by retracting lower lip and apply rim of mask over chin to keep mouth open. Apply entire mask over mouth and nose.

C, Clamp mask to face with both thumbs (thenar eminences) on top of mask and fingers 2–5 of both hands grasping both ascending rami of mandible in front of earlobes. Pull forcefully upward (forward) so that lower teeth are in front of upper teeth and chin juts out. Mouth must remain open under mask. Front of neck must be maximally stretched. Do not pull on the chin, as this tends to close the mouth. Sustain this triple airway maneuver as long as the patient is unconscious or until a pharyngeal or tracheal tube can be inserted. (In infants apply mask upside down and cover the entire face.) Take a deep breath, blow into mask until chest moves, take mouth off, and let him exhale passively. Strap mask to face. When available deliver oxygen via nipple of mask; 10–15 liters per minute flow results in about 50 per cent O_2 inhaled. With higher flows, artificial ventilation with 100 per cent O_2 is possible by intermittently occluding port with tongue and opening it when the chest rises. (From Safar, P.: Crit. Care Med. 2:273, 1973.)

mouth-to-mask ventilation is more easily performed than mouth-to-mouth, since with the former the operator can remain positioned at the patient's vertex. The Laerdal pocket mask with oxygen nipple also provides *spontaneous* inhalation of 50 to 80 per cent oxygen with 15 liters per minute of oxygen flow (Figure 13).

Masks used for exhaled air ventilation should be transparent (to permit recognition of cyanosis, vomit, mucus, and blood, and clouding with spontaneous exhalations for monitoring), and have a well-sealing cuff, head strap, oxygen insufflation nipple, and breathing port with a standard 15/22 mm. connector. These masks should fit adults, children, and infants. The Laerdal pocket mask fits all ages. For infants it covers the entire face and should be applied with the nose part of the mask over the chin.

In a recent study (Breivik, 1977) use of the pocket mask enabled families to learn to perform exhaled air ventilation on each other without manikins and facilitated learning of the triple airway maneuver (Step A-4) by the lay public. The latter is particularly desirable for use in accident victims in lieu of maximal head-tilt.

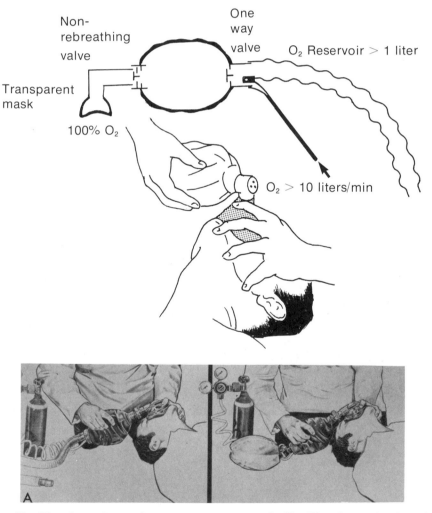

Figure 14   Self-refilling bag-valve-mask unit. *A, top,* Diagram of self-refilling bag with inlet valve and oxygen tube reservoir, and non-rebreathing valve (see text). *Bottom,* Laerdal Resusci-Folding Bag II: *Left,* with large-bore tube oxygen reservoir; *right,* with bag oxygen reservoir, for 50 to 100 per cent O_2 delivery during spontaneous inhalation and artificial ventilation.

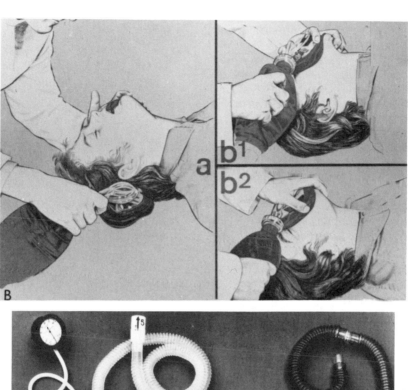

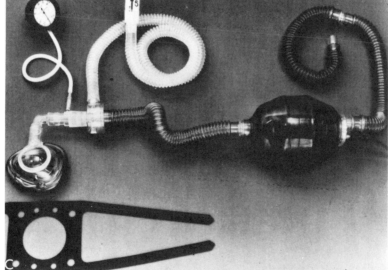

Figure 14 (Continued) B, Ventilation with self-refilling bag-valve-mask unit (Laerdal RFB II). (*a*) In relaxed unconscious person, insert pharyngeal tube and tilt head backward. (*b1*) Apply mask and clamp it to face as shown; firm pressure particularly at the nose is required to prevent leakage when squeezing the bag for ventilation. (*b2*) An alternative way of clamping the mask to the face, i.e., with fingers hooked to chin for sustaining head-tilt, and with palm of hand over top of mask pressing downward. If triple airway maneuver is required, use both hands and ask a helper to squeeze the bag. (From A. Laerdal, CPR Flip Charts.)

C, Modification of self-refilling bag-valve-mask unit (Laerdal RFB II) for CPPV (IPPV plus PEEP) with 100 per cent O_2. A special attachment of the non-rebreathing valve permits collection of exhaled air and attachment of PEEP valve (this Boehringer valve must be held upright). Airway pressure gauge for monitoring PEEP pressure. (Spontaneous O_2 breathing with CPAP is not possible, since the required inflow into the bag under pressure would distend the bag, lock the non-rebreathing valve in the inflation position, and cause lung rupture.)

BAG-VALVE-MASK OXYGEN

The self-refilling bag-valve-mask unit (Ruben, 1958) (Figure 14) followed the bellows-valve-mask devices (Kreiselman, 1943), which are no longer recommended. Obtaining a tight seal at the mask proved difficult with the bellows device—there was a tendency to push the chin down and obstruct the airway when the bellows was squeezed, and the operator could not feel the resistances encountered.

The self-refilling bag-valve-mask unit is not easy to use with a mask in the nonintubated patient, but is particularly valuable and effective for ventilation and oxygenation of the intubated patient. Its 1 to 1.5 liter size bag provides less reserve gas volume in case of leakage than does mouth-mask-oxygen, and does not leave both hands free for performing the triple airway maneuver. Therefore, the operator must be prepared to insert a pharyngeal tube and must be experienced with the provision of mask fit (e.g., trained in anesthesiology).

The bag-valve-mask unit consists of a self-refilling bag with an inlet valve to which an O_2 reservoir (tube or bag) is attached and a non-rebreathing valve at the mask or tracheal tube. In order to deliver 100 per cent O_2, the reservoir must be at least as large as tidal volume (bag volume) and the O_2 inflow rate at least as high as minute volume (Saklad, 1963; Safar, 1975). The non-breathing valve must have an expiratory valve to permit delivery of the gas mixture from the bag during spontaneous breathing. The device should be easy to clean and disinfect; have a nonsticking valve that does not permit backward leak (Loehning, 1964) and that does not lock in the inflation position during delivery of O_2; have transparent, well-fitting face masks of various sizes; and standard 15-mm. female/22-mm. male fittings. Among the commercially available units now, the Laerdal RFB II unit fulfills these specifications. The bag-valve-mask units' main advantage is their ability to deliver 100 per cent O_2, which, however, is also possible with use of the pocket mask with O_2 nipple (Figure 13).

Since use of the bag-valve-mask unit usually closes the mouth under the mask, at least one-third of unconscious patients require an oropharyngeal or nasopharyngeal tube to overcome nasal obstruction. The *technique* is as follows: Position yourself at the patient's vertex. Tilt his head backward.

If he is relaxed, insert an oropharyngeal or nasopharyngeal tube (Step A-6). *Spread* the mask, *mold* it over the patient's mouth and nose, *clamp* it to his face with one hand, *tilt* his head backward, and *squeeze* the bag until the chest rises. Release the bag for exhalation. Abrupt bag release is necessary for proper valve function.

There are at least two methods for clamping the mask to the patient's face: (a) press with your thumb over the nose part of the mask and with the index finger over the chin part and use your middle, ring, and little fingers to pull his chin upward and backward; (b) if you use a Laerdal flat cushion mask, hook your fingers around the patient's chin and apply pressure on the top of the mask with the palm of your hand, always maintaining backward tilt. Holding mask and head with one hand and providing additional jaw thrust is almost impossible. You may use your knee, hip, and/or chin for supporting mask fit and head tilt. If you have a helper, one operator can hold the mask and provide the triple airway maneuver with both hands while the other operator squeezes the bag. This method, however, is inconvenient, as it ties up two people.

The self-refilling bag-valve-mask unit also has been used for *anesthesia* with minimal equipment under field conditions (Pearson, 1961); and for bronchodilator *aerosol* administration with a nebulizer interposed between non-rebreathing valve and patient (Milai, 1965). For oxygenation, a modification of the Laerdal unit permits *PEEP* during IPPV (i.e., CPPV) with 100 per cent O_2 (Fig. 14) (Safar, 1975). This may be lifesaving in pulmonary edema, aspiration, near-drowning, or other conditions associated with increased pulmonary shunting. For *spontaneous* breathing with *CPAP*, however, even a modified self-refilling bag-valve-mask unit *cannot* be used because of the danger of the valve's locking in the inflation position and causing lung rupture. For spontaneous breathing with CPAP, a regular bag and non-rebreathing valve with PEEP-valve assembly is needed (Chapter 10).

MANUALLY TRIGGERED OXYGEN POWERED VENTILATORS

Oxygen powered manually triggered ventilation devices (e.g., Elder valve) permit instantaneous manual initiation and termination of positive pressure inflation with oxygen. These units are recommended if they can deliver 100 per cent oxygen; provide instantaneous flow rates of 1 liter per second or more for adults (lower adjustable flow rates for infants and children); have the manual trigger positioned so that both hands of the operator can remain at the mask and provide the triple airway maneuver while triggering inflation (Safar, 1965); have a safety valve to release pressure at about 50 cm. H₂O for adults (with a switch to 30 cm. H₂O for infants and children); have standard 15-mm. female/22 mm. male fittings; and permit spontaneous breathing, i.e., function as a demand O₂ inhalation device. The demand valve (inhalator) should be highly sensitive so that flow rates follow the patient's demand without excessive airway pressure fluctuations, even during tachypnea.

High instantaneous flow rates have been recommended for CPR to enable interposition of ventilations between chest compressions. These high flow rates may cause high pharyngeal pressures and gastric distention. Therefore, these devices are most effective when used with a tracheal tube or an EOA.

The principal disadvantages of these devices in comparison with the bag-valve-mask unit and mouth-mask-O₂ technique are their dependence on compressed gas, inability to feel resistance during inflation, and inability to humidify oxygen delivered (Nobel, 1971A).

AUTOMATIC OXYGEN POWERED VENTILATORS

Most old-style oxygen powered automatically cycling ventilators (resuscitators) used in the past in ambulances are *not* recommended (Safar, 1965a; NAS, 1966A; AHA, 1974A). Reasons include: the fixed cycling pressure does not permit adaptation of inflation volume, pressure, flow, and rhythm to the changing mask leakage, lung-thorax compliance, airway resistance and spontaneous breathing efforts. The "suck-and-blow" units in addition retard exhalation. During external heart compressions, because of inadequate pressure and flow rate, these devices tend to cycle prematurely into exhalation. Their heavy weight, complexity, and cost are added disadvantages.

For prolonged artificial ventilation of the intubated or tracheotomized patient in-

side or outside the hospital, suitable automatic ventilators with adjustable and readable airway pressure, tidal volume, and rate are recommended (Chapter 10). These should be capable of producing IPPV, CPPV, IPPB, and ideally also IMV—with controllable inhaled oxygen concentrations and capability to deliver drug aerosols and warm humidity. The new technique of high frequency positive pressure jet ventilation (Klain, 1977) (Step A-9 above) may simplify mechanical emergency artificial ventilation with or without CPR. This remains to be studied.

OXYGEN INHALATION

For emergency resuscitation, oxygen should replace exhaled air or air as soon as it becomes available (Smith, J., 1968; Safar, 1975). When the patient resumes spontaneous breathing, assisted breathing with oxygen should continue as long as he is unconscious. Even when he recovers consciousness after an anoxic insult, spontaneous inhalation of O₂ is recommended until hospital admission and take-over of his care by personnel experienced in advanced respiratory therapy. If the patient who did not receive CPR is breathing spontaneously but is cyanotic or dyspneic, he should also inhale oxygen enriched atmosphere.

A simple and effective technique for *spontaneous* inhalation of about 50 to 80 per cent oxygen in a nonintubated patient is use of the Laerdal pocket mask (Figure 13); and 100 per cent oxygen can easily be delivered with the self-refilling bag-valve-mask unit. Both techniques offer the advantage of interchangeable use for spontaneous and artificial ventilation with oxygen, which regular semi-open oxygen masks do not provide. The spontaneously breathing intubated patient is best connected to a large-bore valveless T-tube for delivery of oxygen with warm humidity. For long-term oxygen inhalation through mouth, tracheal tube, or tracheostomy tube, the oxygen must be delivered with warm humidity or mist.

C. Circulation Support—External Heart Compressions

CAUSES AND RECOGNITION OF CARDIAC ARREST

Causes of cardiac arrest include: myocardial ischemia, asphyxia, hypoxemia, electric shock, certain drugs, sensitivity reactions, and exsanguination (Chapter 2). Irrespective of cause, in order to prevent cerebral damage or death, the operator must start CPR immediately. In sudden primary cardiac arrest, if the onset of reoxygenation by CPR is delayed beyond about four minutes, the chances of the patient's recovering without brain damage are small (in 1977).

"Cardiac arrest" is defined as "the clinical picture of sudden cessation of circulation in a patient who was not expected to die at the time." Cessation of circulation is diagnosed when *all* the following conditions are present: unconsciousness; apnea or gasps; deathlike appearance; and no pulse in large arteries (e.g., carotid or femoral). Pulselessness of the large arteries is the most important sign. Absence of heart sounds is an unreliable sign. Although dilated pupils are listed as an additional sign, one should not wait for pupils to dilate, since this may take over one minute after cessation of circulation, and in some patients the pupils never dilate. Relative changes in pupil size, however, are valuable in following the efficiency of artificial circulation and the course of postresuscitation recovery.

Pulselessness should be recognized by *feeling for the carotid pulse* (Figure 1), one hand maintaining backward tilt of the head while the other feels for the carotid pulse on the near side of the rescuer (one side only!). Reaching over the patient's neck may occlude his airway. Feel for the pulse by placing your index and middle fingers gently on his larynx (Adam's apple); then slide them off to the side and press gently backward on his neck. Palpate with the flat portion of your fingers rather than with the tips. If you do this correctly, the carotid artery should lie beneath your fingers. When feeling the artery, take care not to occlude it. Interrupt resuscitation as briefly as possible, but feel long enough to make sure that you pick up a slow heart rate. Feeling the carotid pulse is recommended for detecting pulselessness, because the operator is already at the patient's head, his neck is accessible, and more peripheral pulses may be absent in spite of the presence of the carotid pulse. In hospital patients, however, the femoral artery is also acceptable. In infants and small children, the carotid pulse may also be felt, but this easily compresses the airway or causes laryngospasm; thus, pulselessness is best determined by feeling over the precordium, the abdominal aorta, or the femoral artery.

EXTERNAL HEART COMPRESSIONS

The rediscovery of external heart compressions (EHC) (Kouwenhoven, 1960; Jude, 1961), when added to airway control (Step A) and artificial breathing (Step B) has made it possible for any trained person to initiate possible reversal of clinical death, even outside hospitals.

The heart occupies most of the space between the sternum and the spine in the lower chest. Artificial circulation is most readily produced by external heart compressions, i.e., squeezing the heart between the sternum and the spine. Blood is thereby forced out of the left ventricle into the body, including the heart muscle and brain, and is simultaneously forced from the right ventricle into the lungs, where it is oxygenated. When sternal pressure is released, the elasticity of the chest wall causes the thorax to expand and the heart refills with blood.

External heart compressions can produce systolic blood pressure peaks of 100 torr and more, but the diastolic pressure is usually not more than 10 to 40 torr, resulting in a cardiac output and carotid artery flow of only 10 to 40 per cent of normal (Redding, 1961; DelGuercio, 1965). This is enough to prevent cerebral death for one to two hours, but usually not enough to awaken the patient from anoxic coma.

In giving external heart compressions, pressure must be applied at exactly the lower half of the sternum in order to be effective and to avoid injury. The layman will recognize the sternum by feeling the abdomen, which is soft, and the sternum, which is hard. The pressure point is identified by feeling the xiphoid process (lower end of the sternum) and placing two fingers just above the base of the xiphoid process and the heel of the other hand adjacent to the two fingers. This identifies the lower half of the sternum; another way of identifying the correct location for external heart compressions is by dividing in half the distance between the base of the xiphoid and the suprasternal notch (Figure 15).

External heart compression does not produce reliable ventilation and must therefore always be accompanied by artificial ventilation (Safar, 1961). Even this basic fact is not appreciated by many physicians.

The *technique* of external heart compression is as follows: Position yourself to either side of the patient. Place the heel of one hand over the pressure point at the lower half of the sternum and place the heel of the other hand on top of the first hand (Figure 15). Push the sternum downward toward the spine about 1½ to 2 inches (4 to 5 cm.) in adults and hold the sternum down for about one half second (50 per cent of the cycle); then release rapidly. Reapply pressure every second or at a slightly faster rate. Rates slower than 60 per minute do not provide sufficient blood flow. Compress the sternum forcefully enough to produce a good artificial carotid or femoral pulse. Have another member of the team monitor one of these pulses. Compressions should be regular, smooth, and uninterrupted.

In *adults*, apply compression using your entire body weight rather than arm muscles alone to avoid fatigue. Do not lift your hands from the sternum between compressions. Compress with the heels of your hands, keeping your fingers raised to avoid producing rib fracture by pressing against the lateral aspects of the thorax. Pressing below the xiphoid may cause regurgitation or rupture of the liver, and pressing too high may fracture the sternum.

The patient must be in the horizontal position to permit venous return, which may be promoted by raising the legs. The patient must be on a firm surface (ground, floor, hard litter, spine board or — in the hospital — a cardiac arrest bed board). Heart compressions should not be delayed when such hard support is not immediately available. If the patient is in bed, do not waste time moving him to the floor, but slip a bed board or tray between his thorax and the mattress. Never interrupt compressions except for a few seconds, since even optimally performed external heart compressions produce only borderline circulation which is rarely adequate to awaken the patient.

In small *children*, compress the sternum with one hand only; in *infants* with the tips of two fingers. The heart in infants and small children lies higher in the chest, and the danger of injuring the liver is greater; apply EHC over the midportion of the sternum. Press down only about one half inch in infants, and 1 to 1½ inches in small children. In children and infants, rates of 100 to 120 per minute are recommended. Also, backward tilt of their heads lifts the back; this calls for support of the child's back with one of the rescuer's hands, a folded blanket or other support. In small infants, the compressing operator may encircle the chest with both hands and compress the midsternum with both thumbs.

THE CPR SEQUENCE: COMBINATION OF ARTIFICIAL VENTILATION AND CIRCULATION

The sequence of CPR steps is as follows (Figure 16):

(A) If the patient is *unconscious* — tilt his head backward.

(B) If he is *not breathing* — ventilate his lungs rapidly three to five times; then quickly feel for his *carotid pulse*.

(C) If his *pulse is present* — continue ventilation; if his *pulse is absent* — start external heart compressions.

Recommended rates and ratios of ventilation and sternal compressions are a compromise, based on experimental data (Harris, 1967; Safar, 1961; AHA, 1966A). The methods aim at optimal ventilation and circulation, as well as technical feasibility.

The *one-operator technique* is most important to teach the lay public, first responders (police, firemen), and health professionals, because usually only one skilled bystander is present at first. Kneel at the patient's side; stand if he is on a litter, table, or bed. The recommended ratio is alternating two quick lung inflations with 15 sternal compressions. In order to obtain at least 60 sternal compressions per minute, the operator must perform each series of 15 compressions at a rate of at least 80 compressions per minute, and deliver the two deep lung inflations in rapid succession within five seconds, without allowing full exhalation to occur between breaths. Again — maintain the patient's head tilted backward while ventilating and, if possible, raise the shoulders with a rolled blanket or hard object (e.g., special molded EHC board) to aid in maintaining the backward tilt during external heart compressions in case EHC or the patient himself produces some borderline ventilation. Alternate rapidly between ventilation and sternal compressions. When ventilating

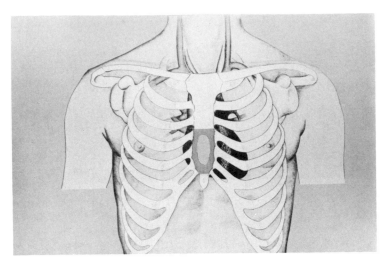

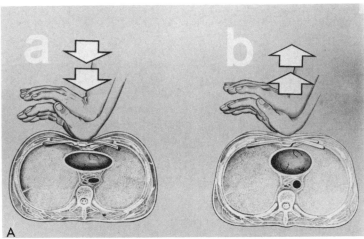

Figure 15   External heart compressions. A, *top,* The correct place for application of EHC, i.e., the lower half of the sternum. *Bottom,* Compression of heart between sternum and spine with heel of hand applied to sternum (*a*). Release of pressure to let heart fill (*b*). Compress and release for 50 per cent of each cycle. Maintain contact between hand and sternum.

by mouth-to-mask or bag-mask, the mask should be strapped to the patient's face to avoid delays due to frequent reapplications.

The *two-operator technique* recommended is continued uninterrupted heart compressions, about one per second (at a rate of at least 60 per minute) with one lung inflation interposed after every fifth sternal compression (Fig. 16). The two operators should be positioned on opposite sides of the victim, which permits easy switching of positions without interruption of the rhythm. Interposing ventilations that quickly is difficult in the patient without a tracheal tube; therefore, some of us favor use of the 2:15 ratio even when there are two operators, as long as the patient's trachea is not intubated. After tracheal intubation, inflations may be

interposed between or simultaneously with EHC. The latter improves blood flow (Harris, 1967; Whiteford, pers. comm.).

The new technique of high frequency positive pressure oxygen jet ventilation (Klain, 1977) (Step A-9 above) may make synchronizing unnecessary, since it could be superimposed ad libitum upon any frequency of heart compressions.

It is important to *check* the effectiveness of CPR. The ventilating operator should do this by (*a*) intermittently palpating the (artificial) carotid pulse; and (*b*) by checking whether a spontaneous pulse has returned, at first after one minute of CPR and every few minutes thereafter, during brief interruptions of heart compressions.

The pupils should also be examined pe-

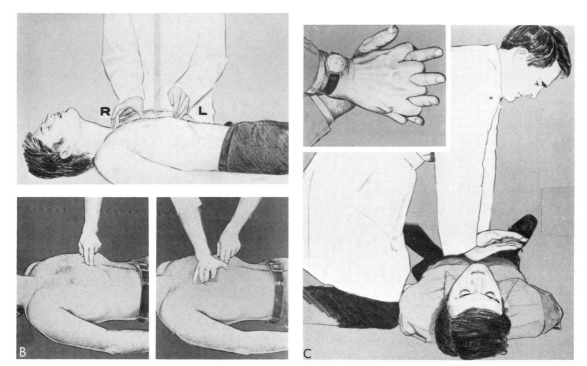

Figure 15 (*Continued*)   *B*, Identification of correct point for EHC. *Top*, Feel for suprasternal notch and base of xiphoid, measure one-half this distance and compress lower half of sternum; R, right hand; L, left hand. *Bottom*, Alternative method; i.e., identify base of xiphoid, measure two fingers cephalad (*left*), and apply heel of hand over lower half of sternum (*right*).

  C, Body and hand position for EHC. Compress straight downward using part of body weight. Keep hands off ribs. *Inset*, Alternative method, locking hands while performing EHC with heel of lower hand. (From A. Laerdal, CPR Flip Charts.)

riodically, as narrowing, and particularly a reaction to light, shows cerebral recovery, whereas widely dilated pupils are an ominous sign as to the brain's status and the efficacy of CPR. Continue CPR until a spontaneous pulse returns; then continue artificial ventilation without sternal compressions until spontaneous breathing returns; and continue artificial ventilation with oxygen until the patient regains consciousness.

In severe *bradycardia* or *asystole* from *complete heart block* (Stokes-Adams syndrome), the still well-oxygenated heart can be made to contract spontaneously by external mechanical stimulation (pacing) via the chest wall, without EHC. Stimulation alone can be accomplished by repetitive blows over the midsternum or to the left of the sternum with a fist, i.e., *fist pacing* (chest thumping) at a rate of about 60 per minute (see "witnessed arrest" below). EHC as described above also stimulates spontaneous contractions and in addition moves blood (a form of assisted circulation). Since EHC is more painful, it is reserved for the unconscious

patient, whereas repetitive thumping is recommended when the patient is conscious. For prolonged external stimulation in the conscious patient with heart block, a mechanical external thumper has been developed (Zoll, in Safar, 1977).

Outside the hospital, effective ventilation and sternal compression should be well established before the victim is moved. The feasibility of restoring spontaneous circulation at the scene or en route to the hospital depends on the availability of advanced life support by paramedics or by physician-staffed ambulance services. Restarting spontaneous circulation at the scene is desirable.

If the patient must be moved for restoration of spontaneous circulation because the spontaneous pulse does not return with CPR, and drugs and defibrillator are not available, CPR must be continued without interruption during transport. This may prove difficult.

The ventilating operator may work from the head end of the stretcher while the chest compressing operator works from the side

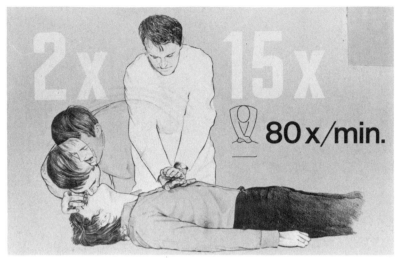

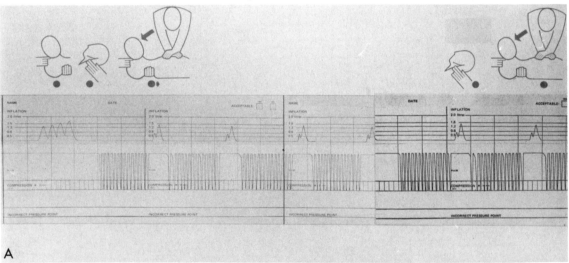

A

Figure 16 CPR sequence (combination of artificial ventilation and circulation). A, CPR single operator without equipment. Technique (*top*) and Recording Resusci-Anne print-out (*bottom*). If unconscious, tilt head back. If not breathing, give four quick lung inflations. Feel for pulse 5 to 10 seconds. If no pulse, give 15 heart compressions, then two quick lung inflations and alternate 15 compressions and two inflations. Perform EHC at a rate of about 80 per minute (slightly faster than one per second) in order to produce at least 60 heart compressions per minute.

and three or more bystanders carry the stretcher. The most experienced should act as team leader.

When moving the patient over narrow stairways and other difficult places, manual CPR will have to be improvised (for instance, when the patient is strapped to a chair), but should not be interrupted for more than about 15 seconds at a time. In the ambulance the usual CPR technique has been with the rescuer kneeling on a pillow near the side of the patient's head and chest, keeping the victim's head tilted backward

with a roll under the shoulder or use of a special backboard. A pharyngeal tube is inserted and a transparent mask strapped to the patient's face to avoid delays from frequent reapplications of the mask. · The 2:15 ratio is used. EHC with the patient in the upright position (e.g., sitting) is ineffective.

A novel technique suggested by Fryer of Pittsburgh is a single operator sitting on a bench which is placed over the patient's hips and fastened to the stretcher; the operator facing cephalad (toward the patient's

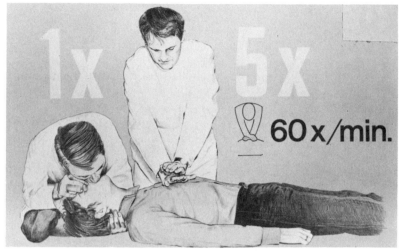

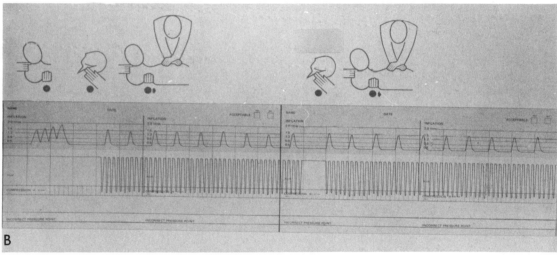

Figure 16 (Continued) B, CPR two-operators without equipment. Technique (*top*) and recording manikin print-out (*bottom*). Interpose one quick lung inflation after every five sternal compressions performed without interruptions at a rate of about one compression per second. (From A. Laerdal, CPR Flip Charts.)

face), performing external heart compressions from this astride position. For ventilation we suggest mouth-to-mask/O₂ breathing from a mouthpiece in the rescuer's mouth via a large-bore tube and non-rebreathing valve attached to the mask. A pharyngeal tube is inserted, the mask is strapped to the patient's face and the operator pushes the chin upward (backward) to maintain head tilt when giving lung inflations.

We do not favor the use of *EHC machines*, some of which have mechanical ventilators attached, over manual CPR for reasons of efficacy (Benson, 1971), but they may be of value during difficult transport situations where they can give more consistently

effective CPR than can the manual technique (Nagel and Birch, in Safar, 1977A). When such devices are used, manual CPR must be started first; and they should be used only by personnel fully drilled in the switch to the mechanical device.

These "chest thumpers" should provide an adjustable stroke of 1½ to 2 inches, be applied rapidly without interruption of manual CPR for more than 5 seconds at a time, support backward tilt of the head, and minimize the danger of accidental malpositioning of the plunger during use. Ventilation should be by the operator or, when a mechanical device is incorporated, it should be a volume- or time-cycled, not a pressure-cycled ventilator (see above, Section B). These devices should only be employed with a cuffed tracheal tube or EOA, since their ventilator component does not adapt to the changing leaks and resistances usually encountered with ventilation by mask. Presently available "chest thumpers" should not be used in infants and chiildren. A rescuer must remain at the patient's head all the time to monitor plunger action and ventilation and to check the pulse and pupils (Nobel, 1973A).

For *open chest heart compression,* see later in this chapter under "Special Considerations."

PHASE II: RESTORATION OF SPONTANEOUS CIRCULATION

Phase II in conjunction with Phase III (Immediate Postresuscitative Life Support) was in the past labeled "Definitive Therapy." Restoration of spontaneous circulation should be as prompt as possible since external heart compressions (EHC) can produce only 10 to 40 per cent of normal carotid blood flow (Redding, 1961). Restoration of spontaneous circulation usually requires administration of drugs, electrocardiographic diagnosis, fibrillation treatment, and sometimes blood volume replacement. These measures certainly are not required if a spontaneous pulse returns promptly following initiation of ventilation and sternal compression, as is often the case in pulselessness secondary to asphyxia.

D. Drugs and Fluids Via Venous Lifeline

VENOUS LIFELINE

During EHC, an intravenous route for the administration of drugs and fluids should be established as quickly as possible without interrupting CPR in order to support blood flow during EHC and to help restore spontaneous circulation. If an intravenous (I.V.) infusion is running, drugs, fluids, and glucose are given via the existing route. If there is no infusion in place, the first I.V. injection of epinephrine may be made via a small-gauge needle into a peripheral vein (e.g., external jugular vein), if establishment of a percutaneous peripheral venous catheter lifeline is not immediately possible. For

the first dose of epinephrine we recommend 0.5 to 1.0 mg. (0.5–1.0 ml. of a 1:1000 solution). Sodium bicarbonate, requiring a larger volume for injection, usually is withheld until a venous catheter lifeline is established. Continuous infusion via metal needles is not recommended, as these are easily dislodged during CPR.

During EHC, when the patient is being bounced, and when priority must be given to ventilation, oxygenation, and circulation, attempts at cannulating subclavian or internal jugular veins for central venous catheterization are contraindicated because of the danger of inducing complications (e.g., pneumothorax) when these measures are attempted in the moving patient, and because the procedure may interrupt effective EHC. Therefore, as soon as possible, members of the team not occupied with ventilation and EHC should start a *peripheral* venous lifeline, preferably using a percutaneously inserted "extracath" or "intracath" plastic cannula in an arm or leg vein. Second choice is the external jugular vein, and third choice is the femoral vein (located in the inguinal region just medial to the femoral artery, which is palpable during EHC). Last choice is a quick venous cut-down.

When a *cut-down* is required for a peripheral venous lifeline during prolonged CPR attempts, it is usually more quickly and easily accomplished on the ankle (saphenous vein) than on the wrist or elbow. Cut-down on the saphenous vein of the ankle, just in front of the internal malleolus, can be accomplished very rapidly by making a 2- to 3-cm. transverse incision, picking up the vein with a hemostat by bluntly spreading tissue, inserting a large bore needle or cannula into the vein, and clamping the vein distally. A large metal cannula is inserted via a small incision in the vein, and a hemostat can be placed over vein and cannula proximally to save time. There is no need initially to use other clamps and sutures.

After spontaneous circulation has been restored (which may include drugs and fluids given directly via intermittent needle injections I.V. or via peripheral venous lifeline) subsequent controlled insertion of a *central* venous catheter is indicated. This may be done safely via the subclavian vein on either side or the internal jugular vein on the right side (which does not require immediate roentgen check of catheter placement, as it readily enters the superior vena cava).

The emergency venous lifeline should be used for rapid infusion of a *plasma substitute* (even in normovolemic arrest), because tissue hypoxia results in dilation of vascular beds and leakage of fluid from the intravascular compartment. For acute initial plasma volume expansion isotonic saline, Ringer's solution, or lactated Ringer's solution with 5 to 10 per cent dextrose and a colloid plasma substitute (human albumin or dextran 40) may be used. There are no good data on the differences between these solutions and their suitability for resuscitation. After restoration of spontaneous circulation, certainly a colloid plasma substitute is more likely to remain in the circulation than a crystalloid solution. Experience has shown that in normovolemic arrest plasma volume expansion by about 10 per cent of estimated blood volume (10 ml./kg. body weight) usually is beneficial. Packed red blood cells or whole blood is rarely required to restart spontaneous circulation, even in exsanguination arrest, provided the source of hemorrhage is controlled. The types and volumes administered are influenced by the cause of the arrest and the patient's response to resuscitative efforts.

The *intracardiac* injection of drugs is contraindicated (except for intracardiac injection under vision during open chest cardiac resuscitation, see below) as it may produce pneumothorax, injury to a coronary artery, and prolonged interruption of EHC (AHA, 1966A, 1974A; Safar, 1968A). Intracardiac injection of epinephrine should be considered only in the rare instance that a vein is inaccessible, and should be done via a long, thin (e.g., 22 gauge) needle through the fifth intercostal space parasternally into a heart chamber.

Intra-arterial pressure infusion (Negovsky, 1962) of blood or plasma substitutes via arterial cut-down is effective in helping restart spontaneous circulation in exsanguination cardiac arrest with smaller volumes of blood or plasma substitute than needed for venous infusion; however, it is a time consuming measure and carries the risk of retrograde air embolism. Moreover, solutions readily available in the emergency situation, which usually are cold, acid, and not oxygenated, are more effective given via vein and circulated through the lungs by EHC (Kirimli, 1965, 1969). (See Exsanguina-

tion Hemorrhage later in this chapter and also Chapter 2.)

DRUGS

As soon as possible after the initiation of CPR-ABC, epinephrine about 0.5 to 1.0 mg. (in adults) should be injected I.V. Dilution of the drug is not necessary. This dose should be repeated, perhaps even in larger doses (1 to 2 mg.) every 2 to 5 minutes if indicated. Even before an I.V. infusion has been started, we prefer to give the first dose of epinephrine via a small-gauge needle into any accessible peripheral vein. Whenever circulatory arrest has lasted two minutes or more or tissue hypoxia had existed prior to shorter periods of arrest, the tissue acidosis and acidemia present tend to counteract the circulatory effect of epinephrine and other catecholamines and depress cardiac contractility. Therefore, the second most important drug required for CPR under such circumstances of suspected acidosis is sodium bicarbonate. Until more reliable studies are available to clarify the use of these drugs in CPR, epinephrine and bicarbonate in rapid sequence during IPPV and EHC are the drugs of choice. *Epinephrine should not be used* when monitored VF is immediately reversed by countershock.

Epinephrine should be given I.V. as the first drug (Crile, 1906) without waiting for an electrocardiographic diagnosis. The alpha-receptor stimulating effect of epinephrine increases systemic peripheral vascular resistance (without constricting the coronary and cerebral vessels), raises diastolic pressure during EHC, and thereby improves myocardial and cerebral blood flow during EHC (Redding, 1962, 1968; Pearson, 1963, 1965). The beta-receptor stimulating effect of epinephrine is not important during EHC, but is advantageous when spontaneous circulation returns, giving a high initial cardiac output and arterial pressure at the beginning of spontaneous reperfusion, which benefits cerebral and other vital organ system blood flow (Ames, 1968; Safar, 1976a).

In asystole, epinephrine helps restart spontaneous cardiac action, as it increases myocardial contractility, elevates perfusion pressure, lowers defibrillation threshold, and often restores a spontaneous pulse in pulselessness with bizarre EKG complexes (electromechanical dissociation). Although epinephrine can produce ventricular fibrillation in the nonfibrillating heart with areas of ischemic anoxia, in the fibrillating heart it facilitates defibrillation by improving myocardial perfusion during EHC and by making the ventricular fibrillation (VF) pattern stronger and thereby more susceptible to defibrillation (Kirimli, 1966). Also, resumption of adequate spontaneous circulation after successful electric countershock is facilitated.

Pure alpha receptor stimulating sympathomimetic amines, such as norepinephrine (Levophed), phenylephrine (Neosynephrine) or methoxamine (Vasoxyl) are also effective in raising diastolic arterial pressure during EHC and in facilitating restoration of spontaneous circulation in asystole (Redding, 1962), but they do not provide the additional cardiac inotropic effect of epinephrine, which is desirable upon return of spontaneous circulation. In contrast, pure beta receptor stimulating sympathomimetic amines, such as isoproterenol (Isuprel) and calcium are *not* effective in supporting restoration of spontaneous circulation during EHC in cardiac arrest, since they lack the ability to increase systemic vascular resistance (Pearson, 1965).

Sodium bicarbonate is the second most important drug to be given during CPR (Mellemgaard, 1960; Stewart, 1964). Restoration of spontaneous circulation in asphyxial arrest and successful electric countershock in ventricular fibrillation are enhanced by epinephrine alone — more so by epinephrine plus bicarbonate — but *not* by bicarbonate alone (Kirimli, 1966). Neither drug is effective without IPPV and EHC. Epinephrine with or without bicarbonate given in asystole may result in VF, which calls for external electric countershock. The small volume of epinephrine is easy to administer quickly, whereas the large volume of bicarbonate (1 ml. per kg.) can and should be given slowly. Therefore, we recommend administering epinephrine first and bicarbonate next during CPR–ABC.

The recommended dose of sodium bicarbonate is approximately 1 mEq./kg. body weight I.V. (epinephrine should not be given in the bicarbonate solution, which may inactivate the catecholamine). Bicarbonate usually is available in a 1 molar solution (1 mEq./ml.) in prefilled syringes or bottles or bags for I.V. infusion. The dose of 1 mEq./kg. should be repeated, preferably

with arterial pH guidance, aiming for pHa values near 7.4 (7.2 to 7.6). When pHa determinations are not available, bicarbonate should be repeated about every 10 minutes of CPR. During the borderline artificial circulation of EHC, there is little washout of acid. Therefore, during hyperventilation, the use of multiple unmonitored doses of sodium bicarbonate has resulted in pHa values of 7.7 to 8.0, which causes VF rather than increases the likelihood of successful electric defibrillation. In contrast, immediately after restoration of spontaneous circulation, washout of acids (H_2CO_3 and lactic acid) from tissues is greatly increased, and therefore more bicarbonate is needed.

Ventilation volumes must be increased during sodium bicarbonate administration, as this drug is a CO_2 donor. During spontaneous circulation, the amount of bicarbonate required may not only be estimated according to arterial pH values, but rather aim at correction of base deficit (Chapters 3 and 10). Assuming an extracellular fluid volume of 25 per cent of body weight in kilograms, one can calculate the bicarbonate dose required for base deficit correction by multiplying the base deficit in mEq./liter with 25 per cent of body weight in kg. to determine the mEq. bicarbonate needed. The first half of this dose should be given rapidly and the other half slowly. This method of correction will not cause excessively high pHa values, provided ventilation is adjusted to keep arterial P_{CO_2} at 30 to 40 torr. Excessive amounts of sodium bicarbonate may be harmful, not only by producing alkalemia but also by causing hyperosmolality.

In witnessed VF, electric countershock must be applied immediately without delay for drug administration or CPR–ABC. If the first countershock is not effective, CPR must be started and epinephrine and bicarbonate given I.V. as soon as possible. The drugs are circulated for about 1 minute by EHC before repeat countershocks are applied. In unwitnessed arrest during CPR, we prefer to give epinephrine first into the running I.V., bicarbonate subsequently, continuing with intermittent doses of epinephrine until restoration of spontaneous circulation.

Tris buffer (THAM) has been used in lieu of and in the same dosage as mEq./kg. sodium bicarbonate; THAM has the advantage of not being a CO_2 donor and thus not requiring excessive hyperventilation (without which bicarbonate produces transient worsening of cerebral acidosis as the CO_2 enters the brain more rapidly than bicarbonate), but has the disadvantage of not being available in a readily usable solution for resuscitation. Also, the concentration required tends to sclerose veins. THAM needs re-study.

Other drugs may be needed to prevent cardiac arrest or for life support after cardiac arrest and restoration of spontaneous circulation. These drugs include atropine, lidocaine, norepinephrine, metaraminol, dopamine, isoproterenol, calcium, propranolol, morphine, and steroids.

Atropine reduces vagal tone, enhances atrioventricular conduction, and reduces the likelihood of ventricular fibrillation triggered by the myocardial hypoperfusion associated with extreme bradycardia. It may increase the heart rate not only in sinus bradycardia but also in high-degree atrioventricular block with bradycardia, but not in complete atrioventricular block. In complete AV block isoproterenol is indicated. Thus, atropine has essentially no place during Phases I and II of CPR. Atropine is indicated during spontaneous circulation when the heart rate has decreased to less than about 60 beats per minute and there are PVCs or hypotension. Atropine is given in 0.2- to 0.5-mg. increments I.V., up to a total dose of about 2 mg. In third degree atrioventricular block larger doses may be tried.

Lidocaine (Xylocaine) is a local anesthetic which raises the ventricular fibrillation threshhold (Carden, 1956). It is an antiarrhythmic agent that, in equipotent antiarrhythmic doses, produces less myocardial depression than other anti-arrhythmic drugs. Lidocaine increases the electric stimulation threshold during diastole. It depresses cardiac irritability in cases of frequently recurring VF. Its greatest value has been in the treatment of PVCs and thereby prevention of their progression to VT or VF. Lidocaine is given in an initial bolus of about 1 mg./kg. body weight I.V., to be followed by a continuous infusion (of a solution of 1 mg. lidocaine/ml., in 5 per cent dextrose in water) at a rate of about 1 to 3 mg./minute, usually not exceeding 4 mg./minute in a 70-kg. adult. The limitations and differences in action of lidocaine and other anti-arrhythmic agents such as procainamide (Pronestyl), quinidine, diphenylhydantoin (Dilantin), and Bretyl-

lium must be understood (Dembo and Resnekov, in Safar, 1977A).

Norepinephrine (Levophed) primarily stimulates alpha-receptors, with little beta-receptor action. Although it is effective in helping to restore spontaneous circulation during EHC in lieu of epinephrine (Smetana, 1961), epinephrine is preferred. Norepinephrine, however, is less likely to produce recurrent tachyarrhythmias and, therefore, is preferred for arterial pressure support *after* restoration of spontaneous circulation. It is the most potent vasopressor available and should, therefore, be given by carefully titrated I.V. infusion, using solutions of 8 to 16 µg./ml. In cardiogenic shock, including post-CPR hypotension without hypovolemia, norepinephrine is not likely to produce dangerous renal vasoconstriction, provided it is not given to the point of producing hypertension. Nevertheless, prolonged administration of norepinephrine is considered ill-advised and, therefore, a milder vasopressor with less likelihood of producing renal ischemia should be substituted (e.g., dopamine) when the more potent norepinephrine is not needed anymore.

Metaraminol (Aramine) has both alpha- and beta-receptor stimulating action, but is less potent than epinephrine. Metaraminol usually causes no tachycardia and may be given as an I.V. bolus of 2 to 5 mg., repeated every 5 to 10 minutes as needed, or by titrated I.V. infusion of a solution containing 0.4 mg./ml.

Dopamine is also a sympathomimetic agent and exerts a dose-dependent vasoconstrictor and cardiac inotropic effect. Its vasopressor potency is less than that of norepinephrine, and it is more likely to dilate than constrict renal vessels. Slow infusion has primarily inotropic and renal vasodilating effects, whereas more rapid infusion or higher concentration exerts an over-all vasoconstrictor effect. Dopamine, given by titrated I.V. infusion in rates between 1 and 50 µg./kg. body weight/minute, in a solution of about 200 mg./250 ml. (800 µg./ml.), is useful for supporting arterial perfusion pressure after restoration of spontaneous circulation (when the more potent agent norepinephrine is not needed anymore). As with all vasopressors, normovolemia or slight blood volume expansion must be established as well.

Isoproterenol (Isuprel) is a pure beta-receptor stimulator which, because of its lack of vasoconstrictor action, does not seem to enhance restoration of spontaneous circulation during EHC (Pearson, 1965). It thus has no place during CPR except in the case of asystole from known heart block (Stokes-Adams syndrome). Even then, epinephrine is preferred to restart the heart and isoproterenol is given immediately after restoration of spontaneous circulation. In post-CPR cardiogenic shock, mixtures of isoproterenol and norepinephrine, both by titrated infusion, have been tried. Isoproterenol alone, although it will increase cardiac output, may do this at the expense of increased myocardial oxygen consumption, and is less likely to maintain the desirable cerebral perfusion pressure than are the other sympathomimetic amines. If isoproterenol is decided upon, it is usually given by I.V. infusion at a rate of 2 to 20 μg./minute, using a solution of 1 mg. in 500 ml. In severe ventricular bradycardia the infusion rate is adjusted to increase the heart rate to about 60/minute, while tiding the patient over the waiting period for a pacemaker insertion.

Calcium also increases myocardial *contractility* without causing vasoconstriction (Kay, 1951) but is not as likely to produce vasodilation and tachycardia as isoproterenol. Calcium, however, also increases myocardial *irritability,* like epinephrine and isoproterenol. In excessive amounts, calcium may cause the heart to contract and stop beating, particularly in the fully digitalized patient. It does not seem to enhance the likelihood of restoration of spontaneous circulation during EHC (Pearson, 1965). Its usefulness has not yet been clarified; it may be a more appropriate agent to use than the sympathomimetic amines in cardiac depression from certain drugs, such as barbiturates. Calcium may be of value in selected cases of profound cardiovascular collapse with severe hypotension or with pulselessness (electromechanical dissociation) and in the rare case where repeated doses of epinephrine have not resulted in restoration of spontaneous circulation when the EKG shows asystole or electromechanical dissocation. The dosage for calcium chloride is not clear, but usually 2.5 to 5 ml. of a 10 per cent solution are given (3.4 to 6.8 mEq. of calcium ion). Such I.V. doses may be repeated every 10 minutes. Calcium gluconate provides less ionizable calcium and therefore must be given in larger amounts, such as 10 ml. of a 10 per cent solution (4.8 mEq.). Cal-

cium must not be given in the bicarbonate infusion, as the two precipitate.

Propranolol (Inderal), a beta-receptor blocker, has no place during EHC, as it may make the heart unresuscitable. Doses of 1 mg. I.V., however, may be useful in rare instances of repetitive bouts of VT or intractable VT or VF, resistant to countershock and lidocaine. Propranolol can cause bronchospasm.

Morphine is not indicated during and immediately following CPR itself, but is one of several adjunctive drugs indicated in acute pulmonary edema, which may occur before, during, or after cardiac arrest (Chapter 3). Morphine seems to act by dilating capacitance vessels, producing a "bloodless (pharmacologic) phlebotomy," and also by depressing the exaggerated breathing movements and anxiety that feed the cycle of developing pulmonary edema.

Steroids have been recommended for their anti-inflammatory and antiedema effect in the immediate postresuscitative period to ameliorate the reaction of the lungs to aspiration, which is common in CPR cases (Chapter 3) and the reaction of the brain to the ischemic-anoxic insult (Chapter 5). Steroid doses, as part of the immediate postresuscitative management, are listed under Step I later in this chapter.

Other useful CPR drugs with which the physician should be familiar and which should be available in the emergency drug kit include 50 per cent dextrose; a rapidly acting digitalis preparation (e.g., digoxin); bronchodilators such as aminophylline, and a beta-2 receptor stimulator (e.g., metaproterenol); muscle relaxants (safe use requires training in anesthesiology), e.g., succinylcholine, curare; a rapidly acting diuretic (e.g., ethacrynic acid, furosemide); an antihistamine (e.g., diphenhydramine, i.e., Benadryl); a narcotic antagonist (e.g., nalorphine or Narcan); a thiobarbiturate (Step H); and the most potent myocardial depressant, potassium chloride.

Routes other than the intravenous should be considered when an intravenous life-line is not possible. Epinephrine can be given with almost I.V.-like rapidity of onset of action, through the *intrapulmonary* route (Redding, 1967), by instilling 1 to 2 mg. of epinephrine, diluted in 10 ml. of sterile distilled water (not saline), via tracheal tube (or even better, via a thin suction catheter inserted into a bronchus) (Elam, in Safar,

1977A). Lidocaine, 50 to 100 mg. in 10 ml. of water, is also effective via the pulmonary route. The endotracheal administration of other drugs for CPR has not yet been established. Sodium bicarbonate must not be given by the pulmonary route, as it can produce tracheobronchial and pulmonary damage.

The *intramuscular* route is effective in producing therapeutic blood levels of atropine (2 mg. I.M.), or lidocaine (300 mg. I.M.) for the *prevention* of arrhythmias (Valentine, 1974). The intramuscular route has *no place* for drug administration during emergency resuscitation because of the unpredictability of absorption and drug action, onset, and dosages.

(E) Electrocardioscopy

As soon as possible after the start of CPR/ABC, the EKG pattern should be determined (Figure 17), primarily to differentiate between: (1) asystole; (2) pulselessness with EKG complexes (also called cardiovascular collapse, electromechanical dissociation); and (3) ventricular fibrillation (VF) or ventricular tachycardia (VT) without pulse. These are the three most common patterns associated with pulselessness. Although epinephrine and bicarbonate are indicated in all three, ventricular fibrillation calls for immediate electric countershock.

The EKG may be determined most rapidly by using defibrillator chest electrodes that incorporate the EKG pickup electrodes, which should be provided with all modern defibrillators. In addition, the EKG monitor should provide needle and/or stick-on electrodes which can be quickly applied to the right arm and left leg (active electrodes) and the left arm or chest (indifferent electrode) for emergency resuscitation.

Techniques, equipment, and training are influenced by the need for: (a) immediate

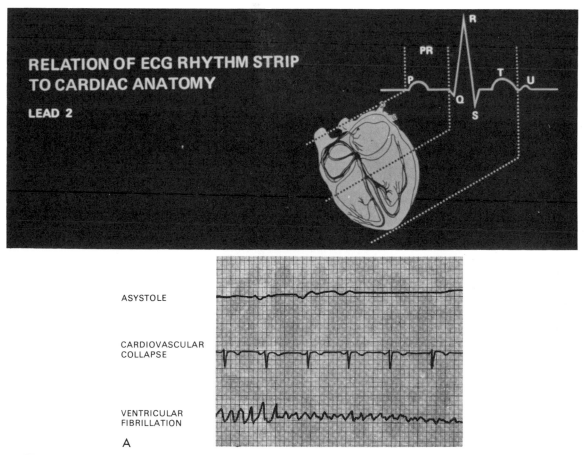

Figure 17 Electrocardiographic patterns. *A, top,* Relation of normal ECG to cardiac anatomy. *Bottom,* The three typical ECG patterns associated with pulselessness; i.e., asystole, cardiovascular collapse (electromechanical dissociation, mechanical without electric asystole), and ventricular fibrillation.

Illustration continued on the following page.

(1) PVC with R-on-T

(2) Frequent PVCs

(3) Multifocal PVCs

(4) PVCs with VT

(5) VT

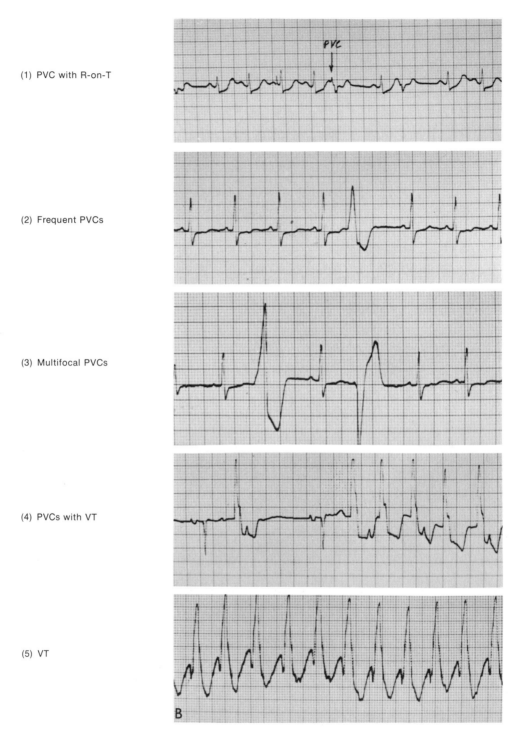

Figure 17 (*Continued*)   *B*, Tachyarrhythmias. (1) PVC with R-on-T, which may lead to VF. (2) Frequent PVCs. (3) Multifocal PVCs. (4) Runs of PVCs with short run of VT. (5) Ventricular tachycardia. All lead 2.

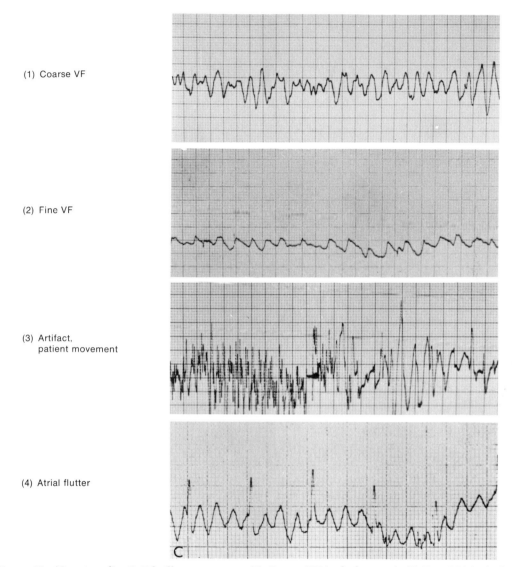

(1) Coarse VF

(2) Fine VF

(3) Artifact, patient movement

(4) Atrial flutter

Figure 17 *(Continued)* C, Fibrillation patterns. (1) Coarse VF (pulselessness). (2) Fine VF (pulselessness). (3) Artifact from patient movement (with pulse). (4) Atrial flutter (with pulse).

Illustration continued on the following page.

recognition of the above three arrhythmias associated with pulselessness; *(b)* more detailed EKG diagnosis throughout CPR Phases I and II by an EKG electrode method that does not hamper external heart compressions and ventilation; and *(c)* long-term EKG monitoring in Phase III that does not limit limb motion and permits detailed EKG diagnosis of myocardial disease by specialized leads. Step *(a)* is best provided for most rapidly by portable battery-powered defibrillator-EKG monitor units with EKG electrodes incorporated into the defibrillator chest paddles. Step *(b)* is provided through the same unit also being equipped with needle and/or stick-on electrodes to be applied rapidly to the right arm and left leg (active electrodes) and the left arm or elsewhere (indifferent electrode). Step *(c)* is provided by stick-on chest electrodes, an EKG recorder that connects to the monitor, and special leads. EKG telemetry equipment has been useful for the prevention of cardiac arrest by early recognition of life-threatening arrhythmias in hospitalized patients, and for physician command of paramedics in the field.

In cardiac arrest, proceed with airway control, artificial ventilation, and EHC; apply the defibrillator-EKG chest electrodes; make a quick diagnosis, and apply an electric countershock in the case of VT or

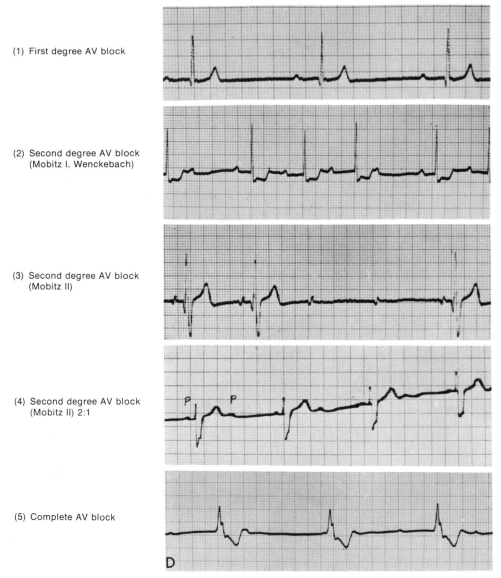

(1) First degree AV block

(2) Second degree AV block (Mobitz I, Wenckebach)

(3) Second degree AV block (Mobitz II)

(4) Second degree AV block (Mobitz II) 2:1

(5) Complete AV block

Figure 17 (*Continued*) D, Bradyarrhythmias. (1) First degree AV block. (2) Second degree AV block (Mobitz type I–Wenckebach phenomenon). (3) Second degree AV block (Mobitz type II). (4) Second degree AV block 2:1 (Mobitz type II). (5) Complete AV block with ventricular rhythm.

VF. Interrupt EHC for a few seconds at a time to allow a clear EKG diagnosis, as EHC produces EKG artifacts. After restoration of spontaneous circulation, when perfusion is stable, switch the leads to the stick-on chest electrodes. For Lead II, place one electrode just below the right clavicle (negative electrode), and the other below the left pectoral muscle (positive electrode). Appreciate the fact that the EKG does not indicate presence or absence of circulation (except for asystole and VF, which are always accompanied by pulselessness) and thus EKG monitoring

must be accompanied by the other steps of CPR including oxygenation, venous infusion, drug administration, and arterial pressure monitoring (first by feeling the pulse and using the regular cuff technique; later, if intensive care is needed, by arterial catheter) (Redding, in Safar, 1977A).

Since most sudden cardiac deaths associated with myocardial ischemia or infarction occur following life-threatening arrhythmias (see later), EKG monitoring should be used as a preventive measure immediately on all patients with suspected heart attack or shock. Cardiac arrest can often be prevented by early detection and prompt treatment of PVCs; ventricular tachycardia (VT); or severe bradycardia. PVCs and VT are treated with I.V. lidocaine (VT without pulse by electric countershock), and bradycardia with atropine, isoproterenol, and pacing.

LIFE-THREATENING ARRHYTHMIAS (FIG. 17)

Health professionals providing advanced CPR life-support must be able to recognize at least the following tachy and bradyarrhythmias:

Premature ventricular contractions (PVCs) are extra beats triggered by an ectopic focus. They are followed by a compensatory pause and may be multifocal and have different forms. If every other beat is preceded by a PVC, it is called "ventricular bigeminal rhythm." Runs of many PVCs become VT. If PVCs fall on a T wave, they can trigger VT or VF (the R-on-T phenomenon). PVCs are treated by lidocaine, which may, for long-term prevention, be changed to procainamide, diphenylhydantoin, propranolol, quinidine, digitalis, or other drugs. If PVCs are triggered by a very slow heart rate in heart block (see below), they can be prevented with the use of atropine, isoproterenol, or pacing. In contrast, atropine itself may result in tachyarrhythmias.

Premature atrial contractions may occur in normal persons, and, if frequent, may indicate heart disease and initiate atrial tachycardia. Therapy consists of sedation. Atrial flutter or fibrillation can also occur occasionally in normal hearts, but is more likely a sign of heart disease. It is best treated by DC countershock cardioversion, and digitalis or propranolol may have a place in treatment.

Ventricular tachycardia usually is a regular sequence of bizarre runs of PVCs and is a precursor of VF. During VT there may or may not be a palpable pulse, depending in part on the rapidity of the rate. In the presence of a pulse, lidocaine I.V. is tried to terminate VT; however, VT with pulselessness is treated like VF, namely, with electric countershock. It is important to differentiate between atrial and ventricular tachycardia, since the former is harmless and the latter is life-threatening. If the differentiation is impossible, attention to the hemodynamic effects (pulse, arterial pressure, CVP) is required.

Ventricular fibrillation is the most common cause of sudden cardiac death, most often due to spotty areas of underperfusion in the myocardium in "hearts too good to die"—that is, capable of producing adequate cardiac output if the VF is reversed (Beck, 1960). The pathophysiology, causes, and reversibility of VF have been discussed in Chapter 2.

Bradycardia is dangerous in the critically ill person when the heart rate is less than 60 per minute. In this case one should attempt to differentiate between sinus and ventricular bradycardia. The *atrioventricular block* may be first, second, or third degree (Figure 17). *First degree A-V block* is merely a delayed passage of the impulse through the A-V node, causing a prolonged PR interval. It serves as a warning, but rarely is treatment needed. *Second degree A-V block* results in dropped beats and may be one of two types—the Mobitz type I pattern (Wenckebach A-V block) and the more dangerous Mobitz type II A-V block. Mobitz type I A-V block is common in myocardial infarction, usually transient, and requires atropine or isoproterenol rather than a pacemaker. Mobitz type II A-V block occurs in large myocardial infarctions as a forerunner of total A-V block. It needs at least a standby pacemaker.

Third degree (complete) A-V block is characterized by an absence of impulses from the atria to the ventricle, with a slow idioventricular rate of 30 to 40 beats per minute, as in Stokes-Adams syndrome. The P-waves are unrelated to the QRS complexes. With a very slow ventricular rate, blood flow may become inadequate to maintain consciousness, and reduced myocardial perfusion can result in congestive heart failure, angina, VT, or VF. Treatment in the patient who tends to become unconscious or whose heart rate is considered dangerously slow should be with external fist pacing (see "Witnessed Arrest" later in this chapter), while an I.V. infusion of isoproterenol is started. With this, the patient's heart rate usually can be supported adequately until an I.V. pacemaker is inserted. During CPR/ABC, when upon restoration of spontaneous circulation there is frequently recurrent VT or VF, one should study the EKG in detail to determine whether the tachyarrhythmia is preceded by third degree (complete) A-V block. In this case, seemingly paradoxic treatment with isoproterenol or epinephrine can keep the heart rate high enough to prevent such recurrent tachyarrhythmias and cardiac arrests. Atropine is more likely to increase the frequency of heart beats when there is sinus bradycardia rather than ventricular bradycardia (complete heart block).

(F) Fibrillation Treatment

Ventricular fibrillation results commonly from coronary insufficiency, adverse drug reactions, electrocution, cardiac catheterization in an irritable heart or, secondarily, during resuscitative efforts for asystole from asphyxia, drowning, exsanguination, and other causes of cardiac arrest (Chapter 2). Whereas VF often can be prevented by appropriate drug therapy, treatment of VF during CPR with depressant drugs (e.g., lidocaine, other local anesthetics, quinidine, potassium chloride, beta blockers) is usually either unable to terminate VF or will transform VF into asytole, which is intractable to CPR efforts, including epinephrine. Therefore, the most rapid, effective and accepted method for fibrillation treatment is electric countershock (Prevost, 1899; Beck, 1947; Zoll, 1956). VF will rarely cease spontaneously without countershock (Stephenson, in Safar, 1977A). Low voltage electric shock can induce VF, whereas high voltage properly applied terminates VF if the current sent through the heart is at least 2 amperes (Hooker, 1933; Kouwenhoven, 1954, 1973). This produces simultaneous depolarization of all myocardial fibers, after which spontaneous cardiac contractions may start if the myocardium is well oxygenated and nonacidotic (Chapter 2). The amount of current passing through the heart cannot be monitored. Techniques for electric countershock that minimize chest wall resistance and optimize electric shock wave patterns, durations, voltage delivered (in AC shock) and energy (watt-seconds) delivered (in DC shock) have evolved semi-empirically (Knickerbocker, in Safar, 1977A). Thus the most effective way to terminate VF and VT without pulse is an *external countershock*, which may be performed by alternating or direct current (Nobel, 1971, 1973A). DC countershock may be more effective in large diseased hearts, as well as in hypothermic patients (Gurvich, 1946; Lown, 1962; Peleska, 1957). In the treatment of VT and VF,

however, the main advantage of DC over AC countershock is irrelevant; namely, the fact that its short duration and ability to be programmed exactly can prevent placement of the electric shock on the upstroke of the T wave of the EKG, which may induce VF in the beating heart. EKG diagnosis (Fig. 17) and electric countershock (Fig. 18) must go hand-in-hand.

For external countershock, standard electrode position is one just to the right of the upper half of the sternum below the clavicle and the other just to the left of the cardiac apex or left nipple (Fig. 18). Electric contact between electrodes and skin must be optimal, without providing a current path between electrodes over the patient's skin (e.g., when the electrode paste is smeared). Applying just enough paste or saline-soaked sponges usually provides an adequate contact. Electrode paste makes the chest slippery for EHC, whereas saline-soaked sponges do not. The sponges have the added advantage of being applied more rapidly, thus minimizing interruption of EHC. Electrodes placed over the sponges should be pressed firmly to the chest, the team asked to stand clear of patient and bed for the moment of shock, and the countershock discharged by the physician pushing the appropriate hand switches (preferably one on each paddle to avoid accidental discharge) — and preferably by the physician who directs the team.

To produce the required energy in the heart, an AC countershock, usually of 500 to 1000 volts (0.1 to 0.25 second), applied directly to the outside of the chest is required in the average adult. Although lower voltage shocks may sometimes succeed, high energy levels are recommended because failure of the first countershock may delay restarting of spontaneous circulation. The same applies to the now more commonly used DC countershock, which has the added advantage of being superior for cardioversion in the beating heart. DC countershock is produced by a capacitance discharge-type defibrillator, delivering 200 to 400 watt seconds of about 0.01 second duration. Although subtle histologic changes in the myocardium are related to the amount and duration of current sent through the heart, and, thereby, to the heat produced in the heart, external application of such high energy or high voltage countershocks does not damage the heart so as to impair resumption of spontaneous contrac-

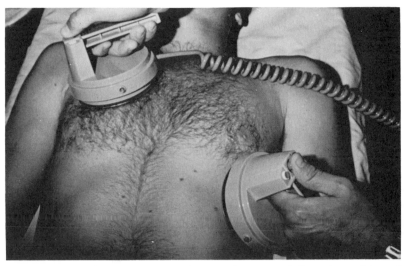

Figure 18 External electric defibrillation via two bimanually triggered chest electrodes applied on conductive jelly or saline-soaked sponge, one electrode just below right clavicle, the other over cardiac apex. Electrodes incorporate defibrillation and EKG leads. (From AHA Advanced Life Support Slide Series, 1975.)

tions. This risk of producing heat damage is greater when low voltage or low energy is used frequently, as in the case when the first attempt fails. In contrast, direct application of the current to the heart (see "Internal Cardiac Resuscitation") is more likely to produce burns on the surface of the heart.

Although the most commonly used energy for external DC countershock is 400 watt seconds for adults, 100 to 200 watt seconds for children, and 50 to 100 watt seconds for infants, lower energies occasionally have been effective in VT and sometimes even in VF. However, the ideal amount of energy required in any given case cannot be determined during CPR in advance. While the above energy recommendations are for the conventional single discharge wave form, other wave forms may call for different energy requirements. For this, one must consult the manufacturer's literature. Defibrillators must be checked frequently to determine the actual energy delivered, since the reading on the dial is not always accurate. Also, a regular maintenance program for defibrillators is essential.

In the argument between AC countershock versus DC countershock technique, the main advantage of the latter is that DC shocks can be applied from portable battery-powered defibrillators (Peleska, 1957), whereas AC shocks depend on wall current.

In witnessed monitored VF, external countershock should be applied immediate-ly, without first giving drugs and starting CPR/ABC. If unsuccessful, CPR must be started promptly to prevent cerebral and myocardial hypoxia and then followed by administration of drugs and repeat attempts at electric defibrillation, adapting the sequence of actions according to variables monitored and the patient's underlying problem. One must appreciate that the countershock is more likely to be successful if given one-half to two minutes following the administration of epinephrine, I.V. during EHC. Countershock should not be withheld until the large volume of bicarbonate is injected. When several countershocks fail to terminate VF, several rapidly repeated (serial) shocks have sometimes been successful; however, such serial defibrillation attempts are only possible with the use of the AC defibrillator since the DC defibrillator does not recharge rapidly enough.

In intractable or recurrent VF, lidocaine I.V. may be of value. In recurrent or protracted VF resistant to electric defibrillation, efforts to reverse VF and appropriate drug therapy should be continued until successful or until reversion to asystole with signs of myocardial death. Some patients have recovered with intact CNS after one to two hours of VF, during which time only EHC produced borderline circulation. After defibrillation, the EKG may show asystole, abnormal EKG complexes, or reasonably normal EKG complexes. EHC must be continued as long as there is no spontaneous carotid pulse. In asystole, CPR is accompanied by administration of epinephrine and bicarbonate.

Experimental semi-invasive defibrillation techniques, such as the use of *esophageal*-chest surface electrodes, reduce the electric resistance between electrodes and, therefore, the total energy required and defibrillator size (Elam, in Safar, 1977A).

Since electric countershock will not add damage in asystole or electromechanical dissociation (although it is not effective in restarting the heart in these conditions), it is justified, in the absence of a cardioscope and the presence of a defibrillator, to employ an *empirical* (unmonitored) *countershock*. Such a single shock, however, should not delay the start of other CPR measures. Unmonitored countershock in children is not recommended. Countershock without EKG diagnosis would rarely be necessary, because of the increasing availability of EKG monitors combined with defibrillators.

PHASE III: IMMEDIATE POST-RESUSCITATIVE LIFE SUPPORT

(G) Gauging

When to start and when to stop resuscitation depends on the physician's judgment and is part of the art and science of resuscitation (Safar, 1963). Modern resuscitation has changed the definition of death (Chapters 2 and 5). *Clinical death* is the absence of circulation and breathing movements with all cerebral activities suspended, but not irreversibly so. In *acute* respiratory and circulatory distress, reoxygenation must be started immediately. There is no time for contemplation and consultation. If restoration of spontaneous circulation proves impossible, cardiac compression may be discontinued when dilated nonreactive pupils, absent breathing movements and areflexia (e.g., stimulation by suction catheter of the carina, the most sensitive reflex) indicate cerebral death for over one hour *and* the heart is in intractable mechanical asystole. However, bizarre EKG complexes without heart beat may go on for many minutes of cardiac arrest and many hours during CPR; i.e., mechanical, but not electrical, asystole.

One must keep in mind that dilated fixed pupils can occur as the result of brain injury or catecholamines given for resuscitation. During emergency resuscitation, particularly during efforts to restart spontaneous circulation, judging the salvability of the central nervous system is difficult if not impossible. Particularly in children one should not give up early. Their CNS picture should not indicate termination of efforts to restart circulation. Therefore, we feel that in patients of any age without incurable lethal disease, emergency CPR efforts should be continued unless there are signs of *cardiac death*. This is likely when there is continuing absence of all ventricular electrocardiographic activity (i.e., electric aystole) for 10 minutes or more of adequate CPR, including appropriate drug therapy. In contrast to asystole, in the presence of recurrent ventricular fibrillation or electromechanical dissociation (pulselessness with EKG complexes) or changing EKG patterns in patients with sick hearts, up to about 2 hours of CPR efforts have sometimes resulted eventually in restoration of spontaneous circulation.

After restoration of spontaneous circulation, most patients who begin to wake up within five to ten minutes of reperfusion recover with a clinically normal CNS (Safar, 1977Aa). Those who are comatose (in the absence of CNS depressant drugs) at about ten minutes often suffer variable degrees of temporary or permanent brain damage. New methods of brain resuscitation (see Chapter 5 and this chapter, Step H) have made recovery of the brain possible even after more than five minutes of circulatory arrest.

If *after* restoration of spontaneous circulation the patient has not regained consciousness, the underlying disorder appears incompatible with survival or it is possible in an orderly fashion to determine and certify "brain death" (Chapter 5), the physician should not hesitate to discontinue long-term resuscitation (intensive care). In general, good prognostic signs are rapid recovery of eye and upper airway reflexes. Progressive deterioration of reflexes, continuing unconsciousness and nonreaction of dilated pupils are poor prognostic signs. In infants and children post-arrest intensive care should be continued longer than in adults, since in children complete neurologic and psychologic recovery have occurred after long periods of coma (Ravitch, 1961), particularly when the arrest was associated with hypothermia (Siebke, 1975). The EEG is only one of several signs and should not be considered decisive in itself.

Survival of a patient with severe brain damage may impose an unbearable financial and emotional burden on the family. The decision to discontinue efforts should be made by the attending physician in consultation with experienced consultants (e.g., anesthesiologist, CCM physician, neurologist). Objective criteria based on scientific facts are needed to prove the irreversibility of coma in the individual patient. Since such methods and criteria have not yet been developed, clinical judgment is still used as the principal guideline.

For discontinuance of long-term life support efforts, Grenvik and associates recommend two sets of *guidelines* (Grenvik, 1978; Loughhead, 1976):

(1) *Brain death* determination and certification (for criteria and methods see Chapter 5). Brain death certification should not be carried out during emergency resuscitative efforts, but should be done after stabilization of the patient in the ICU (see Step I, below) and after sufficient time has been allowed for the course of CNS deterioration to be assessed in an orderly fashion by two licensed physicians (Chapter 5).

(2) *Irreversible coma* or vegetative state *without brain death* (without areflexia and electrocortical silence). At the Presbyterian-University Hospital of Pittsburgh guidelines were designed and approved in 1975 for the degree of care appropriate in hopeless moribund patients. All patients can now be classified in an orderly fashion in the following four categories:

(a) *Total support* These are critically ill or injured patients in whom there is no evidence that survival will be accompanied by severe chronic brain failure. Their vital organ systems frequently are seriously affected, but in these patients everything possible is done to reduce mortality and morbidity.

(b) *All but CPR* These are patients with a functioning brain or at least some hope for brain recovery, who have irreversible cardiopulmonary or other multiple organ failure or are in the terminal stages of incurable disease (e.g., advanced cancer, terminal stages of chronic lung disease, high spinal cord lesions). These patients are often treated vigorously but only to the point of cardiac arrest, which, if it occurs, is not

treated and the patient is permitted to die. Obviously, in the terminal stages of an incurable disease resuscitation should not be attempted. This should be understood by physicians and nurses caring for the patient.

(c) *No extraordinary measures* (i.e., "letting die;" passive euthanasia) In these patients all treatments are meaningless, prolonging death rather than life. Only comforting therapy is given. Examples are patients with minimal brain function without hope for improvement, such as seemingly permanent coma or vegetative state in the post-CPR phase of intensive care. Obviously, CPR is also withheld. Extraordinary measures to be withheld or withdrawn include ICU admission, arrhythmia control, blood infusions, vasoactive drugs, and mechanical ventilation.

(d) *Brain death* In these patients all treatment is discontinued (see 1, above).

The meager data available on the long-term outcome of patients who "survived" CPR attempts are beyond the scope of this chapter; they suggest that wiser use of CPR *is* indicated (Lemire, 1972; Stephenson, 1974) (Chapter 2). Once spontaneous circulation is restored and brain death is not present, *stabilization* with *advanced intensive care* (H and I, below) for at least 48 hours is needed before meaningful reassessment of brain viability is possible.

H. Human Mentation — Cerebral Resuscitation

The urgency with which CPR must be started and the perfection with which near-normal arterial oxygen transport must be restored are determined by the fact that the hypoxia-sensitive brain is the target organ of resuscitation (Chapter 5) (Safar, 1976). Modern postresuscitative intensive care (Step I, below) is essential for normalizing or optimizing extracranial variables in support of cerebral recovery. In addition, however, the following therapeutic potentials have been or are being evaluated for direct postischemic-anoxic therapy to ameliorate the resulting brain damage: hypertensive brain flush; barbiturate loading; hemodilution; heparinization; osmotherapy; hypothermia; and many different drugs.

After review of available experimental and clinical data and drafts of clinical trial protocols prepared by Safar and associates, a group of national resuscitation experts met in October, 1975 (Wolf Creek Conference), and international brain ischemia researchers and clinical leaders met in May, 1976 (International Emergency and Critical Care Medicine Congress, Pittsburgh, PA). The following recommendations resulted (Safar, 1977Aa); (*a*) Brief mild hypertension upon reperfusion, followed by normotension, should be part of post-CPR care; (*b*) barbiturate loading is ready for clinical trial (Chapter 5); and (*c*) other promising therapeutic modalities need further experimental evaluation. An increasing number of institutions have requested involvement in barbiturate loading trials, which should be carried out by experienced physicians trained in anesthesiology, using common protocols. Clinician-scholars favor multi-institutional, controlled, prospective clinical trials with randomization of barbiturate therapy.

There are many published reports of experimental and clinical studies on the mechanisms and amelioration of *focal* brain ischemia (stroke) (Smith, A, 1974) and start of therapy *before* the ischemic anoxic-insult (protection) (Secher, 1968). Since 1970 we have studied *global* ischemia treatment *after* the insult, developed reproducible animal models (Nemoto, 1975) and discovered that reflow promotion (Safar, 1976) and barbiturate loading (Bleyaert, 1975; Nemoto, 1977) can ameliorate postischemic-anoxic brain damage.

The "postresuscitation disease" postulated by Negovsky (1962, 1974) adds to the initial insult to determine outcome (Chapters 2 and 5). Several investigators, including our group, have shown that there is reduced cerebral blood flow postischemia and that increased intracranial pressure postischemia is not a major problem (Snyder, 1975). *Reflow promotion* by a combination of postischemic hypertension, hemodilution, and heparinization greatly ameliorated neurologic deficit and increased survival rate in dogs following 12 minutes of VF and restoration of spontaneous circulation by CPR (Safar, 1976). These three therapeutic modalities however, which were studied together, are still to be separated by controlled experiments. One short period of moderate *arterial hypertension* shortly after the start of reperfusion, can ameliorate the no-reflow phenomenon (Ames, 1968; Hossmann, in Plum, 1974). However, not only hypotension but also prolonged (or repeti-

tive) severe hypertension must be avoided, as it can worsen cerebral edema and outcome (Bleyaert, 1977).

In monkeys, *thiopental*, 90 mg./kg., given immediately *after* 16 minutes of global brain ischemia greatly ameliorated the ensuing neurologic deficit and histologic changes (Bleyaert, 1975; Nemoto, 1977). The mechanisms of thiopental protection are unknown and probably numerous (Chapter 5) The equianesthetic dose in man is not known, but is suspected to be about one third the dose for the Rhesus monkey. Several types of barbiturate seem to protect the brain. Optimal doses are not known.

The new *protocols* summarized in this chapter under Steps H and I will undergo periodic changes, but are presently recommended for multi-institutional *studies* (Safar, 1977Aa). These detailed protocols and other background materials are available from the author upon request. The objectives of this clinical study are: (1) to give victims of ischemic-anoxic insults an optimal chance to recover with little or no neurologic-intellectual-behavioral deficit; (2) to determine the efficacy in man of new measures for brain resuscitation after their efficacy has been proved in controlled animal experiments; (3) to determine the duration of "clinical death" in man; and (4) to improve standard CPR practices. *The following Pittsburgh protocols (1977) may change with new evidence.*

PROTOCOL #1: BASIC POSTRESUSCITATIVE MANAGEMENT

Included are all patients who require emergency resuscitation; they should be treated by this protocol if they are comatose or stuporous as the result of an ischemic-anoxic insult. Patients in the prehospital setting who meet the above criteria should receive as many components of this protocol as the physician who directs paramedics considers feasible. Physician control of paramedics by radio must be continuous. Most of the measures listed in this protocol are *not* for "standing orders." *Excluded* are all patients for whom the decision "all but CPR" or "no extraordinary measures" has been made.

(*a*) *Restoration of oxygenation and spontaneous circulation* should be accomplished according to the 1973 National Standards (AHA, 1974A) as outlined in this chapter under Phase II.

(*b*) *Immediately after restoration of*

spontaneous circulation, until recovery of consciousness, life support of extracranial vital organ systems should be carried out meticulously, as recommended in this chapter under Phase III, Step I, subsequently.

(c) "Hypertensive brain flush" should be accomplished as soon as feasible after restoration of spontaneous circulation, unless absolutely contraindicated. Systolic arterial pressure should be raised to 130–150 torr (in the previously normotensive person) once for 1–5 minutes. Thereafter, as long as the patient is unconscious, normotension (mean arterial pressure of 90–100 torr) should be maintained. Hypertension and normotension can be accomplished by titrated I.V. infusion of norepinephrine and/or dopamine and slight expansion of plasma volume (see Phase II, Step D). Epinephrine given during CPR may result in a hypertensive bout upon resumption of spontaneous circulation. Repetitive and more severe hypertension and hypotension must be avoided or immediately corrected.

PROTOCOL #2: CLINICAL (RESEARCH) TRIAL OF BARBITURATE LOADING

Only patients who have suffered a *severe* global ischemic-anoxic insult without prompt awakening should be *included* for clinical trials (experimental use) of immediate postresuscitative barbiturate loading. Examples include primary cardiac arrest with no circulation for five minutes or more and continued coma from the ischemic-anoxic insult (not from CNS depressant drugs) 5–10 minutes following restoration of oxygenation and circulation (excluding the time of external heart compressions). "Comatose" means that the patient does not respond to painful stimuli with movements, or responds merely with reflex posturing without localization. Ischemic-anoxic insults include primary and secondary cardiac arrest (Chapter 2) and severe decrease of arterial oxygen transport without cardiac arrest, resulting in coma (shock).

Patients outside the hospital meeting the rough criteria may be treated with Protocol #1 by paramedics under physician direction by radio; but receive barbiturate loading (Protocol #2) only upon arrival in the Emergency Department. If the ambulance physician is trained in anesthesiology and is personally present during prehospital management of the patient, he may start barbiturate loading outside the hospital.

Protocol #2 requires (in most institutions) approval by a Human Experimentation Committee, which can give approval for randomization and act as the patient's advocate, since informed consent obviously cannot be obtained during emergency resuscitation conditions. This thiopental treatment patient study protocol will be modified after initial experiences. We suggest randomized use with controlled data collection to determine the advisability of future routine use of this treatment. The final decision as to whether the patient meets the criteria for being *randomly* selected for barbiturate loading should be made by the most senior *anesthesiologist* present among the resuscitation team members. Since the administration of thiopental in the manner required and described for brain protection in an unconscious patient constitutes deep anesthesia, it should be under the direction of a physician trained in anesthesiology. These physicians should then become team leaders for all patients selected for the barbiturate loading trial. Upon the patient's admission to the ICU, the anesthesiologist may delegate continuance of barbiturate loading and life support to another adequately trained ICU-based physician. The team coordinator should be receptive and responsive to suggestions of other team members.

In patients selected for barbiturate loading, *thiopental* should be administered as early and as rapidly as possible after the insult—in cardiac arrest cases, preferably immediately upon restoration of spontaneous circulation. Thiopental seems ineffective when started later than two hours following restoration of spontaneous circulation and oxygenation. Thiopental will be administered while the patient is receiving artificial ventilation and other life support measures (see Protocol #1 and Step I, subsequently). Thiopental should be administered as rapidly as the patient's circulatory system will tolerate until either a total maximum of 30 mg./kg. has been given or about six hours have elapsed since the beginning of thiopental infusion (less than 30 mg./kg. may be the total dose in this case).

An I.V. loading dose of thiopental, 10 to 20 mg./kg., may be given if possible within the first 10 minutes, or within 30 minutes if the circulation does not tolerate more rapid administration. This is followed by administration of the remainder of the total dose of 30 mg./kg. as tolerated. Concentrations of thiopental used are 2 per cent for the loading dose and 0.4 per cent for the remaining infusion, both best administered by "piggy back" I.V. infusion. Thiopental should be administered at least to the point of silencing the EEG, or if the EEG is already silent, the drug is superimposed upon the silent EEG.

One of the main factors limiting the administration of thiopental is its *cardiovascular depressant effect*. Mean arterial pressure, preferably monitored via arterial catheter, should be maintained at 70 to 100 torr (higher in the previously hypertensive person), with vasopressor and slight plasma volume expansion. One may start with norepinephrine and switch to dopamine infusion not later than about one hour after beginning vasopressor therapy. Thiopental infusion should be discontinued temporarily when large amounts of vasopressor are needed for blood pressure support. EKG monitoring will permit discontinuance of thiopental infusion when the drug seems to provoke life-threatening arrhythmias. Thiopental infusion should be discontinued when the CVP or pulmonary artery wedge pressure (PAWP) (to be monitored after the patient returns to the ICU) rises to levels considered unsafe. Barbiturate loading, vasopressor infusion, and volume expansion should be stopped when signs of pulmonary edema occur, e.g., a significant relative decrease in PaO_2 with 100 per cent O_2 tests, rales, or roentgenographic evidence of pulmonary edema. Once thiopental has been initiated and stopped because of circulatory intolerance, it may be restarted and continued after stabilization of the circulation. The total time from beginning to discontinuing the infusion should not exceed six hours, regardless of interruptions.

Clinical investigators who decide to use this or a similar protocol are urged to obtain detailed protocols and forms from the author. Data collection should be initiated during emergency resuscitation, including the scoring of the depth of coma, e.g., using the Glasgow Coma Scoring System (Teasdale, 1974). After ICU admission, a more detailed neurologic examination scoring system will be used by our group (e.g., Pittsburgh Coma Score). A summary data form should be prepared upon discharge of the patient from the ICU by the physician coordinating the brain resuscitation project, and should be augmented at the time of discharge from the hospital and again during follow-up. Trials of the Pittsburgh barbiturate protocol in about 25 patients (1976–1977) in several hospitals proved its feasibility and gave encouraging results.

(I) Intensive Care

The patient's outcome, particularly that of his brain function, depends on the duration and intensity of the initial insult, the quality of emergency resuscitation, and immediate postischemic-anoxic secondary changes and their amelioration by advanced intensive care. This should follow the now well-established concepts of life support in multiple vital organ system failure. These changes, the "postresuscitation disease" (Negovsky, 1962, 1974), occur in all vital organ systems and feed on each other (Kampschulte, 1969; Smith, T, 1968). For example, hypoxemia, hypercarbia, and hypotension add cerebral ischemia and edema (Chapter 5). Intensive care is long-term resuscitation. Although methods for long-term resuscitation (i.e., optimizing respiratory, circulatory, metabolic, renal, hepatic and cerebral function) go beyond the scope of this chapter, the following *guidelines* are listed here since this subject has received little attention in the past (Safar, 1977Aa):

(1) *Control of arterial perfusion pressure*. Arterial normotension should be maintained as long as the patient is unconscious, for up to seven days post-insult, since even slight hypotension may hurt the brain with impaired autoregulation and spotty ischemic changes. Arterial normotension is a mean arterial pressure of 70 to 100 torr—higher in the previously hypertensive person. This can be accomplished by careful titration of, first, norepinephrine and then dopamine I.V. infusion (see Phase II, Step D) and slight plasma volume expansion (most tolerate 10 per cent of estimated blood volume in addition to normovolemia). Severe or repetitive hypertension can add vasogenic cerebral edema and worsen neurologic deficit.

(2) *Moderate hypocarbia* should be maintained ($PaCO_2$ 25 to 35 torr) by mechanical ventilation or spontaneous breathing, but exhaustion from spontaneous hyperventilation must be avoided.

(3) *Acid-base homeostasis* should aim for a pHa between 7.3 and 7.6. The base excess/deficit should be controlled if and when it appears indicated.

(4) *Normoxia or hyperoxia* should be maintained, namely PaO_2 as high as possible above 100 torr, with a safe inhaled O_2 concentration, i.e., for the first few hours 100 per cent, reduced after about six to 12 hours to 50 per cent. Optimized IPPV-CPPV should be used as indicated. Periodic 100 per cent O_2 tests (Chapters 3 and 10) should be continued throughout to recognize and reverse pulmonary shunting.

(5) If the patient is comatose, an *arterial catheter* should be inserted as soon as feasible after initial arterial PO_2, PCO_2, and pH determinations by arterial puncture. The arterial catheter permits direct arterial pressure monitoring and frequent arterial blood gas and pH determinations.

(6) A *central venous lifeline* should be established. Central venous pressure changes should be treated to consider not only cardiac but also cerebral homeostasis. In the absence of intracranial pressure (ICP) monitoring, which would permit calculation of cerebral perfusion pressure (mean systemic arterial pressure minus ICP), cerebral perfusion should be estimated from mean arterial pressure minus central venous pressure, and mean arterial pressure adjusted to keep cerebral perfusion pressure at 70 torr or higher. A *pulmonary artery catheter* may also be inserted for monitoring pulmonary artery pressure, pulmonary artery wedge pressure, and mixed venous O_2 values.

(7) *Normothermia* (37°C. core temperature) should be maintained unless hypothermia is used as therapy (see later). Hyperthermia must promptly be reversed.

(8) *Stabilization through relaxation* may be necessary for immobilizing the patient to control ventilation, oxygenation, shivering, and convulsions. Paralysis may be intermittently discontinued to permit neurologic evaluation. Curare, pancuronium, or other muscle relaxants may be used—preferably under the guidance of an anesthesiologist. In post-CPR patients who are in need of controlled ventilation (e.g., flail chest, shunting, cardiogenic shock) and brain protection and are not on large-dose thiobarbiturate trials, conventional doses of a short-acting barbiturate (e.g., pentobarbital, Nembutal) I.V. by titration, in addition to or instead of curarization, for at least 48 hours

post CPR, may enhance chances of recovery. Restlessness and "bucking" post CPR must be prevented or blocked.

(9) Unless contraindicated, *steroid medication* may have a beneficial effect on brain, heart, and lung lesions (aspiration). Suggested drugs and doses are: dexamethasone, 1 mg./kg., or methylprednisolone, 5 mg./kg. first, followed by dexamethasone, 0.2 mg./kg., or methylprednisolone, 1 mg./kg., every six hours until the state of consciousness improves. The steroid should be discontinued at three to four days.

(10) *Control of convulsions* by peripheral neuromuscular block (relaxants) should be extended to control of EEG convulsions by conventional doses (e.g., 1 mg./kg. per individual dose) of pentobarbital or phenobarbital.

(11) *Blood variables* should be controlled: Hematocrit between 30 and 40 per cent; serum electrolyte concentrations at normal values; plasma oncotic pressure at or above 15 torr (or serum albumin at or above 3 gm. per cent); serum osmolality between 280 and 330 mOsm./L.; and blood glucose between 100 and 300 mg. per cent.

(12) *Fluids and alimentation* are first administered through dextrose, 5 to 10 per cent in 0.25 to 0.5 per cent sodium chloride I.V. (30 to 50 ml./kg. per 24 hours in adults and children; 100 ml./kg. per 24 hours in infants), with potassium added as needed. Fluid therapy should be adjusted according to overall clinical circumstances and also when increased diuresis or sodium and water retention occur. About 2000 to 4000 calories/24 hour per 70 kg. body weight should be administered by vein or gastric tube as early as feasible after the first postresuscitative day. Antacids shall be administered via gastric tube. Monitoring of body weight is important.

(13) Starting as early as possible, the *neurologic status* should be assessed and monitored by use of a scoring system. Opthalmoscopy should be performed as soon as feasible and periodically thereafter—not only to look for papilledema (which is rare post-global ischemia-anoxia), but to observe the filling of retinal vessels, hemorrhage, spasm, and segmentation that may occur with impaired perfusion, as in approaching brain death.

(14) *Psychiatric status* should be assessed and monitored, beginning with the patient's first response to verbal command.

(15) *Secondary deterioration* of some patients after initial neurologic improvement, seen particularly after severe ischemic-anoxic insults, calls for modern heroic trials in an attempt to prevent brain death and learn more about this condition. When treated in insitutions where advanced brain monitoring to achieve homeostasis is possible, these patients may have ICP monitoring (by hollow skull screw or intraventricular catheter); continuous computerized EEG monitoring with evoked potentials; perhaps superior jugular bulb catheterization for determining arteriovenous cerebral gradients for oxygen, glucose, and lactate; and monitoring of CSF, pH, lactate, and other values for clinical research (Chapter 5).

In *intracranial hypertension* (ICP above 15 torr), therapeutic actions are recommended in this chronologic order: hyperventilation below $PaCO_2$ 25 to 35 torr; CSF drainage (if ventricular catheter is in place); osmotherapy; barbiturate in therapeutic doses (e.g., thiopental or pentobarbital, 1 mg./kg., as needed); and hypothermia.

Osmotherapy has been described in Chapter 5. *Hypothermia*, the last resort for ICP control, is best performed under barbiturate anesthesia plus muscle relaxant to produce poikilothermia during surface cooling (Shapiro, 1974). Core temperature can be reduced to about 30°C. Deliberate hypothermia should be directed by a staff physician experienced with this technique (Chapter 5).

Most of the above recommendations have experimental and/or clinical bases. For neuronal survival, however, much remains to be learned about optimizing variables that reflect extracranial vital organ functions.

SPECIAL CONSIDERATIONS

WITNESSED ARREST

In patients *with* ongoing *EKG monitoring*, sudden witnessed cardiac arrest due to VT or VF must be treated with immediate electric countershock, without delays by attempts at airway control, ventilation, and EHC. This immediate countershock technique is common in cases of VF in coronary care units. Immediate countershock usually is effective as long as the heart is oxygenated, i.e., for about 30 to 60 seconds after the onset of pulselessness. In the cardiac catheterization laboratory this period has been ex-

tended by making the still-conscious patient with VF cough vigorously. This can provide a form of self-administered "cardiac massage" and may keep enough blood flowing to maintain consciousness for a few minutes until countershock can be applied (M. Sones, Cleveland Clinic). It is unfortunate that most defibrillators presently available are not designed and priced low enough to be placed in immediate readiness at the bedside of all patients in risk of arrest.

The *technique* of CPR in monitored witnessed arrest is as follows: Feel for the carotid or femoral pulse; if absent, apply one electric countershock (see Phase I, Step F, above); immediately recheck the pulse; if he is still pulseless, tilt his head backward; give four quick lung inflations; check the pulse again; and begin EHC and standard CPR.

In case of witnessed asystole or bradycardia with consciousness, apply repetitive chest thumping (see below) at a rate of about 60 per minute. When the patient becomes unconscious, resume EHC and standard CPR. EHC both stimulates the heart into spontaneous contractions in complete heart block (if the myocardium is still oxygenated) and also moves blood.

In witnessed cardiac arrest *without EKG monitoring* and/or immediate availability of a defibrillator, the presently recommended technique is as follows: Tilt the patient's head backward to open the airway; simultaneously palpate the carotid pulse; if the pulse is absent give a precordial *thump*; in the absence of breathing give four quick lung inflations; feel the pulse again, if it is still absent, resume EHC and standard CPR.

The *precordial thump* (Fig. 19) has been introduced by the AHA as a compromise measure for monitored or suspected VT or VF in the absence of a defibrillator. Unfortunately there is no evidence that the electric current produced in the heart by the thump is strong enough to terminate VF (Yakaitis, 1973; Redding, in Safar, 1977A). There is some experimental and clinical evidence that runs of VT have been changed to sinus rhythm with a precordial thump (Pennington, 1970). No such evidence exists for the conversion of VF to sinus rhythm. In contrast, the thump applied to a person in any rhythm other than VF can induce VF, particularly when the heart is asphyxiated. In spite of this negative evidence concerning the thump, the AHA has recommended the above-mentioned sequence for wit-

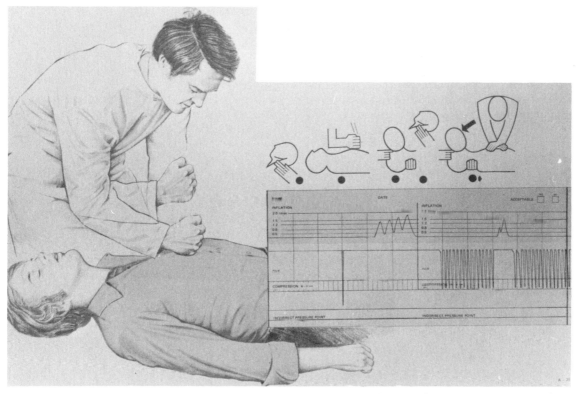

Figure 19 Precordial thump (see text). Bottom tracing of inset shows thump as first measure in witnessed sudden arrest, followed by regular CPR. For repetitive thumping (for external mechanical pacing in severe bradycardia or asystole from heart block), see text. (From A. Laerdal, CPR Flip Charts.)

nessed cardiac arrest, except for not recommending the use of the thump in children (AHA, 1974A). The precordial thump cannot start cardiac contractions in anoxic asystole and cannot be depended upon to convert an established VF. It is not a substitute for EHC.

Repetitive thumping by fist or by external mechanical pacer (Zoll, in Safar, 1977A) is recommended for asystole or severe bradycardia in heart block (Adams-Stokes Syndrome) while the patient is conscious. Thumping is less painful than EHC. In coma from heart block, however, EHC is preferred since this not only stimulates the oxygenated heart into spontaneous contractions, but also moves blood. No synchronization between EHC and the spontaneous contractions is necessary.

The *technique* of *thumping* is as follows (Fig. 19): From a height of 8-12 inches above the chest, deliver a sharp, quick single blow over the midportion of the sternum, using the fleshy bottom portion of the fist. Deliver the thump within the first minute of cardiac arrest. If there is no immediate response, begin CPR (AHA, 1974A).

INFANT RESUSCITATION

Special considerations of CPR in infants and small children have been listed with the description of the various techniques above. *Fetal* and *neonatal* monitoring and resuscitation are specialized fields beyond the scope of this chapter (Evans, in Safar, 1977A; Hook, 1974). The following few comments are made more for emphasizing priorities than for teaching special techniques. In *newborn infants,* resuscitation techniques and their evaluation have been greatly enhanced through the now almost routine use of Apgar scoring at one and five minutes following delivery (Apgar, in Abramson, 1960A). Emergency *respiratory* resuscitation usually can be accomplished effectively by bag-mask-oxygen, using either a to-and-fro semi-open bag-valve unit (which requires an anesthesiologist's skills) or the infant version of a self-refilling bag-valve-mask unit with oxygen. When this fails, early tracheal intubation by skilled personnel should be performed in infants with persistently low Apgar scores. Mouth-to-tracheal tube puffing via a tapered Cole endotracheal tube, with oxygen enrichment, has become a readily available and recommended technique. Neonates born with asphyxia and/or in shock benefit from umbilical artery pressure and pH monitoring, pHa normalization with bicarbonate and prophylactic continuous positive pressure breathing (spontaneous breathing with CPAP). This should be used more often to prevent the development of full-blown respiratory distress syndrome.

The place of *cardiac* resuscitation in newborn infants is controversial. Obviously in transient pulselessness (no palpable and audible heartbeat) following a complicated delivery, a brief period of EHC may turn the tide and is therefore justified. Sudden VF in newborns is almost unheard of. If pulselessness lasts for more than a moment, irreversible CNS damage (cerebral palsy) is almost certain to follow, because cardiac arrest in the newborn infant occurs secondary to prolonged asphyxia and/or shock, usually associated with prolonged traumatic labor. Therefore some, including this author, feel that, in newborns at risk, respiratory resuscitation and fluid and acid-base control should be carried out vigorously; but prolonged cardiac resuscitation efforts are contraindicated, as they may result in the survival of a severely brain-damaged child.

In *infants and children* beyond the first few hours of life, and in the absence of birth defects incompatible with ultimate survival, sudden pulselessness must be treated with all-out CPR. Differences in technique for CPR Phase I were described above with the techniques for adults (Figure 20). Phase II

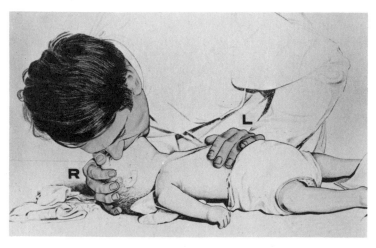

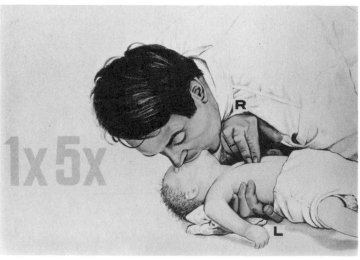

Figure 20 Infant resuscitation. *Top*, Mouth-to-mouth plus nose ventilation. Right hadn holding head tilted backward (R). Shoulders elevated. Left hand (L) preventing gastric distention. Ventilate with puffing from your cheeks.

Bottom, In pulselessness CPR with fingers at midsternum. Chest support with other hand. Interposed or superimposed ventilation 1:5. (From A. Laerdal, CPR Flip Charts.)

may require *drug therapy,* in which case dosages must be adjusted. Epinephrine should be given in 1:10,000 dilution (1 mg./10 ml.), 0.1 ml./kg. Sodium bicarbonate is given in a 1 mEq./kg. body weight dose as in the adult, repeated as indicated by monitored pHa and base déficit values. Lidocaine, when needed, is given I.V. in 0.5 mg./kg. doses in infants and 5 mg. doses in children (until the desired effect is reached); it may be continued by I.V. drip, 6 mg./kg./4 hours, not to exceed 100 mg./hour. Calcium chloride, 10 per cent, may be given in 1 ml./5 kg. doses I.V. Catecholamines are best titrated by I.V. infusion in 5 per cent dextrose in water; e.g., norepinephrine, 1 mg./500 ml. for infants and 2 mg./500 ml. for children; metaraminol, 25 mg./100 ml.; and isoproterenol, 1 to 5 mg./500 ml. (AHA, 1974A).

OPEN CHEST CARDIAC RESUSCITATION

For most cases of cardiac arrest, EHC has replaced internal cardiac compression because it can be started without delay and without producing life-threatening injury. In the hands of physicians with the necessary skills, equipment, and facilities, however, the open chest approach to the treatment of cardiac arrest is safe and sometimes indicated (Beck, 1947; Dripps, 1948; Stephenson, 1974A). This is particularly true in circumstances for which it may be the only effective method of restoring life (Stephenson, in Safar, 1977A). These indications include: (1) When one suspects intrathoracic pathology such as tension pneumothorax or hemorrhage, particularly from penetrating wounds of the chest, crushing chest injury or following cardiothoracic surgery. (2) When one cannot produce a palpable femoral or carotid pulse with external cardiac compression, as is occasionally the case in patients with chest or spine deformities or severe emphysema with barrel-chest. (3) When repeated external defibrillation attempts have failed, as may be the case in deep hypothermia when the heart would have to be rewarmed directly in order to be defibrillated.

Thoracotomy should be performed by a physician skilled with the technique. This procedure not only permits hemostasis by compression of the site in intrathoracic exsanguination, but also in abdominal hemorrhage permits compression of the descending thoracic aorta. Sometimes, direct cardiac compressions can produce better artificial blood flow than EHC (DelGuercio, 1965). Direct observation of the heart also helps guide drug therapy and electric countershock.

The *technique* of open chest heart resuscitation is as follows (Figure 21): Cut through skin and muscles under the left breast at approximately the fourth intercostal space. Pierce the intercostal structures bluntly with a knife handle or bandage scissors and tear the intercostal space open with your fingers. Insert a rib spreader when available. Compress the heart immediately before opening the pericardium by placing the fingers of one hand behind the heart and the thenar and thumb in front of the heart. Take care not to pierce the atrium with your thumb. Compress large hearts with one hand behind and one hand in front of the heart. If you suspect ventricular fibrillation, open the pericardium for diagnosis. Take care not to injure the heart, and do not interrupt compressions for more than a few seconds.

Inject drugs, if necessary, into the cavity of the left ventricle. Perform internal defibrillation by placing two large paddle electrodes with saline soaked pads directly on the heart, one behind the left ventricle, the other over the anterior surface of the heart. Have control over the switch that releases the countershock. Internal DC countershocks can be effective with as little as 50 watt seconds energy. Internal AC countershock, which should deliver 110 to 120 volts with 0.1 to 0.25 seconds' shock duration, although rarely used, can be improvised by connecting two metal spoons (held in rubber gloved hands!) to a regular wall outlet which is briefly plugged in by a helper (Jude, in Safar, 1977A). Internal DC (or AC) countershock should start with low energy (voltage), since high energy shocks applied directly to the heart are more likely than external countershocks to produce heat damage, including myocardial burns.

In suspected cardiac tamponade, if time permits and the patient is not yet pulseless rapid drainage of the pericardial sac by needle puncture (alongside the xyphoid) plus EHC in case of pulselessness may obviate the need for thoracotomy. If the diagnosis is uncertain, the chest should be opened. Patients with crushed chest with a pulse usually require only oxygen inhalation and perhaps artificial ventilation (with

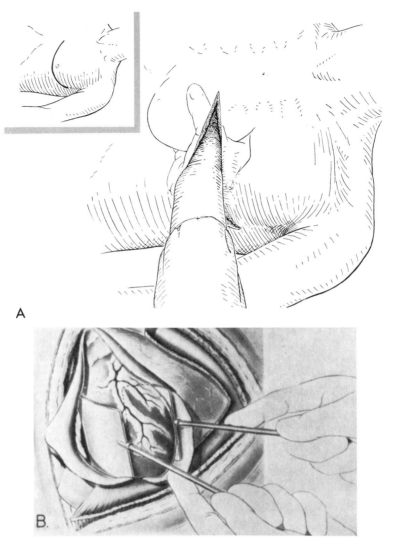

A

B.

Figure 21 *A,* Open chest via fifth left intercostal space (inset). Grasp and rhythmically compress heart as described in the text. (From Johnson, Surgery of the Chest, Chicago, Year Book Medical Publishers, 1952.)

B, Internal direct electric defibrillation. When you feel fibrillation, open the pericardial sac, apply internal electrodes as illustrated (wearing rubber gloves), and apply countershock (see text). (From Stephenson, H.: Cardiac Arrest and Resuscitation. St. Louis, The C. V. Mosby Co., 1974.)

pleural drainage standby because of the likelihood of pneumothorax); in cardiac arrest, however, EHC should be tried first (although it may compound internal injuries) unless intrathoracic bleeding is suspected. In suspected tension pneumothorax a large-bore needle is inserted on the side of the suspected pneumothorax, through the second intercostal space in the midclavicular line. If pneumothorax is confirmed, the needle should be replaced with a large-bore chest tube (Chapter 10).

EXSANGUINATION CARDIAC ARREST

Exsanguination usually leads to an agonal state (no pulse, gasping) and finally clinical death in asystole (Chap. 2) (Negovsky, 1962). Resuscitative efforts may provoke VF (Kirimli, 1965).

Resuscitation consists of the *simultaneous* application of the following (Kirimli, 1965): IPPV-CPPV with 100 per cent O_2. EHC and continued CPR as described under Phase I. Massive venous infusion through large-bore catheter or needle of the most immediately available plasma substitute (sodium chloride or Ringer's solution, dextran, hydroxyethyl starch or albumin) with epinephrine, 1 mg., and bicarbonate, 1 mEq./kg., added. Surgical hemostasis of the bleeding site. EKG monitoring and external electric countershock if VF occurs.

When massive volume replacement is started with salt solutions, it must at some point be continued with a colloid, since salt solutions do not remain in the intravascular compartment (Takaori, 1967). If hemostasis accompanies resuscitative efforts, restoration of spontaneous circulation in exsanguination cardiac arrest is possible without bank blood or red blood cell infusion as, usually at the point of cardiac arrest, about 40 per cent of the total red cell mass is still in the body. If the hematocrit is low after restoration of spontaneous circulation, this can be corrected with red blood cells under controlled conditions. Hemostasis of bleeding extremity wounds can be performed with direct pressure and tourniquet; of intra-abdominal bleeding (e.g., abdominal aneurysm rupture), with open chest cardiac resuscitation and compression of the lower thoracic aorta. Intrathoracic bleeding requires direct compression of the bleeding site during cardiac compressions via thoracotomy.

Although *arterial* pressure *infusion* of the shed, warm, oxygenated heparinized blood with epinephrine can restart the heart even without EHC, through retrograde perfusion of the coronary circulation (Negovsky, 1962), this cannot be relied upon when using clinically available plasma substitutes or bank blood, which are cold, non-oxygenated, and acid (Kirimli 1969). Therefore, *venous infusion* with CPR is recommended (Chapter 2). When an artery is readily available—for example in a large open wound or during surgery—exsanguination cardiac arrest may be treated with direct intra-arterial pressure infusion during cardiac compressions, as smaller volumes are required to restart the heart than with venous infusion. See also Phase II, Step D above.

NEAR-DROWNING

When starting resuscitation in victims of near-drowning, there may or may not be water in the lungs, as laryngospasm may have prevented aspiration. Inhalation of fresh water causes hemodilution and pulmonary shunting from surfactant failure; inhalation of sea water causes plasma loss into the lungs and pulmonary edema. Both require sophisticated respiratory care with CPPV-O_2. When cardiac arrest develops during submersion, resuscitation is also possible (Redding, 1961a, 1962) (Chaps. 2, 39F).

Do not delay reoxygenation by attempts to drain fluid from the lungs. A good swimmer can start mouth-to-mouth or mouth-to-nose resuscitation while treading water. Most trained rescuers can start mouth-to-mouth while standing in shallow water. In contrast, effective EHC is not possible until the victim is removed from the water. Teaching general water rescue is as important as teaching resuscitation (ARC, 1974A).

In general one should follow the principles of CPR as outlined above (AHA, 1974A). Clear the pharynx as needed. Water and vomitus may drain by gravity before and during resuscitative efforts. If after removal from the water the victim's abdomen is distended, turn him briefly on his side and compress the upper abdomen to expel water and gas, or into the prone position, lifting him with your hand under his stomach to force water out ("breaking" the victim). These efforts should not be routine as they may delay reoxygenation and, if performed, should be rapid. Switch ventilation from exhaled air to 100 per cent O_2 as soon as possible, as pulmonary changes occur with even small amounts of inhaled water (Chapter 2, 3, and 10). Hospital admission is mandatory, even if the victim recovers consciousness at the scene or during transportation. Blood electrolyte changes vary with the fluid and salt inhaled. They occur with massive inhalation of water and dissipate within one-half to one hour. While the pulmonary lesion is now reversible with sophisticated respiratory intensive care (and other life support measures) (Chapters 2, 3, and 10), the limiting factor remains postischemic-anoxic brain damage. Thus brain resuscitation (see Phase III, Step H above) is important in patients who do not begin to wake up within about ten minutes of restoration of spontaneous circulation. Usually these are victims with healthy hearts in whom, for instance, barbiturate therapy may not be hazardous. Do not give up resuscitative efforts, since recovery from near-drowning with complete CNS restoration has been reported even after prolonged periods of submersion, particularly when drowning occurred in cold water (Siebke, 1975). Blood electrolyte changes are evanescent and no obstacle to resuscitation (Modell, 1971).

If neck injury is suspected following diving into shallow water, try to float the victim onto a backboard before removing him from the water. If mouth-to-mouth ventilation is needed, use the triple airway maneuver with moderate backward tilt of the head, asking a helper to keep head, neck, and chest aligned to avoid aggravating spinal cord injury.

MISCELLANEOUS RESUSCITATIVE CONDITIONS

Electric shock (Chapter 2) may occur on the top of an electric pole. If cardiac arrest develops in this situation, deliver a precordial thump and mouth-to-mouth breathing and then lower the victim as quickly as possible to the ground. CPR in the upright position is not effective, as it does not permit venous return. The many other special resuscitative problems posed by conditions leading to cardiopulmonary failure include tension pneumothorax, aspiration, status asthmaticus, cardiac tamponade, pulmonary embolism, electrocution, anaphylactic shock, carbon monoxide poisoning, hypoglycemia, etc. The principles of modern CPR described under Phases I, II and III above prevail in all of them. The special additional measures required are discussed in Chapters 2, 3, 4, 5 and 10.

PITFALLS OF CPR

CPR can cause iatrogenic complications. Some are minor compared with certain death if CPR is not started; others leave residuals (Evans, in Safar, 1977A).

Backward tilt of the head and positive pressure inflation attempts of the lungs, correctly performed, do not produce serious complications, even if performed unnecessarily. There are some exceptions however. For instance, if the airway is inadequate or inflations are too forceful, gastric insufflation may occur and may provoke regurgitation and inhalation of gastric contents. Lung rupture with tension pneumothorax is possible when excessive volumes are blown into infants or when the patient's lungs are diseased. Prolonged attempts at tracheal intu-

bation may produce asphyxia and cardiac arrest. In the aged with atherosclerosis, sustained maximal backward tilt of the head plus turning the head to the side, can cause circulatory impairment of the vertebral artery–basilar artery system, resulting in brain stem failure. In accident victims, moderate backward tilt of the head and the triple airway maneuver are recommended, since maximal backward tilt, turning the head to the side, and ante-flexion of the head, may aggravate a spinal cord injury and cause paralysis.

EHC may result in costochondral separation or multiple rib fractures, especially in elderly patients, even if performed correctly. This is not a serious complication. Should a flail chest result, prolonged controlled ventilation is necessary after resuscitation. Pressure applied too high on the sternum may fracture it. Pressure applied too low may rupture the liver or cause regurgitation. Pressure applied laterally may break ribs and contuse lungs. Bone marrow emboli are possible but are not considered to be an obstacle to recovery. Incorrectly placed subclavian catheters have commonly caused complications such as pneumothorax, hemothorax, or mediastinal infusion.

The AHA enumerates "points to remember" (AHA, 1974A): (1) Do not interrupt CPR for more than 5 seconds, except for tracheal intubation and moving the victim over stairways, which may necessitate longer interruptions but which, however, should not exceed 15 seconds each. (2) Do not move the patient until stabilized; restoring spontaneous circulation at the scene has resulted in higher survival rates than transporting the patient with CPR and restarting spontaneous circulation in the Emergency Department. (Stabilization includes ventilation, oxygenation, venous lifeline, EKG monitoring, and communications for consultation and arrangement for hospital admission.) (3) To avoid injury to the liver, do not maintain pressure on the abdomen to decompress the stomach while EHC is being performed. (4) Pay attention to details of techniques.

TEACHING OF CPR

STUDENTS AND TRAINEES

Our recommendations on who should be taught which phases and steps of CPR

(Tables 1, 2, 4) conform in general to AHA recommendations (1974A), except that we give more specifics concerning what should be taught to various types of medical personnel. We also recommend use of self-training methods for teaching the lay public CPR basic life support without equipment by single operator technique only. We have suggested exploration of mass training via television; a teachability test in school children showed not only that the self-training system is at least as effective as the instructor-coached methods, but also that repeated film viewing alone results in a higher proportion of satisfactory test performance than no training at all and no greater potentially hazardous performance than do self-training or instructor's training with the use of manikins (Berkebile, 1973A, 1976A).

The AHA recommended that CPR courses be required as part of the curriculum of all medical, dental, nursing, osteopathic, respiratory therapy, and other allied health schools, and that a demonstration of proficiency in performance of CPR be part of the requirements for medical school graduation. The AHA also recommended that all nurses and physicians, including hospital house staff, be competent in all phases of CPR. To accomplish this it is recommended that annual staff reappointments at all hospitals require all physicians either to demonstrate proficiency in CPR basic life support through participation in resuscitation efforts or teaching or to agree to attend an approved course. Also, physicians and nurses working in Emergency Departments must be trained and certified in basic *and* advanced life support. It is further recommended that the above requirements be included in standards for accreditation by the Joint Commission. Annual retraining is recommended unless the trainee is frequently exposed to actual resuscitation cases.

Physicians to become CPR instructors should seek AHA certification and should be thoroughly familiar with the teaching materials and standards listed in the first section of the bibliography of this chapter. All other physicians should candidly reassess their capability to perform the steps of resuscitation needed in emergencies they might encounter (Table 4). Although in recent years the interest in CPR teaching and learning by nonphysician health care personnel has intensified, many physicians are still incapable of performing even the most rudimentary CPR skills (Phase I, without equipment); their own misjudgment concerning their capabilities often causes them to avoid further training (Safar, 1974Aa).

The ability to teach mouth-to-mouth breathing effectively (Safar, 1958B; Elam, 1961; Lind, 1961) and CPR Phase I without equipment (Winchell, 1966A) to all types of personnel, including the lay public, was proved long ago. Recent data also indicate that performance rates are more than doubled by practice-to-perfection on realistic manikins. This has been made more feasible through the introduction of basic life support self-training systems (Berkebile, 1973A; Safar, 1974Aa). In communities where a large proportion of the lay public was trained in CPR (e.g., in Seattle where the instructor method was used), an increased salvage rate in cases of prehospital cardiac arrest was observed (Crampton, 1972; Cobb, in Schaffer, 1975)

All these developments have led to the recommendation by national organizations that not only head-tilt and mouth-to-mouth ventilation but also CPR Phase I without equipment be taught to as many members of the lay public as possible. Phase I (basic life support) without equipment, when taught to the lay public, does not carry a substantial risk of producing unnecessary injury (Winchell, 1966A; Berkebile, 1973A). Therefore, all school children should be required to have annual training in artificial ventilation, beginning with the fifth grade, and in CPR, starting with the eighth grade. Additional target groups for CPR basic life support without equipment should be those seeking drivers' licenses and family members of cardiac patients. Obviously all health care personnel, from first responders (e.g., police, firemen, lifeguards) through physician specialists, should be trained in basic life support without equipment and, depending on their involvement and needs, in basic life support with equipment and advanced life support. In addition, all physicians, dentists, nurses, inhalation therapists, and paramedics–ambulance should learn CPR advanced life support (Phase I with equipment and Phase II). Nurses working in Emergency Departments and ICUs should be trained in definitive therapy and be permitted to defibrillate and administer drugs as preordered by physicians (Table 4).

TABLE 4   CPR Basic Life Support Self-Training System°

(A) *Instructor-Coordinator:* Obtain and set up equipment in Learning Laboratory; announce program; schedule trainees; and debrief, test (knowledge and skills) and certify trainees.

(B) *Procedure:* Trainees in groups of two or more use learning laboratory until able to pass debriefing test.
    (1) Study text-picture *handouts* (manuals).
    (2) View *film* demonstration of CPR/ABC.
    (3) Familiarize yourself with Laerdal Recording Resusi-Anne *manikin* (see instructions).
    (4) Set up flip charts (or slides).

		LAY PUBLIC	POLICE, FIREMAN, LIFE-GUARD	EMT, HOSPITAL TECH-NICIAN	GENERAL RN	ICU-ED RN, RESP. THER., PARA-MEDIC	MED. STUD., MD, DDS	ECCM MD
(5) Select appropriate audio tapes (see types of trainees) and use for coached manikin practice-to-perfection.								
Tape 1a	Introductory Information	X	X	X	X	X	X	X
b	CPR-A, B without equip.	X	X	X	X	X	X	X
c	CPR-A, B, C without equip. one person	X	X	X	X	X	X	X
d	CPR-A, B, C without equip. two persons	–	X	X	X	X	X	X
e	Witnessed Arrest (thump)	–	X	X	X	X	X	X
f	Infant CPR without equip.	X	X	X	X	X	X	X
g	Special airway control, non-medical personnel	X	–	–	–	–	–	–
Tape 2a	Special airway control, Medical personnel	–	X	(X)	X	X	X	X
°°b	Pocket Mask-O_2	–	X	(X)	X	X	X	X
°°Tape 3a	O_2 and suction equip.	–	X	(X)	X	X	X	X
b	Bag-valve mask O_2, pharyngeal tubes, hand O_2 ventilator	–	–	(X)	–	X	X	X

(6) Before tapes 2–3, study *O_2 admin. handouts* and programmed text.

(7) Complete written (knowledge) *self-test* for procedures (1) and (6).

(8) See *instructor-coordinator* for debriefing, testing (knowledge of procedures (2)–(5) above; and manikin skill test) and certification.

°Developed by and available from Department of Anesthesiology/CCM, University of Pittsburgh, 1060 C Scaife Hall, Pittsburgh, PA 15261 and the A. Laerdal Corp., 1 Labriola Court, Armonk, N.Y. 10504.

In collaboration with the Laerdal Company; and, in part, supported by NIH Heart-Lung Institute, Contract Number NOI-HR-42965. Can be used with or without instructor. Slides optional.

°°Training in use of O_2 equipment should be individually initiated and supervised by the instructor-coordinator. He should use (*a*) demonstrations (large groups); (*b*) coached practice-to-perfection (small groups); (*c*) refresher-type self practice with tapes 9–11 in learning lab.; (*d*) testing and certifying.

(X) for EMT's–ambulance, but not hospital technicians.

TEACHING METHODS FOR CPR

Historically, basic life support training started with practicing on each other and on anesthetized patients and volunteers at Baltimore City Hospitals in 1958–61, and continued with slide lectures, film viewing, and instructor-coached manikin practice-to-perfection as soon as the Laerdal resuscitation manikins became available in 1960 (AHA, 1968A; 1975A, 1976A; Safar, 1958a; 1974Aa). More recently, a self-training system has proved at least as effective and certainly more cost-effective than instructor dependent teaching (Berkebile, 1973A). The fol-

lowing training systems are presently available: (1) The Laerdal self-training system for lay personnel (AHA, 1976A). (2) The University of Pittsburgh self-training system, which is an extension of the Laerdal system to include basic life support techniques with and without equipment for lay and all health care personnel (Table 4) (UHCP, 1973–1977A). (3) The ARC semi-self-training system with films (ARC, 1975A). (4) The AHA system, which requires instructors (AHA, 1975A).

Training aids must include a realistic manikin—preferably the new Laerdal recording Resusci-Anne manikin (Figure 22)

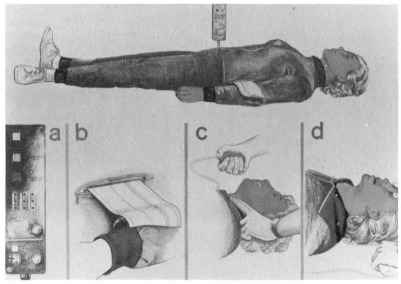

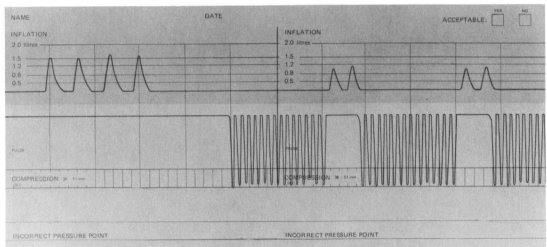

Figure 22 *Top*, Recording Resusci-Anne heart-lung resuscitation manikin (Laerdal). (*a*) Control panel (top to bottom, green light, 0.8 L ventilations; yellow light, adequate heart compressions; red light, incorrect heart compressions; metronome switch; battery power indicator; paper recorder switch). (*b*) Paper record of ventilations and heart compressions. (*c*) Carotid pulse controlled by bulb squeezing. (*d*) Pupil size controlled by bulb squeezing (not recommended).

Bottom, Ideal paper record as it emerges from manikin's side. First minute of CPR by single operator (top tracing, ventilations; bottom tracing, sternal compressions).

in which the force of heart compressions (pulse) and volumes of ventilations are automatically recorded on a paper strip which the instructor/coordinator uses for evaluating the trainee's performance. The regular or recording Resusci-Anne manikin should have a carotid pulse which co-trainees or instructors can make appear and disappear by using a bulb attached to the carotid artery tubing. In regular manikins, pulse and lung inflation pressure gauges are available to monitor performance.

The traditional instructor method includes demonstration of each step and sequence of the procedure by the instructor and then coaching each trainee's performance to perfection on the manikin. Finally, the instructor tests the trainee's final performance of the entire sequence without coaching. Tests must include the ability to differentiate between the presence and absence of the carotid pulse.

The teaching of basic life support with or without equipment using the new self-training system (Figure 22, Table 4) (UHCP, 1973–77A) is best organized by an instructor/coordinator. The materials come in two suitcases containing an introductory training film, recording Resusci-Anne manikin, flip charts, coaching audio tapes with audio tape player, and ventilation equipment. Handouts and sound tapes describe use of the system. It can be made available for schools, hospitals, and other institutions on a permanent or temporary basis and set up in a learning laboratory for which the instructor/coordinator can organize individualized usage. At least two trainees at the same time should use the system in order to help each other. Finally, the instructor/coordinator should debrief the trainee when presented with the recording manikin's record, and should apply knowledge and skill tests for certification.

Self-training is as follows: New trainees should first see a motivational film (e.g., Gordon, in AHA, 1975A), then study handouts with texts and pictures; next, view a technique demonstration film of Phase I, Steps A, B, C without equipment (e.g. Safar, in UHCP 1973A); finally, use the recording Resusci-Anne manikin and flip charts while being coached by the appropriate audio tape, selected according to Table 4.

Both the instructor-dependent (AHA, 1967A) and self-training systems require instructor/coordinators—for self-training merely to organize and test. Both methods must teach with simplicity, clarity, and repetition and must *insist* on perfection in details. They should, in teaching mouth-to-mouth ventilation, point out the most common causes of failure—namely inadequate head-tilt, inadequate force of blowing, and leakage. In the performance of EHC they should stress the common cause of failure—excessive periods of interruption of compressions. They should point out the importance of starting EHC only in proved cardiac arrest, and that, with proper use of the technique, the likelihood of serious complications is minimal in comparison with the alternative (death).

Certification in CPR-Phase I (basic life support) as "doers" or "instructors" has been introduced by the AHA to foster uniform standards. AHA certification is based on cognitive (written or oral) and performance examinations. For details consult your local or national Heart Association.

There are many *criteria* for passing the CPR knowledge and performance test. We have introduced lenient criteria for lay personnel and stringent criteria for health care personnel (Winchell, 1966A; Berkebile, 1973A). The AHA applies different criteria for passing in different regions. For assessing adequacy of lay performance of CPR Steps A, B, and C, the manikin test is more important than the written knowledge test. We recommend that the performance test on manikins reveal, at least in general terms, the correct sequence of action (head-tilt, ventilate, feel pulse, circulate); at least four lung inflations over 0.5 liter and 30 sternal compressions over 2 inches in the first minute of the performance test, and eight lung inflations plus 50 sternal compressions during the second minute.

Teaching *Phases II and III* (advanced and postresuscitative life support) proved difficult, since no universally applicable self-training mechanisms are available. Historically, Phase II of CPR has been taught by the groups of Beck and Leighninger, Jude and Kouwenhoven, and Safar and Redding in the animal laboratory since the 1950s to hundreds of medical personnel (Safar, 1974Aa). This is no longer practical because of the greater number of trainees and the cost and unavailability of laboratories, animals, and time. The dog, moreover, is not suitable for practicing Steps A, B, C because his airway does not obstruct with flexion of the neck and neither EHC nor exhaled air ventilation can be practiced realistically. The anterior/posterior diameter of the thorax is greater than in the human, and the heart is relatively free in the non-fixed mediastinum, which makes practice of EHC unrealistic. The dog is suitable, however, for demonstrating various patterns of dying and their reversal, the effect of drugs, open chest cardiac compression, ventricular fibrillation, external and internal defibrillation, the time factor in resuscitation, and the use of the hospital crash cart and other equipment. Since dog laboratory demonstrations are not feasible in most hospitals, they must be considered merely an optional part of CPR training. A good film may replace the animal demonstrations.

Human subjects can be used for parts of CPR training. Exhaled air ventilation cannot be practiced properly in conscious human volunteers, since the airway either does not obstruct with flexion of the neck or the volunteer resists inflation attempts. However, positioning the head and mandible can be demonstrated and practiced. Sternal compression should not be carried out on a conscious human subject. However the exact point of application of pressure on the lower sternum can be indicated and the instructor can demonstrate proper positioning of the hands. Anesthetized patients may be used for practicing airway control and various methods of artificial ventilation and tracheal intubation; this must be under the strictest control of a staff anesthesiologist, who assumes responsibility for possible injuries. For selected hospital personnel, the pathology department may assist in providing an opportunity for the practice of tracheal intubation on corpses.

Newborn resuscitation has been effectively practiced on the baby Laerdal manikin for Steps A, B, C without equipment. Tracheal intubation may be practiced on the infant intubation manikin, on stillborn infants, and on anesthetized cats or primates.

Tracheal intubation should be taught to all medical and paramedical personnel (Table 1). For use under emergency situations it can be taught reasonably effectively, even without the use of anesthetized patients, provided there is supervised practice on the job (Benson, 1971; DeLeo, 1975). Training should start with the acquisition of knowledge from texts and pictures, and should be followed by video tape or film demonstration and continued by supervised practice to perfection on intubation manikins. The only presently available, reasonably realistic intubation manikins are those by Laerdal (adult and infant manikins), which are now under revision (AHA, 1976A). Ideally, patient practice in the anesthesia setting of the operating room should follow. The goal should be passing a test consisting of intubating the trachea in the anesthetized, curarized, or comatose patient within 30 seconds from the go-ahead time.

Rapid "crash" intubation (Stept, 1970A) should be practiced on patients scheduled for elective anesthesia, since the emergency patient may be hurt by failure to intubate. Every Emergency Department should have experienced intubation personnel available in the house, around the clock, capable of performing crash intubation when needed. In the hands of the novice this technique is hazardous. In the absence of skilled personnel, airway control steps short of tracheal intubation should be used since difficulties, delays, and complications during unsuccessful attempts at tracheal intubation have led to asphyxia and cardiac arrest.

HOSPITAL-WIDE ORGANIZATION

The AHA recommends that every hospital with acute care facilities assign to a specific committee the responsibility for providing CPR teams on a 24-hour per day basis. These teams, which must be capable of performing CPR and all aspects of emergency life support, should consist of nurses, technicians, respiratory therapists, house staff, and on-call attending staff physicians. Wherever possible, the CPR hospital committee should be composed of at least a surgeon, a cardiologist, an anesthesiologist, an in-service nurse, and an administrator. The committee should be responsible for providing a written plan of action (protocol), CPR training and practice sessions, and a record of CPR occurrences available for periodic audit and review.

The AHA also states that "every general hospital with acute care facilities should provide in its emergency department an advanced life support station so that any patient who has symptoms suspicious of myocardial infarction or other cardiopulmonary emergency will be placed immediately on monitoring and surveillance, until a definite decision is made regarding his management. ... if there is strong suspicion that the patient has had an acute myocardial infarction he should be transferred to a coronary care unit.... During transfer he should be connected to a battery operated monitor-defibrillator and should be accompanied by appropriate drug administration en route, if necessary" (AHA, 1974A).

Organization and mobilization of hospital personnel for CPR calls will depend on local circumstances (AHA, 1968A). One method is a *general response*, i.e., to have all physicians and nurses who hear the alert respond to it. The physician present who is most experienced in resuscitation (which is often difficult to determine or agree on) must take charge, since lack of team leadership is the most common cause of ineffective, incompetently carried out CPR efforts. The team leader must indicate which personnel are needed and make the responsibilities clear.

Another plan is to use a designated *team response*. The committee should appoint a team leader who will exercise decisive team leadership. In large hospitals with 24-hour coverage by physicians of various disciplines, members of one discipline can be chosen on the basis of their experience and availability to assume the role of team leader. This avoids the confusion on the scene that occurs when one discipline is not in charge. The team usually is composed of representatives from anesthesiology, medicine, and surgery, a crash cart technician or respiratory therapist, and at least two nurses from the arrest location. One problem with the designated team leader approach is the variability in training and experience of house staff of various departments serving on CPR teams. In special care units, like Emergency Departments, team function is easier to organize, as most team members work together most of the time on non-emergency cases. Lack of skilled, knowledgeable team leadership (because of departmental territorialism) and delegation of CPR efforts to inexperienced house staff in many teaching hospitals of this country have led to a deterioration of the quality of CPR efforts.

One type of *team function* is as follows: The person recognizing the emergency starts resuscitation and calls for a helper, who in turn calls the telephone operator by a prearranged alert number that overrides all other calls. The telephone operator pages "alert" or "code blue," and gives the room number. This is essential to avoid delay caused by calling back for the location. The team members respond to the alert and rush to the scene. The team leader takes over ventilation or checks the adequacy of ventilation started by another person and monitors the effectiveness of EHC. The cart technician who has rushed the crash cart to the scene prepares the defibrillation–EKG monitoring paddles and later attaches the EKG limb electrodes. One nurse assists with intravenous infusion and draws up medications. The second nurse keeps records. The team leader reads the EKG, determines drug therapy, and applies the countershock as needed. If help is scarce, he will insert the intravenous needle or perform a cut-down. Intubation should be attempted by a staff member who is skilled in the technique and who can perform it quickly.

Special nurses, particularly those assigned to the Emergency Department and ICUs, should be trained and authorized to defibrillate and give special drugs, as preordered.

The patient should be transported from the scene of the resuscitation to the ICU only after he has been stabilized. The person who initiates emergency resuscitation must see to it that the patient receives *post resuscitative intensive care*. If complex postresuscitative intensive care (e.g., brain resuscitation) is indicated, hospitals without this expertise available should seek *consultation* advice by phone or call a resuscitology "flying squad" rather than transfer patients from one hospital to another at a time when every minute of sophisticated life support counts.

EQUIPMENT

The hospital resuscitation equipment listed subsequently (AHA, 1974A) should be provided on at least one mobile crash cart for hospital-wide use and, in addition, on crash carts for strategic locations such as the Emergency Department, ICU, coronary care unit, operating suite, recovery room, roentgen department, cardiac catheterization laboratory, etc. Each nursing station or floor should have this equipment available for use within one to two minutes.

The *basic equipment* that should be available for *Phase I, Steps A and B*, should include (AHA, 1974A): Oropharyngeal and

nasopharyngeal airways of all sizes (Fig. 6);
S-tubes (optional); esophageal obturator airway (optional) (Figure 7); tracheal intubation and suction equipment (see Steps A-5, 8) (Figure 8); cricothyrotomy set (Figure 11); translaryngeal oxygen jet insufflation equipment (optional) (Figure 12); Mouth-to-mouth pocket mask with oxygen nipple (Figure 13); acceptable bag-valve-mask unit with oxygen reservoir (Figure 14); nosogastric tubes; oxygen supply, at least in the form of two small (size E) cylinders with reducing valve and delivery tube, capable of supplying at least 15 liters per minute of oxygen (Chapter 10).

The *basic equipment* that should be available for *Phase I Step C* and for *Phase II* should include (AHA, 1974A): A battery powered portable defibrillator-ECG monitor (oscilloscope) with the EKG electrodes incorporated into the external defibrillator paddles (with sterile internal defibrillator paddles for children and adults, and with extra EKG needle and stick-on electrodes); a portable EKG recorder with connection to the defibrillator monitor; I.V. infusion sets with regular and micro drips; "extracath" and "intracath" plastic cannulas, sizes 14 to 22 gauge, for I.V. infusions; infusion stopcocks and venous extension tubes; a venous cut-down set; pressure infusion equipment; I.V. solutions in plastic bags, which should include 5 per cent dextrose in water, in Ringer's solution, and in 0.5 per cent sodium chloride, and a colloid such as dextran-40 or 5 per cent albumin; a pleural drainage set; an open cardiac resuscitation set (thoracotomy); sterile gloves; tourniquets; adhesive tape; scissors; and urinary catheters. For the administration of drugs (see Phase II, Step D above), an assortment of syringes and needles and (for occasional use only), a long, 22 gauge intracardiac needle should be available. Backboard and folded towels are needed for EHC.

COMMUNITY-WIDE ORGANIZATION

CPR capability must be built as a standard setter into all components of the emergency and critical care medicine (ECCM) delivery system (Table 5) (Safar, 1968, 1974A; Frey, 1975; HEW, 1973–77). This system is only as good as its weakest component. The regional system must be coordinated by an EMS operations center with experienced paramedical dispatchers, backed up by ECCM-experienced physicians on the radio. This center (Components 8 and 9, Table 5) appraises everyday medical emergencies as well as disasters and serves as a communications and ambulance-dispatching center. It mobilizes resources

TABLE 5 *Emergency and Critical Care Medicine System*

	PHYSICIAN MANPOWER		
	SERVICE COMPONENTS		COORDINATION
COMPONENTS	EMERGENCY PHYSICIAN	CCM PHYSICIAN	EM PLUS CCM PHYSICIANS
(1) Scene: Recognition, aid by bystanders°	—	—	
(2) Scene: Initiation of system†	(+)	—	
(3) Scene: Resuscitation, stabilization°	+	(+)	(8) Organization, Communization
(4) Transportation with life support°	+	(+)	(9) Planning, Education, Evaluation
(5) Emergency Department, <5% of patients critical	+ Clinical Base of EM physician	(+) Resus. only	(10) Research
(6) Operating Room, Surgery, Anesthesia	—	(+)	
(7) Intensive Care Unit, 100% of patients critical	—	+ Clinical Base of CCM physician	

°Prehospital physician advice and radio control of EMT's and paramedics. Presence of physician optional.
†Call mobile ICU ambulance, phone 911 or dial operator.
+Required; (+) optional.
For abbreviations, see Glossary.

outside of hospitals and directs the flow of patients. The dispatching center, all ambulance and rescue vehicles, and all major emergency hospitals should be linked by two-way radiotelephone. The dispatching center should be empowered to select hospitals and ambulance services according to the needs of the patient.

The national and international recommendations, guidelines, and standards for all components of the ECCM system, which we and others helped initiate and develop, are not fully implemented in any region of the U. S. because of lacking or unclear authorities and responsibilities, politics, providers' vested interests, and inadequate physician leadership. We are looking toward emergency and critical care medicine physicians' resuscitation knowledge and capability to lead EMS out of an atmosphere of politics and mediocrity and to re-establish the critically ill patient as the target of EMS efforts.

For prevention of prehospital cardiac arrest and provision of advanced life support if resuscitation is needed, extra-hospital advanced life support units are required. They must be able to provide Phases I and II of CPR. They should be located in sport arenas, convention centers, stadiums, civic auditoriums, industrial plants, large office building complexes, areas with large in-transit populations, etc. (AHA, 1974). Mobile ICU ambulances staffed by paramedics can be used for mobile life support units. A physician knowledgeable and skilled in the management of basic and advanced CPR must assume the medical responsibility for the life support unit. The AHA also recommends that his responsibility include direct or remote supervision under the physician's continuous or intermittent direction; nurses and paramedics must be familiar with the use of voice and EKG telemetry equipment if the station is so equipped; and specialized continuing education programs for all life support unit personnel are required. Non-physician staff (paramedics and/or nurses) of these units must be in constant radio communication with the physician director—for example, the one staffing the EMS operations center (Nagel, 1970). The equipment in the unit should include at least that listed for hospital crash carts (see preceding section of this chapter).

These life support units must be able to provide advanced life support by: (1) identifying patients with cardiopulmonary emergencies; (2) instituting immediate monitoring and establishing an I.V. lifeline prior to obtaining a detailed medical and administrative history; (3) providing continued surveillance until a professional decision on management is made; (4) stabilizing the patient's condition prior to transfer to the hospital; and (5) following guidelines on referrals, record keeping, and communication (AHA, 1974A).

For treatment at the scene and during transportation, public education in CPR can save an estimated thousands of lives (Crampton, 1972; Lund, 1976; Schaeffer, 1975; Nagel, 1970; Safar, 1974A). Results of CPR-ABC during transportation by regular ambulances have been poor (Wilder, 1964). Therefore, advanced life support at the scene and during transportation should be provided by mobile ICU ambulance services (Frey, 1975A), which should be equipped and staffed by physicians (Pantridge, 1967; Grace, 1974) or paramedics (Safar, 1972) trained according to national standards (Caroline, in USDOT, 1976A).

Life-threatening emergencies, particularly resuscitation cases, should be taken to the nearest hospital that has comprehensive emergency facilities, i.e., a Category 1 or 2 hospital (Safar, 1968, 1974A). These major emergency hospitals should be established on a regional basis. They should be staffed around the clock by teams of specialists available within minutes and should conform to the highest standards attainable within the community. Unless the patient is beginning to wake up at the scene or during transportation, it is desirable to transfer resuscitation cases to Category I hospital ICUs. Since coronary disease is recognized as the principal cause of sudden death, patients suspected of myocardial infarction should be admitted to the nearest hospital that can provide emergency cardiac care, not necessarily a Category 1 facility.

The use of helicopters or aircraft for the transport of acutely ill and injured patients from isolated or otherwise inaccessible sites and from smaller hospitals to major emergency hospitals should be developed (Frey, 1973A, 1974A). Heliports should be established at major emergency hospitals close enough to the emergency department to obviate the need for transfer between helicopter and hospital special care unit by ambulance. Helicopter ambulances and aircraft for patient transport should have the same equipment as recommended for mobile ICU-type ambulances (Dortmann, 1970).

LEGAL CONSIDERATIONS

The law does not lead but follows events occurring in practice. Thus, medico-legal considerations and recommendations concerning CPR have always been in a state of flux (AHA, 1974A; Huber, in Safar, 1977A). The AHA standards "do not intend to limit or inhibit persons inside or outside of hospitals from providing emergency medical treatment.... Since it may be unrealistic to expect immediate compliance with these standards in some circumstances, a reasonable time for implementation should be allowed."

The AHA recommends legislative action at state levels to clarify what nonphysician health care personnel can and should do; to clarify the medical practice act accordingly; to give immunity (for acts done in good faith and not involving gross negligence or willful, wanton, or reckless misconduct) for those certified in basic or advanced life support; to make training and certification in CPR a job requirement for key health care personnel; and to prevent law enforcement officers from interfering with qualified persons' resuscitation efforts. Restriction of hospital staff privileges to those who have shown the ability to render CPR basic life support, although recommended by national organizations, is not yet a widespread practice. The AHA also published statements on initiation and termination of resuscitation efforts and orders not to resuscitate.

The physician should know the doctrine of *"res ipsa loquitur"* (The thing speaks for itself); e.g., when cardiac arrest occurs in the operating room it must be assumed that someone was negligent and that the professional must explain if it did not happen through negligence. The physician also should know about the *Good Samaritan Law,* adopted by about 40 states, which is meant to protect medical and paramedical persons from civil liability when, acting in good faith, they attempt to resuscitate a person. (This includes the physician, not a CPR team member, who walks into a hospital and is suddenly called upon to help.) The physician should also know about *informed consent* as it applies to surgical and other therapeutic procedures that may result in cardiac arrest. It has been shown to be impossible to

state specifically what "informed consent" should include. The physician should also know about the legal aspects of discontinuing life support (see Phase III, Step G above) and should familiarize himself with *"natural death acts"* as passed recently in California and in some other states.

Huber (in Safar, 1977A) states that "hospitals and ambulance services must live up to the standards of care and practice in the community, and if a hospital or ambulance service lacks appropriate equipment and/or resuscitation procedures, it can be held liable for falling below this standard." Community standards are increasingly interpreted by law as accepted practices beyond the local level, even at national and international levels.

CONCLUSIONS

The phases and steps of cardiopulmonary-cerebral resuscitation, including the steps of emergency airway control, represent the *sine qua non* in the knowledge and skill requirements for emergency and critical care physicians and nonphysician personnel. Resuscitation capability depends also on common sense, an artistic flexible approach to the emergency situation, and some rapid, almost reflex-like actions employed in a titrated fashion, with a sound mix of scientific and artistic attitude. These can be acquired only with experience and objective evaluation of one's practices. Resuscitation calls for appreciation of the time factors (the attitude of speedy action) and attention to technical details. Those involved in resuscitation must be able to function as team members and/or team leaders. Patient outcome after resuscitation attempts depends in part on the correct employment of many of the steps described in this chapter, and on life support throughout all components of the emergency and critical care medicine delivery system (prehospital and intrahospital)—with the outcome often being determined by the weakest step or component. Thus, physicians in general and emergency and critical care medicine physicians in particular must concern themselves with the educational and organizational aspects of resuscitation services within the hospital and community-wide. Knowledge of the literature does not guarantee the ability to resuscitate effectively.

Abbreviations and Definitions

ABBREVIATION	DEFINITION	ABBREVIATION	DEFINITION
AC	Alternating Current	HLR	Heart–Lung Resuscitation (Cardiopulmonary Resuscitation)
AHA	American Heart Association		
ALS	Advanced Life Support (CPR, D–I)	ICU	Intensive Care Unit
ARC	American Red Cross	IMV	Intermittent Mandatory Ventilation (Spontaneous Breathing + Controlled Ventilation)
A-V	Atrioventricular		
BLS	Basic Life Support (CPR, ABC)		
CCM	Critical Care Medicine	IPPB	Intermittent Positive Pressure (Assisted) Breathing
CNS	Central Nervous System		
CPAP	Spontaneous Breathing with Continuous Positive Airway Pressure	IPPV	Intermittent Positive Pressure (Controlled) Ventilation
CPCR	Cardiopumonary–Cerebral Resuscitation	IV	Intravenous
		kg.	Kilogram(s)
CTMP	Cricothyroid Membrane Puncture	M.D.	Medical Doctor (Physician)
CPPV	Continuous Postive Pressure (Controlled) Ventilation (IPPV + PEEP)	mEq./L.	Milliequivalents per Liter
		mg.	Milligram(s)
CPR	Cardiopulmonary Resuscitation	MM	Mouth-to-Mouth
CVP	Central Venous Pressure	MN	Mouth-to-Nose
DC	Direct Current	NAS/NRC	National Academy of Sciences/National Research Council
ECC	Emergency Cardiac Care (System)		
ECCM	Emergency and Critical Care Medicine	NATO	North Atlantic Treaty Organization
		$PaCO_2$	Arterial Carbon Dioxide Pressure
ED	Emergency Department	PaO_2	Arterial Oxygen Pressure
EEG	Electroencephalogram	PAP	Pulmonary Artery Pressure
EHC	External Heart Compressions	PAWP	Pulmonary Arterial Wedge Pressure
EKG	Electrocardiogram	PEEP	Positive End-Expiratory Pressure
EM	Emergency Medicine	pHa	Arterial pH
EMS	Emergency Medical Services	PLS	Postresuscitative Life Support
EMT-A	Emergency Medical Technician–Ambulance (Basic Life Support capability), i.e., EMT-I	PVC	Premature Ventricular Contraction
		RP	Respiratory Therapist
		TLJV	Translaryngeal Jet Ventilation
EMT-P	Emergency Medical Technician–Paramedic (Advanced Life Support capability), i.e., EMT-II	UHCP	University Health Center of Pittsburgh
		USDOT	United States Department of Transportation
EOA	Esophageal Obturator Airway		
FRC	Functional Residual Capacity	VF	Ventricular Fibrillation
HEW	United States Department of Health, Education, and Welfare	VT	Ventricular Tachycardia
HFJV	High Frequency (positive pressure) Jet Ventilation		

Selected Books, Reviews, Recommendations and Teaching Materials (A)
(Materials Recommended for CPR Instructors)

Available from Agencies and Organizations

AHA (American Heart Association): 7320 Greenville Avenue, Dallas, TX 75231:

CPR Instructors Manual (EM 408), *1967* (A); 1977. Emergency Resuscitation Team Manual: A Hospital Plan (EM 439), *1968* (A).
Standards Conference for CPR and Emergency Cardiac Care, May 1973. (a) Proceedings, published by the A.H.A. in 1975. (b) Recommendations: J.A.M.A. Suppl. 227:833, *1974* (A).
Materials on CPR and emergency cardiac care, including standards, texts, slide series, study guides, manuals, and information on motivational films (e.g., Gordon, A.: Pulse of Life; Prescription for Life, second editions) — for basic and advanced life support. (CPR committee chairman, *1975* (A); 1977 (write for a list).
Information on training manikins (e.g., Laerdal Resusci-Anne; Recording Resusci-Anne; basic life support self-training system; infant CPR; infant intubation; adult intubation, and others). Laerdal Corporation, 1 Labriola Court, Armonk, New York 10504, *1976* (A); and others (e.g., Ambu).

ARC (American Red Cross): National Headquarters, Washington, D.C. 20006:

Basic and Advanced First Aid and Instructors Manuals and multi-media systems, *1973* (A).
Life saving, rescue, and water safety manuals and instructor manuals, *1974* (A).
CPR Instructors Manual with Modular System and Hand-Operated Films, *1975* (A).
Statement on emergency treatment of foreign body obstruction of the airway, *1976* (A).

HEW/EMS (U. S. Department of Health, Education and Welfare, Division of Emergency Medical Services): Information Center, Presidential Building 320, Hyattsville, MD 20782:

Recommendations, standards and guidelines on EMS organization, communication, evaluation, and education, *1973-1977* (A).

NAS/NRC (National Academy of Sciences/National Research Council): 2101 Constitution Avenue, Washington, DC 20418:

CPR Conference, May 1966. (a) Proceedings, published by the N.R.C. in 1967. (b) Statement of ad hoc committee. J.A.M.A. *198*:372, *1966* (A).
Ambulance recommendations—(a) Medical requirements for ambulance design and equipment; Publications USGPO 0-3810725. (b) Training of ambulance personnel and others responsible for emergency care of the sick and injured at the scene and during transportation; Publication USGPO 0-381-726. (c) Advanced training program for emergency medical technicians-ambulance. *1970* (A).
Report on emergency airway management conference June 1976 (workshop chairmen—D. Benson, A. H. Goldberg, A. Sladen, P. Safar), *1976* (A).

U.H.C.P. (University Health Center of Pittsburgh): Center for Instructional Resources, Hillman Library, University of Pittsburgh, Pittsburgh, PA 15260:

Documentary and historic training film, "Introduction to Respiratory and Cardiac Resuscitation," by Safar, P. Produced by the U. S. Army, Walter Reed Institute of Research, film PMF 5349, *1958-60* (A).
ICU life support training films by Grenvik, A. and Safar, P., *1972* (A).
CPR training film, "Public Education in Heart-Lung Resuscitation." By Safar, P., Berkebile, P., and Benson, D. Produced in conjunction with WTAE-TV Pittsburgh, PA, *1973* (A).
CPR basic life support self-training system (Table 4, Figure 20). By Safar, P., Scott, M. A., and Hritz, R., *1973-1977* (A). Available through A. Laerdal (see AHA).

USDOT (U. S. Department of Transportation): Headquarters, Washington, DC 20590:

Basic training program for emergency medical technicians (EMT's)—ambulance. (a) Concepts and recommendations (USGPO 0-372-388), 1970 (A). (b) Course guide and course coordinator orientation program (USGPO 0-372-389), 1970 (A). (c) Instructors lesson plan (USGPO TD 2-208:EM3/3 1969), *1970* (A).
Advanced training program for emergency medical technicians (EMT's—paramedics). Prepared by Caroline, N., and McClintock, J. (University of Pittsburgh Department of Anesthesiology) under D.O.T. contract HS-5-01207. (a) Ambulance course guide. (b) Ambulance instructor lesson plans. (c) Emergency care in the field—a manual for paramedics. *1976* (A). DOT (HSA) Publ. No. 75-2013.

Miscellaneous Teaching Materials

Abramson, H.: Resuscitation of the Newborn Infant. St. Louis, C. V. Mosby Company, 1960 (A).
Applebaum, E. L., and Bruce, D. L.: Tracheal Intubation. Philadelphia, W. B. Saunders Company, 1976 (A).
Berkebile, P., et al.: Public Education in Heart-Lung Resuscitation. (a) Crit. Care Med. *1*:115, 1973 (A). (b) Evaluation of three self-training methods in teenagers. *In* Proceedings of the National Conference (May 1973) on Standards for CPR and ECC. Washington, DC, AHA, 1975 (A). (c) Crit. Care Med. *4*:134, 1976 (A).
Frey, R. (chairman): International Symposium on Mobile Intensive Care Units and Advanced Emergency Care Delivery Systems. Mainz, Germany, September 24-27, 1973 (A). Gutenberg University Press, Mainz, 1973 (A), J. Am. Coll. Emerg. Phys. *4*:60, 1975 (A).
Grenvik, A.: Discontinuance of life support in brain death and vegetative state. *In* Symposium on brain resuscitation. Crit. Care Med. May 1978.
Hook, R., and Davis, C. D.: Resuscitation of the Newborn Infant. *In* Stephenson, H. E. (ed.): Cardiac Arrest and Resuscitation. St. Louis, C. V. Mosby Company, 1974 (A).
Jude, J. R., and Elam, J. P.: Fundamentals of Cardiopulmonary Resuscitation. Philadelphia, F. A. Davis Company, 1965 (A).
Nobel, J., et al. (Emergency Care Research Institute, 5200 Butler Pike, Plymouth Meeting, PA 19462): Papers on evaluation of resuscitation equipment. In the journal, Health Devices: (a) Manually operated resuscitators (*1*:13, 1971 (A)). (b) Defibrillators (*1*:109, 1971; *2*:87, 1973; *2*:117, 1973 (A)). (c) External heart compressors (*2*:136, 1973 (A)).
Safar, P. (chairman): Community wide emergency medical services. Recommendations of the Committee on Acute Medicine, American Society of Anesthesiologists. J.A.M.A. *204*:595, 1968 (A).
Safar, P., et al.: Emergency and Critical Care Medicine: Local Implementation of National Recommendations. *In* Safar, P. (ed.): Public Health Aspects of Critical Care Medicine and Anesthesiology. Philadelphia, F. A. Davis Company, 1974 (A) (Chapter 4).
Safar, P., et al.: Teaching and Organizing Cardiopulmonary Resuscitation. *In* Safar, P. (ed.): Public Health Aspects of Critical Care Medicine and Anesthesiology. Philadelphia, F. A. Davis Company, 1974 (Aa) (Chapter 7).
Safar, P. (ed.): Advances in Cardiopulmonary Resuscitation. (Wolf Creek Conference on CPR, October 1975). New York, Springer-Verlag, 1977 (A).
Safar, P.: Postresuscitative Intensive Therapy for Cardiopulmonary-Cerebral Resuscitation. Recommendations and Patient Trial Protocols. Advances in CPR. New York, Springer-Verlag, 1977 (Aa) (Chapter 29).
Safar, P. (ed.): Brain resuscitation. Crit. Care Med. Symposium Issue, 1978 (in press).
Safar, P.: Cardiopulmonary Resuscitation. A Manual for Physicians and Paramedic Instructors (in twelve languages). World Federation of Societies of Anesthesiologists, 1968 (A) (Out of print). Second edition: Cardiopulmonary-cerebral Resuscitation. Philadelphia, W. B. Saunders Co. (Aa), 1978 (in preparation)
Stephenson, H. E. (ed.): Cardiac Arrest and Resuscitation. St. Louis, C. V. Mosby Company, 1974 (A).

Stept, W. J., and Safar, P.: Rapid induction/intubation for prevention of gastric content aspiration. Anesth. Analg. *49*:633, 1970 (A).

Winchell, S. W., and Safar, P.: Teaching and testing lay and paramedical personnel in cardiopulmonary resuscitation. Anes. and Analg. *45*:441, 1966 (A).

References

Adair, J. C., and Ring, W. H.: Management of epiglottitis in children. Anesth. Analg. *54*:622, 1975.

Adair, J. C., et al.: Ten years' experience with IPPB in the treatment of acute laryngotracheobronchitis. Anesth. Analg. *50*:649, 1971.

Ames, A., III, et al.: Cerebral ischemia. II. The no-reflow phenomenon. Am. J. Pathol. *52*:437, 1968.

Asmussen, E., Hahn-Petersen, A., and Rosendal, T.: Air passage through the hypopharynx in unconscious patients in the prone position. Acta Anaesth. Scand. *3*:123, 1959.

Beck, C. F. and Leighninger, D. S.: Death after a clean bill of health. J.A.M.A. *174*:133, 1960.

Beck, C. S., Pritchard, H., and Feil, S. H.: Ventricular fibrillation of long duration abolished by electric shock. J.A.M.A. *135*:985, 1947.

Benson, D. M., et al.: Mobile intensive care by "unemployable" blacks trained as emergency medical technicians (EMT's) in 1967-69. J. Trauma *12*:408, 1971.

Bleyaert, A. L., et al.: Amelioration of postischemic encephalopathy by sodium thiopental after 16 minutes of global brain ischemia in monkeys. Anesthesiology 1978 (in press).

Boehm, R.: Über Wiederbelebung nach Vergiftungen und Asphyxie. Arch. Exp. Pathol. Pharmakol. *8*:68, 1878.

Breivik, H., et al.: Life supporting first aid self-training. (to be published).

Carden, N. I., and Steinhaus, J. E.: Lidocaine resuscitation from ventricular fibrillation. Circ. Res. *4*:640, 1956.

Carroll, R., Hedden, M., and Safar, P.: Intratracheal cuffs: performance characteristics. Anesthesiology *31*:275, 1969.

Carroll, R. G., et al.: Recommended performance specifications for cuffed endotracheal and tracheostomy tubes: a joint statement of investigators, inventors, and manufacturers. Crit. Care Med. *1*:155, 1973.

Crampton, R. S., et al.: Prehospital CPR in acute myocardial infarction. N. Engl. J. Med. *26*:132, 1972.

Crile, G., and Dolley, D. H.: An experimental research into the resuscitation of dogs killed by anesthetics and asphyxia. J. Exp. Med. *8*:713, 1906.

DeLeo, B. C.: Training of Rescue Squads in Endotracheal Intubation. *In* National CPR Standards Conference, May 1973 Proceedings. Dallas, AHA, 1975.

DelGuercio, L. R. M., Feins, N. R., and Cohn, J. D., et al.: A comparison of blood flow during external and internal cardiac massage in man. Circulation *30*:63, 1964; *31*:1, 1965.

Don Michael, T. A., Lambert, E. H., and Mehran, A.: Mouth-to-lung airway for cardiac resuscitation. Lancet *2*:1329, 1968.

Dortmann, C., et al.: Der Mainzer Notarztwagen. Der Anästhesist *19*:212, 1970.

Dripps, R. D., et al.: Cardiac resuscitation. Ann. Surg. *127*:592, 1948.

Elam, J. O., Brown, E. S., and Elder, J. D., Jr.: Artificial respiration by mouth-to-mask method: a study of the respiratory gas exchange of paralyzed patients ventilated by operator's expired air. N. Engl. J. Med. *250*:749, 1954.

Elam, J. O., and Greene, D. G.: Mission accomplished: successful mouth-to-mouth resuscitation. Anesth. Analg. *40*:440, 578, 672, 1961.

Elam, J. O., et al.: Oxygen and carbon dioxide exchange and energy cost of expired air resuscitation. J.A.M.A. *167*:328, 1958.

Elam, J. O., et al.: Head tilt method of oral resuscitation. J.A.M.A. *172*:812, 1960.

Elam, J. O., Ruben, H. M., and Bittner, P. H.: Training laymen in emergency resuscitation. Anesth. Analg. *40*:603, 1961(a).

Eross, B.: Nonslipping, nonkinking airway connections for respiratory care. Anesthesiology *34*:571, 1971.

Esmarch, J. F.: The Surgeons Handbook on the Treatment of Wounded in War. New York, Schmidt, 1878, p. 113.

Fink, B. R.: The etiology and treatment of laryngeal spasm. Anesthesiology *17*:569, 1956.

Gillespie, N. A.: Endotracheal Anesthesia. Madison, University of Wisconsin Press, 1950 (2nd ed.).

Gordon, A. S., et al.: Mouth-to-mouth versus manual artificial respiration for children and adults. J.A.M.A. *167*:320, 1958.

Gordon, A. S., et al.: Critical survey of manual artificial respiration. J.A.M.A. *147*:1444, 1951.

Grace, W. J., Kennedy, R. J., and Nolte, C. T.: Blind defibrillation. Am. J. Cardiol. *34*:115, 1974.

Guildner, C. W.: Resuscitation—opening the airway. J. Am. Coll. Emerg. Phys. *5*:588, 1976.

Guildner, C. W., William, W. B., and Subitch, T.: Airway obstructed by foreign material: the Heimlich maneuver. J. Am. Coll. Emerg. Phys. *5*:675, 1976(a).

Gurvich, N. L., and Yuniev, S. G.: Restoration of a regular rhythm in the mammalian fibrillating heart. Am. Rev. Sov. Med. *3*:236, 1946.

Harris, L. C., Kirimli, B., and Safar, P.: Ventilation–cardiac compression rates and ratios in cardiopulmonary resuscitation. Anesthesiology *28*:806, 1967.

Haugen, R. K.: The café coronary. Sudden death in restaurants. J.A.M.A. *186*:142, 1963.

Hedden, M., et al.: Laryngotracheal damage after prolonged use of orotracheal tubes in adults. J.A.M.A. *207*:703, 1969.

Heiberg, J.: A new expedient in administering chloroform. Medical Times and Gazette, January 10, 1874. (Abstract from Zentralbl. Chir. *9*:141, 1874.)

Heimlich, H. J.: A life-saving maneuver to prevent food choking. J.A.M.A. *234*:398, 1975.

Heimlich, H. J., Hoffmann, K. A., and Canestri, F. R.: Food choking and drowning deaths prevented by external subdiaphragmatic compression. Ann. Thorac. Surg. *20*:188, 1975(a).

Hooker, D. R., Kouwenhoven, W. B., and Langworthy, O. R.: Effect of alternating electrical currents on the heart. Am. J. Physiol. *103*:444, 1933.

Ikada, S., Yanai, N., and Ishikawa, S.: Flexible bronchofibre scope. Keio J. Med. *17*:2, 1968.

Jackson, C., and Jackson, C. L.: Bronchoscopy, Esophagoscopy and Gastroscopy: A Manual of Peroral Endoscopy and Laryngeal Surgery. Philadelphia, W. B. Saunders Company, 1965 (4th ed.).

Jacobs, H. B.: Emergency percutaneous transtracheal catheter and ventilator. J. Trauma *12*:50, 1972.

Jacoby, J. J., et al.: Transtracheal resuscitation. J.A.M.A. *162*:625, 1956.

Johnson, K. R., Genovesi, M. G., and Lassar, K. H.:

Esophageal obturator airway: use and complications. J. Am. Coll. Emerg. Phys. 5:36, 1976.

Jordan, W. S., Graves, C. L., and Elwyn, R. A.: New therapy for postintubation laryngeal edema and tracheitis in children. J.A.M.A. 212:585, 1970.

Jude, J. R., Kouwenhoven, W. B., and Knickerbocker, G. G.: Cardiac arrest: report of application of external cardiac massage on 118 patients. J.A.M.A. 178:1063, 1961.

Kampschulte, S., Marcy, J., and Safar, P.: Simplified physiologic management of status asthmaticus in children. Crit. Care Med. 1:69, 1973.

Kampschulte, S., Smith, J., and Safar, P.: Oxygen transport after cardiopulmonary resuscitation. Anäs. Resuscit (Germany) 30:95, 1969.

Kay, H. J., and Blalock, A.: The use of calcium chloride in the treatment of cardiac arrest in patients. Surg. Gynecol. Obstet. 93:97, 1951.

Kirimli, B., Harris, L. C., and Safar, P.: Drugs in cardiopulmonary resuscitation. Acta Anaesth. Scand. (Suppl.) 23:255, 1966.

Kirimli, B., Kampschulte, S., and Safar, P.: Resuscitation from cardiac arrest due to exsanguination. Surg. Gynecol. Obstet. 129:89, 1969.

Kirimli, B., King, J. E., and Pfaeffle, H. H.: Evaluation of tracheobronchial suction techniques. J. Thorac. Cardiovasc. Surg. 59:340, 1970.

Kirimili, B., and Safar, P.: Arterial versus venous transfusion in cardiac arrest from exsanguination. Anesth. Analg. 44:6, 1965.

Klain, M., and Smith, R. B.: Fluidic technology. Anaesthesia 31:25, 1976.

Klain, M., and Smith, R. B.: High frequency percutaneous transtracheal jet ventilation. Crit. Care Med. 5:280, 1977.

Kouwenhoven, W. B., Jude, J. R., and Knickerbocker, G. G.: Closed chest cardiac massage. J.A.M.A. 173:1064, 1960.

Kouwenhoven, W. B., and Langworthy, O. R.: Cardiopulmonary resuscitation. An account of forty-five years of research. J.A.M.A. 226:877, 1973.

Kouwenhoven, W. B., and Milner, W. R.: Treatment of ventricular fibrillation using a capacitor discharge. J. Appl. Physiol. 7:253, 1954.

Kreiselman, J.: A new resuscitation apparatus. Anesthesiology 4:603, 1943.

Kuhn, F.: Die perorale Intubation. Mit einen Vorwort von O. Hildebrand. Berlin, S. Karger, 1911.

Lemire, J. G., and Johnson, A. L.: Is cardiac resuscitation worthwhile? A decade of experience. N. Engl. J. Med. 286:970, 1972.

Liberthson, R. R., et al.: Prehospital ventricular fibrillation. Prognosis and follow-up course. N. Engl. J. Med. 291:317, 1974.

Lind, B.: Teaching mouth-to-mouth resuscitation in primary schools. Acta Anesth. Scand. (Suppl.) 9:63, 1961.

Lind, B., and Stovner, J.: Mouth-to-mouth resuscitation in Norway. J.A.M.A. 185:933, 1963.

Lindholm, C. E.: Prolonged endotracheal intubation. Acta Anaesth. Scand. (Suppl.) 33, 1969.

Lindholm, C. E., et al.: Flexible fiberoptic bronchoscopy in critical care medicine. Crit. Care Med. 2:250, 1974.

Loehning, R. W., Davis, G., and Safar, P.: Rebreathing with non-rebreathing valves. Anesthesiology 25:854, 1964.

Loughhead, M., et al.: ICU patient categorization. Crit. Care Med. 4:108, 1976.

Lown, B.: Comparison of AC and DC electroshock across the closed chest. Amer. J. Cardiol. 10:223, 1962.

Lund, I., and Lind, B. (eds.): International Symposium on Emergency Resuscitation, Oslo, Norway, 1967. Acta Anaesth. Scand. (Suppl.) 29, 1968.

Lund, I., and Skulberg, A.: Cardiopulmonary resuscitation by lay people. Lancet 2:702, 1976.

Maass: Die Methode der Wiederbelebung bei Herztod nach Chloroformeinathmung. Berlin Klin. Wochschr. 29:265, 1892.

McGinnis, G. E., et al.: Engineering analysis of intratracheal tube cuffs. Anesth. Analg. 50:557, 1971.

Mellemgaard, K., and Astrup, P.: The quantitative determination of surplus amounts of acid or base in the human body. Scand. J. Clin. Lab. Invest. 12:187, 1960.

Milai, A. S., Davis, G., and Safar, P.: Simplified apparatus for IPPB/aerosol therapy. Anesthesiology 26:362, 1965.

Modell, J. H.: The Pathophysiology and Treatment of Drowning and Near-Drowning. Springfield, Ill., Charles C Thomas, Publisher, 1971.

Morikawa, S., and Safar, P.: Shortened Guedel airways (discussion). International symposium on emergency resuscitation. Acta Anaesth. Scand. (Suppl.) 9, 1961.

Morikawa, S., Safar, P., and DeCarlo, J.: Influence of head position on upper airway patency. Anesthesiology 22:265, 1961 (a).

Muendich, K., and Hoflehner, G.: Ventilation bronchoscopy. Der Anaesthesist 2:121, 1953.

Nagel, E. L., et al.: Telemetry—medical command in coronary and other mobile emergency care systems. J.A.M.A. 214:332, 1970.

Negovsky, V. A.: Resuscitation and Artificial Hypothermia. New York, Consultant's Bureau, 1962.

Negovsky, V. A.: Introduction: Reanimatology—The Science of Resuscitation. In Stephenson, H. E.: Cardiac Arrest and Resuscitation. St. Louis, C. V. Mosby Company, 1974 (4th ed.).

Nemoto, E.: Amelioration of Post-Ischemic-Anoxic Brain Damage by Thiopental. In Safar, P. (ed.): Advances in Cardiopulmonary Resuscitation (Proceedings of the Wolf Creek Conference, October 1975). New York, Springer-Verlag, 1977, Chapter 28.

Nemoto, E. M., et al.: A long-term global brain ischemia monkey model for therapy evaluation. Fed. Proc. 34:384, 1975 (abstract); and Stroke, 8:558, 1977.

Pantridge, J. F., and Geddes, J. S.: A mobile intensive care unit in the management of myocardial infarction. Lancet 2:271, 1967.

Pearson, J. W., and Redding, J. S.: The role of epinephrine in cardiac resuscitation. Anesth. Analg. 42:599, 1963.

Pearson, J. W., and Redding, J. S.: Influence of peripheral vascular tone on cardiac resuscitation. Anesth. Analg. 44:746, 1965.

Pearson, J., and Safar, P.: General anesthesia with minimal equipment. Anesth. Analg. 40:664, 1961.

Peleska, B.: Transthoracic and direct defibrillation. Rozhl. Chir. 26:731, 1957.

Pennington, J. E., Taylor, J., and Lown, B.: Chest thump for reverting ventricular tachycardia. N. Engl. J. Med. 283:1192, 1970.

Plum, F. (ed.): Symposium on Brain Ischemia. Arch. Neurol. 29, 1973.

Poulsen, H. (chairman): International symposium on emergency resuscitation, Stavanger, Norway, 1960, Acta Anaesth. Scand. (Suppl.) 9, 1961.

Prevost, J. L., and Battelli, F.: On some effects of electrical discharges on the hearts of mammals. Compt. Rend. Acad. Sci. (Paris) *129*:1267, 1899.

Proctor, D. F., and Safar, P.: Management of Airway Obstruction. *In* Safar, P. (ed.): Respiratory Therapy. Philadelphia, F. A. Davis Company, 1965 (out of print).

Ravitch, M., et al.: Lightning stroke. Recovery following cardiac massage and prolonged artificial respiration. N. Engl. J. Med. *264*:36, 1961.

Redding, J., and Cozine, R.: A comparison of open-chest and closed-chest cardiac massage in dogs. Anesthesiology *22*:280, 1961.

Redding, J., et al.: Resuscitation from drowning. J.A.M.A. *178*:1136, 1961 (a).

Redding, J. S., and Pearson, J. W.: Resuscitation from asphyxia. J.A.M.A. *182*:283, 1962.

Redding, J. S., and Pearson, J. W.: Resuscitation from ventricular fibrillation. J.A.M.A. *203*:93, 1968.

Redding, J. S., Asuncion, J. S., and Pearson, J. W.: Effective routes of drug administration during cardiac arrest. Anesth. Analg. *46*:253, 1967.

Rock, J. J., et al.: High pressure jet insufflation used to prevent aspiration and its effect on the tracheal mucosal wall. Crit. Care Med. *4*:135, 1976.

Rosen, M., and Hillard, E. K.: The use of suction in clinical medicine. Brit. J. Anaesth. *32*:486, 1960.

Ruben, H.: Combination resuscitator and aspirator. Anesthesiology *19*:408, 1958.

Ruben, H., Knudsen, E. J., and Carugati, G.: Gastric inflation in relation to airway pressure. Acta Anaesth. Scand. *5*:107, 1961.

Safar, P.: Mouth-to-mouth airway. Anesthesiology *18*:904, 1957.

Safar, P.: Ventilating bronchoscope. Anesthesiology *19*:407, 1958.

Safar, P.: Ventilatory efficacy of mouth-to-mouth artificial respiration. Airway obstruction during manual and mouth-to-mouth artificial respiration. J.A.M.A. *167*:335, 1958 (b).

Safar, P.: The failure of manual artificial respiration. J. Appl. Physiol. *14*:84, 1959.

Safar, P. (chairman): International Symposium (Vienna): Resuscitation: Controversial Aspects. Heidelberg, Springer-Verlag, 1963.

Safar, P.: Emergency Resuscitation. *In* Safar, P. (ed.): Respiratory Therapy. Philadelphia, F. A. Davis Company, 1965 (out of print).

Safar, P.: Pocket mask for emergency artificial ventilation and oxygen inhalation. Crit. Care Med. *2*:273, 1974.

Safar, P.: Humanizing resuscitation and intensive care. Advances in life saving open new problem areas. J.A.M.A. *235*:2182, 1976.

Safar, P., Aguto-Escarraga, L., and Chang, F.: A study of upper airway obstruction in the unconscious patient. J. Appl. Physiol. *14*:760, 1959 (a).

Safar, P., Benson, D. M., and Esposito, G.: Ambulance design and equipment for mobile intensive care. Arch. Surg. *102*:163, 1971.

Safar, P., and Brose, R. A.: Ambulance design and equipment for resuscitation. Arch. Surg. *90*:343, 1965 (a).

Safar, P., et al.: Ventilation and circulation with closed chest cardiac massage in man. J.A.M.A. *176*:574, 1961.

Safar, P., Escarraga, L., and Elam, J.: A comparison of the mouth-to-mouth and mouth-to-airway methods of artificial respiration with the chest-pressure arm-lift methods. N. Engl. J. Med. *258*:671, 1958 (a).

Safar, P., Esposito, G., and Benson, D. M.: Emergency medical technicians as allied health professionals. Anesth. Analg. *51*:27, 1972.

Safar, P., and Lind, B.: Triple airway maneuver, artificial ventilation and oxygen inhalation by mouth-to-mask and bag-valve-mask techniques. Proceedings of a national conference on standards for CPR, May 1973. Dallas, American Heart Association, 1975, p. 49.

Safar, P., and McMahon, M. C.: A Manual for Emergency Artificial Respiration. Baltimore City Fire Department, 1957. Subsequent editions: Resuscitation of the Unconscious Victim. Springfield, Ill., Charles C Thomas, 1959 and 1961 (1957-1961).

Safar, P., and Penninckx, J.: Cricothyroid membrane puncture with special cannula. Anesthesiology *28*:943, 1967.

Safar, P., and Redding, J.: The "tight jaw" in resuscitation. Anesthesiology *20*:701, 1959 (b).

Safar, P., Stezoski, S. W., and Nemoto, E. M.: Amelioration of brain damage after 12 minutes' cardiac arrest in dogs. Arch. Neurol. *33*:91, 1976 (a).

Saklad, M., and Gulati, R.: Adaptation of Ambu respirator for high oxygen concentration. Anesthesiology *24*:877, 1963.

Schaffer, W. A., and Cobb, L. A.: Recurrent ventricular fibrillation and modes of death in survivors of out-of-hospital ventricular fibrillation. N. Engl. J. Med. *293*:259, 1975.

Schellinger, R. R.: The length of the airway to the bifurcation of the trachea. Anesthesiology *25*:169, 1964.

Schiff, M.: Über direkte Reizung der Herzoberfläche. Arch. Ges. Physiol. *28*:200, 1882.

Schofferman, J., Oill, P., and Lewis, A. J.: The esophageal obturator airway. A clinical evaluation. Chest *69*:67, 1976.

Secher, O., and Wilhjelm, B.: The protective action of anesthetics against hypoxia. Canad. Anaesth. Soc. J. *15*:423, 1968.

Sellick, B. A.: Cricoid pressure to control regurgitation of stomach contents during induction of anesthesia. Lancet *2*:404, 1961.

Shapiro, H. M., Wyte, S. R., and Loeser, J.: Barbiturate-augmented hypothermia for reduction of persistent intracranial hypertension. J. Neurosurg. *40*:60, 1974.

Shoemaker, W. C.: A patient care algorithm for cardiac arrest. Crit. Care Med. *4*:157, 1976.

Siebke, H., et al.: Survival after 40 minutes submersion without cerebral sequelae. Lancet *1*:1275, 1975.

Smetana, J., et al.: Resuscitation of the heart; experimental study and clinical experience. Rev. Czech. Med. *7*:65, 1961.

Smith, A. L., Hoff, J. T., and Nielson, S. L.: Barbiturate protection against cerebral infarction. Stroke *5*:1, 1974.

Smith, R. B.: Transtracheal ventilation during anesthesia. Anesth. Analg. *53*:225, 1974.

Smith, J., et al.: Need for oxygen enrichment in myocardial infarction, shock, and following cardiac arrest. Acta Anaesth. Scand. (Suppl.) *29*:127, 1968.

Smith, R. B., Schaer, W. B., and Pfaeffle, H.: Percutaneous transtracheal ventilation for anesthesia and resuscitation: a review and report of complications. Canad. Anaesth. Soc. J. *22*:607, 1975.

Snow, R. G., and Nunn, J. F.: Induction of anaesthesia in the foot-down position with a full stomach. Br. J. Anaesth. *31*:493, 1959.

Snyder, J. V., et al.: Global ischemia in dogs: intracranial pressures, brain blood flow and metabolism. Stroke *6*:21, 1975.

Spoerel, W. E., Narayanan, P. S., and Singh, N. P.: Transtracheal ventilation. Br. J. Anaesth. *43*:932, 1971.

Stewart, J. S.: Management of cardiac arrest with special reference to metabolic acidosis. Br. Med. J. *1*:476, 1964.

Takaori, M., and Safar, P.: Treatment of massive hemorrhage with colloid and crystalloid solutions. J.A.M.A. *199*:297, 1967.

Teasdale, G., Knill-Jones, R., and Jennett, B.: Assessing and recording "conscious level." J. Neurol. Neurosurg. Psychiatr. *37*:1286, 1974.

Tossach, W. A.: A man dead in appearance recovered by distending the lungs with air. *In* Medical Essays and Observations. London, Cadell and Balfour, 1771, pp. 108-111.

Valentine, T. A., et al.: Lidocaine in the prevention of sudden death in the prehospital phase of acute infarction. N. Engl. J. Med. *291*:1327, 1974.

Vesalius, A.: De corporis humani fabrica. Libri Septem, 1543.

Visintine, R. E., and Baick, C. H.: Ruptured stomach after Heimlich maneuver. J.A.M.A. *234*:415, 1975.

Wiggers, C. J.: The physiological bases for cardiac resuscitation from ventricular fibrillation. Method for serial defibrillation. Am. Heart J. *20*:413, 1940.

Wilder, R. J., et al.: Cardiopulmonary resuscitations by trained ambulance personnel. J.A.M.A. *190*:531, 1964.

Yakaitis, R. W., and Redding, J. S.: Precordial thumping during cardiac resuscitation. Crit. Care Med. *1*:22, 1973.

Zoll, P. M.: Development of electric control of cardiac rhythm. J.A.M.A. *226*:881, 1973.

Zoll, P. M., et al.: Treatment of unexpected cardiac arrest by external electric stimulation of the heart. N. Engl. J. Med. *254*:541, 1956 (a).

Zoll, P. M., et al.: Termination of ventricular fibrillation in man by externally applied electric countershock. N. Engl. J. Med. *254*:727, 1956.

Chapter 10

RESPIRATORY CARE TECHNIQUES AND STRATEGIES*

Peter Safar and Nancy Caroline

INTRODUCTION

Emergency and critical care medicine cannot be practiced by leisure contemplation. On the contrary, it requires that its practitioners be capable of rapidly applying a variety of skills in often difficult and changing clinical circumstances. In this chapter, we shall deal with some of the *techniques and strategies* applicable to the care of patients with acute respiratory insufficiency. (Techniques specifically relating to emergency airway control and emergency artificial ventilation have been covered in Chapter 9.) It should be emphasized that techniques are best learned through the following sequence: (1) *seeing;* (2) *doing,* first on manikins or fellow students and finally on patients, under the supervision of skilled instructors whose duty includes protecting the patient; (3) *practicing;* and (4) *teaching.* This chapter therefore is intended to provide only an introduction and guidelines for the acquisition of skills that ultimately must be mastered through performance.

Techniques are not solutions to problems; they are the concrete expression of theoretical solutions, and usually represent compromises with the ideal. The intelligent application of skills in appropriate circumstances requires a thorough understanding of

basic pathophysiology. We have attempted to provide the framework for such understanding in Chapters 2 and 3 and will not reiterate fundamental concepts here; the reader is also directed to the Glossary in Chapter 3 for definitions of terms and abbreviations and tables of normal values. In this chapter, however, we shall try to identify strategies of assessment and treatment and to provide an orderly approach to the patient with acute respiratory insufficiency.

We begin this chapter with a discussion of some general diagnostic techniques which have applicability over a range of clinical problems. We turn our attention next to specific techniques and strategies for providing optimal oxygenation, ventilation and acid-base balance, respectively. Along with these elegant physiologic maneuvers, however, there must be some rather mundane considerations of plumbing and housecleaning, without which patients may die of entirely preventable asphyxia. Therefore, subsequent sections deal with techniques of long-term airway care and pleural drainage.

Finally, it is important to recognize that every therapeutic intervention for respiratory disorders must be assessed in terms of its over-all impact on multiple systems. For this reason, in the concluding section of this chapter, we deal briefly with the monitoring of other vital organ systems as it applies to respiratory care.

The constraints of organizing and writing a chapter require that some rather artificial divisions be imposed. Thus, while in a textbook we may deal separately, for example, with ventilation and acid-base balance, in practice these are not independent variables and cannot be manipulated in isolation

*Acknowledgments: Drs. Ake Grenvik, Michael Loughhead and Arnold Sloden, and Mr. Bela Eross, A.R.I.T., provided material and valuable suggestions for this chapter. Ms. Vicki Shidel typed the manuscript.

This chapter has been used for the Western Pennsylvania Acute Respiratory Care Training Project of 1974–77, supported by the National Heart-Lung Institute (Contract No. HR42965).

from one another. The human body, like any other art masterpiece, represents a whole greater than the sum of its parts. Although for didactic purposes it may be convenient to separate those parts for detailed scrutiny, in the clinical setting it is the interaction among the parts that ultimately determines the success or failure of therapeutic intervention.

DIAGNOSTIC TECHNIQUES

In the present section, we shall describe some of the techniques which are applied in the diagnosis and monitoring of respiratory insufficiency. These are important techniques, but they should not be employed to the exclusion of clinical evaluation (including history taking, inspection, palpation, percussion, and auscultation) and ancillary measures, such as chest roentgenograms and other diagnostic methods. Careful clinical assessment and reasoning based upon a knowledge of pathophysiology must provide the criteria for selection of more sensitive diagnostic methods in any given instance.

Measurement of Arterial Blood Gases and pH

ARTERIAL PUNCTURE AND CATHETERIZATION

Arterial Po_2, Pco_2, and pH provide the most sensitive measurement of a patient's state of oxygenation, ventilation, and acid-base equilibrium. Samples of these measurements are obtained from a peripheral artery, either by direct arterial puncture or through an indwelling arterial catheter.

Arterial Puncture. Arterial puncture may be readily accomplished through a radial, femoral, or brachial artery — listed in order of preference. The equipment required for this procedure includes a 2 ml. syringe, a short 25 to 26 gauge needle, an antiseptic swab, a dry gauze swab, and tape. Use of a glass syringe permits spontaneous filling under arterial pressure and thus enables more accurate differentiation of inadvertent venous puncture; however, disposable plastic syringes are adequate if glass syringes are not available. In either case, the syringe should be prepared by drawing about 0.2 ml. of heparin into the syringe to wet the inside of the barrel, then emptying the syringe by holding it vertically to remove air and to leave only that heparin remaining in the "deadspace" of the needle and syringe.

For *radial artery puncture,* an assistant should hold the patient's hand supinated and in moderate dorsiflexion; a folded towel placed beneath the wrist helps maintain this position. The operator preps the patient's wrist with the antiseptic swab. The point of maximal pulsation of the radial artery is palpated, usually a few centimeters proximal to the thenar eminence, and the tips of the operator's index and middle fingers are placed slightly over the artery to indicate its course. Holding the syringe in the other hand as one would hold a pencil, the operator punctures the skin and aims the needle toward the maximal pulsation of the radial artery. When the artery is entered, a resistance will be felt and, if a glass syringe is used, arterial pressure may push the barrel of the syringe upward. If a plastic syringe is used, *gentle* aspiration is required. When moving the fingers from the pencil-holding position to the aspirating position, displacement of the needle can be prevented by moving the palpating fingers upward to hold the bevel of the needle. Repeated insertions in different planes, while the needle remains subcutaneous, may be attempted until the artery is entered.

After about 1 ml. of blood has been obtained, the needle is smoothly withdrawn and firm pressure is applied on the puncture site with dry gauze for at least five minutes, or a temporary pressure dressing may be used. The syringe should be immediately inverted and any air expelled from it, and the needle then sealed with a protector or stopper or by bending it. Gentle rotation of the syringe will ensure that the blood is fully heparinized. If there is to be any delay in analyzing the sample, the syringe should be placed in ice. The sample should be sent to the laboratory for Po_2, Pco_2 and pH analysis, and in some cases also hemoglobin; the patient's name, time of sampling, and FIO_2 at the time of sampling must be entered on the label. PaO_2 values without FIO_2 values are meaningless.

If the radial arteries cannot be used for sampling, arterial blood may be obtained from a *femoral artery.* This site is less desirable because it is more difficult to ensure both adequate surface antisepsis and hemostasis by pressure in the inguinal region. The same equipment is used, except that the 25 to 26 gauge needle must be somewhat longer. The skin over the femoral artery is meticulously prepped and the artery palpated such that the index and middle fingers straddle the area of maximal pulsation. The skin is punctured between the two fingers and the needle aimed at the maximal pulsation of the artery. The remainder of the procedure is the same as that described for radial artery puncture. After withdrawing the needle, firm manual pressure must be applied to the inguinal area for a full five minutes; a pressure dressing is not effective.

When neither the radial nor femoral arteries are available, the *brachial, axillary, dorsalis pedis,* or *temporal artery* may be used, although their lack of stable fixation sometimes renders puncture difficult. The procedure is similar to that described for femoral artery puncture.

Several *errors* in arterial puncture may lead to inaccurate blood gas determination. The *inadvertent sampling of venous blood* is one of the most common of these errors and will yield a specious reading of lowered PO_2 and slightly elevated $PaCO_2$. A venous sample should be suspected when the results of the blood gas determination are inconsistent with the patient's clinical picture. When in doubt, repeat the test with a fresh arterial blood sample taken from another site. *Air left in the syringe* may be expected to alter both the measured $PaCO_2$ and PO_2 through diffusion of gases between the air pocket and the blood samples; thus, all air should be expelled from the syringe before it is sealed and sent to the lab. A spurious decrease in pH may result if *excess heparin* is left in the syringe prior to arterial sampling, since heparin solutions are quite acidotic. Thus, the plunger should be pushed to the bottom of the barrel prior to sampling.

Potential *complications* of arterial puncture may be avoided by meticulous care in techniques. *Hematoma* results from inadequate compression over the puncture site, while *thrombosis* is favored by excessive compression. Excessively frequent punctures at the same site also lead to arterial thrombosis.

Arterial Catheterization (Fig. 1). Placement of an indwelling arterial catheter may be desirable in circumstances in which there is a need for (*a*) frequent and repeated arterial sampling; (*b*) direct, continuous monitoring of arterial blood pressure; or (*c*) cardiac output determination by dye dilution. The wider the lumen of the artery in relation to the thickness of the catheter, the less likely will be the occurrence of thrombosis secondary to the blood stasis. Either the radial (for no longer than three to four days) or the femoral artery may be used; the latter is preferred because it is less prone to clotting and thrombosis, even when the catheter is left in place for over a week, and it can be secured in place more easily without having to immobilize the patient's limb.

For *femoral artery catheterization,* the equipment and techniques used may vary. One example which was found to be satisfactory in our institution is presented here. The following equipment should be assembled (Fig. 1):

Razor, Betadine solution, sterile gloves and drapes

1 per cent lidocaine in a 2 ml. syringe (for conscious patients); 25 gauge needle for skin puncture

An 18-inch 19 gauge through-the-needle catheter with a 2- to 3-inch 17 gauge thin-walled needle (either commercially available as Intracath or separately assembled needle and catheter)

Sterile gauze, 4 × 4 inches

Silk suture, 5–0, on curved needle, with needle holder, scissors, and hemostat

Betadine skin ointment, 3-inch adhesive tape

Strain gauge, pressure monitor, compatible tubing with Luerlok connections, three-way stopcocks, diluted heparin solution (10 mg or 1000 U/500 ml isotonic saline) with flushing set-up (optionally with Sørensen continuous flushing valve), as illustrated in Figure 1.

The femoral artery of the puncture site (i.e., near the inguinal ligament) lies between the femoral vein (medially) and the femoral nerve (lateral to the artery). The femoral artery is palpated and the overlying skin shaved and disinfected with Betadine solution, using sterile technique. The oper-

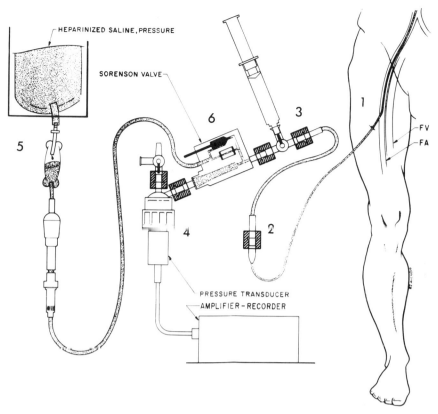

Figure 1 Arterial catheter system. Femoral artery catheter (1) connected via nonslipping connections (2) and three-way stopcock with sampling syringe (3) to pressure transducer (4). Interposed flushing system (5) with heparin (10 mg./500 ml. saline) under pressure and Sorenson valve (6), permitting slow, continuous flush plus intermittent manual flush (see discussion in text).

ator then dons sterile gloves and isolates the inguinal area between sterile drapes. In the conscious patient, the skin overlying the femoral artery is infiltrated with lidocaine. A 17 gauge needle from the Intracath set is introduced and advanced at a 45 degree angle until the femoral artery is entered—signaled by pulsatile flow through the needle. The catheter is then fed through the needle into the lower abdominal aorta, held firmly in place, and the needle is withdrawn over it. Continued pulsatile flow through the catheter indicates that it is properly seated within the lumen of the artery. The catheter is then flushed with heparinized saline via a stopcock, hooked up to the strain gauge via sterile tubing with nonslipping connections, and secured in place with a skin suture. Betadine ointment is used to seal the skin puncture site, and sterile gauze is applied over the puncture site and securely taped with adhesive to form a pressure dressing.

For a *radial artery catheterization*, the equipment used is basically the same, except that a short (2-inch) 20 gauge over-the-needle catheter (Extracath) is used rather than an Intracath.

If the radial artery is selected for catheterization, the integrity of the ipsilateral ulnar artery should first be assured, to lessen the risk of ischemic damage to the hand in the event of subsequent radial artery thrombosis. The patient is asked to make a tight fist to blanch the hand, and the operator then applies occlusive pressure over the patient's radial and ulnar arteries. The patient opens his hand, which should now be fully blanched, and the operator releases pressure on the ulnar artery. If normal color is restored to the hand within seven seconds, ulnar circulation may be considered adequate to maintain the hand in the event of radial artery thrombosis. If the patient is unconscious and cannot make a fist, pulsations of the ulnar artery should be ascertained or both arteries occluded to blanch the hand.

After assuring the patency of the ulnar artery, the wrist is splinted on an arm board in a position of supination and moderate dorsiflexion, leaving the area from the thenar eminence to mid-forearm free of tape. An 18 gauge needle is used to make a small hole in the anesthetized skin. The 20 gauge Extracath needle, held at about a 30 degree angle to the wrist, is passed through the hole in the skin into the radial artery, puncture of the radial artery being signaled by the appearance of blood in the catheter hub. The needle is advanced another 2 to 3 mm. and then held motionless while the catheter is advanced over the needle into the artery. The needle is withdrawn while holding the catheter securely in place, and the catheter is taped in position and attached to the strain gauge via sterile tubing.

In small children and infants in whom percutaneous puncture is not successful, a radial or temporal artery catheterization is used via a small skin incision, with catheter insertion through a puncture hole in the artery under direct vision, without ligating the artery.

When *sampling* arterial or venous blood via catheter for gas and pH determinations, one must first withdraw slightly more than the deadspace volume of fluid and then blood (which may later be reinjected) using a separate syringe; and follow this immediately by sampling into the heparinized sampling syringe. Sampling must avoid entry of air bubbles into the sampling syringe as well as into the patient's arterial system by handling stopcocks and syringes correctly and skillfully, which includes the use of gravity to control air bubbles. When a continuous flush device is used (Sørensen device, Fig. 1), sampling is done via a stopcock on the patient's side of the flush. The sampling errors from bubbles, clots, or excess heparin are similar to those associated with arterial puncture.

Although the *complications* of arterial catheterization are potentially greater and more severe than those of arterial puncture, meticulous technique has made safe use of indwelling catheters, in the femoral artery for weeks and the radial artery for days, quite the routine. Thick indwelling catheters in small arteries (e.g., radial) have resulted occasionally in thromboses, and arterial line flushing with bubbles and thrombi has caused embolization, both of which may lead to loss of limb.

LABORATORY MEASUREMENT OF BLOOD GASES AND pH

Once obtained, whether by direct arterial puncture or via an indwelling arterial cannula, bubble-free heparinized arterial blood samples are sent immediately to the laboratory for analysis. Any facility caring for the critically ill and injured should have the capability of providing rapid blood Po_2, Pco_2 and pH determinations, preferably by competent technicians on call in the hospital on a 24-hour seven-day basis. Modern laboratory equipment permits these measurements to be made from as little as 0.2 ml. of blood within three to five minutes. Since it is often desirable to obtain hematocrit and sometimes blood oxygen content values as well, at least 1 ml. of arterial blood should be sent to the laboratory. For sampling conditions see 100 per cent O_2 test (Fig. 5).

Instruments used to measure arterial blood Po_2, Pco_2 and pH are essentially analog devices, relating a measured change in current or potential to the concentration of ion or gas in the unknown solution. Most *oxygen electrodes* now in use are based upon the "polarographic principle" developed by Clark, utilizing a membrane-covered platinum cathode in KCl solution and a silver/silver chloride anode. Oxygen from the unknown solution (the arterial blood sample) permeates the membrane and is reduced to OH^- by the voltage between cathode and anode. The conductivity of the KCl solution is thereby altered, and the current change so produced is proportional to the Po_2. The *carbon dioxide electrodes* in use are based on the work of Severinghaus. They consist of a glass pH electrode with a reference electrolyte jacket on which a CO_2-permeable membrane is mounted. As CO_2 diffuses across the membrane, it combines with water to form carbonic acid, which in turn rapidly dissociates into bicarbonate and hydrogen ions:

$$CO_2 + H_2O \rightleftharpoons H_2CO_3 \rightleftharpoons H^+ + HCO_3^-$$

The resulting pH of this solution is directly proportional to the Pco_2 of the sample. Finally, the *pH electrode*, which has long been in use in industry and medicine, comprises a glass membrane with a solution of known pH inside. The hydrogen ion gradient between the known solution inside and the sample outside the electrode establishes a potential that is directly proportional to that gradient and is measured on a potentiometer. With careful maintenance and operation by trained technicians, these electrodes provide highly accurate measurements.

The PO_2, PCO_2 and pH electrodes have been refined and combined into a *trielectrode* system by Severinghaus. Various commercial versions are marketed with detailed instructions on use, calibrations, maintenance, checking accuracy and reliability, and servicing. These units usually serve patients better in the hands of specially trained technicians, nurses, or respiratory therapists as part of an accurate ICU laboratory arrangement, than in the hands of clinical pathology laboratory personnel or of changing untrained house staff without quality control. Unreliable blood gas services are a greater hazard to patient care than no blood gas services at all.

For determinations of cardiac output, oxygen consumption, shunting, and oxygen utilization coefficient (see Chapter 3), it is necessary to determine, in addition to the PO_2, the actual *oxygen content* of arterial blood (CaO_2) and of mixed venous or central venous blood ($C\bar{v}O_2$). This measurement is still in the realm of semi-investigative patient management in most hospitals. Oxygen content may be measured by a variety of instruments using chemical, chromatographic, and photoelectric techniques; the more recently introduced apparatus permit determination of oxygen content from blood samples as small as 0.5 ml. in 5 to 10 minutes. The Van Slyke-Neill and Natelson apparatus, now largely out of date, relied on volumetric measurement of oxygen gas released from the sample by addition of potassium ferricyanide. A similar chemical-releasing system is the underlying principle behind gas chromatographic methods of measuring oxygen content. Photoelectric *oximetry* employs a photometer for measuring the fraction of hemoglobin in oxygenated form, which absorbs less visible red light (620 to 770 nm)—and therefore reflects more light at this wavelength—than does reduced hemoglo-

bin. As in the case of samples for arterial blood gases, venous and arterial samples drawn for determination of oxygen content must be handled without exposure to air and stored in ice if analysis is to be delayed.

Simple Spirometry

In this section, we shall deal briefly with some of the measurements that may be applied to patients who are conscious and able to cooperate. Variables to be measured are defined in the Glossary of Chapter 3 (p. 99). Measurements of pulmonary functions specifically applicable to patients being treated with mechanical ventilation will be covered in subsequent sections of this chapter.

Measurements of *vital capacity* (total and timed) and *increased airway resistance* are perhaps the most useful and readily available in the emergency room (Figs. 2 to 4). A variety of portable, electronically activated *spirometers* that are now available permit bedside assessment of vital capacity in the form of forced expiratory volume (FEV, total and timed) and maximum mid-expiratory flow rate (MMFR). Using such a spirometer, the patient is asked to inhale maximally and then exhale as hard and completely as possible. Leakage can be prevented with a tight-fitting oronasal mask or a mouthpiece with nose clip. Coaching toward obtaining the maximal values with repeat performances is important.

The total volume exhaled, i.e., the vital capacity or total FEV, is compared with the normal (predicted) value of the particular patient (Fig. 3) and is considered abnormal if it is less than 80 per cent of the predicted volume. The volume exhaled in the first second constitutes the $FEV_{1.0}$. The flow rate measured over the middle half of exhalation is the MMFR, usually closely related to the $FEV_{1.0}$. Figure 2 illustrates representative spirograms obtained with a "bell-in-water" spirometer. In the normal pattern (the solid black line), normal $FEV_{1.0}$ is 4 liters, yielding an $FEV_{1.0}/VC$ ratio of 80 per cent, and the MMFR is approximately 3.5 liters per second. In *restrictive pulmonary disease*, both $FEV_{1.0}$ and VC are characteristically reduced, while the $FEV_{1.0}/VC$ ($FEV_{1.0}$ in per cent of VC) and the MMFR remain normal. In

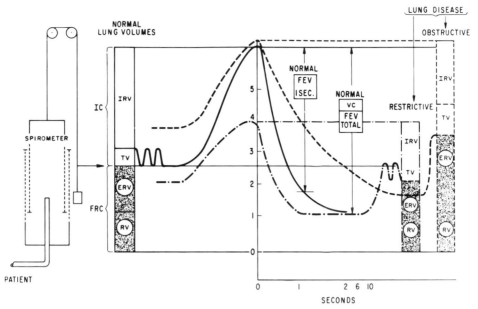

Figure 2 Normal and abnormal lung volumes and idealized spirometry tracings. TV: tidal volume. FRC: functional residual capacity. IC: inspiratory capacity. IRV: inspiratory reserve volume. ERV: expiratory reserve volume. RV: residual volume. VC: vital capacity. FEV: forced expiratory volume (expiratory vital capacity). Solid lines: normal. Dashed lines: primarily obstructive derangement. Dotted lines: primary restrictive derangement. FEV (VC) starting at zero seconds.

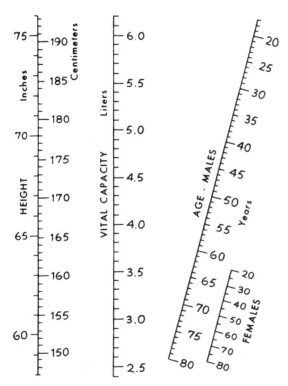

Figure 3 Nomogram for prediction of normal vital capacities in males and females, ages 17 to 80 years. (From Miller, W.: J. Appl. Physiol., *14*:157, 1959.)

obstructive pulmonary disease, on the other hand, $FEV_{1.0}$ is reduced out of proportion to any reduction in VC, yielding a decrease in $FEV_{1.0}/VC$; MMFR is accordingly diminished. Most patients with pulmonary disease have a combination of restrictive and obstructive abnormalities.

Such measurements are of considerable value in following the progress of an asthmatic or chronic bronchitic patient in response to bronchodilator and other acutely effective therapy. If a spirometer is not available, total VC can be estimated with a Wright ventilation meter, which is pocket size; or a Draeger Respirometer, which is portable but not pocket size. Both of these devices measure gas *volume* through a clockwork mechanism connected to a rotating vane. Air passing through the devices is diverted through slots in the vane, the rotation of which is thus directly proportional to the volume of air traversing the instrument, and this volume can be read on the dial. Using this type of respirometer, the patient is asked to inhale through it (after maximal exhalation) as fully as possible (VC in inhalation) or exhale after maximal inhalation (VC in exhalation). These ventilation meters or respirometers are

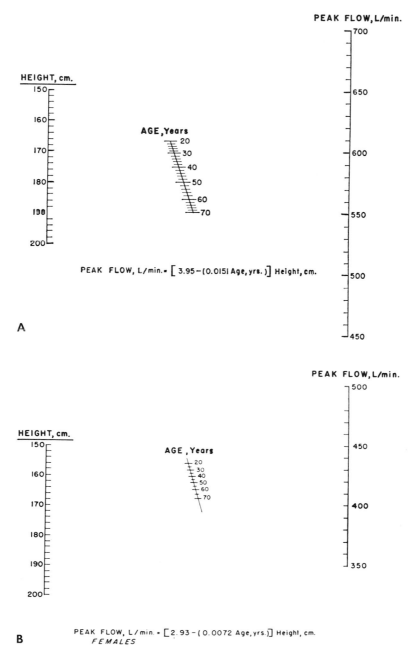

Figure 4 Nomogram for prediction of peak expiratory flow rate (with Wright peak flow meter) from age and height for males (*A*) and females (*B*). (From Leiner, G. C. et al.: Am. Rev. Resp. Dis., 88:644, 1963.)

widely used in recovery rooms and intensive care units to measure the inspiratory capacity (sighing volume).

The Wright *peak flow meter* can be used to follow changes in airway resistance by comparing the maximal expiratory flow rate (MEFR) values obtained with predicted values (Fig. 4). As the patient exhales through

this instrument, a vane closing an internal orifice in the device is deflected to a degree directly proportional to the rate of the gas *flow*. This deflection may be read directly from the dial in units of flow and is proportional to resistance (thus, inversely proportional to the radius of the airway). Finally, if a peak flow meter is not available, a Wright ventilation meter can be used to estimate airway resistance by comparing the forced vital capacity values obtained during inhalation with those during exhalation. Since the inertia of this instrument makes it over-read the volume at high flow rates and under-read it at low rates, one can find that the readings for exhaled VC values are smaller than those measured during inhalation when there is significant (expiratory) airway obstruction.

Whatever measurements are used, they must be repeated at frequent intervals, for what matters is not the absolute number obtained at a single measurement but rather the *trend* among a series of measurements. The acute asthmatic whose airway resistance is steadily improving during a period of therapy in the emergency room may be able to go home, while one whose resistance is unchanged or increasing may require hospital admission.

Measurements of lung volumes involve more sophisticated equipment than is usually at hand in the emergency room or ICU, and most require a conscious, cooperative patient. These are the additional measurements usually provided by pulmonary function laboratories. The information they provide is generally less crucial in the acute management of critically ill or injured patients. *Total lung capacity* (TLC) and *functional residual capacity* (FRC) are most accurately measured in a *body plethysmograph*, which is a large airtight chamber in which the subject sits and makes respiratory efforts against a closed mouthpiece. As he does so, his lung volume decreases (from compression of the gas in his lungs) while the gas volume in the chamber increases (as the pressure inside the chamber falls). Using Boyle's law, which states that pressure times volume is constant, and knowing the pressure and volume in the box, one can then calculate the change in volume of the lung (ΔV). With this information, one can further determine the FRC as follows:

$$P_1 V = P_2 (V - \Delta V)$$

where P_1 and P_2 are pressures measured at the mouth, and V = FRC.

FRC may also be measured using the *helium dilution technique*, in which the subject is connected to a spirometer containing a known concentration of helium (chosen because it is essentially insoluble in blood). The patient takes several breaths until equilibration between the helium in the lungs and the helium in the spirometer is complete. Since the system is closed and no helium loss has occurred, the amount of helium present prior to equilibration (helium concentration times volume, or $C_1 \times V$) must be equal to the amount present after equilibration: $C_2 \times (V_1 + V_2)$. One then solves the V_2 to obtain the FRC. Unlike the body plethysmograph, which measures the total volume of gas in the lungs (including any which might be trapped behind closed airways), the helium dilution technique measures only ventilated lung volume. This is true also of the *nitrogen washout technique,* in which the subject breathes 100 per cent oxygen rather than helium and the calculations are made on the basis of nitrogen concentrations and volumes. FRC measurements are now being introduced into the routine bedside monitoring of selected patients in some advanced ICU's.

In concluding this section, we should mention a few words about *closing volume* and *closing capacity*, measurements which are still under clinical trial to determine their precise significance in the early detection of airway diseases, such as asthma and emphysema. Closing volume is the volume of vital capacity exhaled during the last phase of exhalation from the point of beginning closure of any airways to residual volume. Closing capacity is closing volume plus residual volume. These measurements make use of the fact that there are topographical differences in normal ventilation. The subject is asked to take a full inhalation from residual volume, at the beginning of which helium is injected into the inhaled mixture. Since near the residual volume, the bases of the lungs are relatively unventilated, this bolus of helium will go preferentially to the lung apices. As the subject exhales, the concentration of expired helium is plotted against time, revealing four discrete phases of exhalation: (1) exhalation of pure deadspace gas; (2) exhalation of mixed deadspace and alveolar gas; (3) exhalation of pure alveolar gas; and (4) exhalation of a high concentration of helium. This rapid increase in the concentration of helium at the end of exhalation indicates the lung volume (closing capacity) at which some airways begin to close, i.e., usually at the base of the lungs, with consequent preferential emptying of the apices.

In healthy young subjects, the closing volume is about 10 per cent of the vital capacity above residual volume (i.e., closing capacity is residual volume plus 10 per cent of VC) and increases steadily with age to around 40 per cent by the age of 60. Closing volumes are increased above these values by even small degrees of airway disease, such as early asthma or emphysema, and closing capacity is greater than FRC in ARDS.

OXYGENATION TECHNIQUES

Rationale and Indications

The various techniques of providing supplemental oxygen all aim at ensuring adequate tissue oxygenation, with particular reference to the brain and myocardium (Chapters 3 to 5). Provision of adequate oxygen at the tissue level requires efforts to establish (1) an adequate *arterial* PO_2 (PaO_2), i.e., at least 60 torr (the knee of the hemoglobin-oxygen dissociation curve) and preferably 100 torr for full saturation of hemoglobin with oxygen; (2) an arterial blood *hemoglobin concentration*, usually of 13 to 15 gm./100 ml. blood, to ensure normal arterial oxygen content (about 20 ml./100 ml. blood); (3) an adequate *blood flow*, through maintenance of blood volume and perfusion pressure; and (4) an appropriate *distribution of blood flow*, sufficient to meet the varying metabolic demands of different tissues.

There is a tendency in the care of the critically ill to focus primarily on achievement of "normal blood gases." It is clear from the foregoing, however, that normalization of arterial PO_2 and PCO_2 does not in itself provide any guarantee that optimal tissue oxygenation has been accomplished. Indeed, pursuit of high arterial PO_2 to the exclusion of other mechanisms of tissue oxygenation may in fact lead to unsuspected increases in tissue hypoxia. The uncritical use of positive pressure ventilation is a case in point: in some instances, positive pressure ventilation may effect a very gratifying improvement in PaO_2, but at the same time it may lower cardiac output (through an increase in intrathoracic pressure) to such an extent that the salutory effects of a higher arterial oxygen tension are entirely negated. Thus the potential benefit of any given intervention aimed at improving arterial blood gases must be weighed in terms of its over-all impact on the many other variables affecting tissue oxygenation. The same may be said of any therapeutic intervention along these lines. It is customary, for example, to try to counteract the blood sludging and diminished oxygen carrying capacity of hypovolemia with blood volume expansion; if, however, the hematocrit rises above 45 per cent, oxygen transport may be decreased in spite of increasing arterial oxygen content because of increased viscosity and reduced blood flow.

We return, then, to the prerequisites for adequate tissue oxygenation. Regarding (1), provision of an *adequate arterial* PO_2, we shall have more to say later in this section. When we consider (2), an *adequate blood hemoglobin concentration*, we must take into account not only the absolute levels, in gm./100 ml., of hemoglobin, but also the affinity of that hemoglobin for oxygen. Has oxygen release been impaired in our patient by a shift of the oxygen-hemoglobin dissociation curve to the left, as may occur through excessive mechanical hyperventilation, or through a decrease in 2,3-DPG (with the use of bank blood or intravenous hyperalimentation)? Concern for (3), *adequate blood flow*, requires us to examine local perfusion pressures and autoregulatory mechanisms. Perfusion pressure for the coronary arteries, for example, derives from the mean diastolic arterial pressure minus right atrial pressure; in the brain, it is the mean (or, under certain circumstances, systolic) arterial pressure minus cerebral venous pressure or intracranial pressure (whichever is higher) that determines perfusion pressure. In addition, vasodilatation caused by local H^+ ion concentration in the extracellular fluid may have a profound effect on local blood flow. (4) The *appropriate distribution of blood flow* involves additional considerations of arterial and capillary patency, optimal blood viscosity, and efficient oxygen utilization by the cells. In short, there is more to tissue oxygenation than the maintenance of a "normal" PaO_2.

Some of the respiratory care techniques to be described subsequently have an additional rationale, besides that of promoting optimal oxygenation, and that is to support the healing of injured airways and lungs. Techniques of this genre include humidification of inhaled gas to prevent ciliary damage; sterile precautions to minimize further insult from iatrogenic respiratory tract infection; expiratory retardation of gas flow to provide "splinting" of airways in chronic obstructive pulmonary disease; and optimal application of continuous positive airway pressure to increase alveolar recruitment and stabilization in conditions of increased alveolar surface tension or pulmonary edema.

When oxygen is provided to a patient in concentrations of over 21 per cent, it must be regarded as a drug, having indications, contraindications, and potential benefits and dangers like any other pharmaceutical agent. The techniques of oxygen administration are expensive and complex; they may be hazardous if applied improperly. Thus, oxygen therapy should be undertaken only by trained personnel on specific indications, with appropriate concentrations and safe equipment.

The principal *indication* for increasing the FIO_2 above 0.21 is *arterial hypoxemia*, i.e., a PaO_2 of less than 75 torr. Hypoxemia occurs in most critically ill or injured patients (see Fig. 3 in Chapter 3); thus it should be almost routine to provide enriched oxygen mixtures to these patients without waiting for PaO_2 confirmation. *Tissue hypoxia*, as it occurs in various shock states, cerebral edema, severe anemia (reduced hemoglobin concentration), carbon monoxide poisoning, and hypermetabolism (e.g., convulsions, high fever, burns), provides another indication for enriched oxygen mixtures. In these conditions, raising the PaO_2 *above* 100 torr may in part ameliorate tissue hypoxia by increasing the PO_2 *gradient* from the arterial side of the capillary to the tissue mitochondria. Although arterial oxygen content is increased only slightly by this mechanism through oxygen physically dissolved in blood (0.3 ml. oxygen per 100 ml. blood per 100 torr PO_2 rise), even this small rise in oxygen content (e.g., 1.5 ml. oxygen per 100 ml. blood added when the PaO_2 is raised from 100 torr to 600 torr) may be important in severe anemia or shock.

Further indications for significantly raising FIO_2 are those conditions which might benefit from *denitrogenation* of the alveoli and blood. In this instance, 100 per cent oxygen breathing from a leak-free non-rebreathing system may reduce the volume of air in tissues and body cavities. Whether an FIO_2 of 1.0 for several hours reduces interstitial emphysema, air embolism, pneumo-

thorax, and gaseous distention of the intestines more rapidly than does the safer FIO_2 of 0.6 has not been studied (see p. 282).

Finally, oxygen administration is indicated as *prophylaxis* in conditions which can readily lead to airway obstruction, hypoventilation, apnea or other causes of hypoxemia: Poorly controlled, recurrent seizures or conditions predisposing to seizures (e.g., the dehydrated child with infection and high fever); muscle weakness with reduced vital capacity; and depression of upper airway reflexes (e.g., in recovery from anesthesia). In these circumstances, denitrogenation of the patient's alveoli with 50 to 100 per cent oxygen provides a margin of safety, giving medical personnel more time to correct the respiratory emergency when it occurs, before the PaO_2 decreases to dangerously low levels. Positive pressure added to FIO_2 values of 0.6 to 1.0 is a further prophylactic measure. As described later in this chapter a slight continuous increase in alveolar pressure may protect against development of hypoxemia from pulmonary edema or increased alveolar surface tension, both of which are common in shock, trauma, sepsis, chest injury, exsanguinating hemorrhage with massive infusions, and other conditions that cause lung injury.

Key Measurements

In trying to assess the efficacy of any given oxygenation technique, we must ask three basic questions:

(1) How much oxygen is being delivered, to the alveoli?

(2) What proportion of the oxygen delivered to the alveoli actually reaches the arterial blood?

(3) How well is the arterial oxygen distributed to the tissues?

The answer to the first question requires an accurate determination of the fraction of oxygen in the delivered gas, i.e., the FIO_2. To answer the second question, we must know the arterial PO_2, particularly under circumstances in which the effects of ventilation-perfusion mismatching can be minimized or eliminated. The third question, that of oxygen distribution to the tissues, requires that we examine cardiac output, regional blood flow, the affinity of hemoglobin for oxygen, and a variety of other factors. In this section, we shall be concerned chiefly with the answers to the first two questions; the third question is taken up in other chapters of this book.

DETERMINATION OF FIO$_2$

FIO$_2$ may be directly ascertained by intermittent or continuous sampling of oxygen at the mouth, nose, or tracheal tube through an oxygen analyzer. While modern oxygen-air mixers permit one to set the FIO$_2$ delivered from a compressed gas source at a known level, these devices are not fully reliable. Their accuracy must be checked with periodic FIO$_2$ determinations, lest toxic oxygen concentrations be inadvertently administered (see p. 282).

ARTERIAL OXYGEN TENSION AND THE 100 PER CENT OXYGEN TEST

The oxygen tension of a sample of arterial blood (PaO$_2$) is meaningful only if examined in terms of the inhaled FIO$_2$. For example, a PaO$_2$ of 100 torr has a very different significance in the patient breathing room air and the patient breathing 100 per cent oxygen. In the first instance, one may assume that the patient has healthy lungs and good matching of ventilation and perfusion; in the second instance, a profound shunt is present, and the patient is in trouble. Thus, it is not the PaO$_2$ per se which is a measure of the patient's pulmonary status, but rather the alveolar-arterial oxygen tension *difference* [P(A − a)O$_2$, or D(A − a)O$_2$] that is significant

here, provided that the net alveolar ventilation is normal (i.e., PaCO$_2$ is normal or low). The P(A − a)O$_2$ is increased when ventilation is either diminished (mismatching) or entirely absent (shunting) in perfused lung units or when there is impaired diffusion of gases across the alveoli, the latter situation — diffusion block — being distinctly rare. One can sort out the various possible causes of an increased P(A − a)O$_2$ through the use of the *100 per cent oxygen test* (Fig. 5), by which the components of the P(A − a)O$_2$ due to ventilation-perfusion mismatching or impaired diffusion are eliminated. Thus, using an FIO$_2$ of 1.0, the P(A − a)O$_2$ reflects solely alveolar shunting (venous admixture). Such shunting is most often caused by collapsed, compressed or fluid-filled alveoli, and its progress can be followed by frequent determinations of the PaO$_2$ with an FIO$_2$ of 1.0.

Normally, during breathing of air (FIO$_2$ = 0.21), the alveolar PO$_2$ is about 100 torr and the PaO$_2$ 75 to 100 torr, thus the P(A − a)O$_2$ gradient is minimal. With the FIO$_2$ at 1.0, a shunt of 2 to 5 per cent of cardiac output in a healthy person produces a P(A − a)O$_2$ of only 50 to 100 torr, i.e., a PaO$_2$ of about 550 to 600 torr (atmospheric pressure minus PACO$_2$ minus PAH$_2$O minus a gradient of not more than 50 to 100 torr).

The *100 per cent oxygen test* is repeated here in detail because of its importance and is carried out in two to three steps (Fig. 5):

Step 1: The PaO$_2$ is determined after at least 10 minutes of *air* breathing at *atmospheric* (barometric) pressure (BP) if the patient can be safely kept on air. This will indicate whether hypoxemia exists (PaO$_2$ less than 75 torr).

100 Per Cent Oxygen Test: D(A − a)o$_2$ Test (Shunt Equivalency Test)

Step	FIO$_2$	Airway Pressure	PaO$_2$ (torr)	
			Normal Values	Examples of Abnormal Values
(1)	0.21	BP (atm. pr.)	75–100	40
(2)	1.0	BP (atm. pr.)	500–600	500 ⟍ ⟋ 100°°
(3)	1.0	Positive pressure°	500–600	300°° ↓ 100 ⟍ 80

°For alveolar recruitment with SB–CPAP; IMV; IPPV or CPPV. Oxygen via bag-valve-mask (or tracheal tube) or ventilator-tracheal tube.

°°Indicates shunting partially reversible with positive pressure.

Figure 5 100 per cent oxygen test (see text).

Step 2: The patient breathes *100 per cent oxygen* for 5 to 10 minutes at *atmospheric* (barometric) pressure (BP) in the airway to wash out nitrogen from alveoli, using any of the leak-free non-rebreathing type O_2 delivery systems (Figs. 6 and 7; see also Chapter 9). Then, the PaO_2 is determined. If it is near 500 to 600 torr, the hypoxemia encountered with Step 1 can be assumed to be due to ventilation-perfusion mismatching without shunting, or to hypoventilation if the $PaCO_2$ is high. The lower the PaO_2 below about 500 torr on FIO_2 1.0, the greater the proportion of shunting. Quantitating the amount of shunt requires mixed venous blood, venous and arterial oxygen content measurement, and extensive calculations (Chapter 3). Such semi-investigational methods are not needed for most patients' therapy. The clinician should know, however, that with normal cardiac output and oxygen consumption (i.e., a normal venous-arterial oxygen content difference of 4 to 6 ml./100 ml. blood), a PaO_2 of about 100 torr on FIO_2 1.0 means a shunt of about 22 per cent of cardiac output; and if the PaO_2 on FIO_2 of 1.0 were 40 to 50 torr, the shunt would be about 50 per cent.

Step 3: The patient breathes *100 per cent oxygen* with some form of *positive pressure,* either spontaneous positive pressure breathing (Figs. 8 and 9) or assisted or controlled positive pressure ventilation (Figs. 10 and 11). After at least two to five minutes of positive pressure breathing with an FIO_2 of 1.0, the PaO_2 is again determined. If it is higher than at Step 2, we can assume that positive pressure was capable of reducing the shunt (as common in acute pulmonary edema or alveolar atelectasis from increased surface tension) (see Fig. 3 in Chapter 3). If the PaO_2 is the same or lower than in Step 2, we must assume that the shunt cannot be ameliorated by positive pressure at this time. Further, if the PaO_2 is lower than in Step 2, we may assume that the positive pressure in itself did something to decrease PaO_2, either by increasing the shunt flow, by decreasing cardiac output or by increasing oxygen consumption (see Fig. 4 in Chapter 3).

The easiest way under emergency conditions to perform Steps 2 and 3 of the 100 per cent oxygen test is to use the self-refilling bag-valve-mask unit with oxygen reservoir, which permits spontaneous breathing at atmospheric pressure as well as assisted and controlled positive pressure ventilation with and without PEEP (Chapter 9).

We mentioned earlier that it is the $P(A - a)O_2$ that is significant in assessing the patient's pulmonary status rather than the PaO_2 alone. This is true in circumstances in which the inhaled oxygen concentration is less than 100 per cent. However, when the FIO_2 is 1.0, the *relative changes in* PaO_2 provide the most useful data. In this instance, the $P(A - a)O_2$ with $PAO_2 = BP - PH_2O - PACO_2$) gives little additional or practical information over the use of PaO_2 alone. Further, the use of $P(A - a)O_2$ is often poorly understood, since its value increases as the shunt worsens. Finally, the value of $P(A - a)O_2$ does not permit assessment of the actual PaO_2, which must be known for therapeutic reasons, since the PaO_2 should be kept at least at 60 torr, and preferably at 100 torr, for full saturation of hemoglobin with oxygen.

The 100 per cent oxygen test is more sensitive than physical examination and roentgenogram in the early detection of diffuse alveolar edema or collapse and is a useful tool for following relative changes in shunting with therapeutic measures. However, one must also appreciate the fact that the 100 per cent oxygen test tends to *overread* the shunt somewhat, due to the vasodilatation produced by high PO_2 in shunted areas and possible absorption atelectasis in areas which might be intermittently obstructed. Some, therefore, favor 90 per cent O_2 over 100 per cent for this test; however, the advantage of this modification has not yet been documented. While therapeutic administration of 100 per cent oxygen is safe in emergency conditions (with the exception of premature newborns), FIO_2 should be reduced to 0.6 for long-term therapy as early as possible after the 100 per cent oxygen test has been accomplished to forestall the development of pulmonary oxygen toxicity.

Methods of Oxygen Administration

OXYGEN DELIVERY SYSTEMS

Oxygen for medical use is provided in cylinders of various sizes, filled to approximately 2200 pounds per square inch (psi) pressure. The manufacturer is responsible for periodic checking and re-certifying of the cylinders. There are three commonly used oxygen delivery systems:

Portable (Fig. 6). The portable oxygen delivery system consists of a small portable

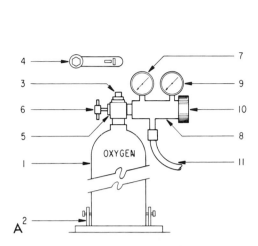

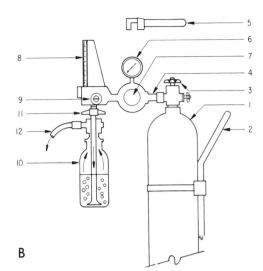

Figure 6 A, Portable oxygen delivery system. (1) Small cylinder, (2) stand, (3) cylinder valve, (4) wrench, (5) yoke, (6) yoke handle, (7) cylinder pressure gauge, (8) reducing valve, (9) flow meter, (10) needle valve, and (11) delivery tube.

B, Movable oxygen delivery system. (1) Large cylinder, (2) movable cart, (3) cylinder valve, (4) yoke, (5) wrench for fastening yoke, (6) cylinder pressure gauge, (7) reducing valve, (8) flow meter, (9) needle valve, (10) bubble humidifier, (11) wing nut for humidifier, and (12) delivery tube.

oxygen cylinder (e.g., an "E" cylinder, with a capacity of 659 liters) attached to a cylinder base or small, wheeled cart to prevent it from toppling over and a yoke, reducing valve, flow meter, and oxygen delivery tube. A humidifier is desirable but rarely found on portable oxygen units, as it makes them top heavy. Its use is less crucial because the portable unit is meant primarily for emergency resuscitation.

Setting up this oxygen delivery system should be practiced under the guidance of an instructor and is done as follows:

(1) Place the tank securely upright and position yourself to the side.

(2) For "E" or "D" size cylinders, remove seal from cylinder outlet. "Crack" the cylinder by briefly turning the cylinder valve on and off with the wrench, to clean the valve of debris.

(3) Inspect the yoke to be certain that it is of the right type for an oxygen cylinder. Remove washer from cylinder and place on oxygen inlet nipple of yoke.

(4) Engage nipple into the cylinder outlet while also engaging the pin index nipples into the appropriate holes. Tighten the yoke securely with the handle.

(5) Close the needle valve flow control.

(6) Turn on the cylinder valve slowly until cylinder pressure on the content gauge is maximal. Note cylinder pressure on gauge and assure absence of audible leaks.

(7) Attach desired oxygen administration equipment to delivery tube.

(8) Turn on needle valve to desired oxygen flow.

Whenever turning a compressed gas cylinder on, *do not* hold your face over the outlet, lest a malfunctioning yoke cause severe injury.

Movable (Fig. 6). The movable oxygen delivery system consists of a large oxygen cylinder (e.g., an "H" cylinder, with a 6900 liter capacity), wheeled cart, reducing valve, flow meter, and humidifer or nebulizer.

Stationary. In hospitals and ambulances, stationary oxygen delivery systems are used, as they provide a large, continuous supply of oxygen. A bank of large cylinders or a tank of liquid oxygen is connected to multiple wall outlets by pipes (in ambulances, sometimes only one large cylinder is connected via pipe to a single outlet).

All the systems should be capable of delivering oxygen at both low flow/low pressure (as required for bags and masks) and high flow/high pressure, usually 30 to 50 psi (as required for ventilators). All systems with large cylinders or wall outlets for long-term use in critically ill patients, as seen in emergency departments and ICU's, should ideally have oxygen-air mixers to permit FIO_2 control (e.g., Veriflo, Bird). These mixers should be equipped with flow meter (low pressure) and high pressure (50 psi) outlets. Since the continuous accuracy of these units is not fully reliable, periodic FIO_2 checks with an oxygen analyzer are required. Furthermore, periodic checks of cylinder pressure (which reflects oxygen cylinder content) in standby cylinders must be part of the maintenance program of all life support stations, including ambulances, emergency departments, and ICU's.

HUMIDIFICATION AND NEBULIZATION

Humidification of oxygen is strongly recommended whenever oxygen is administered for more than about 10 minutes, since dry oxygen damages the lining of the lower air passages, particularly if the patient is breathing through his mouth or through a tracheal tube. During normal nose breathing, air in the trachea is at 100 per cent humidity at 37°C. The delivery system should aim for that. Humidification produces molecular water in its gaseous form (vapor), whereas nebulization means droplets of water suspended in gas.

The bubble humidifier (Fig. 6) passes oxygen through a system with multiple openings into a water reservoir. Even if this provides a relative humidity of 100 per cent at room temperature in the humidifier, the relative humidity drops to about 50 per cent when the gas is warmed to 37°C. in the patient. Thus, for 100 per cent humidity at body temperature delivered into the patient, either the water has to be heated above body temperature, since the gas cools on its way to the patient, or water must be delivered in the form of droplets (mist, aerosol).

Heating a jet-capillary junction nebulizer (Fig. 6) is probably unnecessary, since the mass of water delivered is increased only minimally. The nebulizer delivers millions of tiny droplets of water, usually with a spectrum of droplet sizes approximately 1 to 20 μ, and thus is capable of providing 100 per cent relative humidity at body temperature, even when unheated. The droplets give off water vapor as they are warmed by the patient's airways.

The principle of nebulization by the *jet-capillary junction* principle is as follows: the rapid gas flow from the jet creates a negative pressure (Venturi effect) which sucks liquid through a thin tube from the saline reservoir, breaks the solution into fine droplets and throws them against a ball-shaped baffle, and with the oxygen, flows out the delivery tube (Fig. 7A). Baffle and delivery tube cause the large droplets to condense out and flow back into the container. All nebulizing equipment (Fig. 7A) should have large-bore delivery tubes, as the narrow tubes may plug with condensed water, and should be connected, usually via an open aerosol mask, to the patient's face or via a large-bore T-tube or ventilator to the intubated or tracheotomized patient.

Ultrasonic nebulizers do not require a nebulizing stream of gas, and are thus used mainstream; they deliver a more constant size of droplets than standard nebulizers. Since irritation of the tracheobronchial tree by ultrasonic mist as well as overhydration (particularly in infants) is possible, most ultrasonic nebulizers should be used only intermittently in selected cases.

Humidifiers and nebulizers should contain sterile 0.45 per cent saline (humidifiers may also use sterile water). The equipment should also be sterile and is changed every 12 to 24 hours. Hazards of humidification include interference with the mechanism of heat loss, excessive water retention, and increased risk of infection from contamination. The iatrogenic infection risk is greater with the use of nebulizers than with humidifiers, since the droplets can carry bacteria which are apt to grow in nebulizer bottles. Disposable equipment adds to the measures designed to prevent iatrogenic pulmonary infection.

BACKGROUND OF OXYGENATION TECHNIQUES

In the not-so-remote past, oxygen was administered chiefly via tents, semi-open masks, and nasopharyngeal catheters, which increased inhaled oxygen concentration at atmospheric pressure to a variable and largely unmeasured degree. Since, however, inhaled oxygen above 21 per cent must be administered as "a drug," the appropriate "dosage" (FIO_2) should be prescribed and controlled. The open or semi-open continuous flow oxygen delivery systems, with unpredictable air dilution depending on O_2 flow and breathing pattern, although simple and inexpensive, do not permit FIO_2 control. Such control is now possible, however, with leak-free systems and oxygen-air mixers (e.g.,

Veriflo, Bird). As to positive pressure techniques, Barach demonstrated in the 1940s that *spontaneous breathing* with 100 per cent oxygen at *continuous positive airway pressure* improved oxygenation in patients with pulmonary edema, and the technique he described was employed in aviation medicine. However, it was not until 1971, through the work of Gregory and associates with neonatal respiratory distress syndrome, that spontaneous breathing with positive airway pressure (SB-PAP) became accepted as a useful therapeutic modality (Figs. 8 and 9). Immediately following Gregory's report, we began using SB-PAP also in adults, again with satisfactory results.

Intermittent positive pressure *controlled ventilation* (IPPV) had been used until the late 1960s primarily for artificial ventilation, but not primarily for oxygenation (Fig. 10). IPPV (controlled ventilation) was used largely to ventilate patients paralyzed by poliomyelitis or by curarization for anesthesia. IPPB (assisted breathing) was introduced in the 1950s by Miller and others for use via mouthpiece or mask for improved delivery of bronchodilator aerosols. Notably, Miller also found that IPPB was effective in raising arterial oxygen saturation in pulmonary edema; similar observations were made by many anesthesiologists who applied various positive pressure patterns with 100 per cent oxygen, using the "educated hand" on the breathing bag.

Moerch in the 1950s treated crushing chest injury for the first time with prolonged controlled ventilation by IPPV. He and others, including these authors, who have used this technique since its inception, found that controlled mechanical hyperventilation with oxygen enabled improved oxygenation in patients who developed pulmonary consolidation. Using volume-set ventilators and (inadvertently) increasing airway pressures throughout the respiratory cycle, they actually produced *positive end-expiratory pressure* (PEEP), thus changing IPPV to continuous positive pressure ventilation (CPPV) (Fig. 10). However, IPPV with PEEP (CPPV), although used before, did not become a systematically applied respiratory care technique until after Petty and Ashbaugh demonstrated its effectiveness in pulmonary edema and consolidation (ARDS) in the late 1960s.

Thus, the presently available conventional oxygenation techniques have expanded from spontaneous breathing of oxygen without positive airway pressure to spontaneous breathing of oxygen with positive airway pressure (SB-PAP) either during expiration alone (EPAP) or continuously (CPAP) (Figs. 8 and 9); to assisted and controlled ventilation with oxygen (Figs. 10 and 11). In this fashion, emergency artificial ventilation techniques (Chapter 9) and long-term mechanical ventilation techniques have become also oxygenation techniques.

SPONTANEOUS BREATHING OF OXYGEN WITHOUT POSITIVE PRESSURE

The *Laerdal pocket mask with oxygen nipple* is a simple, semi-open system permitting the patient to breathe through the open mask port while a continuous flow of oxygen is delivered via the valved mask nipple (see Fig. 13 in Chapter 9). There is neither a valve nor a bag. The mask may be strapped to the face to deliver oxygen during spontaneous breathing, or it may be held to the face manually (in the unconscious patient, using the triple airway maneuver). It permits mouth-to-mask artificial ventilation through the open mask port when needed. When using the pocket mask for oxygen inhalation, the exact inhaled oxygen concentration cannot be predicted, as it depends not only on the oxygen flow rate, but also on the dilution with air (during spontaneous breathing) or with the operator's exhaled air (during mouth-to-mask ventilation). However, an approximate inhaled oxygen concentration during spontaneous breathing of 30 per cent can be expected with an oxygen flow rate of about 5 liters per minute, 50 per cent with an oxygen flow of about 10 liters per minute, and 80 to 100 per cent with an oxygen flow of over 20 liters per minute (in the adult).

During mouth-to-mask artificial ventilation, the operator can produce ventilation with 100 per cent oxygen by using an oxygen inflow of at least 20 to 30 liters per minute and by intermittently occluding the mask port with lips or tongue until the chest rises. However, the operator must then guard against overinflation by taking his mouth off the port as soon as the patient's chest rises. For short-term use, the pocket mask may be used with the portable oxygen delivery system; for long-term use, humidification should be added.

The *self-refilling bag-valve-mask unit,* described previously for artificial ventilation (see Fig. 14 in Chapter 9) permits increase of delivered oxygen to about 50 per cent when 10 to 12 liters per minute of oxygen is delivered distal to the intake valve without reservoir. With addition of an oxygen reservoir (tube or bag with a volume to equal or exceed tidal volume), the inspired oxygen concentration can be increased to 100 per cent. The Laerdal Resusci-Folding Bag II is suitable for spontaneous breathing, assisted respiration, and controlled ventilation (artificial ventilation) and has a tightly fitting, inflatable mask rim, transparent mask to permit visualization of the face, and a strap. For emergency purposes, the bag-valve-mask unit may be used with the small portable oxygen delivery system. For long-term use, a humidifier should be part of the delivery system. This device is unsuitable for use with a nebulizer.

The *hand-triggered oxygen resuscitator* (Chapter 9) (e.g., Elder valve, Robertshaw valve) only permits delivery of 100 per cent oxygen without humidification, making it unsuitable for long-term use. For spontaneous breathing, a demand valve mechanism in this resuscitation valve permits the patient to draw 100 per cent oxygen from the cylinder via the reducing valve, using only slight negative pressure. In rapid and deep breathing, however, the demand valve may offer excessive resistance during inhalation or exhalation. This is another factor against its long-term use in the spontaneously breathing patient.

The *oronasal oxygen mask without bag* (Fig. 7A) works on the same simple principle as the pocket mask; it contains no valves, only side holes through which exhaled air is vented and through which air is also drawn in during inhalation and mixed with a continuous flow of oxygen delivered via narrow

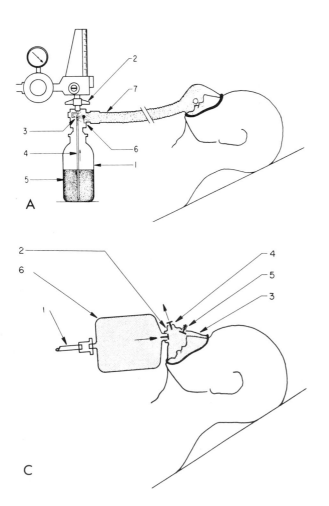

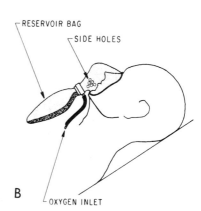

Figure 7 *A,* Aerosol (mist) oronasal oxygen mask, usually made of transparent plastic. (1) Nebulizer bottle, (2) wing nut for nebulizer, (3) jet-capillary junction for nebulizer, (4) capillary tube, (5) nebulized fluid, (6) baffle, and (7) large-bore delivery tube.

B, Oxygen mask for administration of oxygen at atmospheric pressure. Partial rebreathing oxygen bag-mask unit, usually made of transparent plastic, valveless.

C, Nonrebreathing oxygen bag-mask unit, usually made of transparent plastic. (1) Oxygen inlet with delivery tube, (2) inhalation valve, (3) oronasal face mask, (4) exhalation valve, (5) safety air inlet valve, and (6) reservoir bag.

tube. With the oronasal oxygen mask without bag, as well as with other open systems, it is impossible to predict the precise oxygen concentration inspired because of the mixing of oxygen flow and air dilution, which depends on the patient's tidal volume, rate, flow, and pattern. However, using this mask, one can roughly gauge inspired oxygen concentration as follows: for about 30 per cent oxygen inhaled, use approximately 5 liters per minute; for about 50 per cent inhaled, use approximately 10 liters per minute. It is difficult to achieve an FIO_2 greater than 0.5 with this type of mask.

The *partial rebreathing oxygen bag mask unit* (Fig. 7B) also has no valves, but has a reservoir bag that provides higher inhaled oxygen concentration with the same flow rates as those used with the oronasal oxygen mask without a bag. It results in more rebreathing of exhaled air, although this can be minimized by increasing the oxygen inflow rate. The mask has side holes for drawing air in and for exhalation. For 30 per cent or less inhaled oxygen, this mask is not recommended, since it results in too much rebreathing of exhaled air at low flow rates. For about 50 per cent oxygen inhaled, use about 5 to 10 liters per minute, and for about 80 to 100 per cent oxygen inhaled, use over 15 liters per minute oxygen flow.

The *non-rebreathing oxygen bag-mask unit* (Fig. 7C) also has a reservoir bag into which the oxygen flow is delivered. However, unlike the partial rebreathing mask, it is equipped with one-way valves to prevent rebreathing of exhaled air. An inhalation valve between bag and mask allows one-way flow from bag to mask, a leak-free mask prevents air admixture, and an exhalation valve permits one-way flow of exhaled air from inside the mask to the outside. There is a safety air inlet valve which lets air in when the patient empties the bag with inhalations.

Whenever the flow rate is sufficiently high that the bag does not collapse at the end of inhalation (flow rate exceeding minute volume), there is no dilution of the oxygen with air from the safety inlet valve. This mask is used for 100 per cent oxygen inhalation without positive pressure, as indicated as a first step in the treatment of pulmonary edema, following smoke or carbon monoxide inhalation or near-drowning, or for the second step of the 100 per cent oxygen test (Fig.

5). However, for all these purposes under emergency conditions, the self-refilling bag-valve-mask unit with oxygen reservoir (see Fig. 14 in Chapter 9) is preferable.

In hospitals where oxygen/air mixing devices can be incorporated into the oxygen delivery system, any oxygen concentration between 21 and 100 per cent may be administered with greater accuracy using a non-rebreathing mask rather than a semi-open system.

The *aerosol (mist) oronasal oxygen mask* (Fig. 7A) is suitable for relatively uncontrolled oxygen administration, as with the oronasal oxygen mask without bag. The aerosol mask, however, has a large-bore oxygen port, and air holes in the sides are larger in order to prevent condensation of mist. Oxygen with nebulized sterile 0.45 per cent saline solution is indicated in special conditions such as severe asthma, acute worsening of bronchitis, and other conditions in which loosening of secretions is required. Nebulization should be used only under special circumstances. When the nebulizer is equipped with an air entrainment device, 40 or 70 per cent oxygen may be delivered from the nebulizer but at higher flow rates than those read on the flow meter. Variations of inhaled oxygen concentrations are still considerable, since breathing volumes, rates, and patterns vary.

The *two-pronged nasal cannula* is a narrow-bore oxygen delivery tube ending with two nipples, one for each nostril. It is useful for oxygen inhalation in chronic lung disease patients but not in those with acute respiratory insufficiency, since control of inhaled oxygen concentration is difficult to achieve with this device and flow rates over 5 liters per minute are uncomfortable.

The *nasopharyngeal oxygen catheter* was commonly used in the past but has been largely abandoned because of the difficulty in placing the tip of the catheter into the oropharynx, patient discomfort, gas swallowing, and poor control of inhaled oxygen concentration.

The *oxygen tent* has also been largely abandoned because of fire hazard and difficulty in controlling inhaled oxygen concentration, heat accumulation, and difficult access to the patient for general and resuscitative care. However, "croup tents" are still used for children with subacute or chronic respiratory disorders.

Most above-mentioned devices are suitable for oxygen enrichment in spontaneously breathing conscious compensated patients with COPD.

The "Venturi mask" is a semi-open oronasal mask which, through relatively precisely controlled high-flow air entrainment and low exact oxygen flows, provides relatively correct, known inhaled oxygen concentrations ranging from 24 to 40 per cent. In compensated COPD, it may have a slight advantage over the standard semi-open techniques in guaranteeing that the FIO_2 will not exceed the preset value and thereby will not produce oxygen-induced hypoventilation. In acutely decompensated COPD and other causes of acute respiratory insufficiency, however, 50 to 60 per cent oxygen is preferred; and in CPR, pulmonary edema, near-drowning, carbon monoxide poisoning, and smoke inhalation, 80 to 100 per cent oxygen is desirable.

SPONTANEOUS BREATHING OF OXYGEN WITH POSITIVE PRESSURE

During normal breathing there is slight negative airway pressure during inhalation and slight positive airway pressure during exhalation. Positive end-expiratory pressure (PEEP) is commonly used to refer to airway pressure maintained *above* atmospheric during the expiratory phase of the breathing cycle. However, PEEP is primarily applied to MV; and when it is added to IPPV, it becomes CPPV (Fig. 10). SB-PAP, i.e., spontaneous breathing-positive airway pressure, does not require a ventilator and can be applied with or without a tracheal or tracheostomy tube (Figs. 8 and 9). IPPV or CPPV by mechanical ventilation (MV) usually requires a tracheal or tracheostomy tube.

The function of SB-PAP is to increase the pressure gradient between alveoli and pleura (transpulmonary pressure), i.e., the pressure tending to distend alveoli. This may recruit and splints alveoli, maintaining an increased volume of gas in the lungs; through this increase in FRC and the attendant reduction in shunting, the PaO_2 in hypoxemic patients is increased. Furthermore a continuous slight increase in airway pressure, by stabilizing alveoli and their perfusion, may promote regeneration of surfactant.

The relatively new technique of spontaneous breathing of oxygen with SB-PAP

plays a major role in the treatment of hypoxemia due to reduced FRC, usually from collapsed or fluid-filled alveoli (Figs. 8 and 9). Acute pulmonary edema, for example, when it has not yet progressed to the stage where tracheal intubation is required, may benefit from this approach. SB-PAP via face mask, nasal prongs, or head box has replaced mechanical ventilation (MV) as the initial, usually effective, respiratory care for neonates with respiratory distress syndrome. The method also merits more frequent trial in adults, as it sometimes obviates the need for tracheal or tracheostomy tube with their associated complications.

Prerequisites for use of SB-PAP include (1) a conscious, cooperative patient with intact upper airway reflexes (when used via mask); (2) A high gradient between PaO_2 and FIO_2; (3) adequate spontaneous tidal volumes of at least 10 ml./kg. body weight; and (4) normal or low $PaCO_2$.

The required *assembly* (Fig. 8) includes a threshold resistance in the form of a PEEP valve, which may be a simple water bubbler, a compact mushroom spring or magnetic valve, or a floating ball PEEP valve (which must be held vertically) (Fig. 9).* The level of IPAP (CPAP) is determined by the initial level of pressure in the circuit when the inspiration is begun, and the relationship between gas flow from the source and the patient's peak inspiratory flow rate (Fig. 8B). Delivered gas from the source must be FIO_2-controlled (oxygen-air mixer), humidified (heated humidifier) and—at least in adults—passed through an elastic reservoir bag (Fig. 8A). Finally, the equipment must include a transparent tight-sealing face mask (e.g., Laerdal cushion mask or new anatomic mask) which should be fastened to the patient's face via a head strap (we have also recommended strapping the mask to the head with an elastic head net made for holding wound dressings). A highly cooperative patient can also use SB-PAP via a mouthpiece, at least for brief periods.

While no data are available to provide clear guidelines for *levels* of SB-PAP, most patients receiving this treatment via face mask benefit from and tolerate peak pres-

---

*Some of the manufactured PEEP valves are the Laerdal (water bubbler), Emerson-Bennett (mushroom), Eross (Instrumentation Laboratories, Pittsburgh) (magnetic), and Boehringer (floating ball) (Fig. 9).

SPONTANEOUS POSITIVE PRESSURE BREATHING
SB - EPAP/CPAP

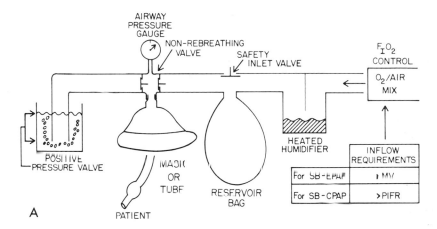

PATTERNS OF PRESSURE BREATHING
Spontaneous Breathing

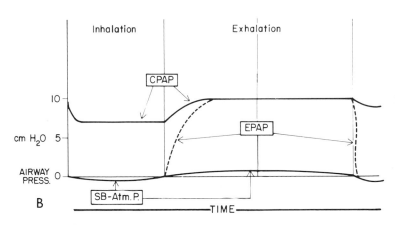

Figure 8 A, Oxygen set-up for spontaneous positive pressure breathing via mask, tracheal tube, or tracheostomy tube. MV: minute volume. PIFR: peak inspiratory flow rate. For SB-EPAP, continuous inflow rate of O_2/air mixture must be at least minute volume; for CPAP, it must be at least PIFR (over 25 liters per minute during quiet breathing). Bubble PEEP valve at left could be replaced with "dry" valves (mushroom, magnetic, ball, or other, Fig. 9).

B, Airway pressure patterns with spontaneous positive pressure breathing. CPAP: continuous positive airway pressure. EPAP: expiratory positive airway pressure only. These patterns are achieved with the equipment outlined in 8A.

sures of 3 to 5 cm. H_2O, which can be used almost prophylactically in certain conditions of alveolar disease. Pressures may be increased to about 12 cm. H_2O if the patient tolerates it. High pressures should be administered only via tracheal or tracheostomy tube, since esophageal opening pressure is 15 to 25 cm. H_2O. With higher pressures applied via face mask, dyspnea, hypoventilation, gas swallowing, and gastric distention are common. Therefore, a gastric tube should

always be used with SB-PAP by mask, unless only very low prophylactic pressures are applied. For adjusting SB-PAP, one should monitor patient comfort, respiratory frequency and effort (to estimate the work of breathing), airway pressure, $PaCO_2$, and circulatory variables.

Oxygen administration by SB-PAP has several *advantages* over other oxygen administration techniques: (1) the iatrogenic infection often associated with tracheal in-

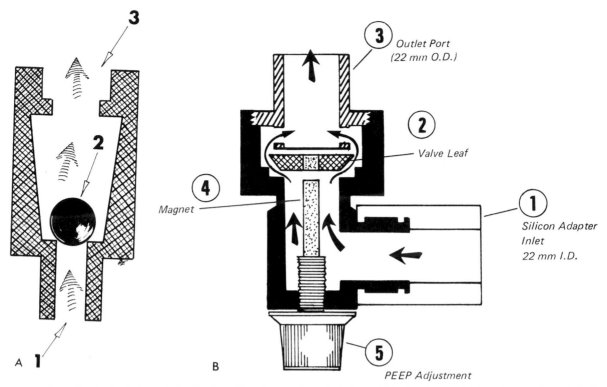

Figure 9   A, Boehringer PEEP valve. (1) Inlet port for exhaled air, (2) ball valve, and (3) outlet port for exhaled air. Keep valve perpendicular! (From Boehringer Laboratories, P.O. Box 337, Wynnewood, PA 19096.)

    B, Eross magnetic PEEP valve. (1) Inlet port (22 mm. I.D. silicone connector) for exhaled air, (2) valve leaf (plastic with metallic pole), (3) cap, (4) outlet port (22 mm. O.D.) for exhaled air, (5) magnet (standard or stronger than standard for super PEEP), and (6) PEEP adjustment knob. (From Instrumentation Industries, Inc., 215 Thomas Drive, Pittsburgh, PA 15236.)

tubation may be avoided when SB-PAP is used via face mask; (2) FRC is increased (shunting decreased) over that obtained with SB-atmospheric pressure; (3) SB-PAP enables perhaps better ventilation-perfusion matching and better cardiac output than does MV (CPPV) because of lower mean intrathoracic pressure (which also requires less fluid loading to maintain cardiac output); (5) patients tolerate SB-PAP better than they do MV (CPPV) and thus require less sedation; (6) SB-PAP probably entails less barotrauma because alveolar stretch is controlled by the patient; and (7) the simplicity and low cost of SB-PAP makes that technique readily available in a variety of circumstances.

    However, SB-PAP with face mask does have some *disadvantages* in comparison with CPPV. To begin with, the patient must cooperate, and this is not always feasible with the critically ill. Furthermore, even in the cooperative patient, there is a risk of gastric distention, aspiration, and facial is-

chemia, as well as the possibility of otitis media due to increased nasopharyngeal pressure. Finally, SB-PAP may increase the work of breathing to the point of dyspnea and CO_2 retention, requiring a switch to CPPV.

    SB-PAP with face mask is contraindicated in patients with stupor-coma, nausea or vomiting, small spontaneous tidal volumes, circulatory instability, or CSF leak (basal skull fracture).

ASSISTED AND CONTROLLED VENTILATION WITH OXYGEN AND POSITIVE PRESSURE

    When SB-PAP FIO_2 0.5 to 0.6 cannot maintain PaO_2 above 60 torr, or does so only at the expense of a rising $PaCO_2$, mechanical ventilation (MV) with continuous elevation of airway pressure (IPPV with PEEP; i.e., CPPV) is indicated (Fig. 10). This is best accomplished via tracheal or tracheostomy tube. CPPV further decreases venous admixture (shunt) and may thereby be life-saving,

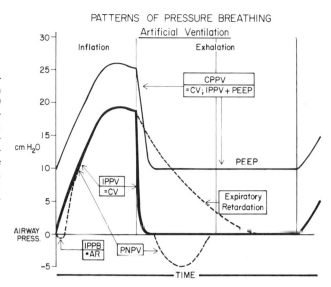

Figure 10 Airway pressure patterns with assisted and controlled positive pressure ventilation IPPV: intermittent positive pressure (controlled) ventilation. CV: controlled ventilation. IPPB: intermittent positive pressure (assisted) breathing. AR: assisted respiration. PNPV: positive negative pressure ventilation (also called NEEP, negative end-expiratory pressure). CPPV: continuous positive pressure ventilation, i.e., controlled ventilation with IPPV plus PEEP (positive end-expiratory pressure). PEEP for alveolar recruitment. Expiratory retardation for splinting airways.

particularly in cases of pulmonary edema and consolidation, as it increases PaO_2 and permits a reduction of FIO_2 to safe levels (0.5 to 0.6). However, too high PEEP may reduce cardiac output, arterial pressure, and thus arterial oxygen transport to tissues, particularly in patients with heart disease or hypovolemia.

The presently accepted, standard technique of artificial ventilation in patients with ventilatory failure is controlled intermittent positive pressure ventilation (IPPV), i.e., an increase in airway pressure until the lungs are inflated with the desired tidal volume, followed by an abrupt decrease of airway pressure to atmospheric to allow for passive exhalation (Fig. 10). IPPV can be accomplished by manual compression of a bag or bellows via appropriate valving or by ventilator, using MV. IPPV is controlled *ventilation*—i.e., ventilation rate, rhythm, and flow are dictated by the operator's hand or by the ventilator, the patient being rendered apneic from disease, breath-holding, low $PaCO_2$, or drug depression. When the patient triggers inhalation, IPPV becomes "assisted ventilation," i.e. intermittent pos. press. *breathing* (IPPB). A mix of SB and CV is IMV (Fig. 11).

Indications for MV by IPPV include (1) inability of the patient to maintain a normal $PaCO_2$; (2) excessive work of breathing; (3) metabolic acidemia when the patient cannot hyperventilate enough spontaneously to normalize pHa without becoming exhausted; and (4) severe flailing of the chest wall.

When hypoxemia persists on mechanical ventilation, the addition of positive end-expiratory pressure is desirable. IPPV plus PEEP is referred to as continuous positive pressure ventilation, or CPPV. Its use is indicated in circumstances similar to those which call for SB-PAP, i.e., when the patient demonstrates an inability to maintain PaO_2 above 60 torr with FIO_2 at 1.0 (short-term) to 0.5 (long-term). Thus, the switch from SB-PAP to MV with CPPV is primarily indicated when a further increase in PaO_2 without invoking toxic FIO_2 is needed and when hypoxemia occurs in unconscious, confused, or otherwise uncooperative patients who require tracheal or tracheostomy tubes.

PEEP is produced by attaching a threshold resistance to the expiratory port of the non-rebreathing valve of the manual or mechanical ventilator (PEEP valve, Fig. 9). PEEP allows an abrupt decrease of airway pressure to a sustained elevated plateau. This technique must be strictly differentiated from expiratory retardation, which ends with airway pressure at atmospheric level (Fig. 10). Like SB-PAP, *PEEP* is employed for alveolar recruitment and stabilization (particularly in pulmonary edema and consolidation); PEEP also helps to increase PaO_2 and thereby permit reduction in FIO_2 to nontoxic levels (0.5 to 0.6) by increasing FRC (which also increases lung compliance) and decreasing shunt. *Expiratory retardation,* on the other hand, is used for splinting intrapulmonary airways during exhalation (particularly in emphysema and asthma).

Pulmonary compliance varies with lung

volume, and compliance can be improved by increasing FRC from abnormally low values. This improvement in compliance in turn enables the patient to be ventilated at lower pressures. However, in some patients, such as those with overwhelming viral pneumonia, severe shunting may not improve even with very high PEEP levels; and safe reduction of FIO_2 to 0.6 is not possible when this occurs. A vicious circle of pulmonary oxygen toxicity, barotrauma, and further shunting ensues, with reduction in PaO_2 progressing to anoxic death. For patients in this group, extracorporeal membrane oxygenation may be considered (p. 279).

The *level of PEEP* must be selected carefully and adjusted to an optimal range in a titrated fashion. Levels of PEEP may be classified along the following spectrum: (1) prophylactic PEEP (1 to 5 cm. H_2O), used to prevent atelectasis and increase FRC above closing volume; (2) conventional PEEP (5 to 20 cm. H_2O), indicated if FIO_2 at 0.6 cannot maintain PaO_2 at or above 60 torr; and (3) high PEEP (20 to 50 cm. H_2O), employed in extreme hypoxemia. Perhaps more useful than this schema, however, is the concept of *optimal PEEP*, which may, depending upon the circumstances, fall anywhere along the spectrum.

In examining the concept of *optimal PEEP* (Suter), it is important to understand that PaO_2 reflects only *arterial* oxygenation of the blood. Since the ultimate goal is adequate *tissue* oxygenation, a more sensitive guide for the adjustment of PEEP may be to monitor not only PaO_2 but also changes in mixed venous (pulmonary artery or superior vena cava) PO_2 or preferably even oxygen content. These figures will indicate whether arterial oxygen transport is keeping pace with oxygen consumption. CPPV in general increases PaO_2 with each increment of PEEP. However, when high levels of PEEP are needed for maximal reduction in shunting, by opening closed or fluid-filled alveoli, a concomitant reduction in cardiac output may occur. Furthermore, when excessive PEEP decreases systemic arterial pressure, coronary and cerebral blood flow may decrease and the resulting myocardial ischemia may reduce cardiac output further. This untoward effect can be at least in part counteracted by blood volume expansion, together with the use of a cardiac inotropic agent (e.g., Dopamine) to maximize pulmonary flow of unshunted blood and maintain arterial perfusion pressure.

Fortunately, the stiffer the lungs, the lower the positive airway pressure transmitted to the pulmonary circulation and venae cavae. Thus, in the patients who truly need PEEP, higher levels are less likely to decrease cardiac output from increased pulmonary vascular resistance and reduction in venous return. Nevertheless, PEEP should not be pushed to the point of decreasing mixed venous PO_2, but rather adjusted to optimize compliance, i.e., lung volume change per unit pressure change (tidal volume divided by the pressure difference between inspiratory airway pressure and PEEP). High PEEP (20 to 50 cm. H_2O) should be used only for patients with ARDS in whom careful blood volume expansion does not improve PaO_2 to the desired level,

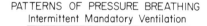

PATTERNS OF PRESSURE BREATHING
Intermittent Mandatory Ventilation

IMV = SB-Atm. P or SB-CPAP + IPPV (slow rate)

I = Inhalation

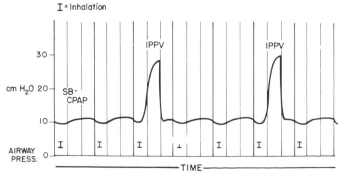

Figure 11 Airway pressure patterns with intermittent mandatory ventilation (IMV). SB-CPAP: spontaneous breathing with continuous positive airway pressure (see text).

and for patients with left ventricular failure in whom diuretics fail to improve oxygenation. Both patient groups should have colloid osmotic pressure normalized. Once high PEEP is chosen, it should be optimized as described above, combined with normalized $PaCO_2$ and pHa, preferably by intermittent mandatory ventilation (IMV). The monitoring of cardiac output (by thermodilution catheter) and intrapleural pressure (Kirby et al., 1975; Downs, 1976) should be considered in these circumstances. Furthermore, compliance, PaO_2, $P\bar{v}O_2$, and the other variables mentioned should be determined frequently, since ARDS is a dynamic state which requires frequent adjustment of ventilator techniques. As the lung condition improves, PEEP values of 5 to 10 cm. H_2O usually become adequate.

Possible *complications* due to CPPV include those associated with prolonged tracheal intubation, circulatory depression from increased intrathoracic pressure, and lung rupture (pulmonary barotrauma). When PEEP is used, there should always be pleural drainage "standby," and personnel must be alert to recognize and promptly treat tension pneumothorax by insertion of chest tube and reduction in airway pressure. Weaning from and discontinuance of MV ideally should be accomplished before removal of the chest tube.

EXTRACORPOREAL OXYGENATION

When pulmonary oxygenation failure is resistant to CPPV with high PEEP and supportive measures, the final available oxygenation method, which is also the most expensive and is still hazardous, is extracorporeal membrane oxygenation (ECMO). This technique entails long-term (from days to weeks) partial pumping of unsaturated venous or arterial blood into an oxygenator and back into a large artery or vein. ECMO requires 24-hour standby and coverage by a highly trained, multidisciplinary critical care team, which must provide bedside vigilance. For this reason, ECMO is appropriate only in large regional centers, i.e., Category I referral hospitals.

At this time, the results with ECMO are inconclusive. A multi-institutional trial of ECMO has so far given disappointing results (18 survivors among 150 patients). Most of the deaths were from hemorrhage, particularly intracranial hemorrhage in cases of trauma, related to the heparinization required to keep the extracorporeal circuit open. Research on improved technology of ECMO, particularly a search for nonthrombogenic surfaces and studies on lung healing, may result in a wider and earlier application of ECMO. At this time, increasingly sophisticated respiratory care without ECMO, including IMV with high PEEP, has reduced to a very small figure the number of patients in whom ECMO might be justified. For this reason, and because of the uncertain benefits of ECMO, the technique is warranted only in very carefully selected patients.

According to the recommendations of the National Institutes of Health, ECMO is indicated in (1) patients in whom, despite MV with optimized PEEP over 5 cm. H_2O and FIO_2 at 1.0, PaO_2 has been less than 50 torr for more than two hours; and (2) patients like those in (1), but in whom PaO_2 has been less than 50 torr for more than 12 hours on FIO_2 of 0.6 or more and a shunt of over 30 per cent has developed. Also, $PaCO_2$ must be 30 to 45 torr when the indication is considered, the lung failure must be potentially reversible, and the patient must have a reasonable chance for quality survival without severe brain damage. Indications for ECMO must be based on good clinical judgment, and it must not be undertaken until optimized CPPV, diuresis, colloid osmotic pressure normalization, chest physiotherapy, antibiotics, steroids, normothermia, sedation, paralysis, and optimal circulatory, metabolic, acid-base, and fluid balance have all been tried. Obviously, these stringent indications will change when the technique becomes safer in the future. *Contraindications* to ECMO include sepsis; irreversible obstructive and destructive lung disease; and irreversible severe central nervous system damage or cardiac function impaired to the extent that a worthwhile existence after recovery from lung failure is impossible.

It is beyond the scope of this chapter to teach detailed methods of ECMO. Institutions in need of an ECMO service should study the literature and send a team to an existing ECMO program before selecting the most appropriate equipment and designing treatment protocols. Our purpose here is merely to acquaint the reader with the technique. In terms of equipment, since the disc and bubble oxygenators used for open heart surgery destroy blood elements, prolonged ECMO requires a membrane oxygenator (Bramson et al., 1965). Among the circuits tried, pumping from the venae cavae (nonocclusive drainage via femoral vein) into the aortic arch (via the femoral artery) results in better cerebral oxygenation and pulmonary decongestion (required for lung healing) than veno-venous pumping or veno-femoral artery pumping. Bypass flows up to 60 to 70 per cent of cardiac output are possible with nonocclusive techniques. Full heparinization is still required, and the lungs are ventilated with FIO_2 at 0.5 and slight PEEP. Hematologic effects other than heparinization are harmless, since the ECMO-induced thrombocytopenia, denaturation of proteins, and hemolysis are mild and reversible.

HYPERBARIC OXYGENATION

Hyperbaric oxygenation (HBO) is the administration of oxygen at more than one atmosphere pressure. Understanding the present state of HBO requires extensive knowledge of hyperbaric medicine, which is beyond the scope of this book. For our purposes, it is sufficient to know that in the normal person in whom arterial hemoglobin is fully saturated when breathing 100 per cent oxygen at one atmosphere, HBO will add only *dissolved* oxygen, i.e., 0.3 ml. of oxygen per 100 ml. blood per 100 torr PO_2. Thus, at two atmospheres, arterial blood can contain in physical solution not more than 4.3 ml. of oxygen per 100 ml. blood ($1520 - 40 - 47$ torr $\times 0.003$); and at four atmospheres (3040 torr), 8.8 ml. of oxygen per 100 ml. blood. This small increase in arterial oxygen content is bought at a cost of significant hazard, for HBO may precipitate pulmonary oxygen toxicity, cerebral oxygen toxicity (convulsions within a few hours with three atmospheres and an FIO_2 at 1.0), fires, explosions, and "bends" or arterial air embolism during decompression.

Following extensive and clinical investigations of HBO 10 to 20 years ago, the complications and the enormous expense of maintaining HBO facilities have limited use of this method to research and to treatment of occasional cases of anaerobic bacterial infections, ischemic gangrene, CO poisoning, and diving accidents. Renewed research of HBO is warranted, since the therapeutic usefulness of this technique is still controversial and its potential in the treatment of post-ischemic states, particularly of the brain and heart, remains to be fully evaluated.

Selection of Oxygenation and Ventilation Techniques

In the foregoing section, we have described a broad and perhaps bewildering spectrum of oxygenation techniques. The problem for the clinician remains, however, which techniques should be selected and in what sequence for any given clinical circumstances. Clearly, the random application of any technique in the wrong clinical setting may not achieve the desired results, and a technique that is valuable in one circumstance may be useless or even dangerous in another. Thus, there should be an orderly, step-wise approach to the application of oxygenation methods.

The following guidelines for the selection and progression of oxygenation and ventilation techniques (Fig. 12) are based on the experience of the authors' groups and on knowledge of pathophysiology (for techniques, see Figs. 7 to 11, 13, and 14). These deliberately simplistic guidelines should be used with clinical judgment and considered separately for oxygenation failure and ventilation failure, although both conditions often coexist.

In patients with *acute hypoxemia* (PaO_2 less than 75 torr) during air breathing, the first step is a trial of an FIO_2 of 0.3 to 0.6 at atmospheric (barometric) pressure (BP). If this inhaled oxygen concentration is insufficient to maintain an arterial PO_2 of at least 60 torr (ideally over 100 torr), a brief trial of FIO_2 at 1.0 with BP is justified. Should the PaO_2 still remain at 60 torr or less on an FIO_2 of 1.0, SB-PAP with an FIO_2 of 1.0 (short-term) to 0.5 (long-term) via mask should be tried next. Finally, if for any reason the patient needs tracheal intubation or if his PaO_2 cannot be maintained above 60 torr with SB-PAP, controlled or intermittent mandatory ventilation via tracheal or tracheostomy tube should be started, using CPPV with optimized PEEP. These steps are summarized in Figure 12. Notably, assisted respiration with IPPB is *not* considered an appropriate choice of therapy in patients with hypoxemia from alveolar shunting.

Whatever step in the oxygen sequence is

A. Failure of Oxygenation

Alveolar Dysfunction
$PaO_2 < 60$ torr ($FIO_2 \geq 0.6$)

FIO_2 0.6 to 1.0

(1) SB with BP
(2) SB with CPAP/EPAP
(3) IMV (i.e., SB + CV) with CPAP + CPPV
(4) CV with CPPV (IPPV + PEEP)
(5) Optimize circulation, metabolism, COP, osmolality, fluids, electrolytes renal function (diuretic dialysis?)
(6) ECMO

Weaning

B. Failure of Ventilation

Airway or Neuromuscular Dysfunction
$PaCO_2 > 45$ torr
IC < 15 ml./kg. BW
IF < 30 cm. H_2O

FIO_2 0.3 to 0.6

(1) SB with BP
(2) IMV (i.e., SB + CV) with BP + IPPV
(3) AR with IPPB
(4) CV with IPPV
(5) Expiratory retardation

Weaning

Figure 12 Guidelines for selection of oxygenation and ventilation patterns for oxygenation failure (A) and ventilation failure (B). (Abbreviations are explained in the Glossary and in the text.)

found most suitable, the FIO_2 at 1.0 should be reduced as soon as feasible to about 0.5 for long-term use.

Meanwhile, circulation, metabolism, blood composition (including hematocrit, colloid osmotic pressure, and osmolality), fluid and electrolyte balance, and renal function should all be optimized. In pulmonary edema and consolidation, this effort calls for a trial of diuresis (in cardiogenic pulmonary edema and other types when pulmonary artery wedge pressure is increased) and albumin (when the colloid osmotic pressure is reduced), and in infection it includes appropriate antibiotic therapy. If all this fails to sustain PaO_2 at least at 50 to 60 torr, with optimal CPPV and an FIO_2 at 1.0 (short-term), ECMO is the only remaining alternative and might be considered in those centers equipped to undertake this modality.

During the initial phases of weaning, IMV with CPAP plus CPPV, with FIO_2 at 0.5 is recommended (Fig. 11). Weaning may then proceed back down the same steps that led to mechanical ventilation.

In contrast, in patients whose problem is primarily *ventilatory failure* ($PaCO_2$ more than 45 torr; inspiratory capacity less than 15 ml./kg. BW; or inspiratory force less than 30 cm. H_2O) or exhaustion from increased work of breathing, the airway should be optimally secured and ventilation patterns should be chosen to permit airway pressure to become atmospheric during exhalation (see later). These conditions include neuromuscular dysfunction (i.e., postoperative curarization,

polyneuritis, myasthenia gravis) and lower airway obstruction (e.g., severe asthma, bronchitis, and emphysema). When SB with BP and only slight oxygen enrichment (FIO_2 at 0.3 to 0.6) cannot maintain a normal $PaCO_2$, IMV with IPPV or assisted respiration with IPPB may be started. If these measures fail to maintain $PaCO_2$ normal, or if spontaneous initiation of breaths is impossible (as in curarization), controlled ventilation with IPPV is preferred. In airway disease with air-trapping and wheezing (asthma, emphysema), *expiratory retardation*, using a controlled narrowing of the expiratory port of the non-rebreathing valve of the ventilator should be used and adjusted during auscultation of the lungs in an attempt to minimize wheezing. Usually, assisted respiration with IPPB is favored in patients with COPD, while in patients with paralysis, controlled ventilation with IPPV is preferred.

IPPB treatment sessions (in contrast to continuous assisted respiration with IPPB) are widely over-used for "improved" bronchodilator aerosol administration. Such sporadic "treatments" probably have little use in the care of the critically ill and injured.

In patients with blunt chest injury and severe flailing, treatment of the pulmonary consolidation (hypoxemia) with continuous positive pressure techniques should have priority over treatment of flailing with controlled ventilation by IPPV; assisted respiration with IPPB has no place in the treatment of flail chest. IMV including SB-CPAP should be tried, and severe flailing may require controlled ventilation with CPPV.

Potential Hazards and Complications of Oxygen Therapy

The benefits of increasing FIO_2 above 0.6 or elevating airway pressure must be weighed against the risk of pulmonary damage inherent in higher oxygen concentrations or higher airway pressures. In premature newborns, *arterial* PO_2 greater than 80 torr carries the additional risk of blindness. Increasing the *airway pressure* more than absolutely necessary in any patient entails risk of lung rupture and circulatory embarrassment.

The risk of *pulmonary oxygen toxicity* depends on the *inhaled* oxygen tension, specifically on the dose of oxygen (alveolar PO_2 greater than 400 torr, i.e., FIO_2 greater than 0.6 at atmospheric pressure) and the duration of uninterrupted exposure. Volunteers inhaling 100 per cent humidified oxygen have experienced slight but reversible changes (e.g., tachypnea, reduced vital capacity) starting at 6 to 12 hours. Extensive animal research work and recent observations in man have shown that uninterrupted inhalation of 100 per cent oxygen leads within about 48 hours to irreversible hemorrhagic pulmonary edema and consolidation, starting with destruction of pulmonary capillary walls and alveolar lining cells. These changes are delayed or ameliorated (but not prevented) when severe shunt is the cause of hypoxemia. At the safe side of the spectrum is the observation in poliomyelitis patients that an FIO_2 of about 0.5 for many months with only brief interruptions (e.g., for suctioning) did not cause clinically detectable irreversible pulmonary damage. Thus, in patients with pulmonary disease and hypoxemia, an FIO_2 of 1.0 is safe for emergency resuscitation and for several hours to follow, and an FIO_2 of about 0.5 is safe over a long-range period.

Systemic oxygen toxicity depends on *arterial* oxygen tension. There is no evidence that raising PaO_2 values from 75 to 100 torr to about 500 to 600 torr, as is achieved with an FIO_2 of 1.0 in the presence of normal lungs, is harmful in itself. In *adults,* apparently only PaO_2 values over 1000 torr, a level reached only under hyperbaric conditions, can damage the brain (causing seizures) (see p. 280).

The *premature newborn infant* is a very different creature, however, and reacts to a PaO_2 rise above about 80 torr with spasm of the retinal vessels, which may lead to retrolental fibroplasia and blindness. The degree of ocular damage depends upon the degree of hyperoxia (PaO_2) and its duration, as well as on the degree of the baby's prematurity.

Certain patients with COPD constitute another group with special vulnerability to increased inhaled oxygen concentrations. In the past, occasional patients with COPD were found dead after having been left unattended in oxygen tents. It should come as no surprise that these patients, whose respiratory drive primarily depends on a reduced PaO_2 (the respiratory center being adjusted to a high $PaCO_2$) will hypoventilate when given oxygen to breathe. They thereby develop further increases in $PaCO_2$, with somnolence, coma, and secondary asphyxia (from upper airway obstruction and apnea) and cardiac arrest. Thus, they first become better oxygenated due to oxygen inhalation, but later succumb to the complications of hypoventilation-induced coma. This problem is entirely preventable by not leaving the oxygen-breathing COPD patient unattended. The problem must *not* be prevented by withholding oxygen when it is needed. *Compensated* COPD patients rarely need FIO_2 values greater than 0.3 to keep their PaO_2 above 60 torr, as hypoxemia is primarily due to ventilation-perfusion mismatching without shunting. Some may benefit from this minimal FIO_2 enrichment on an outpatient basis during exercise. *Decompensated* COPD patients, however, need an increase of FIO_2, often to 0.6 to 1.0, as they may have additional shunting from pneumonia or pulmonary edema. In this case, spontaneous hypoventilation can be avoided during oxygen breathing by close attention and verbal or pharmacologic stimulants to breathing. If such patients have a tracheal or tracheostomy tube in place, hypoventilation can be averted by mechanical ventilatory assistance. Sustained PaO_2 values in the 30s and 40s, commonly seen during breathing of air by decompensated COPD patients, are life-threatening, since the slightest further decrease of PaO_2 may lead to cerebral edema, arrhythmias, and cardiac arrest. There is no excuse for withholding oxygen therapy from any patient who requires it.

Increased airway pressure, often required for improved oxygenation, carries the potential hazards of lung injury and circulatory depression. Sustained increases in airway pressure with excessive accompanying increases in intra-alveolar pressure may lead to lung *rupture* with interstitial emphysema, pneumothorax, or arterial air embolism (rare). The likelihood of multiple alveolar rupture is enhanced by necrotizing lung disease and continuous application of increased alveolar pressure.

The mechanisms of *circulatory depression* by increased airway pressure are essentially threefold: (a) In the normal person, an increase of mean intrathoracic pressure to 5 to 10 cm. H_2O or more reduces venous return to the heart, thereby reducing cardiac output and (sometimes) arterial pressure. During intermittent positive pressure ventilation (IPPV), when the expiratory pause at atmospheric pressure is at least as long as the inflation phase, mean intrathoracic pressures are usually less than 10 cm H_2O and do not impair cardiac output because of a compensatory sympathetic discharge, unless the patient is oligemic or there is sympathetic blockade. (b) Increased mean alveolar pressure with sustained alveolar distention not only may "squeeze" the venae cavae but may also produce a form of pneumatic tamponade effect on the heart, impairing its filling and thereby reducing stroke volume. (c) Alveolar distention increases pulmonary vascular resistance by stretching and compressing pulmonary vessels and capillaries. In normal lungs, the optimal (lowest) pulmonary vascular resistance seems to be present at a mid-state of lung inflation, which in sick lungs is enhanced by slight continuous increase in alveolar pressure. Vascular resistance again is increased in collapsed lung units, in part due to pulmonary vasospasm from low tissue Po_2, in part due to mechanical factors.

The ability of increased intrathoracic pressure to decrease cardiac output (by decreasing venous return) and the ability of increased alveolar pressure and distention to increase pulmonary vascular resistance and to produce pneumatic cardiac tamponade are all reduced by pulmonary changes that make the lungs less compliant. This is a fortunate circumstance, for the principal indications for continuous positive airway pressure techniques are the very stiff lung conditions which reduce FRC. Apparently, stiff lungs can "buffer" to some extent the transmission of pressure from the alveolar lumina to the

vascular system. Nonetheless, in stiff lungs as well as more compliant ones, positive pressure breathing techniques (particularly spontaneous breathing with CPAP and controlled ventilation with CPPV) must be carefully titrated for optimal conditions.

VENTILATION TECHNIQUES

Rationale and Indications

While the previous section dealt primarily with methods of improving arterial blood oxygenation, this section focuses on methods of treating ventilatory failure. We may define ventilatory failure as the patient's inability to spontaneously maintain an alveolar ventilation (minute volume minus deadspace minute volume) adequate for removal of CO_2 (i.e., inability to maintain $Paco_2$ less than 45 torr), an inspiratory capacity (IC) adequate for lung expansion (at least 15 ml./kg. BW); or an inspiratory force of 30 cm. H_2O (tested during brief airway obstruction).

$Paco_2$ is determined by over-all alveolar ventilation, CO_2 production, and deadspace (anatomic plus alveolar deadspace)/tidal volume ratio. In order to maintain a normal $Paco_2$, alveolar ventilation must be increased when CO_2 production is increased (e.g., from fever, restlessness, convulsions, infection), or when deadspace is increased (e.g., from emphysema, pulmonary embolism, shock). When the patient himself cannot increase alveolar ventilation by increasing tidal volumes or frequency of breathing, artificial means of augmenting ventilation must be sought. These include coaching, respiratory stimulants, and mechanical ventilation (MV).

Ventilatory failure frequently coexists with oxygenation failure—the patient who is unable to take deep breaths, for example, as in partial paralysis after anesthesia or from coma (ventilatory failure), may develop miliary atelectasis (oxygenation failure). Probably, periodic deep breaths (about every 15 minutes) or large tidal volumes in general (15 ml./kg. BW) are required to maintain most alveoli open most of the time, particularly in damaged lungs with increased surface tension. Large spontaneous breaths are also required for effective airway clearance by coughing. Ventilation with small tidal volumes without periodic sighing, on the other hand results in progressive (miliary) atelectasis, decreased lung compliance, shunting, hypoxemia, and perhaps secondary infection. If the patient is unable to sigh himself (which can be objectively determined by measuring IC with a ventilation meter via mouthpiece, mask, or tracheal tube), artificial means of sighing must be instituted, even if he can maintain normal $PaCO_2$ by increasing the frequency of his small tidal volumes (see later).

Methods of improving ventilation without MV are indicated in decompensated COPD without exhaustion or severe secretional obstruction (which may require tracheal intubation). Coaching or analeptics can sustain respiratory volumes in selected COPD patients and thereby prevent a rising $PaCO_2$ in spite of oxygen inhalation. These techniques, which are used to avoid tracheal intubation and MV, may be useful in COPD patients without pulmonary consolidation who must have hypoxemia corrected but should not be relied upon to control hypoxemia in COPD decompensated with pneumonia or pulmonary edema. When possible, MV should be avoided in patients with COPD, since some of these patients, once deprived of the necessity of breathing spontaneously, are difficult to wean from the ventilator.

Increased work of breathing, usually the result of increased lung-chest compliance or increased airway resistance, constitutes another reason for providing ventilatory assistance or control. Clinical judgment is required to determine which patients need ventilatory help. The conscious patient will be able to indicate dyspnea leading toward exhaustion; in the stuporous or unconscious patient, rising $PaCO_2$ levels may be the only sign of a need for ventilatory support. In either instance, increased work of breathing sets up a vicious circle of increased energy requirement, CO_2 production, and ventilation requirement; when the ventilation requirement so produced cannot be met, hypercarbia worsens. These and other considerations make it obvious that in the critically ill or injured patient who may have difficulty maintaining normal $PaCO_2$ or PaO_2, or who has severe metabolic, acid-base, circulatory, or fluid volume imbalance, controlling pulmonary ventilation and oxygenation with MV is the key to life support (Figs. 10 to 14).

The uses of PEEP and expiratory retardation have been mentioned earlier. Another adjunctive technique, rarely used now, is *positive-negative pressure ventilation* (PNPV) (Fig. 10). PNPV was originally introduced to lower the mean intrathoracic pressure during controlled ventilation with IPPV for two purposes: (1) to prevent or reverse the circulatory depression (hypotension, decreased cardiac output) caused by the increased intrathoracic pressure of IPPV, particularly in cases of hypovolemia or sympathetic paralysis; (2) to reduce cerebral venous pressure and thereby promote drainage of blood from the cranium in patients with intracranial injury.

Currently, the indications for PNPV are few, if any. The method may increase airway collapse and air-trapping and perhaps promote pulmonary edema as well. Thus PNVP must be adjusted with auscultation to ensure that it does not induce wheezing or rales. Hypotension induced by IPPV or CPPV in the presence of oligemia is best treated by correcting the oligemia, rather than by PNPV. Furthermore, while increased intrathoracic pressure does cause increased intracranial pressure, in most patients with intracranial injury who need IPPV because of ventilatory failure, an expiratory pause at atmospheric pressure at least as long as the inflation phase will prevent ICP rise. In patients with intracranial injury requiring CPPV because of lung failure, the increased intrapulmonary pressure is not necessarily transmitted to the venae cavae and jugular veins if there is reduced lung compliance. Therefore, carefully adjusted IPPV or CPPV is safe, even in patients with intracranial injury, particularly if airway pressure is optimized according to monitored intracranial pressure.

Measurements in Critically Ill Patients on Mechanical Ventilation

Critically ill or injured patients, particularly those treated with MV via tracheal or tracheostomy tube, are deprived of the means of communication, and are often, when sedated, curarized or comatose, deprived of their protective reflexes. While MV stabilizes and controls ventilation and oxygenation, and thereby permits the team to focus on the underlying disease, it also introduces certain hazards unless safeguards are introduced.

These safeguards include intensive monitoring (from *monēre,* Latin, meaning "to warn"). The most important monitors are the senses—primarily sight, touch, and sound—of the physicians or nurses staying with the patient, and their feedback actions through intelligent use of their "cerebral computers."

The critically ill patient admitted to the Emergency Department, operating room, or ICU and found to be in need of MV should immediately be monitored by one person who can maintain continuity of observations through bedside vigilance. This "baby-sitter" should first observe (in order of priority) chest movements, carotid pulse, state of consciousness, color of mucous membranes, breath sounds, heart rate, arterial pressure (first using the cuff technique), skin temperature, and eye reflexes, including the size and reactions of the pupils. When feasible, *heart and breath sounds* should be monitored by precordial or esophageal stethoscope, as customarily used in the operating room. This gives more immediate and usually more meaningful information about ventilation and circulation than continuous or intermittent monitoring of tidal volumes and EKG. In conscious patients, inspiratory capacity should be determined. During MV, tidal volumes, airway pressure, and respiratory frequency should be monitored, adjusted, and controlled.

Reliable *tidal volume* monitoring requires a leak-free (cuffed) tracheal or tracheostomy tube, or a tight-fitting face mask. Expiratory tidal volume measured by ventilation meter during MV is more accurate than inspiratory volume, which will be unreliable when measured during positive airway pressure in the presence of a leak. *Airway pressure* should be determined as near as possible to the tracheal or tracheostomy tube. Tidal volume and airway pressure (end-inspiratory minus end-expiratory pressure) then permit calculation of lung-chest compliance (in ml./cm. H_2O), which should be determined frequently during MV when the patient's abdominal muscles are relaxed. Determination of dynamic ("effective") lung-chest compliance during MV is easy with use of a volume-set ventilator and merely recording changes in airway pressure.

As soon as possible, arterial and central venous catheters should be introduced to record pressures, and continuous *EKG* monitoring should be initiated. For blood gas and pressure monitoring, a superior vena cava catheter is preferred over an inferior vena cava or right atrial catheter. *Arterial blood gases* (PaO_2 with FIO_2 stated; $PaCO_2$; pHa; hemoglobin; and calculated bicarbonate and base excess) should be determined frequently. Intermittent *100 per cent oxygen tests* are desirable for guidance of MV. Finally, the superior vena cava or pulmonary artery catheter is used to determine changes in venous oxygen values (mixed venous PO_2 or oxygen content), since determination of these venous values, particularly their relative changes whenever PaO_2 is determined, permits estimation of changes in arterial oxygen transport in relation to demand (oxygen consumption) as influenced by changes in MV settings.

Blood gas values and other immediately required variables should be determined in a laboratory which can provide results within five minutes; experience has shown that routine laboratories are not set up for such rapid response, and that their charges become prohibitive for monitoring critically ill patients.

In addition to the above variables, life support of patients with multiple organ failure on MV is guided by intermittent monitoring of urine flow; fluid intake and output; serum and urine osmolality; serum electrolytes, protein, and colloid osmotic pressure; hematologic values; central body temperature; body weight; sputum culture; and chest roentgenograms.

Insertion of a *pulmonary artery balloon catheter* (Swan-Ganz) is indicated for monitoring of pulmonary artery wedge pressure (a reflection of left atrial pressure) in left ventricular failure; to titrate major fluid (particularly colloid) therapy in patients with membrane leakage or renal failure; to determine whether increased pulmonary artery pressure and perhaps right-sided heart failure is the result of increased pulmonary vascular resistance or rather left atrial pressure rise due to left-sided heart failure. In addition, the pulmonary artery catheter (more accurately than the superior vena cava catheter) permits monitoring of $P\bar{v}O_2$, a reduction of which indicates decreased cardiac output and/or increased oxygen consumption. In addition, $P\bar{v}O_2$ may decrease with hemodilution (reduced arterial oxygen content), left shift of the hemoglobin-oxygen dissociation curve, and whenever PaO_2 decreases below that required for full saturation of hemoglobin (about 90 torr). Relative changes in $P\bar{v}O_2$ are valuable for monitoring arterial oxygenation/circulation/metabolism interactions. The oxygen utilization coefficient (oxygen consumption/transport) can be calculated.

The technique of pulmonary artery catheterization should be learned after study of the appropriate literature and from individuals experienced with its use. Pitfalls with $P\bar{v}O_2$ readings include spuriously high $P\bar{v}O_2$ values despite worsening of the patient's condition in certain phases of septic shock or cirrhosis of the liver. Spurious values may also be obtained with forceful aspiration of left atrial blood with the catheter in the wedge position. Erroneously high pulmonary artery *pressure* readings may occur with the catheter displaced into the right ventricle and during positive pressure ventilation. Pulmonary artery and pulmonary artery wedge pressures ideally should be monitored as transmural pressures, i.e., subtracting intrathoracic pressure (esophageal balloon or intrapleural pressure when monitored) from mean pulmonary artery or wedge pressure. If these measures are not available, pressures should at least be read during the exhalation phase at atmospheric pressure.

Improving Lung Inflation and Ventilation Without Mechanical Assistance

In some conscious patients, MV attempts may be postponed in spite of ventilatory failure, and more conservative methods that do not require tracheal intubation may be tried first. Patients for whom such a strategy is sometimes appropriate include those demonstrating an inability to sigh, status asthmaticus without coma, or decompensated COPD.

While lack of coughing is an expiratory failure leading to inadequate clearing of tracheobronchial secretions, lack of *sighing* is an inspiratory failure leading to miliary atelectasis. In situations such as abdominal or chest wall pain, as well as recovery from anesthesia or intoxication, patients who can maintain a normal $PaCO_2$ may nonetheless be unable to sigh with an IC of at least 15 ml./kg. BW. Such patients should first be *coached*

verbally to take deep breaths, and the depth of their inhalations checked by a ventilation meter. The patient should further be taught to hold his breath for two to five seconds to fully expand his alveoli. If he is able to sigh with coaching, the coach can be supplanted with an *"incentive spirometer,"* a device which indicates to the patient whether he has succeeded in inhaling a pre-set sighing volume. Exhaling from FRC into a resistance (e.g., the traditional "blow bottle") produces a form of EPAP that is less effective in expanding alveoli than the deep breaths the blow bottle procedure occasionally provokes prior to blowing. However, sighing above FRC cannot be reliably achieved with EPAP by blow bottle.

If coaching fails to produce the required IC, the available methods for passive sighing, all of which are dependent upon the skill of the nurse or respiratory therapist administering them, include the following:

(1) Use of the CO_2 *deadspace rebreathing tube:* a 1-liter deadspace tube with oxygen at 3 to 5 liters per minute added into the distal end of the tube can stimulate the conscious patient into doubling his tidal volume with about 5 minutes of deadspace breathing, without decreasing FIO_2. This CO_2 therapy is contraindicated in patients with arrhythmias, stupor-coma, COPD, or intracranial disorder.

(2) *Manual sighing* with a self-refilling bag-(valve)-mask unit by a skilled operator. This is a volume-set inflation (most self-refilling bag-valve-mask units have a 1.5-liter capacity) that may also be used in the stuporous or comatose patient.

(3) *IPPB treatment sessions* using a pressure-set assistor ventilator. Such IPPB inflations can be made reliable for sighing only by monitoring exhaled tidal volumes, since the pressure-set ventilator can be prematurely cycled by the patient resisting the inflation with closure of the larynx or tightening of the abdominal or chest wall. Nonetheless, IPPB by mask or mouthpiece has not been shown statistically to reduce postoperative pulmonary complications, when given either prophylactically before surgery or routinely afterward. Furthermore, there is no proof that bronchodilator application via IPPB is any more effective than that via spontaneous breathing at atmospheric pressure. Individualized, titrated IPPB treatments, however, skillfully administered, may

help selected patients with secretions, bronchospasm, or pulmonary congestion.

Passive sighing maneuvers can usually be discontinued when postoperative patients become ambulatory, as exercise stimulates deep spontaneous breathing.

Manual assisted respiration with IPPB by *bag-mask* without a ventilator has proved effective in cases of croup and status asthmaticus without coma, to oxygenate and ventilate while administering drugs for decongestion of the mucosa, bronchodilatation, and normalization of pHa. At the Children's Hospital of Pittsburgh, prolonged manual IPPB by mask has significantly reduced the need for tracheal intubation in status asthmaticus. Although manual controlled ventilation ordinarily is used for emergency resuscitation only, its use has been extended for hours and, with ventilators connected to conscious patients' tight-fitting face masks, even for days. This obviously is contraindicated in the stuporous or comatose patient. In general, mechanical controlled ventilation via mask is discouraged because of its tendency to produce gastric insufflation and other complications.

In patients with COPD who require oxygen inhalation but who do not yet require tracheal intubation (i.e., exhaustion, coma, or inordinate secretions have not supervened), verbal coaching or IV analeptics have been tried. Coaching has already been discussed. In regard to *analeptics,* the artificial stimulation of breathing in ventilatory failure—as has been recommended with the use of doxapram or earlier with the use of nikethamide or ethamivan—can be criticized on physiologic grounds. Although an increase in $PaCO_2$ can sometimes be avoided during oxygen administration, these analeptics may cause increased oxygen consumption and thereby worsen the acidemia or even cause convulsions. In any event, their titration requires a "baby-sitter," who might just as well direct his efforts toward coaching, without pharmacologic agents. Furthermore, attempts to use analeptics in the stuporous patient whose airway has not been protected by a tracheal tube may result in aspiration. When there are inadequately cleared secretions and decreased lung compliance, stimulating the already exhausted patient may intensify the exhaustion and lead to secondary apnea. Thus, if analeptics are tried at all, their use should be limited to the "dry" COPD patient without tracheobronchial secretions whose decompensation, in terms of hypoxemia, is mild. Even in this instance, analeptics should be regarded merely as a stopgap measure. If doxapram is used, the recommended initial infusion rate is between 0.5 and 0.6 mg./min. in adults, titrated against arterial blood gas values. The concentration of doxapram should be selected to avoid fluid overloading.

Doxapram stimulates the respiratory center and thereby decreases $PaCO_2$ and may increase PaO_2; it also tends to increase cardiac output and oxygen consumption. When given too rapidly, it may give a feeling of warmth, produce sweating, restlessness, hallucinations, hypertension, and tachycardia and may even result in cardiac arrhythmias and convulsions. Obvious contraindications to doxapram include hypertension, hyperthyroidism, epilepsy, cardiac failure, and arrhythmias.

A carbonic anhydrase inhibitor, dichlorphenamide, was found to be a useful adjunct in the therapy of patients with COPD and severe CO_2 retention. A daily dosage of 200 mg. produced rapid improvement in clinical status and $PaCO_2$ and PaO_2 levels. The drug should not be used for the acutely decompensated COPD patient but rather for long-term maintenance.

Techniques of Mechanical Ventilation

TYPES OF ARTIFICIAL VENTILATION

The airway pressure patterns, physiology, and physics of modern positive pressure artificial ventilation are the same for emergency (manual) and long-term (mechanical) ventilation. Historically, in the 1950s the chest-pressure arm-lift methods of emergency artificial ventilation were found ineffective and IPPV-CPPV was introduced as the most effective mode of emergency artificial ventilation, in the form of mouth-to-mouth and bag-valve-mask ventilation. Similarly, for long-term ventilation (MV) the iron lung (tank ventilator) used extensively for poliomyelitis patients was replaced by IPPV-CPPV via tracheal or tracheostomy tube in the early 1950s in Scandinavia and later in the United States, starting in Baltimore and Chicago. Controlled ventilation of IPPV via tracheal or tracheostomy tube thus has become the basic mode of modern MV at this time.

The iron lung (body box, tank ventilator) encases the patient, except for his head, with a tightly fitting collar around the neck. Intermittently applied negative pressure around his body creates a pressure gradient from the upper airway (atmospheric pressure) to the atmosphere surrounding the chest and abdomen (negative pressure), which tends to expand the thoracic cavity and draw air into the lungs. In contrast, IPPV produces this pressure gradient by increasing airway pressure in relation to atmospheric pressure around the chest and abdomen. The effect on venous return to the heart is the same in both, except that the tank ventilator tends to decrease cerebral venous pressure, since the head is outside the box; this decrease, however, is offset by the pressure of the neck collar. Thus, the iron lung offers no hemodynamic advantages over intratracheal positive pressure ventilation but rather the disadvantages of rendering the patient inaccessible and immobile. The iron lung is also bulky, expensive, and incapable of raising the high-pressure gradients required to ventilate adequately with decreased lung compliance or increased airway resistance. A recent attempt was made to utilize the tank respirator for newborn infants with respiratory distress syndrome in order to avoid the use of a tracheal tube. However, the body box soon became obsolete even for this relatively limited and questionable indication, with the introduction of SB-CPAP via mask, hood, or nasal prongs.

There are now three *modes for prolonged MV* by intermittent positive pressure via tracheal or tracheostomy tube: (1) controlled ventilation (CV); (2) assisted ventilation (AV); and (3) intermittent mandatory ventilation (IMV) (Figs. 10 and 11).

In *controlled ventilation* (CV), ventilatory rate, rhythm, flow, and volume are set by the operator or machine. With pressure-set ventilators, tidal volumes may change when the patient's lung-chest compliance or airway pressures change (unless the pressures are readjusted according to monitored tidal volumes), but the patient can do nothing to alter the ventilatory frequency. In patients with ventilatory drive, competition between a volume-set ventilator and the patient (e.g., when the patient exhales while the ventilator

inflates) can lead to an excessive rise in airway pressure and to the risk of barotrauma. Fighting ("bucking") the ventilator may also cause arrhythmias and a rise in intracranial pressure and should therefore be suppressed.

Indications for *controlled ventilation* (CV) (IPPV) by MV are: (1) inability of the patient to maintain a normal $PaCO_2$ (hypoventilation); (2) excessive work of breathing; (3) metabolic acidemia in which normalization is required; and (4) severe flailing of the chest wall.

Controlled ventilation has advantages over AV and IMV in patients with depressed respiratory center (e.g., drug overdose, head trauma), paralysis (e.g., curarization for surgery, poliomyelitis, myasthenia gravis), and severe chest flailing. CV is also associated with the lowest work of breathing. However, its disadvantages compared with AV and IMV include a higher mean intrathoracic pressure, lower cardiac output, underutilization of respiratory muscles and respiratory center, resulting in more weaning difficulties, lack of $PaCO_2$ control by the patient, and the possibility of discoordination with spontaneous movements.

In *assisted ventilation* (AV) (IPPB), the patient's efforts trigger the ventilator and thus the respiratory frequency, while inflation is in part achieved by the ventilator. Most assistor ventilators have a mechanism to take over automatically with CV if the patient's efforts stop. AV has the advantage over CV of patient control in activating his respiratory center and enabling use of his respiratory muscles, and sometimes greater patient tolerance with less need for sedation. However, with pressure-set assistor ventilators, the patient has no control over tidal volume, and often the ventilator is not sufficiently sensitive to the patient's efforts. A negative airway pressure of not more than 1 to 2 cm. H_2O should be sufficient to trigger the ventilator. For obvious reasons, curarization is contraindicated with AV.

While AV is a ventilatory mode still used in decompensated COPD patients and asthmatics from the outset and during weaning from CV of any type, it is increasingly replaced by IMV.

In *intermittent mandatory ventilation* (IMV), spontaneous breathing with airway pressure atmospheric or elevated (SB-PAP) is augmented by superimposed CV with IPPV or CPPV, permitting adjustment of rate and volume (Fig. 11). IMV has several significant advantages, for it permits activation of the respiratory center and muscles without the discoordination commonly seen with CV. Furthermore, IMV entails less psychologic dependence on the ventilator; permits patient control of minute volume, frequency, and PaCO₂; allows control of SB-PAP and PEEP; and enables lower mean airway pressures (with higher cardiac output and less barotrauma) than with CV by CPPV. There is less need for sedation than with CV, less danger of asphyxia in case of disconnection, and—most important—easier weaning with identical FIO₂, reducing the IMV rate while the patient simultaneously increases his spontaneous breathing rate.

The main *disadvantage* of IMV derives from the fact that the ventilator cycles automatically with a preset, although often very slow, rate, which may interfere with the patient's inhalations. However, most patients spontaneously adjust their own breaths with the inflations from the ventilator. New variations of IMV permit patient triggering of the mechanical inflations, such as intermittent assisted ventilation (IAV) or synchronized IMV (SIMV), and control of the ratio between mechanical inflations and spontaneous breaths, as in intermittent demand ventilation (IDV). Still, mechanical inflations may occur at any point during inhalation. With IDV total ventilation volumes vary with the patient's spontaneous breathing rate. IAV (or SIMV) and IDV require complicated equipment and have little conceptual advantage over regular IMV.

The equipment required for IMV (Fig. 14) is a combination of that described above for SB-PAP (Fig. 8) and a pressure-set (Fig. 13) or volume-set (Fig. 14) ventilator. A knowledgeable respiratory therapist can set up an IMV arrangement for most commonly used ventilators. Respiratory gas for both ventilation modes of IMV (SB and CV) should pass through the same air-oxygen mixer and humidifier. Usually, at first the patient is treated at an inflation rate of 8 to 12 breaths per minute and an inflation volume of 10 to 15 ml./kg. BW. When he begins breathing spontaneously, the frequency of CV is gradually reduced according to the patient's clinical condition, blood gas values, CNS and circulatory status, and the usually steadily improving spontaneous tidal vol-

umes and rates (see discussion of weaning below).

When administering positive pressure artificial ventilation, the operator must clearly understand the interactions between tidal volumes (inflation volumes), airway pressure, ventilatory rate and rhythm, and flow rates during inflation and exhalation (Figs. 10 and 11). In patients with normal lungs in whom increased airway pressure is not buffered by reduced lung compliance, the IPPV pattern least injurious to cardiac output and arterial pressure is the "waltz rhythm," i.e., a time ratio of 1:2 of positive pressure inflation/exhalation at atmospheric pressure.

In general, increased airway resistance calls for decreased flow rates to deliver the same tidal volume with the same peak airway pressure; air-trapping from bronchial collapse during exhalation calls for expiratory flow retardation; alveolar atelectasis or fluid filling with shunting calls for continuous elevation of airway pressure (PEEP); reduced lung compliance calls for increased airway pressures; and oligemia or sympathetic paralysis with hypotension calls for the least rise in mean airway pressure, or even negative end expiratory pressure (NEEP).

Fluidic technology developed in industry has been adapted to various experimental methods and machines for artificial ventilation (Klain and Smith, 1976). While the avoidance of mechanical valves increases reliability and simplicity, fluidic gas valves require very high, wasteful gas flows and make humidification and volume control of MV difficult. Fluidic technology is still in the developmental stage so far as artificial ventilation is concerned.

A novel method of artificial ventilation, found effective for special anesthesias, is *high-frequency jet ventilation* (Klain and Smith, 1977). This method provides oxygenation via translaryngeal oxygen jet, while a special fluidic ventilator produces IPPV with rates as high as 100 to 300 per minute, with tidal volumes even less than estimated deadspace capable of CO₂ removal. The exact mechanism of this is not understood, but CO₂ removal probably occurs through channeled streams of gas, which can wash out CO₂ even if individual inflation volumes are small, in contrast to the mass movement of gas conceived as the mode of exchange during low-frequency ventilation. While high-frequency jet ventilation can be superimposed on spontaneous breathing as a mode of assisted ventilation and is capable of reducing elevated $PaCO_2$, its ability to decrease shunting (recruit alveoli) without sighing and with a very low airway pressure has not yet been studied.

CHARACTERISTICS AND CLASSIFICATIONS OF VENTILATORS

The external body ventilator (tank, iron lung) was mentioned previously for historical reasons. It has been abandoned because of its bulk and cost; the inaccessibility and immobilization it imposes on patients; the limitation of its ventilation pressure reserve; and its lack of advantages over tracheal IPPV in terms of venous return. A variant of the tank ventilator is the *cuirass* ventilator, a rigid shell covering the anterior thorax and abdomen. This device still has a place in selected patients with residual paralysis and compliant lungs in whom tracheal intubation should be avoided. Its effect is no more than assistance of spontaneous breathing. The same applies to the "raincoat ventilator" which has the additional disadvantage of causing the patient to accumulate heat inside the plastic cover. Abdominal belts are sometimes used in COPD patients to help lift the diaphragm during exhalation, while inspirations remain active. There are several other rarely used ventilation devices of limited value. The *rocking bed,* used extensively for weaning of poliomyelitis victims, was designed to move the diaphragm up and down by moving the abdominal contents; however, the rocking bed fails to move gas when the patient does not breathe with the ventilator or has airway obstruction (coma), increased airway resistance, or decreased compliance. The *electrophrenic ventilator* is an electrode placed near the phrenic nerve in the neck, stimulating contraction of the diaphragm and thus inspiration. Although theoretically this device would reproduce normal ventilatory movements without need for tracheal intubation, the practical effectiveness of this approach has never been demonstrated.

Presently used *mechanical ventilators* for IPPV and its variants are designed to drive gas into the lungs and to let the patient exhale with or without assistance. The differences among these ventilators in airway pressure and gas flow characteristics are more important for patients with sick lungs than those with normal lungs. When classifying ventilators according to the method of inspiratory phase initiation, we must differentiate between *controller* (fixed-rate) ventilators (the inspiratory phase is initiated at a predetermined rate independent of patient effort); *assistor* ventilators (the ventilator initiates the inspiratory phase only in response to the patient's inspiratory efforts); and *assistor-controller* (demand) ventilators (the inspiratory phase is ventilator initiated either in response to or independently of the patient's inspiratory effort). When the rate of the controller mode is set below the patient's rate, controlled inflations occur only when the patient's respiratory rate falls below that of the ventilator setting.

Secondary classifications can be made according to the method of inspiratory phase initiation: *IMV ventilator, synchronized IMV ventilator, intermittent demand ventilator,* and *intermittent assistor ventilator* (see p. 298). Some also have introduced a basic classification according to the pressure required to produce inflation, namely, *positive pressure ventilator,* i.e., one attached to the patient's airway (the most common modern ventilator), and *negative pressure ventilator,* i.e., one producing transpulmonary pressure by creating negative pressure around the thorax and abdomen (tank, body, cuirass ventilators; all of very limited value).

The most important classification is that of the *inspiratory phase termination.* Here, we differentiate between *pressure-cycled* (pressure-set or pressure-fixed), i.e., one which terminates the inspiratory phase at a predetermined pressure (inspiratory time and volume vary with changes in airway resistance and compliance); *volume-cycled* (volume-set or volume-fixed), i.e., one which terminates the inspiratory phase after a predetermined volume of gas is delivered (airway pressure and inflation time vary with changes in airway resistance and compliance); and *time-cycled* (time-set or time-fixed), i.e., one which terminates the inspiratory phase after a predetermined inflation time lapse (inspiratory airway pressure and volume vary with airway resistance and compliance). Several ventilators incorporate a combination of the above three features, and the mode for terminating the inspiratory phase may change under different circumstances. For example, a volume-cycled ventilator—the recommended and most popular—at times may cycle before the preset volume is delivered if a safety pop-off pressure is reached.

Ventilators may be classified according to the method by which their force is generated. There is the *pressure generator,* characterized by an unchanging source of pressure which produces variable flows in response to changes in airway resistance; a *flow generator,* which gives a linear flow output at a preset level, producing fluctuating pressures in response to changes in airway resistance; and *pressure-flow generator hybrid units,* producing curvilinear wave forms approximating one-half of a sine wave. These produce increasing pressure or nonconstant flow, e.g., Emerson, Engstrom, or Moerch volume-set piston ventilators.

Finally, ventilators may be classified according to gas flow transmission, namely, *direct gas flow,* i.e., the driving gas for the ventilator is also the gas delivered to the patient (e.g., Bird) (Fig. 13); or *indirect gas flow,* i.e., a power circuit with its driving gas or electric motor merely squeezing a bag or bellows which is connected to the patient (e.g., Bennett MA-1) (Fig. 14).

The *ideal ventilator* should reliably provide the following:

(1) (volume set) tidal volumes between 0 and 2 liters

(2) inflation frequencies between 0 and 40 per minute

(3) airway pressures between 0 and 70 cm. H_2O

(4) an end-inspiratory pause

(5) an end-expiratory positive pressure (PEEP) of 0 to 50 cm. H_2O

(6) adjustable time and flow rates during inflation and exhalation

(7) assistor, controller, mixed, and IMV modes

(8) an SB-CPAP/EPAP mode for IMV

(9) an automatic sighing mechanism (optional)

(10) an adjustable safety pop-off pressure valve

(11) means for controlling inhaled oxygen and CO_2 concentrations (ideally through servo control)

(12) an optional negative end-expiratory pressure (NEEP) mode

(13) a heated humidifier with airway temperature and humidity controls

(14) a drug aerosol nebulizer

(15) a device to permit drainage of condensed water in tubings

(16) an air intake bacterial filter

(17) an exhaled air scavenger or bacterial air filter

(18) lightweight, nonslipping, nonkinking connections to the patient

(19) an alarm to indicate volume, pressure, or cycling failure; extremes of gas temperature; and disconnection

(20) a reliable inexpensive power source

(21) readable tidal volumes, rate, minute volume, airway pressure, and FIO_2 (for monitoring)

At this time, there is no ventilator which provides all these features.

In patients with healthy lungs (such as those in postanesthesia recovery rooms), a simple pressure-set ventilator is adequate (e.g., Fig. 13). However, patients with abnormal lungs may require sophisticated adjustments of pressure, volume, flow, rate, and mode of ventilation. Thus, one of the more advanced volume-set ventilators (e.g., Fig. 14) should be employed. Most important is the fact that with increased airway resistance or decreased lung compliance, a ventilator of the pressure-set type will produce a decreased tidal volume; while the volume-set ventilator will maintain the tidal volume. Thus, the volume-set ventilator is preferable in critically ill or injured patients. In the presence of small leaks, however, the volume-set ventilator cannot compensate, and the tidal volume will decrease; whereas the pressure-set ventilator will continue insufflating the lungs until the peak pressure is reached in spite of a small leak. With large leaks, the pressure-set ventilator will not cycle unless it has a time-cycled mechanism. All types of ventilators should have the means to continuously monitor airway pressure (as close as possible to the patient) and tidal volume. As some of the gases are compressed by the increased pressure within the tubing, a ventilation meter attached to the expiratory port will measure not only the volume coming from the patient but also the compression volume, which is about 3 ml./cm. H_2O with a typical tubing setup of the volume-set ventilator. If accurate tidal volumes are needed, a double exhalation valve is required.

THE BIRD MARK VII
VENTILATOR

The Bird Mark VII ventilator is a popular pressure-cycled, gas-powered assistor-controller (Fig. 13) that delivers adjustable inspiratory flow rates at 1 to 80 liters per minute (with arbitrary numbers on the dial). It produces a cycling rate up to 80 per minute, an airway pressure controllable between 5 and 60 cm. H_2O, and expiratory retardation when needed. The assistor mode provides sensitivity control between 0.5 and

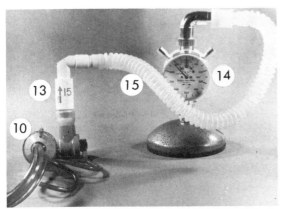

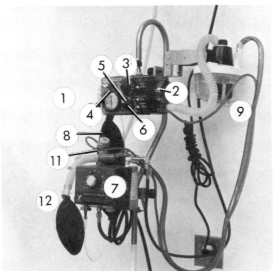

Figure 13   (1) Bird Mark VII pressure-set ventilator modified for long-term mechanical ventilation. (2) Pressure control setting. (3) Flow control setting. (4) Sensitivity setting. (5) Air mix setting. (6) Apnea control knob. (7) Air-oxygen mixer (Veriflo). (8) Ventilator-O_2 mixer kit. (9) Heated Puritan cascade humidifier. (10) Drug aerosol nebulizer. (11) Exhalation valve with retard attachment. (12) Patient connection to test lung. (13) PEEP valve. (14) Ventilation (volume) meter. (15) Large-bore tubing from exhalation and PEEP valves to ventilation meter.

5 cm. H_2O negative pressure to trigger inflations. FIO_2 control requires an oxygen-air mixer, with the ventilation setting on 100 per cent oxygen, unless a special reservoir bag is attached to the air inlet portion of the ventilator and is fed with gas from the oxygen-air mixer. When the ventilator is set on air dilution, higher inspiratory flow rates are possible. However, when powered by oxygen without an air mixer, instead of the intended 40 per cent oxygen delivered it can deliver FIO_2 values greater than 0.6, which makes long-term use of this ventilator without an oxygen-air mixer unsafe. In the air dilution mode, this ventilator functions as a constant pressure generator; in the 100 per cent oxygen mode, it functions as a constant flow generator. Therefore, the Bird Mark VII, when used with an oxygen-air mixer and reservoir bag plus "air-dilution" setting, becomes more functional and flexible.

The Bird ventilators have excellent drug aerosol nebulizers. In addition, a heated humidifier or nebulizer should be interposed mainstream.

Prior to use on a patient, the ventilator and its components should be carefully assembled, inspected, and tested with a test lung. One may initially set pressure, flow rate, and sensitivity all on reference numbers 15. The assistor mode cycling should be set for a negative pressure of 1 cm. H_2O. These settings are readjusted after the ventilator is connected to the patient. Clinical assessment of ventilation volume should be done with a volume meter if available but otherwise by observing chest movement. Expiratory retardation (when needed in asthma or emphysema) should be adjusted until wheezes are minimized; the retard cap must never completely occlude exhalation! To monitor tidal volumes when expiratory retardation is used, connect the inlet port of the ventilation meter to the expiratory port of the exhalation valve, and attach a special expiratory retard cap to the outlet port of the ventilation meter. A PEEP valve may be interposed (Fig. 13, *top*).

For *controlled ventilation*, the apnea control (expiratory timer, rate) is turned counterclockwise to activate the ventilator automatically. Then the apnea control knob must be adjusted until the desired rate is achieved. A ventilation meter attached to the expiratory port of the non-rebreathing valve will help determine whether a given pressure delivers the desired volume (usually 12 to 15 ml./kg. BW). The inspiratory/expiratory ratio should be set initially at 1:2, for controlled ventilation at a frequency of about 12 per minute. For *assisted ventilation,* set the automatic cycling on the ventilator to a respiratory frequency that is lower than the patient's spontaneous breathing frequency. Since the tidal volume will change with compliance, resistance, and patient position, the volume should be monitored frequently and airway pressure adjusted accordingly. The humidifier should also be checked routinely, since dry gas can hurt the lungs quickly.

If the ventilator fails to cycle into the expiratory phase, it should be disconnected and checked by test lung while the patient is ventilated by bag-valve unit. The most common cause of this malfunction is leakage; the most common sites are at the tracheostomy tube cuff, nebulizer jar, or exhalation valve. Sometimes, the ceramic shaft of the internal valving may stick.

When the inspiratory time is too short or is excessively long, the situation can usually be corrected by simply readjusting the inspiratory flow rate. This adjustment will vary with the pulmonary condition; the higher the flow rate, the faster the peak airway pressure will be achieved, resulting in a shorter inspiratory time and smaller tidal volume. Slow flow rates are needed to treat obstructive disease and to improve distribution of ventilation in pulmonary shunting. However, flow rates should not be so slow that the patient overrides the inspiratory flow rate of the ventilator and does not receive positive pressure.

When the sensitivity control is set for the *assistor mode,* oversensitive settings may cause automatic cycling, excessive flow rates, and low tidal volumes. For assisted ventilation, the apparatus should be set for a controlled ventilation rate of about 10 per minute, which would take over when the patient is unable to trigger the ventilator.

THE BENNETT MA-1 VENTILATOR

The Puritan Bennett MA-1 ventilator is an electrically driven, volume-set, assistor-controller ventilator (Fig. 14). An air pump compresses a bellows, which in turn intermittently inflates the patient via appropriate tubings. The non-rebreathing valve is on the ventilator with double tubings to and from the patient, connected by a Y tube.

This ventilator provides tidal volumes up to 2000 ml., airway pressures up to 80 cm. H_2O, inspiratory flow rates up to 100 liters per minute, respiratory cycling rates from 6 to 60 per minute (special IMV rate card is optional), sensitivity (negative triggering pressure) between 0.1 and 10 cm. H_2O, and FIO_2 control adjustable from 21 per cent up to 100 per cent oxygen. The ventilator also provides a built-in sigh mechanism with special controls for pressure, volume, and frequency. While expiratory resistance is a standard control on the ventilator, PEEP and NEEP are optional attachments. With these, a negative pressure of up to 10 cm. H_2O and a PEEP pressure of up to 20 cm. H_2O may be achieved. For high PEEP, the manufacturer, upon request, will increase the capability of the PEEP device to the desired level. Ventilation is monitored by a bellows-type monitoring spirometer, which is an integral part of the ventilator. The ventilator also provides a variety of visual and audible signals and alarms. Humidification is accomplished by a heated cascade humidifier with variable temperature setting and monitoring capabilities at the airway. Prior to use, the ventilator must be carefully assembled, inspected, and tested with a test lung. Frequent monitoring of parameters such as FIO_2, temperature, airway pressure, and tidal volume is essential.

Even though the standard MA-1 ventilator is not equipped with intermittent mandatory ventilation, the manufacturer now has available a special modification kit which permits the lowering of the ventilatory rate to accommodate IMV. This kit, however, does not include the special valving system and reservoir bag necessary for IMV. Such special IMV attachments are available from other manufacturers. When the Bennett MA-1 is used in the IMV mode, the monitoring spirometer must be disconnected from the system unless a special modification is utilized to divert the gas from the spirometer during spontaneous breathing. *Every hospital* providing acute respiratory intensive care should have a volume-set ventilator with IMV attachment (Fig. 14), and a *PEEP mechanism* with water bubble valve (Fig. 8A), magnetic PEEP (Fig. 9B) floating ball valve (Fig. 9A) or mushroom PEEP valve (e.g., Emerson, Bennett).

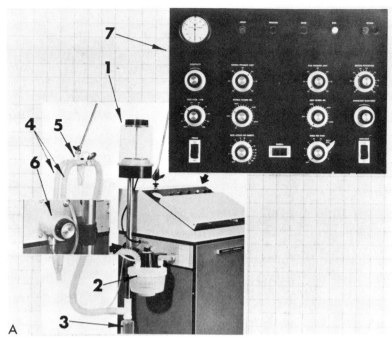

Figure 14 A, The Puritan Bennett MA-1 Ventilator, an example of a volume-set ventilator. (1) Spirometer (exhaled tidal volume monitor, bellows type) and alarm. (2) Cascade humidifier with manual temperature knob. (3) Water trap in exhalation tubing. (4) Inspiratory and expiratory tubings with Y connector to patient. (5) Exhalation manifold with small drug aerosol nebulizer, exhalation valve and inhaled gas temperature gauge. (6) PEEP valve (optional). (7) Control panel with airway pressure gauge; and controls for pressure, volume, rate, flow, sensitivity, mechanical sighing, delivered oxygen concentration and expiratory resistance; nebulizer; and visual and audible signals and alarms.

For *testing* ventilator with test lung prior to connection to patient: (1) power switch off, insert electric plug. (2) Power switch on. (3) Connect properly indexed oxygen supply hose to back of ventilator and to properly identified outlet. Oxygen supply pressure should be 50 p.s.i., unrestricted by flow meter. (4) Fill cascade humidifier jar with sterile distilled water and reassemble tightly. (5) Set temperature to #6. (6) Sensitivity, turn knob clockwise until ventilator starts cycling and the assist light illuminates. At this point, turn counterclockwise until cycling stops. (7) Set flow control knob at 40 to 60 liters per minute. (8) Set normal pressure limit control knob at 80 cm. H_2O. (9) Set normal volume control at desired volume level (15 ml./kg. BW). (10) Set rate control to desired inflations per minute (e.g., 12/minute). (11) Sighing: Set mechanical sighing safety pressure limit at 80. If sigh is not desired, set it at 20. Set sighing volume approximately at 1.5 to 2 times tidal volume. If sighing is not desired, turn sighing volume knob to zero. Set sighing frequency per hour. If sighing is not desired, turn to "off" position. Set number of multiple sighs (e.g., 2 to 3); if sighing not desired, set control to 1. (12) Set oxygen concentration desired. (13) Turn expiratory resistance off. Adjust it once the patient is connected to the ventilator, with auscultation. (14) Set nebulizer switch at "off." (15) Set pressure limit warning buzzer to full "up" position. This may be readjusted later. (16) Test spirometer alarm, set calibrated spirometer stick at desired tidal volume. (17) Attach sterile test lung to Y connector of ventilator. (18) Squeeze and release test lung to generate negative pressure to test assist mode. (19) Note inflation of bag, rise of pressure, and termination of inspirations. Note tidal volume recorded on spirometer versus tidal volume at control setting. Check breathing tubes and connections for air leak. Test alarms. (20) Connect to patient. (21) Readjust periodically desired ventilation volumes and patterns.

Initiation of CV by MV in critically ill patients with a volume-set ventilator can be done quite simply: Before connecting the ventilator, adjust it with a test lung to a tidal volume of 15 ml./kg. BW (thus, sighing is not needed), 12 inflations per minute, FIO_2 1.0 and no PEEP (IPPV) or a PEEP of only 5 cm. H_2O (CPPV). Connect the ventilator to the patient. Readjust the rate of inflations according to $PaCO_2$. Minimize wheezing with the appropriate degree of expiratory retardation, guided by auscultation, if necessary. Readjust PEEP (if necessary) to obtain the desired PaO_2 (60 or 100 torr), eventually with FIO_2 0.5 to 0.6. In severe oxygenation problems, optimize PEEP according to com-

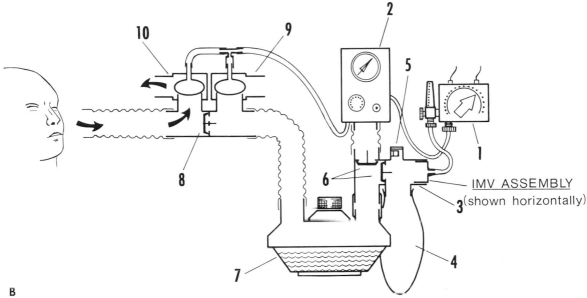

B

Figure 14B (*Continued*) B, IMV-CPAP. (1) Air-oxygen mixer. (2) Ventilator. (3) IMV-CPAP assembly. (4) Reservoir bag. (5) Variable leak. (6) One-way valves. (7) Humidifier. (If a cascade humidifier is used, the incoming flow should be greater than the patient's peak inspiratory flow. The tower from the cascade is removed to permit resistance free inhalation.) (8) One-way valve for double manifold. (9) Manifold used during IMV to exhaust continuous gas flow from air/O₂ mixer. (This valve is not used during CPAP unless it is equipped with PEEP attachment.) (10) Exhalation valve where VT is monitored. A PEEP valve (Fig. 9) is connected here when CPAP is desired. (From Instrumentation Industries, Inc., 215 Thomas Drive, Pittsburgh, PA 15236.)

pliance (minimize end-inflation pressure minus PEEP difference) and cardiac output (avoid a sharp decline of mixed venous (O_2). For IMV, start similarly but with a slower rate of inflations. For PEEP over about 5 cm. H_2O reduce tidal volume to 10 to 12 ml./kg. BW.

OTHER VENTILATORS

The Bird Mark VII and Bennett MA-1 ventilators have been listed and illustrated, since they are the most commonly used pressure- and volume-set ventilators in the U.S. at this time. New brands and models, however, appear and disappear from the scene, and many old proven brands are still around. Personnel responsible for MV should familiarize themselves with each ventilator they use by studying the literature (e.g., Mushin's book on mechanical ventilation; manufacturers' literature) and practice all settings and adjustments first on a test lung and on themselves.

Other *pressure-set* assistor-controllers include, among others, the Bird Mark VIII, the Bennett PR-2, and the Monaghan 225.

Other *volume-set* ventilators include the Emerson piston ventilator; its predecessor, the Moerch piston ventilator (one of the first long-term volume-set ventilators in the world); the Engstrom ventilator (used widely abroad; expensive); and the Ohio 560 ventilator. Most of these are electrically powered and dependable and permit separate adjustments of volume, rate, and flow. They are actually volume-set and time-cycled, as well as pressure and volume readable. In some (Emerson, Moerch), the electric motor directly drives the piston which delivers the gas into the patient's circuit; in others (Ohio 560, Engstrom), the electric motor drives a turbine or piston that delivers gas in the primary circuit, which in turn compresses a bag or bellows that is connected to the patient's circuit. The volume-set ventilators mentioned and several others are acceptable alternatives to the Bennett MA-1.

MONITORING AND ADJUSTING MECHANICAL VENTILATION

Once it has been decided that the patient requires MV, he is ventilated by bag-valve-O_2 while the physician, nurse, or therapist checks and presets the ventilator, using a test lung. For initiation of controlled ventilation, we recommend a cycling pressure of 20 cm. H_2O (for pressure-set ventilators) and a tidal volume of 15 ml./kg. BW (for volume-set ventilators) at a rate of about one inflation every five seconds, with a ratio of inflation/exhalation of 1:2 or 1:1. First, with such a setting the ventilator is connected to the patient, to start with FIO_2 at 0.5 to 1.0 (e.g., 0.9). All settings are readjusted later. Inflation time should be at least one second to permit adequate gas distribution. In abnormal lungs, optimum distribution is probably achieved by a rapid inflow rate initially and holding the gas in the lungs for about one second (end-inspiratory plateau). In patients with normal lungs, exhalation to atmospheric pressure is sufficient. In patients with airway disease, expiratory retardation is subsequently introduced with adjustments to minimize wheezing; and in patients with alveolar shunting, PEEP is added and optimized.

Tidal volumes (monitored during exhalation), airway pressures, and cycling rates must be prescribed, monitored at all times, and recorded. For controlled ventilation, tidal volumes and rates must be ordered and controlled; and with use of a volume-set ventilator, the airway pressures will vary. Volumes and pressures should be monitored and recorded in the form of dynamic (effective) lung-thorax compliance in ml./cm. H_2O. In addition, intermittent blood gas monitoring is mandatory with frequency of determinations depending on circumstances. Patients on MV must have heart rate, arterial pressure, EKG, CVP, temperature, and state of consciousness monitored as well.

For long-term MV, intermittent $PaCO_2$ monitoring can be augmented effectively by continuous end-tidal PCO_2 monitoring, which is valuable in reflecting relative changes in $PaCO_2$, although end-tidal PCO_2 and $PaCO_2$ are not identical in patients with abnormal lungs. The former is lower than the latter when there is an increase in dead-space.

When using large tidal volumes, e.g., 12 to 15 ml./kg. BW for IPPV, periodic sighing is probably not necessary, since each inflation is a sigh. With PEEP, tidal volumes of 10 to 12 ml./kg. should be the limit to avoid alveolar rupture. The desired $PaCO_2$ (usually 30–40 torr) is then achieved by increasing or decreasing the ventilatory frequency. With assisted ventilation (AV) (IPPB) and IMV, the patient regulates total alveolar ventilation himself; the operator prescribes, sets, and controls the peak airway pressure, sensitivity and rate for IPPB; and the rate and tidal volume of the CV mode and the PEEP (CPAP) for IMV.

Experience has shown that ventilation volume nomograms cannot be relied upon to give tidal volumes and rates required to achieve normocarbia under clinical conditions, particularly in patients with abnormal lungs. Therefore, there is no substitute for adjusting the initial minute volume setting according to $PaCO_2$ or at least end-tidal PCO_2, best by changing the ventilation rate.

Progression and weaning of ventilation techniques are shown in Figure 12.

Weaning from Mechanical Ventilation

Weaning the patient from MV to spontaneous breathing, and finally from a tracheal or tracheostomy tube to a natural airway must be individualized and is a clinical art, although it should be based on as much physiologic data as possible. Usually, weaning from MV is followed by extubation or, in the case of a tracheostomy tube, a switch to an uncuffed tracheostomy tube; and finally from supplemental oxygen—in that order.

Historically, weaning by trial and error according to clinical judgment and perhaps vital capacity (inspiratory capacity) measurements was followed by adherence to strict criteria, such as blood gas values, inspiratory force, inspiratory capacity, and other variables. More recently, weaning from controlled ventilation via IMV to spontaneous breathing has simplified this procedure considerably and has mitigated the tendency toward dangerous fluctuations in blood gas and pH values during weaning. While the Boston criteria call for an inspiratory force of at least −20 cm. H_2O, a vital capacity of at least 15 ml./kg. BW, and a PaO_2 of at least 70 torr on an FIO_2 of 0.4, it may be impossible to measure some of these parameters accurately in the stuporous patient. Moreover, some patients who never fulfill these criteria can be weaned safely from CV via AV or IMV to spontaneous breathing.

In patients with *normal lungs* and only hours of MV (e.g., after anesthesia with curarization), weaning from controlled ventilation can be safely performed by abruptly switching to spontaneous breathing via tracheal tube using a T-tube with warm, humidified oxygen at an FIO_2 of about 0.5; at the time of weaning, inspiratory capacity with coaching or painful stimuli should be at least 15 ml./kg. BW. Criteria for determining recovery of muscle power besides the IC include the patient's ability to raise his head, squeeze a hand, and move both chest and abdomen upward when asked to breathe deeply. A switch to spontaneous breathing in these cases may be accomplished when the patient responds to verbal command. In the intubated stuporous or comatose patient with "normal lungs," spontaneous breathing may be via T-tube, with periodic deep lung inflations (15 ml./kg.) about every 10 minutes until coached sighing is possible; in patients with "abnormal lungs," spontaneous breathing with prophylactic PEEP (SB-PAP) (e.g., 3 to 5 cm. H_2O) is often beneficial to increase FRC. Extubation must wait until the patient is conscious (responds to verbal command) and has recovered protective upper airway reflexes.

In patients with abnormal lungs, chest wall, respiratory muscles, or nervous system, weaning from MV, particularly after long periods of MV, is difficult. Earliest possible weaning is desirable to avoid atrophy of respiratory muscles. On the other hand, too early weaning may lead to hypoxemia, asphyxia, and cardiac arrest, or at least to resumption of controlled ventilation. The main obstacles to early weaning are increased deadspace/tidal volume ratio, as commonly encountered in COPD; inspiratory capacity less than 15 ml./kg. BW; increased work of breathing; and low PaO_2. Therefore, the disease states causing these derangements should be corrected before weaning is started. In general, patients who cannot maintain an IC of at least 10 ml./kg. BW and a PaO_2 above 60 torr with FIO_2 of 0.6, or a $P(A-a)O_2$ under 350 torr with FIO_2 at 1.0, during spontaneous breathing trials, cannot be weaned safely. In addition, trials of spontaneous breathing must be interrupted

when tachycardia (heart rate over 120 per minute), severe cardiac dysrhythmias, hypertension, hypotension, decreased cardiac output, tachypnea (respiratory rate over 40 per minute), increased pulmonary artery wedge pressure, increased CVP, decreased venous PO_2 and excessive anxiety, apprehension, agitation, fatigue, somnolence, and/or restlessness occur. Under any of these circumstances, the patient should be returned immediately to CV or IMV with higher frequency.

Critical (dangerous) blood gas levels include PaO_2 of less than 100 torr on FIO_2 of 1.0; mixed venous PO_2 of less than 25 torr; progressive rise in $PaCO_2$ over 45 torr; and a decrease in pHa to 7.2 or less. Although cardiac output and oxygen consumption usually are lowest under controlled ventilation, with cardiac output increasing over oxygen consumption when switching to assisted ventilation or IMV and increasing even further when switching to spontaneous breathing, patients with cardiac disease or pulmonary consolidation may at times experience a decrease in cardiac output when MV is discontinued and an improved circulatory state when it is resumed. In patients in whom shunt can be quantitated, a shunt of over 25 per cent usually makes weaning impossible.

Basic criteria for initiating weaning include absence of primary initiating cause for MV; response to verbal command; stable circulatory state; acceptable chest roentgenogram; absence of severe abdominal distention; and absence of medication with muscle relaxants for over 12 hours. For COPD patients narcotics are also contraindicated. Ideally, there should also be an acceptable hematocrit, a near-normal plasma protein concentration, adequate intravenous or parenteral nutrition, and psychologic preparation of the patient prior to weaning.

The *techniques of weaning* depend on the duration of MV, the patient's pulmonary status and general condition, and other factors:

(1) After short-term CV in patients with normal lungs (e.g., after recovery from residual anesthesia and curarization in the recovery room), weaning is abrupt to spontaneous breathing.

(2) After moderate periods of CV or IMV or in patients with abnormal lungs, a switch from CV to spontaneous breathing is done via T-tube with "prophylactic" PEEP (3 to 5 cm.

H_2O) to avoid decrease in FRC; if blood gas and other variables are acceptable in about one hour, the patient is extubated if conscious.

(3) After long-term MV (CV or IMV) gradual weaning with IMV is recommended. This includes a gradual individualized switch from controlled ventilation to IMV by reducing the CV rate by about two inflations each hour, eventually to one CV inflation every two minutes and then, if blood gas values are acceptable, to consider extubation if the patient meets the criteria for extubation.

Weaning should be with FIO_2 at 0.5 to 0.6 and warm humidity. When switching directly from CV to spontaneous breathing, periods of five minutes per hour of spontaneous breathing may be interposed and either the duration or the frequency of these periods increased gradually.

Weaning should not be begun at night, since it requires continuous bedside attendance by knowledgeable personnel. In general, the priorities in discontinuing respiratory care modes are as follows: (1) reduce FIO_2 to 0.5 to 0.6; (2) reduce respiratory frequency of MV with IMV; (3) reduce PEEP to 2 to 5 cm. H_2O; (4) reduce expiratory retardation when applicable; (5) reduce sighing; and (6) extubate.

Weaning can often be facilitated by having the patient in a semi-sitting position and coaching by a knowledgeable, compassionate individual. Vital signs and blood gases must be taken frequently with each step-wise change. The EKG should be monitored, and a bag-valve unit must be in readiness. Discoordination of respiratory muscles should be detected and weaning slowed, although weaning will be ultimately possible in such circumstances.

Hazards and Complications

"FIGHTING THE VENTILATOR"

With current IMV techniques, "fighting the ventilator" is rare, but occasional patients either on IMV or on CV may "fight the ventilator," i.e., breathe spontaneously with CV or react with bucking (coughing) to the tracheal or tracheostomy tube. Asynchronous breathing during CV may worsen ventilation-perfusion mismatching, may lead to excessive airway pressures when the ventilator inflates during spontaneous exhalations, and thus may be harmful to the circulation and lungs (risk of barotrauma). In addition, reacting to the tracheal tube or the ventilator may cause arrhythmias and a rise in intracranial pressure, which must be avoided particularly in patients with intracranial injury. The most common reasons for a patient's drive to breathe more deeply or faster than the ventilator are lung disease, CNS disease, shock, or hypoventilation by MV because of inappropriate settings or airway leaks.

Synchronization is best achieved through the following orderly, sequential approach: (1) hyperventilate, manually or mechanically, to reduce $PaCO_2$ slightly and thereby remove the drive from the respiratory center; (2) oxygenate fully (raise PaO_2 over 90 torr) through FIO_2 control and optimal PEEP if necessary to abolish hypoxemic respiratory drives; (3) apply a smooth rhythm of CV in order to "fatigue" the pulmonary stretch receptor reflexes; (4) rule out or eliminate tracheobronchial irritation by secretions or too deep insertion of the tracheal tube (the carina is most sensitive) as a source of bucking; (5) recognize and treat multiple factors which stimulate respiratory drive, such as atelectasis (e.g., insertion of the tracheal tube into the right main bronchus), acidemia, tissue acidosis (shock), hypotension (carotid sinus reflex), CSF acidosis (brain damage), moderate rise in intracranial pressure, hyperthermia, pulmonary edema-consolidation, or pleural fluid.

Severe hyperventilation ($PaCO_2$ less than about 25 torr) to achieve synchronization should be used only briefly when necessary, but not long-term, since alkalemia (hypocarbia) increases tissue oxygen consumption, reduces cardiac output, may impair oxygen delivery to tissues by shifting the oxygen-hemoglobin dissociation curve to the left, may cause arrhythmias, and can reduce cerebral blood flow. Moderate hypocarbia ($PaCO_2$ 25 to 35 torr) is usually safe, aids in establishment of smooth CV without patient asynchronization, and may even be desirable in cases of intracranial injury.

In conscious anxious patients, small doses of a sedative [e.g., diazepam (Valium)] and in patients in pain, titrated doses of a narcotic are certainly justified. However, only after the above factors (1) through (5) have been ruled out, or attempts have begun to correct them, would it be rational to seek synchronization by heavy sedation with hypnotics or narcotics or by using neuromuscular blocking agents. Softening doses of neuromuscular blocking agents are sometimes necessary when spontaneous respiratory drive is very strong (for instance, in fulminating pulmonary edema) and are essential when bucking and fighting the ventilator can be instantaneously destructive to the brain or can induce hypoxemia (e.g., in patients following head injury or brain surgery). Under such circumstances, full curarization in skilled hands should permit prompt, smooth CV with a search for a correction of the factors underlying asynchronization.

Muscle relaxants used may be of the depolarizing type (succinylcholine) or nondepolarizing (curare, pancuronium). These drugs partially or completely paralyze all skeletal muscles, including the respiratory muscles, depending on the dose and mode of administration. When needed in the conscious person, their use should be preceded by a sedative or narcotic, since paralysis in the conscious state is at best unpleasant, and with succinylcholine it is painful. Because of its rapid onset of action, succinylcholine is commonly used to facilitate endotracheal intubation, to terminate laryngospasm, and to promptly block excessive diaphragmatic movements or convulsions.

Since succinylcholine induces muscle fasciculations prior to paralysis, and thus may cause life-threatening arrhythmias from acute hyperkalemia and postparalysis muscle pain, its use is often preceded by a small dose of curare (3 mg.), which can block these fasciculations. An apneic dose of succinylcholine is approximately 0.5 mg./kg. BW. Because it is short-acting, its use in resuscitation and intensive care is commonly via intermittent intravenous infusion of a solution containing 2 mg./ml.

Curare (approximate single "softening" dose 0.1 mg./kg. BW; fully apneic dose 0.5 mg./kg. BW) and pancuronium (approximate single "softening" dose 0.02 mg./kg. BW; fully apneic dose 0.1 mg./kg. BW) have longer duration of action (about one-half hour or more). Curare tends to lower arterial pressure because of its ganglionic blocking effect and possible histamine release; whereas the use of pancuronium is sometimes associated with hypertension and tachycardia. Myasthenia, aminoglycoside antibiotics, and acidosis augment the effect of nondepolarizing relaxants.

The most important factor in treating the conscious patient who is fighting the ventilator is *coaching* by an understanding, sympathetic physician, nurse, or therapist. Sometimes "bucking" the tube can be ameliorated with a topical anesthetic (e.g., lidocaine 4 per cent, 3 ml.) instilled into the tracheobronchial tree.

HYPOVENTILATION, HYPERVENTILATION

Spontaneous *hypoventilation* is the principal indication for artificial ventilation. Patients on mechanical ventilation can unexpectedly hypoventilate and thereby develop hypoxemia and hypercarbia, because of ventilator malfunction, accidental disconnection, or tube obstruction. Other causes of unexpected hypoventilation include sudden increase in ventilatory demands without change in minute volume, as for instance, in fever, convulsions, restlessness, or increase in deadspace from pulmonary embolism. Furthermore, patients on pressure-set ventilators hypoventilate when airway resistance increases or lung-chest compliance decreases. Therefore, chest movement, FIO_2, PaO_2, and $PaCO_2$ should be monitored as continuously as possible. With presently available technology, the best continuous monitoring available is a "baby-sitter," who could be an instructed, intelligent lay person; a "baby-sitter" should be provided for every patient on MV and should be instructed to call for help and switch to ventilation by bag whenever there is any question about chest movements, constancy of minute volume, tidal volume, or oxygenation.

The final determinant of hypoventilation, namely, increased $PaCO_2$, can be evaluated intermittently. End-tidal PCO_2, which can be monitored continuously with an infrared CO_2 analyzer, closely approximates arterial PCO_2 in normal lungs and is usually lower in abnormal lungs. However, even in patients with abnormal lungs, end-tidal PCO_2 changes in the same direction as $PaCO_2$ and therefore end-tidal PCO_2 is a useful tool for continuous monitoring of alveolar ventilation, at least in patients on MV who are not yet stabilized. Manufacturers should provide us with alarm systems triggered by extremes of end-tidal PCO_2.

Spontaneous *hyperventilation* resulting in hypocarbia occurs frequently in critically ill patients whose breathing movements are driven by CNS acidosis (e.g., head injury, post-ischemic brain damage), over-all tissue acidosis (shock), various external stimuli, anxiety, or other factors. Moderate spontaneous hyperventilation ($PaCO_2$ 25 to 35 torr) may be permitted to persist unless there is a clinical picture of excessive work of breathing, in which case mechanical ventilation should be instituted, since spontaneous ventilatory efforts themselves may add to the acidosis or result in exhaustion with sudden apnea. $PaCO_2$ values much below 25 torr may be harmful in themselves. Severe hypocarbia caused by controlled ventilation should be avoided, not only because it is usually produced by high ventilation volumes and airway pressures which may result in circulatory depression but because of the effect of hypocarbia itself. On the other hand, moderate hypocarbia ($PaCO_2$ 25 to 35 torr) is often advantageous, at least transiently, to initiate controlled ventilation for the patient "fighting the ventilator" and in patients with increased intracranial pressure.

The *disadvantages* of hypocarbia include decreased cardiac output; respiratory alkalemia with a shift to the left of the oxyhemoglobin dissociation curve and impaired oxygen release in the capillaries; decreased cerebral blood flow; increased oxygen consumption and an increase in cardiac dysrhythmias, probably related to the high pHa. There is a high mortality in ICU patients with prolonged alkalemia.

CIRCULATORY EFFECTS

While controlled ventilation with IPPV has been around since the fifteenth century (Vasalius, Paracelsus), the ability of IPPV to decrease cardiac output has not been reported until this century (Moore et al., 1935; Werko, 1947; Cournand et al., 1948). There is, however, no decrease in cardiac output when IPPV is carried out with return of airway pressure to atmospheric during an expiratory phase that is maintained at least as long as the inflation phase. Further, as the elevated intrathoracic pressure reduces venous return to the heart, there is a compensatory venous pressure rise due to constriction of capacitance vessels tending to reverse the original alteration toward normal. This effect can, if necessary, be artificially induced with the use of vasopressors.

The tendency of increased mean intrathoracic pressure to decrease cardiac output is greater when there is hypovolemia. Also, the critically ill patient may react differently to positive pressure than the normal individual, and some critically ill patients with stiff lungs may actually increase their cardiac output during positive pressure ventilation (Beach et al., 1973). Reduction of cardiac output due to a decrease in pHa itself is rare, unless the acidosis is severe (pHa 7.1 or less). However, $PaCO_2$ changes in themselves, independent of pHa changes, may alter cardiac output (Prys-Roberts et al., 1968). Moderately increased $PaCO_2$ results in increased cardiac output, probably due to catecholamine release.

Most early ventilators could produce negative end-expiratory pressure (NEEP) to compensate for the net increase in intrathoracic pressure during IPPV. NEEP results in an increase in central blood volume, stroke volume, and cardiac output. However, applying negative pressure to the airway often leads to a decrease in PaO_2, probably as a result of closure of small airways with air-trapping and perhaps pulmonary edema. Therefore, NEEP is rarely indicated or used today.

The deleterious circulatory effects of MV can easily be avoided by adhering to the principle that IPPV in patients with normal lungs should permit an expiratory pause at atmospheric pressure of at least as long as the inflation phase; and in patients with abnormal lungs, IPPV should optimize positive pressure patterns, particularly PEEP.

The prevention and treatment of *hypocarbia* during MV should focus on decreasing the respiratory rate rather than the tidal volume, which should not be below 8 ml./kg. BW and preferably should be 10 to 15 ml./kg. (10 to 12 ml./kg. should be the limit with PEEP). However, decreasing the rate of the ventilator may provoke the patient to escape from controlled ventilation, with the subsequent necessity of using heavy sedation or curarization to restore CV. In ARDS patients, further rate decreases may lead to undesirable decrease in PaO_2. If decreasing ventilator minute volume cannot be performed safely because it would also decrease PaO_2, then one may add *mechanical deadspace* to the ventilator tubing, increase the PCO_2 in the inspired gas, or switch to IMV. Slow, gradual addition of mechanical deadspace to the ventilator tubing is the most common way of controlling PaCO$_2$. Up to 500 ml. of deadspace tube may be necessary, placed between the ventilator's non-rebreathing valve (or Y tube) and the tracheal or tracheostomy tube, to increase PaCO$_2$ to the desired level. The desired PaCO$_2$ in part depends on the need to normalize arterial pH. The deadspace added should not exceed 50 per cent of tidal volume.

An elegant method for *PaCO$_2$ normalization* is use of the CO$_2$ mixer for control of FICO$_2$, usually available as an adjunct to the air-oxygen mixers (Veriflo, Bird). This is a simple and less hazardous technique (Breivik et al., 1973). CO$_2$ concentrations of 0.5 to 3 per cent are bled into the inspired gas to *optimize* PaCO$_2$. Notably, the optimal PaCO$_2$ may be above normal values in patients with COPD and in those with metabolic alkalemia; and somewhat below "normal" in patients with metabolic acidema or intracranial problems.

In patients with hypocarbia on MV, PaCO$_2$ optimization or normalization is particularly indicated in cases of ARDS, COPD, and metabolic alkalemia. Adding deadspace or FICO$_2$ is contraindicated in patients with intracranial hypertension, CSF acidosis, severe cardiogenic shock, metabolic acidemia and in those on spontaneous breathing, assisted ventilation, or IMV. Like oxygen, CO$_2$ should be used as a drug, whether administered passively by rebreathing or actively by admixture, the dose carefully titrated according to blood gases and the clinical picture (ideally to cardiac output). CO$_2$ normalization often increases cardiac output (both heart rate and stroke volume), probably through the mechanism of sympathetic discharge. CO$_2$ is also a bronchodilator and a vasodilator. Overdosage leads first to hyperventilation in the spontaneously breathing patient (who may fight the ventilator) and later to respiratory depression. The heart initially will be stimulated but with higher doses of CO$_2$ may fail. Cardiac failure is not in itself a contraindication to PaCO$_2$ normalization, but one must bear in mind that patients in cardiogenic shock may react paradoxically with a decrease rather than an increase in cardiac output.

The best results with PaCO$_2$ normalization have been seen in hypoxemic patients with ARDS who are on MV with PEEP; PaCO$_2$ normalization counteracts the circulatory depressant effects of PEEP and by increasing cardiac output, in turn increases PaO$_2$ and makes a reduction of FIO$_2$ to safe levels possible.

BAROTRAUMA

If a pneumothorax occurs in a patient on MV, it may rapidly become a tension pneumothorax with severe decrease in venous return and cardiac output. If not treated immediately, this complication is usually lethal. Barotrauma may also lead to interstitial emphysema with or without secondary effects on the cardiovascular system. In addition, ruptured alveoli may permit gas to enter the pulmonary veins and left side of the heart, causing systemic arterial air embolism; this in turn can cause sudden ventricular fibrillation from coronary gas embolism and coma, convulsions, apnea, arrhythmias, and hypotension from cerebral gas embolism. In infants, interstitial gas may dissect into the pericardial sac and cause tamponade. The likelihood of barotrauma is enhanced by abnormal lungs (particularly ARDS and COPD), high airway pressures, and ventilatory patterns that promote excessive alveolar distention. Gas can also dissect from the mediastinum or the pleural space into the peritoneal space, either through small holes in the diaphragm (congenital abnormality) or by breaking through pleural and peritoneal surfaces, causing pneumoperitoneum and abdominal distention.

Interstitial gas under pressure can compress intrapulmonary airways and vessels, cause ventilation-perfusion mismatching, and together with tension pneumothorax and atelectasis, result in cardiac arrest from hypoxemia plus "obstructive shock." Prevention and treatment include rapid pleural drainage and a compromising reduction in airway pressure with short-term FIO$_2$ 1.0 to give the leaking lung tissue a chance to seal.

ACID-BASE BALANCE

General Considerations

The modest hydrogen ion exerts a quiet tyranny over the organism, dictating a myriad of complex interactions among lungs, kidneys, and a retinue of chemical buffer systems. The surveillance of hydrogen ion concentration, and the attendant maintainance of acid-base equilibrium, are therefore one of the grandest cooperative ventures of the body.

Even under normal conditions of primarily aerobic metabolism, the body produces an excess of acid which must be neutralized or eliminated in order to maintain the internal environment at a near constant pH. Normally the body produces two forms of acid: volatile carbonic acid (H_2CO_3, about 20,000 mEq. produced every 24 hours) and fixed, nonvolatile organic acids (50 to 70 mEq. produced every 24 hours). To deal with this acid load, the body employs three principal mechanisms: buffering, pulmonary excretion, and renal excretion.

The most rapidly acting of these defense mechanisms is the *buffer system* in the extracellular fluid, which acts within seconds; intracellular buffering occurs within hours. The *respiratory mechanism*, through which excess carbonic acid is excreted in the form of CO_2, works within minutes, while the *renal mechanism*, which accounts for excretion of bicarbonate and fixed acids (40 per cent titratable acids, 60 per cent ammonia) requires hours to days. Clearly, any dysfunction of the lungs or kidneys thus implies potential disruption of acid-base equilibrium.

The interactions among participating organ systems have their physiochemical basis in the relationship expressed by the Henderson-Hasselbalch equation:

$$pH = pK + \log \frac{[HCO_3^-]}{[H_2CO_3]}$$

where K is the dissociation constant of carbonic acid. In solving this equation for its various unknowns, we learn a great deal about the state of both respiratory and metabolic components of the acid-base system.

To begin with, the *pK* is assumed to be that of the predominant buffer system in the body, bicarbonate; i.e., pK = 6.1. Thus, the equation becomes:

$$pH = 6.1 + \log \frac{[HCO_3^-]}{[H_2CO_3]}$$

The *pH* is measured directly, via electrode, from a sample of arterial blood, as previously described. We are left then with the carbonic acid and bicarbonate concentrations.

Carbonic acid cannot be readily measured. However, its equilibrium with carbon dioxide and water lies far to the right, most carbonic acid in the body being in the form of dissolved CO_2 (the usual H_2CO_3/CO_2 ratio is about 1:100). Therefore, we do not err significantly by rewriting our equation as follows:

$$pH = 6.1 + \log \frac{[HCO_3^-]}{[CO_2]}$$

Notably, the concentration of CO_2 dissolved in the blood bears a constant relationship to the P_{CO_2}:

$$[CO_2] = a \times P_{CO_2}$$

where a = 0.031.
Again rewriting our equation, then:

$$pH = 6.1 + \log \frac{[HCO_3^-]}{0.031 \times P_{CO_2}}$$

We now have an equation we can solve, for the pH and P_{CO_2} are both readily measured in a sample of arterial blood, and the bicarbonate can then be calculated. The equation also provides a useful way of examining the metabolic and respiratory components of acid-base problems, for it is clear from the equation that an isolated decrease in bicarbonate will lower pH (metabolic acidemia), and an increase in bicarbonate will raise the pH (metabolic alkalemia) — while an isolated increase in P_{CO_2} will lower the pH (respiratory acidemia) and a decrease in P_{CO_2} will raise the pH (respiratory alkalemia).

The only drawback to this way of looking at things is that P_{CO_2} and HCO_3^- are not independent variables; the latter reflects changes in the former and this is not, in itself, a reliable measure of solely the metabolic component of an acid-base problem. In evaluating any given stage of acid-base equilibrium, what we would really like to know is, "What would the bicarbonate be if the P_{CO_2} were normal (P_{CO_2} = 40 torr)?" Under these circumstances, an abnormality in bicarbonate could clearly be ascribed only to a metabolic aberration. In clinical situations of complex acid-base disturbances, it is rarely possible to normalize the patient's arterial PCO_2 for the purpose of making such measurements. However, we *can* normalize the PCO_2 of an aliquot of the patient, i.e., his arterial blood sample. In a method known as the Astrup technique, the patient's arterial blood is equilibrated against known gas standards of high and low PCO_2. From these measurements, the bicarbonate at $PCO_2 = 40$ torr, i.e., the *standard bicarbonate* (SB) is derived, and it reflects solely the metabolic component of the patient's acid-base problem, since the respiratory component has, on paper at least, been entirely corrected. A clinically useful estimate of the standard bicarbonate can be made, without invoking the Astrup technique, by using the Sigaard-Andersen curve nomogram, which relates standard bicarbonate to measured pH, PCO_2 and hemoglobin (Fig. 15).

A useful derivative of the standard bicarbonate, reported in lieu of the latter by many laboratories, is the so-called *base deficit*, which is essentially an expression of how many milliequivalents of bicarbonate would be required to bring 1 liter of blood back to normal pH.

Let us examine for a moment the manner in which these values are used in practice. Given only three parameters from the laboratory—the arterial pH, arterial PCO_2 and standard bicarbonate (or base deficit)—one can reliably diagnose any acid-base disorder, without recourse to complex diagrams or tables. The pH, to begin with, tells us whether the patient has an acidemia or alkalemia. We next examine the PCO_2 and standard bicarbonate (base deficit) to determine which of these would account for the observed alteration in pH. If the direction of change in the PCO_2 is consistent with the change in pH, the site of the lesion is respiratory (in which case physiologic compensation will be renal). If, on the other hand, the pH change can be accounted for by the change in standard bicarbonate (base deficit), the site of the lesion is metabolic (and physiologic compensation will be respiratory).

A few examples will demonstrate the use of this approach:

Patient 1: pHa = 7.55; $PaCO_2$ = 22; standard bicarbonate (SB) = 23; base deficit (BD) = +1 (base excess, BE, = -1).

The pH is elevated; therefore, the patient has an alkalemia. The only value which will account for this alkalemia is that of the PCO_2, which is depressed. Furthermore, the standard bicarbonate and base deficit are normal, indicating there is no metabolic compensation. *Conclusion*: Uncompensated respiratory alkalemia.

Patient 2: pHa = 7.49; $PaCO_2$ = 20; SB = 20; BD = 5 (BE = -5).

The pH is slightly elevated; thus, the patient has an alkalemia. Again, this alkalemia can be accounted for by the depressed PCO_2, hence the site of the lesion is respiratory. The standard bicarbonate is slightly depressed (the base deficit is increased), indicating metabolic compensation. *Conclusion:* Compensated respiratory alkalemia.

Patient 3: pHa = 7.45; $PaCO_2$ = 80; SB = 46; BD = -17 (BE = +17).

The pH is normal. However, the patient has a markedly elevated PCO_2 and thus, by all accounts, should have a respiratory acidemia. The standard bicarbonate is elevated (base deficit is negative; i.e., there is a base excess), perhaps reflecting metabolic compensation. *Conclusion:* Compensated respiratory acidemia? WRONG! This was a trick. You must not be seduced by numbers into forgetting fundamental principles of physiology. Physiologic regulation is based on servomechanisms that require an imbalance in the system to be activated; thus, compensation is never perfect. The normal pH in this patient reflects a combined respiratory acidemia and metabolic alkalemia.

Patient 4: pHa = 7.06; $PaCO_2$ = 39; SB = 10; BD = +19 (BE = -19).

The pH is markedly depressed; therefore, the patient is acidemic. The acidemia can be accounted for by the decrease in standard bicarbonate (increase in base deficit), hence it is a metabolic acidemia. Since the PCO_2 is in the normal range, there is no respiratory compensation. *Conclusion:* Uncompensated metabolic acidemia.

That is fine, as far as it goes, but one has to ask *why* a patient with such a profound acidemia is not hyperventilating. Is there some reason for respiratory depression as well? Again, it is a matter of not letting the

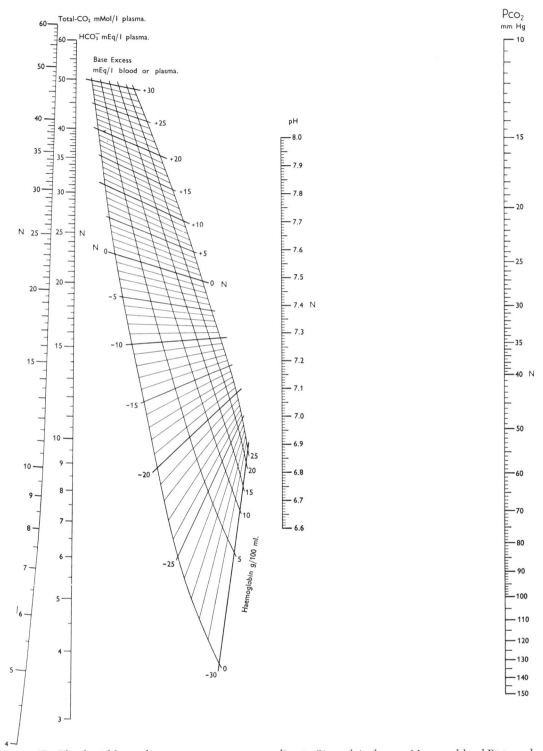

Figure 15   Blood acid-base alignment nomogram according to Sigaard-Andersen. Measure blood P_{CO_2} and pH with appropriate electrodes. Connect values and read bicarbonate concentration in milliequivalents per liter (left). Determine hemoglobin and read base-excess where P_{CO_2}–pH–bicarbonate line crosses the base-excess nomogram at the appropriate hemoglobin concentration. N: normal. This nomogram is designed for use with blood 38°C. (From Sigaard-Andersen: Scand. J. Clin. Lab. Invest., *15*:211, 1963; also see Severinghaus, J.: Chapter 61 in Handbook of Physiology, Vol. II, Sec. 3, Respiration. American Physiology Society, 1965.)

TABLE 1 Disturbances of Acid-Base Balance

Condition	pHa	PaCO$_2$	Standard HCO$_3^-$	BD	Compensatory Mechanism	Treatment	Examples
1. Metabolic acidemia						Buffers	Shock–cardiac arrest Diabetic ketoacidosis Diarrhea
uncompensated	↓↓	normal	↓↓	↑↑			
compensated	↓	↓	↓↓	↑↑	Respiratory	(hyperventilation?)	Renal failure
2. Respiratory acidemia						Increase minute ventilation	Hypoventilation
uncompensated	↓↓	↑↑	normal	none			
compensated	↓	↑↑	↑	↓	Renal		
3. Metabolic alkalemia						Administration of acids Prevention of Cl loss Modest hypoventilation	Vomiting Bicarbonate administration
uncompensated	↑↑	normal	↑↑	↓↓			
compensated	↑	slightly ↑	↑↑	↓↓	Minimal respiratory		
4. Respiratory alkalemia							Hyperventilation
uncompensated	↑↑	↓↓	normal	none			
compensated	↑	↓↓	↓	↑	Renal	PaCO$_2$ normalization by controlled ventilation, addition of deadspace, or FICO$_2$	

Note: Box indicates site of lesion.

numbers obscure the physiology. A patient with profound metabolic acidemia should be hyperventilating; if not, something else is profoundly wrong as well.

In the remainder of this section, we shall deal with specific disturbances in acid-base equilibrium (Table 1).

Specific Disturbances in Acid-Base Equilibrium

It is perhaps helpful to preface our discussion of specific acid-base disturbances with a few general *rules of thumb:*
• When the site of an acid-base lesion is respiratory, *physiologic compensation* is renal; when the site of the lesion is metabolic, physiologic compensation is respiratory.
• *Therapeutic intervention,* on the other hand, is usually undertaken in the same mode as the pathophysiologic disturbance; i.e., metabolic lesions are treated with metabolic interventions, while respiratory lesions are corrected by manipulation of ventilation.
• When the numbers reported by the laboratory are at variance with the *clinical*

impression, take another look at the patient and, if necessary, repeat the laboratory determination. Even derangements of acid-base equilibrium proceed from logical mechanisms and should therefore be amenable to logical explanation. If they are not, something is wrong with the measurement or the reasoning process or both.

METABOLIC ACIDEMIA

Metabolic acidemia arises when there is excessive accumulation of acids, loss of bicarbonate, or some combination of the two. Its multiple etiologies may be conveniently classified according to the scheme of Kassirer, which is based upon the unmeasured anions: "anion gap" = $Na^+ - (Cl^- + CO_2$ content).

Normal unmeasured anions
(8–12 mEq./liter)

Serum K$^+$ typically low:
   diarrhea
   carbonic anhydrase inhibition
   renal tubular acidosis
Serum K$^+$ typically high:
   ammonium chloride administration
   chronic pyelonephritis
   obstructive uropathy

Increased unmeasured anions
(> 12 mEq./liter)

Serum K+ normal or increased:
  diabetic ketoacidosis
  alcoholic ketoacidosis
  lactic acidosis
  salicylate intoxication
  methanol poisoning
  paraldehyde ingestion
  ethylene glycol poisoning
  renal failure

Metabolic acidemia is *diagnosed* when the arterial pH is depressed and the base deficit elevated (standard bicarbonate depressed). $PaCO_2$ may or may not be depressed, depending on the state of compensation. To be more explicit, etiologic diagnosis requires a careful history as well as measurement of blood sugar, ketones, lactate, creatinine, and electrolytes and calculation of the anion gap. These ancillary measurements have considerable importance, since identification of the cause in metabolic acidemia strongly influences the choice of therapeutic strategies (Table 2).

The intact human machine attempts its *compensation* of metabolic acidemia first through a rapidly acting respiratory mechanism, i.e., hyperventilation. Indeed, the presence of hyperventilation in a critically ill or injured patient should always prompt investigation of that patient's acid-base status and not be merely written off as due to anxiety or respiratory embarrassment. More long-range physiologic compensation of metabolic acidemia falls to the kidneys, which increase both their reabsorption of bicarbonate and their excretion of titratable acid and

TABLE 2   *Types of Metabolic Acidemia*

TYPE OF ACIDEMIA	HISTORY	CLINICAL	LABORATORY	THERAPY
diabetic ketoacidosis	• often insulin-dependent • antecedent stress, illness, missed insulin	nausea, vomiting dehydration Kussmaul breathing coma polyuria	hyperglycemia ketonemia/ketouria hyperkalemia ↑ anion gap	• hydration, vigorous • titrated insulin • rarely, bicarbonate
alcoholic ketoacidosis	• young chronic alcoholics • drinking binge • anorexia, hyperemesis • usually seen about 48 hr. after cessation of drinking	vomiting semicoma	near-normal blood sugar marked ketosis ↑ anion gap	• glucose • vigorous hydration • insulin not necessary • occasionally bicarbonate
lactic acidosis	• r/o phenformin • r/o underlying malignancy	toxic	elevated serum lactate and lactate/pyruvate ↑ anion gap	• massive doses of bicarbonate • hydration with diuresis • may need dialysis
salicylate intoxication	• 80% pediatric • suicide attempt	early hyperventilation hyperthermia dehydration delirium, seizures	salicylate level over 50 mg./100 ml. ↑ anion gap	• hydration with forced diuresis • cautious bicarbonate • external cooling • gastric lavage/emesis
methanol poisoning	• usually chronic alcoholic	asymptomatic latent period 8–36 hr. headache, vertigo vomiting abdominal, back pain dyspnea, apnea peripheral vasoconstriction coma blindness	methanol/formate in blood and urine mild ketonemia albuminuria ↑ anion gap	• vigorous bicarbonate • hydration • ethanol • dialysis
ethylene glycol poisoning	• chronic alcoholic • pediatric	euphoria followed by deepening coma tachycardia paralysis respiratory distress renal failure	↑ anion gap	• emesis/lavage • oxygen • titrated bicarbonate

ammonia. Blood buffering through exchange of H$^+$ and K$^+$ ions is minimally effective, although it may induce profound changes in serum K$^+$ concentrations.

Therapeutic intervention in metabolic acidemia is directed principally at the metabolic side of the equation, through replacement of bicarbonate lost directly or consumed in buffering. In general, efforts to augment respiratory compensation, by increasing the patient's minute ventilation, are ill-considered, since they fail to deal with the underlying problem and indeed may exacerbate the metabolic acidemia.

The treatment of choice for metabolic acidemia is sodium bicarbonate. There are exceptions and modifications to this—some of which we shall deal with shortly—but as a general rule of thumb, it is a good one. Sodium bicarbonate directly replenishes the body's base deficit, which is fundamentally a bicarbonate deficit, and has no significant disadvantages when compared with other alkalinizing agents. The volume and rate of bicarbonate administration will depend upon the etiology and severity of the acidemia. Lactic acidemia, for example, may require enormous doses of bicarbonate administered over a short period of time, while the acidemia of decompensated diabetes may require little or no bicarbonate therapy. In general, however, plasma bicarbonate levels below 5 to 8 mEq./liter are very dangerous since, at these levels, compensatory hyperventilation will be strained to its maximum limits, and therefore any further fall in plasma bicarbonate will be attended by a severe pH reduction. Thus, in severe metabolic acidemia from whatever cause, sodium bicarbonate should be administered with the aim of raising the plasma bicarbonate to around 10 to 14 mEq./liter within the first several hours. A more rapid, acute correction of plasma bicarbonate is unnecessary and may, indeed, have adverse consequences, such as acidification of the spinal fluid with deterioration in neurologic status and overcorrection, with subsequent metabolic alkalemia.

The mEq. of bicarbonate required to bring base excess to zero equals the base deficit (in mEq./L.) times 1/5 of body weight (which approximates the ECF in liters):

$$\text{mEq. } HCO_3^- \text{ required} = BD \times \frac{BW}{5}$$

For example, with a base deficit of 20 mEq./L. in a 60-kg. adult, 20 × 60/5 (i.e.,

240) mEq. of $NaHCO_3$ given intravenously (best in a 1 mEq./ml. solution) will usually bring the base deficit to zero, at least transiently. Bicarbonate infusion should be slow to minimize red blood cell damage and hyperosmolality. Caution should also be exercised to correct hypokalemia, if present, before administering a bicarbonate load. In existing hyperventilation, overbreathing should be slowed down after the initial CO_2 load from bicarbonate has been exhaled, lest an overshoot of pHa occur. In most cases of metabolic acidemia treatment of the cause (e.g., shock) and pHa normalization (in the presence of moderate hyperventilation, i.e., $PaCO_2$ 25–35 torr) should receive priority over correction of calculated base deficit. Even with the best of calculations, however, the results of alkali therapy are not reliably predictable; thus arterial pH, $PaCO_2$ and base deficit or standard bicarbonate must be measured frequently after initiation of bicarbonate treatment and further therapy *titrated* accordingly. Once the plasma bicarbonate has reached the level of 10 to 14 mEq./liter, a somewhat more leisurely approach may be taken in further correction, assuming that the underlying cause of excess acid production has been brought under control.

Special problems arise when bicarbonate therapy must be undertaken in patients with certain underlying pathologic conditions—most notably patients with pre-existing volume overload (e.g., cardiac failure) or patients with severe potassium deficiency. In the first instance, the additional sodium load which administration of sodium bicarbonate imposes may precipitate severe cardiac decompensation and must therefore be offset by counterbalancing interventions. Peritoneal dialysis often provides an effective solution to this problem, for dialysis not only induces a contraction of intravascular volume but also, through absorption of lactate across the peritoneal membrane, yields an immediate source of bicarbonate. Hemodialysis and plasmapheresis (using sodium bicarbonate to replace sodium losses) have also been used successfully in this situation. In the second instance, i.e., patients with coexisting severe acidemia and severe hypokalemia, correction of acidemia requires the most delicate titration; for administration of bicarbonate without adequate potassium replacement can lead to highly arrhythmogenic degrees of further hypokalemia, while potassium replacement without correction of acidemia can provoke equally lethal degrees of hyperkalemia. For this reason, bicarbonate and potassium should, in these circumstances, be administered simultaneously (through separate infusions), with careful monitoring of the electrocardiogram as well as serum K^+ and arterial blood gases.

A word about alkalinizing agents other than sodium bicarbonate. *Sodium lactate* has been used effectively in the treatment of metabolic acidemia. However, it offers no advantages over sodium bicarbonate and has the potential disadvantage that it requires an intact cellular mechanism for oxidation of the lactate anion; thus sodium lactate may be minimally effective in patients with lactic acidosis, hepatic dysfunction or low flow states. Tris(hydroxymethyl)aminomethane *(THAM)* is an amine proton acceptor which has been advanced for the treatment of a number of acidemic states. In the context of metabolic acidemia, tris buffer probably offers no advantage over sodium bicarbonate, and the alkalinity of intravenous solutions of tris buffer carries certain hazards in terms of local tissue reaction. Because it contains no sodium, tris buffer may have a role in the treatment of metabolic acidemia coexisting with states of sodium and water retention. When used, tris buffer must be administered through a large-bore needle or catheter in 0.3 molar solution. Average dose used is 0.14 ml./kg./min. Careful titration, with monitoring of arterial pH and PCO_2, is required. THAM is available as a powder, which must be dissolved just before use; this limits its value in emergencies.

RESPIRATORY ACIDEMIA

Respiratory acidemia is seen in the context of hypoventilation, with consequent accumulation of carbonic acid. Clinically, it arises in any circumstance in which minute ventilation is insufficient to remove carbon dioxide generated by metabolism — most commonly in pathologic conditions that impair central control of respiration, respiratory muscle function, or integrity of the airways.

Respiratory acidemia is *diagnosed* when the arterial pH is depressed and the $PaCO_2$ is elevated. Base deficit may or may not be reduced (standard bicarbonate elevated), depending on the degree of metabolic compensation.

The acute *compensatory response* to hypercapnia consists almost entirely of tissue buffering, which is minimally effective in raising plasma bicarbonate levels; thus, in the acute phases of severe hypercapnia, rapid rises in $PaCO_2$ may be associated with severe acidemia. Hypercapnia developing over a more prolonged period, however, as in patients with COPD, is compensated through renal mechanisms (decreased excretion of bicarbonate; increased excretion of titratable acid, ammonium, and chloride) and thus may be associated with only modest degrees of acidemia.

Therapy in acute respiratory acidemia is primarily aimed at *improving ventilation*, the techniques of which have been described in an earlier section. Adjunctive alkali therapy is generally not warranted, but may be appropriate and even life-saving in extreme respiratory acidemia, severe mixed (respiratory and metabolic) acidemia, and in acidemia associated with status asthmaticus. In these circumstances, modest doses of sodium *bicarbonate* may transiently elevate the arterial pH to safer levels until the respiratory lesion can be repaired (Chapter 3).

Because of its ability to buffer carbonic acid, THAM has been advanced as an effective means of treating respiratory acidemia. However, in chronic pulmonary insufficiency, tris buffer depresses ventilation, leading to further hypoxemia and an increase in $PaCO_2$, which offsets the tris-induced fall in carbonic acid. Thus, tris buffers can be safely used in this context only if ventilation is mechanically assisted or controlled.

METABOLIC ALKALEMIA

Metabolic alkalemia reflects a relative or absolute increase in the plasma bicarbonate and may have multiple causes, including the following:
- iatrogenic (overzealous administration of bicarbonate)
- loss of chloride as HCl (vomiting, nasogastric suction)
- increased urinary acid excretion
- severe potassium deficiency
- endocrine disorder (hyperaldosteronism, Bartter's syndrome, Cushing's syndrome)

Metabolic alkalemia is *diagnosed* by an elevated arterial pH and base excess (elevated standard bicarbonate). Arterial PCO_2 may show modest elevation if compensatory mechanisms are active. However, the respiratory *compensation* for metabolic alkalemia is usually quite limited, for in general the organism, because of concomitant hypoxemia, is disinclined to cease breathing merely in order to correct an acid-base disturbance. Nonetheless, there are exceptions, and several hundred cases of respiratory failure secondary to metabolic alkalemia have been reported in the literature (cf., for example, Steer et al., Tuller et al., Lifschitz et al.).

Therapy of metabolic alkalemia requires repletion of *chloride ion*. In mild cases, slow correction may be accomplished by administration of chloride as sodium chloride and potassium chloride, which correct alkalemia by suppressing renal acid excretion and promoting renal alkali excretion. In cases of extreme metabolic alkalemia, however, these measures are too slow, and the administration of mineral acid is also required. If available, L-arginine monohydrochloride is the parenteral preparation of choice, and several hundred milliequivalents can be given intravenously over 24 hours. Ammonium chloride or dilute (0.1 N) hydrochloric acid may also be used, although the rate of administration is limited in the former case by CNS toxicity and in the latter by local tissue reaction. The dose of mineral acid required may be estimated according to the following equation:

mEq. acid required =
    0.25 × body weight (kg.) × base excess

Again, as in the treatment of metabolic acidemia, this is just an estimate, and electrolytes and arterial blood gases must be closely monitored. In cases in which significant losses of gastric juice play a role in the alkalemia, the composition and volume of these losses should also be measured and appropriately replaced.

Patients with severe metabolic alkalemia usually have marked *potassium* and *volume* depletion as well—sometimes requiring as much as 4 to 6 liters of isotonic saline and 400 to 600 mEq. of potassium chloride during the first 24 hours.

In patients being treated with mechanical ventilation and oxygen, extreme degrees of metabolic alkalemia may be transiently mitigated by introducing a component of respiratory acidemia. This is best accomplished by adding mechanical deadspace to the ventilator apparatus or by increasing the inspired concentration of carbon dioxide

(see pp. 300–301); and raise FIO_2. Such deliberate hypercarbia is a stop-gap measure only, and definitive correction of metabolic alkalemia will still require chloride repletion.

RESPIRATORY ALKALEMIA

Respiratory alkalemia is the result of hyperventilation, which in turn may come about from anxiety, central nervous system impairment, attempts to compensate metabolic acidemia, or excessive minute ventilation on a mechanical ventilator. It is *diagnosed* when the arterial pH is elevated and the $PaCO_2$ depressed. Acute *compensation* is minimal, but over several hours to days, renal compensatory mechanisms may lead to a base deficit (depression of standard bicarbonate).

Therapy of respiratory alkalemia depends in part upon the cause but in general it is aimed at normalizing the arterial PCO_2. In anxious patients, who often present to the emergency room with circumoral paresthesias and carpopedal spasm, rebreathing into a bag or deadspace tube with oxygen may be all that is required to enable reaccumulation of CO_2. When patients being maintained on MV demonstrate marked respiratory alkalemia and high ventilation volumes are required for oxygenation, addition of mechanical deadspace or an increase in the inspired concentration of CO_2 ($FICO_2$) may be required (see pp. 300–301). Reductions in minute ventilation should be undertaken with caution, and usually at the expense of rate rather than tidal volume, since extreme reductions in tidal volume may lead to atelectasis, hypoxemia, and all the complications thereof.

LONG-TERM AIRWAY CARE

Natural Airway, Physiotherapy

A patent airway is the first prerequisite to respiratory care. One of the most significant threats to a patent airway is coma. Thus, in the unconscious patient, the steps of emergency airway control should be pursued as quickly as possible until the airway is open (Chap. 9). These steps include noninvasive methods from backward tilt of the head to the triple airway maneuver and cannulating techniques through tracheal intubation. The comatose patient should eventually receive a tracheal tube unless he has intact protective upper airway reflexes and can be attended by a knowledgeable "baby-sitter" at all times. If he is to be observed for long periods, the nonintubated, stuporous or comatose patient may be placed in the stable side (NATO) position, with the head tilted backward in order to promote drainage of liquid foreign matter from the mouth. He should not be placed prone. If he is an accident victim, he is better maintained in a horizontal position, supine, with head, neck, and chest in alignment, moderate backward tilt of the head, and if necessary, forward displacement of the mandible; turning may aggravate a spinal injury.

A conscious patient with a natural airway may need clearing of tracheal secretions. This may be aided by humidification (particularly if he is a mouth breather), coughing, suctioning, and physiotherapy.

Coughing may be voluntary (if necessary by coaching) or by reflex. The normal cough mechanism includes a deep inhalation, closure of the glottis, intrapulmonary pressure build-up (as high as 100 torr) through contraction of abdominal and intercostal muscles, and sudden opening of the vocal cords, allowing an expulsive air jet to carry secretions and other foreign matter upward. With reduced vital capacity (lack of pre-cough deep inhalation), the cough becomes less effective. Also, in COPD in which the retractile force of elastic fibers on the intrapulmonary airways is lacking, expulsive coughing should be practiced at very high lung volumes and with short bursts. Obviously, stupor from disease or drugs impairs reflex coughing, and pain during deep inhalation or exhalation impairs voluntary coughing. The latter calls for carefully titrated analgesia; teaching the patient to cough with manual support of the surgical incision is also helpful. In patients with CNS depression short of deep coma, clearing of tracheobronchial secretions by coughing can be stimulated by finger pressure against the trachea just above the sternal notch.

The effect of coaching may be augmented by *sighing* methods that force deep breaths, such as inflations by bag-mask, CO_2 rebreathing tube, or properly applied IPPB. Additional methods to be considered include blind nasotracheal suctioning, instillation of saline solution into the trachea via nasotracheal or cricothyroid cannula, and brief tracheal intubation for suctioning only.

Blind *nasotracheal suctioning* consists of insertion of a well-lubricated, curved-tip suction catheter through the topically anesthetized nasal passage toward and (hopefully!) through the larynx, in the cooperative conscious patient. He should be in the sitting position with the head tilted backward and the chin forward (sniffing position) and the operator should maneuver the tube through the nose into the larynx.

In blind nasotracheal suctioning, the tongue may be pulled forward to lift the glottis out of the way. Entry into the trachea is recognized by air flow or coughing. Two to 3 ml. of saline injected through the catheter may soften secretions. Suctioning must be brief, as it may produce hypoxemia in spite of pre-oxygenation. Often the effect of this technique is merely stimulation of the laryngeal entrance, resulting in reflex coughing. If this is effective, one should not pursue suctioning further. If the trachea is intubated with a suction catheter, suction should be applied only briefly and the tube partially withdrawn for pharyngeal suctioning before it is fully withdrawn. Do not suction while inserting or withdrawing the tip of the tube through the nasal passage, as this may cause epistaxis.

In the stuporous or debilitated patient who is not intubated because of intact reflexes, blind suctioning techniques can lead to arrhythmias, intractable laryngospasm with asphyxia, or regurgitation and aspiration. The direct insertion of a laryngotracheal catheter through the larynx without preliminary tracheal intubation also may empty the lungs during suction when the larynx closes around the suction catheter and may cause hypoxemia. In such cases, therefore, when clearing of secretions is necessary, a tracheal tube should be inserted for suctioning.

For *cricothyroid membrane* puncture and insertion of a polyethylene catheter (about 7 cm. long) through an Intracath needle, local anesthesia and sterile technique must be used. Two ml. of sterile saline injected into the trachea may produce coughing and soften secretions.

Finally, *chest physiotherapy* for tracheobronchial clearing, sighing, and improved ventilation and oxygenation has become a valuable adjunct in respiratory care, particularly in combination with inhalation of mist, administration of bronchodilator drugs, coughing, and IPPB therapy. The methods encompassed by the term "chest physiotherapy" include breathing exercises for lung expansion, coughing, percussion, vibration, and postural drainage. Detailed description of these techniques is beyond the scope of this text. Chest physiotherapy should be performed by trained personnel.

Breathing exercises include optimal position, coaching on the use of the diaphragm, and expansion of certain lung regions with the operator using touch and persuasion. Coached coughing was described previously. Percussion and vibration are used in conjunction with postural drainage to mobilize and remove secretions. Percussion is performed at a slow rate with the hands cupped. Vibrations can be done manually or mechanically. Postural drainage requires knowledge of a variety of positions optimal for the drainage of the lung area involved, and should be combined with breathing exercises, coughing, percussion, and vibration. For details on chest physiotherapy, we encourage study of detailed texts and practice under the supervision of physiotherapists (Bushnell, 1973).

Tracheal Intubation Versus Tracheotomy

Tracheal intubation is the method of choice for providing an airway in emergencies or for anesthesia. In recent years, *translaryngeal intubation* has been used increasingly in place of tracheostomy for prolonged airway care and mechanical ventilation. This trend has decreased the potentially lethal airway complications following incorrectly performed tracheotomies, such as accidental displacement of the tracheostomy tube, erosion of a large artery by the tube in too low tracheostomies, pneumothorax, and tracheal stenosis at the site of the tracheal window. The literature regarding complications of tracheotomy is too large to be quoted here. Prolonged translaryngeal oro- or nasotracheal intubation, however, is also associated with long-term complications— usually of less serious nature. Refinements in tracheal tube design have minimized laryngotracheal damage (Fig. 17), but retention of even a regular tracheal tube

for less than 72 hours is rarely followed by serious lesions. The need for a tracheal tube beyond this time may be a factor in considering early tracheotomy.

While translaryngeal intubation is the procedure of choice for the emergency situation and for long-term airway care in conditions reversible within about one week (some patients of all ages have tolerated translaryngeal tubes for up to one month without serious long-term sequelae), *tracheotomy* offers the following *advantages* over long-term use of translaryngeal tubes: (1) easier access to the tracheobronchial tree for suctioning; (2) ease of nursing care and patient nutrition; (3) ease of tube change; (4) less coughing and bucking, which should be avoided in intracranial pathologic states; and (5) in the conscious patient, preservation of the ability to talk and reduction of discomfort.

In conscious patients requiring long-term mechanical ventilation, talking is possible with the use of the minimal cuff leak technique or with a novel "speaking tracheostomy tube" (Safar, 1965). Phonation is impossible for a patient if a translaryngeal tube is in place. With use of a tracheostomy tube, on the other hand, the vocal cords are not traversed and the minimal cuff leak technique during use of volume-set time-cycled mechanical ventilators enables understandable speech during lung inflation. With this technique, however, speech is intermittent and limited to the lung inflation phase. Aspiration is possible during exhalation, tidal volumes vary because of the variability of translaryngeal leaks, and the air rushing through the pharynx with each inflation bothers some patients. Therefore, a speaking cuffed tracheostomy tube has been designed which not only meets many of the national and international specifications for general tube and cuff design but also permits fair communication in spite of leak-free cuff inflation by delivering a low flow of air or oxygen into the trachea just above the cuff.

Tracheostomy

In contrast to cricothyroid membrane puncture, tracheotomy is an *elective* procedure for establishing the long-term airway—"tracheostomy." Tracheotomy should be performed in the intubated, well-ventilated, well-oxygenated patient, with the head tilted backward, in circumstances when it appears that a tracheal airway will be necessary for longer than about one week.

The technique of tracheotomy (Fig. 16) should include:

a horizontal or vertical (midline) incision;

ligation of the thyroid isthmus if it is in the way;

an opening in the trachea at the level of the second and third tracheal rings, using a cut, a window, or an inverted U-shaped flap (merely a cut in small children!);

stay sutures (for at least two days after fresh tracheotomy), to enable immediate securing of the tracheal opening if the tube becomes dislodged;

use of a carefully checked atraumatic tube of appropriate size (see Chapter 9), with soft cuff in adults.

During tracheotomy the translaryngeal tracheal tube should be withdrawn at first only partially, with its tip remaining in the larynx until the tracheostomy cannula is inserted, its cuff inflated, the tracheobronchial tree suctioned, and ventilation and oxygenation via the tracheostomy tube well established.

Cuff Trauma and Its Prevention

Early long-term mechanical ventilation via uncuffed tracheostomy tubes did not produce tracheal damage (except at the tracheal window and when the tip of the tube impinged against the tracheal wall). This technique of deliberate upward air leakage permitted exsufflation of secretions but made control of ventilation volumes and prevention of aspiration impossible. Therefore, when intratracheal positive pressure ventilation replaced the iron lung, large atraumatic latex cuffs were mounted on the metal tracheostomy tubes. After months of continued use of these large-cuff tubes, tracheoscopies revealed no major tracheal wall damage. In contrast, the "newer" narrow, high-pressure, small contact area, unilaterally bulging cuffs, introduced by manufacturers in the 1960s, resulted in necrosis of the tracheal mucosa at the cuff site, and in tracheoesophageal fistulas.

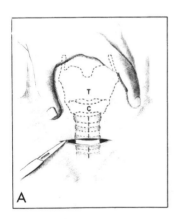
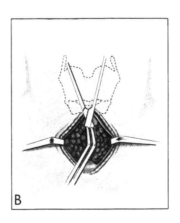
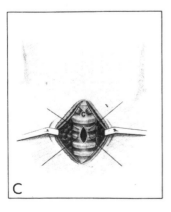
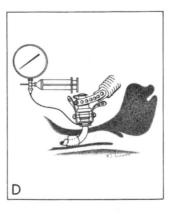

Figure 16 Tracheotomy technique. *A*, Horizontal or vertical skin incision. *B*, Ligation and division of thyroid isthmus (if necessary) for access to tracheal rings 2 and 3. *C*, Tracheal window at tracheal rings 2 and 3 (slit without excision of tissue in small children) with stay sutures for immediate access to tracheal opening in case of tube dislodgement. *D*, Plastic tracheostomy tube with large soft cuff, cuff inflation pressure and volume control, swivel adaptor and nonslipping connections.

In an attempt to clarify these discrepant observations, Carroll studied performance characteristics of endotracheal cuffs. He found directly measured *pressure* by the cuff against the tracheal mucosa (lateral tracheal wall pressure) to be *lowest* (at the point of preventing leaks during IPPV) with cuffs with large residual volume (air that can be withdrawn from the cuff after it has been allowed to assume its normal shape with inflation tube exposed to atmospheric pressure), large surface contact area, even inflation, a small additional volume required to seal the cuff, and minimal cuff pressure increase when the cuff was inflated 1 ml beyond the no-leak inflation volume. With these baggy large-volume cuffs, intracuff pressure almost equalled the pressure exerted by the cuff against the tracheal mucosa, and fluctuated parallel with intratracheal pressure during IPPV. An intracuff pressure (i.e., tracheal wall pressure) of 15 to 20 torr is recommended at intratracheal pressure being atmospheric; cuff pressures lower than 15 torr may not protect against aspiration, and cuff pressures higher than 30 torr may cause necrosis of the tracheal mucosa. These authors also determined, in dogs and human patients, the need for the cuff to position the tube in the center of the tracheal lumen; for the tip of the tube to be smooth, soft, and non-protruding; for swivel adaptors to minimize traction on the tube; and for special connectors to prevent accidental disconnection (Fig. 17).

Use of these safe cuffs nevertheless requires the following *precautions:* (1) The cuff should be inflated only to the point of abolishing audible leakage, but not less, in order to prevent aspiration. (2) The cuff must be large enough to drape freely over the tracheal mucosa and provide a seal with an intracuff pressure of about 20 torr or less. (3) Roentgenographic check should rule out overstretching the cuff beyond its unstretched diameter. (4) Intracuff pressure should be monitored (using a three-way stopcock and a 20-ml. syringe and manometer) and kept at 15 to 20 torr, because overinflation is common and often leads to serious tracheal wall damage. (5) In tracheal dilatation, the cuff should be positioned in the undilated portion of the trachea. (6) Manufacturers' instructions should be followed. Modifications of the above concepts evolved in the form of the cuff pressure-limiting balloon (Fig. 17), and the foam-filled

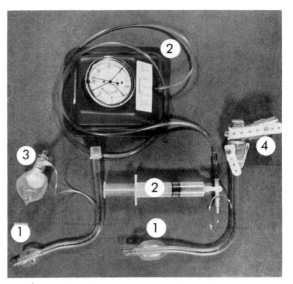

Figure 17 (1) Large-volume low-pressure cuff on either regular plastic tracheal tube or Lindholm mod ification of Dwyer S-shaped plastic tracheal tube (from National Catheter Corporation, New York). Cuff inflation system with pressure limitation by either three-way stopcock – cuff inflation syringe – cuff pressure gauge (2) or McGinnis cuff pressure-limiting balloon (3) (from Lanz Medical Products, Wilmerding, PA 15148). (4) Eross swivel adaptor with nonslipping connections (from Instrumentation Industries, Inc., Pittsburgh, PA 15236).

cuff. The latter must be deflated by aspirating with a syringe; it inflates when the cuff pilot tube is exposed to atmospheric pressure. The foam cuff produces safe tracheal wall pressures and a leak-proof fit, provided that the correct size tube and cuff is chosen.

Intracuff pressure and tracheal wall pressure may increase during anesthesia with nitrous oxide. This is due to rapid diffusion of the soluble nitrous oxide into the cuff and the very slow diffusion of nitrogen out of the cuff (when the cuff was inflated with air). High inhaled concentrations of oxygen over a prolonged period will also increase the tracheal tube cuff gas volume and increase the tracheal wall pressure. All this can be prevented by monitoring the cuff pressure, periodically aspirating the gas from the cuff, and reinflating until a seal is achieved. Another factor that can increase tracheal wall damage, even with use of the safe cuffs described above, is arterial hypotension, either in shock states or deliberately induced during surgery. In these cases, cuff pressure may more readily exceed arterial perfusion pressure, resulting in tracheal necrosis.

Tube Trauma and Its Prevention

There are many reports on various types and degrees of damage caused by prolonged tracheal intubation. Hedden et al. (1969) reported on complications occurring in 116 patients who had tracheal tubes in place for up to ten days in an intensive care unit. Laryngoscopy upon extubation of survivors revealed varying degrees of inflammation and edema of the aryepiglottic folds, epiglottis, and vocal cords in those who had the tube in place for less than 48 hours; and ulcerations of the posterior aspect of the laryngeal entrance in those intubated longer than 48 hours. In those who died, the same types of ulcerations were seen at autopsy, but they were of a much more severe degree than in the survivors. The damage was more severe in females than in males, probably because of the larger size of the tracheal tube in relation to larynx size in females. The lesions in the posterior aspects of the larynx entrance can be explained on the basis that the regular tracheal tube in the larynx is forced posteriorly by the triangular shape of the laryngeal hiatus and by the lordosis of the cervical vertebral column, which forces the cricoid forward. Thus, the tube is deformed into an S-shape, causing it to pass from the posterior pharyngeal wall anteriorly into the larynx, with the posterior laryngeal wall acting as a fulcrum. In addition, there were ulcers of the tracheal mucosa that was in contact with the tracheal tube cuff, particularly the mucosa overlying the tracheal rings. The authors alluded to the possibility that improved tube design could reduce laryngotracheal trauma.

Similar types and distributions of lesions were found in the extensive study by Lindholm (1969) of 457 patients of all ages who had translaryngeal tracheal tubes in place longer than 24 hours.

Based on the above studies, Lindholm and Carroll (1975) evaluated the force exerted on the larynx by 23 commercially available orotracheal tubes. Conventional tubes proved highly injurious. The regular red rubber tube generated forces of 700 to 1000 gm. against the larynx. Plastic and Silastic tubes and nonkinking latex-reinforced spiral tubes (anode tubes) were much less injurious. Least traumatic was the Lindholm modification of the Dwyer tube (Fig. 17), i.e., the anatomically S-shaped plastic tube. This S-shaped tube, although less traumatic, is more difficult to insert and requires a stylet for insertion. Either type of tube, if made of nontoxic plastic and with the large soft cuff, has made prolonged tracheal intubation relatively noninjurious.

Tracheobronchial Suctioning

Inability to clear pulmonary secretions is a common problem in patients who need artificial ventilation via tracheal or tracheostomy tube. This necessitates effective aseptic and atraumatic suctioning of the tracheobronchial tree when needed. Routine suctioning is not encouraged, as it tends to be associated with subsequent iatrogenic infection or ulceration of the mucosa.

Straight suction catheters usually enter the right main bronchus. Therefore, we recommend use of curved-tip suction catheters, which can be directed specifically into one or the other main bronchi, irrespective of head position. Turning the head to the right in tracheotomized patients in order to make the suction catheter enter the left main bronchus is an unreliable technique.

In patients with acute respiratory insufficiency, tracheobronchial suctioning is often accompanied by periods of hypoxemia unless the lungs are filled with 100 per cent oxygen just prior to suctioning and suctioning is brief. Oxygenation during suctioning can be maintained longer and more reliably with use of the intratracheal jet insufflation technique.

Bronchoscopy

Open rigid tube bronchoscopy may be the best method for assuring a clear airway in rare or special cases of pharyngolaryngeal disease or of solid obstructive materials in the tracheobronchial tree. Anesthesiologists, otolaryngologists, and others practicing bronchoscopy should be skilled and experienced in passing the rigid open bronchoscope in the awake patient under adequate oxygenation. Fiberoptic bronchoscopy is more suitable for diagnosis than for clearing of large amounts of tenacious asphyxiating tracheobronchial material.

Humidification and Nebulization

Bypassing the nasal air passage by tracheal or tracheostomy tube results in drying of the tracheobronchial mucosa, blockage of the ciliary escalator clearing mechanism, secondary infection, and necrotizing tracheobronchitis. Therefore, humidification of administered gas is important. In order to deliver 100 per cent relative humidity at 35 to 37°C. into the trachea, the water in the humidifier must be warmed to above 37°C., depending on the cooling taking place between the humidifier and the trachea. Thus, unheated humidifiers are inadequate. Heated humidifiers such as the presently popular Cascade humidifier used extensively in recovery rooms and ICUs, can be improved even further with use of a thermometer near the patient's airway and servo-control of the humidifier heating element. In contrast to humidifiers, nebulizers deliver water in the form of droplets. These droplets form a mist which represents gas supersaturated with water. Although heating a jet-capillary junction-type nebulizer is unnecessary, heated mainstream nebulizers give maximal humidification. Ultrasonic nebulizers do not require a nebulizing stream of gas, and thus are used mainstream; they deliver droplets of a more constant size than standard nebulizers.

For humidification techniques, see the section *Oxygenation Techniques* in this chapter and Figures 6 and 7.

PLEURAL DRAINAGE

Emergency pleural drainage is required when air, fluid, or blood collects in the pleural cavity with such rapidity or in such volume that ventilation is progressively impaired. Perhaps the most acute such emergency is *tension pneumothorax,* in which a leak in the lung parenchyma, acting as a one-way valve, results in increasing compression of lung, airways, and vena cava. Tension pneumothorax should be suspected when there is a consistent history (chest trauma, COPD, patient on MV), evidence of respiratory distress, and circulatory embarrassment. Progressive distention of the chest and resistance to positive pressure ventilation should also arouse suspicion. Physical examination may reveal tympanism and ab-

sent breath sounds on the side of the pneumothorax, with tracheal shift toward the contralateral lung. Subcutaneous emphysema may or may not be present. The abdomen may be distended from downward displacement of the diaphragm and secondary pneumoperitoneum.

Tension pneumothorax is a dire emergency that requires immediate treatment. Diagnosis may be confirmed, while affording moderate relief, by inserting a 14 gauge angiocath into the pleural cavity through the second intercostal space, in the midclavicular line. Escape of air under pressure confirms the diagnosis and also permits some decompression. A finger cot, slit at the distal end and secured to the angiocath with a rubber band, provides an adequate flutter valve against retrograde movement of air; this angiocath plus flutter valve allows continuing decompression, enabling the physician and staff to prepare less hastily for placement of a chest tube.

As soon as circumstances permit, the Angiocath device should be supplanted by *large-bore tube drainage* (Fig. 18). The necessary *equipment* for this may include:

  sterile gloves and drapes
  "prep" solution
  1 per cent Xylocaine
  10 ml. syringe; 22- and 25-gauge needles
  scalpel with No. 11 blade
  sterile forceps, Kelly clamps, and scissors
  sterile 4 × 4 gauze
  No. 1 and No. 2 Nelson trocars and Nos. 14, 16, and 20 French 16-inch Bardic catheters, or Argyle plastic thoracostomy tube with enclosed trocar
  4–0 silk suture
  collection bottle system (see below)
  sterile drainage tubing and connectors

In suspected pneumothorax, a site in the second intercostal space in the midclavicular line is widely prepped. A wheal of local anesthetic is raised, using the 25-gauge needle, and the injection is carried deeper with the 22-gauge needle—hitting the rib and then passing immediately superior to it in order to avoid the intercostal vessels and nerves. The syringe is withdrawn as the needle penetrates the pleura to confirm position, and the pleura is then thoroughly anesthetized. *If air cannot be withdrawn into the syringe, the pleural catheter should not be introduced at that site.*

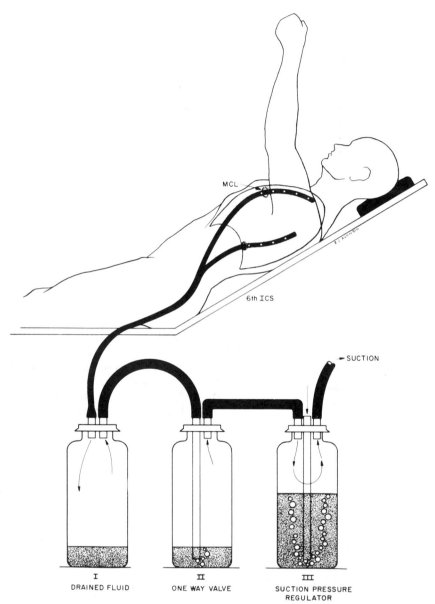

Figure 18 Pleural drainage system. Chest tubes with multiple holes are inserted through the second inter-costal space anteriorly for draining gas, and through approximately the sixth to eighth intercostal space just behind the midaxillary line posteriorly for draining liquid. They are connected via a Y tube to the bottle system consisting of bottle (1) for collection of fluid; bottle (2) a one-way valve; and bottle (3) to keep a constant controllable negative pressure. When connected to wall suction or a commercially available high flow suction apparatus, negative pressure can be maintained in the presence of lung leaks only with a suction flow higher than the flow through the leak. The appropriate size chest tube is inserted through a stab incision in the skin and into the pleural cavity with the open technique (blunt Kelly clamp pierced through the intercostal space and pried open for tube insertion) or the closed technique (using trocar). For transportation a one-way valve instead of the three bottle system is used.

The catheter is prepared by cutting several additional side holes over the first 4 inches and testing it for ease of passage through the appropriate trocar (Bardic catheters often require removal of an ellipse from the end to permit passage through a trocar). A silk tie, placed around the tube 1 to 2 inches from the most proximal hole (estimated thickness of the chest wall) serves as a useful marker to ensure that the tube is advanced until the last side hole is intrapleural and not subcutaneous.

There are three acceptable techniques for actual placement of the thoracostomy tube—the chosen technique depending on available equipment and a given physician's experience:

(1) If a *trocar and plastic* (Bardic or other) *catheter* are being used, a Kelly clamp should be placed on the catheter in such a way that the catheter will protrude from the trocar to the point where the last side hole is visible. The skin is nicked with scalpel and a stitch is placed—to be used later for securing the catheter. The trocar is then introduced through the incision, perpendicular to the skin, and advanced with a gentle rotary motion. Once again, one aims for the superior rib margin; entrance into the pleural space is signaled by a definite "give." When this occurs, the trocar is removed and the sleeve is advanced about 1 cm.; the catheter is then inserted through the sleeve up to the previously placed Kelly clamp. The clamp is removed and shifted to the area of the catheter between the metal sleeve and the skin, allowing the sleeve to be removed. The chest tube is advanced about 2 to 5 cm., to the silk suture marker, and immediately secured with the skin stitch.

(2) The *Argyle* plastic thoracostomy tube with enclosed trocar is much simpler to use than the above system but requires meticulous care lest overzealous attempts to penetrate the chest wall lead to parenchymal lung damage. As in the previously described technique, a small incision is made in the anesthetized skin and a stitch is placed. The argyle catheter is advanced through the incision, at right angles to the skin, just superior to the rib. When the sharp inner trocar enters the pleural space, the tube is advanced over it to the previously placed silk suture marker. After the tube has been secured to the skin, a Kelly clamp is placed between the skin and the tip of the trocar, and the trocar is removed.

(3) Perhaps the safest technique for chest tube placement involves *blunt puncture* with a Kelly clamp. Once again, an incision is made through the skin wheal and a stitch for securing the catheter is placed. With a Kelly clamp, blunt dissection is carried down to the rib. The pleura is penetrated just above the rib with the tip of the closed Kelly, and the thoracostomy tube, with one end clamped off, is then rapidly introduced between the spread jaws of the clamp. The tube is then secured as previously described.

Once the thoracostomy tube has been correctly positioned in the pleural space and secured, it is connected to a valved drainage system and the occluding clamp is removed.

Patients with known or suspected *hemothorax, hydrothorax,* or *empyema* will require a second thoracostomy tube for adequate drainage. The technique for placement of the tube is the same as that described above, but the tube is inserted in the sixth intercostal space at the midaxillary line. The positioning of any thoracostomy tube should be checked as soon as possible with appropriate chest roentgenograms.

There are several *closed drainage systems* which may be set up to evacuate fluid and air from the pleural cavity. As noted earlier, for patients with tension pneumothorax, a flutter valve will prevent retrograde movement of air and be especially useful when the patient must be transported to or within the hospital. Definitive treatment, however, requires a closed chest drainage system (Fig. 18):

(1) *One-bottle water-seal drainage* is the simplest of these systems and works by gravity. It consists of a bottle with two tubes passing through the cap; the first tube passes just through the cap, and acts as an air vent; the second, connected proximally to the patient, extends down into the bottle so that its tip lies 2 cm. beneath the water surface. (The water level in the bottle should be marked before the patient is connected to the system.) When positive pressure in the pleural space exceeds 2 cm. H_2O, air or fluid will be driven through the tubing into the bottle.

(2) When gravity alone is insufficient to provide adequate drainage or enable lung re-expansion, suction may be required. This can be effected using a *two-bottle water-seal system.* The first bottle is essentially the same as that described above and acts as the

water seal. However, the vent tube, rather than being open to air, is connected to a second bottle which serves as the suction control. This second bottle has two additional tubes penetrating its cap—a short tube, connecting the bottle to a suction source, and a long, open tube submerged 10 to 20 cm. in water. The depth of submersion of this tube determines the amount of negative pressure applied, for if suction pressure exceeds the height of the water column in this bottle, air will bubble through the open tube.

(3) Patients draining large quantities of fluid from a hydrothorax or hemothorax are often more easily managed using a *three-bottle chest suction system*. In this set-up (see Fig. 18), a drainage bottle is interposed between the patient and the water-seal bottle.

Many hospitals now employ commercial disposable plastic units, such as Pleur-Evac, which can be used as a one-, two-, or three-bottle system. Calibrations on the various chambers enable accurate suction control and measurement of fluid drainage; furthermore, air flow meters indicate the volume of air being drawn from the chest.

Whatever system is used, there are certain general principles which apply to the care of all patients connected to water-seal drainage:

(1) Each thoracostomy tube requires a separate closed drainage system.

(2) All connections between chest tubes and drainage tubing should be securely taped.

(3) The water level in the water-seal bottle must be closely monitored. If the level is too high, especially in one-bottle systems, adequate drainage will require higher and perhaps unfeasible levels of intrapleural pressure; if the level is too low, evaporation of water may result in loss of the water seal and a sucking chest wound.

(4) The water-seal bottle should be placed at least 50 cm. below the patient's chest, lest the negative pressure generated during deep inhalation pull air from the bottle into the chest.

(5) The water level in the suction control bottle must also be closely monitored and adjusted to provide the desired amount of negative pressure.

(6) Thoracostomy tubes should be secured in a manner to prevent kinking and traction. Connecting tubing should be long enough to permit the patient to sit up or turn 180 degrees laterally.

(7) Tubing and bottles must be checked frequently for patency; the water column in the water-seal tube should oscillate with ventilation; if it does not, a chest film should be taken to determine whether full lung re-expansion has occurred or whether the tube is simply obstructed.

(8) Kelly clamps should always be immediately available at the bedside, in case of inadvertent disconnection of any part of the system.

CONCLUDING COMMENT

During the past decade, respiratory care techniques—concepts and equipment—have improved to the point of safer and more effective management, particularly of the critically ill patient with very sick lungs. The basic concepts, however, are the same as those which evolved in the 1950s and earlier. While better tools for monitoring and life support have made control of respiratory parameters more objective and scientific, there is still no substitute for clinical judgment and humane care, with bedside vigilance of every critically ill patient who requires artificial support of oxygenation or ventilation. Emergency and critical care physicians, nurses, and respiratory therapists must keep abreast of ongoing developments in emergency resuscitation (Chapter 9) and respiratory care techniques (this chapter), which are constantly undergoing changes, which these personnel must learn to appraise. Thorough knowledge of respiratory physiology and physics of respiratory care should help in differentiating between those changes based on relevant new knowledge and found by critical tests to be effective in patients (i.e., changes worth adopting) and those merely pushed for commercial reasons, "fashions," and local customs. The final tests are acceptance by knowledgeable clinicians and improved patient care outcome.

Selected References: Films for Demonstration of Some Respiratory Care Techniques

Respiratory Care Advanced Life Support

1: Endotracheal Intubation (for manikin practice) (A. Sladen), 1977.

2: Esophageal Obturator Airway Insertion (for manikin practice) (A. Sladen), 1977.

3: Respiratory Failure (A. Grenvik, P. Safar), 1973.

4: Arterial Puncture and Catheterization (A. Grenvik, P. Safar), 1973.

5: Central Venous Catheterization (A. Grenvik, P. Safar), 1973.

6: Pulmonary Artery Catheterization (A. Grenvik, P. Safar), 1973.

7: Mechanical Ventilation (A. Grenvik, P. Safar), 1973.

8: Ventilators (A. Grenvik, P. Safar), 1973.

Prepared for the Resuscitation/Acute Respiratory Insufficiency Teaching Program of Western Pennsylvania, National Institutes of Health, Heart and Lung Institute (contract number NO1-HR-42965).

These films (5-15 minutes each) are available with hand-outs and printed narrations; they are on 16 mm. color/sound and are available from the Center for Instructional Resources, Hillman Library, University of Pittsburgh, Pittsburgh, PA 15261.

Bibliography

American Physiological Society: Handbook of Physiology. Section 3, Volumes I and II, Respiration. Washington, D.C.: American Physiological Society, 1964.

Anthonisen, N. R., Danson, J., and Robertson, T. C., et al.: Airway closure as a function of age. Resp. Physiol. 8:58, 1969.

Ashbaugh, D. G., Petty, T. L., Bigelow, D. B., and Harris, M. T.: Continuous positive-pressure breathing (CPPB) in adult respiratory distress syndrome. J. Thorac. Cardiovasc. Surg. 57:31, 1969.

Barach, A. L., Bickerman, H. A., and Petty, T. L.: Perspectives in pressure breathing. Resp. Care 20:627, 1975.

Barach, A. L., Martin, J., and Eckman, M.: Positive pressure respiration and its application to the treatment of acute pulmonary edema. Ann. Intern. Med. 12:754, 1938.

Barber, R. E., Lee, J., and Hamilton, W. K.: Oxygen toxicity in man: a prospective study in patients with irreversible brain damage. N. Engl. J. Med. 283:1478, 1970.

Bates, D. V., Macklem, T. T., and Christie, R. V.: Respiratory Function in Disease: An Introduction to the Integrated Study of the Lung. 2nd ed. Philadelphia, W. B. Saunders Company, 1971.

Beach, T., Millen, E., Grenvik, A., et al.: Hemodynamic response to discontinuance of mechanical ventilation. Crit. Care Med. 1:85, 1973.

Beecher, H. K., Bennett, H. S., and Bassett, B. L.: Circulatory effects of increased pressure in the airway. Anesthesiology 4:612, 1943.

Behnke, A. R., Johnson, F. S., Poppen, J. R., and Motley, H. P.: The effect of oxygen on man at pressures of from 1 to 4 atmospheres. Am. J. Physiol. 110:565, 1935.

Bendixen, H. H.: Rational ventilator modes for respiratory failure. Crit. Care Med. 2:225, 1974.

Bendixen, H. H., Egbert, L. D., Hedley-Whyte, J., et al.: Respiratory Care. St. Louis, The C. V. Mosby Company, 1965.

Bendixen, H. H., Hedley-Whyte, J., and Laver, M. B.: Impaired oxygenation in surgical patients during general anesthesia with controlled ventilation: a concept of atelectasis. N. Engl. J. Med. 269:991, 1963.

Brain, J. D., Proctor, D. F., and Reid, L.: Respiratory defense mechanisms. In Lenfant, C. (ed.): Lung Biology in Health and Disease. New York, M. Dekker, 1974.

Bramson, M. L., Osborn, J. J., Main, F. B. et al.: A new disposable membrane oxygenator with integral heat exchange. J. Thorac. Cardiovasc. Surg. 50:391, 1965.

Brecher, G. A.: Venous Return. New York, Grune & Stratton, 1956.

Breivik, H., Grenvik, A., Millen, E., and Safar, P.: Normalizing low arterial CO_2 tension during mechanical ventilation. Chest, 63:525, 1973.

Broennle, A. M.: New light on pediatric respiratory problems. Crit. Care Med. 2:221, 1974.

Bushnell, S. S.: Respiratory Intensive Care Nursing. Beth Israel Hospital. Boston, Little, Brown and Co., 1973.

Cady, L. D., Jr., Weil, M. H., Afifi, A. A., et al.: Quantitation of severity of critical illness with special reference to blood lactate. Crit. Care Med. 1:75, 1973.

Campbell, E. J. M.: The management of acute respiratory failure in chronic bronchitis and emphysema. Am. Rev. Resp. Dis. 96:626, 1967.

Carroll, R., Hedden, M., and Safar, P.. Intratracheal cuffs: performance characteristics. Anesthesiology 31:275, 1969.

Carroll, R. G., Kamen, J. M., Grenvik, A., et al.: Recommended performance specifications for cuffed endotracheal and tracheostomy tubes: a joint statement of investigators, inventors, and manufacturers. Crit. Care Med. 1:155, 1973.

Cheney, F. W., and Butler, J.: The effects of ultrasonic aerosols on the total respiratory resistance of intubated patients. Anesthesiology 32:456, 1970.

Civetta, J. M., Barnes, T. A., and Smith, L. O.: "Optimal PEEP" and intermittent mandatory ventilation in the treatment of acute respiratory failure. Resp. Care 20:551, 1975.

Civetta, J. M., Brons, R., and Gabel, J. C.: A simple and effective method of employing spontaneous positive-pressure ventilation. J. Cardiovasc. Surg. 63:312, 1972.

Clements, J. A.: Pulmonary surfactant. Am. Rev. Resp. Dis. 101:984, 1970.

Clemmesen, C., and Nilsson, E.: Therapeutic trends in the treatment of barbiturate poisoning. Clin. Pharmacol. Ther. 2:220, 1961.

Clowes, G. H. A., Jr., Jopkins, A. L., and Neville, E. W.: An artificial lung dependent upon diffusion of oxygen and carbon dioxide through plastic membranes. J. Thorac. Surg. 32:630, 1956.

Comroe, J. H., Dripps, R. D., Dumke, P. R., and Deming, M.: Oxygen toxicity: the effect of inhalation of high concentrations of oxygen for 24 hours on normal men at sea level and at a simulated altitude of 18,000 feet. J.A.M.A. 128:710, 1945.

Coryllos, P. N., and Birnbaum, G. L.: Studies in pulmonary gas absorption in bronchial obstruction. Am. J. Med. Sci. 183:317, 1932.

Cournand, A., Morley, H. L., Werko, L., and Richards, D. W.: Physiological studies of the effects of intermittent positive pressure breathing on cardiac output in man. Am. J. Physiol. 152:162, 1948.

Davenport, H. W.: The ABC of Acid-Base Chemistry. Chicago, University of Chicago Press, 1969.

Desautels, D. A., and Bartlett, J. L.: Methods of administering intermittent mandatory ventilation (IMV). Resp. Care 19:187, 1974.

Dorsch, J. A., and Dorsch, S. E.: Understanding Anesthesia Equipment. Baltimore, The Williams & Wilkins Co., 1975.

Downs, J. B.: A technic for direct measurement of intrapleural pressure. Crit. Care Med. 4:207, 1976.

Downs, J. B., Kleir, E. F., Desautels, D., et al.: Intermittent mandatory ventilation: a new approach to weaning patients from mechanical ventilators. Chest 64:331, 1973.

Draper, W. B., and Whitehead, R. W.: The phenomenon of diffusion respiration. Anesth. Analg. 28:307, 1949.

Egan, D. I.: Fundamentals of Inhalation Therapy. St. Louis, The C. V. Mosby Co., 1969.

Engstrom, C.-G.: The clinical application of prolonged controlled ventilation. Acta Anaesth. Scand., Suppl. 13, 1963.

Eross, B.: Nonslipping, nonkinking airway connections for respiratory care. Anesthesiology 34:571, 1971.

Ersoz, C. J., Hedden, M., and Lain, L.: Prolonged femoral arterial catheterization for intensive care. Anesth. Analg. 49:160, 1970.

Fishman, A. P.: Pulmonary edema. The water-exchange function of the lung. Circulation 46:390, 1972.

Frumin, M. J., Epstein, R. M., and Cohen, G.: Apneic oxygenation in man. Anesthesiology 20:789, 1959.

Greenbaum, D. M., Millen, J. E., Eross, B., et al.: Continuous positive airway pressure without tracheal intubation in spontaneously breathing patients. Chest 69:615, 1976.

Gregory, G. A., Kitterman, J. A., Phibbs, R. H., et al.: Treatment of idiopathic respiratory distress syndrome with continuous positive airway pressure. N. Engl. J. Med. 284:1333, 1971.

Grenvik, A.: Acute respiratory failure. In Conn, H. F. (ed.): Current Therapy. Philadelphia, W. B. Saunders Company, 1973, pp. 92–103.

Grenvik, A.: Respiratory, circulatory, and metabolic effects of respirator treatment: a clinical study in postoperative thoracic surgical patients. Acta Anaesth. Scan., Suppl. 19:1, 1966.

Grillo, H. C., Cooper, J. D., Geffin, B., and Pontoppidan, H.: A low pressure cuff for tracheostomy tubes to minimize tracheal injury: a comparative clinical trial. J. Thorac. Cardiovasc. Surg. 62:898, 1971.

Hedden, M., Ersoz, C. J., Donnelly, W. H., and Safar, P.: Laryngotracheal damage after prolonged use of orotracheal tubes in adults. J.A.M.A. 207:703, 1969.

Hedden, M., Ersoz, C. J., and Safar, P.: Tracheosophageal fistulas following prolonged artificial ventilation via cuffed tracheostomy tubes. Anesthesiology 31:281, 1969.

Hedley-Whyte, J., Burgess, G. E., III, Feeley, T. W., and Miller, M. G.: Applied Physiology of Respiratory Care. Boston, Little, Brown and Co., 1976.

Hill, J. D., deLeval, M. R., Fallat, R. J., et al.: Acute respiratory insufficiency. Treatment with prolonged extracorporeal oxygenation. J. Thorac. Cardiovasc. Surg. 64:551, 1972.

Hodgkin, B. G. (ed.): Respiratory Care. A Guide to Clinical Practice. Philadelphia, J. B. Lippincott Co., 1977.

Ibsen, B.: The anaesthetist's viewpoint on treatment of respiratory complications in poliomyelitis during the epidemic in Copenhagen, 1952. Proc. R. Soc. Med. 47:72, 1954.

Jonzon, A., Oberg, P. A., Sedin, G., and Sjostrand, U.: High frequency low tidal volume positive pressure ventilation. Acta Physiol. Scand. 80:21, 1970.

Kamen, J. D., and Wilkinson, C. J.: A new low pressure cuff for endotracheal tubes. Anesthesiology 34:482, 1971.

Kim, S. I., Winnie, A. P., Carey, J. S., and Shoemaker, W. C.: Use of doxapram in the critically ill patient: does increased oxygen consumption reflect an oxygen dividend or an oxygen debt? Crit. Care Med. 1:252, 1973.

Kirby, R. R., Downs, J. B., Civetta, J. M., et al.: High level positive end-expiratory pressure (PEEP) in acute respiratory insufficiency. Chest 67:156, 1975.

Kirby, R. R., Robison, E. J., and Schultz, J.: A new pediatric volume ventilator. Anesth. Analg. 50:533, 1971.

Klain, M., and Smith, R. B.: Fluidic technology. A discussion and description of a fluidic controlled ventilator for use with high flow oxygen techniques. Anaesthesia 31:25, 1976.

Klain, M., and Smith, R. B.: High frequency percutaneous transtracheal jet ventilation. Crit. Care Med. 5:280, 1977.

Kumar, A., Pontoppidan, H., Falke, K., et al.: Pulmonary barotrauma during mechanical ventilation. Crit. Care Med. 1:181, 1973.

Leith, D. E.: Barotrauma in human research (editorial). Crit. Care Med. 4:159, 1976.

Lenfant, C.: Measurement of ventilation/perfusion distribution with alveolar-arterial differences. J. Appl. Physiol. 18:1090, 1963.

Lindholm, C. E.: Prolonged endotracheal intubation. Acta Anaesth. Scand. suppl 33:1, 1969.

Lindholm, C. E., and Carroll, R. G.: Evaluation of tube deformation pressure in vitro. Crit. Care Med. 3:196, 1975.

Lindholm, C. E., Ollman, B., Snyder, J., et al.: Flexible fiberoptic bronchoscopy in critical care medicine. Diagnosis, therapy and complications. Crit. Care Med. 2:250, 1974.

Macklin, M. T. and Macklin, C. C.: Malignant interstitial emphysema of the lungs and mediastinum as an important occult complication in many respiratory diseases and other conditions: interpretation of clinical literature in light of laboratory experiment. Medicine 23:281, 1944.

McGinnis, G. E., Shively, J. G., Patterson, R. L., and Magovern, G. J.: An engineering analysis of intratracheal tube cuffs. Anesth. Analg. 50:557, 1971.

Mead, J., and Collier, C.: Relation of volume history of lungs to respiratory mechanics in anesthetized dogs. J. Appl. Physiol. 14:669, 1959.

Milai, A. S., Davis, G., and Safar, P.: Simplified apparatus for IPPB/aerosol therapy. Anesthesiology 26:362, 1965.

Miller, W. F.: Aerosol therapy in acute and chronic respiratory disease. Arch. Intern. Med. 131:148, 1973.

Miller, W. F., and Sproule, B. J.: Successful use of intermittent inspiratory positive pressure oxygen breathing in pulmonary edema. Dis. Chest 35:469, 1959.

Moerch, E. T., Avery, E. E., and Benson, D. W.: Hyperventilation in the treatment of crushing injuries of the chest. Surg. Forum 6;270, 1956.

Moerch, E. T., Saxton, G. A., Jr., and Gish, G.: Artificial respiration by the uncuffed tracheostomy tube. J.A.M.A. 160:864, 1956.

Moore, R. L., Humphreys, G. H., and Wreggit, W. R.: Studies on the volume output of blood from the heart in anaesthetized dogs before thoracotomy and after thoracotomy and intermittent or continuous inflation of the lungs. J. Thorac. Surg. 5:159, 1935.

Mushin, M. W., Baker, L. R., Thompson, P. W., and

Mappleson, W. W.: Automatic Ventilation of the Lungs. 2nd ed. Philadelphia, F. A. Davis Co., 1969.

Osborn, J. J.: Monitoring respiratory function. Crit. Care Med. 2:217, 1974.

Pautler, S., Cimons, I. M., Cauna, D., et al.: Pulmonary oxygen toxicity at one ATA. Acta Anaesth. Scand., suppl. 24:51, 1966.

Petty, T. L., and Ashbaugh, D. G.: The adult respiratory distress syndrome. Chest 60:233, 1971.

Pierce, A. K., and Saltzman, H. A. (eds.): Conference on the scientific basis of respiratory therapy. Rev. Resp. Dis. 110(6):1, 1974.

Pierson, D. J.: Respiratory stimulants: review of the literature and assessment of current status. Respiratory stimulants. Heart & Lung 2(5):726, 1973.

Pontoppidan, H., Geffin, B., and Lowenstein, E.: Acute Respiratory Failure in the Adult. Boston, Little, Brown and Co., 1973.

Powner, D. J., Snyder, J. V., Morris, C. W., and Grenvik, A.: Retroperitoneal air dissection associated with mechanical ventilation. Chest 69:739, 1976.

Prys-Roberts, C., Kelman, G. R., and Greenbaum, R.: The influence of circulatory factors on arterial oxygenation during anesthesia in man. Anaesthesia 22:257, 1967.

Prys-Roberts, C., Kelman, G. R., Greenbaum, R., et al.: Hemodynamics and alveolar-arterial PO_2 differences at varying $PaCO_2$ in anesthetized man. J. Appl. Physiol. 25:80, 1968.

Rice, D. L., Aive, R. J., Grasch, W. H., et al.: Wedge pressure measurement in obstructive pulmonary disease. Chest 66:628, 1974.

Robin, E. D., Cross, C. E., and Zelis, R.: Pulmonary edema. N. Eng. J. Med. 288(5):239 (part I) and 288(6):292 (part II), 1973.

Rotherman, E. B., Safar, P., and Robin, E. D.: CNS disorder during mechanical ventilation in chronic pulmonary disease. J.A.M.A. 189:993, 1964.

Safar, P.: Postresuscitative intensive therapy for cardiopulmonary-cerebral resuscitation. Recommendations and patient trial protocols. In Safar, P. (ed.): Advances in Cardiopulmonary Resuscitation. New York, Springer-Verlag, 1977, Chap. 29.

Safar, P. (ed.): Respiratory Therapy. Philadelphia, F. A. Davis Co., 1965 (out of print).

Safar, P., Abraham, R., DeKornfeld, T. J., et al.: Intensive care unit and the anesthesiologist. South. Med. J. 54:8, 1961.

Safar, P., Berman, B., Diamond, E., et al.: Cuffed tracheotomy tube versus tank respirator for prolonged artificial ventilation. Arch. Phys. Med. 43:487, 1962.

Safar, P., and Grenvik, A.: Speaking cuffed tracheostomy tube. Crit. Care Med. 3:23, 1975.

Safar, P., Grenvik, A., and Smith, J.: Progressive

pulmonary consolidation: review of cases and pathogenesis. J. Trauma 12:955, 1972.

Sanford, J. P.: Infection control in critical care units. Crit. Care Med. 2:211, 1974.

Severinghaus, J. W.: Blood gas concentrations. In Handbook of Physiology. Washington, D.C., American Physiological Society, Section 3 Volume II, 1964, page 1475.

Severinghaus, J. W., and Bradley, A. F.: Electrode for blood PO_2 and PCO_2 determinations. J. Appl. Physiol. 13:515, 1958.

Shoemaker, W. C.: Pattern of pulmonary hemodynamic and functional changes in shock. Crit. Care Med. 2:200, 1974.

Siggard-Andersen, O.: Blood acid-base alignment nomogram. Scales for pH, PCO_2, base excess of whole blood of different hemoglobin concentrations, plasma bicarbonate and plasma total CO_2. Scand. J. Clin. Lab. Invest. 15:211, 1963.

Sladen, A., Aldredge, C. F., and Albarran, R.: PEEP vs. ZEEP in the treatment of flail chest injuries. Crit. Care Med. 1:187, 1973.

Sladen, A., et al.: Pulmonary complications in water retention in prolonged mechanical ventilation. N. Engl. J. Med. 270:448, 1968.

Slonim, N. B., and Hamilton, L. H.: Respiratory Physiology, 2nd ed. St. Louis, The C. V. Mosby Co. 1971.

Spoerel, W. E., and Chan, C. K.: Jet ventilation for tracheobronchial suction. Anesthesiology, 45:450, 1976.

Suter, P. M., Fairley, H. B., and Isenberg, M. D.: The optimum end-expiratory airway pressure in patients with acute pulmonary failure. N. Engl. J. Med. 292:284, 1975.

Sykes, M. K., McNicol, M. W., and Campbell, E. J. M.: Respiratory Failure. Blackwell Scientific Publications. Philadelphia, F. A. Davis Company, 1969.

Weil, M. H., Morissette, M., Michaels, S., et al.: Routine plasma colloid osmotic pressure measurements. Crit. Care Med. 2:229, 1974.

Werko, L.: The influence of positive pressure breathing on the circulation in man. Acta Med. Scand., Suppl. 193, 1947.

West, J. B.: Pulmonary gas exchange in the critically ill patient. Crit. Care Med. 2:171, 1974.

West, J. W.: Respiratory Physiology—The Essentials. Baltimore, The Williams & Wilkins Co., 1975.

Winter, P. M., Gupta, R. K., Michalski, A. H., et al.: Modification of hyperbaric oxygen toxicity by experimental venous admixture. J. Appl. Physiol. 23:954. 1967.

Zapol, W. M., Schneider, R., Snider, M., and Rie. M.: Partial bypass with membrane lungs for acute respiratory failure. Int. Anesthesiol. Clin. 14(1):119, 1976.

GLOSSARY

See also glossary in Chapter 3 (pp. 99–103) for terms, definitions, and normal values.

ARDS	Adult respiratory distress syndrome
AV	Assisted ventilation
BD	Base deficit
BP	Barometric (atmospheric) pressure
BW	Body weight
COP	Colloid osmotic pressure
COPD	Chronic obstructive pulmonary disease
CPPV	Continuous positive pressure (controlled) ventilation, i.e., IPPV plus PEEP
CPR	Cardiopulmonary resuscitation
CSF	Cerebrospinal fluid
CV	Controlled ventilation
ECMO	Extracorporeal membrane oxygenation
FIO_2	Inhaled oxygen fraction (concentration)
FRC	Functional residual capacity
FEV	Forced expiratory volume (vital capacity)
Hb	Hemoglobin
HBO	Hyperbaric oxygenation
IAV	Intermittent assisted ventilation
IDV	Intermittent demand ventilation
IF	Inspiratory force
IMV	Intermittent mandatory ventilation
IPPB	Intermittent positive pressure (assisted) breathing (ventilation)
IPPV	Intermittent positive pressure (controlled) ventilation
MEFR	Maximum expiratory flow rate (same as peak expiratory flow rate)
mEq./L.	Milliequivalent(s) per liter
MV	Mechanical ventilation
$NaHCO_3$	Sodium bicarbonate
NEEP	Negative end-expiratory pressure
$P(A - a)O_2$	Alveolar-arterial oxygen tension difference
$PaCO_2$	Arterial CO_2 pressure
$PACO_2$	Alveolar CO_2 pressure
PAH_2O	Alveolar water vapor pressure
PaO_2	Arterial oxygen pressure
PEEP	Positive end-expiratory pressure
PET	End-tidal CO_2 pressure
pHa	Arterial hydrogen ion concentration, negative logarithm
PNPV	Positive negative pressure ventilation (same as IPPV plus NEEP)
RV	Residual volume
SB	Spontaneous breathing
SB-CPAP	Spontaneous breathing with continuous positive airway pressure
SB-EPAP	Spontaneous breathing with expiratory positive airway pressure
SB-PAP	Spontaneous breathing with positive airway pressure (EPAP and/or CPAP)
TLC	Total lung capacity
torr	Unit of pressure equal to 1 mm. Hg (named after Torricelli, an Italian mathematician)
VC	Vital capacity
VT	Tidal volume
ZEEP	Zero end-expiratory pressure

Chapter 11 CARDIAC PROCEDURES

A. Synchronized Cardioversion of Arrhythmias
B. Pericardiocentesis
C. Insertion of a Temporary Transvenous Pacemaker
D. Utilization of a Flow-Directed Balloon Tipped Catheter

A. SYNCHRONIZED CARDIOVERSION OF ARRHYTHMIAS

John H. Stone

DEFINITION

The term "synchronized cardioversion" refers to the delivery of a direct-current shock across the chest for the reversion of supraventricular or ventricular dysrhythmias (other than ventricular fibrillation, for which a synchronized shock is *not* used). In this procedure, release of the electrical charge on the capacitor is synchronized with and triggered by the patient's own R wave of the electrocardiogram, thereby avoiding the "vulnerable zone" of the T wave and minimizing the possibility of ventricular fibrillation. Cardioversion may be used in either elective or emergency clinical situations.

INDICATIONS FOR CARDIOVERSION

As in other approaches to the patient who has an arrhythmia, the clinical adage applies—treat the patient, not the arrhythmia. In other words, treatment must be directed by the clinical context in which the rhythm disturbance occurs. Cardioversion may be used *electively* for the reversion of many supraventricular arrhythmias, notably atrial fibrillaton and atrial flutter, but also for paroxysmal atrial/paroxysmal junctional tachycardias and arrhythmias associated with the Wolff-Parkinson-White syndrome (WPW), if these are resistant to the simpler standard approaches. *Elective* cardioversion is undertaken only after careful analysis of the patient's entire clinical situation, current drug regimen, and duration of the dysrhythmia, and after consideration of anticoagulant therapy prior to the procedure.

Indications for *emergency* cardioversion include the following.

(1) Ventricular tachycardia.

(2) Supraventricular tachycardias in which the presence of co-existing heart disease results in serious deterioration of the patient's clinical status, including, e.g.,

(*a*) coronary atherosclerotic heart disease with angina pectoris or acute left heart failure;

(*b*) rheumatic mitral stenosis with pulmonary edema (the latter secondary to the shortened diastolic filling period accompanying the tachycardia);

(*c*) compromised cardiac status in patients with hypertrophied left ventricles in whom the normal atrial transport function of sinus rhythm is critical: idiopathic hypertrophic subaortic stenosis, aortic stenosis, hypertensive cardiovascular disease.

(3) Ventricular *versus* supraventricular tachycardia with pre-existing bundle branch block or aberration.

TECHNIQUE OF EMERGENCY CARDIOVERSION

(1) Start intravenous infusion.

(2) Establish good oxygenation—a separate operator is desirable to ensure this.

(3) Select that lead of the patient's EKG with large R wave for synchronization (the capacitor discharge *can* be triggered by large T waves, which of course, could be catastrophic).

(4) Test synchronization circuit for correct function (the shock is timed to be delivered approximately 10 msec. after the peak of the R wave and on its downslope).

(5) Administer diazepam (Valium) intravenously for amnesia in a dosage of 5 to 15 mg. The patient should be asked to count backward from 100 until the count becomes

erratic or garbled (usually four to five minutes). Administration of diazepam may not be necessary, of course, if the patient is stuporous as a result of decreased cerebral blood flow (especially true in some instances of ventricular tachycardia, for example).

(6) Paddle placement. Two types of paddles are available: (*a*) one anterior, one posterior; or (*b*) *both* anterior. In using anterior–posterior paddles, the anterior paddle should be placed between the left lower sternal border and the cardiac apex; the posterior paddle is placed beneath the patient between the vertebral column and the tip of the left scapula. In the second instance, with two anterior paddles, one paddle should be placed just to the left of the cardiac apex in the left anterior axillary line, and the other at the right upper sternal border. In either case, firm pressure of about 20 lbs. of force on the anterior paddle(s) is required for good electrical contact. Electrode jelly should be used in amounts enough to ensure electrical conduction (but not in such excess that "bridging" or arcing of current may occur between the paddles). Saline-soaked 4 × 4 gauze pads also may be used (alcohol-soaked pads should not be used because they may catch fire).

(7) Energy setting. This is variable depending on the arrhythmia. Ventricular tachycardia and atrial flutter often are responsive to low energy settings (10 to 100 watt-seconds). Atrial fibrillation may well require higher levels, with the initial shock at 150 to 250 w.-sec. In children (or adults weighing < 50 kg.), use 3.5 to 6.0 w.-sec./kg. of body weight.

(8) Observe usual precautions: no one in contact with patient or bed; all other electrical equipment removed from the patient.

(9) Deliver synchronized shock(s). If ectopic beats follow the first shock, give 50 to 100 mg. lidocaine intravenously. The amount of energy delivered on successive shocks is increased by 50 to 100 watt-second increments until conversion or the highest setting on the machine is reached. Check lead V_1 for sinus rhythm after each shock.

(10) Should ventricular fibrillation occur as a complication of the synchronized shock, the machine should immediately be placed in the defibrillator mode (*synchronizer circuit off*), recharged, and another shock administered.

(11) Maintain good oxygenation at all times; observe for depressed respirations secondary to the diazepam. The patient may have to be reminded to take deep breaths. Supplemental oxygen should almost always be given.

(12) Arrange for monitoring of the patient (24 hours is optimum).

(13) Consider institution of maintenance antiarrhythmic therapy, which may help to prevent recurrence of the arrhythmia (lidocaine, quinidine, procainamide, etc.).

(14) Look for treatable causes of the arrhythmia (pulmonary emboli, electrolyte imbalance, hypoxemia, valvular heart disease, thyrotoxicosis, unrecognized myocardial ischemia, alcohol, etc.).

GENERAL SUGGESTIONS

(1) Use the minimum amount of energy necessary for conversion. This is especially important in patients known to be taking digitalis (in patients on heavy doses of digitalis, the first shock might well be 5 to 10 w.-sec.). The combination of digitalis in high doses and higher cardioversion settings may predispose to serious postcardioversion arrhythmias.

(2) Assure adequate oxygenation of the patient at all times, especially several minutes before, and from 30 to 60 minutes after, the shock is given.

(3) Some clinicians prefer to give a bolus of lidocaine (50 to 100 mg.) intravenously just before the shock, in order to minimize ventricular irritability in the immediate postconversion period.

(4) Data are not conclusive as to whether quinidine in maintenance doses (or in combination with other drugs such as propranolol) helps prevent recurrent atrial fibrillation. Institution of such therapy varies with the clinician and the individual patient's situation.

GENERAL CONTRAINDICATIONS
TO CARDIOVERSION

(1) Advanced A–V block.

(2) Slow ventricular rate in atrial fibrillation/flutter.

(3) Drug-induced arrhythmias, particularly those secondary to digitalis intoxication.

(4) Patients with known "sick sinus syndrome" (in which atrial arrhythmias with rapid ventricular responses *alternate* with profound sinus bradycardia). If cardioversion is to be attempted during the tachycardia phase of this syndrome, pacemaking capability should be immediately available, because the abnormal sinus node may not take over immediately after the shock.

(5) Recent arterial embolus.

COMPLICATIONS OF CARDIOVERSION

(1) Possible electrical damage to myocardium (especially in cases requiring repetitive high energy shocks).

(2) Skin burns.

(3) Systemic emboli (1 to 3 per cent incidence in patients with atrial fibrillation; likelihood increased in patients with mitral stenosis).

(4) Failure of sinus node to capture after cardioversion; asystole; serious ventricular arrhythmias.

(5) In 1 to 3 per cent, pulmonary edema (secondary to transient left ventricular dysfunction or left atrial "paralysis"). The incidence of this complication, as of others, increases directly with the amount of energy used in the procedure.

Suggestions For Further Reading

Dorney, E. R.: The Use of Cardioversion and Pacemakers in the Management of Arrhythmias. *In* Hurst, J. W., et al. (eds.): The Heart, 3d ed. New York, McGraw-Hill Book Co., 1974, p. 559.

Parker, M. R.: Defibrillation and Synchronized Cardioversion. *In* Advanced Cardiac Life Support (manual). Dallas, American Heart Association, 1975.

Resnekov, L.: Theory and practice of electroversion of cardiac dysrhythmias. Med. Clin. North Am. *60:*325, 1976.

B.   PERICARDIOCENTESIS

John H. Stone

DEFINITION

Pericardiocentesis is the introduction of a needle into the pericardial space for removal of fluid. The procedure is done either: (1) for relief of pericardial tamponade; or (2) to obtain fluid for diagnostic purposes. Because of its inherent hazards, aspiration of the pericardial space should be considered a major procedure.

INDICATIONS

The prime indication for this procedure in the Emergency Department is *cardiac tamponade,* the most common causes of which are trauma, infections, and neoplastic disease (see Pericarditis, p. 465). Cardiac compression may be rapid or insidious, depending on the etiology. The clinical picture is dictated not by the absolute *amount* of fluid, but by the rapidity with which it accumulates. Rapid accumulation of relatively small amounts of fluid (e.g., in patients with blunt or penetrating chest trauma) may result in fatal tamponade; on the other hand, under circumstances of more gradual fluid accumulation, the pericardial sac may slowly stretch to accommodate a liter or more of fluid without overt signs of tamponade. Decreased ventricular filling, decreased cardiac output, elevation of venous pressure, a shock-like state, and impaired cerebral function are the end-results of tamponade. The major diagnostic clues include: (1) elevation of the venous pressure, accompanied by (2) falling systolic blood pressure; (3) narrow pulse pressure; (4) tachycardia; and (5) paradoxic pulse (inspiratory decline in systolic blood pressure greater than 10 mm./Hg). Tachypnea usually is present. Heart tones may be either normal or faint. The heart size on chest x-ray depends entirely on the amount of fluid present.

The other major indication for pericardiocentesis arises when it is necessary *to obtain fluid for diagnostic purposes.* Under these (usually) more leisurely circumstances, the major differential diagnosis is between accumulated pericardial fluid and cardiomegaly secondary to heart disease, both of which may present with a similar cardiac silhouette on x-ray. In this instance, *echocardiography* is a very useful and sensitive way to confirm the presence of pericardial fluid and at the same time make inferences about myocardial wall contractility.

TECHNIQUE

The paraxiphoid subcostal approach is the usual one and is preferred by this author (Fig. 1). The patient is positioned with the head and thorax elevated 45 to 60 degrees above horizontal. An intravenous line is placed; equipment for resuscitation, including essential drugs, endotracheal tube, defibrillator, and EKG machine, should be immediately available.

Usual aseptic preparation of the skin is employed, and the paraxiphoid area is draped if circumstances permit. The area between the left costal margin and the xiphoid is infiltrated with 2 per cent lidocaine (Xylocaine). A long (12- to 18-cm.) cardiac needle with a short bevel (to minimize cardiac laceration) is attached to a 50-cc. syringe via a three-way stopcock. One of a pair of bulldog (alligator) clamps connected by a sterile insulated wire is attached to the hub of the needle; the other clamp is attached to the V lead of a grounded EKG machine.

The needle is advanced, with EKG monitoring of the V lead, through the skin just below the costal margin; then, moving cautiously under the ribs and parallel to the inner aspect of the rib cage, the needle tip is directed superiorly and advanced toward the left midclavicle a few millimeters at a time. The characteristic resistance of the pericardium may be felt at the needle tip. When fluid is encountered, the needle should be

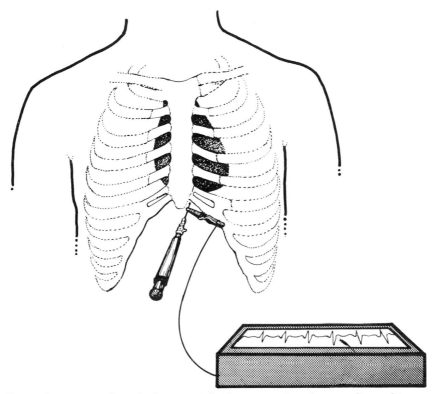

Figure 1 Pericardiocentesis through the paraxiphoid route, using electrocardiographic monitoring. (From Symbas, Panagiotis N.; Traumatic Injuries of the Heart and Great Vessels, 1972. Courtesy of Charles C Thomas, Publisher, Springfield, Illinois.)

stabilized by attaching a Kelly clamp at the skin surface.

The V lead of the EKG should be monitored throughout the procedure (Bishop, et al., 1956). Elevation of the ST segment in a typical "current of injury" pattern (or elevation of the P-R segment if the atrium is entered), or the occurrence of ventricular ectopic beats, indicates that the myocardium has been reached; withdrawal of the needle a few millimeters may prevent laceration of the heart.

Removal of as little as 25 to 50 cc. of fluid in the patient with acute cardiac tamponade may result in almost immediate improvement of his condition, with a decrease in venous pressure and a rise in blood pressure. If the fluid is bloody, a microhematocrit should be performed on it and compared with the patient's venous hematocrit. A sample should also be observed to see whether clotting occurs (the beating heart usually defibrinates blood that has been in the pericardial space; clotting should suggest that a cardiac chamber may have been entered inadvertently).

In acute traumatic tamponade, if no improvement occurs or if symptoms and signs recur after initial improvement, thoracotomy is required (Symbas, 1972). Some thoracic surgeons feel that pericardiocentesis to remove bloody fluid resulting from trauma should be considered a temporary measure, to be followed by thoracotomy in almost all cases.

COMPLICATIONS

Complications include: (1) laceration of the myocardium or coronary artery; (2) ventricular arrhythmias, including ventricular fibrillation; (3) vasovagal reactions; and (4) fatality secondary to injection of air (for diagnostic purposes) into a cardiac chamber rather than the pericardial space.

Electrocardiographic monitoring of the procedure is of great value in minimizing the possibility of myocardial laceration. Under certain unusual circumstances, however (e.g., electrically-silent myocardium due to infiltration of the heart with tumor, or possibly with scarring after transmural myocardial infarction), laceration has been reported in spite of this safeguard (Sobol, et al., 1975).

Pericardiocentesis is of unquestioned value and often is life-saving in acute cardiac tamponade. For *diagnostic* purposes, since fatalities have been reported despite the exercise of great care during the procedure, some clinicians feel that open surgical drainage and biopsy of the pericardium may often be safer and at the same time may yield more clinically useful information (Fowler, 1974).

References

Bishop, L. H., Estes, E. H., and McIntosh, H. D.: The electrocardiogram as a safeguard in pericardiocentesis. J.A.M.A. *162*:264, 1956.

Fowler, N. O.: Pericardial Disease. *In* Hurst, J. W., et al. (eds.): The Heart, Arteries, and Veins, 3d. ed. New York, McGraw-Hill Book Co., 1974, p. 1384.

Sobol, S. M., Thomas, H. M., and Evans, R. E.: Myocardial laceration not demonstrated by continuous electrocardiographic monitoring occurring during pericardiocentesis. N. Engl. J. Med. *292*:1222, 1975.

Symbas, P. N.: Cardiac Tamponade. *In* Traumatic Injuries of the Heart and Great Vessels. Springfield, Ill., Charles C Thomas, 1972.

C. INSERTION OF A TEMPORARY TRANSVENOUS PACEMAKER

Gerald F. Fletcher

INDICATIONS

Indications for insertion of a temporary transvenous ventricular pacemaker in an Emergency Department setting are limited to basic pathophysiologic problems that affect cardiac output and performance. These usually involve maintenance of heart rate and blood pressure with adequate tissue perfusion in patients who present with Stokes-Adams attacks or intractable heart failure. These are often seen in the setting of acute myocardial infarction. The most common indication for pacing in acute infarction is a bradyarrhythmia, such as complete atrio ventricular block, sinus bradycardia, or atrial fibrillation with a slow ventricular rate. These may occur either with an inferior or anterolateral infarction. Occasionally, patients present with degenerative diseases of the fascicular conduction system of the heart with gradually deteriorating heart rate (bilateral bundle branch block), sometimes in the range of 16–20 beats per minute, during which time angina pectoris may be accelerated and manifestations of heart failure or hypotension may develop. Certainly, these problems are indications for emergency temporary transvenous ventricular pacing.

Indications for temporary transvenous *atrial* pacing are sinus node disease, sinus arrest, digitalis intoxication (with both atrial and ventricular arrhythmias), situations in which atrial contractility is necessary for enhancement of cardiac output, and conditions when ventricular ectopic beats and other subsidiary pacemakers need to be "overdriven" by more rapid atrial rates. An atrial pacemaker also may be indicated, in rare instances, for a rapid supraventricular tachycardia (perhaps with Wolff–Parkinson–White syndrome) such as atrial flutter with 2-to-1 or 1-to-1 conduction that requires pacing for interruption of the atrial cycle. Also, at times,

pacing is indicated for a fast sinus tachycardia to slow the ventricular rate by inducing 2-to-1 or 3-to-1 atrioventricular block.

These latter indications for pacemakers are quite rare in an Emergency Department setting and probably would be utilized only after more extensive cardiovascular evaluation. Therefore, the most common indication for a pacemaker (namely a ventricular pacemaker) is complete atrioventricular block in the setting of acute myocardial infarction or, perhaps, in degenerative fascicular diseases of the conduction system of the heart.

TECHNIQUE

The technique for insertion of a temporary transvenous pacemaker may be either percutaneous or by venous cut-down. These surgical techniques are described elsewhere (p. 336). The venous sites commonly used are external jugular, cephalic, basilic, and subclavian—the latter percutaneously. In addition, some authors have described a percutaneous transfemoral approach. Various types of catheters may be utilized after entering the vein. If a percutaneous method is used, the pacing wire is passed through the needle lumen, then the needle is withdrawn over the pacing wire, leaving only the pacing catheter in the vein. If a cut-down method is used, the pacing catheter is passed with direct vision into the vein and advanced. Pacing catheters may be unipolar or bipolar, either one of which is effective for temporary pacing, although the voltage needed for capture may vary.

Advancing of a pacing catheter through a cut-down or percutaneously via an arm vein usually involves manipulation of the arm and twisting of the catheter within the vein to advance it through the vessels in the superior neck, chest, and into the right

329

atrium. This is best done from an approach through the left arm, as the curvature of the catheter is best followed through the left subclavian vein into the superior vena cava, and then to the right atrium. This, however, can be done through a vessel in the right arm if the arm is moved in order to straighten the venous route to the right atrium. Premeasuring of catheter length and estimation of distance of advancement may facilitate the placement of the catheter. Advancing of the catheter via the external jugular or subclavian route is a more direct route to the atrium and involves little manipulation. If the pacing catheter is to be left in the right atrium (which would be unusual in an emergency setting), the tip should be positioned near the junction of the superior vena cava and atrium for effective capture. Electrocardiographic monitoring, if fluoroscopy is not available, will help in placing the catheter in that large atrial waves will be present which would denote the presence of the catheter in the right atrium when that point is reached.

Further advancing of the catheter is similar with both percutaneous and cut-down techniques. Fluoroscopy is strongly advised. After the catheter is advanced into the right atrium a loop should be made in the catheter, and by counterclockwise rotation with slight movement forward and backward, the catheter should "flip" across the tricuspid valve. At this point, the catheter should be advanced to the apex of the right ventricle which is anterior and inferior, as noted on fluoroscopy. The catheter may go beyond the apex and into the outflow track of the right ventricle, and adequate pacing can occur at this point. However, the stability of the catheter is optimal when it is lodged in the apex of the right ventricle. Posteroanterior and lateral chest radiographs following catheter insertion are essential to verify the anterior and inferior placement of the catheter in the right ventricle. Figure 1 shows the proper position for a transvenous right ventricular pacing catheter. An alternate method confirming adequate placement involves connection of the catheter to a pacing box (with pacer setting faster than the intrinsic rate). This will confirm adequate placement in the ventricle by capture of rhythm. Figure 2 shows precordial electrical activity confirming pacemaker capture—each wide QRS complex is preceded by a pacemaker "spike."

COMPLICATIONS

Complications of the transvenous catheter procedure are *multiple but occur in-*

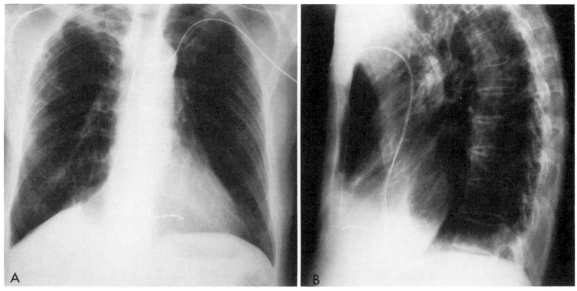

Figure 1   A, Posteroanterior chest x-ray view of transvenous pacemaker catheter in proper position in apex of right ventricle.
B, Lateral x-ray view of same pacing catheter in proper position anterior and inferiorly.

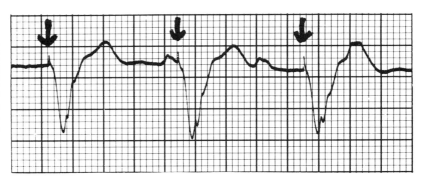

Figure 2 Precordial scalar electrocardiographic record showing typical configuration of 1 to 1 pacemaker conduction of a transvenous, endocardial catheter in the apex of the right ventricle. Note that each QRS complex is preceded by a "pacer spike" indicated by arrows.

frequently. Perforation of the free wall of the right ventricle or the right atrium causing hemorrhagic pericarditis may occur. This problem may be detected only by a transient pericardial rub or pericardial sound with the catheter tip rubbing against the epicardium. This can usually be managed conservatively by observation of the catheter and the patient, making sure that no hemodynamic deterioration occurs. In addition, perforation of the interventricular septum and movement of the catheter tip into the left ventricle may occur. This may cause difficulty with inadequate capture by the catheter.

Catheter tip movement may occur into the right atrium, back across the tricuspid valve, into the superior vena cava, hepatic vein, inferior vena cava or coronary sinus. Absence of effective pacing and changing of configuration of ventricular depolarization on ECG by the pacing catheter should reveal changes to help document this. Of course, manipulation or replacement of the catheter is necessary when this occurs, and confirmation of the correction can be made by chest x-ray.

Ineffective capture by the pacemaker when properly placed may occur in massive myocardial infarction, extreme electrolyte disturbance, and, of course, ineffective pacing electrical apparatus. The latter may result from catheter tip malfunction, breakage of the catheter wire, or malfunction of pacing box.

Phlebitis and thrombosis locally at the site of catheter insertion into the vein are not uncommon. This may necessitate removal of the catheter and utilization of another vein; however, warm soaks and antibiotic creams may be utilized and prove effective. With subclavian puncture problems with arterial perforation, pneumothorax, vein tearing, and air embolus should always be considered.

References

Cheng, T. O.: Atrial pacing: its diagnostic and therapeutic application. Prog. Cardiovasc. Dis. *14*:230, 1971.

Flannagan, J. P., et al.: Air embolism—a lethal complication of subclavian vein puncture. N. Engl. J. Med. *281*:488, 1969.

Kaltman, A. J.: Indications for temporary pacemaker insertion in acute myocardial infarction. Am. Heart J. *81*:837, 1971.

Pryor, R.: Fascicular blocks and the bilateral bundle branch block syndrome. Am. Heart J. 83:441, 1972.

Stillman, M. T., and Richards, M.: Perforation of the interventricular septum by transvenous pacemaker catheter. Diagnoses by change in pattern of depolarization on the electrocardiogram. Am. J. Cardiol. *24*:269, 1969.

Weinstein, J., et al.: Temporary transvenous pacing via the percutaneous femoral vein approach. A prospective study of 100 cases. Am. Heart J. 85:695, 1973.

Yuceoglu, Y. Z., Lunger, M., and Dresdale, D. T.: Transvenous electrical pacing of the heart. Results of 96 insertions in 78 patients. Am. Heart J. *71*:5, 1966.

D. UTILIZATION OF FLOW-DIRECTED BALLOON TIPPED CATHETER

George I. Litman

Development of the flow-directed balloon tipped catheter (Swan–Ganz) has provided a safe and feasible means of rapidly determining the right atrial, right ventricular, pulmonary arterial, and pulmonary wedge pressures in the critically ill patient, either with or without the aid of fluoroscopy. Pulmonary arterial wedge pressure accurately reflects left atrial mean pressure so that, in the absence of mitral valvular disease, it represents a reliable indicator of left ventricular dynamics. The recording of pressures from the pulmonary artery and pulmonary wedge positions, along with samples of blood from right heart chambers, aids in the differentiation of mitral valve regurgitation from an interventricular septal defect. Special modifications of the flow-directed balloon tipped catheter have provided for cardiac output determination by the thermodilution technique and emergency cardiac pacing.

INDICATIONS

Pulmonary wedge pressure measurement has replaced central venous pressure determination in many clinical situations since studies have clearly demonstrated that the central venous pressure does not accurately reflect left ventricular filling pressure. The following presently are considered indications for utilization of the flow-directed balloon tipped catheter:

(1) Assessment of left ventricular filling pressure in patients with acute myocardial infarction, especially those who evidence congestive heart failure or cardiogenic shock.

(2) Decompensated valvular heart disease.

(3) Noncardiac conditions where fluid replacement is necessary, such as septicemia, extensive trauma, peritonitis, acute pancreatitis, severe blood loss, etc.

(4) Intraoperative monitoring in procedures where fluid shifts or major blood loss is expected.

(5) As an aid to the differential diagnosis of the "white lung syndrome" where the possibilities are pneumonitis, pulmonary edema, adult respiratory distress syndrome, or severe interstitial fibrosis—all of which have similar radiographic appearance.

TECHNIQUE

Insertion of the Swan-Ganz catheter has been described utilizing the percutaneous internal jugular, antecubital, or femoral technique. The venous cut-down method is described below. A size 7F catheter is used.

(1) Initially, the integrity of the balloon is tested by inflating with 1.2 cc. of air under water. Where there is a possibility of producing a dangerous air embolus, CO_2 should be utilized in the procedure.

(2) Via a cut-down, the catheter is inserted into the right or left antecubital vein utilizing a Hohn vessel dilator or disposable vein guide so as not to damage the balloon.

(3) After advancing the catheter to the vein in the area of the shoulder, inflate the balloon to half volume (0.4 to 0.6 cc.), thus facilitating the further passage to the right atrium. Gently advance the catheter until a right atrial pressure recording is obtained (approximately 40 cm. from the right and 50 cm. from the left antecubital fossa). Accurate and electrically safe electrocardiographic and pressure recording equipment must be available for this procedure.

(4) The balloon is now completely deflated and then reinflated to full volume (1.2

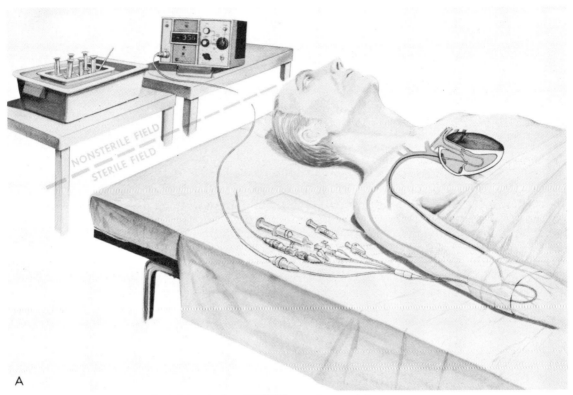

A

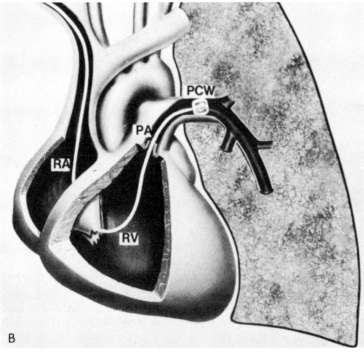

B

Figure 1 A, Demonstration of insertion of Swan-Ganz catheter through median basilic vein in the right arm. Note catheter which has passed through the superior vena cava, right atrium, and right ventricle and into the pulmonary artery.

B, A demonstration of the flow-directed balloon tipped catheter inserted in the pulmonary capillary wedge position. (RA: right atrium, RV: right ventricle, PA: pulmonary artery, PCW: pulmonary capillary wedge.) The right upper tracing is of a normal pulmonary artery pressure. The right lower tracing demonstrates a pulmonary wedge pressure tracing demonstrating large V-waves of mitral valve regurgitation in a patient with an acute myocardial infarction.

cc.). Keep a syringe with air or CO_2 constantly attached to the lumen of the balloon to prevent inadvertent instillation of any other material.

(5) During continuous EKG and pressure monitoring, advance the catheter through the right atrium, right ventricle, pulmonary artery, and into the pulmonary wedge postion (Fig. 1). This should take no longer than 10 to 20 seconds. If more than 15 cm. of catheter is advanced without obtaining wedge position, kinking should be considered and, after deflating the balloon, slow withdrawal should be performed. Attempt to reinsert after corroborating a right atrial pressure tracing.

(6) Once the wedge pressure has been obtained, the balloon is deflated, allowing for continuous pulmonary artery pressure monitoring. The balloon should be reinflated for only short intervals each time a wedge pressure recording is necessary and deflated immediately to avoid prolonged occlusion of the pulmonary segment. Inflation should be done slowly under continuous pressure monitoring and stopped as soon as the change to wedge pressure configuration is noted. Inflation of the balloon produces a feeling of resistance so that on release of pressure the barrel of the syringe slips back. If no resistance is encountered, the integrity of the balloon is in question and inflation should be discontinued.

(7) A chest x-ray should be obtained soon after insertion to check the position of the catheter.

(8) Continuous infusion (D5W with 10 I.U. of heparin per ml.) is essential to maintain patency of the catheter. Inability to withdraw blood can indicate either clotting or inadvertent wedging. Failure to recognize wedging may lead to serious pulmonary infarction.

The catheter will successfully enter the pulmonary artery in 95 per cent of attempts. Failure usually is associated with pulmonary hypertension or low cardiac output states, e.g., cardiogenic shock. The normal mean pulmonary artery pressure is up to 15 mm. Hg while the normal mean pulmonary wedge pressure is up to 10 mm. Hg. When ready to withdraw the catheter (it has been left in place for as long as seven to ten days), it should be done with the balloon deflated to half volume to prevent arrhythmias and to avoid damage to valvular supporting structures.

COMPLICATIONS

As with any indwelling catheter, thrombophlebitis, infection, and catheter clotting can occur. Reported complications include minor atrial and ventricular arrhythmias, rupture of the balloon (without significant sequelae), and rare occasions of thrombus formation on the tip of an indwelling cath-

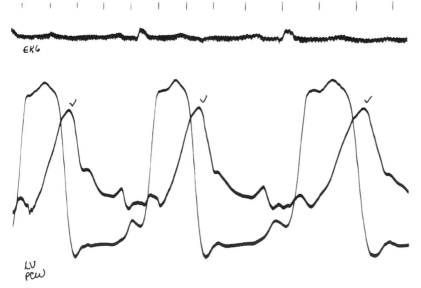

Figure 2 Simultaneous left ventricular and pulmonary wedge pressure recordings. Note large V waves recorded utilizing a flow-directed balloon tipped catheter in wedge position in a patient with acute mitral valve regurgitation following myocardial infarction.

eter after several days. Other complications include knotting of the catheter, perforation of the pulmonary artery with associated hemoptysis, and one reported case of fatal pulmonary hemorrhage while the patient was receiving anticoagulants. Ischemic damage to the lungs has occurred secondary to vascular occusion by the catheter itself, since it may wedge peripherally or the pulmonary artery may be obstructed by the balloon.

To prevent complications, the catheter should be floated into place with the balloon filled each time wedge pressure measurements are needed. Extra precautions should be utilized in patients with pulmonary hypertension and the time in wedge position kept to a minimum. Constant infusion is necessary to prevent thrombosis within the catheter lumen. Frequent chest x-ray evaluation of tip and balloon, especially during the first 24 hours, should be obtained.

The catheter probably should be removed when consistently damped pressure tracings are observed in association with hemodynamic or pulmonary function abnormalities. This would be consistent with pulmonary occlusive disease, e.g., cor pulmonale, shock, increased dead space ventilation, and increasing hypoxemia with fixed inspired O_2 concentration.

References

Chun, G. M. H., and Ellestad, M. H.: Perforation of the pulmonary artery by a Swan-Ganz catheter. N. Engl. J. Med. *284*:1041, 1971.

Civetta, J. M., and Gabel, J. C.: Flow-directed pulmonary artery catheterization in surgical patients: indications and modifications of technique. Ann. Surg. *176*:753, 1972.

Foote, G. A., Schabel, S. I., and Hodges, M.: Pulmonary complications of the flow-directed balloon tipped catheter. N. Engl. J. Med. *290*:927, 1974.

Forrester, J. S., et al.: Filling pressures in the right and left sides of the heart in acute myocardial infarction. N. Engl. J. Med. *285*:190, 1971.

Geha, O. G., Davis, N. J., and Lappas, D. C.: Persistent atrial arrhythmias associated with placement of a Swan-Ganz catheter. Anesthesiology *39*:651, 1973.

Gold, H. K., Leinbach, R. C., and Dunkman, W. D.: Wedge pressure monitoring in myocardial infarction. N. Engl. J. Med. *285*:230, 1971.

Golden, M. S., et al.: Fatal pulmonary hemorrhage complicating use of a flow-directed balloon tipped catheter in a patient receiving anticoagulant therapy. Am. J. Cardiol. *32*:865, 1973.

Lapin, E. S., and Murrey, J. A.: Hemoptysis with flow-directed cardiac catheterization. J.A.M.A. *220*:1246, 1972.

Lipp, H., O'Donoghue, K., and Resnekov, L.: Intracardiac knotting of a flow-directed balloon catheter. N. Engl. J. Med. *284*:220, 1971.

Swan, H. J. C., et al.: Catheterization of the heart in man with use of a flow-directed balloon tipped catheter. N. Engl. J. Med. *283*:447, 1970.

Yona, F. H., et al.: Massive thrombosis associated with use of the Swan-Ganz catheter. Chest *65*:682, 1974.

Chapter 12

VASCULAR PROCEDURES

Jonathan E. Rhoads, Jr.

PROCEDURES ON VEINS

The Value of Veins

In modern medical and surgical care, veins are of extreme importance in diagnosis, evaluation, and therapy. In the immediacy of dealing with sick patients, it behooves all physicians to think in terms of preserving veins for future needs. Veins are used for drawing blood for determinations of blood counts, electrolytes, enzyme and liver function studies, and immunologic and other sophisticated studies in which a sample of blood is needed for the determination. Veins are the place where intravenous cannulas are inserted for administering fluids, blood, and medications that cannot be administered by any other route, e.g., amphotericin B and certain chemotherapeutic agents. Veins also are used to reconstruct arterial systems when they become diseased by arteriosclerosis or lost by trauma. The value of veins for the patient's future medical care cannot be underestimated. A list of the diagnostic and therapeutic uses of veins can be found

TABLE 1
Diagnostic and Therapeutic Uses of Veins

A, Venipuncture
B, Intravenous infusion of blood, fluids, medications
C, (1) Central venous pressure measurement
    (2) Introduction of Swan-Ganz catheters
    (3) Right heart catheterization
D, Insertion of transvenous pacemakers
E, Venous grafts as arterial substitutes
F, Intravenous alimentation
G, Insertion of vena cava umbrella filter
H, Site of creation of AV fistula for hemodialysis
I, Site of cut-down
Optimal veins for these purposes are noted in Figure 1, using the letters above.

in Table 1. These veins are diagrammatically illustrated in Figure 1.

Veins may be destroyed or rendered useless by the abuse of certain drugs such as impure narcotics by the patient, or by the prolonged use of indwelling intravenous cannulas by the physician. In addition, they sometimes are destroyed by cutdowns or by trauma. Probably every house officer has the experience of spending a great deal of time searching for a suitable vein when many obvious, prominent thrombosed veins present themselves but cannot be used.

Certain veins are particularly useful for various specific purposes. For example, the antecubital vein is perhaps the easiest one for drawing blood for diagnosis and evaluation of the patient's changing condition. Certain of the veins in the hand and forearm are the optimal sites for starting intravenous infusions. The veins in the legs should not be tampered with, for the most part, except under urgent and desperate circumstances, because of the risk of provoking thromboembolic complications. The saphenous veins are the major source of grafts for arterial reconstruction because of their length and thick walls. The cephalic vein in the arm is second choice for arterial replacement.

The ultimate in destruction of the venous system is the point at which the patient dies either because veins cannot be cannulated or because one or the other of the venae cavae becomes thrombosed. When the author was a first-year resident, he was informed that "there is always a vein." With the passage of time one learns that occasionally a point is reached when the last veins become consumed, or vena caval thrombosis occurs, and the outcome is fatal. It behooves physicians to take care of the veins as they manage patients.

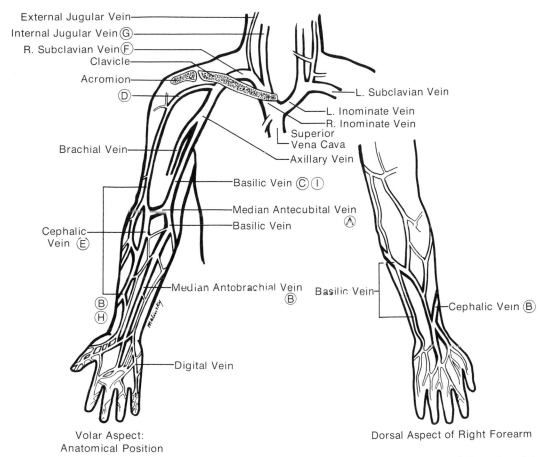

Volar Aspect:
Anatomical Position

Dorsal Aspect of Right Forearm

Figure 1 Major veins of the upper half of the body. The diagram shows the major veins of clinical usefulness. The circled letters indicate the optimal sites for the purposes listed by these letters in Table 1. These sites are by no means mutually exclusive. There is a great deal of overlap. In this drawing, the external jugular vein is not indicated for any function but may in fact be very useful for drawing blood, starting an I.V., inserting a CVP, performing a cut-down, or inserting a transvenous pacemaker or hyperalimentation catheter. Although the author has on occasion used this vein for all these procedures, it is not the optimal vein for any of them.

The cephalic vein is listed as a source of venous graft for arterial reconstruction. In the upper extremity, it is the optimal vein for this purpose, but in the leg, the greater saphenous vein is preferable.

Venipuncture

Venipuncture is the standard method of obtaining a blood sample for determination of laboratory values. It is illustrated in Figure 2. Any vein may be used for venipuncture, but the veins of the antecubital fossa usually are the easiest place at which to perform this procedure; attempting it at other sites may be more painful for the patient, and in some veins leads to hematoma formation. Veins that are punctured repeatedly will develop thickened walls, but may be used over and over again if treated well.

TECHNIQUE

Venipuncture is best accomplished with the patient either sitting or recumbent with his arm supported. A tourniquet is applied to the upper arm and tightened sufficiently to occlude venous return from the extremity, but not so much as to stop arterial inflow. If the veins do not distend immediately, the patient is asked to open and close his fist several times, which places a demand for blood supply on the muscles of the forearm so that, as the muscles contract, venous blood is pumped out of them, distending

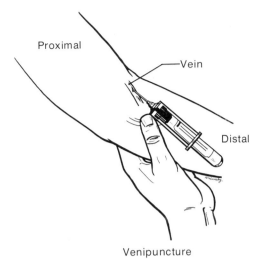

Venipuncture

Figure 2   To perform venipuncture, a tourniquet is first applied proximally (not shown); at the site of venipuncture the skin is wiped with an alcohol swab, and the skin is pulled away from the site of entry by the operator's thumb so that the force of the needle against the skin does not cause the point of entry to slide away from the underlying vein. The operator's other hand, manipulating the Vacutainer, is not shown.

them for venipuncture. Sometimes if a vein is not readily distended it is helpful to massage it, or pat it gently with the hand. Placing warm packs on the extremity for some minutes before attempting venipuncture frequently causes peripheral vasodilation, and facilitates venipuncture.

The site for venipuncture is cleansed. This frequently is accomplished with a swab soaked in alcohol. For higher degrees of sterility, a formal surgical preparation with a potent antibacterial agent such as iodine or Betadine is recommended. Wiping the skin with alcohol removes loose dirt, particulate matter, and desquamated epithelium, but alcohol is not completely effective immediately as an antibacterial agent. It is satisfactory in the vast majority of venipunctures made for the purpose of drawing blood. The vein is identified either visually, or by palpation if it cannot be visualized. On gently feeling the region where it is thought to exist, a cystic cylindric structure may be encountered. The skin is then tensed and fixed, one hand pulling the skin away from the site of venipuncture distally in the line of the direction of the vein, while the other hand takes the needle and syringe and inserts it first through the skin and into the vein. Usually the wall of the vein offers a

certain amount of resistance, which diminishes as the needle enters the lumen. A sample of blood then is obtained. If the needle is for the purpose of intravenous infusion, it is taped in place and appropriate tubing is applied.

Various types of test tubes for collecting specimens are delineated in Table 2. When blood is drawn, several samples may be required for different purposes, such as one for hematology, one for chemistry, and one or more for various serologic studies. In addition, different samples of blood require different anticoagulants, which are detailed in Table 2.

When a patient is first seen, blood samples may be required for a variety of purposes. In the average emergency, blood tubes for hematology, electrolytes, type- and cross-match for blood transfusion are the usual routine needs.

Depending on circumstances, one also may want blood for SMA12, amylase determination, or prothrombin time and partial thromboplastin time.

BLOOD CULTURES

These may be obtained through the same needle used to take blood for other tests, but special sterile precautions are indicated. The skin must be prepared more thoroughly. The appropriate bottles for accepting the cultured blood must be readied in advance, and the physician should wear gloves and a mask, taking as much sterile precaution as possible.

If intravenous fluids are being infused into the same extremity from which blood is drawn, the sample obtained may represent a mixture of blood and I.V. solution, and thus is not representative for laboratory purposes. For example, blood has a glucose concentra-

TABLE 2
Evacuated Tubes For Blood Samples

COLOR OF RUBBER STOPPER	ANTICOAGULANT	PURPOSE
Red	None	Electrolytes Enzymes Serologic studies
Lavender	EDTA	Blood counts
Black	Citrate	Prothrombin time Partial thromboplastin time

tion of 80 to 100 mg. per cent, but D5W has glucose concentration of 5,000 mg. per cent. A small amount of 5 per cent dextrose in water mixed with the blood sample will produce falsely elevated blood sugar levels. The same argument can be applied to electrolyte and hematocrit levels, leading to either high or low values depending on circumstances, but the errors are of less magnitude than those for glucose.

Patient comfort and satisfaction can be enhanced by planning all the necessary tests in advance, sticking the patient once, and obtaining all the necessary blood samples. Sometimes, in dealing with a new or acutely ill patient, it is wise to draw an extra tube of blood, label it, and refrigerate it, in case the need arises for an additional test. Most patients will tolerate a second venipuncture without much complaint, but are likely to complain more than a little at a third.

When a large vein is available, blood samples may be drawn with the Vacutainer equipment illustrated in Figure 3. This allows a needle with a point at either end to be inserted into the vein, and a vacuum test tube is applied to the needle at the other end, allowing the blood to be drawn into the test tube by the suction of the vacuum in the tube. By changing tubes, blood can be drawn for any one of a number of purposes and sent to the appropriate laboratories in separate tubes. At the time of changing tubes, blood is prevented from leaking from the open needle into the barrel of the Vacutainer system (and subsequently spilling onto the patient's arm and surrounding furnishings) by a rubber cover over the short needle on the Vacutainer end. If the double-pointed needle lacks this cover, spill of blood may be prevented by pressing over the tip of the needle in the vein with a finger to occlude the inflow into the needle at that point.

If a good vein is not available, it is sometimes easier to withdraw blood from a small vein with a conventional syringe and needle arrangement, and then to transfer the blood from the syringe into the Vacutainer test tube.

Rapid flow of blood may break red blood cells, releasing potassium ions. After centrifuging, the serum is colored pink by free serum hemoglobin. Falsely elevated potassium levels may be obtained in this manner. To prevent hemolysis during blood

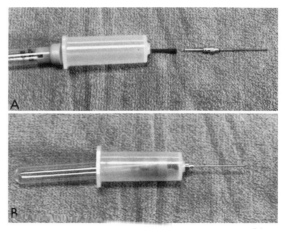

Figure 3 The elements of the Vacutainer blood drawing equipment.

A, From left to right: vacuum tube, plastic barrel, rubber needle cover, and double-pointed needle. The long point on the right of the needle enters the vein; the short point on the left enters vacuum tube and has a rubber cover over it. The double-pointed needle is supplied in a sterile package and is disposable. The needle screws into the barrel, which is not sterile and is reusable.

B, The equipment is assembled and ready for venipuncture. The short needle is pushed partially into the rubber of the cap. A faint circumferential line in the plastic barrel may be seen in the photograph. The Vacutainer is pushed up to this point in assembling the equipment, and it springs back slightly owing to the elasticity of the rubber. After the long needle has been introduced into the vein, the Vacutainer is pushed into the barrel as far as it will go. The short needle then pierces the rubber, and the vacuum in the tube draws the blood out of the vein.

drawing, the blood may be drawn slowly through a large bore needle into a syringe, and then transferred gently from the syringe (after removing the needle) into the Vacutainer after taking the rubber stopper off the top of the Vacutainer. The rubber stopper then is reapplied to keep the blood from spilling out.

There are virtually no contraindications to venipuncture, although some bleeding may be encountered in patients with clotting disorders.

FEMORAL VENIPUNCTURE

In patients in whom suitable superficial veins for obtaining blood samples cannot be found, blood may be drawn from a large vein such as the femoral, the subclavian, or the internal jugular. Major complications are associated with venipuncture of any of these, so they should be resorted to only when there is no alternative. Complications associated with needling the subclavian and internal jugular veins are described later in this chapter. Venipuncture of the femoral vein (Fig. 4) may cause thrombosis of the vein, with the possibility of pulmonary embolism, and all the long term complications of a postphlebitic leg. The femoral artery may be injured by attempts at needling the adjacent vein, leading either to hematoma or thrombosis. Legs have become gangrenous following attempts at femoral venipuncture. This procedure may be of great value, but carries significant risk. Patients in whom it is required once are likely to require it repeatedly. Therefore, if it is required, all conceivable necessary blood samples should be obtained with a single puncture: blood culture (including appropriate skin preparation), hematology, electrolytes, type- and cross-match, etc.

Technique. The femoral pulse is palpated. The needle is inserted 1 to 2 cm. medial to the pulsation. The syringe is aspirated at various depths. When venous blood returns, a sufficient quantity is drawn off, and the needle is withdrawn. (If arterial blood is inadvertently withdrawn, it will serve most purposes for which venous blood was desired, except a venous O_2 saturation.)

Gentle pressure is applied to the groin for several minutes to prevent hematoma.

Intravenous Infusions

One of the greatest advances in medical care has been the ability to insert cannulas into the vein and to infuse a variety of fluids, blood products, and drugs. Thomas Latta was first to use intravenous saline therapy in 1831, to treat cholera. Essentially, all our ability to resuscitate patients from shock, serious injuries, and other medical emergencies depends on intravenous infusions. Anesthesia also relies on it very strongly, as does the management of patients in intensive care units.

CANNULAS

A variety of cannulas may be used; originally, only hypodermic needles were available or cut-down was required. With the advent of plastics, plastic tubes became available for use with a cut-down to expose a vein. The two have now been combined into a wide array of commercially available, efficacious products, some of which are illustrated in Figure 5. The selection of an appropriate cannula depends on the situation. In

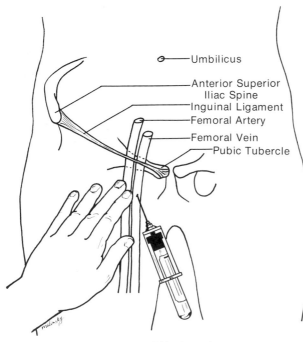

Umbilicus

Anterior Superior
Iliac Spine
Inguinal Ligament
Femoral Artery
Femoral Vein
Pubic Tubercle

Figure 4 The femoral vein is just medial to the femoral artery. The artery is located by feeling its pulsation, and the vein is located by inserting the needle just medial to it. A sterile preparation is required if a blood culture is desired. The author usually prefers to use a syringe rather than a Vacutainer for femoral venipuncture. Complications and hazards of this procedure are described in the text.

Femoral Venipuncture

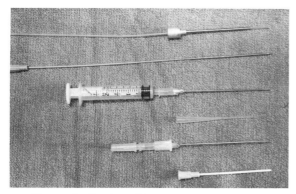

Figure 5 Devices for percutaneous intravenous cannulation. Shown from top to bottom are a 14-gauge Intracath, an E-Z Cath (both made by the Deseret Co.), a Medicut with the plastic cannula removed from the needle, the cannula of the Medicut, a Bard-a-cath unit with the plastic cannula removed from the needle, and the plastic cannula of the Bard-a-cath.

Notice that the Intracath needle fits over the catheter. At the other end (not shown) it has a hub to accept I.V. tubing. The needle will not fit over this hub. Therefore, the tip of the needle must be protected to keep it from cutting the tubing after insertion because it is not possible to remove the needle from the tubing. Note also that the needle is larger than the tubing, and blood may leak out of the vein around the tubing.

In all the other units shown, the needle is withdrawn from the lumen of the cannula so that the fit into the vein is snug and there is no needle left to injure the tubing. Finally, the size of the unit is the size of the cannula. With the Intracath, an 18-gauge catheter fits through a 14-gauge needle. This distinction is important in situations in which large volumes must be infused rapidly (see Table 3).

All these units come in a variety of gauges, and the Intracath and E-Z Cath come with varying lengths of tubing for placing central venous pressure lines.

situations in which blood transfusion may be required, it is important to use a large-bore needle: typically, a No. 16 or No. 14 Medicut or Intracath would be appropriate. In emergencies, or in situations in which a patient may be moving around considerably, one of the plastic cannulas is less likely to infiltrate and lose the intravenous route for administration of drugs and fluids. For short term infusions of a single drug, as in a weekly administration of a chemotherapeutic agent, a simple needle inserted into a vein is satisfactory and is the least expensive method of establishing an I.V. infusion. In certain circumstances, the scalp vein needle or butterfly needle (see Figures 6 and 7) is very advantageous because of its ability to remain in place and because it is less likely to cause thrombophlebitis. The

scalp vein needle comes attached to a medium length of small-gauge polyethylene tubing. As such, it is easy to tape into position securely, and the extra tubing can be taped so that there will be no tension on the needle if there is a tug on the I.V. tubing.

Likewise, the choice of the vein into which to start the I.V. depends on the situation and the purpose for which the I.V. is being started. For traditional I.V.s, the cephalic vein in the forearm and the veins of the back of the hand perhaps are best suited (and readily demonstrable) in most individuals, since these do not roll excessively as you approach them with a needle. The area is relatively stable, and the I.V.s started in these veins last quite a while and are not likely to compromise the antecubital vein, which is the most desirable vein for obtaining blood samples. The cephalic vein, as it courses along the biceps muscle, is sometimes a useful site; it is more mobile than the veins of the forearm, but serves quite

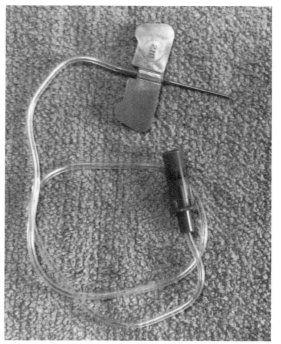

Figure 6 The scalp vein needle—also known as a butterfly needle—is a short needle with flexible plastic handles that fold together for insertion and flatten out to be stabilized with tape. The name "scalp vein needle" comes from its use in starting I.V.s in the veins of a baby's scalp—the best site in an infant. They are also useful in adults in a stable situation because they are slow to develop thrombophlebitis.

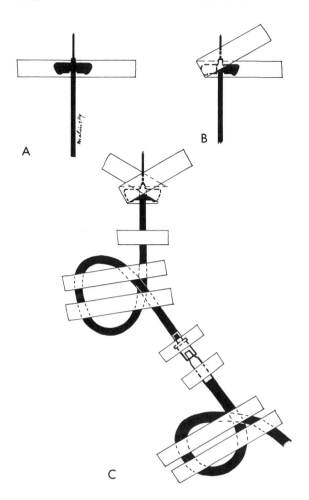

Figure 7 Taping of a butterfly needle.

A, A strip of ½-inch adhesive tape about 4 inches long is passed under the flattened plastic handles, adhesive side up, so that it sticks to the back of the plastic handles.

B, Each end of the tape is folded across the front of the handle obliquely in the direction of the needle so that it sticks to the front of the handle and to the skin. Applying the tape in this way reduces the tendency to elevate the tip of the needle against the underside of the dermis, which might result in perforation of the vein by the needle point or in occlusion of the channel of efflux of fluids entering the vein from the needle.

C, The criss-cross taping of the needle is completed. The tubing is stabilized with a strip of tape close to the needle. A loop is placed in the butterfly tubing and secured with tape. The hub of the butterfly tubing and the tip of the I.V. tubing are each taped to prevent separation of the junction. Finally, a separate loop of I.V. tubing is taped to the patient. The loops are placed so that an inadvertent tug on the tubing will not dislodge the I.V., but will tear the loop of tubing free from the patient first.

The criss-cross method of taping the needle is stable because any tension on the tape will have a component parallel to the direction of the needle, which helps to prevent dislodgement. All tubing and loops should be taped with a low profile so that the tubing is not inadvertently caught by an instrument, an attendant's hand, or the patient's hand, with resulting dislodgment.

well. The external jugular veins are useful if arm veins or hand veins cannot be found. Cannulas inserted into the external jugular vein may be hard to maintain in position owing to the motion of the neck. Veins of the lower extremity should rarely, if ever, be used for intravenous infusions because of the greater risk of thrombophlebitis in the lower extremity. In an urgent situation, one would want to start an I.V. most expediently, and it probably is justifiable to use the lower extremity veins under these circumstances in order to establish a temporary line for support of the patient. Sometimes, in an emergency situation, the subclavian and the internal jugular are appropriate veins to cannulate; they also are useful sites at which to establish central venous pressure lines.

The size needle or cannula to be used depends on the situation: a small needle will administer crystalloid solution satisfactorily. A large needle is required for rapid administration of blood. Table 3 lists the relative time required for 500 ml. of whole blood to flow through varying sizes of cannulas at a typical pressure. The much more rapid flow through the large cannulas (smaller gauge numbers) is due to the fact that the resistance to flow is inversely proportional to the fourth power of the radius. In situations requiring rapid transfusion, a large cannula should be used.

When blood pressure is being moni-

TABLE 3
Time Required for 500 cc. Blood to Pass Through Cannulas of Different Sizes Against No Resistance

GAUGE	MINUTES
20	35
18	15
16	10
14	8
12	4

tored during the administration of fluids, blood, or drugs, the blood pressure cuff should be on the opposite arm from the I.V., because the cuff will obstruct the flow from the I.V. every time the pressure is taken.

TECHNIQUE OF STARTING AN I.V.

The equipment is assembled. This equipment should include appropriate cannula(s), I.V. tubing, I.V. solution, and a pole on which to hang the I.V. Tape is required for securing the I.V. as soon as it is inserted, so that it is not dislodged; the tape is prepared in segments of appropriate length and width so that they can be applied immediately. The skin is prepared as described in the section under "Technique of Venipuncture." If the I.V. is expected to remain in place for more than 24 hours, a careful antiseptic preparation is recommended. The needle is inserted into the vein, and blood is seen to return into the needle or syringe; then, if a plastic cannula is used, it is advanced into the vein and the needle is withdrawn. It usually is secured in position with tape; antibiotic ointment may be placed over the point of entry into the skin; a dressing is applied to the point of entry; and the tubing is taped in such a way that a small loop is made near the point of connection of the tubing to the cannula (Fig. 8). The connection should be fastened so that it cannot easily pull apart. The author usually tapes the cannula and tubing to the skin immediately adjacent to one another, leaving the connection itself visible for observation purposes. It is more difficult to do this when one inserts a simple needle on the end of the I.V. tubing to the vein. An arm board frequently is required to stabilize the arm in position. The tape should be applied in such a way that the joint is immobilized, to prevent dislodgment of the cannula. Patient comfort should be taken into account in the placement of an I.V. cannula and in the appropriate measures taken to immobilize the part (Fig. 9). Arm boards that maintain the elbow extended for long periods of time are uncomfortable (Fig. 10). A comfortable position for an arm board is one that holds the wrist straight or slightly extended, allows the fingers to curl around the edge of the arm board (approximating the position of function), and does not interfere significantly with elbow motion.

Several niceties may be included for

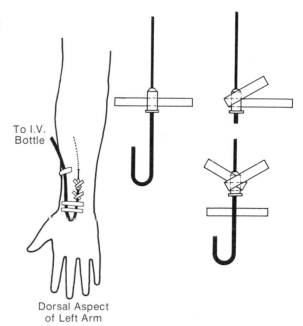

To I.V. Bottle

Dorsal Aspect of Left Arm

Figure 8 Taping of I.V. cannula. The criss-cross method of taping is used here, both on the hub of the cannula and on the I.V. tubing. A turn is placed in the tubing and is taped twice. The junction of the tubing and the cannula is visible. Additional tape is applied to the tubing farther back, and frequently an extra loop of tubing is incorporated. Not shown is a dressing over the point of entrance of the needle into the skin.

increased patient comfort when starting an I.V., such as shaving the arm to remove hair so that the tape will not pull the hair when it is removed. If a large cannula is to be inserted, the point of insertion can be anesthetized with 0.1 to 0.2 cc. of intradermal local anesthetic. These extra measures take a little more time and require a little more organization, but can be accomplished efficiently if the necessary preparations are made. Health professionals who have suffered illness and undergone these procedures are more appreciative of the efforts made.

TECHNIQUE OF SUBCLAVIAN VEIN CANNULATION

The subclavian vein courses up through the axilla and passes posterior to the medial third of the clavicle, where it joins the ipsilateral internal jugular vein to form the innominate vein. The two innominate veins join to form the superior vena cava. The patient is placed in a supine position with his feet

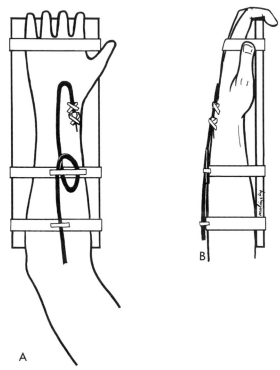

Figure 9 Comfortable position of arm board. The fingers curl around the tip of the board, and the thumb is free at the edge of the board and can move easily; the board is short and does not interfere with elbow flexion. Three strips of tape are needed to hold the board to the hand and forearm — 1½-inch tape is optional on the adult forearm, and 1-inch tape is used on the hand. The loop in the tubing is taped to the tape holding the arm board, not to the patient's skin. Note the low profile of the tubing so that it will not be inadvertently caught by a hand or instrument, dislodging the I.V.

TECHNIQUE OF SUBCLAVIAN CATHETERIZATION

A cannula with a long needle is selected (such as an Intramedicut) (Fig. 11, *A*). A syringe is applied to the needle and, starting at a point 3 cm. inferior to the middle of the clavicle, the needle is advanced toward the sternal notch (Fig. 11, *B*). It must be passed deep to the clavicle; the needle can be felt to pierce a layer of fascia, after which the subclavian vein should be entered (Fig. 11, *C*). It should be possible to withdraw blood into the syringe as soon as the tip of the needle is in the vein. If the bevel is

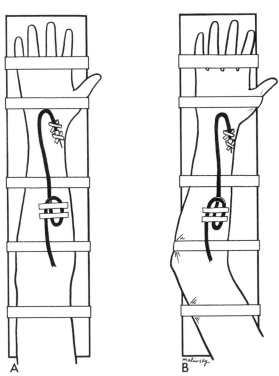

Figure 10 Uncomfortable application of arm board. The fingers are taped out straight — they will feel stiff in this position, and the patient will then have an urge to bend them. The thumb is restricted in its motion by tape across the first metatarsal — this will pull on the skin as the patient attempts to move the thumb. The loop is taped to the skin, not to the tape holding the board.

A, The elbow is straight and feels stiff. To relieve the stiffness, the patient will want to bend it, but if he does, the proximal piece of tape will cut into his arm.

B, The patient rotates the arm at the shoulder back and forth until the elbow can be bent a little. Now the tape pulls against the skin above and below the elbow. It may on occasion pull long enough and hard enough to slide some of the epidermis off, producing a partial thickness skin injury.

elevated, or possibly in Trendelenburg position. This drains blood from the lower extremities and engorges the venous system superiorly, including the subclavian vein. The skin is prepared with an appropriate antiseptic solution. Subclavian and internal jugular cannulas have the potential for being in place a long time, so it is necessary to prepare the skin carefully, first defatting it with alcohol, ether, or acetone, then cleaning it with Betadine, and maintaining a sterile field.

If subclavian cannulation is required under urgent circumstances, and appropriate sterile precautions are omitted, plans should be made to pull it out in a day or two when the patient's condition has stabilized, to prevent sepsis. If the patient is expected to be transferred to another physician, he should be so advised.

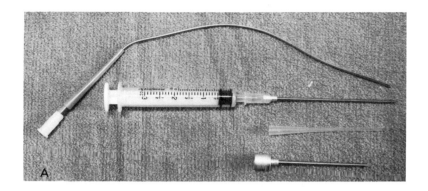

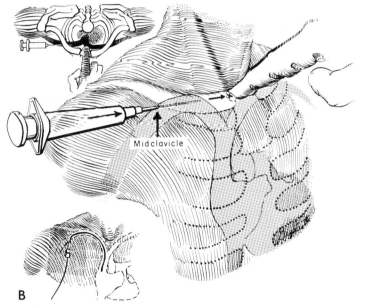

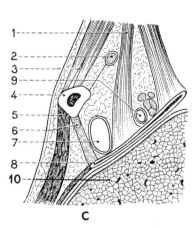

Figure 11 Intramedicut for subclavian venous cannulation.

A, The subclavian vein is cannulated with the large bore (16-gauge) Medicut shown in the picture (see text for technique). The needle is withdrawn, leaving the cannula in the vein, and the 20-gauge radiopaque catheter is advanced through the cannula and into the vena cava. The cannula is then withdrawn to the plastic hub, I.V. tubing is connected, and the catheter is sutured in position.

The cannula is shown alongside the needle. For comparison, the needle of a 14-gauge Intracath is also shown. Note the additional length of the Intramedicut needle. Occasionally it is possible to reach the subclavian vein with an Intracath needle in thin individuals, but in many persons the longer needle is required. For internal jugular cannulation, the Intracath is long enough.

B, Technique of percutaneous infraclavicular subclavian catheterization. The needle, inserted under the midclavicle and aimed in three dimensions at the top of the posterior aspect of the sternal manubrium (indicated by the fingertip in the suprasternal notch), lies in a plane parallel with the frontal plane of the patient and will enter the anterior wall of the subclavian vein. (From Dudrick, S., et al.: Intravenous hyperalimentation. Med. Clin. North Am. *54*(3):579, May 1970.)

C, Subclavian area, sagittal section. 1. M. scalenus anterior. 2. M. omohyoideus. 3. M. sternocleidomastoideus. 4. Clavicular. 5. M. pectoralis major. 6. Tendosubclavious and lig. costoclaviculare. 7. V. subclavia. 8. Costa I. 9. A subclavia et plexus brachialis. 10. Lung. After the ligament (6) is punctured, the subclavian vein will be entered. Note the close relationship of the pulmonary parenchyma (10), which makes a complication of pneumothorax possible. (Modified from Aubaniac, R.: Sem. Hop. Paris 28:3445, 1952.)

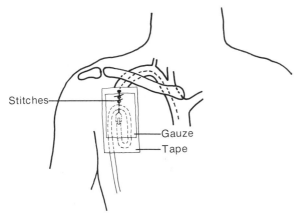

Figure 12 Taping of subclavian I.V. line. The catheter is doubly sutured to the skin. Antibiotic ointment is applied to the point of entrance into the skin. A small piece of gauze covers this area. A loop of tubing is made over this gauze and is covered with another piece of gauze. The entire assembly is then dressed occlusively with adhesive tape. An additional piece of tape (not shown) anchors the tubing to the dressing. The tape is applied to a limited area of the anterior thorax, so as not to limit motion of the arm or neck.

plastic cannula in place, and tubing is advanced through the cannula into the vein. The cannula then is withdrawn along the tubing, which is sutured in place. Antibiotic ointment is applied to the point of entry into the skin, the I.V. tubing is attached, and the infusion commences. The cannula and point of entry are dressed as illustrated in Figure 12.

The tubing is taped neatly on the anterior chest wall, incorporating a loop into the dressing. The tape is applied to a limited area so as not to limit motion of either the neck or the shoulder.

It is important not to allow air to enter this cannula, or significant (even fatal) air embolism may occur. It is valuable to take a chest x-ray following insertion of a subclavian venous catheter, *(a)* to check the position of the catheter tip, and *(b)* to confirm that no significant internal injury has occurred, such as a pneumothorax (Figs. 13 and 14).

pointed toward the patient's feet, it then is feasible to advance a cannula through the needle into the subclavian vein and have it pass into the vena cava without injury to the cannula from the point of the needle. The needle then is removed, and the tubing is sutured in place. Some authors advocate suturing it with two sutures. Using the Intramedicut, the needle is withdrawn leaving a

COMPLICATIONS

The complications of subclavian venous cannulation by this technique include laceration of the subclavian artery; local hematoma, hemothorax; infusion of the intravenous solution into the thorax; infusion of the intravenous solution into the mediastinal tissues; air embolism; thrombosis of the subclavian vein and/or vena cava; and sepsis. Subclavian venous cannulation should not

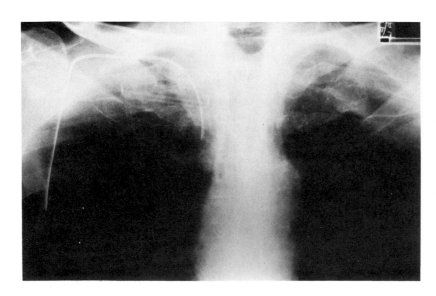

Figure 13 X-ray of a subclavian catheter in good position following placement. The Intramedicut catheter is not long enough to reach the right atrium, but satisfactory central venous pressure can be recorded from the superior vena cava.

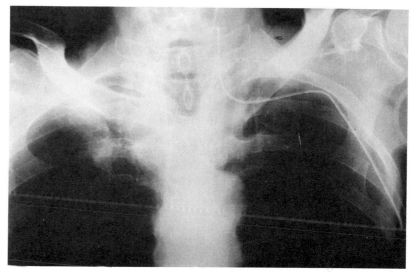

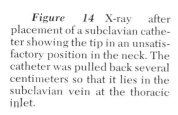

Figure 14 X-ray after placement of a subclavian catheter showing the tip in an unsatisfactory position in the neck. The catheter was pulled back several centimeters so that it lies in the subclavian vein at the thoracic inlet.

be attempted unless one is also prepared to deal with these complications.

TECHNIQUE OF INTERNAL JUGULAR CANNULATION

An appropriate cannula is selected and the skin is prepared. The patient's head is turned slightly away from the side where the internal jugular vein will be cannulated. The point of entry of the needle is between the heads of the sternocleidomastoid muscle. The internal jugular vein lies immediately beneath. The needle is directed at about a 45-degree angle to the skin down into the direction of the thoracic inlet between the clavicular and sternal heads of the sternocleidomastoid muscle. Very soon, it may be felt to enter the carotid sheath and the subclavian vein. When blood is withdrawn, one knows one is in the vein. The same precautions for filling the vein with blood and for preventing infection should be observed with this cannulation as with subclavian venous cannulation. The cannula then is advanced into the vein and secured. Antibiotic ointment and an appropriate dressing are applied.

Figure 15 Retention of plastic tubing in a vein. If difficulty is encountered in placing a catheter into a vein through a needle, one is sometimes tempted to pull the catheter back and try again. However, the catheter must not be withdrawn through the needle because it is possible for the needle to cut the catheter off in the vein, as illustrated. The piece of catheter can then embolize to the heart and lungs. If one is unsuccessful in placing a catheter, the needle and catheter must be withdrawn together, or the needle can be withdrawn first.

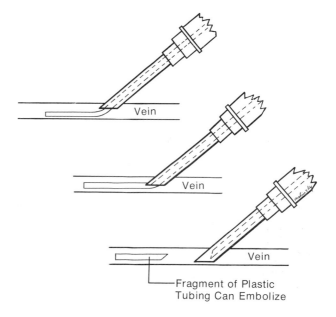

COMPLICATIONS

These include perforation of the carotid artery; cannulation of the trachea or esophagus; and most of the complications listed under "Subclavian Venous Cannulation." The dressing should incorporate the features of the dressing for a subclavian line: it should be occlusive and not limit motion of the neck, and should secure the line. It is technically easier to insert an internal jugular cannula, but it is much more difficult to maintain because the objectives of the dressing cannot be achieved so well in this anatomic location.

COMPLICATIONS OF STARTING AN INTRAVENOUS INFUSION

Some cannulas are designed in such a way that the plastic catheter fits through the needle. In these cases, if one inserts the needle, pushes the catheter through it, and attempts to draw the catheter back through the needle, it is possible for the point of the needle to catch the catheter, cut it off, and leave a foreign body in the vein that can then embolize to the heart or pulmonary artery (Fig. 15). When using such a cannula one must be very careful never to draw the catheter back through the needle. If it needs to be withdrawn, the needle and the catheter should be removed together without pulling the catheter back against the needle. The Intracath, made by the C.R. Bard Company, is an example of such a device.

Cut-Downs

In cases where it is not possible to place an intravenous cannula percutaneously for want of veins, or because they are sclerosed or in spasm and the situation is urgent, a cut-down may be performed. Essentially, any peripheral vein may be used for the pur-

---

Figure 16 Techniques of venous cut-downs.

1. Any identifiable vein may be used. However, usually no peripheral vein can be identified, and that is the reason for the cut-down. If no vein can be identified because of obesity, the cephalic vein at the wrist is a good choice of location. If no vein is visible because of many previous I.V.s, the basilic vein is a likely spot. This location is also a good site if a central venous pressure catheter, Swan-Ganz catheter, or temporary pacemaker is needed because it is possible to advance the catheter easily from this point into the right side of the heart. The skin of the selected site is shaved and cleansed with an appropriate antiseptic solution (such as Betadine), and sterile drapes are applied. The operator wears gloves, a cap, and a mask.

2. A transverse incision is made through the dermis into the subcutaneous tissue. (Some physicians prefer a longitudinal incision because it allows easy exposure of a greater length of vein. The author prefers a transverse incision because it heals better and it may facilitate finding a vein in an area where no vein is initially demonstrable.) The subcutaneous tissue is spread with a hemostat in the direction of the vein to dissect the subcutaneous tissue away for the vein. This process is one of finding the vein and simultaneously freeing it from adjacent tissue.

3. A hemostat is passed under the vein to complete its dissection and to pull two ligatures around the vein. A curved hemostat works best. The distal ligature is tied securely (but not cut); the proximal ligature is left untied.

4. Using the tied distal ligature for control and traction, the vein is incised about halfway across. The author prefers fine pointed scissors for this purpose, but a scalpel may be used.

5. The venotomy incision is oblique. After it is made, the lip retracts and can be grasped with forceps. Toothed Adson forceps are well suited for this purpose because of their small size and strength. If the vein is too small to pick up with forceps, the lip may be controlled with 6–0 silk traction suture(s).

6. The plastic cannula sometimes enters a vein better if it is beveled, but a sharp point on the end of the cannula may perforate the vein above the site of cannulation. Therefore, the point of bevel is cut off secondarily. Heavy gauge scissors are used for cutting the plastic, not the fine pointed scissors that were used to open the vein.

7. Using traction on the distal ligature, the cannula is inserted into the venotomy and advanced a sufficient distance: 3 to 4 cm. is adequate for purposes of infusion, but it is advanced into the vena cava if it is intended to be a central venous pressure line. The lip of the venotomy may be picked up with forceps (not shown).

8. The proximal ligature is tied around the cannula tightly enough to prevent back-bleeding around it but not to prevent removal of the catheter when the time comes. The excess suture material is cut off.

9. The skin is closed around the catheter and the catheter is sutured to the skin, either directly, as illustrated, or by tying one of the skin sutures around it. A drop of antibiotic ointment may be used, and a dry, sterile occlusive dressing is applied. The cannula is attached to the I.V., and infusion commences promptly to prevent thrombosis of the cannula. If the connection is made before the skin is closed, particular care must be taken to avoid contaminating the open wound.

The cannula may always be withdrawn after its insertion, but once the sterile field is broken, it cannot be advanced without contaminating the wound.

See illustration on opposite page.

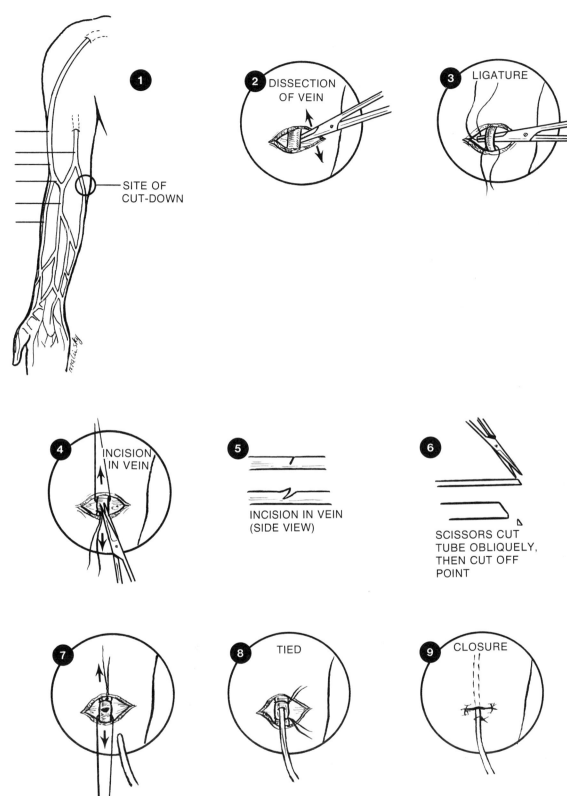

Figure 16 See legend on opposite page.

pose: the cephalic vein at the shoulder, or in the upper arm, or at the wrist are good spots. The basilic vein just above the elbow on the medial aspect of the arm is also an excellent vein for cut-down purposes. In very urgent situations, the saphenous vein at the ankle is perhaps the easiest vein to reach and gain access to the circulation. The saphenous vein at the ankle has two major disadvantages: (1) the risk of significant phlebitis in the leg vein with subsequent thromboembolic phenomena must be considered; (2) it is a long way from the ankle to the central venous system, and infusion of cold fluids may cause the vein to go into spasm and make it difficult to obtain rapid infusion of fluids and drugs through this route.

The external jugular vein in the neck also is a satisfactory vein for cut-down, and on occasion the saphenous vein, or one of its branches, at the groin may be employed—again with the possible complication of thromboembolic phenomena in the leg. Any time a cut-down is performed, that vein must be considered as sacrificed forever. Any one of a number of cannulas may be used for a cutdown: various polyethylene tubes, the tubing from an Intracath, or in some cases a sterile pediatric feeding tube is available in size No. 5 or 8 French when a very large line is required.

EQUIPMENT

A scalpel will be necessary; usually several hemostats; several pairs of scissors, including a small pair of fine pointed scissors; suture; small retractors, and possibly a self-retaining retractor; syringe and needle for injecting local anesthesia; sponges; and antiseptic solution.

TECHNIQUE

The skin over the area of the cut-down is shaved and washed with the antiseptic solution, and sterile drapes are applied around the area to prevent contamination of the instruments, and subsequently of the surgical field. The region of the incision is infiltrated with local anesthetic (this may be omitted in the unconscious patient or the neonate). The author usually prefers transverse incisions, as these ultimately heal more quickly and with less scarring. In addition, it is easier to find the vein through a

transverse incision than it is through a longitudinal incision, as usually the vein is not readily in evidence (if it were, one would probably start an I.V. in the usual manner, rather than do a cut-down). The incision then is made through the anesthetized skin. The incision must be carried down through the dermis so that the fat protrudes and the dermis is completely separated. At this point it is possible to separate the fat bluntly with a hemostat, spreading longitudinally in the direction in which the vein is expected to run. When the vein is identified, it can be dissected by spreading bluntly on either side of it with a hemostat and sutures passed around it. A sufficient length (about 1½ to 2 cm.) is cleared of adjacent tissue. Some veins (e.g., the greater saphenous vein at the ankle) may have a small sensory nerve accompanying them, and it is important to dissect this nerve off the vein, otherwise it will be injured in the subsequent manipulations leading to sensory changes and possibly long-lasting pain in the extremity. The vein is tied off distally; this thread is not cut, but is retained for traction. A ligature is passed loosely around the vein proximally and the vein is opened. The author prefers to open it with a small oblique incision halfway across the circumference of the vein, using a pair of fine-pointed scissors. Others use a scalpel. The lumen then is identified with a probe if necessary, and spread with a mosquito or small hemostat to accommodate the cannula. A new disposable vein dilator that simplifies this process is available.

It sometimes is helpful to bevel the tip of the cannula beforehand so that it may be advanced into the vein easily. If the cannula is about the same size as the vein, so that it is difficult to advance it, it sometimes helps to place tiny traction sutures of 6–0 silk in the lip of the vein, where it is cut to open the vein wide enough to advance the cannula. After the cannula is in place, blood should be seen to come back through it (it may not if there are valves immediately above the cannula preventing the return of blood, or if the vascular tree is empty). I.V. tubing is attached to the cannula, and the infusion is commenced. Care must be taken that the cannula is not dislodged by the weight of the I.V. tubing at this point. On the other hand, the operator's hands must remain sterile, to complete the procedure; if the operator touches the unsterile I.V. tubing, bacteria may be carried into the wound. The proximal ligature then is tied around the cannula snugly, but not enough to occlude the cannula. The distal ligature is tied around the cannula for additional support. The wound is closed with two or three sutures, and one or more of these is used to tie the cannula to the skin. A dressing is applied with antibiotic ointment over the point of the entrance of the cannula into the skin, and the tubing is looped on the patient's skin and secured with tape in such a way that a tug will not pull it loose.

COMPLICATIONS

These include injuries to adjacent structures such as tendons, nerves, and arteries; embolization of the cannulas (although this is unlikely); air embolism; and perforation of the veins somewhere above the site of cannulation, with subsequent administration of fluids into the surrounding tissues.

Most cut-downs can be expected to last two to three days before the vein becomes inflamed and the cannula will have to be removed. An inflamed vein is quite painful and may lead to fever and sepsis. Some solutions containing high potassium and some medications (e.g., cephalothin) are extremely irritating to veins. Some physicians use a very small amount of heparin in each I.V. bottle to reduce thrombosis (e.g., 500 units per bottle of 1000 cc.).

Central Venous Pressure Lines

A measurement of central venous pressure provides information about the filling pressure of the right ventricle. Under many circumstances, it is presumed when the filling pressure of the right ventricle rises that the circulating blood volume is full. Exceptions to this may be found in cases of pulmonary embolism in which there may be right ventricular overload, and in certain other types of right heart failure. In such cases, a relatively small blood volume may be associated with a high CVP reading. On the other hand, sometimes the left ventricle may fail before the right ventricle does, and pulmonary edema may develop before CVP rises significantly. A CVP measurement is one of many parameters that may be used to assess a patient's blood volume and cardiac status, and should not be relied on as a sole indicator of the patient's condition. For example, if there is evidence of tachypnea and rales in the lung bases even when CVP is low, the patient must be presumed to be going into pulmonary edema, and appropriate steps should be taken. Conversely, if CVP is high, blood pressure is low, and urine output is low, the circulation is failing despite a high CVP reading.

Indications for insertion of a CVP line include the management of shock; massive hemorrhage or major trauma; certain patients with sepsis; those in poor condition undergoing major or intermediate surgical procedure; and those with myocardial infarction. Whenever there is major derangement of the cardiovascular system in a patient with multiple system disease, or in whom there is uncertainty about how much fluid to administer, CVP is useful as a parameter to help evaluate ongoing needs for fluid and blood. There is much room for physicians' judgment as to which patients need a central venous pressure line and at what time in their treatment it should be inserted.

The normal range of CVP is up to 15 cm. of water.

A variety of catheters and cannulas are available that can be advanced into a central vein. The measurements may be read off a water manometer, using as zero a point 2 inches below the angle of Lues on the sternum almost regardless of what position the patient is in, either supine or sitting. In the adult, the tricuspid valve will be about 2 inches below this point in either position. As a matter of routine, it is wise to measure CVP in the same position every time, usually a recumbent position, always using the same zero point. An alternative to a water manometer is a pressure transducer and appropriate measuring equipment such as a calibrated oscilloscope or a digital electronic read-out.

TECHNIQUE OF INSERTING A CENTRAL VENOUS PRESSURE LINE

A variety of techniques may be used that involve either inserting a long intravenous cannula through a needle into the vein, or performing a cut-down and inserting the cannula through a cut-down into the vein. In either case, the distance to the region of the superior vena cava or the right atrium is estimated, the cannula is advanced that far, and then is attached to an I.V. tubing with a slow infusion of fluid to keep the tube patent; a three-way stopcock is used to attach the column of fluid to a pressure manometer or to a pressure transducer.

Suitable veins for insertion of the CVP line by percutaneous cannulation are the antecubital vein at the elbow, the external jugular, and the subclavian and internal jugular veins. Useful veins for inserting it by cutdown are the cephalic vein at the shoulder, the external jugular vein, and the basilic vein at the elbow. The external jugular and cephalic veins enter the subclavian vein at such an angle that it sometimes is difficult to pass the catheter into a central vein. Movement of the arm over the head sometimes straightens out the vein and allows the catheter to pass. The catheter passed into this vein frequently will pass smoothly into the central venous system without meeting resistance.

The internal jugular and subclavian veins are almost ideal for inserting venous pressure lines, as the catheter enters the central venous system almost immediately. After the CVP line is inserted, it is important to obtain a chest x-ray to check the position of the catheter and ensure that it is in the area intended.

In placing a CVP line, great care should be taken to assure good sterile technique so that the catheter does not become infected and require early removal.

MAINTENANCE OF CENTRAL VENOUS PRESSURE LINES

If blood is allowed to flow back into a CVP line, a clot will form in the line and it will become unusable within a few hours. Therefore, in measuring the pressure, the optimal technique is to turn the stopcock and allow fluid to enter the manometer from the infusing bottle, and then to turn the stopcock so that the fluid runs from the manometer into the patient. In this way, blood is not allowed to return into the tubing except as the pressure fluctuates toward the end of the reading. A small amount of heparin (e.g., 1000 units in a liter of solution) will help to prevent clotting of the catheter. Usually, the

fluid running through the CVP line runs at a slow speed to keep it open, perhaps 20 cc. an hour. In this way, the flow of fluid into the patient is not interrupted when CVP readings are taken. If the patient is receiving drugs through the CVP line, their flow will be altered or interrupted during measurements.

In administering certain drugs intravenously, the CVP line should be used; vasoconstrictors such as norepinephrine and epinephrine administered into a peripheral vein may cause slough of regional tissue. Also, if concentrated potassium (>40 mEq./liter) must be administered, the CVP line is an optimal line for the purpose because the potassium is immediately diluted in a large flow of blood and does not irritate the vein at that level. (The total number of milliequivalents administered must remain small enough so that potassium intoxication does not occur.) Concentrated potassium administered into a peripheral vein is very painful. Cold blood should *not* be administered by this route, as it may cool the heart.

Central venous pressure lines may be inserted through the saphenous system into the inferior vena cava. This usually requires a cut-down, and carries certain amount of risk of thrombosis and thromboembolic phenomena; therefore, this route generally is not recommended.

Phlebotomy*

Emergency phlebotomy may be carried out in certain patients in pulmonary edema as a way of relieving dyspnea caused by congestive heart failure with pulmonary edema. The indications for this procedure are limited because in most cases there are methods of treating pulmonary edema with cardiotonic drugs, diuretics, rotating tourniquets, bronchodilators, and narcotics. However, in an occasional patient who is hypervolemic, it may provide some immediate relief of dyspnea. It is particularly useful in

---

*The reader may notice that the word "phlebotomy" means cutting a vein. In medieval times bloodletting was accomplished by nicking a vein, and allowing the blood to flow. This therapy is now accomplished with a needle, tubing, and collection bag; but the name remains.

patients who have been overtreated with blood or fluids. It also is helpful in anemic patients, for whom the blood can be removed, plasma separated from the cells by centrifugation, and the cells returned to the patient (i.e., plasmapheresis).

The obvious disadvantage of phlebotomy for the treatment of pulmonary edema or fluid overload lies in the possibility of precipitating hypovolemic shock. The technique of phlebotomy is the same as that commonly used for obtaining blood from blood donors. A single bag or vacuum bottle will take off about 500 cc. of blood. The blood then may be preserved and may be reinfused into the patient at a future time.

PROCEDURES ON ARTERIES

Arterial Punctures

Arterial blood samples are required to study the oxygenation of the blood, and to gain over-all assessment of cardiopulmonary function and acid-base balance. Knowledge of the body's PO_2, PCO_2, pH, as well as bicarbonate and base excess, provides very essential information in planning therapy for the acutely ill or injured. A full discussion of acid-base distribution is beyond the scope of this chapter. Blood ammonia levels also are obtained from arterial blood samples.

TECHNIQUE

The necessary equipment is assembled first.

(1) A small (2 or 5 cc.) sterile glass syringe rinsed with heparin from which all air has been expressed.* (Gases such as O_2 and CO_2 diffuse through plastic faster than through glass.)

(2) A small needle: 22 gauge; larger needles cause more trauma to the artery.

---

*To prepare the syringe, draw up a small amount of heparin (1000 U. per cc.), draw the plunger back the full length of the barrel, filling the syringe with air so that all surfaces are exposed to the heparin; then carefully express the air and excess heparin out through the needle in such a way that no air bubbles are left behind and that the tip of the syringe and needle are filled with heparin. Heparin is expensive and is in short supply, and excessive amounts of it should not be wasted in heparinizing syringes for blood gas samples.

(3) A small container full of ice chips to cool the specimen.

(4) A rubber stopper to place over the end of the needle.

(5) Alcohol sponges.

(6) An appropriate laboratory requisition and label for the specimen.

After assembling the equipment, a suitable artery—usually the radial or brachial artery—is selected. The course of the artery is mapped by palpation, the skin is cleansed with alcohol, and the needle attached to the syringe is advanced briskly into the artery. Arteries tend to be mobile and to roll away from the needle. Sometimes it is better to transfix the artery with the needle, and then withdraw the needle slowly with very gentle negative pressure on the barrel of the syringe. Blood will come up into the syringe under pressure and push the plunger of a glass syringe up. (Plastic syringes have a rubber-plastic surface that is not easily pushed up by arterial pressure.) One can

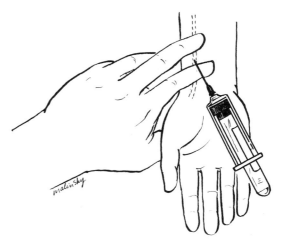

Figure 17 Technique of arterial puncture. The operator palpates the artery with the index and middle fingers of the nondominant hand. A mental outline of the artery's course is formulated. Using the dominant hand, the syringe (prepared as described in the text) is inserted quickly and firmly into the artery. Frequently it pierces the back wall. (Arteries are often mobile and roll away from a probing needle, so insertion with conviction and decisiveness is indicated.) The plunger is withdrawn gently; if no blood comes, the entire needle and syringe may be withdrawn together slowly until blood appears in the syringe. Usually arterial pressure will raise the barrel of the heparinized glass syringe with virtually no traction on the part of the operator. Venous blood will not produce this effect.

1

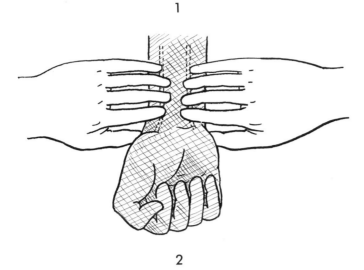

2

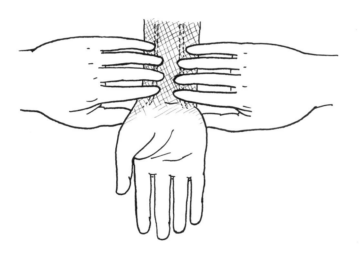

3

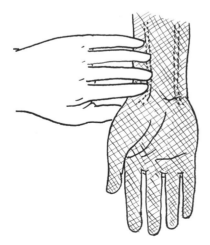

Figure 18 Allen's test. Before instrumenting the radial artery it is important to be sure that a competent ulnar artery is pesent. This can be done as follows:

1. The examiner compresses both arteries and the patient makes a tight fist to squeeze all the blood out of the hand.

2. The patient then extends the fingers, and the examiner observes the blanched hand.

3. Compression of the ulnar artery is released, and the examiner observes the hand fill with blood. If filling does not occur, the ulnar artery is presumed to be nonfunctional.

This sequence of events may be varied to test the adequacy of the radial artery as well.

distinguish between venous and arterial blood by the pressure. In cyanotic patients, arterial blood may be dark enough to be confused with venous blood. When a suitable volume (1 to 2 cc.) is obtained, the syringe and needle is capped with the rubber stopper so that no air can enter. The syringe is labeled and immersed in the ice chips, and taken promptly to the laboratory for analysis. Pressure is maintained over the site of puncture for five minutes by the clock—longer if the patient is anticoagulated or has a coagulopathy. The pressure should be firm enough to keep blood from leaking through the needlehole, but not enough to occlude the artery. There must be a flow of blood to bring platelets and clotting factors to the hole to plug it.

HAZARDS

Instrumentation of any artery can tear the intima and lead to thrombosis of the artery; the danger is greater if the artery is the seat of arteriosclerotic change. Therefore, the femoral artery, although larger and readily accessible, is a poor choice of source for arterial blood gases because it frequently is involved with arteriosclerosis in older patients, and thrombosis of it may lead to loss of the leg. The author knows of cases in which instrumentation of the femoral artery has resulted in amputation. Similarly the carotid artery, although large and palpable, should not be needled to obtain arterial blood samples, because thrombosis here may lead to stroke. Arteries suitable for drawing blood gas samples include the radial, brachial, and superficial temporal. Note, however, that if the brachial is used, subsequent blood pressure determinations on that arm may be in error.

A hematoma should not be allowed to form. The use of a small diameter needle, and the immediate application of pressure for five minutes by the clock following withdrawal of the needle, will minimize hematoma formation. The arteries may be punctured repeatedly if necessary in the management of a patient, but once a hematoma has formed the artery may not be palpable, and so may be unavailable for repeat determination of the blood gases. In addition, hematomas are uncomfortable and unsightly; they may result in significant blood loss (requiring transfusion); and they may become secondarily infected.

Large needles are more likely to tear the intima and leave a larger hole for hematoma formation; therefore, small caliber needles should be used.

Arterial Cannulas

A cannula may be inserted into an artery in a manner similar to venous cannulation. This procedure is valuable for frequent determinations of arterial blood gases, for electronic measurement of blood pressure, and for cardiogreen dye cardiac output determination.

HAZARDS

The obvious complications can be expected: thrombosis and hemorrhage. If the cannula is left in more than a few hours, the artery may thrombose and (it is hoped) recanalize after several weeks, although its lumen will never be what it was originally. If the radial artery is used, the ulnar artery usually will supply the hand.

In a small percentage of patients the ulnar artery is inadequate, absent, or previously thrombosed. In these, radial artery cannulation may result in an acutely ischemic hand, and ultimately in necrosis of the hand. The author has observed this sequence of events in a 14-year-old girl. An Allen's test should always be performed prior to cannulating the radial artery (testing for ulnar artery adequacy).

Moreover, the indwelling arterial cannula will obstruct and thrombose any branches whose orifice it covers over; therefore, only short cannulas should be used. Arterial thrombosis may even threaten the limb.

Finally, if an arterial pressure line is dislodged, profuse bleeding under arterial pressure will occur. It can be easily controlled by direct pressure, but if it is not detected immediately, hypotension and exsanguination may result.

Chapter 13

ABDOMINAL PROCEDURES

Ellen E. Anderson

ABDOMINAL TAP

The examination of the abdomen in a patient who has sustained head trauma, blunt abdominal trauma, or multiple injuries is notoriously difficult. A recent prospective study of 500 blunt abdominal trauma patients treated at the Naval Hospital in San Diego noted that 40 per cent of those thought on the initial physical examination to have a "surgical" abdomen had no intra-abdominal injury (Parvin, et al., 1975). Another study of 232 patients with blunt abdominal trauma noted that 21 per cent of those with initially obvious signs and symptoms of abdominal trauma did not have significant injuries (Olsen, et al., 1972). It is desirable to avoid unnecessary laparotomies on these patients. The converse situation, probably one of greater significance, involves patients with equivocal or absent signs of intra-abdominal injury or hemorrhage who have sustained significant abdominal injuries that one would like to identify and treat promptly. Wilson et al. (1965) noted that the mortality rate was four times greater when blunt abdominal injury was associated with head injury.

Various forms of peritoneal aspiration by needle or catheter have been advocated since 1906, when Solomon described his technique of abdominal tap. Although the use of the peritoneal tap has largely been superseded in recent years by peritoneal lavage, it is carried out so rapidly that some surgeons advocate its use prior to lavage, since a positive tap will save the 20 to 30 minutes necessary for lavage.

Indications

Current indications for peritoneal tap include patients with:

(1) blunt abdominal trauma;

(2) blunt abdominal trauma *in association with* head injury, thoracic injury, extremity injury, alcoholic intoxication, or drug overdose (McCoy, et al., 1971);

(3) acute pancreatitis where serum amylase is not elevated (Morris, 1966); and

(4) primary peritonitis in infancy and childhood where associated disease (cirrhosis, nephrosis) makes the risk of surgery prohibitive (McDougal, et al., 1975).

(5) postoperative peritonitis, as with ruptured duodenal stump (Morris, 1966).

Contraindications

There are no definite contraindications to peritoneal tap. However, it is ill-advised to use it on the occasional patient unable to hold or be held still (e.g., one with severe alcoholic intoxication). Drapanas and McDonald (1961) suggested avoiding abdominal tap in patients with distended bowel. Previous studies have shown, however that intestine will not be punctured by a spinal needle unless the gut is held fixed, and that even if it is punctured, leakage will not occur until high intraluminal pressures are reached (McCoy, et al., 1971).

Technique

The technique of peritoneal tap is simple and quick (Fig. 1). The preferred tech-

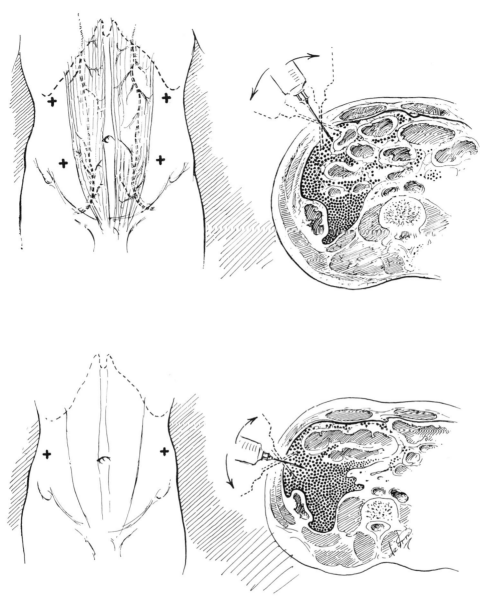

Figure 1. Sites for four-quadrant and bilateral flank taps. Note that the site for bilateral flank taps is midway between costal margin and iliac spine. (From Drapanas, T., and McDonald, J.: Surgery 50:744, 1961.)

nique is that advocated by the late Dr. Drapanas in 1961. After voiding or being catheterized, the patient is placed in a supine position. The sites for proposed tap are cleansed with Betadine solution. One may choose a four quadrant tap or bilateral flank tap. Drapanas preferred the bilateral flank tap, believing that aspiration laterally along the peritoneal gutters would increase the chances of a successful tap if only small amounts of fluid were present. Other reasons cited for preferring the flank approach are the decreased chance of needling gas-filled loops of bowel (which float more anteriorly when the intraperitoneal space is filled with fluid and blood), and the decreased risk of needling the inferior epigastric vessels. Care is taken to avoid areas of previous surgical incisions or other areas where the bowel could be fixed to the abdominal wall in the vicinity of a mass. A skin wheal of local anesthetic is made at the tap sites, using a No. 25 gauge needle. The peritoneum below this also is infiltrated. A No. 20 or 18 gauge spinal needle with stylet in place is then inserted until one feels the peritoneum "give" before the needle. The stylet then is removed, and a 10-ml. syringe attached. Gentle suction is applied initially and as the direction of the needle is carefully changed. The best location for aspiration is just within the peritoneal cavity. If no fluid is obtained, the opposite flank (or other three quadrants) are tapped.

Interpretation

As little as 0.1 ml. of fluid has been considered a positive tap. When blood is aspirated, it must be watched for clotting. Blood from a hemoperitoneum will not clot, and the test is considered positive. Blood drawn from the abdominal wall, omentum, or mesentery will clot and gives no information (negative test). If fluid other than blood is aspirated, it is examined grossly, smeared on a slide for microscopic examination, cultured, and a serum amylase test performed where indicated. Aspiration of bile or frank pus is considered a positive test. If fluid on microscopic examination has many differing organisms with no leukocytes, the aspirate is most likely to be from within the bowel (Morris, 1966).

Complications

The only complication reported was a consequence of improper technique: puncture through the rectus sheath lacerating the inferior epigastric artery. This created a hematoma that had to be drained subsequently (Drapanas and McDonald, 1961). Other series reporting large numbers of peritoneal taps did not have complications (McCoy, et al., 1971; Olsen, et al., 1971).

Discussion

The greatest value of the abdominal tap is its indication of hemoperitoneum when nonclotting blood is aspirated. A positive tap is an indication for immediate laparotomy. It must be stressed that a negative tap is meaningless and cannot be interpreted as ruling out serious intra-abdominal problems. The over-all accuracy of the tap is about 80 per cent (Drapanas and McDonald, 1961).

ABDOMINAL LAVAGE

One of the chief drawbacks to the abdominal tap is that its accuracy is directly related to the quantity of blood in the abdomen. In an effort to overcome this disadvantage, the peritoneal lavage was devised by Root, et al. in 1965. Its sensitivity is so great that 30 to 50 cc. of intra-abdominal blood can be detected (Olsen, et al., 1971). The modifications that this test has undergone to help reduce the number of complications, false positives, and unnecessary laparotomies will be discussed. It is important to realize that the test is intended primarily to reflect intraperitoneal traumatic injuries. It may or may not reflect trauma to extraperitoneal structures—duodenum, pancreas, kidney, bladder, and blood vessels. For these injuries, Gastrografin duodenogram, arteriogram, intravenous pyelogram, or cystogram may be needed (Parvin, et al., 1975; Engrav, et al., 1975).

Indications

Olsen and Hildreth (1971) recommend lavage at the time of admission to the Emergency Department in all patients in whom an experienced examiner questions the possibility of an intra-abdominal injury. This would include patients who have sustained sufficient force to have caused such injury, regardless of abdominal findings. Root (1975), in discussing a paper presented at the American Association for the Surgery of Trauma, mentioned that he used as one of his indications for lavage the fact that a person had been killed in an accident or that the vehicle had been totally wrecked. He felt this indicated massive deceleration force.

Contraindications

The most commonly accepted contraindications for peritoneal lavage are:
(1) an unstable patient requiring immediate surgery;
(2) a pregnant patient (because of the risk of injuring the fetus in the lower abdomen or injuring the displaced viscera in the upper abdomen); and

(3) a patient with multiple previous abdominal operations (because of the danger of damaging bowel fixed by adhesions, and the probability of loculation of lavage fluid) (Thal and Shires, 1973; Parvin, et al., 1975).

Thal and Shires feel that gunshot and stab wounds of the abomen or the presence of dilated bowel, are further contraindications. Root (1975), however, does use lavage in selected patients with stab wounds of the abdomen.

Technique (Figs. 2, 3, 4, and 5)

As for peritoneal tap, the patient is supine, and the urinary bladder is empty (by voiding or catheterization). The lower abdomen is prepared with Betadine solution, and draped. Local anesthesia is given about 6 cm. below the umbilicus. If the patient has had a previous surgical incision in this area, the linea alba above the umbilicus may be used instead. A short skin incision is made and carried down to the fascia. Good hemostasis in the skin and subcutaneous tissue must be achieved to avoid false-positive lavage. The fascia is elevated with hemostats, and a small incision is made in the fascia with a knife blade. The peritoneum is visualized and opened. A catheter—between 11 and 18F.—with multiple side-openings (such as a standard peritoneal dialysis catheter) is inserted in the direction of the pelvis until all the side-holes are within the abdominal cavity. Next, the catheter is aspirated. If 20 cc. of blood returns, the test is considered positive and is concluded at that point. If less than 20 cc. of blood returns, 1 liter of normal saline solution in

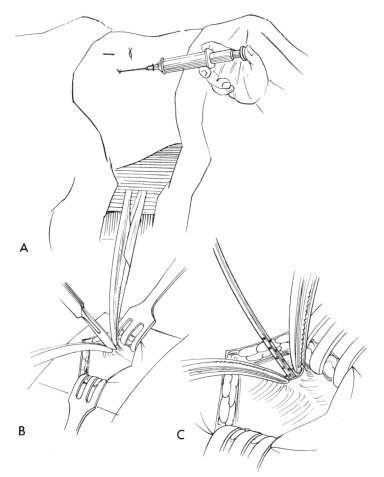

Figure 2. The urinary bladder is first emptied by catheter.

A, The abdominal wall is prepared, draped, and infiltrated with a local anesthetic containing epinephrine. A small incision is made in the midline just below the umbilicus with careful hemostasis.

B, The fascia of the abdominal wall is incised in the midline, and the peritoneum is visualized and opened.

C, A peritoneal dialysis catheter then is inserted into the peritoneal cavity. (From Perry, J. F., Jr.: Curr. Probl. Surg., May 1970.)

A

B   C

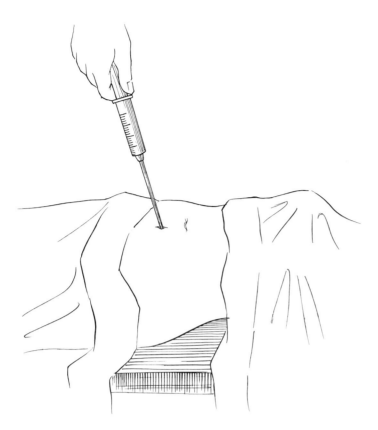

Figure 3. Aspiration of the peritoneal cavity is carried out next. Recovery of gross blood constitutes a positive test and is an indication to proceed with laparotomy. (From Perry, J. F., Jr.: Curr. Probl. Surg., May 1970.)

adults, or 15 to 20 cc./kg. in a child, are infused via the catheter. The patient then is turned side-to-side if at all possible. This mixes the infusate with intraperitoneal fluid. The infusion blottle is placed on the floor to allow fluid to return to the bottle. The gross appearance is noted. An aliquot is removed for red and white blood cell counts, amylase concentration, and gram stain. The catheter is removed if the test is positive, and a single suture is placed in the fascia. The subcutaneous tissue and skin are closed routinely. If the test is negative, the catheter is left in place, and the lavage may be repeated after one to two hours (Engrav, et al., 1975).

Interpretation

The test is positive if greater than 20 cc. of blood returns from the catheter with initial syringe aspiration, or if newsprint cannot be read through the tubing of returning red fluid. The test also is grossly positive if the infusate returns via a chest tube or Foley catheter. These criteria are gross by design so that the surgeon may give prompt care to

the patient. Perry (1970) also regards as positive lavage fluids containing more than 100,000 RBC/cu. mm., more than 500 WBC/cu. mm., more than 200 Karoway units amylase/100 cc. (Engrav, et al., 1975). This quantitation of RBCs correlates with the grosser test of reading print through the tube of returning fluid (Olsen, et al., 1972). Olsen, Redman, and Hildreth in 1972, and a group at the San Diego Naval Hospital in 1975, have done studies that help with the interpretation of weakly positive studies—pink lavage where print can be read through the tubing, or where the counts are less than those mentioned previously. In this group, the Naval Hospital reports 9 per cent with significant injury. Of the same group, Olsen, et al. (1972) report 24 per cent with significant injury. It is suggested that patients with weakly positive lavages undergo abdominal echography and, if this is positive, visceral arteriography.

In view of their experience, the group reporting from San Diego felt that an elevated lavage fluid amylase in a clear aspirate was not an indication for laparotomy unless the patient had progressively increasing

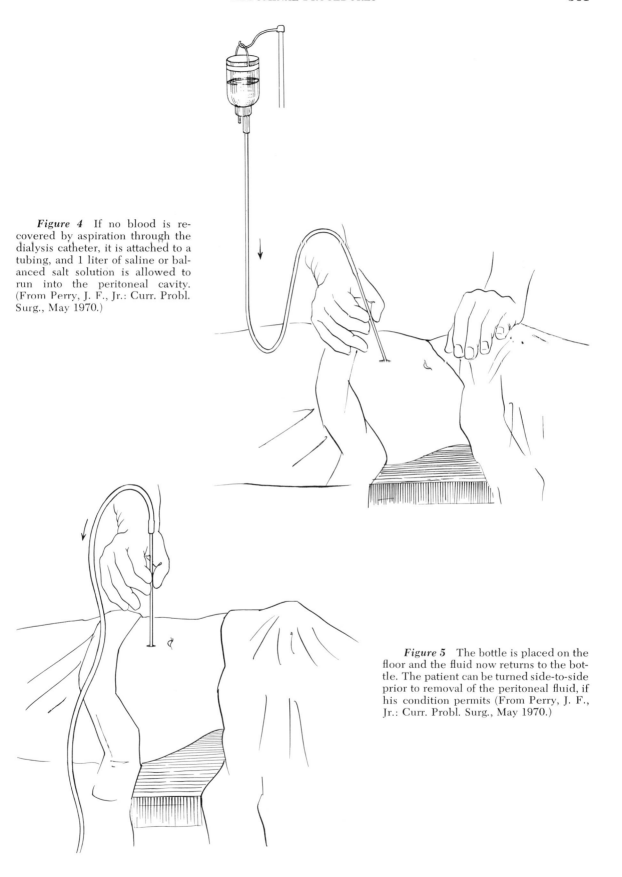

Figure 4 If no blood is recovered by aspiration through the dialysis catheter, it is attached to a tubing, and 1 liter of saline or balanced salt solution is allowed to run into the peritoneal cavity. (From Perry, J. F., Jr.: Curr. Probl. Surg., May 1970.)

Figure 5 The bottle is placed on the floor and the fluid now returns to the bottle. The patient can be turned side-to-side prior to removal of the peritoneal fluid, if his condition permits (From Perry, J. F., Jr.: Curr. Probl. Surg., May 1970.)

serum amylase and persistent abdominal findings (Parvin, et al. 1975), not felt to represent pancreatitis.

Regarding WBCs, it is helpful to remember that the lavage fluid should not be centrifuged and that an automatic counter should not be used. Both can give falsely high values (Root, 1975). Whether or not this could have been the cause, Parvin, et al. (1975) in their series found that only 1 of 18 patients with clear lavage and WBC count greater than 500/cu. mm. had a significant injury.

Complications

The complications of peritoneal lavage generally are related to technique in its performance. Various authors report the following complications:

(1) penetration of the bladder;

(2) perforation of an iliac artery (trocar advanced after entering peritoneum), branch of the right colic artery, and a mesenteric vein, as well as catheterization of an epiploic vein;

(3) perforation of the ileum;

(4) infusion of lavage into the abdominal wall;

(5) penetration of a hematoma created by previous tap;

(6) bleeding from the abdominal wall; and

(7) wound separation.

Some would say the above list illustrates Murphy's Law, i.e., "whatever can go wrong will go wrong." However, it seems clear that by excluding patients with multiple previous abdominal operations, taking care that the patient's bladder is empty, and using countertraction after visualizing the linea alba, most of these complications could be avoided. Parvin, et al. (1975) report an enviable record with this technique: no major complications; 6 per cent incidence of minor complications, including wound separation and wound hematoma.

Discussion

Peritoneal lavage is a rapid, safe, accurate method of determining intraperitoneal injury in patients who have sustained head trauma, multiple injuries, and blunt abdominal trauma. It also may help to diagnose retroperitoneal injuries, but additional tests are advised if these are suspected.

INGUINAL HERNIOGRAPHY

Herniography is a safe, quick method of intraperitoneal injection of radiopaque material to delineate pathologic lesions in the inguinal canal. It was first reported by Ducharme, et al. in 1967. Much of its use has been related to the ongoing controversy regarding bilateral inguinal exploration in repair of pediatric hernias. Since inguinal hernias have nearly a 25 per cent incidence of incarceration in infants, they are repaired as soon as they are diagnosed. This does not allow for observation of the individual patient to see if he will be one of the 10 to 20 per cent of the population who will develop bilateral hernias (James, 1971). Use of the herniogram obviates exploration of the contralateral side with its increased time under anesthesia, risk to the blood supply of the vas deferens or testicle, or both, and destruction of the anatomy of a previously normal area.

Indications

Indications for inguinal herniography can be summarized as follows:

(1) clinically unilateral inguinal hernia, rule out contralateral inguinal hernia;

(2) parental history of inguinal "bulge" not confirmed by physical examination;

(3) questionable physical examination;

(4) hydrocele without palpable hernia;

(5) cryptorchidism;

(6) differential diagnosis of groin mass — inguinal lymph node, hydrocele, inguinal hernia, femoral hernia, incarcerated hernia; and

(7) Possible recurrent hernia (Blau, et al., 1973).

It should be clear that some of these indications refer not only to children, but also to older age-groups — especially items 3, 5, and 6.

Contraindications

Guttman and his associates (1972) mention dehydration, especially in infants and children, as very undesirable. Another contraindication is a known allergy to the contrast material, although this probably would not be known in infants and children. No allergic reactions were reported in the series reviewed (Blau, et al., 1973; Guttman, et al., 1972; Shackelford and McAlister, 1972).

Technique

The basic technique is not dissimilar to that for the peritoneal tap or lavage (see Fig. 3). Those of age are asked to void. Infants probably will void during the procedure. Premedication is not necessary. The patient is placed in a supine position. Ordinarily, adults or cooperative children can be placed on the rotating x-ray table so that they can be turned prone and rotated to 45 degrees after injection. Infants can be placed on a "brat board" or simply held by two people — one holding the arms and head, the other holding the hips and legs. An area in the midline, approximately one-third of the distance from the umbilicus to the symphysis pubis, is cleansed. (Some prefer insertion in right or left lower quadrant, lateral to the rectus sheath; Guttman, et al., 1972.) A skin wheal with local anesthesia may be raised. The

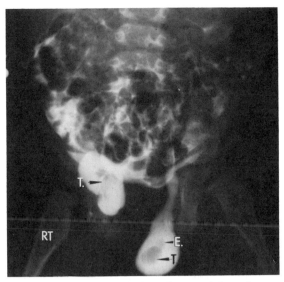

Figure 7 Roentgenogram showing bilateral open peritoneal sacs with an undescended testicle (T) on the right. The testicle (T) and epididymis (E) are identified on the left. (From Blau, J. S., Keating, T. M., and Stockinger, F. S.: Radiologic diagnosis of inguinal hernia in children. Surg. Gynecol. Obstet. *136*:401, 1973. By Permission of *Surgery, Gynecology & Obstetrics*.)

peritoneum is entered with a No. 20 gauge, 1½-inch needle, and aspiration is performed to see if a viscus has been entered. The Renografin-60 or Hypaque-M60 then is injected — 2 cc./kg. for infants up to 7 kg. The dose is increased incrementally up to a maximum of 40 cc. for persons over 50 kg (White, et al., 1970). If there is an apparent hernia, the bowel is gently reduced to prevent "stoppering" the sac. The child is held erect for five minutes at a 45-degree angle with head forward, and is gently shaken. The larger patient lies prone on an x-ray table, which is rotated to a 45-degree angle. An upright anteroposterior film of the pelvis and upper thighs is made five minutes later, followed in 15 minutes by delayed x-ray. At 30 minutes, another film may be taken if a urogram is desired. A satisfactory study is one in which the contrast material outlines the peritoneal cavity both lateral and medial to the inferior epigastric artery on each side (see Figs. 6 and 7).

If the bowel lumen is injected with contrast material, the study can be repeated in another day. Shackelford and McAlister (1972) have routinely reinjected immediately and obtained good studies without side-effects.

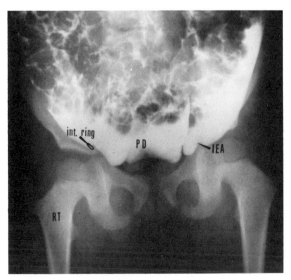

Figure 6 Normal herniogram. The inferior epigastric artery notch (IEA) is the most significant anatomic landmark. The vaginal process starts lateral to this indentation. The posterior cul-de-sac (PD) is demonstrated. (From Blau, J. S., Keating, T. M., and Stockinger, F. S.: Radiologic diagnosis of inguinal hernia in children. Surg. Gynecol. Obstet. *136*:401, 1973. By Permission of *Surgery, Gynecology & Obstetrics*.)

Interpretation

The processus vaginalis is located lateral to the peritoneal identation made by the inferior epigastric artery. Contrast material within the processus or within the scrotum constitutes a positive diagnosis (Blau, et al., 1973). Besides demonstrating a widely open peritoneal sac or a communicating hydrocele, the herniogram may show a hydrocele of the cord or may localize the testicle in a cryptorchid patient. If the processus is less than 1.5 cm. in length and 0.3 cm. in width by x-ray, James (1971) does not feel that removal is justified. He also considers that a positive herniogram is helpful in the presence of suspected incarceration, but that a negative one yields no information. Early exploration is favored in such an instance.

Complications

Complications include:
(1) shocklike episode in dehydrated infants;
(2) pain;
(3) nausea; and
(4) injection of the dye into the colon, small intestine, bladder, or abdominal wall.

Guttman and associates (1972) noted an incidence of 11.2 per cent minor complications in their patients, pain and nausea being the most frequent. Two of their infants who had been fasting manifested a shocklike picture after dye injection. They attributed this to the hydrophilic effect of diatrizoate methylglucamine, as reported by Harris, et al. (1964). The injection of dye into colon, small intestine, bladder, or abdominal wall did not appear to produce any ill effects. Pathologic examination of the hernia sacs did not show acute or chronic inflammatory changes in the series of Blau and associates (1973). White, et al. (1970) in their series noted that the radiation to the gonads was between 50 and 300 mr. for boys, and half of that amount for girls. This is less than the amount used for cystourethrography in children, and is considered to be well below the range that might interfere with spermatogenesis or the blood-forming organs.

Discussion

Inguinal herniography had 95 per cent accuracy in a double-blind study of 100 patients by White (1970). Had surgery in this study been directed by the results of the clinical examination and of the herniogram, no significant errors would have been made. It is felt that herniography is very useful when there is any doubt regarding the bilaterality of an inguinal hernia, or if recurrence or incarceration are under consideration.

BLADDER CATHETERIZATION

Indications

The chief indications for bladder catheterization are as follows:
(1) To monitor urine output in the critically injured patient, during long operative procedures, and during operations on the aorta or its major branches.
(2) To relieve acute urinary retention.
(3) In the patient with severe spinal cord injury.
(4) In patients undergoing pelvic operation.
(5) To obtain urine for diagnostic purposes.

Contraindications

Relative contraindications to catheterization include acute cystitis, urethritis, pyelonephritis, and epididymitis, unless obstruction is the predisposing cause of infection (McDonald, 1974). Stronger contraindications to catheterization include patients in whom several unsuccessful attempts at urethral catheterization have been made, and patients suspected of urethral injury. In either of the latter two cases, there is high risk of iatrogenic injury.

Urethral injury is suspected when:
(1) Blood is present at the urethral meatus;
(2) The patient desires to void but is unable to do so;
(3) A full bladder is palpable;
(4) The prostate is displaced on rectal examination;
(5) A perineal hematoma is present; or
(6) A patient has sustained fracture dislocation of the pelvis or a straddle injury.

Other physical signs suggesting urethral rupture are rigidity and tenderness of the abdomen (intraperitoneal rupture) and ab-

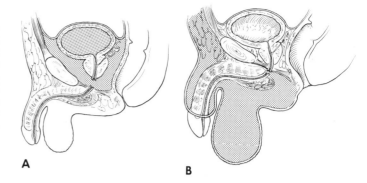

Figure 8 A, Typical location of hematoma and urinary extravasation in injuries to the extraperitoneal portion of the bladder or prostatic urethra. B, Typical route of urinary extravasation and blood collection with injury to the urethra distal to the urogenital diaphragm. (From Committee on Trauma, American College of Surgeons: Early Care of the Injured Patient. Philadelphia, W. B. Saunders Co., 1972.)

dominal muscle spasm, lower abdominal and scrotal swelling, ecchymosis, and bogginess and tenderness on rectal examination (extraperitoneal rupture) (Kaufman, et al., 1972). The typical injuries are well shown in Figure 8.

Technique

Bladder catheterization should be thought of as a sterile operative technique. As the hand that touches the patient becomes immediately contaminated, it is best to have all materials prepared first before touching the patient — cleansing solutions poured, lubricant spread, Foley balloon tested for a leak. For the adult a 16 F. catheter is preferred, as larger indwelling urethral catheters obstruct the drainage of urethral exudates, causing accumulation, infection of secretions, and urethritis (Turner-Warwick, 1975). In children, 8 to 12 F. catheters may be used. The catheter material chosen has not been shown to make a statistical difference in the amount of urethral inflammation caused (Edwards and Trott, 1973). A sterile towel is spread below the urethra. In males, the penis is grasped and the foreskin retracted, both with the left hand. With the right hand, the glans penis is cleansed several times. The catheter then is picked up with the still sterile right hand, holding the distal end tucked between fourth and fifth fingers to avoid contaminating the catheter against unsterile surfaces. (The use of a hemostat for holding the catheter is a further option — see Fig. 9). The catheter tip is well lubricated and inserted gently into the urethra, using a persistent rotary motion when resistance is felt from the sphincter. As this resistance is over-

come, the catheter is advanced completely into the bladder. It then is grasped by the left hand to prevent its slipping out before the catheter balloon can be inflated with 5 to 7.5 cc. of saline or air. The catheter then is pulled forward gently and connected to a sterile closed drainage system (with bacteria-impervious vent near bladder level if possible). The foreskin is drawn forward. If there is great resistance to advancement of the catheter at the level of the prostate, the catheter may be withdrawn and a syringe of 10 cc. sterile lubricant injected into the urethral meatus before a second attempt.

In catheterization of the female patient, the patient is assisted to a frog-leg position if she is not already in dorsal lithotomy. A good light source is important. The left hand is used to spread the labia. The labia and

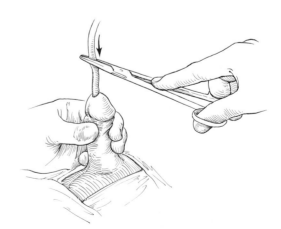

Figure 9 Technique of sterile catheterization. After thorough preparation and draping of the genitalia, a catheter is introduced with a sterile forceps. (From Committee on Trauma, American College of Surgeons: Early Care of the Injured Patient. Philadelphia, W. B. Saunders Co., 1972.)

meatus are cleansed, and the catheter is inserted similarly. If the catheter accidentally enters the vagina, a new catheter is obtained.

In both male and female patients, the catheter is taped securely to the patient to avoid trauma to the urethra or bladder. In the male, the penis is positioned toward the head to minimize discomfort and prevent erosion of the urethra from catheter pressure (Smith and Germain, 1975) (see Fig. 10). Some authors advise gradual bladder decompression after chronic and prolonged bladder distention.

Complications

Problems associated with bladder catheterization can be grouped as follows.
(1) Infection:
    (a) urethritis (with late stricture or fistula);
    (b) bacteriuria;
    (c) epididymitis;
    (d) bacteremia;
    (e) contamination of tissues in urethral tears.
(2) Trauma:
    (a) urethral stricture;
    (b) conversion of a partial urethral tear to a complete one;

(c) creation of a false passage;
(d) bladder lesions secondary to unvented drainage system (Isaacs and McWhorter, 1971).
(3) Paraphimosis (when foreskin is not drawn forward after catheterization).
(4) Hemorrhage and vesical spasm (after rapid decompression in chronic bladder distention) (McDonald, 1974).

SUPRAPUBIC BLADDER DRAINAGE

Indications

Besides the evacuation of urine per urethra, bladder urine also may be obtained from the suprapubic route by simple needle aspiration or by percutaneous catheterization. In pediatric, general, and obstetric practice, suprapubic aspiration is indicated when clean catch urines are inconclusive or contamination is suspected (Cusins, 1973). Suprapubic catheterization is indicated in the following circumstances:
(1) for diagnostic cystometry when one is unable to pass a sufficiently wide catheter per urethra (Nyström et al., 1973);
(2) to relieve urinary obstruction when unable to pass a urethral catheter—the pa-

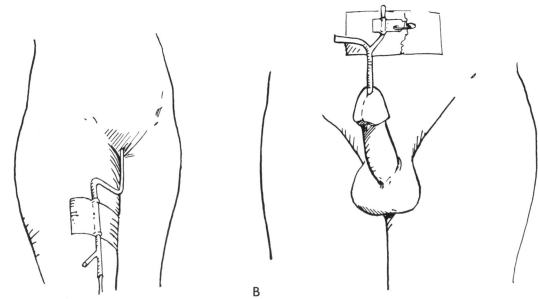

A   B

Figure 10 Anchoring the catheter prevents accidental traction that could result in injury to bladder or urethra. (From Manual of Nursing Procedures, Department of Nursing, Massachusetts General Hospital. Boston, Little, Brown & Co., 1975.)

tient may later need a definitive suprapubic cystostomy (Bonanno, et al., 1970); and

(3) in patients postoperative from bladder surgery and/or gynecologic surgical procedures (Hale and McCorriston, 1969).

Contraindications

Suprapublic catheterization is contraindicated in patients with:

(1) scars from previous lower abdominal or gynecologic surgery;

(2) an abnormal bladder—whether small and shrunken (a capacity less than 200 cc.) or with a thick bladder wall (Nyström, et al., 1973); and

(3) infected urine.

Technique

For suprapubic aspiration or catheterization, the bladder should be at least partially filled with urine. In children, this is achieved by tapping the infant when the diaper is dry. In older children, time should be allowed since the last voiding. In adults, one may try palpating the bladder or pressing with the forefinger 2 cm. above the symphysis pubis to see if that gives the patient the desire to void, or even using ultrasound equipment to locate the bladder wall (Cusins, 1973). The lower abdomen is prepared, and shaved if necessary. A syringe is fitted with a No. 22 gauge 1½-inch needle for children, or No. 20 gauge spinal needle for adults. The needle is inserted in the midline 2 cm. above the symphysis at an angle 10 to 20 degrees to the perpendicular aiming in a slightly caudad direction. A change can be felt when the bladder is entered. Urine is aspirated gently and sent for desired studies.

A similar technique is used for suprapubic catheterization. Commercially prepared suprapubic catheters are available, or one may use a No. 5 infant-feeding tube with the tip cut off and four or five extra holes cut in the side. This latter tube will fit through a No. 13 gauge needle. Passage of the tube through the needle should be tested before insertion of the needle. After the needle is passed in similar fashion to that for tap, urine is aspirated to confirm the needle's position, and the catheter is threaded so that 6 cm. is in the bladder (see Fig. 11). The needle then is removed and the catheter is secured to the skin by suture and tape. A blunt-ended No. 18 gauge needle can be placed in the exterior end of the tubing, and in turn connected to standard intravenous tubing draining to a closed drainage bag. Hale and McCorriston (1969) feel that the cystotomy tube acts as a siphon, and therefore must be kept full of fluid. They recommend injecting the tube with 2 to 5 cc. of 0.25 per cent acetic acid every six hours thereafter to prevent blockage by clots or redundant mucosa. If the cystotomy tubing has been used for postoperative care, it is clamped when the patient has been able to void well on his own. If, after voiding, a residual urine of less than 100 to 150 cc. is found on unclamping, the catheter can be pulled.

Complications

No permanent harm is recorded from the use of suprapubic tap or aspiration. Some temporary problems reported with the catheterization include:

(1) tube kinked;

(2) tip of pediatric tube passed per urethra;

(3) tube removed too early;

(4) hematuria;

(5) leakage around tube of urine or cystography dye;

(6) pain when contrast material was deposited extravesically (one patient); and

(7) suprapubic phlegmon (one patient) (Cusins, 1973).

Discussion

The use of suprapubic tap or catheterization is quick, easy, and free of major complications. Patients who had previously undergone urethral catheterization found suprapubic tap or catheterization much less embarrassing and much more comfortable. It also is noted that patients void earlier with suprapubic drainage than with urethral Foley drainage. It may be the only means of carrying out cystometry on patients with urethral stricture, and is a rapid means of relieving acute urinary retention when a catheter cannot be passed per urethra.

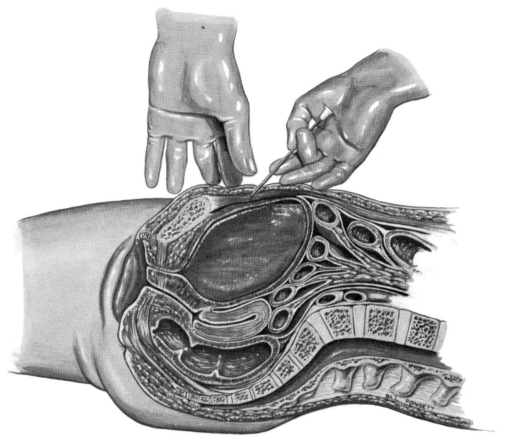

Figure 11   Insertion of trocar for suprapubic catheterization. (Courtesy of Zimmer • USA, Warsaw, Indiana.)

FIBEROPTIC GASTROSCOPY

When Kussmaul in 1868 looked into the stomach of a professional sword-swallower by means of a straight metal-tube gastroscope, a new era had quietly begun. Since that time, endoscopy of the upper gastrointestinal tract has progressed with the inventiveness of man (Tsuneoka, et al., 1973). Currently, the esophagus, stomach, and duodenum are examined simultaneously because of the frequent association of lesions in these areas of the upper gastrointestinal tract (Colcher, 1975).

Indications

Currently, the indications for emergency examination are: (1) *the removal of foreign bodies;* and (2) *investigation of acute*

upper gastrointestinal tract bleeding. Examination in this latter instance frequently is made just prior to abdominal angiography. Location of the bleeding site by endoscopy can facilitate the angiographer's selection of the proper vessel to confirm the bleeding site and begin Pitressin infusion. Colcher reports a 90 to 95 per cent accuracy in correct diagnosis of the source of bleeding when endoscopy is performed during the episode of bleeding, or within four to 12 hours after apparent cessation of bleeding. If the endoscopic examination is postponed for 48 hours, diagnostic accuracy is reduced to 50 per cent. Correct diagnosis early (with appropriate treatment) is particularly important, since many patients will have several potential sources of bleeding—varices, gastritis, ulcer.

In other patients who need endoscopy, most endoscopists prefer barium study of the upper gastrointestinal tract before the procedure. The studies are complementary. The endoscopist does not limit himself to documentation of radiographically demonstrated lesions, but carries out a complete routine study, and the plan for endoscopy is not canceled when the initial UGI barium study appears normal.

Colcher (1975), from the Lahey Clinic, has listed indications for esophagogastroduodenoscopy on two bases, clinical manifestations and radiologic diagnosis. With respect to the former, he has found it most useful in patients with acute upper gastrointestinal tract bleeding, postoperative problems, and dysphagia; and somewhat less useful in patients with chronic blood loss or weight loss when the upper gastrointestinal tract is suspected, persistent abdominal pain or discomfort related to meals. The technique also is less useful in preoperative studies and in the evaluation of resectability of certain tumors, in the evaluation of stomach in patients with blood diseases, some hereditary diseases, and some skin diseases, and in the evaluation of effects of drugs and in problems in pathophysiology.

For the indications based on radiologic diagnosis, Colcher (1975) includes esophageal, gastric and duodenal ulcers; tumors; deformities; malformations; foreign bodies and bezoars; esophageal varices; hiatal hernia with reflux; and postoperative inspection. In emergency practice use would be limited almost exclusively to those patients with: (1) acute bleeding or (2) foreign bodies.

Contraindications

The only absolute contraindication to fiberoptic esophagogastroduodenoscopy is lack of cooperation despite sufficient persuasion and explanation. This includes those with severe psychosis, those with severe ethanol intoxication or cerebral hypoxia, and most children under ten years of age. In some of these patients, examination under general anesthesia will be warranted. Other contraindications are relative. Whether the procedure should and can be carried out depends on the skill of the endoscopist and the strength of need for the procedure. These relative contraindications include:

(1) the period seven to ten days after gastroduodenal surgery (Hedberg, 1974);

(2) marked deformity of the spine secondary to rickets or tuberculosis;

(3) marked deviation of the esophagus due to the presence of aneurysm of the thoracic aorta or mediastinal tumor;

(4) acute stage of acute corrosive gastritis (Tsuneoka, et al., 1973);

(5) cardiac failure, severe coronary artery disease, or recent myocardial infarction;

(6) acute infection (pneumonia, peritonitis, cholecystitis hepatitis); and

(7) obstructive respiratory disease.

Special care is required in patients with Zenker's diverticulum and esophageal diverticulum.

Technique

As with any skilled procedure, technique will vary. However, certain basics always hold. The examiner must know the history and physical findings of the patient, and must view any radiographic studies. The patient needs to understand the basic plan of the procedure and how he can cooperate. When the examination is done electively, the patient is asked to fast from food and drink for the six hours preceding the study, but, as in emergencies, when the study is done for acute upper gastrointestinal hemorrhage, fluid resuscitation should be well under way, the vital signs stable if possible, and the stomach should be evacuated as much as possible. If gastric lavage is not clear, the stomach can be evacuated by an Ewald tube or standard stomach pump tube with several extra holes cut near the tip. Iced saline irrigation is performed, advancing and withdrawing the tube to remove clot from the entire stomach; one should be vigorous in the quantity of irrigant and frequency of irrigation, but gentle in the actual aspiration, to avoid damaging mucosa (Hedberg, 1974).

The pharynx is anesthetized by having the patient gargle viscous Xylocaine. Hedberg (1974) recommends giving all patients 0.5 to 1.0 mg. of atropine sulfate I.M. or I.V. Other premedication varies from nothing to 75 mg. of meperidine (Demerol) I.M. 30 minutes prior to the procedure, and diazepam (Valium) 2 mg. per minute I.V. until the patient is drowsy and has a short delay in response to commands. The average dose of diazepam is 10 mg. (Morrissey, 1972).

The patient is placed comfortably on his

left side. This helps intragastric orientation, allows a right-handed endoscopist to easily feel resistance to insertion, and allows saliva to drain onto a towel by the patient's head. The right hand holds the endoscope as if it were a pencil, guiding it between the left middle and index fingers, which are pushing the base of the tongue forward (see Figs. 12 and 13). The instrument should be advanced in the midline. The patient is asked to swallow. If resistance is met at the entrance to the esophagus, one waits, allows the patient to take several deep breaths, and then begins again to advance the endoscope as the patient swallows. Further resistance may be encountered at the level of the tracheal bifurcation, where again a short wait, allowing the patient to take several deep breaths, usually is sufficient to allow further passage of the instrument. The next site of resistance is the greater curvature of the fundus of the stomach, after the instrument has entered the stomach via the cardia and the posterior wall of the body. The skilled

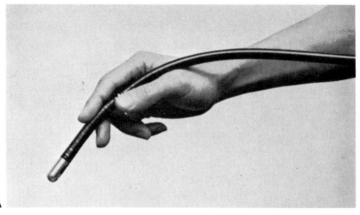

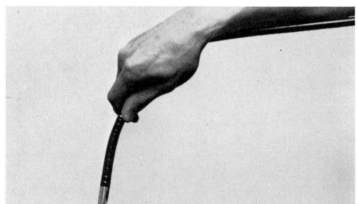

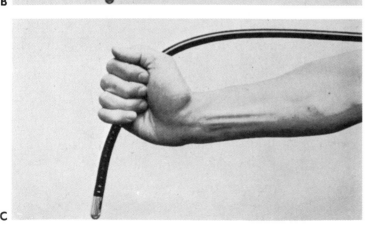

Figure 12 A, Penholder position of the right hand at the beginning of the insertion. B and C, Improper ways of holding the tip of fiberoptic gastroscope. (From Tsuneoka, K., et al.: Fiberscopy of Gastric Diseases. Baltimore, University Park Press, 1973.)

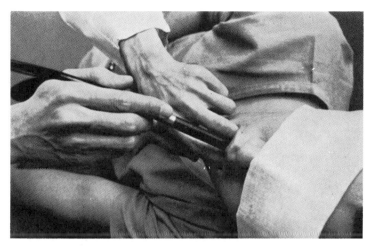

Figure 13 Insertion of fiberoptic gastroscope while pushing the radix of the tongue down with the left hand. Note that the patient is positioned comfortably with left side down. (From Tsuneoka, K., et al.: Fiberscopy of Gastric Diseases. Baltimore, University Park Press, 1973.)

endoscopist can then insert the endoscope into the pylorus with a single movement. Force should not be used during any part of the procedure.

In routine endoscopy, the scope is passed into the duodenum, and the organs are examined as the scope is withdrawn. In the duodenum, the ampulla is of particular interest. Cannulation of the ampulla, with injection of contrast material to show the biliary and pancreatic ductal system, has been one of the advances of endoscopy in the past ten years; it has been a great help in the investigation of the patient with jaundice or intractable upper abdominal pain. The antrum and pylorus usually can be inspected together. Air insufflation produces peristaltic waves. Areas of rigidity or abnormal contours are looked for. Care is taken to visualize all of the stomach. To see the cardia, an inversion maneuver is carried out. The stomach is distended with air in order to nearly efface the folds of the greater curvature. The tip of the endoscope then is slid up the side of the greater curvature to the gastric fundus, visualizing the cardia. The tip of the instrument is straightened before being withdrawn into the esophagus (Wolff and Shinya, 1974).

When a lesion is visualized, it should be biopsied. In ulcerating carcinomas of the stomach, biopsy of both the rim and the slough of the ulcer increased the positive biopsy rate to 95 per cent (Hatfield, et al., 1975). Winawer and his associates (1975) report a correct visual diagnosis of gastric cancer of 90 per cent. Brush cytology gave an over-all yield of 68 per cent, compared to 50 per cent for biopsy alone. Exophytic

tumors were easier to diagnose than infiltrative tumors. Areas of the stomach that were particularly hard to evaluate for tumor were the antrum and cardia. Yamada and associates (1975) advise, in infiltrating lesions, to biopsy the surface with the most eroded area or tiny ulcerations. In the esophagus, Winawer (1975) has reported 97 per cent positive diagnosis of cancer, using direct brush cytology technique.

Other procedures performed with endoscopy include: removal of polyps; breakage of bezoars; dilation of esophageal strictures; placement and cleaning out of endoesophageal palliative prosthesis; extraction of foreign bodies (Wolff and Shinya, 1974), placement of intestinal tubes; and aspiration of basal and stimulated gastric HCl secretion. For these specific techniques, the reader is referred to Demling, et al., 1972; Tsuneoka, et al., 1973; and Wolff, et al., 1974.

The technique for endoscopy in patients with upper gastrointestinal bleeding is well described by Hedberg (1974). Search for the bleeding point is made as the endsocope is first being advanced. Blood in the esophagus is cleared with irrigation and suction via the scope: if this is not possible, the instrument is advanced into the stomach. Observation is made for rivulets of blood, which then are traced back to their source. After the stomach has been seen, reflux from the duodenum is followed up, if present. The fundus and cardioesophageal junction are examined very carefully for a variceal bleeding point or a mucosal tear. In general, biopsy is not advised in the presence of bleeding. At present, the endoscopist's use of electrocoagulation, laser photocoagulation, or cryosurgery in gastrointestinal hemorrhage is under consideration, but further work in the animal laboratory is required before it can be safely used clinically (Katon, 1976).

Complications

Silvis and associates (1976), reporting the results of the 1974 American Society for Gastrointestinal Endoscopy survey, show an over-all complication rate for upper gastrointestinal endoscopy of 1.3/1000 excluding miscellaneous complications, such as drug-induced phlebitis. Breakdown of this showed 2.3/1000 esophagoscopies, 1.2/1000 gastroscopies, and 1.4/1000 duodenoscopies. Endoscopic retrograde cholangiopancreatography (ERCP) had a complication rate of 21.6/1000 examinations, with pancreatitis in 13.4/1000 cases and cholangitis in 6.5/1000 cases. Cholangitis is thought to be related to obstruction of the common bile duct, and probably can be prevented by early operation. The etiology of the pancreatitis is not understood.

The most common complication of esophagogastroduodenoscopy, aside again from the miscellaneous complications of medication reactions (hives, thrombophlebitits), was cardiopulmonary. These reactions possibly were related to the study of a more severely ill population, or to a change in premedication usage (Silvis, 1976). Next in frequency were perforations. These may occur in the esophagus, stomach, duodenum, or jejunum (in postgastroenterostomy patients). The distal esophagus seems more easily injured than the esophageal entrance. Mediastinal and subcutaneous emphysema, pneumoperitoneum, and systemic symptoms may indicate esophageal perforations. In the stomach, Demling and associates (1972) found the most frequent site of perforation 2 to 3 cm. distal to the gastroesophageal junction on the posterior wall. Perforation was suspected whenever the abdomen remained distended for some time after gastroscopy, or if liver dullness to percussion disappeared.

Bleeding, especially after biopsy, was the next most common complication. Other complications after esophagogastroduodenoscopy include: burns from electric bulbs during cinematography; difficulty extracting the endoscope in patients with hiatal hernias; bilateral swelling below the parotid glands after air insufflation in patients with fourth branchial cleft remnants; and submandibular salivary gland swelling secondary to glandular dislocation with ductal obstruction (which resolves in 2 to 24 hours).

Discussion

Kussmaul did indeed open Pandora's box in 1868. The full use of endoscopy probably is yet to be seen and dreamed of, and emergency application of this instrument is in its infancy. As with all procedures, the associated potential complications must be weighed against the benefits of the procedure. Endoscopy has much to offer. It must be hoped that the previously mentioned very high degree of accuracy obtained by biopsy in conjunction with brush cytology of esophagus and stomach cancers will promote earlier treatment of patients with these lesions. The remarkable assistance obtained by the use of endoscopy and angiography in patients with acute upper gastrointestinal bleeding has changed their management markedly. Katon (1976) projects potential sources for endoscopic control of hemorrhage—tissue adhesives, electrocoagulation, laser photocoagulation, cryosurgery, injection of sclerosing agents, and endoscopically placed hemoclips.

PROCTOSIGMOIDOSCOPY

Indications

Protosigmoidoscopy has indications that may be considered acute, as well as those less acute or prophylactic. The more emergent need for proctosigmoidoscopy includes situations of:

(1) gastrointestinal hemorrhage, when endoscopy or nasogastric lavage do not demonstrate the cause proximal to the pylorus; and

(2) sigmoid volvulus.

It also may be considered when a patient has distal large bowel obstruction and sigmoid volvulus should be ruled out.

Other occasions when sigmoidoscopy are indicated include those listed by Turell (1969):

(1) overt bleeding from the anal canal or melena;

(2) protrusion from the anal outlet;

(3) diarrhea, new or recurrent, lasting several days;

(4) mucus or pus discharge from the anus;

(5) pain in the anoperineal region, lower abdomen, or back;

(6) change in bowel pattern;

(7) prior to anorectocolonic surgery;

(8) to observe the progress or regression of colorectal disease;

(9) for bacteriologic and histologic studies of colorectal conditions;

(10) unexplained fever and anemia; and

(11) for treatment of hemorrhoids or polypectomy.

It is recommended that persons over 40 or 45 years of age should have proctosigmoidoscopy annually, even though asymptomatic, to discover significant lesions early. In emergency practice the indications usually would include nos. 1, 3, and 4, and for diagnosis of hemorrhoids and possible treatment, No. 11.

Contraindications

General contraindications to sigmoidoscopy include:

(1) obstruction to the advancement of the sigmoidoscope, whether from severe angulation of the bowel, stricture, or an unremovable object; and

(2) a struggling, nervous, uncooperative patient (Turell, 1969).

Technique

Bowel preparation is required prior to sigmoidoscopy, except for the situations of sigmoid volvulus, perianal abscess, or gastrointestinal hemorrhage in which one is looking for the character and extent of colonic bleeding (Gardner, 1974). Preparation may be as simple as a small enema one hour before the procedure, or as complete as two enemas of 1000 to 1500 cc. of lukewarm water or warm saline solution, the first given 10 to 12 hours prior to procedure, the second three to four hours prior. Turell (1969) notes that 70 per cent of patients do not need preparation.

Mental preparation of the patient is quite important, e.g., assurances that the examination will be discontinued if he becomes too uncomfortable. No sedation or premedication is advised, as the patient's ability to relate discomfort is considered important in preventing inadvertent bowel perforation. If the patient is an infant or small child, or has a painful anal lesion, anesthesia is preferred. If possible, any required surgical procedure is carried out at the same time as anesthetic administration.

The position of the patient can vary. In the elderly, in patients with acute gastrointestinal hemorrhage, in patients with cardiovascular hypertension, and in procedures carried out at the bedside, the left lateral Sims position is preferred, with the pelvis at or beyond the edge of the bed or stretcher, and with Trendelenburg position of the bed if possible. Otherwise, the knee-chest position is preferred. A special table for proctosigmoidoscopy greatly facilitates the procedure, and is well tolerated by the patient (see Fig. 14 for illustration of knee-chest position and an examining table). In the operating room, the jackknife position frequently is used.

The perianal area and buttocks then are examined, and the patient is asked to strain to bring out prolapsing mucosa, internal hemorrhoids, or polyps. A rectal examination is always performed and usually helps sphincteric relaxation. The well-lubricated sigmoidoscope, with obturator in place, is passed gently into the rectum, aiming in the direction of the umbilicus and then toward the sacrum (see Fig. 15). The obturator is removed. Thereafter, the scope is advanced into the visualized bowel lumen. If the scope meets the resistance of the bowel wall, it is withdrawn slightly to visualize the lumen again before further advancement. Small amounts of air can be instilled to aid advancement and to help the physician visualize possible lesions of the bowel wall. At 10 to 12 cm., the bowel angulates, and slight withdrawal and insufflation are repeated with attempts to thread the scope into the visualized lumen (see Fig. 16). In patients with sigmoid resection or other pelvic operations, it may be impossible to do a complete examination. Salazar and Jackman (1969) report inability to examine more than 20 cm. in 50 per cent of women over 70 years old, and in 50 per cent of men over 80 years old. In most adults, the sigmoidoscope can be passed the full 25 cm. length and the bowel just beyond the scope can be visualized. The sigmoidoscope then is withdrawn gradually,

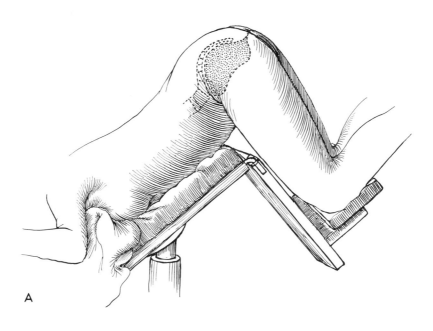

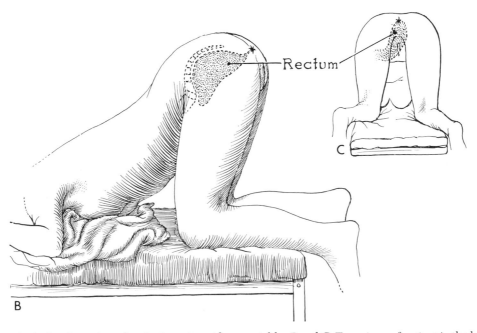

Figure 14   *A*, Good position of patient on sigmoidoscopy table. *B* and *C*, Two views of patient in the knee-chest position for proctosigmoidoscopy. (From Turell, R.: Diseases of the Colon and Anorectum. 2nd ed. Philadelphia, W. B. Saunders Co., 1969.)

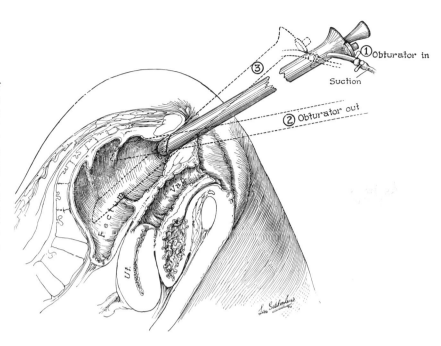

Figure 15 Positions of the sigmoidoscope in the process of endoscopy. *1*, The instrument with the obturator is introduced in a cephalad and anterior direction. *2*, The obturator is removed and the scope is directed posteriorly, and *3*, gently advanced upward under direct vision only. (From Turell, R.: Diseases of the Colon and Anorectum. 2nd ed. Philadelphia, W. B. Saunders Co., 1969.)

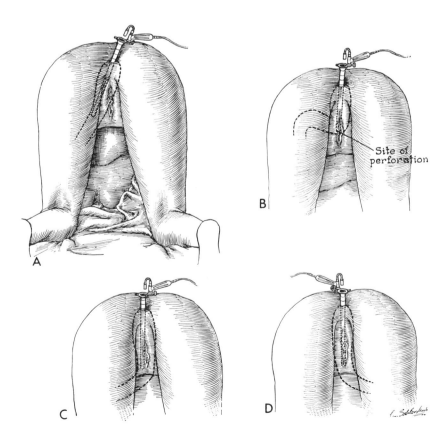

Figure 16 *A*, Easy introduction of the entire length of scope. *B*, Extreme angulation of the bowel and usual site of perforation. *C*, Mild angulation to the left. *D*, Mild angulation to the right side. These can be easily overcome by gentle manipulation. (From Turell, R.: Diseases of the Colon and Anorectum. 2nd ed. Philadelphia, W. B. Saunders Co., 1969.)

taking care to visualize the complete wall, and biopsying any suspicious areas. After any biopsy, the site is watched for bleeding. Pressure can be exerted on the site with cotton-tipped tampons. If necessary, the area may be cauterized.

In patients with sigmoid volvulus, the mucosa at the site of obstruction is inspected for slough, ulceration, or dark blood. These signs indicate strangulation. If these are not seen, the examiner may gently advance a well-lubricated, long, soft rubber rectal tube through the sigmoidoscope into the obstructed sigmoid loop. A rush of air and liquid out of the tube is pathognomonic of sigmoid volvulus, and will douse the examiner unless he steps back quickly. The tube is left in place in the decompressed loop as the sigmoidoscope is withdrawn. The tube is taped securely to the buttocks and left in place for several days until bowel function returns.

Complications

Complications can be listed as follows:

(1) bursting by excessive insufflation of air;

(2) tearing by actual pressure of the instrument;

(3) explosion when colonic gases are detonated by a fulgurating device (Artz and Hardy, 1975);

(4) perforation by biopsy—either too deep a bite, biopsy of a wall already thinned by ulcers, or by pulling down a polyp too far

and taking bowel wall as neck of the polyp (Fielding and Lumsden, 1973); and

(5) bacteremia (LeFrock, et al., 1973).

Despite this formidable list of complications, sigmoidoscopy is a very safe procedure. Gilbert, et al. (1974) report 6500 sigmoidoscopies by trained technicians over a four-year period without complication. Gilbertsen (1974) reported 50,000 consecutive sigmoidoscopies without perforation. Over a 25-year period, with 103,000 examinations, five perforations occurred, or 1 per 20,600 sigmoidoscopies. When they do take place, perforations usually are on the antimesenteric border just above the peritoneal reflection. Early recognition of perforations is paramount in order to facilitate operative intervention. The hole in the gut may be seen by the examiner, or bowel, omentum, or epiploic appendages may be visualized. Pain, shock, or signs of peritonitis may be other manifestations of perforation.

Transient bacteremia was documented by LeFrock and associates (1973) in a group of 200 patients undergoing sigmoidoscopy without biopsy. Bacteremia occurred in 8.5 per cent of patients with no lower intestinal disease, and in 10.6 per cent of patients with active disease of the lower intestinal tract. The difference between the groups was not significant. None of the patients gave clinical signs or symptoms of bacteremia. All the patients had negative blood cultures 30 minutes after sigmoidoscopy. This study raises the question of the possible need of chemoprophylaxis in patients with cardiac valvular disease who are to undergo sigmoidoscopy.

ABDOMINAL ULTRASONOGRAPHY

One of the newer tools of diagnosis is the use of ultrasound. At present there may not be many hospitals in which the emergency physician can obtain the help of ultrasonography at any hour of the day or night. However, as this diagnostic tool becomes more popular, better understood, and refined, it undoubtedly will enter the armamentarium of the acute care physician. The Trauma Service of the Naval Hospital, San Diego has already incorporated abdominal ultrasonography into a portion of its protocol for management of blunt abdominal trauma.

The main benefit of ultrasonography is that it can image abdominal contents not otherwise readily accessible. It indicates

whether they are cystic or solid. This is done noninvasively, without discomfort, and without known side-effects.

The basic principles of ultrasonography are well described in textbooks as well as in the radiologic literature. The *Seminars in Roentgenology*, October 1975 and the *Radiologic Clinics of North America*, December 1975, are devoted to ultrasound. In Table 1, principles of ultrasonography are summarized. The term ultrasound comes from the fact that sound frequencies greater than 20,000 cycles per second cannot be heard by the human ear. Piezoelectric transducers are made to vibrate in response to electric stimulation. They produce short

TABLE 1
Principles of Ultrasonography

FORM OF ENERGY:	Ultrasound—a beam of non-ionizing energy propagated through tissue as a mechanical pressure wave.
PROPERTIES:	Reflection, refraction, diffraction, absorption and scatter.
PRINCIPLE OF ULTRASONOGRAPHY:	Sound reflection occurs at tissue interfaces and depends on: a. Differences in specific acoustic impedance (resulting in differences in velocity of sound propagation) determined by: (1) Density of tissue. (2) Elasticity of tissue. b. Angle of incidence of tissue interface to beam. c. Surface area of tissue interface. d. Surface texture of tissue interface.
PROPAGATION:	Good through liquids and solids. Poor to nil through air or gas (almost 100% reflection)
PRODUCTION:	Pulsed electrical energy is sent to the piezoelectric crystal (transducer) and is converted to ultrasonic pulses, 1 to 5 microseconds duration, 50 to 1000 times per second.
RECEPTION:	Echoes reflected to piezoelectric crystal (transducer), reception during "silent periods."
FREQUENCY:	1 to 15 megacycles per second. With higher frequencies, wavelengths are shorter, resolving power greater, penetration lower. With lower frequencies, wavelengths are longer, resolving power lower, penetration greater.
BIOLOGIC EFFECT:	No significant functional or morphologic effect at energies employed.
METHODS OF DISPLAY:	1. *Mode "A" (Amplitude Modulation) A-Scope Display* Trace intensity constant. Echoes recorded as vertical displacement (spike) of trace. Height of vertical displacement proportional to strength of echo. Horizontal distance along trace proportional to depth (or distance) of reflecting interface. Method—transducer maintained in fixed position. Use—determination of depth of reflecting interface. 2. *Mode "B" (Intensity Modulation) B-Scope Display* Echoes recorded as "dots" along linear trace. Intensity of dots proportional to strength of echoes. Horizontal distance along trace proportional to depth (or distance) of reflecting interface. Method—transducer maintained in fixed position. Use—determination of depth and/or motion pattern of moving reflecting interface. 3. *B-Scan Ultrasonography* Composite image of infinite numbers of Mode B displays. Two-dimensional cross-section structural representation. Method—transducer moves during recording. Acoustical coupling by direct transducer skin contact (contact scanning), or Acoustical coupling, using water bag or water bath (water path scanning). Use—determination of cross-sectional pattern of reflecting interfaces of structures.

Source: Lehman, J. S.: Radiol. Clin. North Am. 9:607, 1966.

bursts of sound of very high frequency in the megahertz range. The total duration of each burst of sound is very short—about a microsecond. During the remainder of the time between pulses of generated sound, the transducer functions as a receiver of echoes returned from interfaces between materials of differing physical density. The strength or intensity of the echo depends on the magnitude of the density change at the interface, and also upon the angle of incidence of the transmitted beam of sound. Distances of objects from the transmitter can be determined if one knows the velocity of sound in the particular medium, and measures the time from emission of sound to its reception back again at the transducer. The method of display of the returning echoes may be as ver-

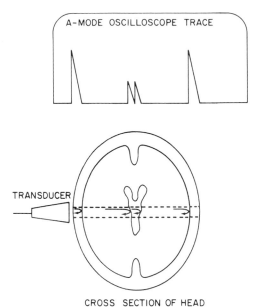

Figure 17 Typical A-mode display. (From Leo, F. P., and Rao, G. U. V.: Radiol. Clin. North Am. *13*:404, 1975.)

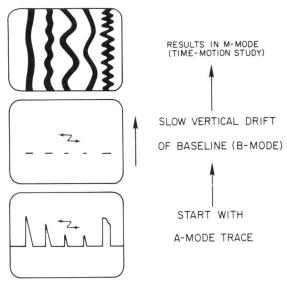

Figure 18 Slow vertical drift of baseline (B-mode) results in M-mode (time-motion study). (From Leo, F. P., and Rao, G. U. V.: Radiol. Clin. North Am. *13*:404, 1975.)

tical spikes of differing amplitude from the horizontal time base (A-mode) or as dots of varying brightness (B-mode). The B-scan is a composite of B-mode displays when the transducer moves during recording. The newer scanners show up to eight shades of gray, instead of only the black-and-white seen on older scanners. The larger echoes appear brighter. The smaller echoes appear less bright (see Figs. 17 to 20). Lower ultrasonic frequencies are needed if deeper penetration is desired.

INDICATIONS

Basically, ultrasonography simply shows reflections from interfaces. It demonstrates echo-free fluid collections as well as solid organs and masses whose echoes depend on their degree of homogeneity. As Doust points out, a nonfunctioning organ is demonstrated as easily as is a normal organ.

Beside the need for demonstrating the size, configuration, and location of organs, abdominal ultrasonography may be indicated in the instances grouped below.

LIVER

(1) To demonstrate ascites.

(2) In the differentiation of jaundice—intrinsic or extrinsic—in difficult

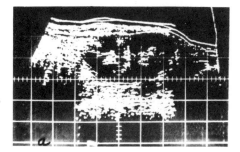
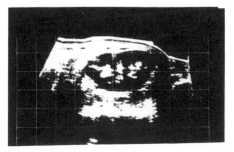

Figure 19 *Left,* Typical B-scan using a bistable cathode ray tube (CRT). Notice the absence of gray scale. *Right,* The same scan obtained using a scan conversion unit and a television monitor. Notice the various gray shades in the image and the additional information resulting therefrom. (From Leo, F. P., and Rao, G. U. V.: Radiol. Clin. North Am. *13*:408, 1975.)

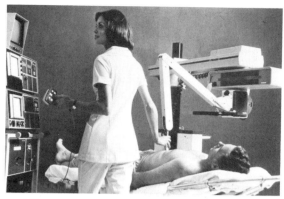

Figure 20 B-scan ultrasonographic equipment. This apparatus is used for contact B-scanning. (By permission of Picker Corporation, Northford, Connecticut.)

cases, or when the patient is pregnant or allergic to iodinated compounds.

(3) To look for cysts, metastases, abscesses.

(4) To check the lung-liver interface and diaphragmatic movement (Carlsen, 1975).

GALLBLADDER

(1) To demonstrate gallstones.

(2) Choledochal cyst.

(3) To confirm dilatation of the gallbladder and help diagnose perforation and abscess formation (Carlsen, 1975; Hublitz, et al., 1972; Leopold and Sokoloff, 1973).

SPLEEN

(1) Ruptured spleen.

(2) Large subcapsular hematoma.

(3) To determine splenic volume.

(4) To differentiate cystic lesions from tumor masses of the spleen (Carlsen, 1975; Holm, 1971).

PANCREAS

(1) Pancreatitis with significant edema.

(2) Pancreatic pseudocyst—diagnosis, measurement of wall, progression or regression.

(3) Carcinoma of the pancreas.

(4) Ultrasonically guided percutaneous fine needle biopsy of the pancreas—still experimental.

(5) To demonstrate intrapancreatic and juxtapancreatic lymph nodes.

KIDNEY

(1) As screening when an azotemic patient is pregnant or allergic to iodinated compounds.

(2) Unilateral nonfunctioning kidney—when intravenous urography and radionuclide studies fail to demonstrate functioning renal parenchyma on one side.

(3) Renal transplantation—to follow size and shape of transplant.

(4) Diagnosis of cyst-tumor deformities when noted on intravenous urography.

(5) Diagnosis of polycystic disease.

(6) Kidney trauma—diagnosis of fracture.

ADRENALS

(1) Diagnosis of tumors.

ABDOMINAL AORTA

(1) Confirmation of an aneurysm.

(2) Evaluation of abdominal calcifications seen on x-ray.

(3) Measure aneurysm and follow up regularly.

(4) Demonstrate aortic dissection.

UTERUS AND ADNEXA

(1) More accurate diagnosis of pelvic masses from knowledge of solid or cystic consistency, presence of septa and papillary projections within cysts, and location in relation to normal pelvic organs.

(2) Diagnosis of pregnancy as early as five or six weeks.

(3) Location of placenta prior to amniocentesis.

(4) Degree of placenta previa.

(5) Determination of fetal maturity by biparietal diameter.

(6) Diagnosis of hydatid moles.

(7) Diagnosis of multiple gestations, cephalic anomalies, polyhydramnios.

(8) Fetal death is suggested if serial scans, three to five days apart, show decrease in the size of the fetal head.

(9) Threatened or inevitable abortion is suspected if an irregular or collapsed gestational sac is lying low in the uterus.

TRAUMA

(1) Suggested if abdominal lavage is weakly positive and patient's condition is stable (Parvin, 1975).

ABSCESSES AND HEMATOMAS OF ABDOMEN AND THE ABDOMINAL WALL

(1) Diagnosis (Jensen and Pedersen, 1974; Leopold and Asher, 1972; Weiner and Diaconis, 1975).

(2) Ultrasonically guided percutaneous aspiration of abscess (Smith and Bartrum, 1974).

RADIOTHERAPY

(1) Planning.
(2) Assessment of response to therapy.

CONTRAINDICATIONS

There are no definite contraindications to abdominal ultrasonography. Since, however, gas and barium sulfate reflect sound strongly, the presence of bowel filled with gas or barium usually precludes a satisfactory study. Patient cooperation is required. The study takes about 20 to 30 minutes. The patient must be able to remain quiet during this time, although he may sit up between intervals. Those unable to lie flat may be placed in a semirecumbent position.

TECHNIQUE

Usually the examination is performed in the supine position, although the prone position is preferred if the kidneys, spleen, or retroperitoneal space are to be examined. The transducer is swept across the area of investigation, keeping in airless contact with the skin. A thin coating of mineral oil or aqueous gel is applied to the patient's skin to facilitate direct coupling with the transducer. A series of eight to ten transverse scans is started at the level of the umbilicus or iliac crests, and continued cephalad at 1 to 2 cm.

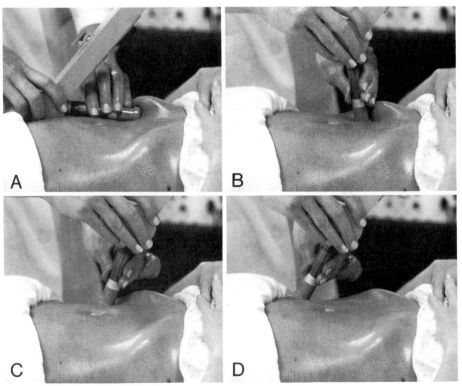

Figure 21   Positions shown in A to D demonstrate proper transducer position necessary to acquire an adequate single pass echogram. Notice the placement of the technologist's hands and the maintenance of a perpendicular beam to the anatomy being demonstrated. The position shown in A is the most critical in acquiring a good image. From this point a slow continuous arc is necessary for an adequate scan. (From Carlsen, E. N.: Radiol. Clin. North Am. *13*:547, 1975.)

intervals. External anatomic landmarks are used to indicate the level of the scan. Longitudinal scans are then performed beginning at the costal margin during suspended respiration. See Figure 21. These are repeated at similar 1 to 2 cm. intervals. If indicated, similar transverse and longitudinal scans of the pelvis can be obtained. Sufficient contact between the transducer and the patient's skin is very important in order to obtain a good scan. When obstacles such as colostomies, wounds, or dressings make it difficult to perform a study, Douct recommends an oblique approach through adjacent intact skin.

For specific organs, particular preparation or techniques may be needed. For example, for examination of the pelvis, the bladder is distended to displace intestine out of the pelvis, serve as a point of reference in identification of other structures, and transmit as a cystic mass. For examination of the gallbladder, the patient is kept fasting overnight. A series of scans along the long axis of the gallbladder is obtained after the limits of the organ have been identified satisfactorily (Carlsen, 1975).

INTERPRETATION

Prime requisites for interpretation of B-scans of the abdomen are good scans, good knowledge of abdominal anatomy and interrelationships of structure, and plenty of experience. Almost all contributors to the literature on ultrasonography give repeated warnings of the pitfalls in interpretation. As a general principle, abnormalities should appear consistently on both longitudinal and transverse scans of the suspect area. Scans at 1 cm. intervals will rule out random noise, whereas real structures will be repeated on two or more scans. Noise echoes within a lesion may occur because of too high an output setting, resulting in the structure being called solid rather than cystic. This can be checked by noting the gain and time gain compensation settings of the instrument, and comparing a known cystic structure such as the bladder or gallbladder (Carlsen, 1975). For the specifics of interpretation of individual organs, the reader is referred to the references at the end of the chapter.

Freimanis and Asher have outlined sev-

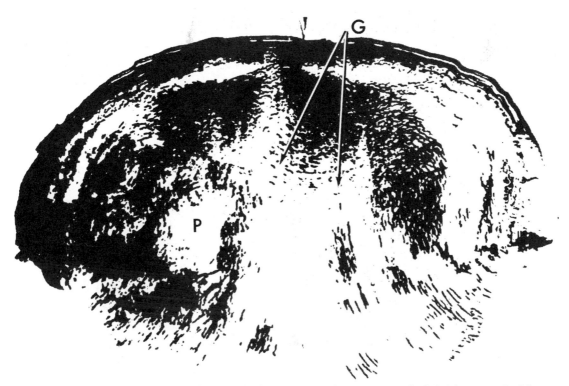

Figure 22   Cross section, lower abdomen. The large paraspinal structure on the left (P) is typical of the psoas muscle seen in the young athlete. Note that the prevertebral area is obliterated by gas (G). This should not be confused with the presence of lymph nodes, provided care is taken to observe through-transmission. (From Leopold, G. R., and Asher, W. M.: Fundamentals of Abdominal and Pelvic Ultrasonography. Philadelphia, W. B. Saunders Co., 1975.)

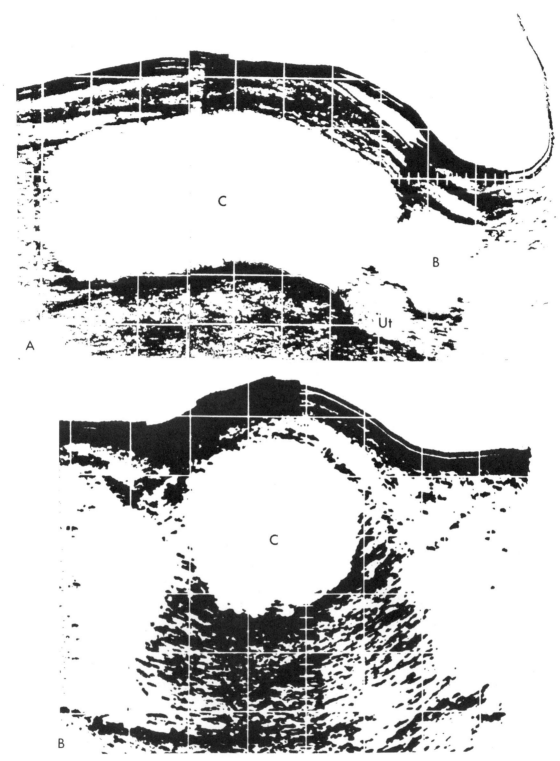

Figure 23 *A*, Sagittal scan. A large ovarian cyst (C) and normal-sized uterus (Ut) are apparent. As sensitivity was increased, the ovarian mass remained sonolucent long after the uterus filled in with echoes. (B = urinary bladder.)

B, Transverse scan, high gain. The cyst has no internal echoes. There is a sharp posterior margin and a large accumulation of sound behind the mass. (From Leopold, G. R. and Asher, W. M.: Fundamentals of Abdominal and Pelvic Ultrasonography. Philadelphia, W. B. Saunders Co., 1975.)

eral principles helpful to diagnosis. They suggest that serial scanning at increasing sensitivities is necessary for adequate depiction and interpretation. Scans in two planes of the entire abdomen, not just of the suspect area, should be the routine. The ultrasonographer must be sure that the beam has really traversed the area in question, i.e., various gain settings should be used so that the structures behind the area are "seen." See Figure 22. They call this the "through transmission sign." In general they feel that physically well defined structures produce well defined outlines, whereas infiltrating lesions, and lesions very closely related to adjacent areas, may be poorly delineated. Fluid collection in confined spaces around organs produces a double contour, one outline being the organ and the second being a wall of the collection. An interruption of a part of the contour may indicate rupture if artifact can be excluded. Their experience also showed a more-than average density and number of echoes returning from behind expanding lesions. See Figure 23. Echoes from within organs represent lack of homogeneity. Many lesions will present a characteristic distribution that helps to identify them, e.g., a preaortic mantle pattern of lymphoma nodes.

COMPLICATIONS

There are no known complications from repeated use of ultrasound at the energy levels currently used in commercially available scanners (Doust, *Gastroenterology* 70:602, 1976).

DISCUSSION

Ultrasound seems like the ultimate—a painless, noninvasive method of "looking around" in an abdomen without complication. It is thought of as a complementary study rather than one eliminating all others. Its biggest problem is that it is in its infancy in all but a few centers, and like any new method it needs to be worked with until it is understood and its methods and limitations are well defined. Perhaps in the future abdominal ultrasonography will be part of the Emergency Department work-up of patients with upper abdominal pain, jaundiced patients, and those with unexplained fever. The panoply of indications previously listed serve as a summary of investigations begun, not of a chapter finally written.

References

Artz, C. P., and Hardy, J. D.: Management of Surgical Complications. 3d ed. Philadelphia, W. B. Saunders Co., 1975.

Baker, R. J.: Newer techniques in evaluation of injured patients. Surg. Clin. North Am. 55:31, 1975.

Blau, J. S., Keating, T. M., and Stockinger, F. S.: Radiologic diagnosis of inguinal hernia in children. Surg. Gynecol. Obstet. 136:401, 1973.

Bolt, R. J.: Sigmoidoscopy in detection and diagnosis in the asymptomatic individual. Cancer 28:121, 1971.

Bonanno, P. J., Landers, D. E., and Rock, D. E.: Bladder drainage with the suprapubic catheter needle. Obstet. Gynecol. 35:807, 1970.

Bradley, E. L., and Clements, J. L.: Implications of diagnostic ultrasound in the surgical management of pancreatic pseudocysts. Am. J. Surg. 127:163, 1974.

Carlsen, E. N.: Liver, gallbladder, and spleen. Radiol. Clin. North Am. 13:543, 1975.

Castle, M., and Osterhout, S.: Urinary tract catheterization and associated infection. Nurs. Res. 23:170, 1974.

Colcher, H.: Gastrointestinal endoscopy. N. Engl. J. Med. 203:1129, 1975

Committee on Trauma, American College of Surgeons: Early Care of the Injured Patient. Philadelphia, W. B. Saunders Co., 1972.

Cusius, P. J.: Urinary tract infections in general practice. The value of suprapubic bladder aspiration with immediate culture plating. S. Afr. Med. J. 47:1707, 1973.

Demling, L., Ottenjann, R., and Elster, K.: translated and adapted by Soergel, K. H., Endoscopy and Biopsy of the Esophagus and Stomach. Philadelphia, W. B. Saunders Co., 1972.

Doust, B. D.: Ultrasonic examination of the pancreas. Radiol. Clin. North Am. 13:467, 1975.

Drapanas, T., and McDonald, J.: Peritoneal tap in abdominal trauma. Surgery 50:742, 1961.

Edwards, L., and Trott, P. A.: Catheter-induced urethral inflammation. J. Urol. 110:678, 1973

Engrav, L. H., et al.: Diagnostic peritoneal lavage in blunt abdominal trauma. J. Trauma 15:854, 1975.

Fielding, J. F., and Lumsden, K.: Large-bowel perforations in patients undergoing sigmoidoscopy and barium enema. Br. Med. J. 1:471, 1973.

Filly, R. A., and Freimanis, A. K.: Echographic diagnosis of pancreatic lesions. Radiology 96:575, 1970.

Freimanis, A. K.: Echographic diagnosis of lesions of the abdominal aorta and lymph nodes. Radiol. Clin. North Am. 13:557, 1975.

Freimanis, A. K., and Asher, W. M.: Development of diagnostic criteria in echographic study of abdominal lesions. Am. J. Roentgenol. 108:747, 1970.

Gardner, B.: Gastrointestinal Bleeding. In Shaftan, G. W., and Gardner, B. (eds.): Quick Reference to Surgical Emergencies. Philadelphia, J. B. Lippincott Co., 1974.

Garibaldi, R. A., et al.: Factors predisposing to bacteriuria during indwelling urethral catheterization. N. Engl. J. Med. 291:215, 1974.

Gilbert, F. I., Jr., et al.: Allied health personnel in cancer detection: utilization of proctosigmoidoscopic technicians in detecting abnormalities of the lower bowel. Cancer 33:1725, 1974.

Gilbertsen, V. A.: Proctosigmoidoscopy and polypectomy in reducing the incidence of rectal cancer. Cancer 34:936, 1974.

Goldberg, B. B.: Vascular Ultrasonography. In Joyner, C. R. (ed.): Ultrasound in the Diagnosis of Cardiovascular-Pulmonary Disease. Chicago, Year Book Medical Publishers, Inc., 1974.

Guttman, F. M., Bertrand, R., and Ducharme, J. C.: Herniography and the pediatric contralateral inguinal hernia. Surg. Gynecol. Obstet. 135:551, 1972.

Hale, R. W., and McCorriston, C. C.: Suprapubic cystotomy with a polyethylene tube. Am. J. Obstet. Gynecol. 105:1181, 1969.

Hancke, S., Holm, H. H., and Koch, F.: Ultrasonically guided percutaneous fine needle biopsy of the pancreas. Surg. Gynecol. Obstet. 140:361, 1975.

The Harriet Lane Handbook. 5th ed. Chicago, Year Book Medical Publishers, Inc., 1969.

Harris, P. D., Neuhauser, E. B. D., and Gerth, R.: The osmotic effect of water soluble contrast media on circulating plasma volume. Am. J. Roentgenol. Radium Ther. Nucl. Med. 91:694, 1964.

Hastings, J. B.: Mass screening for colorectal cancer. Am. J. Surg. 127:228, 1974.

Hatfield, A. R. W., et al.: Importance of the site of endoscopic gastric biopsy in ulcerating lesions of the stomach. Gut 16:884, 1975.

Hedberg, S. E.: Endoscopy in gastrointestinal bleeding, a systematic approach to diagnosis. Surg. Clin. North Am. 54:549, 1974.

Holm, H. H.: Ultrasonic scanning in the diagnosis of space-occupying lesions of the upper abdomen. Br. J. Radiol. 44:24, 1971.

Hublitz, U. F., Kahn, P. C., and Sell, L. A.: Cholecystosonography: an approach to the nonvisualized gallbladder. Radiology 103:645, 1972.

Isaacs, J. H., and McWhorter, D. M.: Foley catheter drainage systems and bladder damage. Surg. Gynecol. Obstet. 132:889, 1971.

James, P. M., Jr.: The problem of hernia in infants and adolescents. Surg. Clin. North Am. 51:1361, 1971.

Jensen, F., and Pedersen, J. F.: The value of ultrasonic scanning in the diagnosis of intra-abdominal abscesses and hematomas. Surg. Gynecol. Obstet. 139:326, 1974.

Joyner, C. R.: The Principles of Ultrasound and Ultrasonic Instrumentation. In Joyner, C. R. (ed.): Ultrasound in the Diagnosis of Cardiovascular-Pulmonary Disease. Chicago, Year Book Medical Publishers, Inc., 1974.

Katon, R. M.: Experimental control of gastrointestinal hemorrhage via the endoscope: a new era dawns. Gastroenterology 70:272, 1976.

Kaufman, J. J., and Brosman, S. A.: Blunt injuries of the genitourinary tract. Surg. Clin. North Am. 52:747, 1972.

LeFrock, J. L., et al.: Transient bacteremia associated wtih sigmoidoscopy. N. Engl. J. Med. 289:467, 1973.

Lehman, J. S.: Ultrasound in the diagnosis of hepatobiliary disease. Radiol. Clin. North Am. 9:605, 1966.

Leo, F. P., and Rao, G. U. V.: The technology of diagnostic ultrasound. Radiol. Clin. North Am. 13:403, 1975.

Leopold, G. R.: Pancreatic echography: a new dimension in the diagnosis of psuedocyst. Radiology 104:365, 1972.

Leopold, G. R., and Asher, W. M.: Diagnosis of extraorgan retroperitoneal space lesions by B-scan ultrasonography. Radiology 104:133, 1972.

Leopold, G. R., and Sokoloff, J.: Ultrasonic scanning in the diagnosis of biliary disease. Surg. Clin. North Am. 53:1043, 1973.

Lillehei, R. C., Dietzman, R. H., and Motsay, G. J.: Shock as Related to Operative Surgery. In Nora, P.

F. (ed.): Operative Surgery. Principles and Techniques. Philadelphia, Lea & Febiger, 1972.

Lim, R. C., Jr.: Surgical Diagnostic and Therapeutic Procedures. In Dunphy, J. E., and Way, L. W. (eds): Current Surgical Diagnosis and Treatment. Los Altos, Lange Medical Publications, 1975.

Lucas, C. E., and Sugawa, C.: Diagnostic endoscopy during laparotomy for acute hemorrhage from the upper part of the gastrointestinal tract. Surg. Gynecol. Obstet. 135:285, 1972.

McCoy, J., and Wolma, F. J.: Abdominal tap: indication, technic and results. Am. J. Surg. 122:693, 1972.

McDonald, D. F.: Urology. In Schwartz, S. I., et al. (eds.): Principles of Surgery. 2d ed. New York, McGraw-Hill Book Co., 1974.

McDougal, W. S., Izant, R. J., and Zollinger, R. M., Jr.: Primary peritonitis in infancy and childhood. Ann. Surg. 181:310, 1975.

Morris, P. J.: Diagnostic paracentesis of the acute abdomen. Br. J. Surg. 53:707, 1966.

Morrissey, J. F.: Gastrointestinal Endoscopy. Gastroenterology 62:1241, 1972.

Neuhof, H., and Cohen, I.: Abdominal puncture in the diagnosis of acute intraperitoneal disease. Ann. Surg. 83:454, 1926.

Nyström, K., Bjerle, P., and Lindqvist, B.: Suprapubic catheterization of the urinary bladder as a diagnostic procedure. Scand. J. Urol. Nephrol. 7:160, 1973.

Olsen, W. R., and Hildreth, D. H.: Abdominal paracentesis and peritoneal lavage in blunt abdominal trauma. J. Trauma 11:824, 1971.

Olsen, W. R., Redman, H. C., and Hildreth, D. H.: Quantitative peritoneal lavage in blunt abdominal trauma. Arch. Surg. 104:536, 1972.

Parvin, S., et al.: Effectiveness of peritoneal lavage in blunt abdominal trauma. Ann. Surg. 181:255, 1975.

Perry, J. F., Jr.: Blunt and penetrating abdominal injuries. Curr. Probl. Surg., May, 1970.

Powers, J. H.: Proctosigmoidoscopy in private practice. J.A.M.A., 231:750, 1975.

Root, H. D., in discussion of paper by Engrav, L. H., et al.: Diagnostic peritoneal lavage in blunt abdominal trauma. J. Trauma 15:854, 1975.

Root, H. D., et al.: Diagnostic peritoneal lavage. Surgery 57:633, 1965.

Salazar, M., and Jackman, R. J.: Reasons for incomplete proctoscopy. Dis. Colon Rectum 12:19, 1969.

Shackelford, G. D., and McAlister, W. H.: Inguinal herniography. Am. J. Roentgenol. Radium Ther. Nucl. Med. 115:399, 1972.

Silvis, S. E., et al.: Endoscopic complications. J.A.M.A. 235:928, 1976.

Smith, D. W., and Germain, C. P.: Care of the Adult Patient. Philadelphia, J. B. Lippincott Co., 1975.

Smith, E. H., and Bartrum, R. J., Jr.: Ultrasonically guided percutaneous aspiration of abscesses. Am. J. Roentgenol. Radium Ther. Nucl. Med. 122:308, 1974.

Solomon, H.: Die Diagnostiche Punction des Bauches. Berl. Klin. Wochenschr. 43:45, 1906.

Storer, E. H., Goldberg, S. M., and Nivatvongs, S.: Colon, Rectum, and Anus. In Schwartz, S. I., et al. (eds.): Principles of Surgery. 2d ed. New York, McGraw-Hill Book Co., 1974.

Stuber, J. L., Tempelton, A. W., and Bishop, K.: Ultrasonic evaluation of the kidneys. Radiology 104:139, 1972.

Thal, E. R., and Shires, G. T.: Peritoneal lavage in blunt abdominal trauma. Am. J. Surg. 125:64, 1973.

Tsuneoka, K., Takemoto, T., and Fukuchi, S.: Fiberscopy of Gastric Diseases. Baltimore, University Park Press, 1973.

Turell, R.: Diseases of the Colon and Anorectum. 2d ed. Philadelphia, W. B. Saunders Co., 1969.

Turner-Warwick, R. T.: Urethral Stricture. *In* Glenn, J. F. (ed.): Urologic Surgery. 2d ed. Hagerstown, Md., Harper & Row, 1975.

Walton, P. D., Jamieson, A. D., and Shingleton, H. M.: The expanding role of diagnostic ultrasound in obstetrics and gynecology. Surg. Gynecol. Obstet. *137*:753, 1973.

Waterhouse, R. K., and Patil, U. B.: Urologic Emergencies. *In* Shaftan, G. W., and Gardner, B. (eds.): Quick Reference to Surgical Emergencies. Philadelphia, J. B. Lippincott Co., 1974.

Weiner, C. I., and Diaconis, J. N.: Primary abdominal wall abscess diagnosed by ultrasound. Arch. Surg. *110*:341, 1975.

White, J. J., Haller, J. A., and Dorst, J. P.: Congenital inguinal hernia and inguinal herniography. Surg. Clin. North Am. *50*:823, 1970.

Wilson, C. B., Vidrine, A., Jr., and Rives, J. D.: Unrecognized abdominal trauma in patients with head injuries. Ann. Surg. *161*:608, 1965.

Wilson, J. P., and Letton, A. H.: Routine sigmoidoscopy. Am. Surg. *33*:143, 1967.

Winawer, S. J., et al.: Endoscopic diagnosis of advanced gastric cancer. Gastroenterology *69*:1183, 1975.

Winawer, S. J., et al.: Endoscopic brush cytology in esophageal cancer. J.A.M.A. *232*:1358, 1975.

Wolff, W. I., and Shinya, H.: Modern endoscopy of the alimentary tract. Curr. Probl. Surg., Jan., 1974.

Yamada, K., Holyoke, E. D., and Elias, E. G.: Endoscopy in patients with malignant conditions of the gastrointestinal tract. Surg. Gynecol. Obstet. *141*:903, 1975.

Chapter 14

MINOR SURGICAL PROCEDURES

Michael E. Ervin

The purpose of this chapter is to help the reader develop basic surgical techniques that can be used as the groundwork for further refining of his or her surgical skills. First to be addressed will be basic suturing techniques, followed by specific problems, such as lip, scalp, and tongue lacerations. The second part of the chapter will concern itself with the various methods utilized in the Emergency Department to obtain anesthesia. This should enable the reader to administer effective nerve blocks and local and regional anesthesia.

SUTURING AND WOUNDS

To develop effective suturing techniques, it is important to understand the principles of wound management. With an understanding of fundamental principles, techniques to handle the variations of wound presentation will follow naturally.

PREPARATION OF THE WOUND

All wounds must be cleaned. This is carried out by one or more of the following: irrigation, antiseptics, and mechanical measures. The most effective modality is a thorough mechanical cleansing using a sponge or soft brush capable of removing devitalized and contaminated tissue. This sponge or brush is usually impregnated with an antiseptic. Concern that vigorous scrubbing will wantonly destroy viable tissue cells is unwarranted in contaminated traumatic wounds in that the prime concern must be directed to the elimination of foreign material and the removal of nonviable tissue.

Prior to mechanical cleansing, the lacer-

ation may be infiltrated with a local anesthetic. This will facilitate a painless and thorough cleansing, which may not otherwise be obtainable, as in the case of a screaming child. Mechanical cleansing is followed by irrigation with about 500 to 1000 ml. of normal saline solution; 150 to 200 ml. of this lavage should be performed as a high-pressure syringe irrigation, since this method has been shown to decrease the bacterial count of the wound and to decrease the rate of infection (Stevenson et al.) (see Fig. 1). To accomplish this, draw up the sterile saline into a 50-ml. sterile syringe and attach a 19 gauge needle. Then, with the needle as close as possible to the wound surface, apply

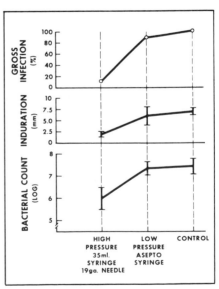

Figure 1 High-pressure syringe irrigation of contaminated wounds displays significant therapeutic merit, while the benefits from low-pressure irrigation are negligible. (From Stevenson, T. R., et al.: Cleansing the traumatic wound by high pressure syringe. J. Am. Coll. Emerg. Physicians 5(1):20, 1976, Figure 7.)

maximal force to the syringe plunger and you will obtain the desired high-pressure stream of saline.

The patient is now draped and is ready for further surgical debridement or repair as indicated.

DEBRIDEMENT OF DEVITALIZED TISSUES

Many wounds are not clean, linear lacerations but involve a crush component. Devitalized tissue rapidly becomes a milieu in which bacteria proliferate. Therefore, the practice of excising crushed and devitalized tissue is one of the strongest weapons against subsequent infection. When in doubt about tissue viability, it is usually best to remove the tissue in question, although if large areas are involved (especially in the face or hands), this decision should be made by the most experienced surgeon or emergency physician available. Also, do not trim or excise tissue when doing so would destroy some irreplaceable structure, such as the philtrum or cupid's bow of the lip (Dushoff, 1974).

Antibiotics cannot be expected to substitute for proper cleansing and debriding of injured tissue.

LAYERED WOUND CLOSURE

For cosmetic healing, wound margins must be free from undue tension. When tension is present, it is important to close the skin in layers, thus minimizing tension on surface sutures, as shown in Figure 2A.

To obtain this type of closure, you must

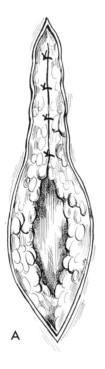

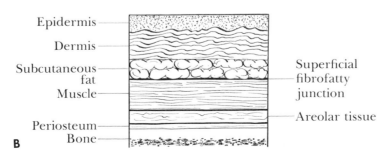

Figure 2 *A*, Close subcutaneous tissue in layers to minimize tension on skin sutures, obtain verticle alignment, and help evert the wound. *B*, Anatomy of the skin.

Epidermis
Dermis
Subcutaneous fat
Muscle
Superficial fibrofatty junction
Periosteum
Bone
Areolar tissue

have a working knowledge of the anatomic layers of the skin. Figure 2B shows the epidermis, dermis, fatty subcutaneous tissue, a superficial fibrofatty layer, muscle, a deep fibrofatty layer, and periosteum or mucous membrane. Ideally, each of these layers, except the muscle, should be sutured. However, in practice, all that is often needed to evert the wound edge and release the surface skin tension is a suture passed through the dermal-fatty junction. If this junction is very close to the skin surface, it may be best to "bury" the knot; i.e., invert the suture so that the knotted end is tied away from the skin surface. Avoidance of deadspace, vertical alignment, and skin eversion are three prime principles that are honored by a layered closure (Dushoff, 1974).

SUTURE PLACEMENT

With a long laceration, divide the wound in half and subsequently bisect the remaining portions. This serves to prevent excess skin remaining at the end of the repair. The needle should enter and exit at points equidistant from the wound margin. Tension is distributed in proportion to the number of sutures placed. In the usual situation, sutures placed every 4 to 5 mm. will approximate margins without tension.

As a result of pre-existing trauma, vasodilatation and oozing due to the local anesthetic, or simply the manipulation of suturing, edema of the wound edge always develops. Sutures that appear to firmly approximate tissues when placed may be the cause of too much tension the following day (see Fig. 3). Therefore, sutures should be placed loose enough to allow swelling without the development of "railroad tracking" or "cross-hatching"—telltale signs of inappropriate wound repair.

In addition to tension, there are five other factors involved in permanent scarring:

(1) The length of time that a skin suture is left in place (see suture removal).

(2) The relationship of the suture to the wound edge. When large areas of tissue are taken with the suture, larger suture marks can result because a larger segment of tissue will be subjected to the constricting effect of the suture. These marks can be avoided by keeping the sutures closer to the wound edge.

(3) Region of the body. "Railroad tracking" is not common on the face, except in areas heavily laden with sebaceous glands. In contrast, the sternal area, trunk, and extremities, with the exception of the hands and soles of the feet, are common sites for such scars.

(4) Infection.

(5) Susceptibility of the patient to form keloids (Grabb and Smith, 1973).

EVERSION OF THE WOUND EDGE

Wounds heal well with a slightly everted margin. An everted wound edge will gradually flatten to form a level wound surface. In contrast, an inverted wound edge, which creates a valley in the skin, will be the cause of an unsightly shadow when a light is cast upon it. This shadow will further accentuate the scar.

Eversion will occur when the course of the suture is deeper than it is wide. A common way to accomplish this is to angle the needle back away from the wound edge, making a bottle-shaped suture pattern (see Fig. 4A). Eversion will also occur if the needle tract is simply passed deeper than its distance from the wound margin (see Fig. 4B). A third way to obtain eversion is to use a vertical mattress suture in which a simple through-and-through stitch is returned, grasping the epithelial margins (see Fig. 4C). Figure 4D indicates what should not be done, since shallow sutures (those which are wider than they are deep) tend to produce an inverted wound margin (Dushoff, 1973–1974). A subcuticular suture is useful when tension is minimal and the wound margins are equal.

EXCESS TISSUE—THE "DOG EAR"

Because of the nature of many wounds, even the best repair may result in an excess amount of skin at one end, i.e., the "dog ear."

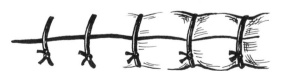

Figure 3 The sutures at the right show the appearance of the wound on the day following repair. Edema has occurred, resulting in excessive tension and increased tendency to form "railroad tracks," which in addition to being unsightly, are difficult to repair.

Sutures must be deeper than wide . . .

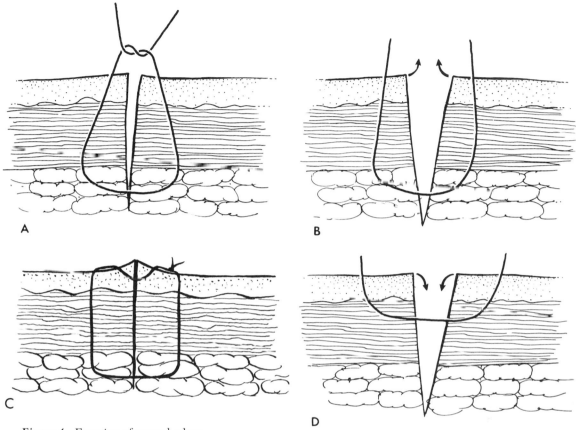

Figure 4 Eversion of wound edges.

A, Angling the needle away from the wound edge will produce eversion. The suture should be wider at the base.

B, Eversion can be accomplished by simply placing the suture deeper than it is wide.

C, Vertical mattress suture.

D, Incorrect! Note that shallow, wide sutures tend to result in *inversion* of the wound margins, causing a poor cosmetic result.

(A, B, and D from Dushoff, Ira M.: A stitch in time. *In* Touching all basics. Emerg. Med. p. 196, Jan. 1973 and Feb. 1974.)

The principle for correction is to selectively shorten the long (excess) side and lengthen the short side. The technique is illustrated in Figure 5A through E (Dushoff, 1973–1974).

SUTURES

Sutures are divided into absorbable [catgut or polyglycolic acid (Dexon)] and nonabsorbable (steel, nylon, Dacron, polypropylene, silk, and cotton). Catgut sutures may be further divided into plain and chromic. Plain catgut will be absorbed faster than that which has been hardened by chromicization (chromic catgut). Therefore, if strength is needed, as in a layered closure, it would be more appropriate to use chromic catgut.

Sutures may be monofilament or may have multiple filaments that are braided or twisted to form the suture. Nonabsorbable sutures may be coated with a medical grade of silicone (on silk), Teflon (on braided Dacron), or other synthetic materials to make them smoother and less reactive. The suture may have a cutting or noncutting needle swaged on one end, or it may have to be threaded through the eye of a needle (Grabb and Smith, 1973).

An absorbable suture should be utilized whenever it is undesirable to accept the presence of a permanent foreign body. Such a situation is most commonly encountered in the contaminated or potentially contaminated traumatic wound seen in the emergency unit. A 3–0 or 4–0 chromic suture is a good, general purpose, absorbable suture for deep placement of layered closure. Some

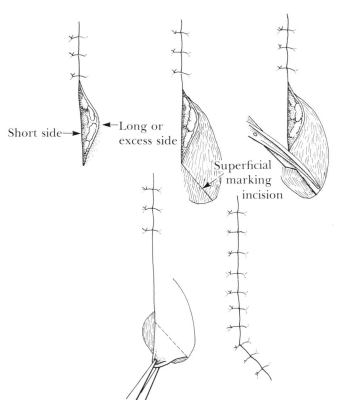

Short side→   ←Long or
                      excess side

                      Superficial
                      marking
                      incision

Figure 5   Correcting the "dog ear."

A, Appearance of "dog ear". Note short side and longer side. Don't try to suture this without modification if a cosmetic result is needed.

B, To correct the "dog ear," make a superficial marking incision at approximately a 45-degree angle to the line of the wound.

C, Cut over your marking incision with a dissecting scissor and undermine the shaded areas.

D, Trim off the excess skin and place the flap so that it matches the previously shorter side.

E, Suture. The result will be to eliminate the raised and unsightly dog ear.

(From Dushoff, Ira M.: A stitch in time. *In* Touching all basics. Emerg. Med. p. 201, Jan. 1973 and Feb. 1974.)

physicians prefer a polyglycolic acid suture because it is easier to handle and causes less tissue reaction.

In the emergency unit, nonabsorbable sutures are used mainly for skin closures. Monofilament wire is the least reactive suture material available but has the disadvantage of expense and nonflexibility. Braided silks and monofilament synthetics are among the most commonly used suture materials. Practical differences between various materials are slight; to a large degree, selection depends on personal preference. The synthetics tend to be stronger but more difficult to manipulate. The braided silk sutures have the theoretical disadvantage of increased rate of infection, but this has not been shown clinically. For routine wound repair, a 4–0 suture generally will suffice. Cosmetic repairs entail the use of 5–0 or 6–0 sutures. When suturing the scalp, 3–0 materials are needed for their strength.

SUTURE REMOVAL

In general, sutures having cosmetic significance should be removed about 72 hours after placement. This early removal greatly reduces the possibility of "cross-hatching." Subsequently, the wound must be reinforced for several days by applying tincture of benzoin to each side of the wound, and placing Steri-Strips across the wound margin. In areas of cosmetic concern, it is best, if a question arises, to err on the side of earlier removal, since cross-hatching is difficult to rectify. You may also opt to remove half the sutures on the third day and the remainder on the fifth day. At that point, you should still Steri-Strip the wound for several days longer.

Sutures located on the extremities may be removed at five to eight days, but if they are over moving parts (e.g., joints), leave them in place for up to 10 days. Scalp sutures are generally removed between the seventh and tenth days while sutures of the trunk may remain for five to eight days. Since wounds of the back and feet take longer to heal, sutures should be left in place for 10 to 14 days. At the earliest sign of wound infection, removal of any suture is indicated.

SPECIAL SITUATIONS

The following situations deserve special attention:

Scalp. The scalp is very vascular and tends to bleed profusely. Bleeding is usually best controlled initially by direct pressure through the aponeurotic layer. Deep through-and-through vertical mattress or simple sutures with 3–0 or larger suture material will produce hemostasis without needing to tie individual vessels. It is not uncommon to find a patient in shock from a moderate-sized scalp laceration because the physician has been trying unsuccessfully to control bleeding by clamping and tying these individual vessels. In addition to better tensile strength, the larger sutures have the advantage of coming with larger and stronger needles. This allows generous, full-thickness sections of scalp to be taken in a single pass without bending or breaking the needle. A layered closure is usually unnecessary. In a screaming child or an uncooperative, intoxicated patient, a running lock suture may be utilized.

Before actually suturing, you must remember to inspect and explore the wound. If the laceration is large, can you see a skull fracture? Do you see glass or other foreign bodies? After inspection, you should put on a sterile glove and palpate the wound with your finger, again feeling for linear or depressed fractures and for foreign bodies. A common error here is to mistake the split edges of the galea for a skull fracture. However, on subsequent inspection you may see the edges of the galea and palpate smooth bone beneath this area.

When suturing is completed, have the patient apply direct pressure with a few 4 × 4 inch gauze pads for five minutes to eliminate suture line bleeding. Do not use commercial sprays, and unless there is continued minor oozing, do not apply dressings. Just allow the repair to dry to the open air and tell the patient that he may wash his hair in 24 to 48 hours. This will result in good wound care and a grateful patient. Have the patient return in 7 to 10 days for suture removal.

Eyebrows. Since it is debatable as to whether regrowth of eyebrows will occur, it is best *not* to shave them when preparing the wound. In some cases, if shaved, they may grow back with a cosmetically displeasing result. Also, shaving the eyebrow eliminates a valuable landmark needed for good wound approximation. Subsequent to suture placement about the face, as with the scalp, direct

pressure over the wound for five minutes will usually eliminate suture line bleeding. Bandages in these areas not only are difficult to apply but also inhibit local care. However, if a local anesthetic agent with epinephrine has been used, a pressure dressing wrapped around the head may be left on for an hour or so, since there may be delayed bleeding.

Lips. Exact approximation of the vermilion border is essential. The initial suture should align this cutaneous junction (see Fig. 6). A minimal difference of even 2 mm. gives a noticeable defect. Suturing progresses along the vermilion surface until the moist mucosal membrane is reached. Suturing of moist buccal surfaces is usually unnecessary and is not indicated in contused

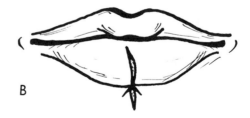

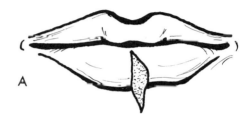

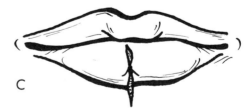

Figure 6 Lip repair.

A, Note laceration extends through the lower vermilion border.

B, The initial suture should realign the vermilion border. To do otherwise can result in mismatching at this crucial juncture which, because of color difference and the elevated nature, gives a result which is noticeably imperfect.

C, This illustrates the *wrong* way. Do not begin at any other point than at the vermilion border!

wounds. When suturing the lower lip, a mental nerve block (see p. 396) and Fig. 9A to C) can be used to eliminate the distortion that would be caused by local infiltration.

Through-and-through lacerations of the oral cavity involve three basic layers — skin, muscle, and mucosa. The muscular layer is approximated with an absorbable suture; the skin is closed with fine nonabsorbable sutures; the mucosal surface can usually be left unsutured. If the mucosal layer is closed, antibiotic prophylaxis should be considered. When suturing mucosal surfaces inside the mouth in an adult, silk sutures should be used, since they are soft and therefore will not cause irritation during movement of the tongue, as would be the case with the stiffer synthetics or catgut. In children, suture removal here may be extremely difficult. For this reason, plain catgut sutures should be utilized to obviate suture removal.

Tongue. In the absence of protracted bleeding, even large lacerations of the tongue will heal without the need for surgical approximation. However, a longitudinal laceration greater than 1 cm. in length involving the tip should be approximated to prevent the development of a forked defect.

Usually, the bleeding ceases spontaneously or with direct pressure. If suturing is needed, one absorbable stitch passed through the bleeding area will usually provide adequate hemostasis.

When the tongue is lacerated, a careful examination of the entire mouth, pharynx, and neck must be performed. One obvious injury may distract an examiner, and others, such as a lacerated Stensen's duct, may be missed.

PRIMARY VERSUS SECONDARY CLOSURE

Any wound that cannot be adequately cleansed or debrided should be considered for secondary closure. In general, if the wound is over 12 hours old or is the result of high-velocity trauma (e.g., gunshot wound), it should not be closed primarily. Stab or puncture wounds generally should not be closed, especially if the base of the wound cannot be seen. Secondary closure is usually carried out between the third and fifth days after injury.

TAPING OF THE SKIN

Microporous surgical adhesive tape (Steri-Strip) can be very advantageous, since it can be applied and removed very quickly, causes little or no skin reaction, avoids the possibility of skin suture marks, and can be left in place for long periods of time under dressings or casts. It is obviously useful in avoiding the pain of obtaining anesthesia, especially in a restless or struggling child. There is one drawback to its easy removal: if a child decides he wants the Steri-Strip off, then it comes off. Nevertheless, these tapes can be used very effectively, especially for repair of small lacerations.

To apply the tapes, first clean and prepare the wound as described previously; then blot dry with sterile gauze. If the wound is deep, a layered closure should be performed. Next, apply tincture of benzoin to each side of the wound margin, taking care not to get the benzoin in the wound itself, as this causes an unpleasant burning sensation. Apply the tape on one side of the wound (keep the tape perpendicular to the wound edge), pull the edges together, and then lay down the tape on the other side. Finally, smooth out the tape to ensure full contact with the entire skin surface. Repeat this procedure with as many tapes as needed.

ANESTHESIA

GENERAL COMMENTS

When selecting any anesthetic agent, use the smallest effective amount of the least toxic substance in the safest possible manner.

Lidocaine and other "-caine" agents are commonly used in local and regional anesthesia. One should be prepared to recognize and treat their complications, and such anesthetics must not be used unless resuscitative equipment and drugs are available. The great majority of these complications are dose-related and may result in drowsiness, coma, or seizure. Cardiac arrest is an uncommon, but potentially lethal complication. The second type of toxicity is allergic in nature, ranging from pruritus and urticaria to frank anaphylactic shock.

If a patient is known to have had a systemic toxic reaction to one specific local anesthetic drug, in most instances a local

TABLE 1 *Classification of Local Anesthetic Agents According to Chemical Structure*

CHEMICAL GROUP	LOCAL ANESTHETIC DRUG
para-aminobenzoic acid ester	procaine (Novocain) tetracaine (Pontocaine) chloroprocaine (Nesacaine)
diethylaminoacet-2,6-xylidide	lidocaine (Xylocaine)
d, 1-N-methylpipecolic acid 2,6,-dimethyl-anilide	mepivacaine (Carbocaine)
beta-diethylamino-cthyl amide	dibucaine (Nupercaine)
benzoic acid ester	cocaine piperocaine (Metycaine)
para-ethoxybenzoic acid ester	diethoxin (Intracaine)
1-cyclohexylamino-2-propyl benzoate	hexylcaine (Cyclaine)

anesthetic agent of another chemical group may be used without producing a reaction (see Table 1). For example, if a patient is allergic to procaine, he will probably not be allergic to lidocaine. However, the usual problem is that the patient does not know positively which agent caused his allergic reaction.

LOCAL ANESTHESIA

A 1 per cent plain lidocaine solution is generally used. Epinephrine may be added when working in vascular areas (e.g., the scalp or face). This not only will aid in hemostasis but will also prolong anesthesia and minimize toxic reactions by delaying entry into the general circulation. Never use epinephrine when anesthetizing fingers, toes, penis, nose, or earlobes, as gangrene may result. It should be used cautiously in the elderly and in patients with hypertension and hyperthyroidism.

Local infiltration should be intradermal and not subcutaneous. The dermal layer may be approached directly from the cut margin of the wound. This method is easier and less painful and has not been shown to have a higher infection rate.

Insert a 25 gauge needle into the dermis.

Aspirate to be certain that the needle is not within a vessel. Raise a skin wheal, and advance the needle; repeat the procedure as many times as needed. Before obtaining anesthesia and attempting a difficult repair in a hysterical child, it is often wise to sedate the child. One of many ways to do this is to administer 1 mg./kg. body weight of Demerol IM, up to 50 mg. A moving target is much harder to repair than a stationary one.

DIGITAL BLOCK

The common digital nerves may be blocked next to the metacarpal heads or as divided branches are encountered at the base of each digit. Epinephrine in the anesthetic agent is absolutely contraindicated, as it may cause digital gangrene. Gangrene may also occur from vascular compression if too large a volume of anesthetic is used when blocking the nerve in the confined space at the base of the first phalanx. If small amounts are used, this problem is not often encountered. However, because of this possible complication, a transmetacarpal approach is safer.

Technique of Transmetacarpal Anesthesia

(1) Cleanse the volar surface of the hand.

(2) Use a 1 per cent lidocaine solution *without* epinephrine.

(3) Palpate the metacarpal head, which is approximately at the level of the distal palmar crease.

(4) Insert a 25 gauge needle perpendicular to the skin just to one side of the metacarpal head. A skin wheal is not needed.

(5) Advance the needle until it is approximately at the same level as the metacarpal head.

(6) Inject 2 to 3 cc. of anesthetic. No paresthesias need be elicited.

(7) Repeat the procedure on the opposite side of the metacarpal head. Anesthesia will be obtained in 2 to 3 minutes.

INTERCOSTAL NERVE BLOCK

Intercostal nerve block is commonly employed for relief of pain due to fractured ribs. Marcaine, a longer acting anesthetic agent, is preferred. Because of cross-over of fibers, it is usually necessary to block the nerves of the ribs above and below the fractured rib.

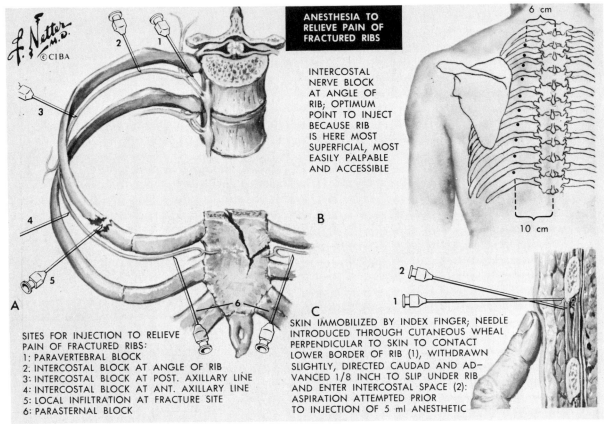

ANESTHESIA TO RELIEVE PAIN OF FRACTURED RIBS

INTERCOSTAL NERVE BLOCK AT ANGLE OF RIB; OPTIMUM POINT TO INJECT BECAUSE RIB IS HERE MOST SUPERFICIAL, MOST EASILY PALPABLE AND ACCESSIBLE

6 cm

10 cm

SITES FOR INJECTION TO RELIEVE PAIN OF FRACTURED RIBS:
1: PARAVERTEBRAL BLOCK
2: INTERCOSTAL BLOCK AT ANGLE OF RIB
3: INTERCOSTAL BLOCK AT POST. AXILLARY LINE
4: INTERCOSTAL BLOCK AT ANT. AXILLARY LINE
5: LOCAL INFILTRATION AT FRACTURE SITE
6: PARASTERNAL BLOCK

SKIN IMMOBILIZED BY INDEX FINGER; NEEDLE INTRODUCED THROUGH CUTANEOUS WHEAL PERPENDICULAR TO SKIN TO CONTACT LOWER BORDER OF RIB (1), WITHDRAWN SLIGHTLY, DIRECTED CAUDAD AND AD- VANCED 1/8 INCH TO SLIP UNDER RIB AND ENTER INTERCOSTAL SPACE (2): ASPIRATION ATTEMPTED PRIOR TO INJECTION OF 5 ml ANESTHETIC

Figure 7 Intercostal nerve block. *A*, Sites for injection.
B, Optimum site at angle of rib.
   C, Technique of blocking right under rib. (From Naclerio, Emil A.: Chest trauma. CIBA Clinical Symposia, 22(3):81, 1970, Plate IV. Copyright © 1970 CIBA Pharmaceutical Company, Division of CIBA-GEIGY Corporation. Reproduced, with permission, from Clinical Symposia, illustrated by Frank Netter, M.D. All rights reserved.)

The intercostal nerve can be blocked at any point between the paravertebral area and the site of injury (Fig. 7A). The best location is often at the posterior angle of the rib (Fig. 7B). At this location, the neurovascular bundle is relatively superficial and the lateral cutaneous branch of the nerve will also be affected. Some authors feel paravertebral block should not be used in the emergency unit since it can cause marked irreversible hypotension due to its effect on autonomic fibers (Naclerio, 1970). Local infiltration of the fracture site is not advised, for it usually produces poor, short-lasting results.

Technique
(1) Cleanse overlying skin.
(2) With a 25 gauge needle, raise a skin

wheal over the lower aspect of the involved rib.
(3) Change to a 22 gauge 1½ inch needle.
(4) Insert the needle through the skin wheal perpendicular to the skin until the lower edge of the rib is contacted (Fig. 7C).
(5) Withdraw the needle halfway and redirect caudally in order to slip just beneath the rib cage (Fig. 7C).
(6) Advance the needle about 3 to 4 mm. past the rib margin. This should place the needle in the area of the neurovascular bundle.
(7) Aspirate to verify that the needle is not in a vessel or the pleural cavity. Then inject 3 to 4 cc. of Marcaine.
(8) Obtain a chest x-ray if there is a

suspicion that the thoracic cavity has been entered (e.g., aspiration of air during procedure).

MEDIAN AND ULNAR NERVE BLOCK

Block of the median and ulnar nerves can provide adequate anesthesia for procedures on the volar aspect of the palm and for reduction of certain fractures. However, the most complete anesthesia is obtained by using intravenous regional anesthesia. (See section on IV anesthesia.) Regional anesthesia also diminishes the possibility of postoperative paresthesias.

Technique at the Wrist
(1) Cleanse the overlying skin.

(2) Locate the position of the nerve in question. The median nerve lies under and just to the radial side of the palmaris longus tendon, and to the ulnar side of the flexor carpi radialis (see Fig. 8A). In the absence of the palmaris longus, the nerve lies about 6 mm. to the radial side of the flexor

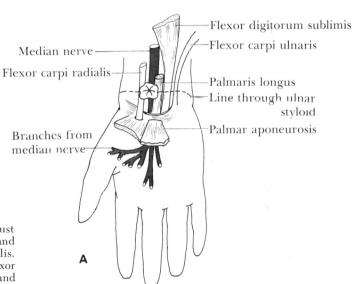

Figure 8 A, Note median nerve and just slightly radial to the palmaris longus tendon and just on the ulnar side of the flexor carpi radialis. If the palmaris longus is absent, use the flexor digitorum sublimus as a reference point and inject approximately 6 mm. to its radial side.

B, Note ulnar nerve lies deep to the ulnar artery and just on the radial side of the flexor carpi ulnaris tendon. When anesthetizing the ulnar nerve, be sure to aspirate first due to the close proximity of the ulnar nerve and artery.

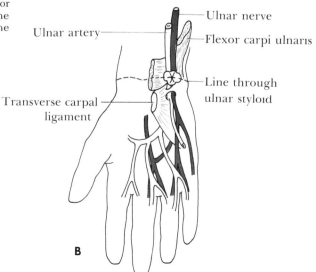

digitorum sublimis. The ulnar nerve lies deep to the ulnar artery and on the radial side of the flexor carpi ulnaris tendon (see Fig. 8B).

(3) Using a 25 gauge needle, raise a skin wheal over the nerve at the level of the styloid process.

(4) Insert a 23 gauge needle perpendicular to the skin. At the depth of about 5 mm., a paresthesia is usually felt.

(5) When paresthesias are obtained, inject 3 cc. of anesthetic agent. If no paresthesia is elicited, inject an additional 2 cc. of anesthetic. When blocking the ulnar nerve, be sure to aspirate before injecting, as the ulnar artery is immediately adjacent to and above the nerve.

If anesthesia is needed in all ulnar distribution, it is preferable to block the ulnar nerve at the elbow instead of the wrist where the ulnar nerve divides into dorsal and ventral branches. To obtain dorsal anesthesia when working at the level of the wrist, extend a field block dorsally.

Technique of Ulnar Nerve Block at the Elbow

(1) Flex the elbow and palpate superficially the cordlike ulnar nerve in the ulnar groove of the humerus.

(2) Cleanse the overlying skin.

(3) With a 25 gauge needle, raise an intradermal skin wheal over the nerve.

(4) Insert a 22 gauge needle through the skin wheal and elicit paresthesias.

(5) When paresthesias are obtained, pull the needle back about 2 mm. so that no anesthetic will be injected into the nerve sheath, which could cause postoperative paresthesias.

(6) Inject 5 cc. of lidocaine.

MENTAL NERVE BLOCK

Unilateral or bilateral mental nerve block provides excellent anesthesia of the lower lip without local tissue distortion. The mental nerve is a branch of the inferior alveolar nerve and is anesthetized as it exits from the mental foramen from the mandible. This foramen lies at the apex and just anterior to the second bicuspid root.

Technique

(1) Identify the first and second premolar teeth (Fig. 9A).

(2) Insert the index finger into the mouth and pull the cheek to the buccal side for exposure (Fig. 9B).

(3) Insert a 1 inch 25 or 27 gauge needle into the mucolabial fold between the premolar teeth (Fig. 9C).

(4) Inject 0.5 to 1 cc. superficially and deep just above the periosteum. This will anesthetize the mental nerve as it exits from the foramen.

The foramen itself should not be entered. This is unnecessary for anesthesia of the lip only and will result in greater frequency of postoperative paresthesia.

INTRAVENOUS REGIONAL ANESTHESIA

Intravenous regional anesthesia is an effective, relatively safe, and easy to perform technique that can be used for fracture reduction, repositioning of elbow dislocations, and repair of multiple lacerations of the upper extremity. It can also be used with some modifications on the lower extremity. It is referred to as the "Bier block," being named after the first person to describe its use in 1908.

Materials:

a. Double cuff sphygmomanometer or single cuff self-contained unit.

b. 1 per cent Xylocaine.

c. 50 cc. syringe.

d. A No. 18 and a No. 23 gauge butterfly needle.

e. One infusion set.

f. Sterile saline.

Technique

(1) The proper dose of Xylocaine is calculated using a 3 mg./kg. dosage schedule. An average adult would receive 200 mg. (e.g., 20 cc. of 1 per cent Xylocaine). This is drawn and mixed with an equal amount (20 cc.) of sterile saline, thus making a 0.5 per cent solution. Some authorities report good results with 1.5 mg./kg.

(2) An IV is started in the unaffected arm, ensuring an accessible intravenous route should signs of toxicity or the need for medication arise. In the past 67 years since its inception, there have been no fatalities in the 10,000 reported cases (Colburn, 1970). However, whenever Xylocaine (lidocaine) is used, routine precautions should be observed.

(3) The double cuff is placed in its usual

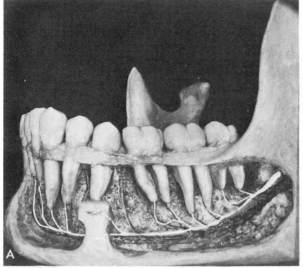

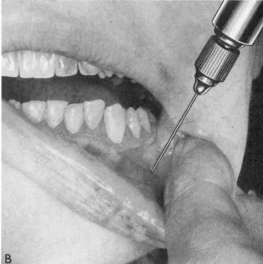

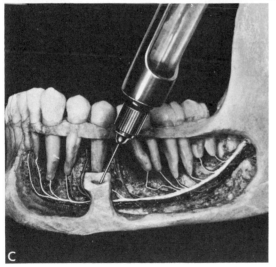

Figure 9 Mental nerve block. *A*, First and second molar teeth identified.

B, Pull cheek with finger for exposure.

C, Insert needle between the premolars at the muco-labial fold. Inject and advance the needle until it touches periostium and inject again approximately 0.5 cc. To enhance accuracy, aim at the apex of the second bicuspid tooth (premolar). However, do not inject into the fora-men directly. (From Manual of Local Anesthesia in General Dentistry, published by Cook-Waite Laboratories, Inc., New York, p. 18.)

position on the affected arm and inflated enough to dilate the veins (30 to 40 mm. Hg). Insert the scalp vein needle as close to the pathologic site as possible, tape it in place, and connect it to the 50 cc. syringe (see Fig. 10).

(4) Deflate the cuff and raise the affected extremity above the chest in order to drain excess venous blood. An Esmark or elastic bandage may be used to aid in exsanguinating the extremity but generally is not needed. While the arm is raised, occasionally aspirate and inject Xylocaine in very small amounts so that blood does not clot in the line. After two minutes of elevation, inflate the upper cuff to well above systolic blood pressure (normally, about 220 mm. Hg). Lower the arm to the patient's side.

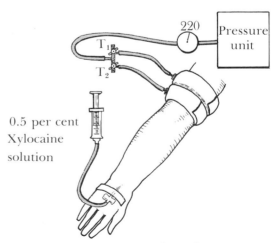

Figure 10 IV regional anesthesia.

(5) Inject the 40 cc. mixture of Xylocaine. Then, remove the butterfly needle and apply pressure with a cotton swab to the puncture site. The skin often becomes blanched and erythematous in patches This is normal and not a toxic manifestation. Complete anesthesia usually occurs in 5 to 10 minutes. Fractures and dislocations can be painlessly reduced saving the patient general anesthesia, a hospital admission, money, and time.

(6) If the patient begins to have tourniquet pain, inflate the lower cuff and then deflate the upper cuff. The tourniquet pressure will now be over an already anesthetized area, alleviating pain. Tourniquet time should normally not exceed 60 minutes and the procedure must absolutely be terminated at 90 minutes.

(7) Upon conclusion of the surgical procedure, the cuff is released for five seconds and then reinflated for about 45 seconds. Repeat this procedure four or five times. This is done to decrease the bolus of Xylocaine released into the general circulation. If no toxic effects are observed, release and remove the tourniquet. If the fracture reduction takes only several minutes, wait 15 minutes before beginning the cyclic tourniquet release so that more Xylocaine may become tissue-bound. After 15 more minutes of observation, the intravenous line on the unaffected side may be removed.

Bibliography

Colbern, Edwin C.: Bier block. Anesth. Analg. Current Res., 49(6):November–December 1970.

Dushoff, Ira M.: About face. Emerg. Med., Nov. 1974.

Dushoff, Ira M.: A stitch in time. Emerg. Med., Jan. 1973 and Feb. 1974.

Grabb, W. C., and Smith, J. W.: Plastic Surgery. 2nd ed. Boston, Little Brown and Co., 1973.

Manual of Local Anesthesia in General Dentistry. New York, Cook-Waite Laboratories, Inc.

Moore, Daniel C.: Regional Block. 4th ed. Springfield, Ill., Charles C Thomas, Publisher, 1975.

Naclerio, Emil A.: Chest trauma. CIBA Clinical Symposia, 22(3):81, 1970.

Stevenson, T. R., et al.: Cleansing the traumatic wound by high pressure syringe irrigation. J. Am. Coll. Emerg. Physicians 5(1):17, 1976.

Chapter 15

EXAMINATION OF THE EYE AND ITS ADNEXA

*George L. Spaeth
and John Purcell*

GENERAL CONSIDERATIONS

The first task facing the emergency physician is the proper determination of the urgency of care (Table 1). *Chemical burns and vascular occlusions constitute the only situations* in which ophthalmic care must be, quite literally, *immediate.* Having first ascertained the relative degree of therapeutic urgency, then the physician should proceed with an orderly, systematic assessment of the ocular system.

Asymmetry is a greatly useful clue that pathology is in fact present. However, the examiner must be on the *qui vive* to keep from being led astray in this regard. The apparently drooping left upper lid may in actuality be normal, the asymmetry being the result of an elevated right upper lid due to thyroid disease. Similarly, for example, the apparently dilated right pupil may be the normal one, the smaller left pupil being a sign of uveitis.

A schema for the examination of the eyes is shown in Table 2.

VISUAL ACUITY

Following assessment of need for instantaneous treatment (as with chemical burns to the eye) and appropriate history taking, the first step in the ocular examination should be the determination and recording of visual acuity. The visual acuity itself may be a valuable aid in diagnosis and prog-

---

TABLE 1   *Urgency of Ocular Emergencies*

By Diagnosis
A. Needing instantaneous therapy*
   1. Chemical burns.
   2. Retinal vascular occlusion.
B. Needing therapy as soon as can be reasonably administered, preferably within the hour.
   1. Acute glaucoma.
   2. Cavernous sinus thrombosis.
   3. Lacerated or ruptured globe.
C. Needing therapy within several hours, although the sooner the better.
   1. Corneal ulcer.
   2. Orbital cellulitis.
   3. Intraocular foreign body.
   4. Adnexal injuries (lid laceration, etc.).
D. Needing evaluation as soon as can be reasonably accomplished; therapy may be urgent or delayed, depending on findings.
   1. Retinal detachment.
   2. Hyphema.

By Symptom†
A. Needing immediate evaluation:
   Sudden loss of vision.
B. Needing evaluation within several hours:
   Sudden "blurring" of vision,
   Ocular trauma.
C. Needing evaluation within 24 hours:
   "Acute red eye."

---

*Routine preparatory history and examination should be modified in these cases.
†General rule: the more acute the symptom the more urgent the evaluation.

TABLE 2   *Methods of Ocular Examination*

1. Assessment of urgency required
2. History
3. Visual acuity
4. External examination
   a. Inspection with flashlight
   b. Palpation
   c. Slit lamp examination (gonioscopy, tonometry)
5. Tonometry
6. Fundoscopy
   a. Direct
   b. Indirect

399

nosis. Moreover, it may in some cases be of great medicolegal importance.

Visual acuity is a test of the whole optical system of the eye. Also, it specifically measures macular function. The measurement of visual acuity should be done prior to manipulation of the eye so that loss of vision caused by an injury will not be incorrectly attributed to the examination and instrumentation. A distance or near test chart may be used, but near vision tests require accommodation, and therefore may be less valid. If the patient cannot recognize the largest letter on the chart, his ability to count fingers or see light should be determined. Since therapy will at least partly depend on the possibility of visual salvage, the comment that the eye is unable to perceive light should not be made unless the examiner is absolutely certain. Glasses should be worn to estimate the best acuity. In elderly patients tested with a near vision chart, proper spectacles must be worn.

When distance vision is less than 20/20, the visual acuity should be checked further by using a pin-hole. If vision does not improve significantly when the chart is viewed through a small hole, the visual reduction probably is *not* due to refractive error, but represents real pathology. Thus, if pin-hole vision is less than 20/20 the physician should be aware that some disease, old or new, probably is present. In children less than 10 years of age the visual acuity may be 20/30 and yet normal. The acuity in the two eyes should be equal.

If standard Snellen charts are used they should be positioned 20 feet from the patient. As this distance is relatively long and therefore difficult to obtain in some Emergency Departments, a near vision testing machine or a projector may be used (with the projector the image size will vary with distance and therefore may be used for distances shorter than 20 feet). Although it is not always necessary to test vision at 20 feet, it *is* essential to test vision at the distance appropriate for the chart being employed at that time.

Lighting conditions are important, but not critically so. There obviously must be sufficient illumination to allow the chart to be seen clearly. The symbols on the chart must be clear. Lights that might dazzle the patient should not be near the chart.

Assessment of visual ability in young children or the uncooperative patient may be difficult. The examiner should test each eye separately for its ability to fixate on a light or a small picture. A complete description of the estimated visual ability should be recorded.

The importance of proper assessment of visual acuity cannot be overstressed. When validly performed the test provides remarkable guidance to the physician who knows its significance.

EXTERNAL EXAMINATION

The external ocular structures (lids, conjunctiva, cornea, sclera) should be examined with a flashlight. If there is a history suggesting possible entry of foreign body into the eye, the upper lid should be everted to examine its undersurface for foreign bodies or signs of trauma. This is accomplished by placing a cotton-tipped applicator above the tarsus of the lid, applying slight pressure against the lid with the applicator while the lashes are grasped by the fingers of the other hand, and then flipping the lid over the applicator as the patient looks down (Figure 1). Careful attention must be paid to signs of trauma, for even small lacerations may indicate serious functional damage. Asymmetry should alert the examiner to search further. The cornea should be crystal clear. The orbital rims and contents may be gently palpated for tumor, fracture, or crepitus.

The depth of the anterior chamber can be estimated by noting, when a light is shined obliquely from the temporal side of the eye, whether the nasal iris is well illuminated or lies in shadow (Figure 2). Material in the anterior chamber should be looked for; this may settle inferiorly and be difficult or, in some cases, impossible to observe without utilization of special techniques such as gonioscopy. A hyphema (layered blood) or a hypopyon (layered inflammatory cells settled inferiorly in the anterior chamber) may be seen between the iris and the cornea.

The pupils should be examined with a flashlight for size, equality, shape, and reaction. This gives an objective sign as to the status of the eye. The size of the pupil can be estimated with a millimeter rule, although the actual measurement is not often necessary to record. A rough estimate usually is adequate. The size of the right pupil in comparison to the left pupil is, however, very important to note. Small differences can signal serious pathology, though asymmetry occasionally may occur in the normal individual's gaze.

The direct response to light of each pupil individually is noted. The light may then be swung from eye to eye to determine the *relative* responsiveness of each eye to light. Normally, constriction should be strongest in the eye into which the light is directly shining. If the pupil of the previously unilluminated eye into which the light is now being directed (eye A) *dilates* immediately after the light has been swung from the other eye (eye B), this demonstrates that the previous consensual constriction of the pupil of eye A was actually stronger than the direct reaction. This "afferent pupillary

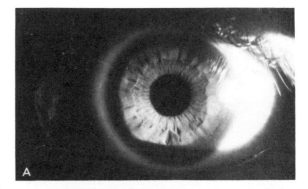

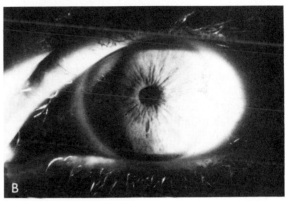

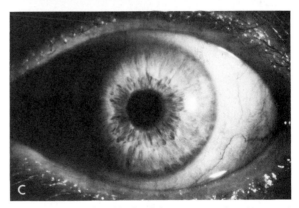

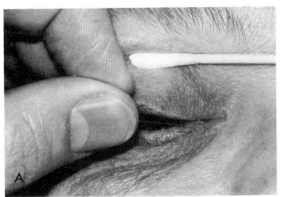

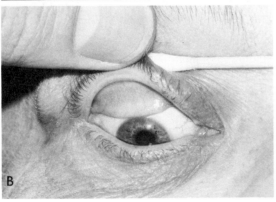

Figure 1 Eversion of the upper lid is essential when there is a complaint suggesting an extraocular foreign body or when the superior tarsal conjunctiva needs examination. This procedure is not uncomfortable if the patient maintains a downward gaze at all times and the flip of the tarsus is done gently. The applicator should be pushed posteriorly just firmly enough to hold it in position. As the lid margin is pulled out and up the applicator exerts pressure primarily in a downward, not posterior, direction. The applicator helps to flip the lid by moving the superior margin of the tarsal plate inferiorly. To restore the lid to its proper position the patient is asked to look up.

Figure 2 The depth of the anterior chamber is of normal depth in A. Note the light reflection at 3 o'clock at the limbus; the light is directed in a plane parallel to the iris. The entire surface of the iris is illuminated; the light even passes into the angle recess, transilluminating the sclera at the limbar border between 6:30 and 11:30 o'clock. In contrast, the prominent shadow of the iris to the left of the pupil in B indicates that the anterior chamber in this eye is shallow. Mydriatic-induced angle closure would be unlikely (though not impossible) in the eye in A. However, dilatation of the pupil is more likely to induce angle closure in the eye with the shallow chamber (B).

In C, the light was directed obliquely rather than parallel to the plane of the iris (note the position of the light reflex in comparison with A and B). The shadow due to the anterior convexity of the iris appears less prominent than in B even though the chamber in C is also pathologically shallow.

TABLE 3   Causes for Unequal Pupils*

1. Congenital variant
2. Disease of the third cranial nerve (oculomotor nerve)
3. Disease of the second cranial nerve (optic nerve)
4. Unilateral blindness
5. Adie's tonic pupil
6. Trauma
7. Glaucoma
8. Topical drugs
9. Horner's syndrome
10. Syphilis
11. Active iridocyclitis
12. Old iridocyclitis

*Only important or relatively common causes are included.

response" (Marcus Gunn) indicates pathology in the afferent pupillary pathways. Causes for this include: retinal detachment, optic neuritis, vascular accident of the optic nerve, glaucoma, and trauma. The major causes for asymmetry of pupil size (anisocoria) are listed in Table 3. Item numbers 1 through 7 are associated with mydriasis. Drugs can cause either mydriasis or miosis. Items numbered 9, 10, and 11 cause miosis. Old iridocyclitis is characterized by irregular pupils due to iris-lens adhesions.

The size, prominence (exophthalmos or enophthalmos) and position (orbital tumor or strabismus) of the eyes should be noted. The position of the eyes in upward, up and out, lateral, out and down, downward, down and in, inward and up and in gaze should be noted as a sign of abnormal motility or the existence of any extraocular nerve disorders (Figure 3). The superior oblique muscle is innervated by the fourth cranial nerve (trochlear), the lateral rectus muscle by the sixth cranial nerve (abducens), and all other extraocular muscles by the third cranial nerve (oculomotor). Lids are closed by the seventh cranial nerve (facial), and opened by the third cranial nerve. Sensation in the entire region is subserved by the fifth cranial nerve (trigeminal); vision is transmitted solely via the second cranial nerve—the optic nerve.

SLIT LAMP EXAMINATION

If a slit lamp biomicroscope is available it can provide much help if one is thoroughly familiar with its use. The layers

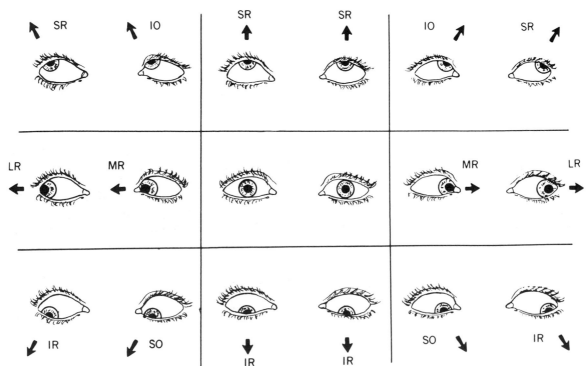

Figure 3   When tested in different positions of gaze the presence of a deviation of movement of the eyes helps to pinpoint which muscle or nerve is involved. Testing the eyes in six positions helps permit determination of the normalcy of the six extraocular muscles: in toward the bridge of the nose—medial rectus (MR); in and down (toward the tip of the nose)—superior oblique (SO); out and down (toward the shoulder)—inferior rectus (IR); out—lateral rectus (LR); out and up—superior rectus (SR); in and up—inferior oblique (IO). (From Van Noorden and Maumenee, Mosby.)

of the cornea, anterior chamber, iris, lens, and anterior one third of the vitreous can be well examined. Its use is indicated when a condition can be better examined or treated with illuminated magnification (i.e., corneal foreign body, trauma, corneal ulcer, or iritis). The examiner views the patient's eyes through the microscope; the light source and microscope can be focused appropriately. Newer models are so made that the light is automatically in focus at the same point as the microscope. This greatly facilitates use of the slit lamp. If this parfocal condition is not present, the oculars may need adjusting or the light may have been moved from its proper position.

The ability to produce a finely focused slit beam permits visualization of otherwise "invisible" portions of the globe, such as the contents of the anterior chamber.

The conjunctiva should be inspected for foreign bodies or absence of tissue. The cornea is checked for foreign bodies, abrasions, or other ocular disease. Sodium fluorescein applied in the lower cul-de-sac will diffuse onto the cornea, and examination with an appropriate blue filter will highlight absent corneal or conjunctival epithelium by virtue of a green stain. As fluorescein solutions are readily infected with pseudomonas, they are probably not suitable for Emergency Department use. Sterile, fluorescein-impregnated paper strips are readily available and are preferred.

The aqueous humor of the anterior chamber is inspected under high magnification for the presence of particulate matter (red cells, white cells, foreign bodies). Visibility of the beam of light as it traverses the anterior chamber is known as "flare" and is a reflection of an outpouring of serum proteins in an inflamed eye. Normally only a faint trace of "flare" can be noted even with the brightest and mostly sharply focused light beam.

The color of the iris and the presence of transillumination or atrophy are noted. The lens and its opacities are easily seen through a dilated pupil.

TONOMETRY

The intraocular pressure can be determined by measuring corneal impressibility with a tonometer. The Schiotz tonometer is a standard instrument, although there are other suitable, even preferable, instruments.

Tonometry should not be performed on any person suspected of having an infected eye, rupture or laceration of the globe, or in an uncooperative patient or a child. The Schiotz tonometer can injure the eye if improperly handled; the applanation tonometers are slightly safer.

Local anesthetic solution (proparacaine) should be instilled in each eye. In Schiotz tonometry the patient lies on his back and is asked to look at a spot on the ceiling or at his outstretched thumb.* The lids are gently retracted with the index finger and thumb, avoiding any pressure on the globe. For determination of pressure accurately, the patient must be relaxed; the lids cannot be forced apart. The tonometer is gently placed on the center of the cornea and is held absolutely vertically. When the weighted unit is floating freely and the pointer oscillating, then the scale reading is taken from the tonometer (Figure 4). The intraocular pressure is determined by referring to a calibration chart which converts the scale reading to millimeters of mercury. Average pressures range from 10 to 20 mm. Hg.

Applanation tonometers are less generally available and are a bit more difficult to

---

*A protective covering (Tonofilm) may be placed over the plunger end to assure sterility and to prevent corneal abrasions. This covering is obtainable from Clini-Tech, 752 Frederick Road, Baltimore, Md. 21228.

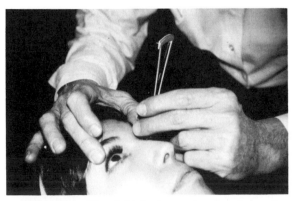

Figure 4 The Schiotz tonometer has been the standard instrument used to determine intraocular pressure in the eye. When used properly it provides a rough estimate of this value. A covering (tonofilm) placed over the plunger makes use of the instrument more difficult, but minimizes the likelihood of producing a corneal abrasion and assures sterility.

TABLE 4   Contraindications to Dilating the Pupil

1. Head trauma.
2. Known or suspected primary *angle-closure* glaucoma*
3. Very shallow anterior chamber angle.

*Open-angle glaucoma is *not* a contraindication to dilating the pupils.

master. They offer definite advantages, however: (1) less chance of producing corneal erosion; (2) less weight on the globe and therefore greater safety; (3) greater ease of cleaning and sterilization; (4) less frightening technique, and (5) more accurate pres-

TABLE 5   Reasons to Suspect a Retinal Tear or Detachment

1. Sudden symptom of "cloud of snowflakes."
2. Symptom of a "rising or falling curtain."
3. Sudden decrease in central vision.
4. Highly myopic person with symptoms #1–3.
5. Direct trauma to the globe.
6. "Low" intraocular pressure (more than 4 mm. Hg lower than other eye).
7. Vitreous hemorrhage.
8. Light flashes.

sure determination. Description of the technique of applanation tonometry is beyond the scope of this text, but is well covered in Duane's Textbook of Ophthalmology.

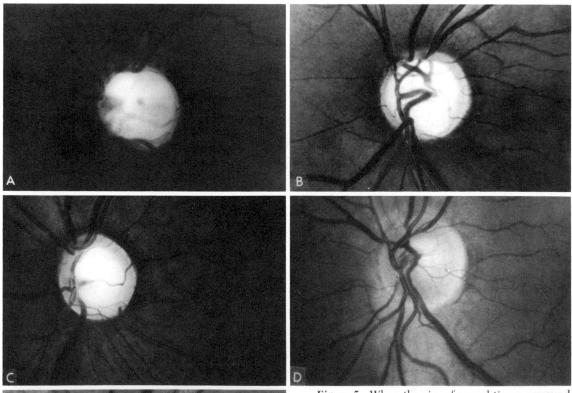

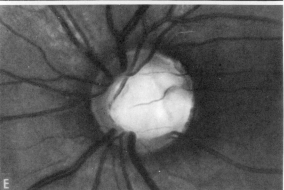

Figure 5 When the rim of neural tissue surrounding the cup of the optic nervehead becomes thinned to the point that the cup reaches all the way to the outer margin of the disk, moderately-advanced glaucoma usually is present, as in *A*. The most frequent location of this tissue loss is inferotemporally (*B*). Contrast this with *C* in which there is a large, deep central cup but preservation of the rim. This appearance can be seen in both normal or glaucomatous patients. The healthy appearing disk in *D* is almost certainly normal; glaucomatous field loss would not be expected in such an eye. *E* is an example of a congenital variant in which the central cup is large; there was no evidence of actual glaucoma in the patient, however. Individuals with such disks deserve careful glaucoma evaluation, but occasionally will be found to be free of any detectable disease.

By and large, no patient having had severe head trauma or in whom neurologic disease is suspected should receive dilating drops. Nor should any patient be dilated without a prior estimate of the depth of the anterior chamber, and if necessary, gonioscopy (Table 4).

The direct ophthalmoscope may be used to examine the optic nerve, macula, and posterior pole of the eye. This is most easily accomplished through a dilated pupil. The peripheral retina is difficult to examine with a direct ophthalmoscope, and the far periphery can not in fact be seen with a direct ophthalmoscope. It is this anterior region that is most likely to be damaged by blunt trauma. Therefore all cases involving trauma to the eye, or suspected of having a retinal tear or detachment, should be thoroughly examined with an indirect ophthalmoscope. In most cases this is best accomplished by referral to an ophthalmologist (Table 5).

The disc size, shape and vascularity should be noted, as well as the presence or absence of defects of the optic nerve known as "cupping" (Figure 5). The retina is examined for hemorrhage, infiltrates, and detachment. The +10.00 lens may be used to inspect the anterior ocular structures (lens and cornea).

More sophisticated techniques of examination probably are not needed by the emergency medicine specialist. If he is familiar with the previous methods of examination a very thorough examination may be performed in the Emergency Department.

Chapter 16

FUNDAMENTAL OTOLARYNGOLOGIC PROCEDURES

William W. Montgomery, Richard L. Fabian, and William G. Lavelle

EXAMINATION OF THE EAR

The medial and lateral surfaces of the auricle and also the mastoid process should be visualized and palpated. The external auditory canal and tympanic membrane are best examined using a head mirror and ear speculum. The battery otoscope is quite satisfactory for examination, although cumbersome when instrumentation is necessary. The pneumatic otoscope is used to test the mobility of the tympanic membrane as well as to provide magnification (Fig. 1, *A*).

The auricle must be pulled upward and backward in order to obtain a good view of the tympanic membrane (Fig. 1, *B*). In infants and small children the auricle is pulled straight back.

The outer third of the ear canal contains hair follicles, sebaceous glands, and cerumen glands. The skin over the inner two-thirds (bony external auditory canal) is quite thin and easily traumatized. At the junction of the middle and inner thirds of the external auditory canal is a narrowing called the *isthmus.* The isthmus is important because exostoses occur at this level and foreign bodies become lodged there.

The tympanic membrane usually is found on a slanted plane with its anterior and inferior quadrant farthest away from the examiner. This accounts for the triangle of light which is reflected anteroinferiorly from the umbo. The various landmarks of the tympanic membrane can be seen in Figure 2.

Testing Procedures in Hearing Evaluation

WHISPERED AND SPOKEN VOICE TEST

The test is performed in a quiet room with the examiner facing the ear to be tested. The other ear is blocked with the patient's hand. The patient should hear conversational voice at 20 feet and whispered voice at 15 feet. This is recorded as 20/20 and 15/15 (a person hearing a whispered voice at 10 feet = 10/15 W.V.). Another rough test is performed 1 foot from the patient's ear. If a patient cannot hear a whispered voice at 1 foot, he has at least a 30 decibel loss. This loss is 60 decibels if he cannot hear a conversational voice at 1 foot.

THE WEBER TEST

This test is accomplished by placing the vibrating tuning fork (512 cps) in the midline at the top of the head, forehead, or front teeth. With a *conductive* loss, the sound lateralizes to the diseased ear. The conductive loss masks some of the environmental noise, and thus the cochlea perceives more efficiently the sound conducted by bone of the diseased side. The lateralization of the sound or vibrations to the good ear signifies *perceptive* hearing loss in the opposite ear.

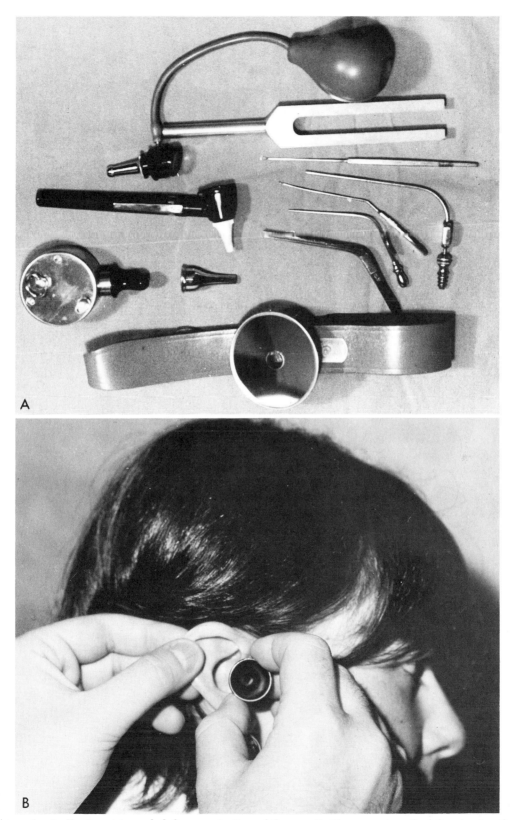

Figure 1　A, Equipment needed for examination of the ear. B, The correct method for viewing the adult tympanic membrane.

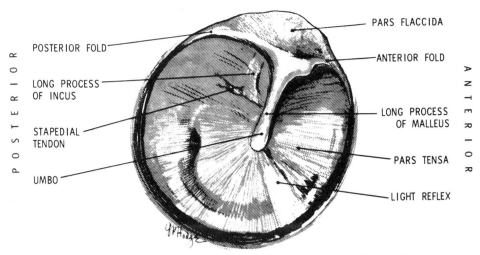

Figure 2   Right tympanic membrane, showing important landmarks.

THE RINNE TEST

This test is a comparison of the duration of air conduction with that of bone conduction. The tuning fork (512 cps) is struck against a rubber object with maximum force so that the results will be consistent. It is first held against the mastoid bone until the patient no longer hears the sound. The fork is then held approximately 1 inch from the ear canal opening until the patient no longer hears the sound. The patient should hear the fork twice as long by air as by bone (air–time duration is, of course, measured from the striking of the fork). A positive but reduced Rinne test indicates perceptive loss. A negative Rinne indicates a conductive hearing loss:

	Air	*Bone*
Normal hearing	100 seconds	50
Conductive loss	50 seconds	50
Perceptive loss	50 seconds	25

Another good test is to strike the tuning fork lightly and compare the patient's air and bone conduction with your own. Other methods are necessary for a complete hearing evaluation, such as pure tone audiometry, speech audiometry, psychogalvanic skin resistance testing, and many others.

AUDIOGRAM

The pure tone audiogram is a more sophisticated method of testing for hearing loss. Basically, it is a test of air and bone conduction from 250 to 4000 cycles. One ear is tested while masking the other ear with loud sound. Another hearing test, using words instead of pure tone, indicates how well the patient discriminates. Generally, if discrimination is very poor, a hearing aid will be of little use to the patient. More complex tests (Bekesy, SISI, and recruitment tests) help distinguish between cochlear and more central lesions.

Procedure to Test Labyrinth

THE CALORIC TEST

This is a measure of labyrinthine function in response to temperature. Water is placed in the external auditory canal and the eyes are observed for onset, direction, and duration of nystagmus. One technique requires 5 cc. of ice water or 20 cc. of tap water irrigation into the ear canal, first making sure there is no cerumen. If there is a perforated tympanic membrane, use 70 per cent alcohol or cold air. Douche the ear canal with ice water with the head in the upright position; press a stopwatch at the onset of douching. Before 15 seconds have elapsed, move the head back 60 degrees from the vertical plane. Twenty-diopter spherical lenses can be used to prevent ocular fixation. Watch conjunctival blood vessels for direction of nystagmus. The normal response is as follows:

(1) Latent period, 15 to 30 seconds.

(2) Duration of nystagmus, 30 to 75 seconds.

(3) Direction of nystagmus is toward the side opposite stimulation for cold fluid, toward the side of stimulation for warm fluid.

Procedure to Test For Fistula

FISTULA TEST

Positive pressure applied to the tympanic membrane and/or the middle ear will cause a sensation of vertigo and objective nystagmus, provided there is a defect in the otic capsule. An example of this is a fistula in the lateral semicircular canal.

PROCEDURE FOR NOSE AND SINUS EXAMINATION

The external nose is examined for defects and palpated for any loss of structure or support. The intranasal examination is accomplished utilizing a standard nasal speculum (Fig. 3). The nasal speculum is directed away from the nasal septum as it is introduced into the external nasal orifice. Contact with the nasal septum and overdilatation of the external nasal orifice is quite painful (Fig. 4). Observe the nasal vestibule for abnormalities; benign and malignant tumors are common in this area. Estimate the adequacy of the airways; observe carefully for deviations of the septum. Determine whether the turbinates are normal, hypertrophic, or atrophic, and note the color of the nasal mucosa.

In order to examine beyond the depth of the nasal vestibule, it is necessary to spray the nose with 0.25 per cent Neo-Synephrine or 1.0 per cent ephedrine solution. Five minutes after spraying, the posterior aspect of the nasal cavities and the superior nasopharynx can be visualized unless the nasal septum is markedly deviated.

The paranasal sinuses can be examined by palpating the roof and floor of the orbit, the ascending process of the maxilla, and the canine fossa. Tenderness may be elicited or masses palpated.

TRANSILLUMINATION OF THE PARANASAL SINUSES

Transillumination of the paranasal sinuses is a useful diagnostic tool for frontal and maxillary sinus disease. A light is placed under the medial aspect of the supraorbital rim for the frontal sinus and above the infraorbital rim for the maxillary sinus. The forehead is observed in the former and the hard palate in the latter. The test is used mostly for following a patient's progress once the clinical and x-ray diagnoses have

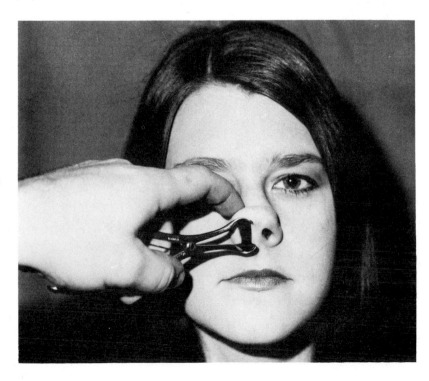

Figure 3 The correct method for intranasal examination.

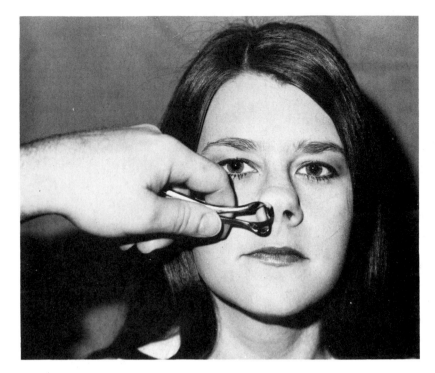

Figure 4 The incorrect method for intranasal examination. Note the orifice is overdilated and the speculum is directed toward the septum, not stabilized.

been established. Decreased transillumination will occur with an underdeveloped sinus or one with unusually thick bony walls. On the other hand, a sinus filled with clear liquid will transilluminate quite well. Transillumination, illustrated in Figure 5, must be carried out in a dark room.

PROCEDURE FOR EXAMINATION OF THE OROPHARYNX

When examining the oropharynx, observe the teeth, gums, palate, floor of mouth, tongue, tonsils, salivary gland orifices, and salivary glands.

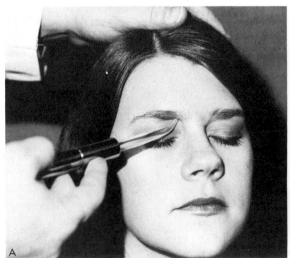
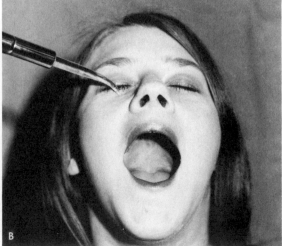

Figure 5 *A*, Method for transillumination of frontal sinus. *B*, Method for transillumination of maxillary sinus.

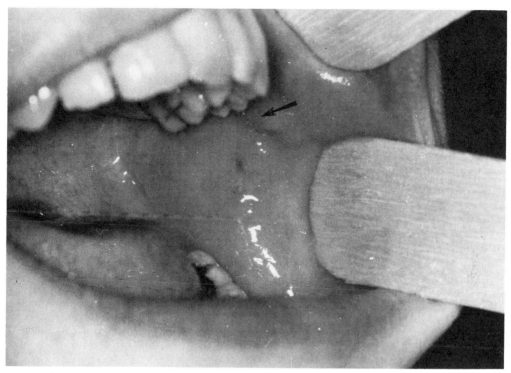

Figure 6 The punctum and orifice of the parotid duct (Stensen's) are found on the lateral buccal mucosa at a point opposite the second upper molar tooth (*arrow*).

The submandibular duct orifice (Wharton's) is visualized as the patient raises the tip of his tongue toward the hard palate (Fig. 7).

The sublingual fold (frenulum) is seen in the anterior midline of the floor of the mouth. On either side of the frenulum is an elevation known as the sublingual papilla. Saliva may be expressed from the duct orifice located in the tip of the papilla by massaging the submandibular gland. The parotid duct orifice (Stensen's) enters the mouth through the lateral buccal mucosa at a point opposite the lateral aspect of the second upper molar tooth. Saliva can be expressed from this duct orifice by massaging the parotid gland in an anterior direction (Fig. 6).

The submandibular gland is palpated directly beneath the ramus of the mandible about halfway between the chin and the angle of the jaw. It has a firm, irregular consistency. The submandibular gland can be more accurately palpated by placing the index finger of one hand on the floor of the mouth between the lateral aspect of the tongue and the teeth while the other hand palpates the gland exteriorly. The submandibular gland descends and becomes more prominent after the age of 40 and is often misinterpreted as an enlargement of the gland or a large lymph node.

The parotid gland is found anterior to, and below, the auricle. It normally extends from the sternomastoid muscle anteriorly to the masseter muscle. If a finger *cannot* be placed medial to the angle of the mandible, the examiner should become suspicious of an abnormal parotid gland (Fig. 8).

The hard and soft palate should be examined; note any weakness or paralysis of the soft palate. The uvula is examined for its size and midline position.

It is very important to examine the floor of the mouth on each side by having the patient move his tongue to the opposite side. At the same time note the function of the tongue. In addition to observing, the examiner should palpate the floor of the mouth for small lesions missed by visual examination (Fig. 9).

The tonsils are visualized between the anterior and posterior pillars. The size of the tonsils is relatively unimportant. If they are cryptic, do their crypts contain debris (pus, foreign bodies, or sebaceous material)? The lingual tonsils should be observed by pull-

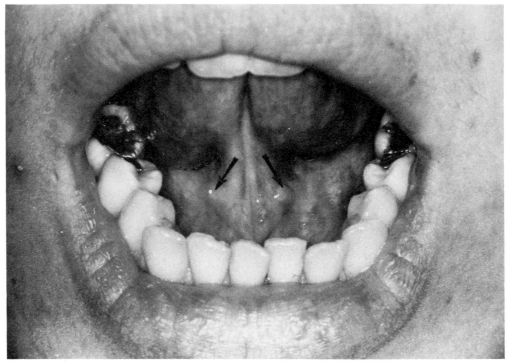

Figure 7   The orifice of the submandibular duct may be found in the region of the sublingual papillae (*arrows*).

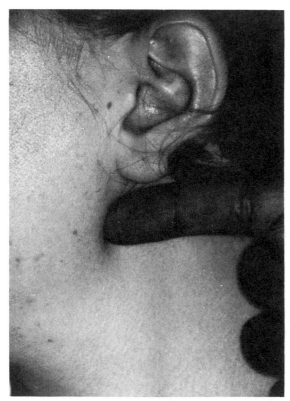

Figure 8   Examination of the parotid gland should include external and bimanual palpation of the parotid region and the region between the mastoid tip and the angle of the jaw.

ing the tongue forward or by examination with a laryngeal mirror. A midline mass in this region may be a lingual thyroid.

The lingual and glossopharyngeal nerves distribute sensory fibers to the anterior two-thirds and posterior one-third of the tongue, respectively. When examining the oropharynx, it is best to keep the tip of the tongue depressor well forward from the posterior third of the tongue in order to avoid stimulating a gag reflex (Fig. 10).

PROCEDURE FOR EXAMINATION OF THE NASOPHARYNX

Examination of the nasopharynx is certainly not part of a routine physical examination. If, on the other hand, symptoms direct the physician to the nasopharynx it should be carefully examined. A size 0-3 mirror is warmed by a flame, hot water, or electric light bulb. The patient must be seated directly in front of the examiner (Fig. 11): both heads must be at the same level. The patient's head is projected slightly forward. The tongue is depressed into the floor of the mouth by the examiner's left hand; his right hand grasps the mirror as one would hold a

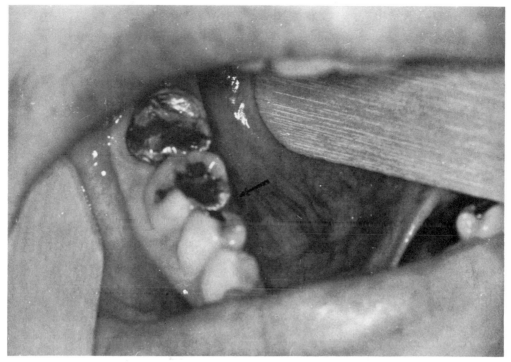

Figure 9 Examination of the lateral floor of the mouth (*arrow*) is best accomplished by retracting the cheek laterally with one tongue depressor and the lateral surface of the tongue medially with a second.

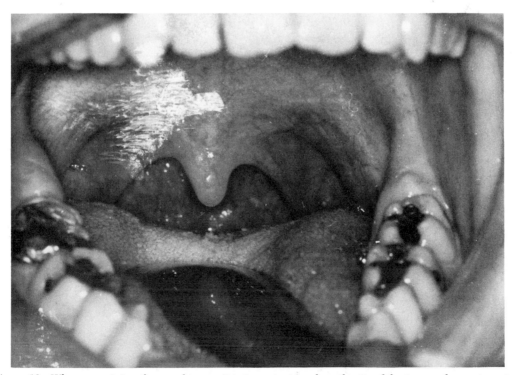

Figure 10 When examining the oropharynx, it is important to place the tip of the tongue depressor anterior to the circumvallate papillae (*arrow*) in order to avoid stimulating the gag reflex.

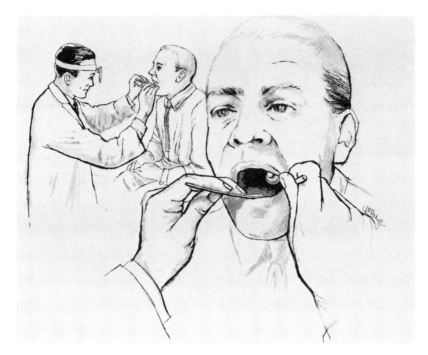

Figure 11 Examination of the nasopharynx.

pencil, and the mirror is slipped behind and to one side of the uvula. Light is reflected to the examining mirror by way of a head mirror. During this examination the patient is encouraged to breathe normally and not to hold his breath. It may be necessary to anesthetize the pharynx with a topical anesthetic agent such as Cetacaine in order to control the gag reflex. The normal structures seen in the nasopharynx are illustrated in Figure 12.

PROCEDURE FOR EXAMINATION OF THE LARYNGOPHARYNX

The laryngopharynx is examined using a size 3 to 6 laryngeal mirror. Fogging is prevented by warming the mirror with a flame, hot water, or electric light bulb. The examiner's and patient's heads should be at the same level. The patient is instructed to sit up straight with his head projected

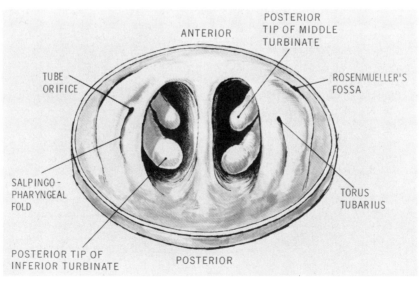

Figure 12 Normal structures in the nasopharynx.

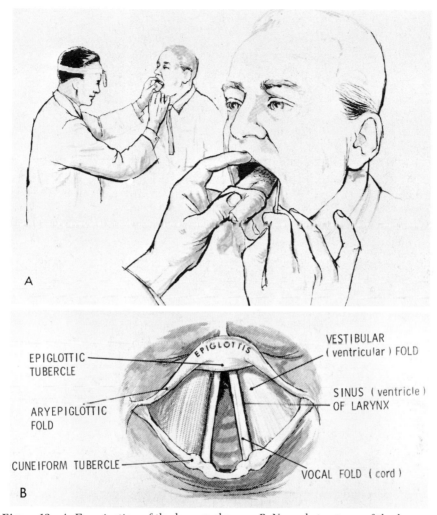

Figure 13 A, Examination of the laryngopharynx. B, Normal structures of the larynx.

slightly forward. The tongue is grasped between a piece of folded gauze. It is important that the examiner's thumb be on top of the patient's tongue and his second finger underneath the tip of the tongue. The index finger is used to elevate the upper lip (Fig. 13, A). The laryngeal mirror is held as one would hold a pencil and inserted in the oropharynx in such a manner that it elevates the uvula without touching the lateral walls of the pharynx or dorsum of the tongue. If the patient has a hypersensitive gag reflex, the examination must be discontinued and the pharynx sprayed with a topical anesthetic agent.

The larynx is visualized in the mirror using reflected light from the headmirror as the patient is instructed to breathe quietly and not hold his breath. He is then asked to say "Ahhh" and "Eeee." These sounds bring the larynx up and backward so that it can be more easily visualized. Observe for the structures shown in Figure 13, B.

PROCEDURE FOR EXAMINATION OF THE NECK

The examination of the neck is conducted with the patient in the sitting position while the examiner faces the side of the neck to be examined.

The submental region is examined by bimanual palpation in addition to the routine external palpation (Fig. 14, A). The index finger of one hand is placed on the an-

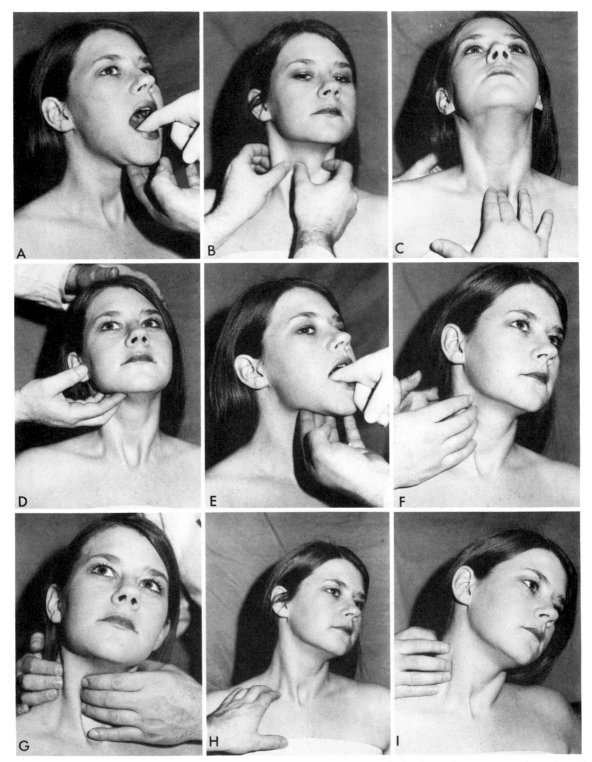

Figure 14 Examinations of (*A*) the submental region, (*B*) the thyroid gland, (*C*) the suprasternal notch, and (*D*) the submandibular triangle.

    E, Bimanual palpation of the submandibular triangle.

    Examinations of the (*F*) right lateral neck from the same side, (*G*) the right lateral neck from the opposite side, (*H*) the supraclavicular region, and (*I*) the posterolateral neck.

terior floor of the patient's mouth to palpate against the fingers of the opposite hand, which have been placed in the submental region. Following this, the laryngeal skeleton and trachea are examined for motility, position, and structures.

To examine the thyroid gland (Fig. 14, *B*), the examiner sits in front of and at the same level as the patient. The patient's neck is rotated slightly to the left when the right lobe is examined. The examiner's right thumb is placed over the lateral cricoid cartilage arch with his fingers extended around the left side of the neck. The cricoid is pressed to the left. The right index finger is placed posterior to the tensed right sternocleidomastoid muscle, pushing the thyroid anteriorly. The right thyroid is then palpated between the index finger and the thumb of the left hand.

The suprasternal notch is palpated with the patient's neck in extension (Fig. 14, *C*). The inferior aspect of the cervical trachea can be palpated unless excessive adipose tissue is present. Enlarged lymph nodes or pulsations in this region are considered abnormal until proved otherwise.

In order to examine the right submandibular region, the patient's neck is slightly flexed and rotated to the left (Fig. 14, *D*). The examiner's fingers are inserted deep underneath the mandible, and its contents are pulled inferiorly.

Bimanual palpation of the submandibular triangle is performed in a manner similar to and usually at the same time as bimanual examination of the submental region (Fig. 14, *E*).

In examining the right lateral neck from the same side, the examiner's fingers are placed anterior and posterior to and along the entire length of the patient's sternocleidomastoid muscle (Fig. 14, *F*). The patient's head is slightly flexed and rotated to the left. The examination of the right lateral neck from the opposite side is similar (Fig. 14 *G*). The background for palpating the lateral neck is the transverse processes of the cervical vertebrae. The carotid bulb can be palpated at the level of the thyroid cartilage notch.

The often neglected supraclavicular region is palpated with the flat surfaces of the fingers (Fig. 14, *H*). This is accomplished with the patient's neck in flexion and extension. Abnormal masses and pulsation may be detected.

To examine the posterolateral neck, the patient's neck is slightly flexed to the right as this region is examined with the flat surfaces of the examiner's fingers (Fig. 14, *I*). The examiner stands to the rear of the patient. The function of the trapezius muscle is evaluated as the patient elevates his shoulder.

PROCEDURE FOR TREATMENT OF EPISTAXIS

Anterior epistaxis usually ceases spontaneously without treatment. Anterior epistaxis often can be controlled by having the patient assume the sitting position with the head slightly forward. He is instructed to breathe quietly through his mouth while firmly compressing the nostrils closed with the index finger and thumb. If this does not work, a piece of cotton moistened with 1:1000 epinephrine solution (if not available, water can be used) is inserted into the nasal cavity. This is compressed against the nasal septum by pressure with a finger against the side of the nose.

When the bleeding of anterior epistaxis has been controlled, the vessel can be cauterized with a silver nitrate bead or a small chromic acid bead placed on the end of a wire. Silver nitrate sticks also may be used. This cauterization can be made painless by moistening a pledget of cotton with 2 per cent Pontocaine or 4 per cent cocaine solution and leaving it in place 10 minutes prior to cautery. Both local anesthesia and temporary control of bleeding can be accomplished by injecting the mucosa in the region of the bleeding with 1 per cent Xylocaine and added epinephrine. Only the bleeding point is cauterized.

If anterior epistaxis cannot be controlled by cautery, a 1-inch Vaseline strip is carefully inserted, as shown in Figure 15, *B*. The anterior end of the gauze packing should be secured in place with string and/or tape in order to prevent its passing into the nasopharynx. This packing should remain in place from one to three days.

Posterior epistaxis can be severe, frightening, and difficult to control. It usually results from a rupture of the sphenopalatine artery or one of its branches. The patient gives a history of blood flowing profusely into the pharynx as well as from the anterior nares.

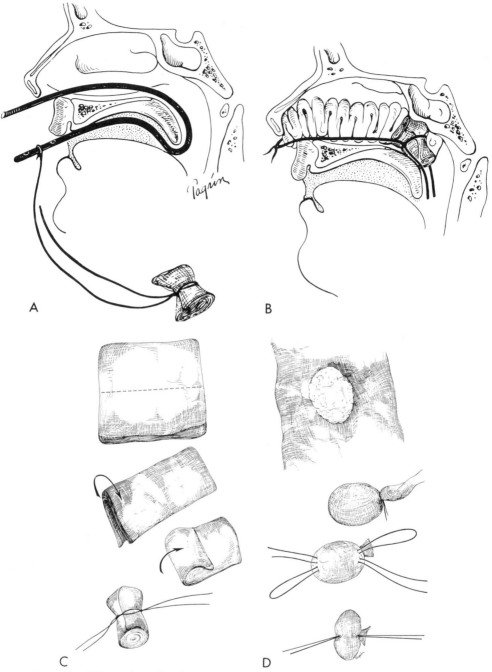

Figure 15 *A*, A soft rubber catheter has been inserted into the pharynx. *B*, The anterior nasal cavity is packed with iodoform gauze. *C*, One type of posterior pack for control of epistaxis. *D*, A more adequate posterior pack.

Unless the patient shows signs of shock, he is placed in the sitting position, and both nasal cavities are packed with cotton strips impregnated with 4 per cent cocaine or a topical anesthetic agent with added epinephrine (1:1000). Often this packing will either slow down or stop the bleeding so that the bleeding site can be visualized or cauterized. Of the numerous techniques for treating posterior epistaxis, that most commonly used is still anterior and posterior packing. After the nasal cavity and pharynx have been anesthetized with a topical anesthetic agent, a soft rubber catheter is inserted into each nasal cavity and down into the pharynx, where it is grasped with a hemostat and pulled out of the mouth (Fig. 15, *A*). Tie the string of the posterior pack around the end of the catheter. Next, pull the catheter from the nose and grasp the string with one hand. Guide the posterior pack coated with Vaseline into the naso-pharynx with the aid of a Kelly clamp or the index finger. Pack the anterior nasal cavity tightly with either 1-inch Vaseline gauze or gauze impregnated with bacitracin ointment (Fig. 15, *B*). An assistant should firmly hold the string of the posterior pack while the anterior packing is being carried out. The two strings protruding from the nasal orifice are tied around a dental roll or a roll of gauze. The strings protruding from the nasopharynx are cut just below the level of the soft palate and are used for removal.

To make a posterior pack, a 4 × 4 gauze pad is impregnated with Vaseline, folded in half, and rolled up (Fig. 15, *C*). Two lengths of heavy silk thread are then tied around the center of the roll, making four ends. Two strands protrude from the anterior nasal cavity and two either hang into the pharynx or protrude from the mouth and are taped to the cheek. The latter strands are for the removal of the pack. A more adequate posterior pack (Fig. 15, *D*) is made by opening a 4 × 4 gauze pad and folding it once. A ball of Vaseline–iodoform gauze or cornish wool, 2 to 4 cm. in diameter, depending on the size of the patient's pharynx, is placed in the center of the folded gauze. The gauze is folded around the packing and tied, as one would a purse, with heavy silk. With a large needle, heavy silk thread is also made to protrude from the bottom of the pack. The advantages are that a small pack is more effective and less uncomfortable because of its shape, is less traumatizing and more hemostatic, and prevents or controls odor. Posterior packs should remain in place approximately four to five days.

Posterior Pack Using a Foley Catheter. A Foley catheter is inserted through the nares into the nasopharynx. The bag is then filled with 5 to 10 cc. of water, and pressure is applied to the end to bring the filled pack to the posterior nasal cavity. With constant pull exerted, the anterior nasal cavity can be packed with Vaseline gauze, using the filled water pack as the back wall.

Gauze can be inserted around the cathe-ter end outside of the nose and a clamp applied. The remainder of the catheter can be taped to the forehead or lateral aspect of the face.

Owing to the dangers of respiratory embarrassment, patients with posterior packing should be admitted into the hospital.

TRACHEOTOMY

Indications for performing a tracheotomy are: (1) respiratory obstruction: (2) secretory retention: and (3) respiratory insufficiency.

RESPIRATORY OBSTRUCTION

Whenever possible, a bronchoscope or endotracheal tube is inserted by way of the intralaryngeal route. Unfortunately, such equipment usually is not at hand at the time this emergency arises. When properly executed, an endotracheal intubation is the most rapid method of establishing an airway, thus avoiding a traumatic, hurried tracheotomy. No anesthesia is required for such an intubation. After intubation, a general anesthetic may be administered while an orderly tracheotomy is performed. The incidence of complications during the tracheotomy is reduced when a bronchoscope or endotracheal tube is present in the trachea.

CRICOTHYROTOMY (LARYNGOTOMY)

The patient's neck is placed in hyperextension by inserting a roll of fabric under the shoulders or by placing the dorsum of the neck over the knee of the squatting surgeon. In so doing, the thyroid notch becomes prominent anteriorly. The surgeon quickly identifies the position of the thyroid notch with the index finger of his right hand (Fig. 16, *A*). This finger descends in the midline to the prominence of the cricoid cartilage. The depression of the circothyroid membrane is identified above the superior margin of the cricoid cartilage. A mark is made in the midline at this level with the fingernail.

A vertical incision is made in the midline over the thyroid and cricoid cartilages (Fig. 16, *B*). Vessels are retracted from the midline with the thumb and index finger of the left hand, as shown.

As the wound is spread apart by finger dissection, the cricothyroid membrane becomes readily apparent and it is incised horizontally as close as possible to the cricoid cartilage in order to prevent bleeding from the cricothyroid artery (Fig. 16, *C*).

The cricothyroid space is widened by inserting either the handle or blade of the knife into the horizontal incision and rotating it 90 degrees (Fig. 16, *D*). This estab-

lishes an airway. A tracheotomy tube is temporarily inserted if one is available. A cricothyrotomy can be accomplished in 15 to 30 seconds. This procedure is very difficult to perform on an infant or young child.

EMERGENCY TRACHEOTOMY

An emergency tracheotomy is indicated when respiratory obstruction is too severe to

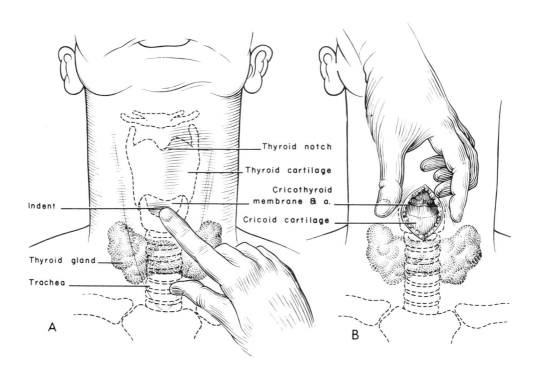

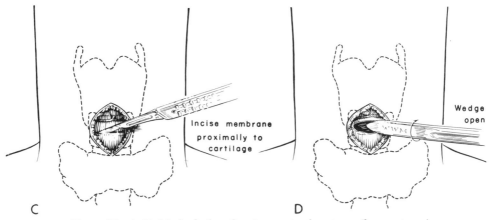

Figure 16   *A–D*, Method of performing a cricothyrotomy (laryngotomy).

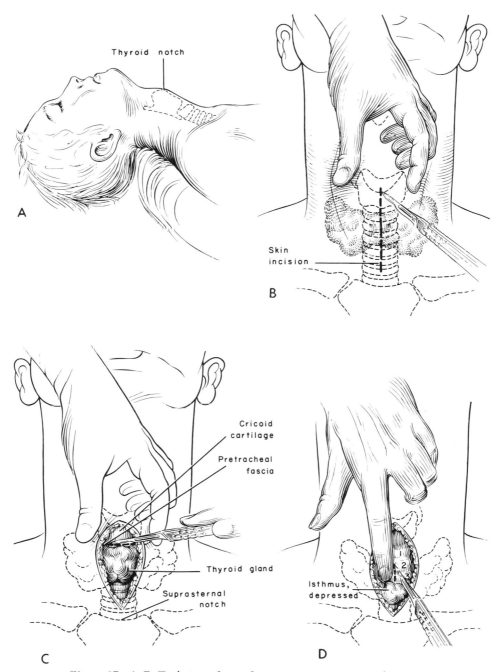

Figure 17 A–D, Technique for performing an emergency tracheotomy.

allow for an orderly tracheotomy, when the facilities are not available for insertion of a bronchoscope or tracheal tube, and when the surgeon believes that the patient cannot survive a few minutes of increasing hypoxia without brain damage.

The patient's neck is placed in hyperextension so that the larynx and trachea will be prominent and to allow the trachea to be elevated in its relationship to the suprasternal notch (Fig. 17, A).

The trachea is placed into prominence and fixed in the midline as the thumb and index finger of the surgeon's left hand push the adjacent musculature and vessels laterally beneath the sternocleidomastoid muscles (Fig. 17, B). The anterior midline positions of the thyroid notch, cricoid cartilage, and cricothyroid membrane are quickly identified. A vertical incision is made in the midline from the level of the cricothyroid membrane nearly to the suprasternal notch. This incision is carried directly through the subcutaneous tissue.

The incision is widened with the surgeon's index finger of his right hand or with the knife handle (Fig. 17, C). The index finger of the left hand identifies the prominence of the cricoid cartilage. A small horizontal incision is made immediately beneath the cricoid cartilage through the pretracheal fascia. The left index finger is inserted into this incision to the space between the thyroid isthmus and the trachea. With firm

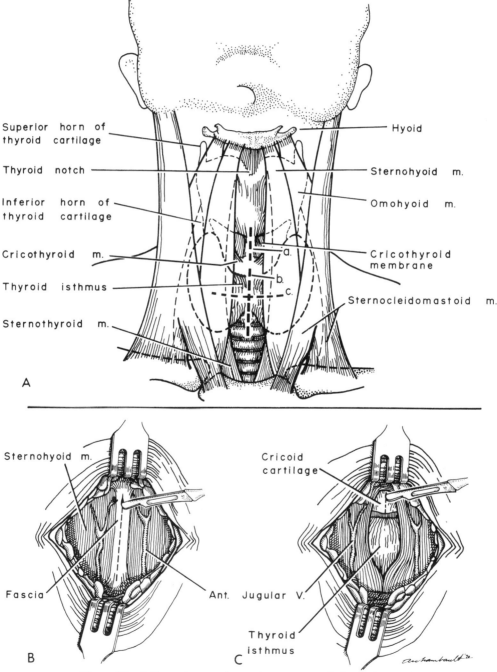

Figure 18   A–P, Technique for performing an orderly tracheotomy.

Illustration continued on opposite page.

pressure, the thyroid isthmus is dissected inferiorly by finger dissection in order to expose the upper three tracheal rings.

The index finger of the left hand is moved slightly to the operator's left so that a midline vertical incision can be made through the second and third tracheal rings (Fig. 17, *D*). A hemostat or tracheotomy dilator is introduced into this incision while a tracheotomy or endotracheal tube is inserted into the tracheal lumen. Once an airway has been established, all bleeding can be con-

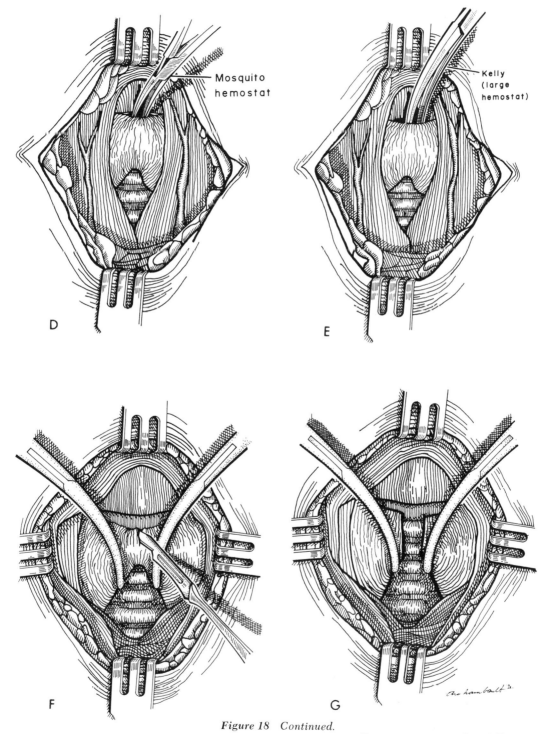

Figure 18 Continued.

Illustration continued on following page.

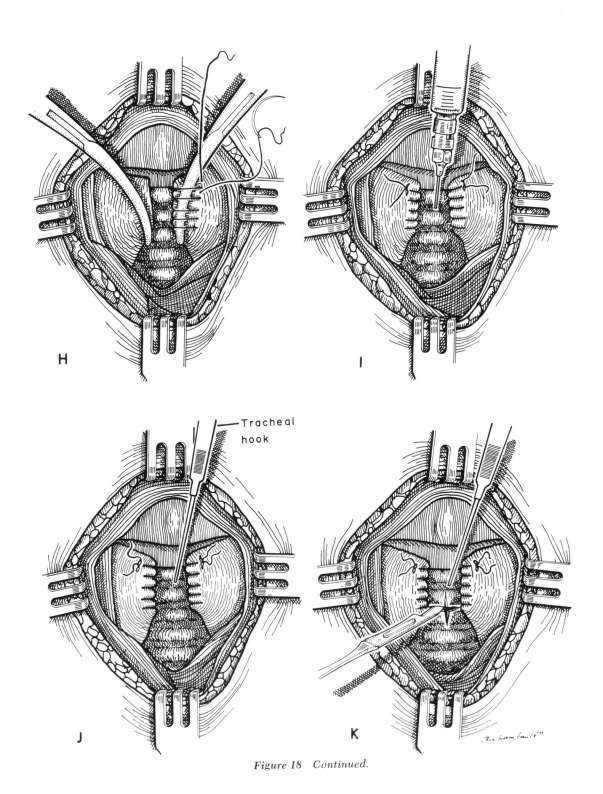

Figure 18   Continued.

Illustration continued on opposite page.

trolled in an orderly fashion. This operation can be accomplished in one or two minutes.

IMPENDING RESPIRATORY OBSTRUCTION

Orderly tracheotomy is the operation of choice for impending asphyxia and other nonemergent indications mentioned previously. The techniques for an orderly tracheotomy are shown in Figure 18.

Figure 18, *A* illustrates the relationships of the various incisions used to approach the upper airway to the thyroid cartilage, cricoid cartilage, thyroid isthmus, and trachea.

A vertical incision (a) is used to approach the cricothyroid membrane and to carry out an emergency cricothyrotomy.

A vertical incision (b) is used for an emergency tracheotomy. This incision extends from the cricothyroid membrane to a point well below the thyroid isthmus in the anterior midline.

A horizontal incision over the thyroid isthmus is used for an orderly tracheotomy (c). This incision is made approximately 2

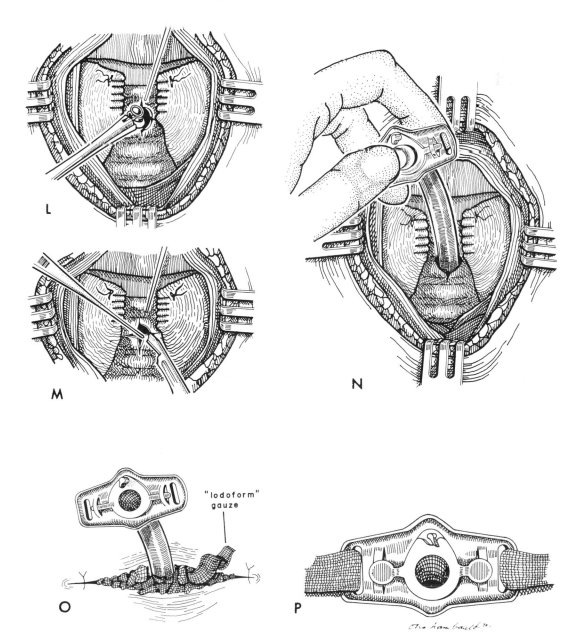

Figure 18 Continued.

cm. below the cricoid cartilage and should be at least 5 cm. in length.

The horizontal incision has been carried through the platysma muscle, exposing the sternohyoid muscles (Fig. 18, *B*). Additional exposure is obtained by undermining superiorly and inferiorly, with blunt dissection, above the fascia covering the sternohyoid muscles. The sternohyoid muscles, median raphe, and anterior jugular veins should be in view. A vertical incision is made in the median raphe between the sternohyoid muscles from the level of the cricoid cartilage to the inferior aspect of the dissection. The sternothyroid muscles are separated in a similar fashion, exposing the inferior aspect of the cricoid cartilage and the thyroid isthmus.

The thyroid isthmus has been exposed (Fig. 18, *C*). Occasionally the isthmus is small and so placed that entrance into the trachea can be gained without division of the isthmus. It is best to approach the thyroid isthmus from above by making a small vertical or horizontal incision through the pretracheal fascia over the cricoid cartilage.

A small hemostat is inserted into the incision over the cricoid cartilage (Fig. 18, *D*). By dissection firmly against the inferior border of the cricoid cartilage and anterior wall of the trachea, a plane can be established between the thyroid isthmus and trachea without producing troublesome bleeding from the thyroid isthmus.

A larger hemostat is inserted to complete the separation between the thyroid isthmus and anterior tracheal wall (Fig. 18, *E*). A large hemostat is then placed on each side of the thyroid isthmus, which is then incised with a knife or scissors (Fig. 18, *F*). The thyroid isthmus is divided at the midline (Fig. 18, *G*).

The thyroid isthmus is suture-ligated on each side with a running stitch of #2–0 chromic catgut sutures (Fig. 18, *H*). Note that the last suture is returned in an opposite direction through the thyroid isthmus in order to facilitate tying it after the hemostat has been removed.

Two milliliters of 4 per cent Xylocaine or cocaine solution are injected into the tracheal lumen with a short #20 hypodermic needle (Fig. 18, *I*). Aspiration of air indicates that the needle has been properly placed into the tracheal lumen.

A tracheal hook is inserted into the tracheal lumen between the first and second tracheal rings (Fig. 18, *J*). The trachea is retracted in an anterosuperior direction.

A cruciate incision through the intercartilaginous membrane and two tracheal rings can be made with a knife unless the tracheal rings are ossified (Fig. 18, *K*).

The four triangular flaps of tissue are removed with a ring punch (Fig. 18, *L*), making certain that this tissue does not fall into the tracheal lumen. The triangular flaps of tissue can also be removed with forceps and a knife or with scissors (Fig. 18, *M*).

A sterile tracheotomy tube with an obturator in place is inserted through the fenestration in the anterior tracheal wall and into the tracheal lumen (Fig. 18, *N*).

The obturator has been removed, and the lateral aspects of the horizontal incision have been loosely approximated with one or two dermal sutures (Fig. 18, *O*). Iodoform gauze is packed in the incision around the tracheotomy tube for hemostasis.

A tracheotomy tape has been passed through each side of the face plate of the tracheotomy tube and secured on either side of the neck with a square knot. The inner cannula has been inserted and locked in place (Fig. 18, *P*). A tracheotomy dressing is then applied and a moist 4 × 4 inch sponge is suspended in front of the tracheotomy tube over a second tracheotomy tape around the patient's neck.

REMOVAL OF CERUMEN AND FOREIGN BODIES FROM THE EXTERNAL AUDITORY CANAL

Cerumen and foreign material should be very carefully removed from the external auditory canal. Irreparable damage to the canal, tympanic membrane and middle ear is not infrequently a complication of unskilled manipulation in this region. The instruments used to cleanse the external auditory canal are shown in Figure 19. General anesthesia may be necessary for this procedure, especially in children.

As has been mentioned, the head mirror and ear speculum are the best way to obtain proper illumination when using instruments in the external auditory canal. The binocular surgical microscope is also extremely useful when removing cerumen or foreign bodies from the external auditory canal.

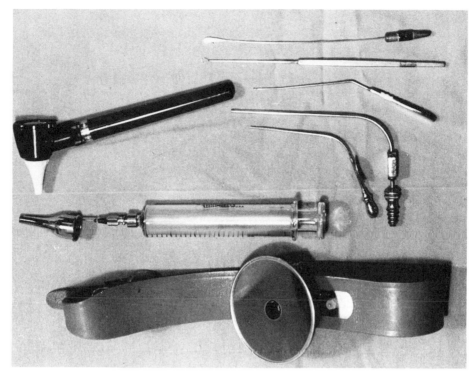

Figure 19 Instruments needed to clean the external auditory canal.

The simplest method for removing cerumen or a foreign body from the ear canal is a wire loop or suction tip, using the technique shown in Figure 20, *A, B*. If the patient is certain that he does not have a perforated tympanic membrane or chronic external canal disease, the ear canal often can be cleansed using a syringe and lukewarm water as shown in Figure 20, *C*. The patient's auricle is held in the posterosuperior direction as the stream of water from the syringe is directed to a wall of the canal. In so doing, the stream of water passes alongside and then behind the cerumen or foreign body, both disrupting it and evacuating it from the external auditory canal.

MYRINGOTOMY

The indications for myringotomy are generally limited to a painful and bulging tympanic membrane. Myringotomy also may be performed as an elective diagnostic procedure for evacuation of serous material and to obtain a biopsy or culture from the middle ear.

A myringotomy performed for acute otitis media is best done using general anesthesia, except in small babies having a high fever. A myringotomy in an adult patient can be performed after infiltrating the posterior aspect of the external auditory canal wall with a local anesthetic agent injected by way of a #25 to #27 hypodermic needle. The procedure is best performed in the posterior inferior quadrant of the tympanic membrane (Fig. 21). Using a myringotomy knife, an incision is made from above downward. If purulent material is obtained, a culture should be taken.

MASTOID PRESSURE DRESSING

The equipment and technique for application of this dressing is shown in Figure 22. 4 × 4 gauze pads and 2-inch roller gauze are used for this dressing. If additional pressure is required, 2-inch conforming type (Kling) gauze can be substituted. A 10-inch strip of 2-inch gauze is placed vertically on each side of the forehead, as shown in Figure 22, *A*. A wad of fluffed 4 × 4 gauze pads is placed over and behind the auricle.

The direction of the bandaging begins

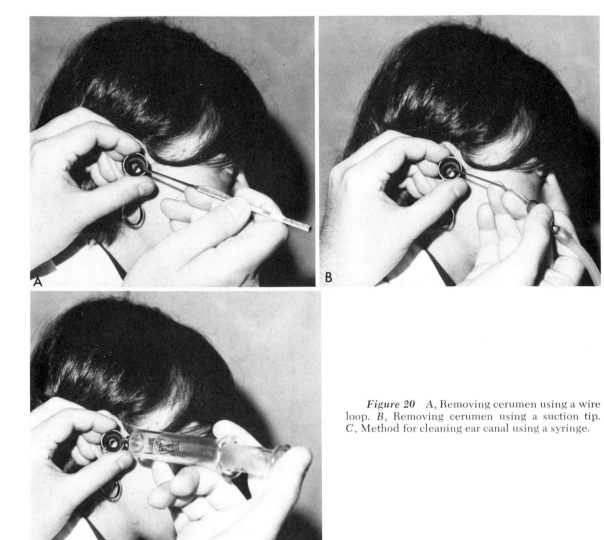

Figure 20 A, Removing cerumen using a wire loop. *B*, Removing cerumen using a suction tip. *C*, Method for cleaning ear canal using a syringe.

Pars flaccida

Post. malleolar fold

Ant. malleolar fold

Long process incus

Stapedial tendon

Round window

Umbo

Incision

Light reflex

Tagrin

Figure 21 Site for myringotomy (right ear).

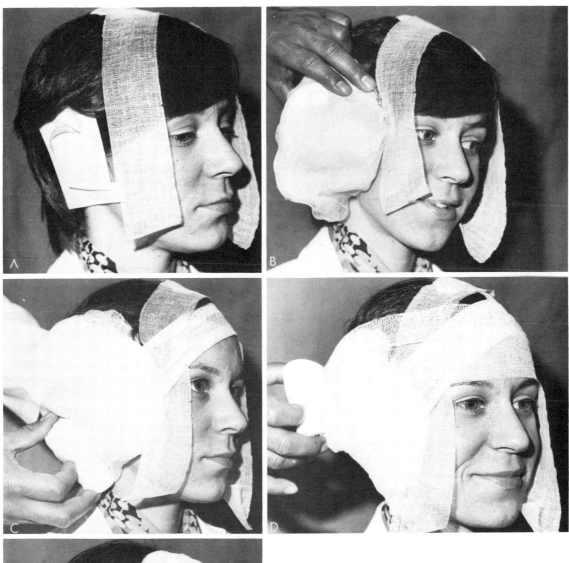

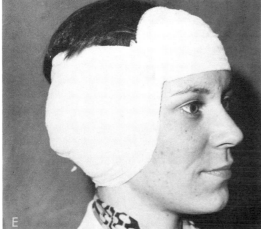

Figure 22 A, Strips of 2″ gauze on each side of forehead. B, Fluffed 4 × 4 gauze. C, Dressing is placed high on forehead, low over ear. D, Dressing placed low on forehead, high on ear. E, Completed dressing.

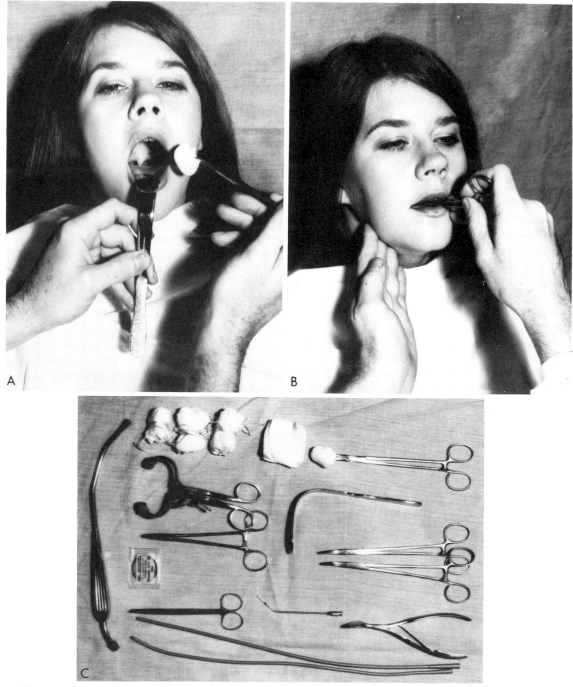

Figure 23   *A, B,* Method for controlling post-tonsillectomy bleeding by pressure. *C,* The equipment needed to control post-tonsillectomy and postadenoidectomy bleeding.

high on the forehead, across the zygomatic arch and over the lower aspect of the auricle. The second wind around the head is low on the forehead and high in relation to the auricle (Fig. 22, B, C). When the bandaging is complete, the vertical strip on each side of the forehead is tied. In so doing, the bandage is further tightened and elevated away from the eyebrows. The end of the bandage is tied to one end of a gauze strip (Fig. 22, D, E).

POST-TONSILLECTOMY AND ADENOIDECTOMY HEMORRHAGE

Hemorrhage following "T & A" most commonly occurs either during the first 12 hours after surgery or on about the fifth postoperative day.

Bleeding at the adenoidectomy site appears from the nostrils as well as from the throat unless the patient is standing or sitting. Ephedrine 1 per cent or Neo-Synephrine 0.5 per cent nose drops may be used to attempt to control mild adenoidectomy bleeding. Persistent or severe bleeding is controlled by inserting a postnasal pack, as described under *Epistaxis*.

Bleeding from the tonsillar fossa often can be controlled by pressure exerted by a small gauze pack on the end of a Kelly type hemostat (Fig. 23). Pressure against this pack can be accomplished by fingers placed externally behind the submandibular gland. Bleeding from a small vessel can be controlled by silver nitrate (stick) cautery.

Usually it is best to suture ligate the offending tonsillar fossa vessels in the operating room and with general anesthesia. On occasion suturing is possible in an adult as an office procedure using local anesthesia. The necessary equipment is shown in Figure 23, C.

Chapter 17

NEUROSURGICAL PROCEDURES

William F. Bouzarth

LUMBAR PUNCTURE IN ADULTS

The principal reason for performing lumbar puncture in the Emergency Department is to differentiate subarachnoid hemorrhage from meningitis. Patients requiring such procedures usually are not cooperative, but the test should be explained to the alert patient in reassuring terms. The patient is placed in the lateral recumbent position. It is advantageous to have the patient at hand's breadth from the edge of the bed so that he is less likely to fall off and the physician can rest his elbows on the mattress. If there is a disproportion between the diameter of the rib cage and the pelvis, a pillow should be placed under the patient to aid in straightening the lumbar spine. Maintain the plane of the back perpendicular to the plane of the bed. The patient should be in a fetal position to flex the spine. Place a soft pillow under the dependent side of the head to add support in maintaining a neutral position. Check to see if the upper shoulder is more forward, a position that may result in rotation of the spine. It is better to have both shoulders in line and sacrifice some degree of flexion, rather than have a rotated spine. With an uncooperative patient, flexion becomes the responsibility of a strong assistant, who places his arm around the patient's upper posterior chest but not around the neck. The other arm should be just under the knees. This takes advantage of leverage without undue flexion of the head (Figure 1).

When a satisfactory position is achieved, the lumbar area is cleansed and painted with an antiseptic solution, avoiding iodinated solutions if a patient is unable to warn of an allergy. Place a sterile towel diagonally across the iliac crest, rather than a large drape with a small hole in the center, which obscures the field. With the hand palpating the iliac crest, select the spinous process that falls on or just below the line between the two crests. This is usually the L4-5 interspace. In an alert patient with no allergies to local anesthetic, a skin wheal can be raised with a 24-gauge needle exactly in the midline between the two spinous processes. An 18-gauge spinal needle is best for a muscular or uncooperative patient; a 22-gauge is used when increased intracranial pressure is suspected. A 20-gauge is a good compromise. Handling the needle near the hub with a sterile glove, the physician inserts the needle point through the midline skin wheal, perpendicular to the plane of the back and to the plane of the mattress. At times the needle must be directed toward the patient's head at a slightly oblique angle. It is then advanced one-half of the distance and released. If the needle is not heading in the proper direction, withdraw it slightly and start again, correcting for the original misdirection. Turn the hub so that the number on the needle gauge is easily read from the top, for now the bevel of the needle will penetrate the transverse fibers of the dura, rather than cut through them. This reduces postspinal leakage of cerebrospinal fluid, but also produces a "pop" when going through the dura. As the needle is advanced, remove the stylet every centimeter. So that the stylet may be reinserted rapidly, never remove the tip completely from the hub (Fig. 1). When fluid is obtained, reinsert the stylet and advance 2 to 3 mm. Check the manometer stopcock so that the fluid will enter the manometer tube. Since most tubes

432

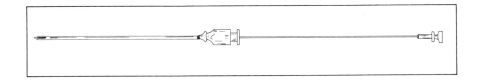

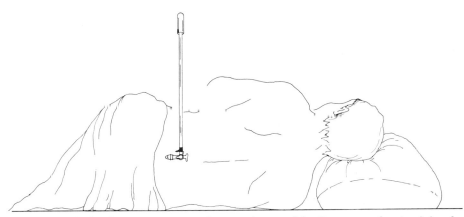

Figure 1 Position for lumbar puncture. Towel covers the top of the iliac crest and patient's head rests on pillow in the neutral position. Note the collection tube at the top of the manometer in case there is increased intracranial pressure. In the insert, note that the end of the stylet remains in the hub for rapid reinsertion.

measure 600 mm. of water, place a collection tube on top. The assistant, even without a sterile glove, can gently support the tube as the physician places the adapter near the needle hub. Remove the stylet and quickly connect the manometer to the needle. With increased intracranial pressure the fluid will rapidly reach the top of the manometer; when this happens withdraw the needle quickly and invert the manometer, allowing the fluid to flow into the collection tube. Usually there is enough fluid for a white blood cell count, gram stain, and culture. With a struggling patient, local anesthesia usually is of no help. Once the point of the needle penetrates the skin, slow advancement, stopping when the patient moves, will generally be successful. Pressure should be measured only when the patient is quiet. The so-called "dry tap" is probably a misnomer, a result of faulty technique.

EMERGENCY TWIST DRILL DECOMPRESSION

Rand et al. (1966) and Burton (1965) have demonstrated relative safety with the use of the twist drill in head trauma, but their success probably depends on extensive knowledge of indications and technique and, more important, on the manipulative skills to perform major brain surgery if a complication develops. However, in isolated hospitals, or when certain conditions require immediate action, twist drill decompression may be the only alternative to death. There is a commercially prepared compact drill (Burton, 1965) with a drill diameter 7/64 of an inch and flat head type that, if purchased, should be used first on a cadaver. The same practice is advised when the bur drills are used (see Fig. 2).

The sites for puncture are 5 cm. from the midline in the frontal area just anterior to the coronal suture, and a second set just over the parietal bosses slightly above and behind the tip of the ears (see Fig. 3). In the temporal area, the drill should be placed 2 fingerbreadths above the zygoma and 2 fingerbreadths in front of the tragus of the ear, keeping in mind that the temporal bone is thin. If time permits, shave the area and apply an antiseptic solution. (If local anesthesia is required, twist drill decompression probably is not indicated.) A small stab wound using a No. 15 Bard-Parker blade 1/2-cm.) is made down to the skull so that the pericranium is incised. The drill end should not be able to penetrate more than 1 cm.

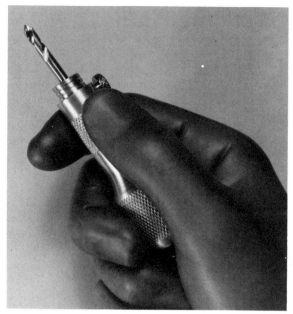

Figure 2   Method of grasp of compact hand drill. The bit length can be varied using set screw. (From Burton, C., and Blacket, H. M.: J. Trauma 5:643, 1965.)

When the drill is completely embedded, it is withdrawn and the opening is palpated with a No. 18 blunt-nose needle. If bone is palpated, the drill is lengthened 0.5 cm. and the above steps are repeated until the inner table has been penetrated. The drill usually gives way, indicating full penetration of the inner table. When the dura is found intact, reinsert the drill a little deeper so that the dura will be shredded and penetrated with more turning. When the hand drill penetrates the dura, the operator usually feels a definite end-point.

SUBDURAL TAPS IN INFANTS

Acute subdural hematoma in infants demands immediate evacuation and in many cases concomitant transfusion. The infant is swaddled in a blanket and the head is placed at the end of the table. All exposed hair is shaved and the scalp prepared with an antiseptic solution. If required, a sugar nipple and local anesthesia may be of value. The coronal suture is palpated at least 3 fingerbreadths lateral to the midline. A short bevel 5-cm. 20-gauge spinal needle is introduced through the scalp slightly anterior to the coronal suture so as to hit the skull. The scalp, with the needle in place, is then pulled posteriorly so that the needle point will be over the coronal suture. It is then advanced slowly until the dura is penetrated, which is indicated by a change in resistance. If no fluid comes out, slowly advance a few millimeters. No more than 20 ml. of fluid or blood should be removed from each side. Sterile dressings are placed over the needle holes, which should seal off spontaneously. Fluid should *not* be aspirated from the needle (see Fig. 4).

SKULL TREPHINATION

Trephination of the skull for acute epidural hemorrhage is a life-saving procedure,

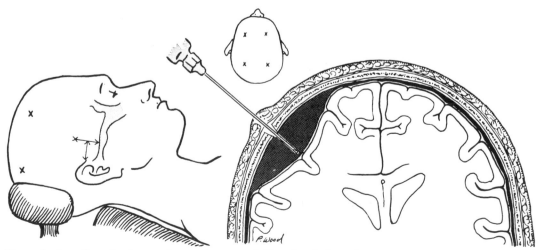

Figure 3   Location of points to place either twist drills or bur-holes. The temporal hole is placed in front of ear. (From Rand, B. O., Ward, A. A., and White, L. E.: J. Neurosurg. 25:410, 1966.)

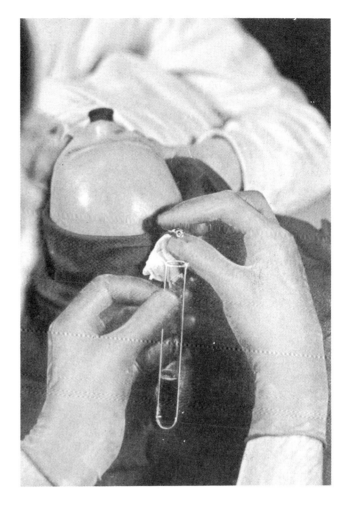

Figure 4 Note that the subdural needle is placed away from the midline. The shaft of the needle is held firmly against the scalp so that it will not wiggle. (From Ingraham and Matson: Neurosurgery of Infancy and Childhood, 1st ed. Springfield, Ill., Charles C Thomas, 1954, p. 195.)

whereas rapid brain dehydration by osmotic diuretics will only "buy" time until a trephine can be placed. If a neurosurgeon cannot operate promptly on the patient with the clinical syndrome of brain herniation (see page 00), it is justifiable for others to do so, preferably in the operating suite where suction and electrocautery are available. The Hudson brace and burs are relatively safe but practice is recommended. When time permits, shave the temporal region and apply an antiseptic solution. The center of the trephine should be 2 fingerbreadths above the zygomatic arch and 2 fingerbreadths in front of the ear. A 6-cm. vertical scalp incision is made and carried down to the skull (Fig. 5). This is most important. The superficial temporal artery should be avoided if possible, and the incision should not go below the superior border of the zygomatic arch. Using the scalpel handle, the pericranium is scraped off the bone, and one or two self-retaining retractors are spread taut until the the scalp and muscle

bleeding is stopped and good visualization of the underlying temporal bone is accomplished. Digital pressure by an assistant may be required to stop bleeding from the superficial temporal artery long enough to allow the operation to continue. Using the 9-mm. Hudson bur, a hole is made until the drill "chucks," i.e., becomes difficult to turn. The hole is enlarged with the 14-mm. bur. At this point it is removed, and either an epidural clot begins to extrude through the hole or the dura is observed. It must be stressed that the drill must penetrate both the outer and the inner table of the skull. If not, the vascular area between the two tables may mimic epidural bleeding. Stuff the hole with bone wax and then remove it. This usually stops bleeding from the bone marrow, but not from the middle meningeal artery. If an epidural hematoma is present, the hole can be enlarged with a rongeur in the radial fashion for the diameter of 4 cm. The clot can then be removed with the aid of suction and irrigation. If it is possible to locate the

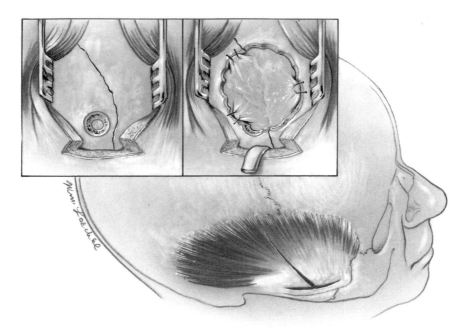

Figure 5   Subtemporal decompression. (From Thomas, L. M., and Gurdjian, E. S.: *In* Youmans, J. R. (ed.): Neurological Surgery. Philadelphia, W. B. Saunders Company, 1973, pp. 960-967.)

bleeding point from the middle meningeal artery, both ends should be clamped with hemostats, ligated, or electrocoagulated. If this is not sufficient to stop the bleeding, a loose dressing is applied over the wound and the patient rapidly transported to a neurosurgical center, escorted by a physician, with adequate blood for replacement from the bleeding wound (Craig and Hunt, 1959).

If epidural hemorrhage is not present, the dura can be opened in a cruciate fashion avoiding the middle meningeal artery, and a liquid subdural hematoma will come out. Once again the trephine is enlarged and the dura opened fully to allow more complete evacuation when the subdural blood is clotted.

If the patient cannot be transferred and the neurosurgeon cannot reach the hospital, the wound can then be closed with three layers (muscle, galea, and skin). If the superficial temporal artery is bleeding, it should be either ligated or electrocoagulated. Remember many intracranial clots are bilateral, so be prepared to operate on the other side.

INSERTION OF SKULL TONGS

There are many ingenious instruments available for skull traction. The Gardner-Wells spring-loaded tongs are simple, effective, and relatively inexpensive (Gardner, 1973). It is preferable, but not necessary, to shave a small area of the head just below the skull equator of the temporal ridges and in

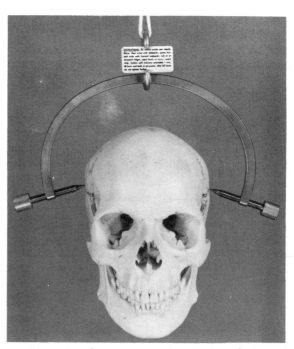

Figure 6   The points are placed above the tips of the ears and below the equator of the skull, and then tightened.

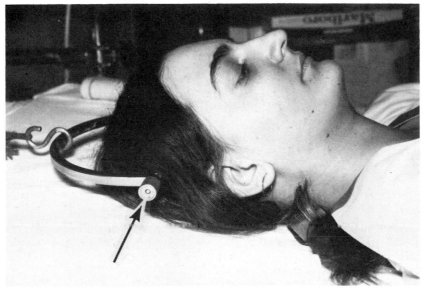

Figure 7 The arrow points to the end of the spring protruding through the small hole, indicating the proper pressure.

line with the external auditory meatus (Fig. 6). After washing the area with soap, antiseptic solution is applied and an anesthetic agent is injected into the scalp, temporalis muscle, and pericranium. The two points are then advanced by turning the knurled ends. When the needle points encounter bone, further tightening will compress the spring inside one unit (Fig. 7). When 30 lb. of "squeeze" is exerted, the metal end of the spring begins to protrude out of the hole. It should be noted that only one needle point has this opening. Next, the tong is lifted up and down a few times to seat the points. The needle point, which is not spring-loaded, is then tightened one-half turn. The lock nuts are tightened with a wrench so that the needle points will not work loose. In psychotic patients two nuts, one on each side of each needle point, may prevent deliberate loosening. It should be pointed out that the set does not come with a wrench.

The desired weight is then applied in 5-lb. increments every 15 to 30 minutes, and monitored by repeated neurologic examination and lateral cervical spine x-ray. This is especially important in the elderly person with spondylosis. A rule of thumb suggests 5

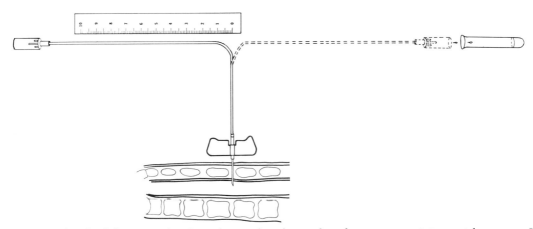

Figure 8 After fluid flows into the clear plastic tube, elevate the tube to measure intracranial pressure. Later lower tube to collect fluid. (From Greensher, J., et al.: J. Pediatr. 78:1035, 1971.)

lb. for each vertebral body. Hence, a dislocation at C5 would require 25 lb. As much as 60 lb. may be needed. Once reduction has occurred, the weight is reduced as the patient is monitored with x-ray. Antibiotic ointment, such as bacitracin, is applied around the needle points twice daily. The next day, loosen the lock units and tighten one needle point one-half turn. The spring-loaded needle points may need to be tightened periodically if the spring end slips back inside.

LUMBAR PUNCTURE IN INFANTS

In infants and children it is imperative that the needle be placed as low as possible, preferably at the L5-S1 interspace, for the spinal cord may not yet have ascended to the adult level at the L1 vertebral body. Penetration of the spinal cord can cause paraplegia. For small infants a thin-walled needle (no stylet) with a 3.5-cm. shaft can be used (Greensher, 1971). To prevent intraspinal epidermoid formation, make a hole in the midline using a 20-gauge spinal needle with stylet. Insert the smaller thin-walled needle in the opening made by the larger needle. The center plastic butterfly grip is attached to the needle and the hub is attached to the 30-cm. plastic tube. When fluid appears, the tube is elevated to measure the pressure and lowered again to collect a specimen (Fig. 8).

References

Burton, C., and Blacker, H. M.: A compact hand drill for emergency brain decompression. J. Trauma. 5:643, 1965.

Craig, T. V., and Hunt, W. E.: Emergency care of extradural hematoma. J.A.M.A. *171*:405, 1959.

Gardner, W. J.: The principle of spring-loaded points for cervical traction. J. Neurosurg. 39:543, 1973.

Greensher, J., et al.: Lumbar puncture in the neonate: a simplified technique. J. Pediatr. 78:1034, 1971.

Rand, B. O., Ward, A. A., and White, L. E.: The use of the twist drill to evaluate head trauma. J. Neurosurg. 25:410, 1966.

Thomas, L. M., and Gurdjian, E. S.: Intracranial Hematoma of Traumatic Origin. *In* Youmans, J. R. (ed.): Neurological Surgery. Philadelphia, W. B. Saunders Company, 1973, pp. 960–967.

Chapter 18 # ORTHOPEDIC PROCEDURES

David P. Simmons
and William R. MacAusland

PROCEDURE 1: SPLINTING

Principles

(*a*) Splinting is advisable for all extremity injuries in order to relieve pain; protect against skin, nerve, or vessel damage; and prevent fracture displacement.

(*b*) Splints should be rigid but well padded.

(*c*) Circumferential wrapping materials should be expansile and applied in a non-constricting manner.

(*d*) Splinting materials should permit penetration by x-rays.

(*e*) Only the necessary parts should be immobilized. In fractures, this includes the joints immediately above and below the fracture.

Types

(*a*) A bulky compression dressing made of circumferential cast padding with several longitudinal plaster strips, wrapped on with an elastic bandage, makes a universal splint for any extremity injury.

(*b*) A pillow, wrapped with elastic bandages, taped or pinned in place is excellent immobilization for knee, tibia, ankle, and foot injuries (Fig. 1, *A*).

(*c*) There are many useful commercial devices of inflatable or molded materials, but simple molded plaster splints are effective, available, inexpensive, and, above all, custom-fit (Fig. 1, *B*).

(*d*) The Thomas ring splint (Fig. 1, *C*) is an essential device for stabilizing femoral fractures, and its application should be practiced.

(*e*) The four-poster cervical brace is the most effective neck immobilizer (Fig. 1, *D*). It is applied in two halves, with an assistant immobilizing the neck by gentle manual traction on the head.

(*f*) Clavicles can be immobilized using a strap (Fig. 1, *E*). Injuries to arm and shoulder require sling and swathe (Fig. 1, *F*) when relatively complete immobilization is needed.

Complications

(*a*) The major difficulty is neurovascular impairment caused by circumferential constriction. Frequent observation as swelling occurs is essential.

(*b*) If an unpadded splint is employed for more than a few hours, especially where there is a neural deficit, local skin necrosis may occur.

(*c*) Many splints do not control rotational forces on the extremity, so that caution is necessary in handling the limb and the patient.

(*d*) A soft cervical collar does not immobilize the cervical spine effectively.

PROCEDURE 2: TRACTION METHODS

Principles

(*a*) Longitudinal tension applied through the soft tissues aligns adjacent structures.

(*b*) Only light weights (5 to 15 lb.) are necessary, as the muscles will lengthen over time through fatigue.

439

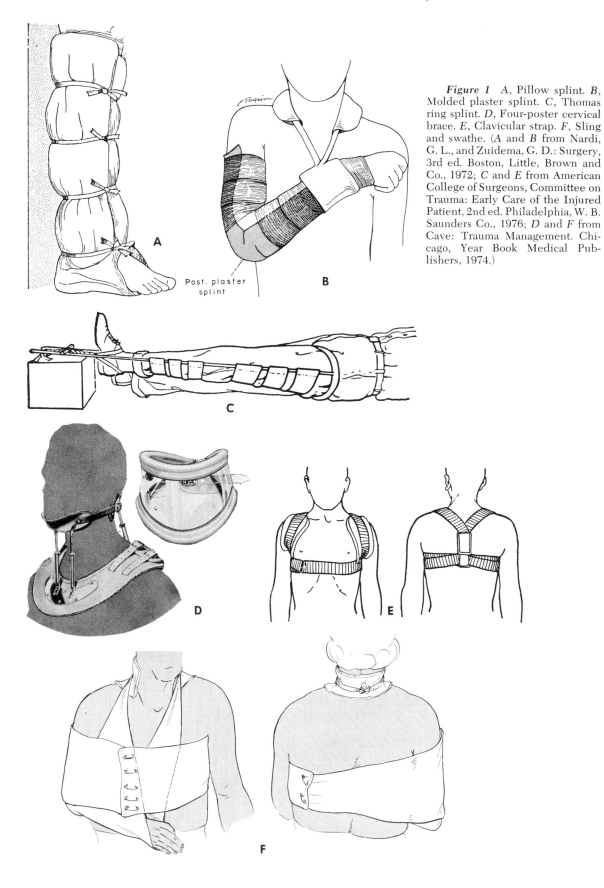

Post. plaster splint

Figure 1 A, Pillow splint. B, Molded plaster splint. C, Thomas ring splint. D, Four-poster cervical brace. E, Clavicular strap. F, Sling and swathe. (A and B from Nardi, G. L., and Zuidema, G. D.: Surgery, 3rd ed. Boston, Little, Brown and Co., 1972; C and E from American College of Surgeons, Committee on Trauma: Early Care of the Injured Patient, 2nd ed. Philadelphia, W. B. Saunders Co., 1976; D and F from Cave: Trauma Management. Chicago, Year Book Medical Publishers, 1974.)

(c) Skin traction is limited by frictional shearing, and thus a skeletal wire is necessary for weights greater than 5 lb.

Technique for Skin Traction (Fig. 2,A and B)

(a) Apply tincture of benzoin locally.

(b) Apply adhesive straps longitudinally, avoiding wrinkles and using padding about bony prominences (e.g., the malleoli, fibular head, and heel cord) to decrease local pressure.

(c) Apply loose circumferential elastic bandage over strapping.

(d) Apply up to 5 lb. of weight to traction cord with metal or wooden spreader to prevent local skin contact from cord.

Technique for Skeletal Traction (Fig. 2,C to G)

(a) Cleanse the skin with an antiseptic solution.

(b) Anesthetize the skin, subcutaneous tissues, and periosteum with 1 per cent lidocaine locally.

(c) Puncture the skin with a scalpel blade.

(d) Select a sterile wire that is threaded, to prevent migration. The approximate wire size is 5/64" for the upper extremity and 1/8" for the lower extremity.

(e) Insert the wire point first, and drill in a direction perpendicular to the long axis of the limb.

(f) Incise the skin over the exiting point of the wire.

(g) Relieve residual skin tension about the wire by further skin incision if necessary.

Complications

(a) Neurovascular impairment may occur if wrapping is too constrictive. Serial observation, with frequent rewrapping, is necessary.

(b) Local skin pressure lesions may occur if bony prominences are not relieved of direct pressure by padding *about*, not *on*, them.

(c) Skin straps will slip and injure skin if the weights are too heavy, or if the elastic wrap is not reapplied frequently to maintain gentle compression.

(d) Traction cords must be kept free, pulleys oiled, and weights kept off the floor to avoid loss of effective traction.

(e) The occurrence of infection with skeletal traction can be diminished by daily inspection and cleansing of the wire sites. The application of antiseptics and antibiotics locally may be effective in preventing infection.

(f) In children, skeletal wires must not be inserted through epiphyseal plates.

PROCEDURE 3: CASTING

Principles

(a) Plaster of Paris is the optimum material for casts because it is available, adaptable, light-weight, porous, inexpensive, removable, and penetrable by x-ray.

(b) Only the necessary parts should be immobilized. In the case of fractures, this includes the joints immediately above and below the fracture.

(c) Casts cannot expand to accommodate swelling. They should be applied only when close observation and treatment are available, i.e., for splitting or removal if necessary.

Technique (Fig. 3, A and B)

(a) Apply adequate soft padding smoothly and circumferentially.

(b) Dip plaster rolls into cool water, which slows the setting and allows time for application.

(c) Lay the plaster on circumferentially, rather than pulling it on, in order to avoid ridging caused by tension.

(d) Apply plaster strips of four to six layers longitudinally to strengthen corners (e.g., the elbow and the ankle) and to prevent sectional weakness in long casts (e.g., the cylinder cast).

(e) Mold the plaster with the palms, not the fingers, to avoid dents that may cause pressure sores, and to strengthen the cast by fusing the plaster layers.

(f) Make the cast look like the part, and it probably will fit without undue local skin pressure.

(Text continued on p. 445)

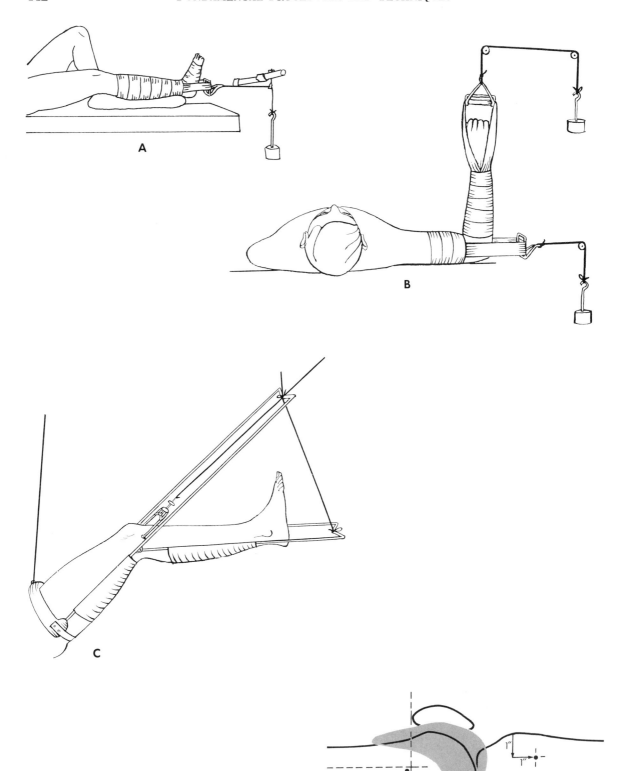

Figure 2 A, Buck's skin traction. *B*, Dunlop's skin traction. *C*, Skeletal traction. *D*, Femoral and tibial wire sites.

Illustration continued on opposite page.

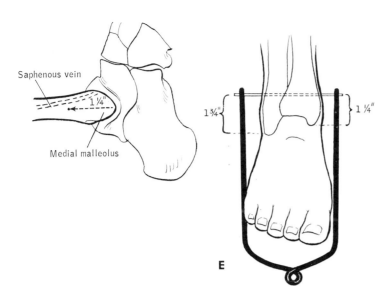

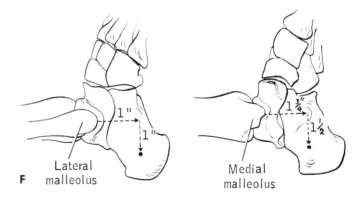

Figure 2 (*Continued*). E, Distal tibial wire. F, Calcaneal wire site. G, Olecranon wire sites. (From Schmeisser, G.: A Clinical Manual of Orthopedic Traction Technique. Philadelphia, W. B. Saunders Co., 1963.)

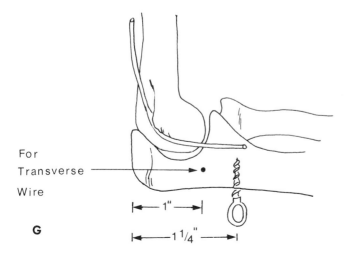

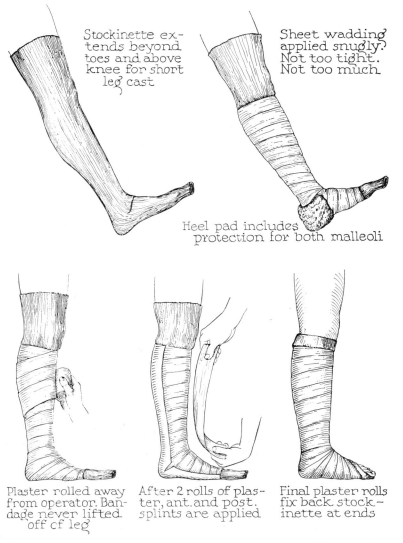

Stockinette extends beyond toes and above knee for short leg cast

Sheet wadding applied snugly. Not too tight. Not too much

Heel pad includes protection for both malleoli

Plaster rolled away from operator. Bandage never lifted off of leg

After 2 rolls of plaster, ant. and post. splints are applied

Final plaster rolls fix back stockinette at ends

A

Figure 3 A, Cast application (stockinette, cast padding, plaster rolls, plaster splints, trimming). (From Compere, E. L.: Handbook of Fracture Treatment, Chicago, Year Book Medical Publishers, 1966, p. 61.)

Illustration continued on opposite page.

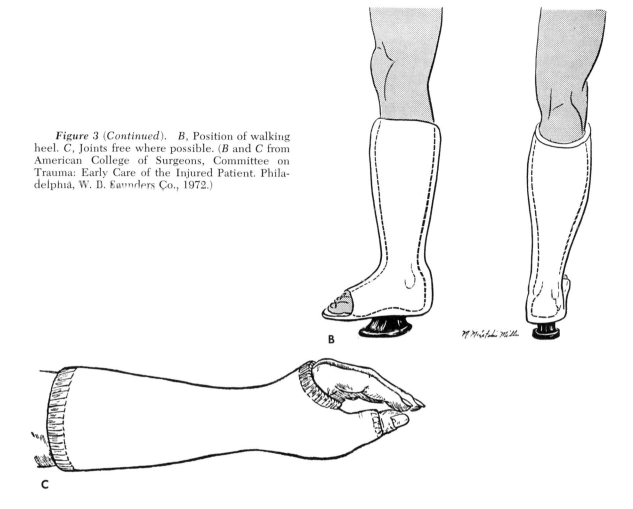

Figure 3 (Continued). B, Position of walking heel. C, Joints free where possible. (B and C from American College of Surgeons, Committee on Trauma: Early Care of the Injured Patient. Philadelphia, W. B. Saunders Co., 1972.)

B

C

(g) Wait for the plaster to set, and it will not have to be too thick or bulky.

(h) Attach a rubber walking heel to the middle of the sole by laying it on a thick plaster splint and binding it to the foot with an additional plaster roll (Fig. 3, B). Weight bearing should be postponed for 48 hours to permit full cast strength to develop.

Complications

(a) Progressive swelling of the limb within the cast can be diminished by elevating the distal part above the level of the heart. Full relief may require splitting and spreading of the plaster. It may be necessary also to cut the entire length of the cast padding with scissors.

(b) Local discomfort under a cast must be regarded as a sign of progressive pressure necrosis, and should be treated by the remov-al of a plaster window over the site, or by changing the cast.

(c) The patient must be instructed not to push any objects between the cast and his skin, or a local pressure lesion may develop. The itching under plaster must be accepted or ignored.

(d) Stiffness of immobilized joints occurs rapidly, so that casts must be trimmed to permit unrestricted motion of uninvolved joints. This is especially true in the hand; thus, short and long arm casts should end proximal to the palmar crease (Fig. 3, C).

PROCEDURE 4: ANESTHESIA

Principles

(a) Adequate analgesia, sedation, and muscle relaxation are essential to accomplish reductions safely, but the choice of an anesthetic must be safe in itself.

(b) Anesthesia should not be administered unless oxygen, suction, endotracheal tubes, and essential supportive drugs are readily available.

Types

I.V. SEDATION

Indications. Generally useful for all ages where only a brief manipulation is necessary.

Relaxation and amnesia are possible, but analgesia rarely is achieved.

Pharmacologic Agents. In adults, diazepam 10 mg., or diazepam 5 mg. and meperidine 50 mg. In children, meperidine 0.5 mg./lb.

Contraindications. A history of sensitivity or allergy to these drugs.

Any compromised respiratory function.

In the very elderly or very young.

Technique. A scalp vein needle or catheter is inserted I.V.

The solution is injected slowly over two to three minutes.

The exact portion of the total maximum dose is titrated by serial observation of the individual patient. Sleeping or respiratory slowing signals the end-points.

Complications. Thes drugs may cause respiratory depression or arrest. Treatment is by support of respiration mechanically while maintaining the airway by position, tubing, and suction as necessary.

INTRAFRACTURE INSTILLATION

Indications. Useful in cooperative patients at individual fracture sites where relaxation of muscle is not necessary.

Pharmacologic Agents. Lidocaine 2 per cent without epinephrine. The maximum dose is 300 mg.

Contraindications. A history of sensitivity or allergy to local anesthetics.

Any contaminated injection sites.

Technique. The skin must be cleansed and sterilized locally.

A local skin wheal of lidocaine is raised.

A needle is introduced into the fracture site, recognized by the aspiration of blood often containing fat globules.

The lidocaine is injected slowly until resistance is felt or the maximum dose is injected.

At least ten minutes should elapse before manipulation is attempted.

Complications. Intravenous injection may result in cardiovascular collapse.

Intra-arterial injection may result in distal necrosis of the limb.

Infection may be introduced into the fracture site.

Too much volume of anesthetic solution may contribute significantly to the swelling.

Convulsions or hypotension may result in cases of allergy.

INTRAVENOUS REGIONAL
(Fig. 4, A)

Indications. Useful for adults and cooperative children where a single limb is involved.

Muscle relaxation and analgesia generally are excellent for periods of up to one hour.

Pharmacologic Agents. Lidocaine 0.5 per cent without epinephrine at a dose of 2 mg./kg.

A 0.25 per cent solution is indicated in the lower extremity.

Contraindications. A history of sensitivity or allergy to local anesthetics.

Significant cardiac disease.

Technique. A proximal tourniquet is applied to the limb, but not inflated.

A scalp vein needle or catheter is inserted into a distal vein of the involved limb.

The limb is exsanguinated by elevation or ace wrapping. The tourniquet is inflated to 200 mm. Hg. The full amount of lidocaine is injected.

Waiting ten minutes prior to manipulating insures a maximum effect.

After the manipulation, the tourniquet should be deflated slowly to minimize the systemic effects.

Complications. The sudden release of a bolus of lidocaine into the systemic circulation may have cardiotoxic effects. Mental changes and bradycardia signal these effects. Monitoring, supportive devices, and drugs should be available.

Intra-arterial injection may result in distal necrosis of the limb.

Convulsions and hypotension may result in cases of drug allergy. Phlebitis may occur after use in lower extremity.

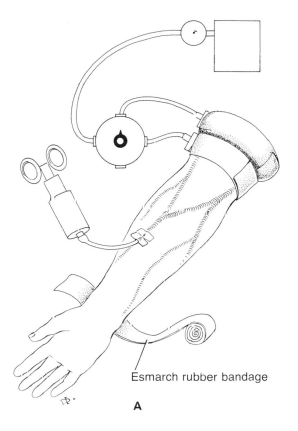

A

Esmarch rubber bandage

Figure 4 A, I.V. regional. B, Axillary block. (From Hill, G., II: Outpatient Surgery. Philadelphia, W. B. Saunders Co., 1973, pp. 37 and 38.)

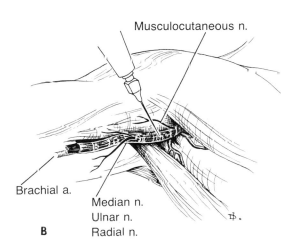

Musculocutaneous n.

Brachial a.

B

Median n.
Ulnar n.
Radial n.

AXILLARY BLOCK (Fig. 4, B)

Indications. Useful for adults and co-operative children where the upper extremity is involved.

Muscle relaxation and analgesia are excellent and prolonged.

Pharmacologic Agent. Lidocaine 1 per cent without epinephrine at dose of 7 mg./kg.

Contraindications. A history of sensitivity or allergy to local anesthetics.

Technique. The skin of the axillary region is cleansed and sterilized locally.

A skin wheal of lidocaine is raised.

The axillary artery is palpated.

A needle is introduced and the solution is injected medially, laterally, and behind the artery. The artery is *not* injected.

Waiting 20 minutes prior to manipulating insures a maximum effect.

Complications. Intra-arterial injection may result in distal necrosis of the limb.

Intravenous injection may result in cardiovascular collapse.

Convulsions and hypotension may result in cases of drug allergy.

All the branches of the axillary plexus may not be anesthetized.

PROCEDURE 5: JOINT ASPIRATION

Principles

(*a*) The technique is useful for the diagnosis of major acute joint injury. The presence of blood in the joint confirms this.

(*b*) The technique may establish the existence of an intra-articular fracture. A mixture of blood and fat confirms this.

(*c*) The technique also is useful in the diagnosis of nontraumatic joint disease. Gross, microscopic, bacteriologic, chemical, and immunologic analysis of the fluid is necessary for this.

(*d*) It is therapeutically useful in relieving the pain of a tense effusion or acute hemarthrosis.

Technique (Fig. 5)

(*a*) The skin must be cleansed and sterilized locally.

(*b*) An approach avoiding neurovascular structures is selected.

(*c*) A skin wheal of lidocaine 1 per cent is raised.

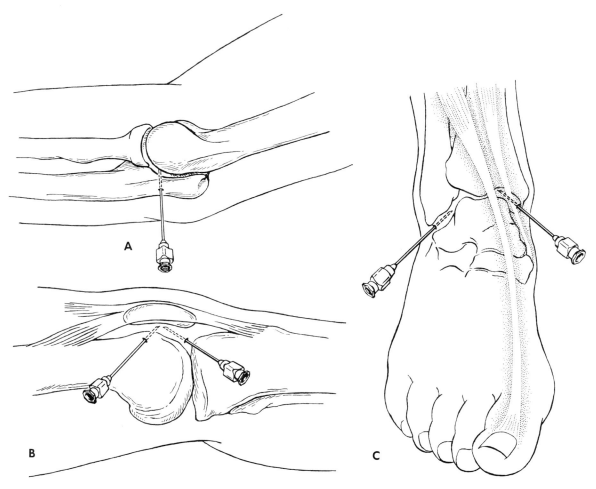

Figure 5   *A*, Elbow joint aspiration. *B*, Knee joint aspiration. *C*, Ankle joint aspiration. (From Steinbocker, O.: Aspiration and Injection Therapy in Arthritis. Hagerstown, Md., Harper & Row, 1972.)

(*d*) A large bore needle (No. 18 or greater) is introduced into the joint. Infiltration of lidocaine while the needle is advanced slowly will reduce the pain.

(*e*) Aspiration of joint contents, or the easy injection of lidocaine and its return, confirms an intra-articular placement. Care should be taken to avoid scoring the articular cartilage.

(*f*) The intra-articular instillation of lidocaine 1 per cent (to a maximum of 300 mg.) may temporarily relieve joint pain and permit stress testing of ligaments (Procedure 7).

Complications

(*a*) An infection may be introduced.

(*b*) The articular cartilage may be damaged by scoring or puncturing.

PROCEDURE 6: INJECTION

Principles

(*a*) The technique is useful for the local treatment of acute and chronic inflammatory conditions of joints, tendons, bursae, and nerves.

(*b*) It should never be used where infection may be present.

(*c*) The injection of lidocaine without steroid may be of diagnostic, as opposed to therapeutic, value.

Pharmacologic Agent

(*a*) Hydrocortisone suspension or its equivalent.

(*b*) 25 mg. in small joints; 50 mg. in large joints.

(c) A small volume should be used in small spaces.

Technique (Fig. 6)

(a) The skin should be cleansed and sterilized locally.

(b) A safe approach, away from neurovascular structures, should be selected. The regional anatomy should be reviewed prior to injection.

(c) A skin wheal of lidocaine 1 per cent is raised.

(d) The needle should be introduced *into* the joint or *adjacent* to the tendon or nerve to be treated. There should be no resistance to injection if the needle is positioned properly. Lidocaine injection prior to steroid instillation will decrease pain acutely.

Complications

(a) An infection may be introduced.

(b) Pre-existing infection may be masked or promoted.

(c) Steroid administration may delay healing of acutely injured tissue.

(d) Local steroids may contribute to the progressive degeneration of tendons and articular cartilage.

(e) Intracutaneous and subcutaneous deposition of steroid may cause permanent damage, such as atrophy or depigmentation.

(f) Frequent steroid injection may have systemic effects.

PROCEDURE 7: STRESS TESTING

Principles

(a) Significant ligamentous tears may be recognized only by manipulative testing. The optimum selection of therapy and its duration in ligament injuries depends on an exact diagnosis.

(b) The patient must be cooperative and relaxed. Anesthesia may be necessary (Procedure 4).

(c) The application of slow, but firm, force is necessary to avoid reflex spasm of muscles, which may mask instability.

(d) Stability is compared to the contralateral normal joint.

(e) Simultaneous x-rays during stress will define and document the extent of instability.

Technique (Fig. 7)

(a) The procedure should be explained to the patient to gain his cooperation.

(b) The regional anatomy should be reviewed prior to manipulation.

(c) Relaxation and analgesia may be insured by sedation or anesthesia.

(d) Slow, but firm, tension is applied to the structure to be tested. Instability is judged by both appearance and feel as compared to the uninjured side.

Complications

(a) Partial ligamentous tears may be completed if force is extreme.

(b) Avulsion fractures may be displaced if force is extreme.

(c) The joint may be dislocated if force is extreme.

PROCEDURE 8: REDUCTION OF DISLOCATIONS

Principles

(a) All acute dislocations should be reduced promptly, as it is safer, easier, and decreases the neurovascular complications.

(b) Open dislocations must be treated immediately and operatively to prevent infection.

(c) Chronic dislocations must be recognized, as closed methods of reduction are unsuccessful and potentially injurious.

(d) Acute distal ischemia may force immediate reduction of a dislocation.

Complications

(a) Neurovascular injuries may accompany the dislocation or its reduction. Observation of the distal neurovascular status is necessary before and after manipulation attempts.

(b) Fractures commonly accompany dislocations. X-rays before and after manipulation are necessary to ensure that there is no

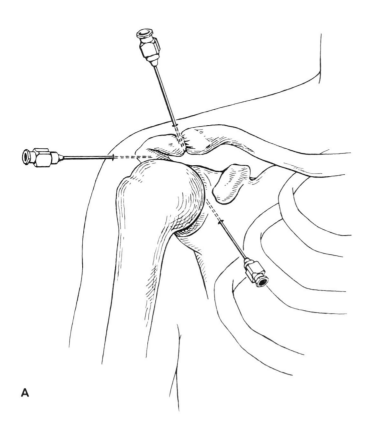

A

Figure 6 A, Shoulder injection (for bursitis/tendinitis). B, Elbow injection (for tennis elbow). C, Wrist injection (for carpal tunnel syndrome). (A and C from Steinbocker, O.: Aspiration and Injection Therapy in Arthritis. Hagerstown, Md., Harper & Row, 1972; B and D from Hill, G., II: Outpatient Surgery, Philadelphia, W. B. Saunders Co., 1973.) D, Wrist injection (for De Quervain's tenosynovitis).

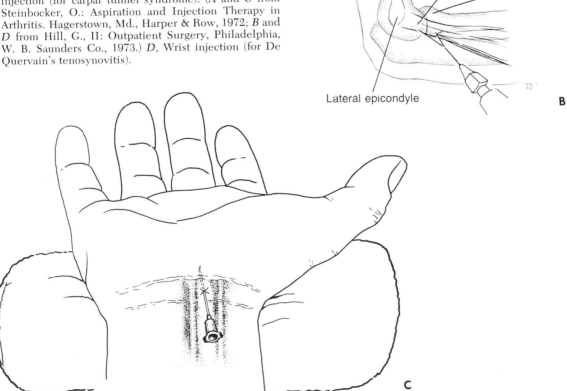

Common extensor tendon

Radial head

Lateral epicondyle

B

C

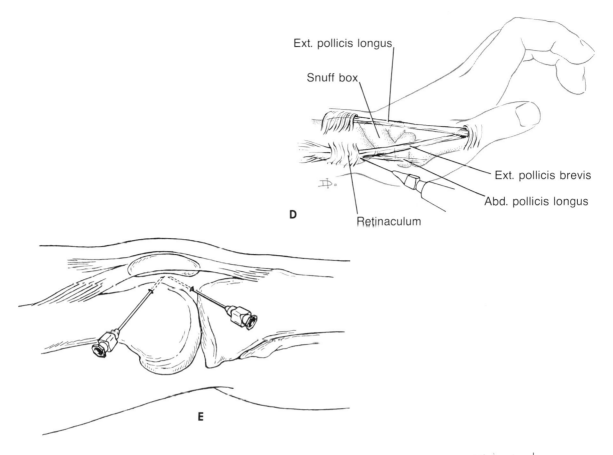

Ext. pollicis longus

Snuff box

Ext. pollicis brevis

Abd. pollicis longus

Retinaculum

D

E

Figure 6 (Continued) E, Knee injection. F, Ankle injection. (E and F from Steinbocker, O.: Aspiration and Injection Therapy in Arthritis. Hagerstown, Md., Harper & Row, 1972.)

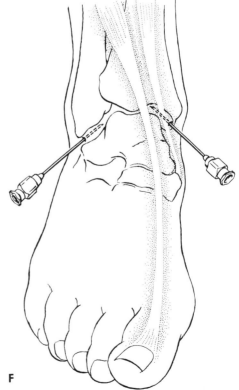

F

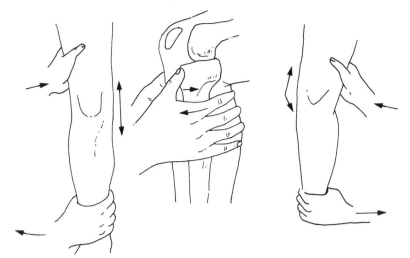

Figure 7. Stress testing knee. (From DePalma, A. F.: The Management of Fractures and Dislocations. Philadelphia, W. B. Saunders Co., 1970, p. 1379.)

fracture. Separate treatment of the fracture may be necessary.

(*c*) Manipulation may result in fracture, but this can be avoided if the reduction is not forced.

(*d*) Recurrent dislocation usually follows where post-injury immobilization is not maintained.

(*e*) Severe joint stiffness secondary to extensive ligamentous disruption ensues if immobilization is prolonged.

(*f*) The complications of failing to reduce a dislocation probably are greater than those that follow reduction.

General Technique

(*a*) Sedation usually is all that is necessary to perform reductions if the patient is informed, the methods are gentle, and adequate assistance in countertraction is available.

(*b*) Dislocations older than a few days should be manipulated under adequate anesthesia, with preparation to proceed operatively if necessary.

(*c*) The usual method is first to apply traction slowly and steadily in the line of the deformity, and then to manipulate to reverse the deformity.

(*d*) Topical tincture of benzoin on the manipulator's hands may reduce skin slippage during traction phase.

(*e*) The patient usually recognizes and reports the success of the manipulation, but it should be proved by x-rays.

(*f*) The position of immobilization should be one to relax the torn capsular and ligamentous tissues.

Regional Technique

SHOULDER JOINT

Axial traction by manual traction (Fig. 8, *A*) or gravity (Fig. 8, *B*) is the safest, gentlest, and least complicating method. Sufficient time (at least 15 minutes) and force (begin at 15 lb.) is necessary for the gravity technique.

After the steady application of traction, gentle rotation of the limb may be necessary to achieve reduction. The Kocher method (Fig. 8, *C*) is faster but always runs the risk of fracturing the humerus. The steps are: (1) traction; (2) external rotation; (3) adduction; and (4) internal rotation.

Sling and swathe immobilization is critical to prevent recurrence.

ELBOW JOINT

Steady longitudinal traction is applied, and adequate counter traction provided (Fig. 8, *D*). Sideways displacement is corrected with the guiding hand.

Traction is maintained while the elbow is flexed.

Splinting the elbow in flexion prevents recurrence.

METACARPOPHALANGEAL JOINT (THUMB)

Adequate anesthesia is necessary. A soft encircling wrap may improve grip on the thumb.

The initial step is hyperextension (Fig. 8, *E-1*). Distal displacement of the phalangeal base is accomplished by direct thumb pressure (Fig. 8, *E-2*). With traction, flexion then achieves and maintains reduction.

The thumb should be splinted in flexion.

INTERPHALANGEAL JOINT

A soft encircling wrap may improve the grip on the finger. Longitudinal traction is applied. Direct manual pressure against the deformity at the base of the middle phalanx reduces the dislocation.

The finger should be splinted in flexion.

HIP JOINT

Spinal or general anesthesia usually is necessary, although reduction attempts could be made using analgesics and muscle relaxants.

Longitudinal traction is applied (note that, in the prone position, gravity assists) (Fig. 8, *F*). Gentle rotation usually completes the more difficult reduction (Fig. 8, *G*).

Skin or skeletal traction is indicated to prevent recurrence.

PROCEDURE 9: REDUCTION OF FRACTURES

Principles

(*a*) All fractures should be considered for prompt reduction. Unlike dislocations, however, many fractures are less complicated if left unreduced, or if reduction is postponed.

(*b*) Open fractures must be treated surgically to prevent infection.

(*c*) Healing or healed fractures must be recognized, as closed methods of reduction are unsuccessful and potentially injurious.

(*d*) Severe distal ischemia may force immediate reduction of a fracture.

Complications

(*a*) Neurovascular injuries may accompany the fracture or its reduction. Observation of the distal neurovascular status is necessary before and after manipulation attempts.

(*b*) Dislocations commonly accompany fractures. Separate reduction of the dislocation usually precedes treatment of the fracture.

(*c*) Incomplete understanding of the

anatomy, or too forceful a manipulation, may result in worsening of the fracture position.

(*d*) Failed reduction attempts aggravate all the potential complications of the fracture, e.g., bleeding, swelling, and skin and neurovascular injuries.

(*e*) The skin and neurovascular hazards of immobilization must be avoided, and it is important to observe the limb serially after reduction.

General Technique

(*a*) The use and choice of anesthesia for reduction depend on the individual requirements of the fracture and the patient (Procedure 4).

(*b*) Fractures older than 10 to 14 days should be manipulated under adequate anesthesia, with preparation to proceed operatively if necessary.

(*c*) The usual method is first to apply traction slowly and steadily in the line of the deformity, and then to manipulate to reverse the deformity.

(*d*) Topical tincture of benzoin on the manipulator's hands may reduce skin slippage during the traction phase.

(*e*) It usually is necessary to have adequate assistance to maintain the reduction while the splints or cast is applied for immobilization.

(*f*) If marked swelling is anticipated, immediate cast splitting may avoid later skin and neurovascular complications.

Regional Technique

HUMERAL SHAFT

Anesthesia rarely is necessary. With the patient upright, longitudinal traction is added to the effect of gravity (Fig. 9, *A*). Correction of angulation usually is accomplished by positioning the elbow. Gentle external molding of the upper arm corrects sideways displacement.

Plaster coaptation splints and a sling provide lightweight, effective immobilization.

FOREARM (BOTH BONES)

Anesthesia usually is necessary.

Traction is best applied by gravity, using finger traps (Fig. 9, *B*) and a weighted

(*Text continued on page 458*)

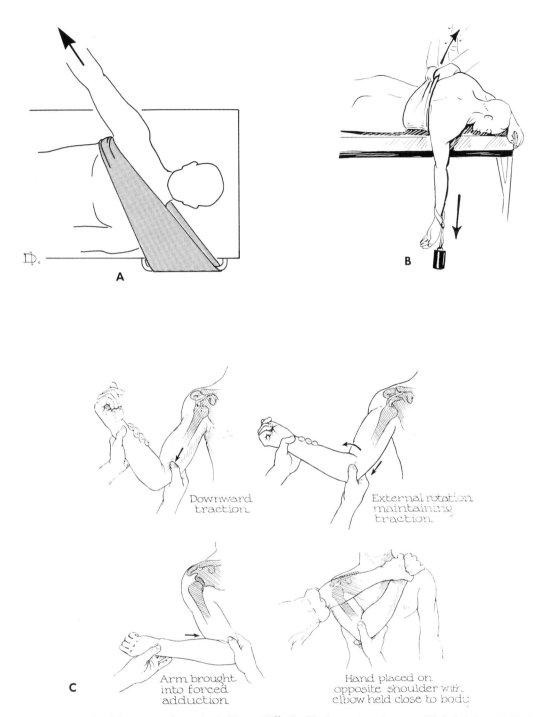

Figure 8 *A*, Shoulder (manual traction). (From Hill, G., II: Outpatient Surgery. Philadelphia, W. B. Saunders Co., 1973, p. 341.) *B*, Shoulder (gravity traction). (From Cave: Fractures and Other Injuries. Chicago, Year Book Medical Publishers, 1958, p. 266.) *C*, Shoulder (Kocher method). (From Compere, E. L.: Handbook of Fracture Treatment. Chicago, Year Book Medical Publishers, 1966, p. 266.)

Illustration continued on opposite page.

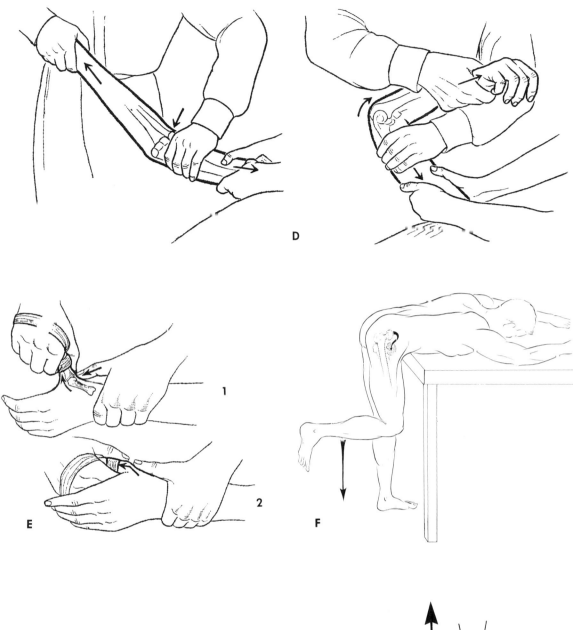

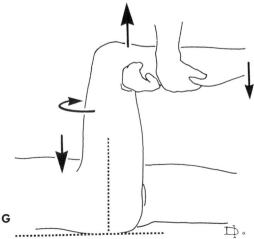

Figure 8 (Continued) *D*, Elbow (longitudinal traction). *E-1*, Metacarpophalangeal thumb (hyperextension). *E-2*, Metacarpophalangeal thumb (direct thumb pressure). (*D* and *E* from DePalma, A. F.: The Management of Fractures and Dislocations. Philadelphia, W. B. Saunders Co., 1970.) *F*, Hip (longitudinal traction). (From Cave: Fractures and Other Injuries. Chicago, Year Book Medical Publishers, 1968, p. 469.) *G*, Hip (gentle rotation). (From Hill, G., II: Outpatient Surgery. Philadelphia, W. B. Saunders Co., 1973, p. 343.)

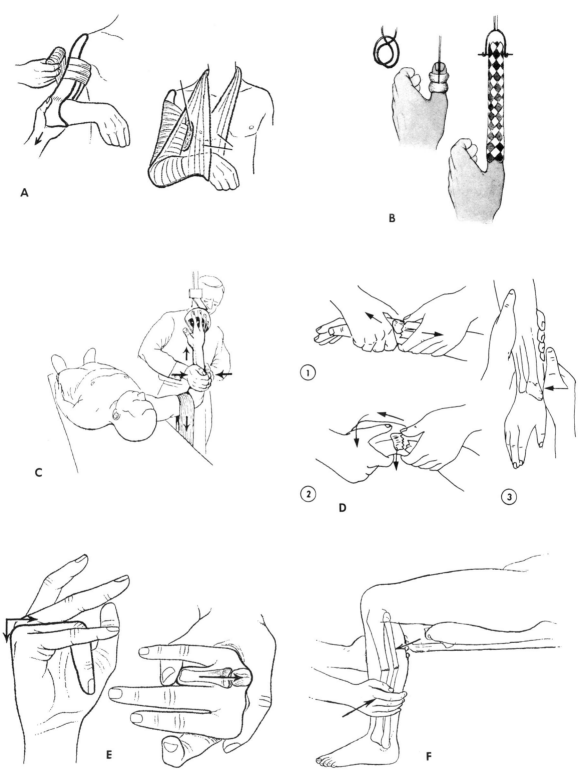

Figure 9 A, Humeral shaft. B, Finger trap traction. C, Forearm. D, Distal forearm (Colles'). (B from Marble, H.: The Hand. Philadelphia, W. B. Saunders Co., 1960, p. 103; A, C and D from DePalma, A. F.: The Management of Fractures and Dislocations. Philadelphia, W. B. Saunders Co., 1970.) E, Metacarpal neck (boxer's). F, Tibial shaft. (E and F from DePalma, A. F.: The Management of Fractures and Dislocations. Philadelphia, W. B. Saunders Co., 1970.)

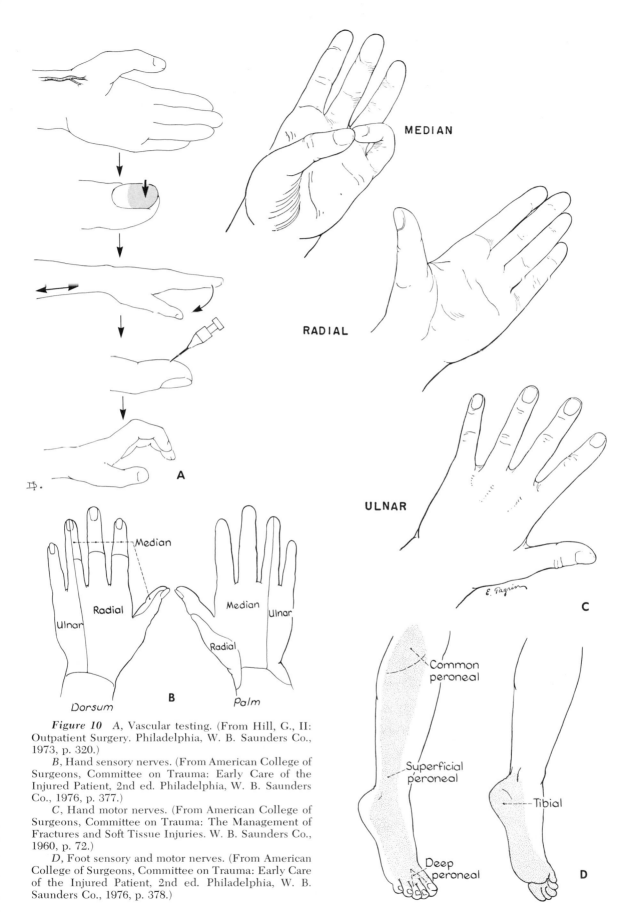

MEDIAN

RADIAL

ULNAR

E. Pagrin

Median

Radial

Ulnar

Median

Ulnar

Radial

Dorsum

Palm

B

C

A

Common
peroneal

Superficial
peroneal

Tibial

Deep
peroneal

D

Figure 10 *A,* Vascular testing. (From Hill, G., II: Outpatient Surgery. Philadelphia, W. B. Saunders Co., 1973, p. 320.)

B, Hand sensory nerves. (From American College of Surgeons, Committee on Trauma: Early Care of the Injured Patient, 2nd ed. Philadelphia, W. B. Saunders Co., 1976, p. 377.)

C, Hand motor nerves. (From American College of Surgeons, Committee on Trauma: The Management of Fractures and Soft Tissue Injuries. W. B. Saunders Co., 1960, p. 72.)

D, Foot sensory and motor nerves. (From American College of Surgeons, Committee on Trauma: Early Care of the Injured Patient, 2nd ed. Philadelphia, W. B. Saunders Co., 1976, p. 378.)

457

sling over the upper arm (15 lb. for ten minutes) (Fig. 9, *C*). Rotation is corrected by positioning the hand. The interosseous space is squeezed to spread the bones.

Long arm immobilization is necessary.

DISTAL FOREARM (COLLES')

Longitudinal traction is applied. The thumbs apply a dorsal force to the distal fragment while the patient's hand is flexed, pronated, and ulnarly deviated (Fig. 9, *D*).

Maintenance of the reduction is accomplished by an ulnarward force on the distal radius, with the hand in slight flexion.

Long arm immobilization usually is necessary initially.

METACARPAL NECK (BOXER'S)

Anesthesia usually is necessary. The metacarpophalangeal joint is flexed to 90 degrees. A dorsal reducing force is applied along the shaft of the proximal phalanx (Fig. 9, *E*).

The digit is splinted in moderate flexion.

PHALANGEAL

Anesthesia usually is necessary.

A soft encircling wrap may improve the grip on the finger. Longitudinal traction is applied. Sideways and rotatory displacement is corrected by manipulation.

The finger is splinted in moderate flexion.

TIBIAL SHAFT

Anesthesia usually is not necessary.

The fracture normally is reduced by simple gravity, with the knee bent over the end of a table. Additional longitudinal traction may be necessary. Sideways molding may be necessary to correct displacement or angulation (Fig. 9, *F*). Rotational alignment may be corrected by positioning the foot.

Long leg immobilization is necessary initially.

TRIMALLEOLAR

Anesthesia usually is necessary. A longitudinal traction force is applied to the foot. The heel is grasped and drawn forward while the foot is strongly rotated internally. The stabilizing hand prevents tibial movement.

Long leg immobilization is necessary.

PROCEDURE 10: NEUROVASCULAR TESTING

Principles

(*a*) Baseline and progressive serial observations of neurologic and vascular function in injuries to the extremities are absolutely critical in selecting the optimum treatment method, and in avoiding its complications (Fig. 10, *A*).

(*b*) It often is better to splint, ice, and elevate a fractured limb than to add the forces of manipulation to the pre-existing injury.

(*c*) The regional anatomy of nerves and blood supply should be reviewed (e.g., in the hand, Fig. 10, *B* and *C*).

(*d*) Comparison with the uninvolved side is important.

(*e*) The circulatory examination includes color, temperature, capillary fill, deficits of sensory and motor ability, and the presence or absence of the peripheral pulse.

(*f*) Light touch and pin prick testing usually is sufficient for sensory testing, but, where spinal cord injury is suspected, a complete neurologic examination of the trunk and extremities is vital. Do not forget perianal sensation, sphincter tone, and the bulbocavernosal reflex.

(*g*) Voluntary active motion is necessary to test motor function fully in the leg and foot (Fig. 10, *D*), but testing the deep tendon reflexes and the withdrawal responses yields some reliable motor information.

(*h*) Severe pain, especially upon passive motion of the fingers or toes, may be the first sign of an ischemic compartment syndrome in the forearm or calf musculature.

Chapter 19

OBSTETRIC AND GYNECOLOGIC PROCEDURES

Elsie R. Carrington

EVALUATION OF PELVIC PROBLEMS

The following data should appear as the lead line in the emergency obstetric–gynecologic evaluation: date, time, age, gravidity, parity, and date of the last menstrual period. These provide immediate orientation with regard to the many problems that affect the reproductive system. They also have a direct bearing on the details of history, the diagnostic possibilities, and the types of examination that should follow. For example, abnormal vaginal bleeding has entirely different implications in the prepubertal child, in the woman in the reproductive years, and in the premenopausal or menopausal woman.

GYNECOLOGIC HISTORY

Following is a suggested outline for the gynecologic history, the necessary details of which are different from those emphasized in the general medical or surgical history. In the emergency setting it may not be possible to get a full history, and attention may have to be directed initially at symptoms, e.g., control of bleeding. However, it is important for accuracy in complex evaluations of undifferentiated acute pelvic problems to proceed with an organized history when circumstance allows.

Chief Complaint: In patient's own words.

History of Present Illness: Pain (pelvic, abdominal, shoulder, genitals, breast), bleeding, amenorrhea, discharge.

Past Medical History and Family History: Often of special significance in relation to the pregnant woman and/or her baby.

Menstrual History: Menarche, regularity, flow. (Date of last menstrual period and previous menstrual period, clots, dysmenorrhea, intermenstrual bleeding, leukorrhea, pruritus, premenstrual distress, hot flashes, hormones.)

Urinary: Frequency, urgency, dysuria, hematuria, stress incontinence, previous infections.

Bowel: Regularity, tenesmus, bleeding, constipation, diarrhea.

Sexual History: Contraceptive method, duration of use, any problems encountered, dyspareunia.

Obstetric History: Date of deliveries, length of gestation, method of delivery, complications during pregnancy, labor or postpartum. Weight and condition of infant at birth. Abortion history.

GYNECOLOGIC EXAMINATION

Vital signs and general screening examination should be recorded in every case, not only in relation to the diagnosis per se but also for evaluation of the risk and influence on management. Because of its direct bearing on many obstetric and gynecologic problems, examination of the breasts, abdomen, costovertebral angles, and lower extremities is considered part of the gynecologic examination. Examination of the external genitalia, speculum examination of the vagina and cervix, bimanual palpation, and rectovaginal examination are essentials of the basic examination of the female pelvis.

459

SPECIAL PROCEDURES

URINE EXAMINATION

The bladder should always be empty before any attempt is made to evaluate the pelvic findings. Because the problem of differentiation of a urinary tract disorder from a gynecologic problem arises so frequently, a catheterized or clean voided specimen serves the dual purpose of eliminating unnecessary difficulties in pelvic examination, smear, and culture as indicated.

SMEARS, CULTURES, AND SUSPENSIONS OF VAGINAL DISCHARGES

Determination of the specific cause for pelvic infections is important in most cases, critical in many. Lower genital tract gonorrheal infection involves the paraurethral and cervical glands predominantly. Cultures should be obtained directly from secretions of these glands. Stripping of the urethra from above downward toward the meatus will evacuate secretions for collection on a cotton swab. A Gram stain showing intracellular diplococci can make the diagnosis of gonococcal infection (see Chapter 43, Fig. 1). Those secretions collected from the cervical glands are too often contaminated with free discharges in the vagina. This problem can be minimized by wiping the cervix and vagina with a dry cotton ball and inserting the swab or small wire loop directly into the cervical canal. The same precautions must be observed in obtaining uterine cultures in cases of postabortal or puerperal sepsis.

WET SUSPENSIONS

The profuse irritating vaginal discharges of Trichomonas infections can be identified in minutes by obtaining a sample of the secretions from the vagina, inserting the swab immediately into a test tube containing 1 or 2 cc. of normal saline solution and examining a drop microscopically without staining. The large motile flagellates are readily identifiable (Fig. 1). Using the same solution and adding two or three drops of 10 per cent aqueous potassium hydroxide makes the mycelia and spores of vaginal Candida readily seen (Fig. 2).

CYTOLOGIC EXAMINATIONS

Contamination of material collected for Papanicolaou smears with vaginal lubricant greatly distorts the cells. Using a speculum moistened with warm water, the cervix and upper vagina may be exposed and smears obtained from three areas. Separate cotton tipped applicators are used to obtain the sample from the vaginal pool in the posterior fornix of the vagina and from the cervical canal. These are rolled individually on clean

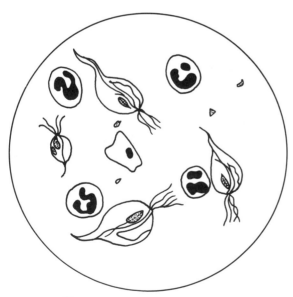

Figure 1 Trichomonas vaginalis.

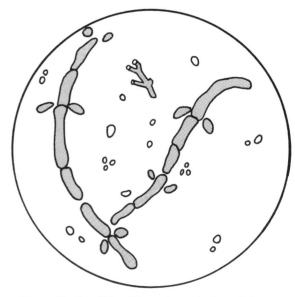

Figure 2 *Candida albicans* in vaginal candidiasis.

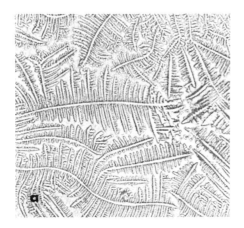

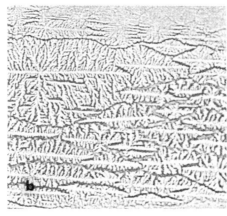

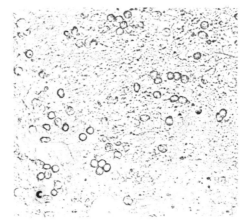

Figure 3 Arborization of cervical mucus. *a*, plus 3 fern; *b*, plus 2 fern; *c*, negative fern.

glass slides. A third sample is obtained by scraping the entire circumference of the cervix with an Ayre spatula or tongue blade. Each of the samples is fixed immediately in equal parts 95 per cent alcohol–ether solution or dry-fixed with a cytologic spray.

RAPID TEST FOR PREGNANCY

A slide test employing immunologic principles is the simplest and most rapid method. One drop of the urine to be tested is added to one drop of the anti-human-chorionic gonadotropin (HCG) rabbit serum and mixed for 30 seconds on a glass slide. Two drops of a suspension of latex particles coated with HCG are added and the slide rocked for 2 minutes. The test is negative if agglutination of the HCG coated latex particles is observed. The HCG in pregnancy urine inhibits agglutination. No flocculations are seen, and the test is positive. The test is somewhat less sensitive than other available methods that require longer periods of time.

EXAMINATION OF CERVICAL MUCUS (FERN TEST)

Rapid assessment of the patient's hormonal status is often possible by examination of the cervical mucus. Arborization or ferning of crystalline materials in the mucus occurs only in the presence of unopposed estrogen stimulation (Fig. 3). Thus it is seen in increasing amounts during the first half of the menstrual cycle, becoming maximal at the time of ovulation, when pain may be the problem (mittelschmerz). It is inhibited in the second half of the cycle by progesterone, and should be negative even during the earliest stages of normal pregnancy.

Mucus secretions are obtained from the cervical canal using a cotton tipped applicator or uterine dressing forceps, spread directly on a clean glass slide and air-dried for about 10 minutes. The microscopic appearance of ferning is unmistakable. The test cannot be performed if the mucus is mixed with blood.

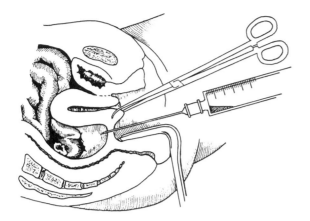

Figure 4 Culdocentesis. (From Willson, J. R., Beecham, C. T., and Carrington, E. R.: Obstetrics and Gynecology, 5th ed. St. Louis, The C. V. Mosby Co., 1975.)

CULDOCENTESIS

Cul-de-sac aspiration may be used to identify peritoneal fluid, blood, or pus within the abdominal cavity (Fig. 4). The cervix is elevated and tension maintained with a tenaculum. A 15-gauge needle is inserted in the midline of the posterior fornix 1 to 1.5 cm. from the cervix. If tension is not well maintained the peritoneum may be pushed ahead of the needle and thus the peritoneal cavity is not entered. A false-negative aspiration is most commonly due to this error.

References

Beller, F. K., et al.: Gynecology: A Textbook for Students. New York, Springer Verlag, 1974.

Green, T. H., Jr.: Gynecology: Essentials of Clinical Practice, 2d ed. Boston, Little, Brown & Co., 1971.

Willson, J. R., Beecham, C. T., and Carrington, E. R.: Obstetrics and Gynecology, 5th ed. St. Louis, The C. V. Mosby Co., 1975.

Part III

CLINICAL EMERGENCY MEDICINE

Section I

EVALUATION OF SELECTED COMMON PRESENTATIONS

Chapter 20

EVALUATION OF ACUTE ABDOMINAL PAIN

Mohammed T. Younis

DECISION TREE

ABDOMINAL PAIN

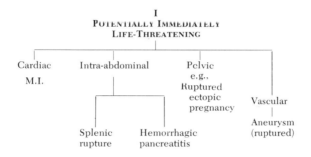

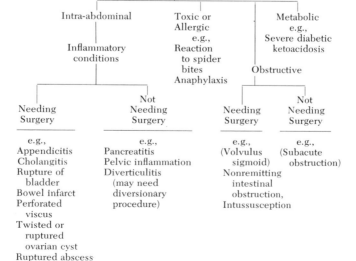

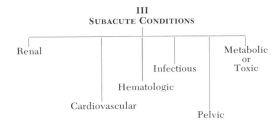

Pain, it has been said, is one of "Nature's earliest signs of morbidity." Few will deny that it stands pre-eminent among all the sensory experiences by which man judges the existence of disease within himself. There are relatively few maladies that will not have their painful phases, and in many of them pain is a characteristic without which diagnosis must always be in doubt.

Abdominal pain is one of the most common conditions calling for speedy diagnosis and treatment. Usually, though by no means always, other symptoms accompany the pain, but in most cases of acute abdominal disease pain is the main symptom and complaint. For accurate evaluation, it is necessary to understand both neuroanatomy and the several types of abdominal pain.

NEUROANATOMY

Both the somatic (or cerebrospinal) nervous system and the autonomic nervous system are involved in the phenomenon of abdominal pain. Sensations can arise from the viscera, skin, or muscle and then be carried via autonomic nervous system fibers (via spinal cord posterior horn), eventually reaching the brain. Neurologic disease involving the cord may alter or even abolish pain sensation (e.g., amyotrophic lateral sclerosis) (Fig. 1).

TYPES OF ABDOMINAL PAIN

Three distinct types of pain may be involved in the symptom complex of abdominal pain. These are: visceral pain (deep), somatic pain, and referred pain.

VISCERAL PAIN

True visceral pain or splanchnic pain is caused by sudden stretch or distention of a viscus, stimulating the autonomic nervous plexus in its wall (e.g., contraction against obstruction) and is interpreted as "crampy" or "gaseous" pain, usually intermittent and referred to the midline of the abdomen. If the viscus involved is derived from the foregut, the crampy pain will be epigastric; midgut pain is periumbilical; and hindgut pain is hypogastric. Visceral pain tends to be rather diffuse and poorly localized, has a high threshold (i.e., usually normal intestinal movements and mild stretch are not perceived), and exhibits an exceedingly slow rate of adaptation (i.e., the individual does not become tolerant to the pain, nor do impulses from the viscera diminish substantially). With severe visceral or deep somatic pain, concomitant responses, presumably due to autonomic or somatic reflexes, may be prominent. These include sweating, nausea (sometimes with vomiting), tachycardia or bradycardia, fall in flood pressure, cutaneous hyperalgesia, hyperesthesia or tenderness, and involuntary spastic contractions of the abdominal wall musculature. The distribution is regional rather than segmental and thus involves sustained reflexes in several segmental nerves. *Most acute intra-abdominal inflammatory diseases requiring operation are preceded by obstruction (whether anatomic or functional) and the earliest clinical symptoms and signs will be related to the visceral pain component.* Examples of intra-abdominal conditions that usually demonstrate this early visceral phase are appendicitis, cholecystitis (biliary colic, or common duct stone), intestinal obstruction, and pancreatitis.

SOMATIC PAIN

This occurs when fibers located in the parietal peritoneum are stimulated by chemical or bacterial inflammation. Pain arising in the abdominal wall, particularly the parietal peritoneum, root of the mesentery, and the

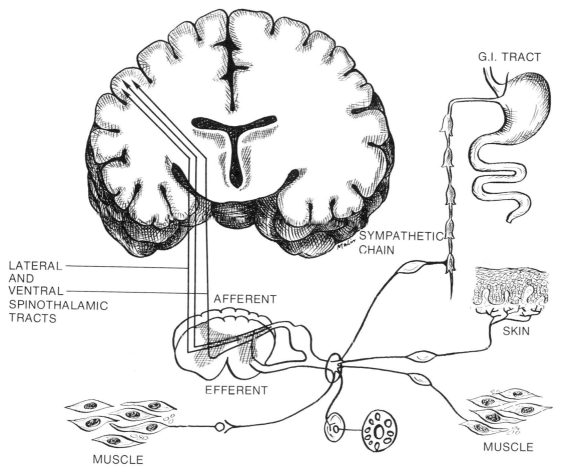

Figure 1 Pathways involved in abdominal pain.

respiratory diaphragm is mediated by somatic afferents in segmental spinal nerves. Pain from parietal structures is for the most part sharper than visceral pain, better localized, and closer to the actual site of stimulation. Any stimulation of the involved peritoneum will produce the pain, so that the patient lies quietly, often with the thighs flexed to relax the peritoneum. Any attempt to palpate the involved area is guarded against by muscular contraction, producing one of the most reliable signs of peritonitis: involuntary guarding. Rebound tenderness is present, as is tenderness to palpation. The peritoneal-intestinal reflex produces cessation of bowel contraction, and therefore bowel sounds may be absent.

Acute appendicitis is a common disease that well illustrates typical visceral and somatic abdominal pain. The visceral pain of early appendicitis is perceived diffusely and dully in the periumbilical and lower epigastric regions, and there is little or no rigidity of the abdominal musculature. Later, when the parietal peritoneum becomes involved in the inflammatory process, the somatic component of pain is more severe and sharply localized in the right lower quadrant. There may also be cutaneous hyperesthesia, tenderness, and muscular rigidity in the right lower quadrant.

REFERRED PAIN

Visceral disease may give rise to pain localized in more superficial areas of the body, often at a considerable distance from the diseased viscus. The reference is usually dermatomic (e.g., neck pain from diaphragmatic irritation). On occasion, pain may be referred to the scar of a previous surgical operation, trauma, or localized pathologic process. This latter is called "habit reference" and implies that pain perception is influenced by the individual's prior pain experience.

The subjective nature of abdominal pain must also be considered. Since pain is a symptom, the patient's reactivity to pain and his pain tolerance become important. Elderly people frequently seem to experience less pain, or perhaps complain less. Certain social cultures encourage more verbal expression of pain, whereas in others a more stoic attitude toward pain is encouraged and thus the magnitude of pain will be underemphasized. In American society, many men feel that the expression of pain is a sign of weakness and, in fact, pain medication is more commonly perscribed for women. The individual's prior reactions to painful stimuli are a good indication of his or her reactivity. Despite this, certain conditions, such as renal colic, produce such intense pain that even the tolerance of stoic men is usually surpassed.

ETIOLOGY

Abdominal pain is the most common presenting symptom associated with intra-abdominal disease. The etiologic classification in Table 1, although not complete, provides a useful frame of reference for the evaluation of patients with abdominal pain.

CLINICAL EVALUATION

The diagnosis of "acute or surgical abdomen" so often heard in Emergency Departments is not an acceptable one because of its often misleading and erroneous connotation. The most obvious of "acute abdomens" may not require operative intervention, and the mildest of abdominal pains may herald the onset of a lesion requiring urgent correction. The general rule can be laid down that most instances of severe abdominal pain in patients who previously have been well lasting as long as six hours are caused by conditions of surgical import. There are exceptions, but the generalization is useful if it serves to call attention to the need for early diagnosis. Any patient with abdominal pain of recent onset requires early and thorough evaluation with specific attempts at accurate diagnosis.

The emergency physician has three decisions to make in approaching this problem, the first being that of appropriate diagnosis—as precise as is possible following a brief period of observation—and, second, that of indicated treatment, particularly deciding whether the patient is a candidate for emergency surgery or whether surgery may be required within days. The third decision is—if an operation is not immediately needed or needed within days—whether deterioration in the patient's condition will likely occur without hospitalization. The evaluation must be sufficient to allow this decision to be made. In some cases observation of the dynamics and serial testing may be needed to arrive at the clinical decision.

Few abdominal conditions require such urgent operative intervention that an orderly approach need be abandoned, no matter

TABLE 1   Some Important Causes of Abdominal Pain

I. Pain originating in the abdomen
  A. Parietal peritoneal inflammation
    1. Bacterial contamination, e.g., perforated appendix, pelvic inflammatory disease, diverticulitis
    2. Chemical irritation, e.g., perforated ulcer, pancreatitis, mittelschmerz
  B. Mechanical obstruction of hollow viscera
    1. Obstruction of the small or large intestine (including incarcerated hernia)
    2. Obstruction of the biliary tree
    3. Obstruction of the ureter
  C. Vascular disturbances
    1. Embolism or thrombosis
    2. Vascular rupture
    3. Pressure or torsional occlusion
    4. Sickle cell anemia
  D. Abdominal wall
    1. Distortion or traction of mesentery
    2. Trauma or infection of muscles
    3. Distention of visceral surfaces, e.g., hepatic or renal capsules
II. Pain referred from extra-abdominal source
  A. Thorax, e.g., pneumonia, referred pain from coronary occlusion
  B. Spine, e.g., radiculitis from arthritis
  C. Genitalia e.g., torsion of the spermatic cord
III. Metabolic causes
  A. Exogenous
    1. Black widow spider bite
    2. Lead poisoning and others
  B. Endogenous
    1. Uremia
    2. Diabetic coma
    3. Porphyria
    4. Allergic factors
IV. Neurogenic causes
  A. Organic
    1. Tabes dorsalis
    2. Herpes zoster
    3. Causalgia and others
  B. Functional

how ill the patient. Only those patients with exsanguinating hemorrhage must be rushed to the operating room, but in such instances only a few minutes are required to assess the clinical nature of the problem. Also, immediate treatment is essential when "third-space" losses produce shock. Immediately life-threatening conditions include splenic rupture, rupture of ectopic pregnancy, and aneurysm. Hemorrhagic pancreatitis is one condition of acute blood loss, however, where operative intervention is not indicated.

Patients with abdominal complaints should be placed in a private cubicle and should not be neglected in the press of other emergencies, as their condition may be dynamic and rapid deterioration can occur. They should be evaluated soon after admission to the Emergency Department and a rapid estimate made of the seriousness of their problem. The patient should be prepared by the nurse; his pulse, blood pressure, and temperature should be taken; and he should be completely undressed. It is a dangerous compromise to try to examine a patient through an aperture in his clothing. In order to come to a conclusion regarding the disposition of the patient, a presumptive diagnosis must be made. Three basic questions should first be answered: Has the patient perforated a hollow viscus? Is he bleeding? Is he obstructed? In essence, how advanced is the inflammatory process, how severe is the hemorrhage, how complete the obstruction? The history and complete physical examination, with the aid of a few laboratory studies and x-rays, should enable the examiner to come to a rapid decision about disposition and further treatment. Nowhere in medicine is a meticulously executed detailed history and physical examination of greater importance.

History

Nothing will supplant an orderly, painstakingly detailed history, which is far more valuable than other laboratory or roentgenologic examination.

CLINICAL VARIATIONS AND THEIR INTERPRETATION

Clinical assessment of abdominal pain requires careful analysis with respect to onset, location, character, and symptoms associated with pain. Particular key findings in the history must alert the examining physician to seek other signs of serious disease. Pain that awakens a person from sleep, onset where the patient can describe when it began almost to the minute, changing abdominal pain (from visceral-type to localized), and pain associated with symptoms of hypovolemia are among these.

Onset of Pain

EXACT TIME AND ACTIVITY AT ONSET

Sudden, abrupt pain in which the patient recalls the precise moment when the pain started is consistent with acute perforation, strangulation, torsion, or vascular accident. Such entities as a ruptured ectopic pregnancy, perforated ulcer, mesenteric vascular occlusion, splenic or renal infarct, and ruptured corpus luteum should all be considered if the onset of pain is abrupt and severe. In case of acute perforation of a hollow viscus, the patient frequently likens this to being struck with a severe blow. Inflammatory lesions and obstructive phenomena generally develop more slowly. Pain that begins suddenly but reaches a maximum more slowly suggests pancreatitis or cholecystitis. Appendicitis must be kept in mind; this is the most common pathologic process seen in patients complaining of abdominal pain in the Emergency Department, and it may present in aberrant patterns. In patients with intestinal obstruction, appendicitis, or diverticulitis, the pain is more likely to have a gradual onset.

SEVERITY OF PAIN AT ONSET

Although not invariably the case, the most acute entities often cause the most intense or severe pain. Notable exceptions involve blood loss where symptoms of hypovolemia may overshadow those of pain. Severe pain that interferes with normal activity is apt to be significant. A perforated peptic ulcer characteristically results in a very severe pain due to the highly irritating nature of the duodenal and gastric content with rapid dissemination throughout the abdomen. On the other hand, the pain of acute pancreatitis is a result of retroperitoneal and

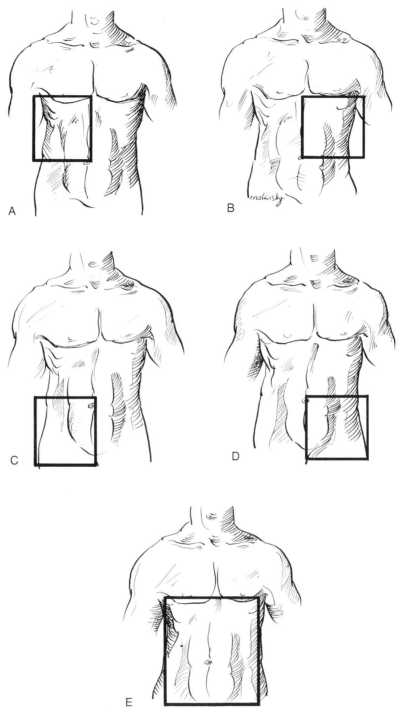

Figure 2. Differential diagnosis of acute abdominal pain by location.

A, *Right upper quadrant pain:*
Acute cholecystitis and biliary colic
Acute hepatitis
Hepatic abscess
Hepatomegaly due to congestive failure
Perforated duodenal ulcer
Acute pancreatitis (bilateral pain)

Retrocecal appendicitis
Renal pain due to acute pyelonephritis
Herpes zoster
Myocardial ischemia
Pericarditis
Pneumonia with pleural reaction
Empyema

Legend continued on opposite page.

intraperitoneal dissemination of enzyme-laden fluid that usually does not cause pain of as great intensity as is experienced in perforated ulcer. Colon perforation (diverticulitis, perforated carcinoma, trauma) is also marked by pain of moderate intensity at first, but the degree of pain increases with time until the patient develops findings quite similar to those of the perforated ulcer patient. Collapse or fainting with onset of abdominal pain testifies to its severity, and is often found with perforation of a viscus, dissecting aneurysm, acute hemorrhagic pancreatitis, or ruptured ectopic pregnancy.

Location of Pain

The location of pain should include a description of original situation, any shifting, and radiation. The initial location may better define the viscera involved, since, once peritonitis occurs, pains become diffuse. Because of variations in location of the organs and the pathologic process plus the vagueness of visceral pain it is difficult to totally exclude diseases on the basis of location, but certain relationships generally pertain. Figure 2 shows the characteristic location of abdominal pain associated with various diseases.

LOCATION AT ONSET

Certain viscera provide reasonably good localization of the pain they generate; others provide little information in this regard. The stomach and duodenum, for example, are quite reliable, and pain localization is invariably in the vicinity of the epigastrium, either to the right or left of the midline. Typically, right upper quadrant pain suggests cholecystitis, right lower quadrant pain acute appendicitis. The pain in pancreatitis localizes reasonably well in the upper abdomen. The appendix classically causes pain in the right lower quadrant. Tube and ovary usually yield pain to the right or left of the suprapubic area, although with extension of inflammation the location may simulate that of typical appendicitis. Other organs such as the small intestines, provide poor pain localization. The pain may be perceived anywhere in the abdomen, although periumbilical pain is most commonly observed.

Figure 2 (Continued)
B, Left upper quadrant pain:
Gastritis
Acute pancreatitis
Splenic enlargement, rupture, infarction, aneurysm
Renal pain due to acute pyelonephritis
Myocardial ischemia
Pneumonia, with pleural reaction
Perforated gastric or marginal ulcer
Ruptured aortic aneurysm
Perforated colon (tumor, foreign body)

C, Right lower quadrant pain:
Appendicitis
Intestinal obstruction
Regional enteritis
Meckel's diverticulitis
Cecal diverticulitis
Cholecystitis
Perforated ulcer
Leaking aneurysm
Abdominal wall hematoma
Ruptured ectopic pregnancy
Twisted ovarian cyst
Acute salpingitis, tube ovarian abscess
Mittelschmerz
Endometriosis
Ureteral calculi
Renal pain
Seminal vesiculitis
Psoas abscess
Mesenteric adenitis
Incarcerated, strangulated groin hernia
Perforated cecum (tumor, foreign body)

D, Left lower quadrant pain:
Sigmoid diverticulitis
Intestinal obstruction
Appendicitis
Leaking aneurysm
Abdominal wall hematoma
Ruptured ectopic pregnancy
Mittelschmerz
Twisted ovarian cyst
Acute salpingitis, tube ovarian abscess
Endometriosis
Ureteral calculi
Renal pain
Seminal vesiculitis
Psoas abscess
Incarcerated, strangulated groin hernia
Perforated descending colon (tumor, foreign body)
Regional enteritis

E, Diffuse pain:
Peritonitis
Acute pancreatitis
Leukemia
Sickle cell crisis
Early appendicitis
Mesenteric adenitis
Mesenteric thrombosis
Gastroenteritis
Dissecting or rupturing aneurysm
Colitis
Intestinal obstruction
Uremia, diabetes mellitus
Diverticulitis, small intestine or colon
Strangulated groin hernia

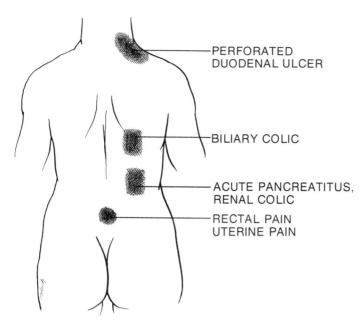

Figure 3. Posterior surface of body showing the sites to which pain is referred in some acute abdominal conditions.

CHANGE IN THE LOCATION OF PAIN

Pain may become localized with abscess formation from inflammatory lesions. It may become generalized with perforation of an abscess. Periumbilical pain that becomes right lower quadrant in location suggests acute appendicitis. Sudden cessation of pain can signal perforation with later development of peritonitis.

RADIATION OR REFERRAL OF PAIN

Certain disorders have typical patterns of pain radiation that may be diagnostic (Figs. 3 and 4).

Biliary tract pain traditionally radiates around the right side to the back and angle of the scapula, whereas pain of pancreatic origin frequently radiates directly through to the back on either side or directly in the

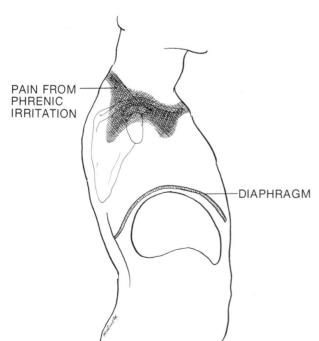

Figure 4. Diagram indicating the area in which phrenic irritation may cause pain.

midline. Posterior penetration of a peptic ulcer also may be referred to the back.

Collection of blood or pus under the diaphragm often will cause aching pain in the top of the shoulder.

Ruptured or leaking aneurysms will give pain in the lumbosacral area and occasionally in the upper thighs.

Renal colic is often referred to the groin and external genitalia.

Appendiceal pain for an entirely different reason occasionally commences in the epigastrium and ultimately migrates to the right lower quadrant. This radiation pattern (the epigastric component) is caused by the reflex pylorospasm that accompanies the onset of appendicitis.

In uterine and rectal disease, pain is referred to the lower back.

Character of Pain

It is not enough to know that the patient has abdominal pain. One must determine its exact character (Fig. 5).

Excruciating pain indicates a vascular lesion, such as massive infarction of the intestine or rupture of an abdominal aneurysm.

Very severe pain readily controlled by medication is more typical of acute pancreatitis or the peritonitis associated with a ruptured viscus. Obstructive appendicitis and incarcerated small bowel without extensive infarction occasionally produce the same type of pain. The intense pain of biliary or renal colic is usually alleviated by medication.

If the pain is dull, vague, and poorly localized, it is also likely to have a gradual onset. These findings suggest an inflammatory process or a low grade infection.

Intermittent pain with cramps and rushes is commonly seen in gastroenteritis. However, if the pain comes in regular cycles, rising in crescendo fashion and then subsiding to a pain-free interval, the most likely diagnosis is mechanical small bowel obstruction. This type of pain occurs occasionally in subacute pancreatitis. If auscultation reveals intermittent peristaltic rushes rising in crescendo fashion and synchronous with pain, small bowel obstruction is very likely. In large bowel obstruction this crampy pain is confined to the lower abdomen and is not as severe as with small bowel

obstruction, which is characteristically periumbilical.

SYMPTOMS ASSOCIATED WITH PAIN

ANOREXIA, NAUSEA, AND VOMITING

Anorexia, nausea, and vomiting are common symptoms of acute abdominal disease, and careful analysis of the character of these symptoms may be of great value in arriving at the correct diagnosis.

When nausea and vomiting are very prominent symptoms, the most likely possibilities are gastroenteritis, acute gastritis, acute pancreatitis, common duct stone, and high intestinal obstruction.

Intractable or fecal vomiting suggests obstruction; pain of high obstruction may be relieved by vomiting.

Presence of blood in the vomitus suggests peptic ulcer disease, or gastritis.

Severe vomiting with retching, particularly following a dietary indiscretion or an alcoholic bout, should immediately suggest laceration of the gastroesophageal junction (Mallory-Weiss syndrome) or an esophageal perforation (Boerhaave syndrome). Massive hematemesis or severe pain radiating into the chest and left shoulder in association with severe vomiting and retching make these critical emergencies very likely.

Pain usually precedes the vomiting in acute appendicitis.

BOWEL HABITS (DIARRHEA, CONSTIPATION, AND OBSTIPATION)

Some alteration of bowel function is common in most cases of acute abdominal emergencies, but the variations are extraordinary.

Diarrhea associated with vomiting is typical of such inflammatory diseases as gastroenteritis.

Often more significant than the history of constipation is the history of failure to pass flatus. If the patient has not passed flatus in 24 hours, he most certainly has profound paralytic ileus or intestinal obstruction.

A history of decreased stool caliber suggests a neoplasm of the distal colon or rectum.

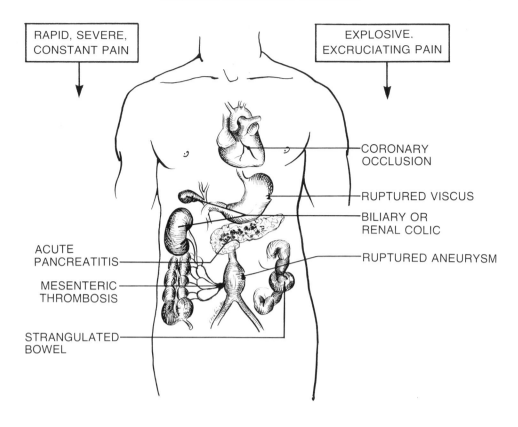

RAPID, SEVERE, CONSTANT PAIN

EXPLOSIVE. EXCRUCIATING PAIN

CORONARY OCCLUSION

RUPTURED VISCUS

BILIARY OR RENAL COLIC

RUPTURED ANEURYSM

ACUTE PANCREATITIS

MESENTERIC THROMBOSIS

STRANGULATED BOWEL

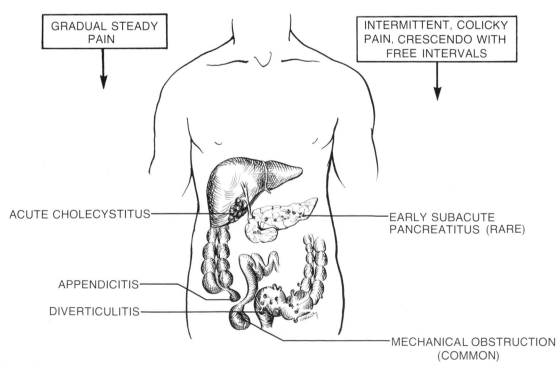

GRADUAL STEADY PAIN

INTERMITTENT, COLICKY PAIN, CRESCENDO WITH FREE INTERVALS

ACUTE CHOLECYSTITUS

EARLY SUBACUTE PANCREATITUS (RARE)

APPENDICITIS

DIVERTICULITIS

MECHANICAL OBSTRUCTION (COMMON)

Figure 5. Differential diagnosis of acute abdominal pain by character.

Clay-colored stools occur with biliary obstruction.

Melena is usually a sign of high intestinal bleeding.

Bright red rectal bleeding occurs in low intestinal lesions.

Bloody and repetitive diarrhea indicates ulceration of the colon. Ulcerative colitis, Crohn's disease, and bacillary and amebic dysentery must be considered. Although bloody diarrhea is often mentioned as a symptom of massive thrombosis, it actually occurs rather rarely in this condition.

CHILLS AND FEVER

Repeated chills and fever characterize pyelonephritis and bacteremia. Their presence in suspected appendicitis strongly suggests perforation.

Repeated chills and fever are most common in infections of the biliary or renal tract. Acute cholecystitis and acute pyelitis usually present with intermittent chills and fever. Chills, fever, jaundice, and hypotension indicate suppurative cholangitis—a surgical emergency.

URINARY SYMPTOMS

Hematuria or dysuria suggests renal colic or a urinary tract infection.

GYNECOLOGIC HISTORY AND SYMPTOMS

An increase in vaginal discharge is frequently associated with pelvic inflammatory disease. A recent untimely menstrual period also suggests pelvic inflammatory disease.

Vaginal bleeding and/or a missed menstrual period should suggest an accident of pregnancy.

CARDIORESPIRATORY SYMPTOMS

Palpitation may indicate the presence of atrial fibrillation and embolic disease. Angina and claudication suggest an ischemic bowel or cardiac disease.

PAST MEDICAL HISTORY, PREVIOUS HOSPITALIZATIONS, AND ABDOMINAL OPERATIONS

It is particularly important to know whether there have been previous episodes of similar pain and what the diagnosis was at that time. Ask specifically about past x-ray examinations—for example, barium enemas, upper gastrointestinal series, and gallbladder x-rays. It is also important to know whether the patient has been hospitalized in the past. Many patients with pancreatitis, pelvic inflammatory disease, kidney stones, or peptic ulcer may have had previous admissions for these recurrent problems. Knowledge of prior abdominal surgery is essential to correct interpretation of the new complaint. Inquiry about previous removal of the appendix is important. A telephone call to the record room of the previous admitting hospital often proves enlightening. Also relatives or friends accompanying the patient to the Emergency Department should be questioned. They may well add to the validity of the history, especially concerning very young or elderly patients. One must not minimize the complaints of patients known to have hypochondriacal tendencies. Drug addicts may be extremely clever in their portrayal of a patient with abdominal pain. The severe symptoms they relate, however, are not in accord with the physical findings. Careful physical examination may also reveal evidence of their addiction, such as scarring of the arm with thrombosis of the superficial veins. Past history of any medical disease may shed light on its possible association with the present abdominal pain.

OTHER DIAGNOSTIC POINTS AND ASSOCIATED EVENTS

1. Gastrointestinal distress in others sharing the same meal suggests gastroenteritis.

2. Recent ingestion of fatty food is associated with acute cholecystitis.

3. With a history of alcoholic excess, pancreatitis must be ruled out.

4. The age of the patient is of considerable consequence, since some diseases are largely limited to certain age groups. Appendicitis is generally a disease of patients between 5 and 50 years; intussusception is primarily seen under the age of 2; cholecystitis is unusual under the age of 20; colon obstruction is uncommon under the age of 35.

5. It is helpful to know whether the patient has taken any medication or used any

other measures to relieve his pain. A history of antacid ingestion suggests peptic ulcer disease. Vomiting (frequently digitally induced) producing relief from pain is indication of ulcer or high obstruction. Relief of pain with passing of flatus or after an enema could indicate incomplete left colon obstruction. Also important is any history of administration of anticoagulants. Moreover, barbiturates may precipitate an attack of porphyria.

6. It is important to inquire about taking adrenal steroids or recent intake of antibiotics. It is well known that adrenal steroid therapy diminishes the symptoms produced by inflammation. Any acute inflammation that may arise, with either localized or generalized peritonitis, without usual symptoms and signs of such inflammation being sufficiently clear could cause alarm. It follows that diminution of abdominal pain in patients being treated by corticosteroids makes it imperative to consider even slight abdominal pain as serious. If the patient has recently taken antibiotics, an allowance must be made for any possible action of these drugs. Antibiotics cannot seal a perforation of the appendix, but they can diminish the symptoms of the ensuing peritonitis.

7. If bleeding is suspected, but the site not apparent, investigate the retroperitoneum.

PHYSICAL EXAMINATION

Thoroughness and a systematic approach are important. An examination pattern rigidly adhered to will pay handsome dividends in these patients. The exception, of course, is with those conditions which upon initial assessment pose an immediate threat to life. In these cases therapy must precede further diagnosis.

General Considerations and Vital Signs

The *appearance* of the patient frequently will give some general clues as to the severity of the illness. The position the patient assumes in order to obtain relief from pain can also be extremely helpful in diagnosis. The patient with pancreatitis characteristically lies on his side, with the vertebral column, knees, and hips flexed. This position relaxes the psoas muscle, which is irritated and in spasm because of the retroperitoneal inflammation. Patients with retrocecal appendicitis occasionally flex the right hip and knee in order to relax the right psoas muscle. The patient with diffuse peritonitis of any etiology commonly prefers to lie in bed in an immobile state. Motion or position change is resisted because of the exquisite pain occasioned by movement of the parietal peritoneum.

Temperature elevation is common in patients with acute abdominal disease, although the temperature is likely to be normal or only slightly elevated early in the course of the disease. It is essential that all the temperatures be obtained rectally and that the thermometer be left in place for a sufficient period of time.

Usually, the temperature in patients with acute appendicitis, acute cholecystitis, uncomplicated intestinal obstruction, ruptured ectopic pregnancy, sigmoid diverticulitis, and other acute surgical emergencies may be close to normal; the initial temperature will rarely exceed 38° C. (101° F.) rectally. When perforation occurs, or intestine becomes gangrenous, the temperature will increase to 39 to 40° C. (103 to 104° F.), but will then fall if shock ensues. Fulminant systemic infections, abscess, or infection involving the central nervous system, lungs, or urinary tract give temperatures over 40° C. (104° F.).

Tachycardia is common in patients with profound illness, such as gangrenous intestinal obstruction, diffuse peritonitis, or ruptured viscus. Serial observations, often after taking the initial pulse, are valuable. However, with acute blood loss, even up to 20 per cent of total blood volume, an initial reflex bradycardia may be seen.

Respiration should be assessed. Grunting, shallow respiration with a relatively motionless abdomen suggests peritonitis. Kussmaul respiration (deep and rapid without sensation of dyspnea) may be due to metabolic acidosis and points to the medical etiology of abdominal pain. Very rapid respiratory rates are observed in patients with peritonitis, pancreatitis, frank hemorrhage, shock, and similar lesions.

Hypotension with abdominal pain should alert one to a surgical emergency or to a hemorrhagic pancreatitis.

TABLE 2 *Routine for Physical Examination of Acute Abdomen*

1. Inspection
2. Cough tenderness; examine hernial rings and male genitalia
3. Feel for spasm
4. One-finger palpation
5. Costovertebral tenderness
6. Deep palpation
7. Rebound tenderness
8. Auscultation
9. Special signs
10. Rectal and pelvic examination

Inspection of the Abdomen (Table 2)

On inspection restrained motion of the abdominal wall during respiration suggests diffuse peritonitis. Maintenance of the hip in a position of flexion is suggestive of psoas abscess, appendicitis, or pelvic abscess. Distention may accompany bowel obstruction or paralytic ileus. Visible peristalsis or visible small bowel loops are clues to intestinal obstruction. Ascites may provide a clue to carcinoma or liver disease. The presence of a pulsatile mass must raise the possibility of an aneurysm. Abdominal distention is best assessed by measuring the abdominal girth at the umbilicus and by viewing the lateral contour of the anterior surface of the abdomen in relation to an imaginary line between the symphysis pubis and the xyphoid process. In patients without distention, the anterior abdominal border usually will be observed to lie below the xyphopubic line. Even in the very obese patient, when the individual lies flat in bed the normal abdominal contour is scaphoid or nearly so. With moderate distention, the lateral appearance of the abdomen on inspection is at or slightly above the xyphopubic line. With more severe distention, a greater disparity exists, until at extreme distention there is marked tightness and gross rounding of the abdominal contour.

Cough Tenderness, Examination of Hernial Ring and Male Genitalia

The next step is to examine the inguinal and femoral canals in both sexes and the genitalia in the male. This must be done very gently, asking the patient to cough but causing as little discomfort as possible. Her-

nias present as acute emergencies when they finally become irreducible. This event may or may not be attended by local pain and tenderness. Regardless of the presence or absence of symptoms and signs suggesting strangulation, an acutely incarcerated hernia must be considered strangulated until proved otherwise. Patients presenting with clinical evidence of acute intestinal obstruction as well as patients with local pain, tenderness, edema, or redness of the skin are surgical emergencies. While the patient is coughing, if he is then asked to point one finger to where he feels the pain one objective localization of the lesion is obtained. With this information in hand the examiner can proceed to examine the abdomen, deliberately avoiding the area he knows to be most tender.

Palpation

Palpation of the abdomen is the most important facet of the physical examination. It should be done gently, as gentle palpation is much more rewarding than is deep palpation. Subtle changes are revealed, and the patient is not stressed into voluntary

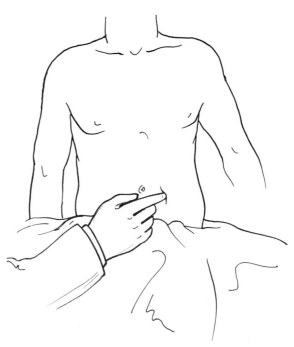

Figure 6 One finger palpation is the best way to localize an area of tenderness.

guarding. It is helpful to distract the patient, especially children, while palpating the abdomen. Observation of the facial expression of the patient during examination often gives a clue to the seriousness of the problem. It is important to examine both sides of the abdomen with both hands, the examiner's right hand examining the left side of the patient's abdomen, his left hand the right side.

SPASM

To establish the presence or absence of true spasm, the hand is placed gently over the rectus abdominus muscle and then depresses it slightly and gently, without causing pain. Properly performed, this manuever is a comforting one to the patient. Now ask the patient to take a long breath. If the spasm is voluntary, the muscle will immediately relax underneath the gentle pressure of the palpating hand. If there is true spasm, however, the muscle will remain taut and rigid throughout the respiratory cycle. This maneuver alone is sufficient to establish the presence of peritonitis. Except for rare neurologic disorders—and for reasons no one understands—only peritoneal inflammation produces abdominal muscular rigidity. In renal colic, the spasm is confined to the entire rectus muscle on one side.

TEST FOR ABDOMINAL TENDERNESS

The test for abdominal tenderness must be done with one finger, not with the entire hand (Fig. 6). It is impossible to accurately localize peritoneal inflammation if palpation for tenderness is done with the entire hand. Careful one-finger palpation, beginning as far away as possible from the area of localized cough-elicited pain and gradually working toward it, usually will enable the examiner to determine precisely the limitation of abdominal tenderness. Abdominal tenderness which is decreased, or disappears when the patient assumes a semi-sitting position—without using his hands for support, thereby contracting his abdominal muscle—suggests an intra-abdominal cause. Conversely, abdominal tenderness originating from the muscular wall itself is intensified by this maneuver. True rigidity or intense bilateral guarding is suggestive of diffuse peritonitis. This impression can be substantiated by the finding of rebound tenderness, in which gentle manual pressure elicits somewhat less tenderness than does the sudden release of that pressure. It is extremely important not to cause excessive or intense pain by injudicious eliciting of tenderness or rebound tenderness. Obviously one tries to reduce the voluntary response and looks for involuntary reflexes secondary to peritoneal irritation. Of greater value is the finding of referred tenderness in which pressure at a distance from the inflamed viscus will cause acute tenderness over the viscus (Rovsing's sign in acute appendicitis). This suggests parietal peritoneal involvement by an inflammatory lesion. Cutaneous hyperesthesia can be demonstrated by stroking the skin with the fingernail, a pen, or some other object. Any area of skin-stroking that causes pain will indicate roughly the spinal segment innervating the area of parietal peritoneum irritated by the acute inflammatory disease.

MASSES

Having established the presence or absence of muscular rigidity and having localized the area of tenderness, the examiner now palpates more deeply for the presence of abdominal masses. Masses that descend with inspiration are related to liver, gallbladder, spleen, or kidney. Stony-hard masses may be evidence of carcinoma. Among the more common lesions identifiable with careful palpation in patients with acute abdominal pain are cholecystitis, appendicitis with early abscess formation, sigmoid diverticulitis, and leaking abdominal aneurysm.

Percussion

Percussion has a limited value in the physical examination in the Emergency Department. Fluid waves and shifting dullness may be difficult to detect and more difficult to interpret. However, the detection of tympany is a sign of intraluminal gas and may represent bowel obstruction or ileus. Massive pneumoperitoneum will also produce these findings. A large area of tympany localized to the left upper quadrant suggests acute gastric dilatation. Distention of the cecum as revealed by percussion should lead the examiner to suspect appendicitis or sigmoid obstruction. Distinguishing ascites

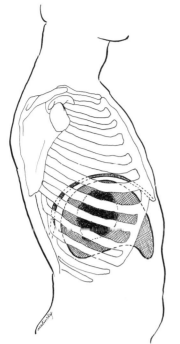

Figure 7. Darker shaded area shows area of decreased liver dullness due to free air in the peritoneal cavity.

other hand, the absence of bowel sounds may be of greater significance. Sounds of intestinal obstruction are usually characteristic, with crescendo waves reaching a maximum, coincident with crampy pain. High-pitched, tinkling sounds may be heard between the intervals of pain. Of considerable importance is the assessment of the frequency of peristaltic sounds, and to do that the abdomen should be listened to for three minutes in either of the two lower quadrants. Normal activity in the fasting state is 10 to 20 sounds per minute. The pitch of intestinal peristaltic sounds is difficult to describe and can be learned best by repeated auscultation of the abdomen. The pitch of bowel sounds depends on the tension of the wall of the intestinal tract and the length of the interface between air and fluid in that particular section of the intestine. The high-pitched bowel sounds are not always indicative of intestinal obstruction unless the other three prime findings of intestinal obstruction are observed: distention; cramping abdominal pain; and obstipation.

from ileus or obstruction is a matter of determining the percussion note as well as the presence or absence of shifting dullness. The presence of the latter sign is an indication of ascites. The presence of fluid with its dull note may signify carcinomatous ascites, portal hypertension, congestive heart failure, hemoperitoneum, or inflammatory ascites. Loss of liver dullness may represent free intraperitoneal air, as in a ruptured viscus (Fig. 7). Suprapubic dullness suggests urinary retention. Tenderness to percussion in the costovertebral angle area may signify primary renal disease, pyelonephritis, or ureteral obstruction.

Auscultation

Much attention has been paid to the presence or absence of peristaltic sounds, their quality and their frequency. Auscultation of the abdomen is probably one of the least rewarding aspects of the physical examination of a patient with acute abdominal pain. Severe catastrophes such as strangulating small intestinal obstruction may occur in the presence of normal peristalsis. On the

SPECIAL SIGNS, EXAMINATIONS, AND LABORATORY TESTS

The following special signs, examinations, and laboratory tests are helpful in diagnosis and have been summarized in Table 3.

Special signs and examinations
Iliopsoas sign (Fig. 8)
Obturator sign (Fig. 9)
Fist percussion signs
Inspiratory arrest (Murphy's sign)
Rectal and pelvic examination
Rectal examination
Pelvic examination
Pulmonary and cardiovascular examination
Laboratory tests
Blood
Serum electrolytes
Urinalysis
Serum and urine amylase
ECG
Abdominal paracentesis

RADIOLOGIC EXAMINATION

Table 4 summarizes the findings of radiologic diagnostic procedures.

TABLE 3   Special Signs and Examinations

SPECIAL SIGNS

There are several maneuvers in physical examination which may elicit confirmatory evidence of an acute abdominal lesion.

SIGN	CHARACTERISTICS
Iliopsoas Sign	The patient flexes his thigh against the resistance of the examiner's hand, (Fig. 8). A painful response indicates an inflammatory process involving the psoas muscle.
Obturator Sign	The patient's thigh is flexed to a right angle and is gently rotated internally and externally (Fig. 9). If pain is elicited, there is an inflammatory lesion involving the obturator internus muscle (pelvic appendicitis, or diverticulitis).
Fist Percussion Signs	Gentle percussion with the fist over the anterior chest wall elicits sharp pain if there is an acute inflammation involving the space between the diaphragm and liver on the right, and the stomach or spleen on the left (Fig. 10). This sign is often positive in acute hepatitis. A negative response is rare in acute cholecystitis.
Inspiratory Arrest (Murphy's Sign)	The patient is asked to take a deep breath as the examiner gently palpates the right upper quadrant. With descent of the diaphragm, an acutely inflamed gallbladder comes in contact with the examining finger, causing the patient pain and arresting the breath.
Rectal and Pelvic Examination	It is important to remember that abdominal signs may be minimal but nevertheless, if accompanied by consistent symptoms, may be exceptionally meaningful when carefully assessed. Signs may be virtually or actually totally absent in cases of pelvic peritonitis, so that careful pelvic and rectal examination are mandatory in every patient with acute abdominal pain.
Rectal Examination	The presence of a pelvic abscess of moderate to great proportion will be detected by finding severe tenderness and cul-de-sac fullness on digital examination. Fullness may be apparent in intestinal obstruction, or paralytic ileus when it is caused by markedly distended and edematous loops of intestine impinging on the pelvic structures.
Pelvic Examination	Tenderness on motion of the cervix is typical of pelvic inflammatory disease. Of great importance is the finding of a unilateral mass or extreme tenderness on one side of the pelvis or the other, most frequently suggesting appendicitis or appendiceal abscess on the right or tubo-ovarian abscess on the left. It can be most difficult to distinguish right-sided tubo-ovarian disease from an appendiceal inflammatory disease, but tenderness on manipulation of the cervix will be extreme in patients with pelvic inflammatory disease. Remember that appendicitis or diverticulitis in close proximity to pelvic organs may give an impression of primary gynecologic disease.

PULMONARY AND CARDIOVASCULAR EXAMINATION

Abdominal pain may be due to disease above the diaphragm. Rales heard on auscultation of the lungs may provide the first clue to the fact that the cause of the abdominal pain is outside the abdomen and/or has extended into the chest. The presence of atrial fibrillation or a prosthetic heart valve makes it important to rule out embolic disease with mesenteric infarction.

LABORATORY STUDIES IN THE DIAGNOSIS OF ACUTE ABDOMINAL PAIN

Laboratory examination may be of enormous value in the assessment of the patient with abdominal pain, yet with but a few exceptions they rarely establish a diagnosis. The number of laboratory tests that can be made is limited essentially by the time of the day and the imagination of the physician. Practically speaking, the diagnostic studies, apart from the examination of the urine, a complete blood count, and a few other relevant tests such as those for serum electrolytes should be accomplished after admission.

STUDY	FINDINGS
Blood	The hematocrit is of critical importance, reflecting in a significant way changes in plasma volume, particularly dehydration due to excessive vomiting or loss of fluids into the peritoneum or intestinal lumen. A low hematocrit may indicate pre-existing anemia or bleeding. The white blood cell count may be helpful if significantly elevated, or if there are serial changes. It can define the presence of an inflammatory process; however, normal or even low counts can be obtained in the presence of established peritonitis especially in the aged debilitated patients, or those taking medi-

TABLE 3 **Special Signs and Examinations** *(Continued)*

STUDY	FINDINGS
	cations which reduce WBC response. Leukocytosis should never be the single deciding factor as to whether or not operation is indicated. A WBC count greater than 20,000 may be observed with perforation of a viscus, but pancreatitis, acute cholecystitis, pelvic inflammatory disease, and intestinal infarct may be associated with marked leukocytosis. A normal white blood count is by no means rare in cases of a perforation of abdominal viscera. A shift to the left suggests an acute inflammatory disease, but does little to differentiate surgical from non-surgical inflammatory conditions. Serial leukocyte counts in patients with obscure or variable findings may be helpful, in that a rising leukocyte count may represent an indication for surgical exploration. The finding of leukopenia, particularly with lymphocytosis with lower abdominal pain, is suggestive of viral infection or gastroenteritis rather than acute appendicitis. Marked leukopenia may suggest a blood dyscrasia or severe sepsis. The leukocyte count is not helpful in differentiating between mesenteric adenitis and acute appendicitis as a cause of abdominal pain. On occasion examination of the blood may be diagnostic (e.g., with malaria—seeing parasites). Mononucleosis may be associated, although rarely, with splenic rupture. The peripheral smear may demonstrate abnormal lymphocytes and mononuclear cells. Sickle cell anemia, with abdominal crisis, may also be diagnosed by a peripheral blood smear.
Serum Electrolytes	Often required to document the nature and extent of fluid losses. Calcium determination is important in pancreatitis. Occasionally hypercalcemia indicative of parathyroid disease may be found with the abdominal pain characteristic of the condition.
Urinalysis	Examination of the urine is of critical importance to exclude urinary tract sepsis and diabetes. This urine analysis is directed toward evaluating diabetes, porphyria, the presence of infection or red cells associated with calculi. The presence of proteinuria, erythrocytes or leukocytes can be significant. Pyonephrosis, perinephric abscess, retrocecal appendicitis, retroperitoneal abscess from rupture of duodenum or colon can lead to the presence of proteins, red blood corpuscles, and white blood corpuscles in the urine.
Serum and Urine Amylase	Serum amylase is an important test in many cases of acute abdomen. A serum amylase test should be made in patients with abdominal pain when diagnosis is obscure; however, a "normal" amylase may be found with active pancreatitis. Also a significant elevation of serum amylase may occur with acute cholecystitis, perforated viscus, strangulated intestinal obstruction, mesenteric thrombosis, high bowel obstruction, and intra-abdominal hemorrhage. Great care must be exercised in denying an operation to a patient solely on the basis of an elevated serum amylase level. The determination of the output of urinary amylase is probably more accurate than the estimation of a serum amylase in the diagnosis of pancreatitis. Lipase values are not widely used in the emergency department, because of the greater ease with which the amylase is performed.
ECG	An ECG should be done routinely in the patient over 40 years of age with abdominal pain since myocardial infarction not infrequently presents in this fashion and it may mimic cholecystitis, or gastritis.
Abdominal Paracentesis	Allows examination of the peritoneal fluid for blood or pus. Safe and effective maneuver in patients with acute abdominal pain. (Rarely a necessity, but when condition is critical, the need for further information is imperative, e.g., in elderly obtunded patients in whom the physical signs are very difficult to interpret, and the presence of peritonitis cannot be excluded. Use caution with distention or previous scars. (See Procedure, Chapter 13.) A study of the paracentesis fluid should consist of test for bile with Smith's reagent, evaluation of the amylase content and microscopic examination of fluid for leukocytes or lymphocytes. The presence of blood, large number of polymorphonuclear cells, or bile usually represents a solid indication for exploratory laparotomy. Determination of the pH of the aspirated fluid is misleading because even high acid gastric juice is rapidly buffered by peritoneal exudate.

TABLE 4 Radiologic Examinations in Diagnosis of Acute Abdominal Pain

CAVEATS:

1. Do not leave gravely ill patient in the x-ray department without constant attendance of a trained person.
2. Diagnosis should not be excluded by a "negative" x-ray.
3. X-rays of use in evaluating abdominal pain are: Plain film, upright, left lateral decubitus, upright chest x-ray.

USEFUL X-RAY FINDINGS:

UPRIGHT CHEST X-RAY
Pulmonary disease
Free air under diaphragm
Air-filled viscera in chest
Mediastinal air

UPRIGHT ABDOMINAL X-RAY
Air fluid levels
Air in stomach, small intestine or colon
Massive dilatation colon (in toxic megacolon)

LEFT LATERAL DECUBITUS
Free air
Air fluid levels

PLAIN FILM OF ABDOMEN
Fluid filled loops
Abnormal densities
Urinary calculi
Gallstones
Pancreas calcification
Air in biliary tree
Obscuration of psoas shadow
Displaced kidney
Enlarged spleen shadow
Displacement of stomach bubble
Displacement splenic flexure

SPECIAL STUDIES

Special contrast studies of use may include barium swallow, barium enema, I.V.P., I.V. cholangiogram.

Studies employing angiography, isotopes, etc., depend upon availability within a specific hospital. These are rarely needed in evaluation of the acute abdomen.

TABLE 5 Summary of Commonly Encountered Conditions Which Cause Acute Abdominal Pain

A. INTRA-ABDOMINAL ACUTE SURGICAL CONDITIONS:

Peritonitis
Perforation of viscus
Bowel infarction
Bowel obstruction
Rupture of an abdominal aortic aneurysm
Appendicitis

Diverticulitis
Cholecystitis
Pancreatitis
Salpingitis
Ruptured ectopic pregnancy
Ureteral stone

B. CHRONIC ABDOMINAL CONDITIONS THAT MAY PRESENT WITH ACUTE ABDOMINAL PAIN:

Reflux esophagitis
Peptic ulcer
Ulcerative colitis

Regional enteritis
Irritable bowel

C. EXTRA-ABDOMINAL DISORDERS:

Myocardial infarction
Pneumonia, pleurisy, and empyema
Acute spontaneous pneumothorax
Acute hepatitis
Rheumatic fever

Acute intermittent porphyria
Lesions of the spine
Diseases of the hip joint
Polyarteritis nodosa
Acute epidemic pleurodynia

DIFFERENTIAL DIAGNOSIS OF ACUTE ABDOMINAL PAIN

Disorders that must commonly be considered in the differential diagnosis of a patient who presents with acute abdominal pain are shown in Tables 5 and 6.

OBSERVATION

Certain patients should be placed in the observation unit until the diagnosis has become clear. In general it is wise to admit the patient to the hospital rather than to send him home if the examining physician is unsure of the problem. Sometimes, even under the best of circumstances, with all available auxiliary aids and with greatest of clinical skill, a definitive diagnosis cannot be established at the time of the initial examination. Nevertheless, despite the lack of clear anatomic diagnosis, it may be abundantly clear to an experienced and thoughtful physician and surgeon, on clinical grounds alone, that operation is indicated, thus emphasizing that exploratory laparotomy may constitute an important tool in the diagnosis of acute abdominal pain. Should that decision be questionable, watchful waiting with repeated questioning and examination often will illustrate the true nature of the illness and indicate the proper course of action. In the majority of cases the problem will be reasonably solved within 24 hours. The lessening of abdominal pain, the return of appetite, and the presence of normal vital signs are encouraging, while the persistence of tenderness, anorexia, and leukocytosis is alarming.

In the "observation area," perhaps better named as "The Emergency Decision-making Unit," additional data may be gathered, including serial hematologic determinations, etc. Charting the factors being followed may be useful in demonstrating disease progression or regression. Also one can provide a trial of intravenous therapy and observe whether oral intake is possible; then try other therapies (e.g., anticholinergics to reduce spasm and secretion, analgesia in probable renal colic, etc.). Observation can help to determine the "slope" of disease course—e.g., a staphylococcal food poisoning may cause severe abdominal pain and vomiting, prostration, and electrolyte imbalance. Although the condition may persist in an acute stage for variable periods, if observation of the dynamics still indicates progressive impairment—e.g., continued vomiting and worsening alkalosis—then the condition requires hospitalization or prolonged observation. Correction of the physiologic derangements is essential. On the other hand, if the clinical state and laboratory test results are progressively improving, one can safely predict continued improvement, and such patients can be discharged.

TABLE 6 Subjective and Objective Findings in Commonly Encountered Conditions That Cause Acute Abdominal Pain

CONDITION	SUBJECTIVE AND OBJECTIVE FINDINGS

A. Intra-abdominal Acute Surgical Conditions

Peritonitis	Pain severe and generalized; prostration; fever/chills; movement worsens pains. Fever; generalized abdominal tenderness with guarding, rigidity and rebound tenderness; decreased bowel sounds; patient lies still; hypotension, tachycardia, pallor and sweating may be present.
Perforation of Viscus	Pain severe and generalized. Signs of peritonitis.
Bowel Infarction	Patient is usually older than 50 years of age (unless arterial embolus is the causative factor). Pain is often diffuse and may not reach maximal intensity for hours; bloody diarrhea occasionally. Hypotension, tachycardia, pallor and sweating may be present; signs of peritonitis; abdominal distention.
Bowel Obstruction	Nausea, vomiting often preceding history of constipation, abdominal distention; pain may wax and wane; history of abdominal surgery. Abdominal distention with generalized tympanetic percussion; high pitched rushing bowel sounds early, decreased later; patient tosses and turns.
Rupture of an Abdominal Aortic Aneurysm	Acute abdominal or flank pain. Pulsatile abdominal mass; hypotension, tachycardia and asymmetric pulses may be present.
Appendicitis	Initially pain is epigastric or periumbilical. Often progresses to right lower quadrant. Onset gradual, progressing over hours. Low grade fever (less than 38° C. 101°F.); right lower quadrant tenderness on abdominal or rectal examination; bowel sounds variable; peritonitis if perforation occurs. Obturator psoas tests are often positive. Rebound tenderness referred to right lower quadrant.
Diverticulitis	Pain in the lower left quadrant; constipation, nausea, often vomiting. Course lasts several days. 25% of patients may have minor rectal bleeding. Fever; lower left quadrant tenderness and fullness or mass; occasional rectal mass and tenderness; decreased bowel sounds. Localized signs of peritonitis may be present.
Cholecystitis	Colicky pain in epigastrium or right upper quadrant. Occasionally radiating to right scapula; colicky with nausea, vomiting, fever; sometimes chills, jaundice, dark urine, light colored stools (obstruction of common duct); may be recurrent. Fever; right upper quadrant tenderness with guarding, occasional rebound; decreased bowel sounds.
Pancreatitis	Upper abdominal pain, occasionally radiating to back; mild to severe; associated with nausea and vomiting; history of alcoholism or gallstones; often recurrent; pain may be eased by sitting up or leaning forward. Periumbilical tenderness; occasionally associated with hypotension, tachycardia, pallor and sweating; bowel sounds decreased.
Salpingitis	Pain initially in lower quadrant but may be generalized; usually severe; fever/chills occasionally; dyspareunia; occasionally vaginal discharge. Fever; tenderness with guarding/rebound in lower quadrant; pain on lateral motion of cervix; adnexal tenderness; purulent discharge from cervix.
Ruptured Ectopic Pregnancy	Last menstrual period more than 6 weeks previous; pain in lower quadrant; acute onset and severe. Adnexal tenderness and mass; postural hypotension and tachycardia may be present.
Urethral Stone	May note a history of previous "kidney stone"; pain may begin in flank and radiate to groin; painful urination and blood in urine are frequently noted. Often unremarkable; flank tenderness may be noted as well as decreased bowel sounds. Fever is noted if urinary tract infection occurs.

B. Chronic Abdominal Conditions Which May Present With Acute Abdominal Pain

Reflux Esophagitis	Burning, epigastric or substernal pain radiating up to jaws; worse when lying flat or bending over, particularly soon after meals; relieved by antacid or sitting upright. Patient often obese; normal abdominal examination.

CONDITION	SUBJECTIVE AND OBJECTIVE FINDINGS
Peptic Ulcer	Burning or gnawing, localized episodic or epigastric pain appearing 1-4 hours after meals; may be made worse by alcohol, aspirin, steroids, or other anti-inflammatory medications; relieved by antacids or food. Deep epigastric tenderness.
Ulcerative Colitis	Rectal urgency; recurrent defecation of small amounts of semi-formed stool; pain worsens just before bowel movements; blood in stools. Low-grade fever; tenderness over colon; rectal tenderness and commonly blood in stools; weight loss may be present.
Regional Enteritis	Pain in the right lower quadrant or periumbilical; usually in young person; insidious onset; may be relieved by defecation; stools are often soft and un-formed. Low-grade fever; periumbilical or right quadrant tenderness or mass; weight loss may be present.
Irritable Bowel	Aggravated by anxiety; rectal urgency; relieved by defecation or passage of flatus. No fever; normal physical examination.

C. Extra-abdominal Disorders

CONDITION	SUBJECTIVE AND OBJECTIVE FINDINGS
Myocardial Infarction	Acute myocardial infarction may simulate perforated ulcer, or acute chole-cystitis, particularly if the pain is epigastric. Abdominal rigidity is absent, and peristalsis is not altered. Other manifestations of coronary occlusion, including EKG changes, should promptly clarify the diagnosis.
Pneumonia, Pleurisy, and Empyema	Any thoracic lesion resulting in diaphragmatic irritation may produce right upper quadrant pain simulating an abdominal condition. Careful history and physical examination together with appropriate x-ray studies clarify the diagnosis.
Acute Spontaneous Pneumothorax	Acute spontaneous pneumothorax has been mistaken for acute cholecystitis. Careful physical examination and chest x-rays are diagnostic.
Acute Hepatitis	Acute hepatitis in its initial phase sometimes presents with severe right upper quadrant pain simulating acute cholecystitis. Diffuse hepatic tender-ness and enlargement together with jaundice are present. Appropriate labor-atory studies will make the diagnosis.
Rheumatic Fever	Rheumatic fever is not infrequently accompanied by vague, ill-defined ab-dominal pain simulating acute appendicitis. A careful history and physical examination will indicate that no acute abdominal lesion is present.
Acute Intermittent Porphyria	Severe abdominal pain may accompany various forms of porphyria. The abdominal findings will usually cast doubt on the diagnosis of abdominal disease, and examination of the urine will reveal the presence of porphobili-nogen.
Lesions of the Spine	Osteoarthritis with compression of the thoracic spine and spinal nerves may produce severe ill-defined abdominal pain simulating a variety of intro-peritoneal lesions, particularly biliary colic. Some degree of involuntary rigidity of the rectus abdominus muscle may present an additional confusing factor. Cord tumors may also produce radiating pain simulating biliary or renal colic. In these conditions, careful analysis of the nature of pain, its radiating character, together with the appropriate x-ray examinations will establish the diagnosis.
Diseases of the Hip Joint	A variety of diseases of the hip may produce pain radiating into the right or left lower quadrant. Acute bursitis, in particular, may simulate pelvic appendicitis. Absence of true abdominal tenderness and rigidity together with examination of the hip will clarify the diagnosis.
Polyarteritis Nodosa	Many types of vasculitis may cause abdominal pain simulating acute sur-gical abdominal disease. Careful examination and skin and muscle biopsy will establish the diagnosis.
Acute Epidemic Pleurodynia	May strongly suggest acute appendicitis. Careful examination of the ab-domen is the surest way of avoiding this error. Tenderness is high and is often present over the lower thoracic wall rather than over the peritoneum.

References

Baker, R. J.: Differential Diagnosis of Abdominal Pain. *In* Condon, R. E., and Nyhus, L. M. (eds.): Manual of Surgical Therapeutics, 3d ed. Boston, Little, Brown and Company, 1975.

Botsford, T. W., and Wilson, R. E.: The Acute Abdomen. Philadelphia, W. B. Saunders Co., 1969.

Campbell, I. W., et al.: Abdominal pain in diabetic metabolic decompensation. Clinical significance. J.A.M.A. 233:166, 1975.

Cope, Z.: The Early Diagnosis of the Acute Abdomen, 14th ed. London, Oxford University Press, 1972.

DeDombal, E. T., et al.: Human and computer aided diagnosis of abdominal pain: Further report with emphasis on performance of clinicians. Br. Med. J. 1:376, 1974.

Dunphy, J. E.: The Acute Abdomen. *In* Dunphy, J. E., and Way, L. W., (eds.): Surgical Diagnosis and Treatment. (2nd Ed.). Los Altos, Lange Medical Publications, 1975.

Gardner, B.: Acute intra-abdominal Inflammatory Disease. *In* Shaftan, G. W., and Gardner, B. (eds.): Quick Reference to Surgical Emergencies. Philadelphia, J. B. Lippincott Co., 1974.

Giradet, L., and Enquist, I. F.: Differential diagnosis between appendicitis and acute pelvic inflammatory disease. Surg. Gynecol. Obstet. 116:212, 1963.

Holdstock, D. J., Misiewicz, J. J., and Waller, S. L.: Observations on the mechanism of abdominal pain. Gut 10:19, 1969.

Lasser, R. B., Bond, J. J., and Levitt, M. K.: The role of intestinal gas in functional abdominal pain. N. Engl. J. Med., 293:524, 1975.

Lim, R. K. S.: Pain. Ann. Rev. Physiol., 32:269, 1970.

Melzack, R., and Wall, P. D.: Pain mechanisms: a new theory. Science 150:971, 1965.

Menaker, G. J.: The physiology and mechanism of acute abdominal pain. Surg. Clin. North Am. 42:241, 1962.

Miller, L. S., Staas, W. E., and Herbison, G. J.: Abdominal problems in patients with spinal cord lesions. Arch. Phys. Med. Rehabil. 56:405, 1975.

Moore, F. D.: The effects of hemorrhage on body composition. N. Engl. J. Med. 273:11, 567, 1965.

Ruch, T. C.: Pathophysiology of Pain. *In* Ruch, T. C., and Patton, H. D. (eds.): Physiology and Biophysics, 19th ed. Philadelphia W. B. Saunders Co., 1965.

Rylen J. A.: The Natural History of Disease, 2d ed. London, Oxford University Press, 1948.

Sasso, R. D., Hanna, E. A., and Moore, D. L.: Leukocytic and neutrophilic counts in acute appendicitis. Am. J. Surg. 120:563, 1970.

Schatazki, R., et al.: Radiological diagnosis in acute abdominal disease of adults. Surg. Clin. North Am., 46: 513, 1966.

Staniland, Jr., et al.: Clinical presentation of acute abdomen: study of 600 patients. Br. Med. J. 2:393, 1972.

Steinheber, F. V.: Medical conditions mimicking the acute surgical abdomen. Med. Clin. North Am. 57: 1559, 1973.

Wasson, J., et al. (eds.): The Common Symptom Guide. New York, McGraw-Hill Book Co., Inc., Blakiston Division, 1975.

White, J. C., Smithwick, R. H., and Simeone, F. A.: The Autonomic Nervous System: Anatomy, Physiology, Surgical Application, 3d ed. New York, The MacMillan Company, 1952.

White, J. C., and Sweet, W. H.: Pain and the Neurosurgeon: A Forty-Year Experience. Springfield, Illinois, Charles C Thomas, 1969.

Chapter 21

THE ACUTELY ANXIOUS PATIENT

Nathan S. Kline and Jean-Pierre Lindenmayer

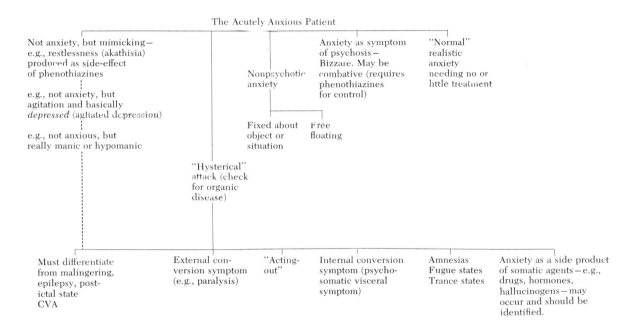

The Acutely Anxious Patient

Not anxiety, but mimicking— e.g., restlessness (akathisia) produced as side-effect of phenothiazines

e.g., not anxiety, but agitation and basically *depressed* (agitated depression)

e.g., not anxiety, but really manic or hypomanic

Nonpsychotic anxiety

Anxiety as symptom of psychosis— Bizzare. May be combative (requires phenothiazines for control)

"Normal" realistic anxiety needing no or little treatment

Fixed about object or situation

Free floating

"Hysterical" attack (check for organic disease)

Must differentiate from malingering, epilepsy, post-ictal state CVA

External con-version symptom (e.g., paralysis)

"Acting-out"

Internal conversion symptom (psycho-somatic visceral symptom)

Amnesias Fugue states Trance states

Anxiety as a side product of somatic agents—e.g., drugs, hormones, hallucinogens—may occur and should be identified.

RECOGNITION

There is usually no difficulty in recognizing an anxiety state: the patient will complain of feelings of panic or impending danger, tenseness, and restlessness. Physical signs of anxiety may be seen, such as hyperactivity, tremor, perspiration, dry mouth, wringing of hands, tachycardia, and possibly hyperventilation. The anxiety is increased under certain circumstances, such as crowded surroundings, and can culminate in a full panic state or as marked agitation. Imminent fear of death or disaster is then not uncommon.

The anxiety can be *fixed* and centered about a particular object or situation, e.g., fear that food eaten for dinner was contaminated, fear that the baby is going to die, fear that the patient is about to be fired from his job the next morning.

The other major type of anxiety is of the *free floating* variety, in which the individual has the same manifestations but cannot relate them to any particular cause. At times, this free floating anxiety is experienced as diffuse bodily sensations with feelings of faintness. In extreme situations, there may be feelings of depersonalization where the patient feels that parts of his body don't re-

487

ally belong to him or somehow are detached from his body.

Anxiety reactions are most of the time related to an imminent danger facing the patient from the outside or to the patient's feeling that his ability to control sexual or aggressive impulses within himself is threatened. As a consequence, the patient is afraid that he may lose control of the situation or himself and that something terrible may happen. An example is the woman with a newborn who feels overwhelmed and resentful of having to take care of her child. She dreads touching the child for fear that she will injure or hurt the child by accident.

Anxiety can also be a manifestation of some other underlying disorder. Persons with phobias and obsessions often will show anxiety if they are unable to deal with their fears and compulsions in the customary way. An individual with a phobia about crossing bridges or handling knives will become acutely anxious if required to cross a bridge or handle a knife.

One of the most frequent confusions in diagnosis is between pure anxiety states and anxious or agitated depressions. If the patient does not relate a history of prior or accompanying depression, the members of the family should be questioned since it is useful to get the patient started on longer term antidepressant treatment as rapidly as possible. The differentiation is of more than academic interest, since long term treatment would be quite different in the two cases. The emergency treatment, however, would be the same.

Very often the first manifestation of an acute schizophrenic episode is anxiety that may mask the more serious underlying disorder. One very typical manifestation of this type of schizophrenic anxiety is *homosexual panic.* The patient is in a great state of agitation, fearing that he or she is homosexual or is being accused of homosexuality. Often this is elaborated into delusions that someone is making approaches toward them or that they impulsively will do something outrageous on their own. Other evidences of schizophrenia should be sought for, such as the delusions just mentioned, auditory or visual hallucinations, irrational thinking, shallow and inappropriate affect. With this group of patients, it is important to begin treatment as early as possible with the major tranquilizers, and therefore it is helpful to make a correct diagnosis. On the other hand, no harm is done except for the delay by treating these patients as though they were suffering from purely anxiety states.

At times a manic state can be confused with anxiety, but usually the manic patient is expensive and euphoric, and this allows for a relatively simple differential diagnosis.

Those patients already in treatment for psychiatric disorders lead to another problem of differential diagnosis. Patients should be carefully questioned as to whether they are receiving any of the major tranquilizers such as phenothiazines, butyrophenones, or thioxanthenes, since these preparations produce akathisia which, at times, is easily confused with anxiety. There is the same restlessness and somatic discomfort plus other symptoms or the anxiety manifestations. Accompanying the akathisia there usually are extrapyramidal symptoms such as dystonia or muscular rigidity. In addition to the masklike facies, one can often elicit muscular resistance up to and including cogwheel rigidity by rapidly bending the arm at the elbow eight or ten times.

Finally, there are normal states of anxiety that do not need specific treatment. Therefore it is important to obtain as adequate a history as possible. In "normal" anxiety, the patient usually is able to relate quite specifically and realistically what the difficulties are. Judgment as to appropriateness of the reaction would show it to be marked but not pathologic in view of the circumstances. As a rule, medication is not indicated.

MANAGEMENT

Frequently the highly agitated or anxious patient arrives with friends or family. A rapid judgment must be made as to whether these companions are contributing to (*a*) the problem, or (*b*) its solution. It probably is useful to try to separate the patient from those accompanying him even if for only a brief period. This will provide an opportunity to reassure those accompanying the patient that the anxiety or agitation can be rapidly controlled and will give at least a few moments' observation as to whether the patient does better with or without his companions. Certainly, if the patient feels more secure with those accompanying him, there is no reason why they should not be present during the interview. However, it is wise under these circumstances to ask the patient whether it is permissible to discuss personal matters freely. This should be noted in the record in case of subsequent medicolegal complications. Often those with the patient can be used constructively, since the patient is apt to forget instructions or recommendations even when these are written down (which they should be). In those cases where the companion seems to be feeding the patient's anxiety, it often is desirable to see if another family member or friend cannot be brought into the picture.

It is obvious that a calm, assured manner on the part of the physician is absolutely essential. On the other hand, the physician should not be totally impassive, but should express verbally awareness of the fact that the patient is suffering, is worried, is anxious, and is frightened, and should indicate that something can be done to relieve the acute symptoms.

On the other hand, in the patient who is extremely agitated to the extent that he is unable to give a coherent history, it is then *appropriate* to keep reassuring the patient "that everything is going to be all right." Except in cases where the patient is so disturbed as to be unable to communicate in a satisfactory manner, it is wise to try to obtain as much of the history as possible at the initial interview before making use of medications. At times, direct physical contact with an anxious patient can be extremely useful; holding the patient by the hand or arm will often assist in producing a calming effect. A human contact is always comforting. Another typical issue frequently brought up by the anxious patient in his first contact with the physician is his fear of either losing control in some way or "going crazy" and having to be sent to a psychiatric hospital. It is helpful briefly to explore the patient's fears about this—particularly what "going crazy" means to him—and then to explain that he is having an anxiety attack and is not becoming insane. If there has been no loss of control in the past, it can be reassuring to point this out to the patient and to add that there is no reason why he should lose control now.

On most occasions, one of the appropriate approaches that often works quite well is to ask the patient to imagine that whatever he or she is fearful about has come to pass, and then to point out that, even should this occur, it would not be a total disaster. Obviously, this does not apply if the patient is concerned about killing his or her child, having a compulsion to jump off the Brooklyn Bridge, or to commit some act which actually would be disastrous. It would be more appropriate when the patient is fearful that a lover may be deserting, a job is about to be lost, or that money has been badly invested.

Once the patient is sufficiently communicative and rapport has been established, a careful history should be taken in order to document the circumstances that were associated with the appearance of the anxiety. There should be search for precipitating events, for situations that worsen or, on the contrary, improve the feelings of anxiety, and for other symptoms associated with the anxiety state. This inquiry will at the same time serve therapeutic purposes since it allows the patient to ventilate and to abreact some of the stronger feelings connected with the anxiety state. It will also allow the physician to help reorganize the patient's usual coping mechanisms by his structured interventions, by his pointing out reality aspects which the patient has distorted, and by his empathic listening. It will be important to find out how the patient has handled similar situations and why his past coping mechanisms were not sufficient this time.

Although the fears of the patient are as a rule exaggerated, the physician should under no circumstances try to minimize or ridicule them. At times, the fears may be real. When the patient reports that he is being pursued by the Mafia, unless the rest of his story is totally disjointed, there may exist a real possibility that he is reporting accurately. Hence it is desirable to try to obtain from the patient some sources whereby the history can be verified and at the same time obtain permission from the patient to check into such sources. At times, the patient's friends or relatives will be eager to contradict what the patient has to say in respect to the justification for the patient's anxiety. It is *not* a good idea to encourage such expressions since, if they were of any use in truly calming the patient, the emergency situation would not exist, and the patient would not be brought to the physician for emergency treatment. It is best to indicate to the others to hold off their story until you have listened fully to what the patient himself has to say. If there is no way of separating the patient from his companions, it is often perfectly acceptable to ask the patient to "hold off" while you listen to what the others have to say, even if the patient does not agree with their accounts. Explain that you will allow time for "rebuttal."

Fortunately there are potent pharmaceutical agents capable of relieving or markedly reducing anxiety in a most dramatic fashion. Consideration should be given to the fact that the patient may be fearful of receiving an injection. Many patients with an anxiety state brought to a physician fear that they will be "doped up" and sent off to a mental hospital. Assurance should be given that the injection will only reduce the level of anxiety and not produce unconsciousness, since a loss of an often tenuous contact with reality is one of the patient's fears. If there is too much resistance to parenteral administration of the medication, it probably is better to use an oral preparation rather than become involved in an altercation that can only provoke the patient's anxiety still more.

The choice of pharmacologic agent depends on the degree of sedation desired. Among the minor tranquilizers (anxiolytic agents) Librium (chlordiazepoxide) is one of the most sedating; meprobamate is slightly less so. Serax (oxazepam) and Tranxene (clorazepate dipotassium) are near the middle in terms of sedation, with Valium (diazepam) usually sedating but sometimes paradoxically acting as a stimulant.

At times, the patient is too agitated to take oral medication and, at other times, rapidity of action is of great importance. Under these circumstances parenteral injections are indicated. Obviously the intravenous route is the most rapid.

In large doses the minor tranquilizers can be respiratory depressants and should be administered with caution under circumstances where this might be a problem—particularly if the patient has been drinking heavily. Using diazepam (Valium) as a standard, the suggested initial parenteral doses are as follows:

> diazepam—5 to 15 mg.
> chlordiazepoxide—50 to 100 mg.

It often is useful to administer an oral dose at the same time since this is a far more convenient form, especially for prolonged use. The suggested initial oral doses, whether alone or used in conjunction with the injectable material, are:

> Valium (diazepam)—10 mg.
> Librium (chlordiazepoxide)—25 mg.
> Serax (oxazepam)—30 mg.

> Tranxene (clorazepate dipotassium)— 15 mg.
> Miltown, Equanil, etc. (meprobamate)—800 mg.

Oral medication usually takes 20 to 40 minutes to start acting and, as a rule, reaches its height of effectiveness in one and one-half to two hours, beginning to dissipate after this. Hence, if a maintenance dose is indicated, it should be given every three to four hours. Although there is danger of drug dependence with long term usage, under the acute circumstances the major focus should be on effectiveness. Prolonged use of high dosage minor tranquilizers is not advised. If such long term use is indicated, the substitution of a phenothiazine or other medication should be considered.

In the case of anxiety resulting from an underlying psychotic process, such as schizophrenia or a manic reaction, the major tranquilizers are the chief therapeutic agents. Since a number of these, particularly chlorpromazine, have a marked sedating action, it usually is unnecessary to make use of the minor tranquilizers. In a patient with acute homosexual panic, for instance, a parenteral dose of 50 mg. of Thorazine (chlorpromazine) accompanied by a 200-mg. oral dose would not be out of line. The 200-mg. oral dose should be repeated every three to four hours as needed, and the same is true of the parenteral preparation. The presence of akathisia as a result of a major tranquilizer administration should not be forgotten, since the restlessness characteristic of this side-effect may be mistaken for anxiety if the differential diagnosis is not taken into account. For patients overly sensitive to the sedating properties of this type of agent, possibly promazine (Sparine) is the mildest medication to use.

The major tranquilizers are also indicated in those patients who have developed a tolerance to minor tranquilizers. Under emergency usage, the following are the usual maximum daily doses for healthy adult males:

> Valium (diazepam)—40 mg.
> Librium (chlordiazepoxide)—200 mg.
> Serax (oxazepam)—120 mg.
> Tranxene (clorazepate dipotassium)— 60 mg.
> Miltown, Equanil, etc. (meprobamate) —2400 mg.
> Thorazine, etc. (chlorpromazine)— 1500 mg.

If the acute anxiety attack does not subside in two to three days or if it recurs when the medication is reduced, psychiatric consultation is definitely indicated. For long term maintenance, the following doses are recommended as daily maximums:

    Valium (diazepam)—20 mg.
    Librium (chlordiazepoxide)—100 mg.

    Serax (oxazepam)—60 mg.
    Tranxene (clorazepate dipotassium)—60 mg.
    Miltown, Equanil, etc. (meprobamate)—1600 mg.
    Thorazine, etc. (chlorpromazine)—1000 mg.

THE HYSTERICAL ATTACK

CONVERSION REACTIONS

Free floating anxiety is an extremely uncomfortable state. Some of this discomfort is removed if the anxiety is attached to a somatic disorder. It also provides an "explanation" which is easier for the patient to handle. Hence, in many cases, anxiety is "converted" into a disorder with somatic manifestations. Indeed, in the process, sometimes the anxiety is so far reduced as to disappear almost totally.

The most common conversion symptoms are those associated with "heart attack." The patient may report precordial pressure, tachycardia and even "pains down the left arm." The symptoms, however, may deviate sufficiently from those of a classic myocardial infarction, e.g., the "pain down the arm" may begin low down and follow an atypical course. Almost any physical disorder can be simulated. If paralyses develop they usually will produce areas of anesthesia or muscular weakness which do not follow the course of any known nerve or muscular grouping but rather a simplified "diagram" of what the patient thinks should occur. Hyperventilation, gastric symptoms, certainly many headaches, urinary frequency, diarrhea, etc., can all be produced on a psychosomatic basis. The term "conversion reaction" is most often reserved for simulation of a neurologic syndrome. In theory the conversion syndrome represents the psychic conflict, including the repressed instinct or drive as well as the defense against it. One of the classic examples is the woman forced to choose between a career as an artist and being a bride who developed paralysis of the arm. Since she "could not" paint any longer, the decision was "made" in favor of becoming a bride. Thus she did not have to reject consciously the choice of a career.

Malingering has to be differentiated from conversion symptoms. Secondary gains, such as protection from work or monetary gains through a lawsuit, usually are always present with malingering.

MANAGEMENT

Obviously the first step is to ensure as far as possible that the patient is *not* suffering from some physical disorder. This presents a special problem in neurotic patients with a past history of physical complaints that eventually evaporated under investigation. In each case serious consideration must be given to the possibility that *this* time the disorder is entirely on a biologic basis or that there is a real disease but that it has been elaborated by the patient's emotional and mental mechanisms.

Even when the physician is reasonably certain that the disorder does not constitute an acute physical emergency, the problem cannot be solved by telling the patient that "there is nothing wrong with you." The patient is actually suffering the pains and discomfort he describes, and being told, in effect, that "they do not exist" is far from a therapeutic approach. Quite the opposite, assuring the patient that you believe the symptoms described actually do exist, helps to establish a more constructive relationship. The patient should be reassured that in any case the pain and dysfunction described do not constitute an acute physical emergency and that no real immediate danger exists. Depending on the situation, the physician may wish to indicate that there may be emotional factors which led to the occurrence of the symptoms described. Exploring psychologic traumatic factors which preceded the syndrome will help clarify the etiology. If there is suspicion of an underlying organic cause, obviously further investigation is in order. It is wise not to "feed" the patient's belief that a physical disorder exists by prolonging examination and investigation. On the other hand, too rapid dismissal may lead the patient to believe that the disease still exists but that the physician in his haste has failed to spend sufficient time to diagnose it.

The anti-anxiety drugs often are quite useful, and an injection of one of the anxiolytic agents, once the diagnosis has been made, often will provide quite rapid relief. At times the relief of symptoms is itself diagnostic and may even be convincing to the patient. Frequently such patients require anti-anxiety (or at times antidepressant) medications over a period of several months and, not infrequently, psychotherapy eventually is indicated. These questions of ultimate treatment and disposition need not be answered in the acute emergent situation. Often in the course of the questioning, the patient will strike on some emotionally charged area of personal concern and, after being given an opportunity to ventilate, will find that the psychosomatic symptoms have been relieved (or made much worse). In the more severe conversion syndromes, relief is not so rapid, and intensive treatment, often by a psychotherapist, is required. Occasionally a prolonged reaction will lead to severe secondary changes such as contractures. Thus physiotherapy to maintain function might be needed.

DISSOCIATIVE STATES

The most dramatic of the dissociative states are amnesias in which the individual may not even be able to identify himself or the cases of multiple personality in which one or more of the personalities is unaware of the others. At other times, there may be erratic types of anesthesias, fugue states, memory loss, and conditions in which there is denial of the existence of certain symptoms. Automatic writing, somnambulism or any independent functioning of a group of mental processes will qualify. Just as the patient with conversion reactions actually does feel the pain which he or she describes, in the dissociative states there is a type of "denial" that allows the patient to ignore pain, "unbearable" situations, and functional disorders even though it is obvious, were it not for the emotional condition, that these would be experienced.

MANAGEMENT

After having ruled out any underlying organic illness (e.g., temporal lobe epilepsy, postictal twilight state, petit mal epilepsy and CVA) and clarified the diagnosis, psychiatric consultation is indicated. By helping the patient to ventilate carefully some of the feelings about the "unbearable" situation from which he has taken flight, the psychiatrist will be able to restore the patient's normal state of consciousness. Sometimes, special techniques, such as hypnosis or an Amytal interview, will be necessary to recover and mobilize lost memories. If the traumatic environmental situation remains unchanged and is too overwhelming to be tolerated by the patient except through a dissociative state, psychiatric hospitalization will be indicated.

ACTING-OUT

On occasion the patient will "act out" some of the emotional and mental states he or she is experiencing. Characteristic of such acting-out is the displacement of the behavior from a situation in which it would be threatening to one in whom it is relatively safe. Partial "discharge" of the emotion relieves the pressure. The patient, frequently a child or adolescent, may assault his or her parents or siblings, attempt to burn down the house, or perform some other antisocial act. The temptation is to be reassuring and pass this off as an isolated incident, since usually the patient is full of remorse afterwards. This will probably work in nine out of ten cases, but in the tenth case there may be a prompt repetition with possibly disastrous results. Unless a psychiatric consultation is *immediately* available, it is best to have the patient dealt with in a "realistic" fashion, by calling in the police and having the patient held until psychiatric consultation is available. Such holding should be very limited and restricted to those severe acting-out problems which threaten others to a significant degree since in some areas juvenile detention centers are extremely frightening places and may produce additional psychic trauma. With lesser degrees of acting-out, psychiatric referral may be delayed somewhat longer, but in any case referral to a psychiatrist is essential since this type of behavior in some cases indicates more serious underlying disease.

Bibliography

Andersen, A. F. R., Jr.: A practical approach to anxiety reactions. N. Y. J. Med. 63:1144, 1963.

Bellak, L., and Small, L.: Emergency Psychotherapy and Brief Psychotherapy, New York, Grune & Stratton, 1965.

Guze, S. B., Woodruff, R. A., Jr., and Clayton, P. J.: Sex, age and the diagnosis of hysteria (Briquet's syndrome). Am. J. Psychiat. 129:6, 1972.

Lader, M., and Marks, J.: Clinical Anxiety. New York, Grune & Stratton, 1971.

Lehmann, H. E., and Ban, T. A.: Pharmacotherapy of Tension and Anxiety. Springfield, Ill., Charles C Thomas, Publisher, 1970.

Meares, A.: The Management of the Anxious Patient. Philadelphia, W. B. Saunders Co., 1963.

Nemiah, J. C.: Neuroses. In Freedman, A. M., Kaplan, H. I., and Sadock, B. J. (eds.): Comprehensive Textbook of Psychiatry, Vol. II. Baltimore, Williams & Wilkins Co., 1975, Chap. 21.

ties should strongly suggest coarctation (especially in the younger patient) or rupture of the aorta in the patient with blunt chest trauma.

Pulse rate, rhythm, amplitude, and character are all important. Alternating weak and strong pulses (pulsus alternans) in heart failure, the small volume pulse of aortic stenosis, and the collapsing and/or bisferiens pulse of aortic regurgitation and idiopathic hypertrophic aortic stenosis may all be helpful. A sinus tachycardia may be one of the few objective findings in pulmonary embolism/infarction. Pulmonary emboli and pericarditis may be accompanied by atrial arrhythmias.

Respiratory rate and amplitude constitute the most frequently overlooked vital sign, but one that is most useful.

Temperature elevations may of course suggest an infectious etiology. The temperature should be taken rectally, unless myocardial ischemia is suspected, since conditions involving dyspnea and tachypnea will result in unreliable oral temperature readings.

The *neck veins* should be inspected with the patient at about 35 degrees above supine, and their level and pulsations recorded with respect to centimeters above the sternal angle. An abnormally increased venous pressure may represent heart failure, acute cor pulmonale, or pericardial disease; in the latter instance, failure of the veins to collapse during inspiration (Kussmaul's sign) may be present.

EXAMINATION OF THE CHEST

A careful examination should include inspection, percussion, palpation, and auscultation of the lungs. Inspection may reveal unilateral differences in chest wall movement or the characteristic rash of herpes zoster. Percussion may disclose abnormal resonance (pneumothorax) or dullness (pneumonia, pleural effusion). Palpation of the chest (including the breasts in the female) can yield important, indeed diagnostic, information about etiology in patients with chest wall pain (see chest wall pain: Tietze's syndrome, costochondrodynia, etc.). Pressure over the costosternal and costochondral joints and above the breasts (especially in women with large, pendulous breasts) may reproduce the patient's pain.

Pulsations of the sternoclavicular joints may be present in thoracic dissecting aneurysm. Auscultation of the lungs is clearly important for the presence of abnormal and/or unilateral findings: rales, rhonchi, pleural rubs.

EXAMINATION OF THE HEART

Inspection may reveal an abnormally located or prominent cardiac impulse, which can be confirmed by palpation. An abnormal systolic parasternal lift should signal underlying right ventricular hypertension of diverse etiologies and may also be found in patients with mitral regurgitation. Clues to the presence of a ventricular aneurysm include impulses located in abnormal areas over the precordium and a late systolic bulge; ectopic impulses occasionally may be felt in the patient with a "fresh" myocardial infarction. Auscultation is especially important: heart tones may be normal, distant, or individually increased in intensity. The presence of an apical S_4 gallop (which can often be felt, as well as heard, in presystole) is an important clue to the abnormal ventricular compliance of both left ventricular hypertrophy and myocardial ischemia. An S_3 gallop confirms heart failure in the proper clinical setting. Tachycardia (which shortens the cardiac cycle at the expense of diastole) or prolongation of the PR interval predisposes to summation of S_3 and S_4 in mid-diastole to produce a loud summation gallop. Abnormalities of the second sound may be found in many clinical situations: *wide splitting* may be seen with acute pulmonary hypertension, such as pulmonary embolism-infarction, and should be expected in right bundle branch block; *reversed* (or *paradoxical*) *splitting* occurs in myocardial ischemia, acute left ventricular dysfunction and left bundle branch block. The pulmonic component of S_2 may be abnormally loud and heard at the apex in acute or chronic pulmonary hypertension. A transient murmur of mitral regurgitation secondary to papillary muscle dysfunction should be looked for in patients with suspected myocardial infarction. A midsystolic click, often followed by a late systolic murmur, is a clue to the etiology of the atypical chest pain seen in patients with the "click-murmur syndrome" ("Barlow's"). The typical three-component (presystolic, systolic, and early diastolic) rub of pericarditis is best appreciated with the patient leaning forward (or even on his hands and knees) in held expiration. In this connection, typical pericarditic pain may be present at a time when *no* rub is present; pericardial rubs are often evanescent, especially in the patient with myocardial infarction.

ASSESSMENT

In many instances, depending on the urgency of the situation, a proper assessment and plan may need to be made almost simultaneously on the basis of available data (see Table 1), thereby dividing the patients along a continuum of priorities. Ancillary data may be needed as noted below, but those patients in the imminently life-threatening category must be triaged quickly—usually without benefit of additional information.

PLAN

The history and physical examination may enable one to arrive at a proper differential diagnosis of the pain and may also suggest further plans, both diagnostic and therapeutic. When time is available, other tests may be done. The chest x-ray, electrocardiogram, blood gas determinations, and other laboratory findings may aid the clinician in arriving at a proper diagnosis. All may be said to exert their greatest diagnostic effect when *positive*, however, and all may be "negative" in instances in which they would, in retrospect, have been expected to be helpful. For example, the chest x-ray often is normal in patients with pulmonary emboli or pleurodynia, but may clearly establish the diagnosis in a patient with a small pneumothorax.

The electrocardiogram may be very helpful, but it should be kept in mind that the resting EKG is *normal* in the majority of patients with stable angina pectoris. It may also be normal early in the course of myocardial infarction; it is especially likely to be nondiagnostic in the so-called "silent" areas of the heart—true posterior, high lateral, and subendocardial. In the Emergency Department situation, an EKG taken during chest pain may be especially valuable (as are other data, including physical examination of the heart made during pain). ST segment depression or ST segment elevation (Prinzmetal variant angina) may be seen *only* during pain in some patients. The diagnosis of chest pain secondary to anxiety must be made with caution after organic causes have been reasonably excluded. Almost every patient with chest pain will have some anxiety, the amount and type of manifestation depending on the patient's personality. Relief of chest pain after administration of a tranquilizer does not necessarily indicate that anxiety was the cause, since pain of anginal or gastrointestinal origin may also be relieved by such therapy.

Arterial blood gases may be helpful when abnormal, and are especially useful in confirming the presence of hypoxia (cyanosis is a notoriously difficult physical finding to be sure of). The finding of hypoxemia with a reduction in the PCO_2 (respiratory alkalosis), although consistent with a diagnosis of pulmonary embolism-infarction, is not specific for it and in fact constitutes the most common blood gas abnormality, regardless of etiology (also seen in pneumonia, pulmonary edema, etc.).

Serum enzymes ("cardiac") are of no diagnostic help for the emergency physician, since their elevation in myocardial ischemia requires the passage of time; decisions as to early management must therefore be made without recourse to such tests.

From a purely pragmatic or operational point of view, it is clear that not all patients will fall into a neat diagnostic category when first seen, but will have to be hospitalized for observation and further tests in order to sort out the cause of their chest discomfort. Efficiency in handling such patients, especially those with suspected myocardial infarction, is critical. In one study of 275 patients transported with a mobile CCU, 10 of the 68 deaths occurred *in the Emergency Department* (Warren et al., 1969). "Delaying patients in emergency areas until the diagnosis is securely founded may result in significant numbers of patients dying from preventable electrical derangements" (Lown and Ruberman, 1970). Such data emphasize the fact that the first few hours after myocardial infarction are the most dangerous. *Early monitoring* of such patients, beginning preferably with ambulance transportation and, certainly in the Emergency Department itself, will facilitate early recognition of danger signals.

The emergency physician has a great responsibility to protect his patient against serious complications and to relieve the patient's pain while trying to determine its etiology.

References

Lown, B., and Ruberman, W.: The concept of pre-coronary care. Mod. Concepts Cardiovasc. Dis. 39(5):97, 1970.

Roberts, R., Henderson, R. D., and Wigle, E. D.: Esoph-ageal disease as a cause of severe retrosternal chest pain. Chest 67:523, 1975.

Warren, J. V., Mattingly, C., and Rand, S.: Design and operation of a mobile coronary care unit (abst.). Circulation 40(Suppl. III):212, 1969.

SUGGESTIONS FOR FURTHER READING

Hurst, J. W.: Symptoms due to Heart Disease. *In* Hurst, J. W., et al.: The Heart, 3d ed. New York, McGraw-Hill Book Company, 1974, p. 140.

Smith, J. R., and Paine, R.: Thoracic Pain. *In* MacBryde, C. M., and Blacklow, R. S.: Signs and Symptoms, 5th ed. Philadelphia, J. B. Lippincott Co., 1970.

Wehrmacher, W. H.: Pain in the Chest. Springfield, Illinois, Charles C Thomas, 1964.

Chapter 23   COMA

Stephen G. Waxman and Thomas D. Sabin

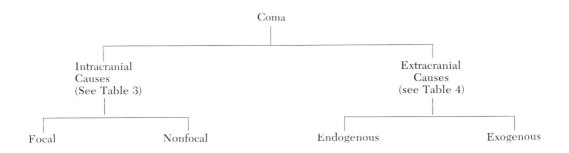

Coma is a frequent and formidable problem in management and diagnosis. Evaluation of the patient is often made more difficult by an absence or paucity of history. The initial diagnostic evaluation must proceed in parallel with supportive and therapeutic measures. In all comatose patients, an oral or endotracheal airway should be inserted immediately and patency of the airway maintained by suction. It is often best to place the patient prone or on his side to prevent aspiration. As described in other chapters in this book, attention should be directed toward maintenance of adequate circulation. In all comatose patients, intravenous glucose (25 gm., usually administered as 50 cc. of a 50 per cent solution) should be administered immediately after blood is drawn for glucose determination to protect the patient from hypoglycemia. Thiamine (50 mg. intravenous) should be administered prior to glucose in any patient in whom there is a question of alcoholism, since a carbohydrate load can precipitate Wernicke's encephalopathy. Urinary catheterization often is necessary. Bedrails should be kept in place and the comatose patient never left unattended.

NEUROPHYSIOLOGIC CONSIDERATIONS

The maintenance of consciousness implies intact function of the ascending reticular activating system (ARAS), located in medial regions of the diencephalon, midbrain, and upper pons. Even small structural lesions may impair consciousness if they interfere with this complex polysynaptic system. Stupor or coma usually supervenes rapidly if damage to the ARAS occurs acutely. Alternatively, the brain stem is subject to compression and secondary dysfunction as a result of mass effects of distant, usually more rostrally located, lesions. In this case there is often a gradual deterioration of consciousness or a latency between onset of illness and development of coma. Often there is an orderly progression of signs as deterioration proceeds along the rostrocaudal axis. Death usually results from impairment of the brain stem mechanisms which maintain respiration. The ARAS also may be functionally depressed in metabolic and toxic encephalopathies. In this case a well defined rostrocaudal progression often is not observed. In contrast to lesions of the brain stem and

501

diencephalon, it is rare for discrete unilateral hemispheric lesions to directly produce coma, since there is no one area in the cerebral hemispheres which is critical for the maintenance of consciousness. Coma as a result of hemispheric dysfunction generally reflects either widespread depression of cerebral activity, most often metabolic or toxic in origin, or herniation due to mass effect with secondary compression of critical brain stem structures.

COMMON HERNIATION SYNDROMES

The two common herniation syndromes most often are a result of the mass effects of intracranial lesions. They occur because the brain, with its blood vessels and meninges, is enclosed in a cranial cavity of fixed dimensions. This cavity is divided by a rigid, fibrous shelf, the tentorium cerebelli, into anterior and posterior compartments. The midbrain extends through a hiatus in the tentorium (the "tentorial notch"). Since the tentorium is fixed to the dura and is relatively rigid, supratentorial mass effects may lead to lateral compression by the adjacent temporal lobe (especially its most medial portion, the *uncus*) and to downward compression through the tentorium. A third type of herniation may occur when the cerebellar tonsils become impacted at the foramen magnum, compressing the adjacent medulla.

Initial diagnostic evaluation should be aimed at differentiating intracranial from

TABLE 1. *Selected Special Diagnostic Tests in Evaluation of Coma*

TEST	MAJOR USE
1. Blood sample	1. Determine hematocrit and WBC count, electrolyte, glucose, urea nitrogen values, toxic screen and arterial blood gases when indicated.
2. Urine sample	2. Test for phenothiazines, aspirin, barbiturates, narcotics, and other substances, depending on laboratory facilities.
3. Gastric aspirate (if overdose suspect)	3. Determine type of intoxication and need for additional lavage.
4. EKG	4. Assess cardiac status.
5. Lumbar puncture	5. Rapid assessment of infection, bleeding.
6. Skull radiography	6. Detect fractures, evidence of midline shift, evidence of chronic changes, particularly of sella turcica or abnormal calcifications.
7. Cervical spine radiography (if trauma suspect)	7. Detect injury to cervical spine
8. Caloric vestibular stimulation and oculocephalic maneuvers	8. Determine level of impairment.
9. Echoencephalography	9. Determine midline shifts.
10. Cerebral arteriography	10. May be indicated to delineate mass lesion or vascular disease.
11. Computerized axial tomography	11. Diagnosis of mass lesions; assessment of ventricular size.
12. EEG	12. May demonstrate seizure activity, differentiate between generalized and focal abnormality.

extracranial etiologies of coma. The intracranial causes of coma may in general be subdivided into those arising as a result of either focal or non-focal pathology. Extracranial causes of coma may reflect dysfunction of homeostatic mechanisms, in which case coma results from metabolic (endogenous) encephalopathy. In other cases, coma may result from toxic (exogenous) encephalopathy.

Table 1 lists special diagnostic tests which can be of aid in addition to a careful and complete examination. Periodic organized examinations are important to detect signs of deterioration and to aid localization.

EXAMINATION OF THE COMATOSE PATIENT

Coma must be differentiated from the "locked-in" syndrome of flaccid tetraplegia and facial paresis, in which there is preservation of consciousness. In this syndrome, which results from destructive lesions of basis pontis, the patient may be able to respond appropriately to questions by eye blink or vertical eye movements. Coma also must be differentiated from the syndrome of akinetic mutism, which occurs in patients with bilateral septal, orbitomedial, frontal, or midbrain lesions. The akinetic mute patient does not speak and is relatively immobile; yet he appears alert, often following the examiner with his eyes.

Every comatose patient should be carefully examined for signs of trauma. These may be subtle, as in the case of blunt head trauma from a sandbag, which may produce only an area of boggy edema. Hemotympanum, bilateral medial orbital ecchymosis, or postauricular ecchymosis ("Battle's sign") suggest basilar skull fracture. The ears and nose should be examined for otorrhea or rhinorrhea. The neck should be carefully examined for asymmetries in the carotid and facial pulses or bruits over the vessels. If there is any possibility of trauma, the neck should be immobilized and a lateral neck x-ray taken prior to other procedures. Nuchal rigidity is strongly suggestive of meningeal irritation. It may also occur as a result of cervical spine pathology or as a result of impaction of the cerebellar tonsils in the foramen magnum. It should be remembered, however, that in the comatose patient nuchal rigidity may not be apparent, so that finding a supple neck has little value in ruling out meningitis. Fever is usually suggestive of infection, but hyperpyrexia (usually greater than 104° F.) may be due to heat stroke, to which patients receiving phenothiazines and anticholinergic medications are predisposed. Low body temperatures may be seen in Wernicke's encephalopathy.

Use the sense of smell to detect alcohol on the breath or the fruity odor of diabetic ketoacidosis. Respiratory patterns should be carefully assessed since a characteristic set appears as dysfunction proceeds along the rostrocaudal axis. Cheyne-Stokes respiration consists of periods of hyperpnea which alternate regularly with periods of apnea. In the comatose patient, this pattern of respiration indicates bilateral hemispheric dysfunction or metabolic coma. *Central neurogenic hyperventilation* is manifested by sustained hyperpnea and indicates dysfunction at the level of upper pons or midbrain. *Ataxic or Biot breathing* consists of irregular inspirations, and suggests dorsomedial medullary dysfunction. In the patient with profound medullary dysfunction due to destructive, compressive, or metabolic depression, spontaneous respirations cease.

The pupils should be assessed (if necessary through the ophthalmoscope, focused on the iris) for size, reaction to light, and, in particular, for asymmetries in size or briskness of response. Midsized (4 to 5 mm.) and unreactive pupils are suggestive of midbrain damage. Pinpoint pupils which are only slightly reactive are classically seen in pontine damage, but are not invariably present. The pupils usually are reactive in metabolic and toxic disorders; exceptions are noted below. A small degree of anisocoria (usually less than 1 mm.) occurs in some 10 per cent of the normal population, but in the comatose patient even minor pupillary asymmetries may reflect early third nerve compression. Funduscopic examination may reveal papilledema, preretinal hemorrhages, or signs of hypertension. It should be noted that papilledema is often not present in the earliest stages of increased intracranial pressure. Extraocular movements should be carefully scrutinized. Moderately dysconjugate gaze has no localizing value. Predilection of gaze to one side may indicate either a hemispheric lesion (usually but not always on the side to which the eyes are directed) or a pontine lesion (contralateral to the direction of gaze). In hemispheric disease, the eyes can often be brought beyond the midline by oculocephalic maneuvers or caloric vestibular stimulation. In the oculocephalic maneuver the head is turned rapidly from side to side. In the lightly comatose patient, if brain stem centers for eye movement are intact, the eyes will conjugately deviate in the direction opposite to the head movement (the so-called "dolls eye" response.) In deep coma, there may be no response to oculocephalic maneuvers.

Caloric vestibular stimulation provides a more potent stimulus for eye movement. The external auditory canal is irrigated with water at least 7° C. below body temperature, with the patient supine and the head elevated 30° above the horizontal. The normal response in an awake person consists of horizontal nystagmus with the rapid phase directed *away* from the side of the irrigated ear. The comatose patient with intact vestibulo-oculomotor pathways will exhibit conjugate eye deviation in the direction of the irrigated ear. If function of these brain stem pathways is depressed, the response to oculocephalic or caloric stimulation will be absent or fragmentary. These maneuvers also may elicit extraocular muscle pareses that were not apparent in the patient with few spontaneous eye movements.

The corneal reflex may be depressed ipsilateral to a brain stem lesion, or, in the acute stages, contralateral to a hemispheric lesion. Asymmetries in facial muscle strength sometimes may be brought out by application of noxious stimuli, such as pressure over the supraorbital ridge. Differences in the palpebral fissures may signify ptosis on the side of the smaller fissure or facial weakness where the fissure is widened.

Examination of the motor system should include assessment of muscle bulk and tone. Multiple myoclonic jerks and fasciculations occur most commonly in coma of toxic or metabolic etiology. Atrophy and spasticity are suggestive of chronic disuse due to upper motor neuron dysfunction. The patient's posture at rest, and in response to vigorous stimulation, should be noted. In *decorticate* posturing, the shoulder is adducted, with the upper extremity flexed at the elbow, wrist, and fingers; the lower extremity may be adducted and extended at the hip and knee, with the foot plantar-flexed. Decorticate posturing occurs with lesions of descending motor pathways above the level

of the rostral midbrain. In *decerebrate* posturing, the arms are adducted, extended at the elbow and hyperpronated; the legs are extended and plantar-flexed. Decerebrate posturing may occur with structural lesions located just rostral to the vestibular nuclei in the midbrain, but more often is seen in the course of herniation from above. It also may occur in toxic or metabolic disorders. Decerebrate or decorticate posturing may in some patients be elicited by sternal pressure, after the arms have been placed semiflexed over the abdomen. The response is in some cases incomplete, but the appearance of even a fragment of the full-blown pathologic posture may be of significance. If the patient moves his extremities spontaneously or in response to midline (e.g., sternal) stimulation or withdraws them from local noxious stimuli, asymmetries should be noted. The deep tendon reflexes and plantar responses should also be assessed, with particular reference to possible asymmetries.

CLINICAL PRESENTATION OF THE COMMON HERNIATION SYNDROMES

The syndrome of uncal herniation results from the expansion of intracranial lesions located in the temporal lobe or the lateral part of the cranial vault. Since progression may be rapid, it is important to make the diagnosis as early as possible. Early in the course, consciousness may be maintained, although some degree of lethargy usually is present. An early clinical sign is unilateral dilatation of the pupil, which results from compression of the intracranial portion of the oculomotor nerve by the herniating medial temporal lobe. The dilated pupil may initially exhibit a brisk response to light, but as the oculomotor nerve is progressively compressed, pupillary reactivity becomes increasingly sluggish and is finally lost. The level of consciousness deteriorates concurrently. Responses to oculocephalic maneuvers and caloric vestibular stimulation initially show oculomotor paresis, but, as herniation progresses, the responses become more difficult to elicit and finally are abolished. Motor signs appear, with a hemiparesis which may be either contralateral to the mass lesion (due to direct hemispheric depression) or ipsilateral to the mass effect (due to compression of the cerebral peduncle against the edge of the tentorium). Further deterioration results in decerebrate posturing and neurogenic hyperventilation.

The central herniation syndrome is usually due to the mass effects of medially located supratentorial lesions. The earliest (diencephalic) stage is characterized by confusion, agitation, or drowsiness. Respirations are regular or of the Cheyne-Stokes types. The pupils are small and reactive, and eye movements are usually full. Cold caloric stimulation usually yields tonic deviation of the eyes toward the stimulated side. Motor signs may be unilateral or bilateral; decorticate posturing is not unusual. As central herniation progresses to produce midbrain dysfunction, the level of consciousness progressively deteriorates, and the patient becomes comatose. Sustained hyperventilation is often seen. The pupils are mid-sized and unreactive, and the responses to oculocephalic maneuvers and cold caloric stimulation are sluggish or incomplete. Decerebrate rigidity may appear first intermittently in response to noxious stimulation and, later, as a sustained posture. In the medullary stage, respirations become ataxic and finally cease. Flaccidity appears as the midbrain structures which mediate decerebrate rigidity fail.

The progression of the two herniation syndromes is summarized in Table 2. In each of the herniation syndromes, there is a characteristic progression as herniation proceeds. Since the clinical picture changes over time as herniation progresses, repeated clinical evaluations of the comatose patient are necessary. It should also be noted that it is not infrequent for the signs in one category, e.g., motor signs or respiration, to be one or more levels "out of register" with other signs signalling herniation.

INTRACRANIAL CAUSES OF COMA

The common focal intracranial causes of coma (Table 3) include cerebral contusion, extraparenchymal and intraparenchymal hemorrhage, infarction, neoplasm and brain abscess. Subarachnoid hemorrhage and meningitis often present a picture of nonfocal dysfunction, although exceptions are not rare.

FOCAL INTRACRANIAL DISEASE

Nonpenetrating head trauma may produce *concussion,* in which there is a transient loss of consciousness lasting only minutes. In concussion there is no gross structural damage. A depressed level of consciousness is often seen in cerebral contusion or laceration. The cerebrospinal fluid

TABLE 2   *Clinical Presentation of Common Herniation Syndromes**

	PUPILS	RESPIRATIONS	EYE MOVEMENT	MOTOR SIGNS
I. *Uncal Herniation* early	ipsilateral pupil; dilated but often reactive	often normal	often full	may be normal
moderate	dilated; sluggish or fixed	Cheyne-Stokes	may see III nerve palsy	hemiparesis; decorticate posturing; contralateral or ipsilateral
advanced	fixed, dilated	central neurogenic	III nerve palsy	decerebration
II. *Central Herniation* diencephalic	small, reactive	normal or Cheyne-Stokes	usually full; caloric stimulation produces tonic deviation	unilateral or bilateral
midbrain/pontine	fixed, midsized	central neurogenic	sluggish and incomplete response to oculocephalic and caloric stimulation	decerebrate posturing
medullary	remain fixed	ataxic	absent	flaccid

*Modified after Plum and Posner, 1970.

*TABLE 3   Common Intracranial Causes
of Coma*

I.   Subdural hematoma
II.   Epidural hematoma
III.   Traumatic intracerebral hemorrhage
IV   Nontraumatic intracerebral hemorrhage — usually
          hypertensive
          a. putamenal (most common)
          b. thalamic
          c. pontine
          d. cerebellar
          e. cerebral white matter
V.   Intraventricular hemorrhage
VI.   Cerebral infarcts
          a. coma uncommon acutely in uncomplicated
             hemispheric infarct
          b. coma present in brain stem infarct if ARAS is
             damaged
VII.   Subarachnoid hemorrhage
          a. ruptured intracranial aneurysm
          b. arteriovenous malformation
VIII. Neoplasm
          a. coma usually supervenes after other present-
             ing signs
          b. sudden onset of coma may result from hemor-
             rhage into tumor or development of acute
             obstructive hydrocephalus
IX.   Pituitary apoplexy
X.   Meningitis
          a. pyogenic
          b. tuberculous
          c. fungal
          d. viral
XI.   Encephalitis
          a. viral
          b. postinfectious
XII.   Brain abscess
XIII. Subdural empyema

may contain a small amount of blood and have a xanthochromic supernatant. Persistent stupor or coma or deterioration of level of consciousness after head injury may be secondary to cerebral edema associated with cerebral contusion or laceration, but should also raise suspicion of subdural or epidural hematoma or traumatic intracerebral bleeding. The "lucid interval" which classically precedes loss of consciousness in subdural and epidural hematoma is not always present, and in fact most patients exhibit a depressed level of consciousness from the outset. There is a wide range in latency between injury and onset of symptoms in subdural hematoma. Subdural hematomas may occur acutely (within hours) or subacutely (within days). Chronic subdural hematomas may become symptomatic months after injury. A history of injury may not be elicited, since even trivial trauma may lead to subdural bleeding, especially in children and in the elderly or alcoholic patient, in whom

bridging veins may be stretched due to cerebral atrophy. Mentation is often dulled, and depression of the level of consciousness may be present without focal signs. Pupillary dilatation, if present, is usually on the side of the hematoma. Hemiparesis, however, may occur either contralateral or ipsilateral to the hematoma. Bilateral subdural hematomas should be suspected if cerebral arteriography demonstrates an extravascular mass, but midline structures are not shifted to a commensurate degree. Epidural hematomas most frequently occur as a result of lacerations of the middle meningeal artery. The clinical picture evolves rapidly, with early development of the pupillary changes associated with uncal herniation. This diagnosis should be considered in any comatose patient with a fracture intersecting the course of the middle meningeal artery.

Nontraumatic intracerebral hemorrhage usually occurs in the context of systemic hypertension, but may also occur in patients with bleeding diatheses, as with anticoagulant therapy, leukemia, and uremia. The most common site is the region of the putamen. The clinical picture of this lateral ganglionic hemorrhage is one of rapid development of hemiplegia and coma, with deviation of the eyes toward the side of the lesion, often heralded by severe headache.

In *thalamic hemorrhage* there is often a contralateral hemiparesis. The eyes deviate downward and inward.

Pontine hemorrhage is characterized by the rapid onset of quadriplegia, with sluggishly reactive pinpoint pupils. The corneal reflexes and the response to oculocephalic and caloric vestibular stimulation are often diminished or absent. Ocular bobbing, consisting of rapid downward deviation of the eyes followed by an upward bobbing movement, occurs in some cases of pontine hemorrhage.

In *cerebellar hemorrhage*, the patient is often conscious at the outset, but coma rapidly supervenes. Initial symptoms commonly include headache, nausea, vomiting, and ataxia. Gaze palsy, irregular respirations, and facial palsy are more variable signs. Since critical brain stem structures are initially depressed by compression rather than intrinsic damage, cerebellar hemorrhage, especially if diagnosed early, may be amenable to neurosurgical intervention.

Intraventricular hemorrhage may occur as a primary event, in which case the patient presents with sudden onset of deep coma rapidly progressing to brain stem failure. Intraventricular hemorrhage may also occur as the result of dissection of an intracerebral hematoma into the ventricles. In this case, a patient with signs of intracerebral hemorrhage will abruptly deteriorate as the hemorrhage dissects into the ventricular system.

Cerebral infarcts often produce lethary or confusion, but unilateral hemispheric lesions uncommonly present with frank coma. Rarely, a patient with sudden and massive hemispheric infarction, as with a carotid embolus, will rapidly lose consciousness and show clinical signs of uncal herniation. More commonly, consciousness is progressively depressed one to three days after infarction, owing to the development of cerebral edema. Brain stem infarctions, on the other hand, may disrupt the reticular activating system and present with coma. Common premonitory signs include transient episodes of vertigo, diplopia, dysarthria, or dysphagia.

Primary or metastatic *neoplasms* of the central nervous system may progress to coma, but usually are diagnosed earlier in their course by virtue of elementary neurologic deficits or changes in mentation. Hemorrhage into an asymptomatic tumor may in rare cases present as an intracerebral mass, which may produce coma. Deep midline tumors (e.g., colloid cyst of the third ventricle, cystic astrocytoma of the cerebellum, pinealoma) may present as acute obstructive hydrocephalus with secondary herniation. The clinical picture may be one of abrupt loss of consciousness and respiratory arrest. *Emergency ventriculostomy may in some patients be lifesaving.*

The syndrome of "pituitary apoplexy" is characterized by sudden headache, visual loss, ophthalmoplegias, shock and obtundation. It may develop as a result of hemorrhage into a pituitary adenoma (in some cases following radiation therapy)." Plain skull films show an enlarged sella turcica, and lumbar puncture often reveals slightly bloody cerebrospinal fluid. This disorder requires immediate steroid replacement. Neurosurgical intervention may be necessary to decompress the optic nerves.

Brain abscess usually presents as an intracranial mass. In some patients there are multiple abscesses. The cerebrospinal fluid may be entirely normal. Common primary sites of infection include the lungs, ears, and sinuses. Abscesses also occur in patients with right-to-left shunts. Fever is often absent, and, when present, usually is due to the primary infection. Subdural empyema most often occurs with acute frontal sinusitis. The clinical picture resembles that of subdural hematoma, but the patient often appears toxic, is usually febrile, and there are frequent focal seizures. There may be swelling ("Pott's puffy tumor") over an infected sinus. The course is usually rapid, and coma supervenes as a result of mass effect or due to secondary meningitis, cerebritis, or cerebral venous thrombosis.

NONFOCAL INTRACRANIAL DISEASE

Subarachnoid hemorrhage most commonly results from a ruptured intracranial aneurysm. Many patients are initially awake and complain of severe headache. Subarachnoid hemorrhage may produce coma by several mechanisms. In many patients, subarachnoid blood depresses cerebral function in the absence of a mass effect. In these patients there is a paucity of localizing signs. In other patients the hematoma may dissect into brain parenchyma, in some cases leading to the development of a pressure cone and herniation. The neck is often, but not invariably, stiff in subarachnoid hemorrhage. Papilledema and preretinal hemorrhages may be seen on funduscopy. If the mass is laterally located, there may be clear lateralizing signs. Aneurysms of internal carotid origin of the posterior communicating artery are often associated with a dilated pupil or third nerve palsy. Hemiparesis may result from hemorrhage into brain parenchyma or from vasospasm. Vasospasm need not be limited to the affected artery.

Both *acute* and *chronic meningitis* may present without focal signs. Although nuchal rigidity is usually seen in the alert patient with meningeal irritation, it need not be present in the comatose patient. When meningitis is complicated by venous thrombosis there may be hemiparesis or focal seizures. Occasionally, cerebral edema and mass effects will punctuate the clinical course. Fever and leukocytosis usually accompany pyogenic infection, but may be absent in the debilitated patient or in the chronic meningitides. The diagnosis of meningitis is made on the basis of careful cerebrospinal fluid examination. Appropriate antibiotic therapy should be instituted as early in the course as possible. In questionable cases a second lumbar puncture 12 hours after the first may be diagnostic. The viral and parainfectious encephalitides may present acutely or subacutely and can progress to coma. The clinical picture may be focal or nonfocal. The cerebrospinal fluid examination usually shows a predominantly lymphocytic pleocytosis.

Postconvulsive coma may also be classed with the nonfocal intracranial causes of coma, since it probably reflects widespread neural inhibition. The postictal patient is most commonly comatose or stuporous for only a brief interval of minutes to hours, although a period of confusion or lethargy may persist much longer. However, the patient with seizures is prone to head injury, so that epidural and subdural hematomas may occur as complications of seizures. Alternatively, seizures and coma may both be precipitated by acute intracranial or toxic/metabolic disorders. Coma following a seizure therefore demands careful evaluation and management.

EXTRACRANIAL CAUSES OF COMA

Extracranial causes of coma (Table 4) may be of metabolic (endogenous) or toxic

TABLE 4   Common Extracranial Causes of Coma

A. *Endogenous*
   I.   Electrolyte disorders
          a. acidosis (metabolic or respiratory)
          b. alkalosis (metabolic or respiratory)
          c. hypo- and hypernatremia
          d. hypo- and hyperkalemia
          e. hypo- and hypercalcemia
  II.   Hypotension, hypertension
 III.   Hypoxia, hypercapnea
 IV.   Hypoglycemia
  V.   Hyperglycemia
 VI.   Hepatic Coma
VII.   Uremic Coma
VIII. Myxedema, thyrotoxicosis
 IX.   Addison's disease
  X.   Wernicke's encephalopathy

B. *Exogenous*
   I.   Toxic encephalopathies
          a. sedatives, barbiturates, tranquilizers
          b. opiates
          c. ethanol/methanol
          d. salicylates

(exogenous) origin. Since there is no primary structural disease, metabolic/toxic coma characteristically presents a picture of symmetric neurologic dysfunction without lateralizing signs. However, in some patients, particularly those with pre-existing but clinically inapparent neurologic deficits, focal signs may appear as a result of a metabolic or toxic disorder. Thus, for example, the patient who apparently has recovered from a cerebral infarct may again manifest his hemiparesis or visual field deficit as a result of electrolyte abnormality, fever, or hypoxia.

Asterixis, tremulousness, and multiple myoclonic jerks usually are seen in the setting of metabolic encephalopathies. Fasciculations may be present. Multifocal seizures also may occur, especially in uremia and nonketotic hyperosmolar diabetic coma.

The metabolic encephalopathies may reflect dysfunction of a number of organ systems and homeostatic mechanisms. Acidosis (metabolic or respiratory), alkalosis (metabolic or respiratory), electrolyte imbalance, hypoxia, hepatic insufficiency, and uremia may cause coma. Consciousness may be depressed in hypo- and hyperglycemia, and in nonketotic hyperglycemia of diabetes mellitus. Hypertensive encephalopathy produces coma, papilledema, increased spinal fluid pressure and protein, and in some cases focal neurologic deficits. Hypo- and hyperthermia also may cause coma; the former sometimes occurs as a result of hypothalamic dysfunction in Wernicke's encephalopathy.

Myxedema, thyrotoxicosis, and Addison's disease are among the more common endocrinopathies causing coma. Diagnosis in each of these cases is often suspected on the basis of the general medical examination and can be confirmed by appropriate laboratory studies.

The toxic (exogenous) encephalopathies may follow the ingestion or infusion of sedatives, narcotics, ethanol or methanol, or salicylates. Coma also may occur in advanced cases of heavy metal intoxication. Pupillary response, although sluggish, is often preserved in toxic and metabolic coma, while other brain stem reflexes (corneal reflexes, responses to oculocephalic and caloric stimulation) may be absent. In opiate-induced coma, however, the pupils may be constricted, and in glutethimide ingestion, the pupils may be fixed in mid-position. Fixed and dilated pupils are seen in atropine poi-

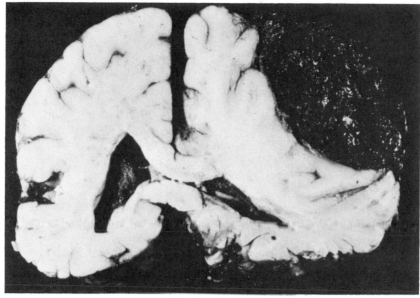

Figure 1. Subdural hematoma from a uremic patient who exhibited signs of the uncal herniation syndrome prior to death. Note the displacement of the brain by this extraparenchymal mass lesion.

soning, in which there is characteristically tachycardia, fever, hypertension, and warm, dry skin. The pupils are not uncommonly unreactive in anoxic encephalopathy. In the acute stage of coma, fixed pupils and absence of brain stem reflexes do not necessarily signal a poor prognosis.

Patients with systemic disorders may be especially vulnerable to certain forms of intracranial pathology. For example, meningitis is not uncommon in diabetes, and chronic renal failure may be complicated by subdural hematomas (Fig. 1) and meningitis. In these cases, lumbar puncture or appropriate radiologic studies may be necessary diagnostic procedures.

LABORATORY STUDIES IN THE ASSESSMENT OF COMA

Initial laboratory studies in the comatose patient should include hemogram, determination of blood glucose (from a sample obtained *before* the patient receives intravenous glucose), serum electrolytes, and urea nitrogen. Urinalysis should be obtained. If oral overdose is suspected, a gastric aspirate should be performed with an endotracheal tube in place. If an overdose of heroin or morphine is suspected, a trial dose of Narcan is warranted. Arterial blood gas determination should be performed if appropriate. In many hospitals, determinations of blood levels of common intoxicants are available. An electrocardiogram should be obtained. Initial radiographic studies should include x-rays of the chest and skull, and, if there is any question of trauma, of the cervical spine, including views of the odontoid process. The skull films should be carefully scrutinized for enlargement of the sella turcica, shift of the calcified pineal away from the midline, or for evidence of skull fracture, infection of sinuses or bone, or abnormal calcifications. Lumbar puncture and careful cerebrospinal fluid examination (see Chapter 49) can only be deferred if a mass lesion is suspected; in this case emergency angiography, ventriculography, or computerized axial tomography may precede and possibly preclude lumbar puncture. The electroencephalogram and echoencephalogram also may provide valuable diagnostic information.

References

Kemper, T. L., and Romanul, F. C. A.: State resembling akinetic mutism in basilar artery thrombosis. Neurology *17*:74, 1967.

Kernohan, J. W., and Woltman, H. W.: Incisera of the

crus due to contralateral brain tumor. Arch. Neurol. Psychiatr. *21*:274, 1929.

Loeser, E., and Scheinberg, L.: Brain abscesses. A review of ninety-nine cases. Neurology 7:601, 1957.

Maccario, M., Messis, C. P., and Vastola, E. F.: Focal seizures as a manifestation of hyperglycemia without ketoacidosis. Neurology *15*:195, 1965.

Magoun, H. W.: The Waking Brain. Springfield, Charles C Thomas, 1963.

McNealy, D. E., and Plum, F.: Brain stem dysfunction with supratentorial mass lesions. Arch. Neurol. 7:10, 1962.

Ott, K. H., et al.: Cerebellar hemorrhage: diagnosis and treatment. A review of 56 cases. Arch. Neurol. *31*:160, 1974.

Plum, F., and Posner, J. B.: The Diagnosis of Stupor and Coma. Philadelphia, F. A. Davis Co., 1970.

Sabin, T. D.: The differential diagnosis of coma. N. Engl. J. Med. *290*:1062, 1974.

Segarra, J. M.: Cerebral vascular disease and behavior. I. Syndrome of the mesencephalic artery. Arch. Neurol. *22*:408, 1970.

Teasdale, G., and Jennett, B.: Assessment of coma and impaired consciousness. Lancet *2*:81, 1974.

Chapter 24　CONFUSION

Arthur P. Safran, and Thomas D. Sabin

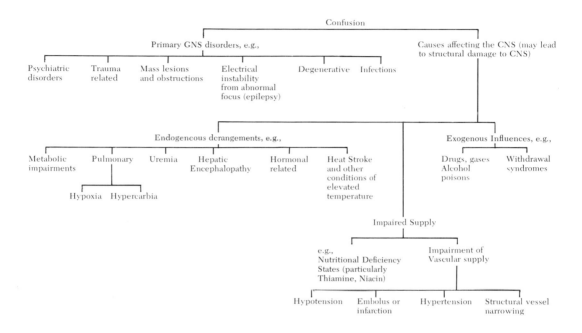

The acutely confused patient suffers a failure in ability to rank the priority of stimuli. A significant environmental stimulus may be unheeded or a trivial one given undue attention. This abnormality is reflected in the patient's behavior and speech as the cardinal feature of confusion—a loss of normal sequential thought. The consequent failure in assignment of behavioral priorities drastically disintegrates this patient's behavioral adaptation to the environment. The confused patient is then brought to the Emergency Department because he is acting and speaking "funny" and cannot care for himself. Some 10 to 15 per cent of patients hospitalized because of acute medical and surgical conditions manifest some form of the confusional syndrome.

Diverse mechanisms, such as brain infarction, displacement of brain tissue by mass lesions, or derangements in brain metabolism, are capable of producing acute confusion. In the elderly or in patients with pre-existing brain disease, an acute episode of confusion most often can be traced to superimposed, non-neurologic illness. Alcohol and drug abuse provide the most common cause of acute confusion in the younger patient population. Since most disorders that cause the confusional syndrome are remediable, prompt diagnosis of such patients is rewarded by cure; but permanent impairment of the patient's higher cortical functions may be the penalty for delay in treatment. Table 1 lists some of the problems entering the differential diagnosis of the acutely confused patient. The major common error of the Emergency Department staff is the transfer of such patients to a psychiatric facility. Comprehensive medical and neuro-

TABLE 1   Some Causes of the Acute Confusional State

I. Central Nervous System Disorders
  A. Conditions Mimicking Confusion
    1. Korsakoff syndrome
    2. Fluent aphasia
    3. Denial syndromes
  B. Conditions Causing Acute Confusion
    1. Mass lesions (tumors, hematomas, granulomas)
    2. Infections (viral, bacterial, parasitic spirochetal, meningitis, encephalitis, or abscess)
    3. Deficiency states (niacin, thiamine, vitamin B_{12})
    4. Epilepsy (postictal states, psychomotor seizures)
    5. Trauma (concussion, contusion; epidural, subdural, or intracerebral hematomas)
    6. Cerebrovascular disease (subarachnoid hemorrhage, infarction of lingual gyrus, nondominant parietal lobe or mesial temporal lobe
    7. Heat stroke
    8. Dementing disorders (especially liable to confusion with even trivial general medical illness, head injury, or simply a change in environment.)
II. Psychiatric Disorders
  A. Acute schizophrenia
  B. Acute manic and paranoid states
  C. Homosexual panic
  D. Ganser's syndrome
III. Extracranial Disorders
  A. Exogeneous intoxications
    1. Alcohol, barbiturates
    2. Tranquilizers
    3. Belladonna derivatives
    4. Psychotomimetics
    5. Others: Ergot, salicylates, caffeine, heavy metals
    6. Withdrawal syndromes
  B. General Medical Diseases
    1. Disturbances of hydration, electrolytes, and osmolarity
    2. Cardiovascular disturbances (hypotension, congestive heart failure, hypertensive encephalopathy)
    3. Pulmonary failure (carbon dioxide narcosis, anoxia)
    4. Hepatic encephalopathy
    5. Uremia and the postdialysis syndrome
    6. Endocrine disorders: Hypoglycemia, thyroid, adrenal, and pituitary syndromes
    7. Porphyria
    8. Vasculitides
    9. Acute infections outside the central nervous system
    10. Toxemia of pregnancy

The police, friends, or family who accompany the patient to the hospital should be questioned concerning the exact circumstances in which the patient was discovered, when he was last known to be well, the occurrence of seizures, the patient's use of alcohol or drugs, and his occupation. Knowledge of any complaint the patient may have mentioned during the weeks prior to his illness, such as headaches, forgetfulness, visual symptoms, and loss of coordination, strength, or sensation, may signify a primary intracranial disease process. Despite the amount of irrelevant information and disordered thinking present, the patient should be asked specifically about hallucinations, drug ingestion, and past health problems.

Neurologic examination of the patient with an acute behavioral change allows separation of the confusional syndrome from other conditions such as the Korsakoff's syndrome or aphasia and the discovery of other neurologic signs that have localizing value. Confusion alone has little localizing value, yet some of the accompanying deficits may be misconstrued as focal signs. Geschwind has noted that confused patients are severely agraphic and that a variable degree of nominal aphasia is also common. Neither of these signs indicate focal disease in the confused patient.

Broca's and Wernicke's aphasia do not occur as part of the confusional state. Denial of illness in some circumstances indicates a parietal lobe lesion, but is another feature of confusion that cannot be used to localize a lesion. Performance on tests of memory is highly variable, but the patient's sporadic production of accurate information regarding orientation and memory suggests that memory defect is not a fundamental feature of confusion. However, the recovered patient is nearly always amnesic for the period of his confusional state. The patient without confusion who has an isolated inability to retain new memories for more than a minute or two with some retrograde amnesia has the Korsakoff syndrome. This state is most often due to trauma, thiamine deficiency, or infarction of the dominant mesial temporal lobe.

The confused patient may perform some tests, such as proverb interpretation and similarities, well; but usually he does poorly with calculations and such problems as copying drawings. Cortical blindness, visual agnosia, or severe aphasia is not seen as part

logic evaluations are required, and these are best performed in the general hospital equipped to treat the acutely ill.

The confused patient often is unable to provide a relevant history and usually has no complaint or insight regarding his problem.

of confusion. Thus the confusional syndrome may be induced by nonfocal lesions and is associated with a variety of deficits, but many cerebral signs are not part of the syndrome. Hence, true focal signs should not be overlooked, and the patient should be given a full mental status examination, including tests for aphasia, agraphia, and apraxia.

The confused patient may be somnolent or excited. The hallmarks of both types are disordered thought sequence and defective attention. In agitated delirium the patient appears "hyperalert," with fleeting attention given to random series of stimuli in his environment; and his speech reflects a rapid succession of unconnected ideas. There are excitement, momentary anger, and alterations in perception manifested by illusions or hallucinations. Visual hallucinations are more common than auditory hallucinations in nonpsychiatric disorders. The patient does not sleep, is restless, and exhibits tremulousness with tachypnea, tachycardia, and diaphoresis. This syndrome is most commonly seen in states of alcohol or drug withdrawal.

The somnolent confused patient must be closely observed for the signs of progressive deterioration in consciousness discussed under Coma (Chapter 23). The general medical examination often will reveal the cause for the acute confusion, since most cases are not due to primary intracranial disease.

CENTRAL NERVOUS SYSTEM DISORDERS

INFECTION

Acute confusion may be the mode of presentation for bacterial, fungal, parasitic, and viral forms of meningitis or encephalitis. A lumbar puncture is warranted in all cases of acute confusion where no obvious contraindication exists. The CSF should be personally examined by the physician. Delirium is also seen in Reye's syndrome and in the postinfectious encephalopathies of childhood.

SEIZURE DISORDERS

A variable period of confusion and abnormal behavior may follow a seizure. This state usually does not persist for more than a few hours and usually shows progressive improvement during a brief period of observation. Hydantoin-induced gingival hyperplasia or the discovery of anticonvulsant medication among the patient's belongings should suggest this diagnosis. In a condition characterized by continuous repeated psychomotor seizures, the patient appears in a dreamlike state, and may have hallucinations, excitement, automatic motor behavior, or even violent and aggressive behavior. The complaint of a very disagreeable odor, or mouthing, chewing, and lip-smacking movements are highly characteristic of psychomotor seizures. An electroencephalogram may reveal abnormal electrical activity in the temporal or nasopharyngeal leads. Herpes simplex encephalitis may present with this syndrome because of the preferential involvement of olfactory and temporal lobe structures by the herpes simplex virus.

TRAUMA

Agitated confusional states are a common sequela to head injury. The confusion usually has a good prognosis, but sometimes gives way to a Korsakoff's syndrome lasting for months. The site of injury may not be obvious, and the scalp should be closely examined. Blood behind the tympanic membranes or a bruise over the mastoid regions indicate a basilar skull fracture. Even trivial head injury in the patient with underlying brain atrophy may precipitate an intense, agitated confusion lasting several weeks. Progressive deterioration in alertness after a head injury should suggest cerebral edema or a subdural, intracerebral, or epidural hematoma.

When large long bones have been fractured, fat emboli may pass through the pulmonary circulation and reach the cerebral circulation, causing severe confusion, obtundation, seizures and showers of petechiae, particularly in the pectoral and inguinal regions. Decompression sickness may also cause confusion related to nitrogen bubbles in the CNS. The history should enable differentiation of this state.

HEAT STROKE

Brain metabolic rate begins to decline at temperatures above 104°F., and confusion with obtundation is seen. Some individuals seem especially liable throughout life to develop confusion and hallucinations, even with slight temperature elevations. Heat stroke is recognized by a history of environmental exposure, dry hot skin, thready pulse, tachycardia, and at times the presence of petechiae. (See Chapter 39.) The temperature in heat stroke may exceed 106°F.

DEFICIENCY STATE

Irritability, insomnia, mania, and profound confusion occur in pellagra. In the U.S., niacin deficiency usually is seen in alcoholics or food faddists. Diarrhea and a rash on skin surfaces exposed to sunlight suggest pellagra.

Thiamine deficiency is much more common than niacin deficiency in the alcoholic, malnourished population and produces Wernicke's encephalopathy. The syndrome is characterized by confusion, nystagmus, ocular palsies (usually bilateral abducens paralysis), and ataxia. The symptoms may develop acutely, especially when the thiamine-deprived patient is given a carbohydrate load. Thus the first heavy meal or an intravenous solution of glucose received with hospitalization may precipitate Wernicke's encephalopathy. This disease is capable of causing sudden death, therefore, thiamine should be administered to all "dedicated" alcoholics when they arrive in the Emergency Department for any reason. The patient with Wernicke's encephalopathy is often severely confused. The confusion, eye signs, and ataxia tend to clear with thiamine therapy, but only then will some patients be found to have residual Korsakoff's syndrome. The prognosis for recovery of the memory defect is poor. In the acute stages the patient "fills in" his deficient recent memory with gross confabulatory responses. Cognitive functions are retained.

MASS LESIONS

Neoplasms, abscesses, granulomas, and blood clots can produce confusional states as a nonspecific effect of distortion of intracranial contents. These diagnoses are uncovered by the associated signs of increased intracranial pressure and the presence of focal deficits in addition to confusion. Tumors involving the frontal lobe are especially apt to cause confusion and severe behavioral changes. Confusion may result from obstruction to cerebrospinal fluid flow with hydro-

cephalus from midline tumors at the base, the posterior fossa, or within the ventricular system. If the confused patient shows progressive obtundation or signs of herniation, urgent neuroradiologic investigation and neurosurgical intervention are required.

DEMENTING ILLNESSES

Most of the diseases associated with dementia are slowly progressive but punctuated by episodes of acute confusion often caused by a second, usually non-neurologic, illness. The most common cause of dementia is Alzheimer's disease, which begins with retentive memory loss, nominal aphasia, and a difficulty with such tasks as copying diagrams. As frontal lobe degeneration supervenes, the patient loses insight into his illness, becomes socially inappropriate, and develops a euphoric apathy which may be interrupted by bouts of irritability and poorly organized, unsustained aggressive behavior. The patient with a history of dementia must be investigated to rule out such treatable conditions as normal pressure hydrocephalus, central nervous system syphilis, certain tumors, vitamin B_{12} deficiency, hypothyroidism, and chronic drug toxicity.

FOCAL BRAIN SYNDROMES

Isolated lesions, most often cerebral infarctions, may produce acute confusion or behavioral changes mimicking confusion. Infarctions of the fusiform or lingual gyri on the undersurface of the occipital lobe may produce acute agitated confusion. The history of acute onset and other signs such as homonymous hemianopia which point to the posterior cerebral artery territory are helpful in making the diagnosis. Some cases of transient global amnesia may be due to bouts of ischemia involving the mesial temporal lobes. Infarctions of the dominant mesial temporal lobe produces a Korsakoff's syndrome for several months, but is permanent with a bilateral lesion. Some patients with infarction of the nondominant parietal lobe present with acute confusion.

Broca's aphasia is nearly always accompanied by hemiplegia. The poorly articulated, effortful, sparse, grammatically incorrect speech accompanied by good comprehension of language allow recognition of this syndrome. Other aphasias are characterized by a flow of well articulated speech, often devoid of meaning, and may be misdiagnosed as confusion or a psychiatric disorder since there may be no associated paralysis. In Wernicke's aphasia there is abundant, fluent speech with severe impairment in comprehension of language. The patient has no insight into his difficulty and is unable to repeat phrases given him by the examiner. The patient produces speech containing neologisms, literal and verbal paraphasias. When there is a fluent aphasia with intact comprehension, but inability to repeat phrases such as "no ifs ands or buts," the lesion has disrupted the connections between Wernicke's area (posterior superior temporal gyrus) and Broca's area (inferior frontal gyrus). This is termed a conduction aphasia. Nominal or amnestic aphasia is a fluent aphasia where comprehension and repetition are both intact. Circumlocutory phrases are common, and there is severe difficulty in naming objects. This form of aphasia is often present in the acutely confused patient without localizing significance. When confusion is not present, nominal aphasia is associated with a focal lesion in the posterior lower temporal lobe or angular gyrus. In all of the aphasias, writing is more severely affected than speech. The schizophrenic with severe thought disorder does not produce paraphasic errors in his speech and his writing may show bizarre use of space and symbols, but, unlike the patient with aphasia, both are often copious. Schizophrenic "word salad" is rare and usually is limited to chronic "back ward" patients who have been allowed to lead isolated existences.

PSYCHIATRIC DISORDERS

The clinical pictures associated with acute schizophrenia and manic-depressive illness are described in Chapter 52. It is very helpful when a past history of psychotic episodes is available. The onset of schizophrenia after the age of 35 is unusual, and the diagnosis should be made with great reluctance after this age. Homosexual panic is suggested by recent exposure to dormitory or barracks life. Patients with severe anxiety or depression may appear on the accident floor in fugue states. Ganser's syndrome occurs in people wishing to escape a stressful situation, often prison. These patients provide incorrect replies to all questions,

but the replies clearly indicate an understanding of the question and often are approximately correct (syndrome of approximate answers). The condition frequently disappears when the patient is confronted with the diagnosis.

TOXIC AND METABOLIC DISORDERS

DRUG INTOXICATION*

The most common agents causing acute confusion are listed in Table 1. The paradoxical ability of the barbiturates to cause excitement in certain patients should be recalled. Belladonna derivatives are present in many medications, and their toxic features have been epitomized as "mad as a hatter, dry as a bone, blind as a bat, and red as a beet." These problems result from the anticholinergic impairment of central nervous system neurotransmission, suppression of sweating, mydriasis with paralysis of accommodation, and widespread cutaneous vasodilatation. The acute confusion occasionally induced by the belladonna family of antiparkinsonian agents can be immediately reversed by intravenous physostigmine. The acute dystonic reactions to the phenothiazines with torticollis, trismus, or swallowing difficulty are often terrifying for the patient, but can be promptly reversed by intravenous Cogentin. The excited confusion of cocaine poisoning is associated with headache, tachypnea, mydriasis, and crawling dyesthesias. The mescaline–lysergic acid derivatives cause perceptual alterations, with visual and tactile hallucinations being most frequent. Caffeine poisoning produces delirium with visual hallucinations, restlessness, tremor, and tinnitus. Ergot derivatives also cause headache with confusion, pruritus, and usually small pupils; but the peripheral arterial constriction with pale, cold, pulseless extremities is the most important clue to the diagnosis. Salicylate toxicity also causes confusion and headache, usually accompanied by hyperventilation and tinnitus. An acneiform rash often is associated with the confusion, memory impairment, or hallucinations of bromidism.

Simple drunkenness is rarely the only problem in persons brought to the Emergency Department in a confused state.

---

*See Chapter 55, Drug and Alcohol Abuse.

Associated signs of head injury, infection, liver failure, and vitamin deficiency should be sought.

WITHDRAWAL SYNDROMES

In alcohol withdrawal, symptoms of confusion, tremulousness, illusions, hallucinations, and restlessness usually begin within 24 to 72 hours of cessation of drinking. Withdrawal seizures consistently occur, and cease before the onset of the mental symptoms. There is marked variation in the severity of alcohol withdrawal syndromes. Some patients have only minor symptoms of irritability, tremulousness, and confusion which last from a few hours to several days. Alcoholic auditory hallucinosis designates a withdrawal state in which thought processes and behavior are normal except for the occurrence of vivid, usually unpleasant auditory hallucinations. The hallucinations commonly disappear within a week, but in rare cases become chronic.

The most severe alcohol withdrawal syndrome is delirium tremens. This constitutes a major medical emergency and has a mortality rate of 10 to 20 per cent. Severe confusion, tremulousness, restlessness, and vivid hallucinations are coupled with fever, rapid pulse, and marked diaphoresis. Onset is often abrupt, lasts one to five days and is terminated after the patient has a prolonged sleep. On awakening he does not recall the episode.

Major withdrawal syndromes with seizures and confusion develop two to eight days after withdrawal of a variety of sedatives and tranquilizers, including the barbiturates, meprobramate, glutethamide, and paraldehyde, when these have been taken chronically in significant dosages. (See Chapters 57 and 58.)

METABOLIC ENCEPHALOPATHIES

These entities are partially listed in Table 1 and discussed in separate chapters of this book. Most of the metabolic encephalopathies produce a somnolent type of confusional state and, with worsening, enter the phases of rostral-caudal progression of central nervous system dysfunction described in Chapter 23. However, acute agitated delirium occasionally may be seen with any of the metabolic encephalopathies and is characteristic of certain others, such as porphyria and hyperthyroidism.

ASSESSMENT

All available history is gathered, and, if necessary, some Emergency Department personnel are assigned the task of locating friends and family or even enlisting the aid of the police to detail the mode of onset of the confusional state, the presence of pre-existing medical conditions, the use of drugs, or toxic exposures. The physician proceeds to an evaluation of the vital signs and a rapid physical examination for evidence of trauma, respiratory or vascular compromise, meningeal irritation, an acute abdomen, papilledema, and gait disturbance. The level of alertness, thought content, memory function, and use of language should be recorded together with any obvious elementary neurologic signs. Skull and chest x-rays, EEG, complete blood count, serum glucose, electrolytes, calcium, blood urea nitrogen, toxic screen, and urinalysis should next be obtained as a minimum initial laboratory evaluation. Arterial blood gases, serum ammonia, liver function studies, serum cortisol, thyroxine, or transaminase levels, antinuclear factor, and urine tests for heavy metals or porphyria (Watson-Schwartz Test) also may be helpful in certain cases.

Lumbar puncture is essential in the evaluation of the acutely confused patient. The lumbar puncture may be deferred in two situations. The first is when diagnosis has been established and the patient is showing rapid improvement, as in a bout of hypoglycemia. If the diagnosis seems clear but immediate improvement is not anticipated, the patient still should have a lumbar puncture. We have seen many patients with alcohol withdrawal syndromes where lumbar puncture revealed evidence of a primary intracranial process, such as subdural hematoma or meningitis, which was the cause for the cessation of alcohol intake. The second circumstance when lumbar puncture may be deferred arises in the patient with signs of increased intracranial pressure due to a mass lesion. An alternate emergency diagnostic procedure is *mandatory* in any instance where the patient's condition is sufficiently omnious to be considered at risk from lumbar puncture. In this situation, neurologic or neurosurgical consultation should be obtained to guide the selection of the alternate procedure, which may require cerebral angiography or ventriculography. Computerized tomography of the brain will clearly be the method of choice for the initial evaluation of patients with mass lesions when this technique becomes available on an emergency basis. The use of other noninvasive examinations such as isotope brain scanning and the electroencephalogram remain a matter of judgment concerning the likelihood of diagnostic yield and whether the rate of progression of the patient's status permits time for such evaluation. Both of these procedures are apt to be technically unsatisfactory in a very restless or combative patient.

PLAN

Certain therapeutic maneuvers must be carried out along with the early phase of diagnostic assessment. Adequate ventilation must be ensured. The patient may require an airway or treatment for shock or hyperthermia. Thiamine (100 mg. parentally) is often given immediately to avoid tragic oversight in the alcoholic or malnourished patient. Initial blood studies are drawn, and intravenous glucose is administered. The sequence of glucose administration following thiamine is intended to avoid the acute precipitation of a thiamine deficiency state. Gastric lavage is also carried out during this early phase in appropriate cases. These preliminary maneuvers usually can be accomplished in 15 minutes by a trained emergency staff.

The specific management of the various disorders is discussed in separate chapters of this text. However, some general principles of management should be mentioned here. The patient should be approached with firm calmness and all procedures explained in detail. His environment should be well lighted. If restraints are necessary these should be applied with the precautions of proper positioning and padding to avoid nerve compression palsies. The patient should be on his side and allowed to assume a comfortable position. The practice of tying the supine patient's limbs to the four corners of a bed promotes struggling behavior and exposes him to the risks of aspiration and brachial plexus palsies. Sedation should be avoided until a diagnosis is established that includes sedation as an appropriate part of treatment. If a family member or friend can stay with the patient, the need for sedation is often minimized. Sedation should be aimed at calming the patient, not at causing a depressed state of consciousness. This practice simply adds the complications of coma to those of the disorder causing the acute confusional state. Orders for sedative medication should, therefore, be written as each dose is needed. Paraldehyde, chloral hydrate, and diazepam are the most widely used sedatives for the delirious patient.

The patient with delirium tremens is so restless that sedation is necessary to prevent exhaustion and cardiovascular collapse. Paraldehyde, 8 to 10 cc. by the rectal or oral route, is still among the most effective and safest agents for delirium tremens. Intramuscular paraldehyde is often complicated by the development of sterile abscesses. The patient should not receive more than 10 cc every two hours. The dosage usually can be reduced after the first eight to 12 hours of treatment. The meticulous maintenance of fluid and electrolyte balance is probably the single most important aspect of the treatment of the DT's. The fever, profuse diaphoresis, and continuous motor activity may raise fluid requirements to 5 to 7 liters per day. Adequate vitamin therapy should be included in the intravenous solutions. Blood urea nitrogen and electrolytes must be closely monitored. The fever should be suppressed with salicylates, sponge baths, or a cooling blanket. These patients require a thorough search for head trauma with intracranial hematoma, meningitis, pneumonia or other infections, liver failure, hypoglycemia, pancreatitis, anemia, and gastrointestinal bleeding which might have caused the patient to stop drinking and precipitated the withdrawal syndrome.

References

Adams, R. D., and Victor, M.: Delirium and other confusional states and Korsakoff's amnestic syndrome. *In* Wintrobe, M. M., et al. (eds.): Harrison's Principles of Internal Medicine, 6th ed. New York, McGraw-Hill, 1970, pp. 184–193.
Chedru, F., and Geschwind, N.: Disorders of higher cortical functions in acute confusional states. Cortex 8:395, 1972.
Geschwind, N.: The aphasias. N. Engl. J. Med. 284:654, 1971.
Gooddy, W.: Orientation. *In* Vinken, P. J., and Bruyn, G. W. (eds.): Handbook of Clinical Neurology. New York, Elsevier, 1969, pp. 202–211.
Lipowsky, Z. J.: Delirium clouding of consciousness and confusion. J. Nerv. Ment. Dis. 145:227, 1967.
McGhie, A.: Psychological aspects of attention and its disorders. *In* Vinken, P. J., and Bruyn, G. W. (eds.): Handbook of Clinical Neurology. New York, Elsevier, 1969, pp. 137–154.
Plum, F., and Posner, J. B.: The Diagnosis of Stupor and Coma. Philadelphia, F. A. Davis Co., 1970.

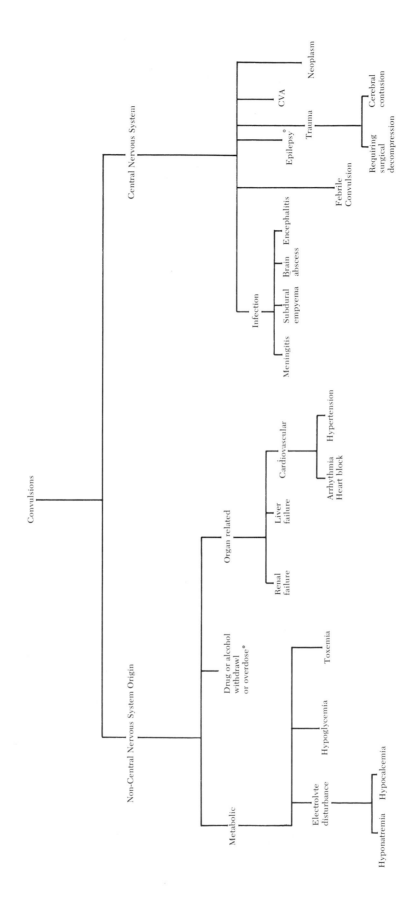

Chapter 25 CONVULSIONS

Leon Menzer and Thomas D. Sabin

The incidence of seizures in the general population is 1 or 2 per cent, so that epileptic patients are often seen in the Emergency Department. Only a few of these patients require urgent emergency treatment, but all require an immediate diagnostic evaluation.

A major motor seizure is startling to witness, but the patient is rarely at risk of death from an isolated convulsion. Such a rare death usually is due to a serious underlying neurologic disease or the mishap of losing consciousness and motor control in a precarious situation (swimming, driving, etc.), rather than to seizure activity itself. It is of the utmost importance to note that a seizure may be but a symptom of cerebral hypoxia, intracranial suppuration, serious head injury, or metabolic derangement.

The nature and tempo of the evaluation is determined by the patient's age, course, the availability of a clinical history, and, most important, by the type of seizures affecting the patient. The first physician who sees the patient often has the best opportunity to obtain crucial historical information from witnesses, friends, or family who have accompanied the patient to the hospital. Was the patient well prior to the seizure? Was the seizure focal in onset? Was there head injury or exposure to toxins? Was this a true seizure or a simple faint? Information concerning previous seizures, drug usage, family history, or the presence of diabetes or hypertension may help clarify the cause of the seizure disorder.

A rapid general and neurologic examination is performed to determine the state of consciousness, the presence of increased intracranial pressure, infection, focal neurologic signs, or obvious general medical disease. When seizures relate to abnormalities such as hypertensive encephalopathy, hyponatremia, hypocalcemia, or toxemia of pregnancy, then the treatment directed toward the primary condition is far more effective than causing progressive obtundation by increasing amounts of intravenous anticonvulsants.

In any circumstance where the cause of the seizure is doubtful and there is no evidence of increased intracranial pressure, the spinal fluid should be examined because of the possibility of meningitis, even if fever is absent. A careful cell count and gram stain are both essential. In certain types of acute purulent meningitis (especially pneumococcal) the gram stain may reveal organisms before there is a cellular response in the spinal fluid. The chronic meningitides, subdural empyema, brain abscess, and encephalitis are other infectious processes which may cause fever and spinal fluid abnormalities. The diagnosis of *febrile seizures* should not be considered until a normal spinal fluid examination is obtained. Febrile seizures commonly occur between the ages of one and six years, and there is often a positive family history. Skull films should be obtained to check for fractures, signs of increased intracranial pressure, or abnormal calcifications. An emergency blood glucose determination should be made to exclude hypoglycemia and to compare with the spinal fluid glucose level. Protein and serology determinations should be made on all CSF specimens, but usually are not immediately helpful. Only rarely does unexpected hypocalcemia account for seizures. The emergency work-up may also include chest x-ray, EKG, CBC, electrolytes, BUN, urinalysis, and anticonvalsant blood levels if the patient has been on anticonvulsant therapy.

519

500 CLINICAL EMERGENCY MEDICINE

The clinical features of seizures are diverse, and some of the problems confronted in the Emergency Department include:

1. Grand mal or major motor status.
2. A conscious or unconscious patient who is said to have had a recent seizure.
3. Focal motor or partial seizure status.
4. Petit mal status.

STATUS

Major motor status or status epilepticus refers to repeated generalized seizures without intercurrent recovery. The incidence of status paradoxically has increased since the introduction of effective anticonvulsants. Most cases of status epilepticus result from drug (including anticonvulsants) and alcohol withdrawal states, severe head injury, or metabolic derangements. Barbiturate withdrawal seizures may be particularly severe. On the other hand, status can occur from drug overdose.

The patient has tonic and/or clonic movements of the limbs and the truncal musculature. Tonic eye deviation during a generalized seizure often has no localizing significance. The patient is unresponsive and may become cyanotic during the tonic phase of the seizure. Motor activity may be continuous or may cease, and the patient may even become responsive to noxious stimuli before the next seizure occurs. Grand mal status must be stopped as quickly as possible when:

1. Severe hypoxia or acidosis develops.
2. There has been a recent surgical procedure and there is danger of wound dehiscence.
3. Recent myocardial infarction or other serious medical conditions are present and place the patient in special jeopardy from hypoxia or vigorous physical activity.
4. Myoglobin appears in the urine owing to muscle necrosis accompanying the extreme exertion.
5. When the body temperature becomes significantly elevated.

Immediate intravenous anticonvulsants are required in these dire circumstances. The physician must be prepared to manage the respiratory arrest, cardiac arrhythmias, or hypotension which may be caused by these drugs.

The administration of drugs, however, must not supersede the simple supportive measures required to maintain ventilation. A secure airway should be rapidly established. An oropharyngeal airway and frequent suctioning often are sufficient, and oxygen should be started if the patient appears hypoxic. A padded tongue blade may be placed between the rear teeth to prevent damage to the tongue and cheeks. A secure route for intravenous administration of drugs is best established with a catheter system since needles are apt to be dislodged during clonic motor activity. If hypoglycemia cannot be promptly ruled out, glucose (50 cc. of 50 per cent dextrose in water) may be administered before anticonvulsants are started. The following anticonvulsant agents are useful in the management of status epilepticus in the adult. In children dosages must be modified depending on weight.

Diazepam (Valium) has the advantage of prompt action and is therefore useful when immediate cessation of seizures is indicated. Diazepam is administered in doses of 5 to 10 mg. intravenously at a rate not to exceed 5 mg. per minute. This dosage may be repeated in 15 minutes. The major side-effects of intravenous diazepam are respiratory depression and hypotension. Seizures tend to recur in 30 to 60 minutes, yet the depression of consciousness and risk of respiratory depression may be cumulative. These effects appear to be potentiated by barbiturates, monamine oxidase inhibitors, and narcotics.

Diphenylhydantoin (Dilantin) is a highly effective anticonvulsant in adults and offers a reasonable margin of safety. It can be used to treat status epilepticus. When a loading dose of 800 to 1000 mg. is given by nasogastric tube, therapeutic levels are achieved in three to six hours. When diphenylhydantoin is administered intravenously, therapeutic levels cannot be safely achieved in less than 20 minutes. Therefore, the drug is not used initially when more immediate seizure control is mandatory. In suitable cases, however, intravenous diphenylhydantoin offers the significant advantage of not severely depressing consciousness, and this permits more complete neurologic evaluation when the seizures have ceased. The drug is infused at the rate of 50 mg. per minute to a maximum dose of 1000 mg. The diphenylhydantoin sodium preparation is highly alkaline, and extravasation of the solution may cause significant local tissue damage. The patient's vital signs and EKG should be monitored closely during the infusion and for some time after to avert or treat the heart block, hypotension, and respiratory depression which have been cited as the causes of the rare fatalities associated with this technique. Intramuscular diphenylhydantoin is not recommended. There is erratic absorption, and local muscle necrosis occurs at the site of the injections.

Phenobarbital is the most commonly used barbiturate in status epilepticus. Respiratory depression and hypotension are the main side-effects of large intravenous doses. An initial dose of 150 to 250 mg. is given at the rate of 25 mg. per minute. Additional doses can be given each 15 to 20 minutes if seizures persist, but the cumulative dose in the first two hours usually should not be greater than 400 mg. All equipment and personnel required to support the patient's respirations fully should be at hand when large doses of phenobarbital are administered. Patients who have been treated previously with intravenous diazepam are more likely to develop apnea during subsequent phenobarbital treatment.

Paraldehyde has been effectively used in the treatment of status epilepticus for several decades. The drug is largely excreted by exhalation and liver metabolism and therefore is suitable for some patients with impairment of renal function. Paraldehyde may be given intravenously (1 to 3 ml. in two minutes), intramuscularly (5 to 10 ml., avoiding sites near nerves) or as an oil-retention enema (0.2 mg./kg. body weight). Paraldehyde is not compatible with most plastics, and glass syringes therefore must be used.

In exceptional circumstances general anesthesia or neuromuscular blockage may ultimately be needed for the patient with persistent status epilepticus. If cerebral edema is present, the use of intravenous mannitol may assist in controlling the seizures.

The important general principles in treating status epilepticus or seizure disorders are:

1. Decide how much danger the seizures represent to the patient.

2. Efforts at establishing the diagnosis for the cause of the seizure must accompany efforts to control the seizures, and these efforts must persist once the seizures are controlled. Treatment of the cause, be it meningitis, hypoxia, or hypoglycemia, must begin as soon as possible.

3. When using agents which may cause respiratory arrest, the physician must be prepared to intubate the patient and control respirations.

4. It is usually best if the physician uses agents with which he is familiar. Overtreatment must be avoided. An awake patient with occasional mild seizures—or even continuous focal seizures that do not endanger life—is certainly safer than a comatose patient requiring artificial ventilation.

5. No known agent is effective in treating all seizures safely, and the choice of agents and dosage must depend on the circumstances of each case.

GRAND MAL

Grand mal status can be a serious, urgent threat to life, but this is not the common situation that arises in the Emergency Department. Most patients are rushed into the hospital after having a single seizure. In this case there is adequate time for history taking and an examination. Immediately after a seizure a patient may be deeply comatose with no response to painful stimuli or plantar stimulation. Deep tendon reflexes and, rarely, the pupillary response to light may be absent. As the patient awakens, he may be agitated, confused, and combative and may complain of headache and muscle pain. If this is the patient's first seizure, or if a previously stable epileptic is developing progressive signs or symptoms, he should be hospitalized for full evaluation and a period of observation. The patient with a first seizure requires a spinal fluid examination and the same laboratory investigations outlined above for the patient in status. An otherwise stable seizure-prone patient may have a seizure triggered because of improper or inadequate drug intake, injudicious alcohol use, sleep or food deprivation, or an emotional crisis. It is very useful to measure blood levels of anticonvulsants to test the patient's compliance with his drug regimen. Patients should be encouraged to record daily drug intake to eliminate inadvertent errors.

Chronic alcohol use can enhance the liver metabolism of diphenylhydantoin and other anticonvulsants and result in low anticonvulsant blood levels, as can phenobarbital. Some drugs like chloramphenicol, isoniazid, and dicumarol may inhibit liver metabolism and lead to elevated anticonvulsant blood levels and toxicity. Conversely, sudden withdrawal of isoniazid from a stable epileptic patient on isoniazid and diphenylhydantoin may result in a lowered blood level of diphenylhydantoin and in seizures.

FOCAL SEIZURES

Focal motor or partial seizure status is manifested by involuntary clonic movements which commence in an extremity or on one side of the face and which spread ipsilaterally. Focal and persistent nonmotor epilepsy may cause a variety of sensory, visual, and auditory experiences or behavioral changes, depending on the areas of cerebral cortex giving rise to the seizures. Seizures of temporal lobe origin or psychomotor seizures are characterized by semi-purposeful movements—so-called "automatisms"—and there often are complex psychic disturbances with feelings of fear, hallucinations, and visceral or olfactory sensations. An occasional patient may become violent. There may be profound confusion during an attack or afterward. Prolonged or continuous psychomotor seizures are not common.

Focal seizures imply the presence of a focal brain lesion. The lesion may be an old scar from trauma or birth injury, a tumor, abscess, cortical phlebitis, or infarction. The precise mode of onset of the seizure may provide an important clue for localizing the lesion. Continuous focal seizures typically are extremely resistant to treatment with anticonvulsants, but fortunately do not usually constitute an urgent threat to life. We have seen patients whose focal status has persisted over a period of weeks despite very vigorous therapy. One of the commonest errors in the management of seizure disorders is to overtreat such patients, and the physician should never trade off the relatively minimal hazards of focal status for the great risks associated with the comatose state. The ward staff must often be reassured on this point, since the appearance of the patient with focal status is disquieting and may lead to overly zealous treatment.

PETIT MAL

Petit mal status occurs in only 2 to 3 per cent of children who have "absence" attacks and bursts of three-per-second spike and wave activity on their electroencephalogram. Both petit mal and petit mal status are extremely rare after adolescence. In petit mal status the patient may appear confused and distracted, and intermittent blinking and mouthing movements may be observed. The patient may occasionally produce or respond to spoken language. This state can persist for hours or days, and sometimes is mistaken for catatonic withdrawal or toxic encephalopathy. The diagnosis can easily be made by demonstrating generalized 3 cps spike-slow wave discharges on the electroencephalogram. Treatment of choice is intravenous diazepam for petit mal status, although ethosuximide appears to be the best agent for the long term treatment of petit mal epilepsy.

References

Lennox, W., and Lennox, M.: Epilepsy and related disorders. Boston, Little, Brown & Co., 1960.

Millichap, J. G.: Drug treatment of convulsive disorders. N. Engl. J. Med. 286:454, 1972.

Penfield, W., and Jasper, H.: Epilepsy and the Functional Anatomy of the Brain. Boston, Little, Brown & Co., 1954.

Schmidt, R. P., and Wilder, B. J.: Epilepsy. (Vol. 2 of Contemporary Neurology Series.) Philadelphia, F. A. Davis Co., 1968.

Wallis, P. T., Kutt, H., and McDowell, F.: Intravenous diphenylhydantoin in the treatment of acute repetitive seizures. Neurology 18:513, 1968.

Woodbury, D. M., Penry, J. K., and Schmidt, R. P.: Antiepileptic drugs. New York, Raven Press, 1972.

Chapter 26

EVALUATION OF DIARRHEA IN THE EMERGENCY DEPARTMENT

C. C. Roussi

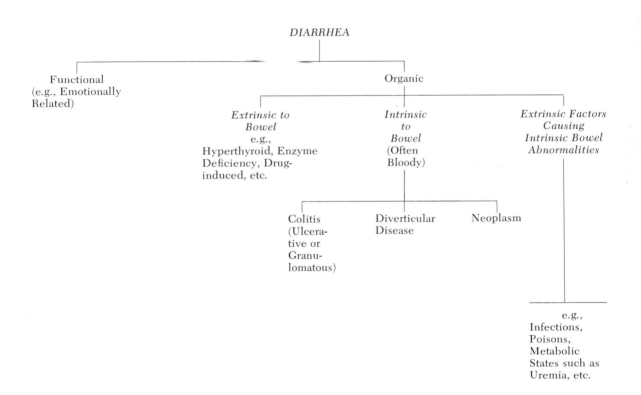

GENERAL INTRODUCTION TO ASSESSMENT

The first step in dealing with the symptom of diarrhea is to determine exactly what the patient means when he uses the term. Most physicians will agree that diarrhea means an increased frequency and/or liquidity of bowel movement. To most patients, however, the term has much broader application, and one soon learns that diarrhea means different things to different people. It is necessary, therefore, to establish the following data in attempting to understand the patient's plight.

(1) *The exact frequency of defecation,* i.e., how many times in a 24-hour period?

(2) *At what time of day?* We may be

523

less concerned about diarrhea that occurs only in the morning and abates after the patient arrives at his place of employment. However, diarrhea that awakens the patient in the middle of the night is much more alarming, and usually proves to have an organic basis.

(3) *Character of the fecal discharge,* i.e., watery, soft, formed, bloody, of what color, and does it float?

(4) *Relationship to meals, specific foods and activities,* i.e., roughage, lactose ingestion, emotional stress. Diarrhea that occurs promptly during or shortly following a meal, and not at any other time, strongly suggests an exaggerated gastrocolic reflex.

(5) *Association with other symptoms,* i.e., abdominal pain, nausea, vomiting, constipation, anorexia, fever, weight loss, and abdominal distention.

(6) *Duration of symptoms.*

This information, combined with a thorough physical examination, usually provides the framework upon which an accurate diagnosis can be based. Although every part of the physical examination is important, the rectal examination deserves special emphasis. It is the most direct means of detecting the presence of a rectal mass, a fecal impaction, or an incompetent anal sphincter; all of these may be causes of diarrhea, particularly in an aging population. In the case of rectal bleeding or bloody diarrhea, the digital examination should be augmented routinely with a proctoscopic examination. This can easily be accomplished with the patient in the left lateral position if a proctoscopic table is not available. No preparation usually is required, and it can provide diagnostic information that is essential in organizing a rational approach to the subsequent disposition and therapy of the patient. The patient with bleeding internal hemorrhoids requires only reassurance and instructions for the local application of an emollient. On the other hand, the finding of a neoplasm or an inflamed and bleeding mucosa clearly indicates the need for hospitalization. If examination of the rectum is negative, but blood is seen to flow antegrade beyond the limits of the scope, one can logically entertain diverticular disease or neoplasm as the cause, and once again justify hospitalization.

There is no ideal or simple way to categorize the myriad of conditions that may provoke the symptom of diarrhea. Regardless of the approach, one usually is left with an exhaustive but cumbersome listing of conditions, the sum total of which constitutes a differential diagnosis of diarrhea. Such a list is useful, but does not lend itself to the unique circumstances and requirements of the Emergency Department, where it is necessary to have a method or systematic approach in dealing with the symptom of diarrhea that satisfies the demand to determine rapidly the underlying pathology, and allows prompt appropriate disposition or initial therapy. The following schema has proved useful to me.

DIARRHEA

(1) Functional.
(2) Organic.
  (*a*) Disease process is intrinsic to the bowel.
  (*b*) Disease process is extrinsic to the bowel.
  (*c*) Disease process is both intrinsic and extrinsic to the bowel.

Functional Diarrhea

This is a common disorder associated with motor dysfunction of the colon, i.e., irritable colon syndrome. Its course is chronic and characterized by recurrent acute exacerbations, precipitated by emotional stress. Abdominal cramping and distention due to aerophagia may be prominent accompanying symptoms, manifested on the physical examination by hyperactive bowel sounds and increased tympany to finger percussion. The stool is watery, and frequently contains increased amounts of mucus. Laboratory data is uniformly normal. It is important to remember that the hallmark of functional diarrhea is that it occurs only during the day, and the patient is remarkably free of symptoms after he retires for the evening.

Organic Diarrhea

DISEASE PROCESS IS INTRINSIC TO THE BOWEL

There is tissue disruption in the bowel itself that produces histologic and structural changes. As a result, one can expect these changes to be reflected in pathologic findings, both on the physical examination and in laboratory data. Included in this group is:

(1) ulcerative colitis;
(2) granulomatous enterocolitis;
(3) neoplastic disease;
(4) diverticular disease.

Although it is less likely in the case of granulomatous enterocolitis, bleeding or bloody diarrhea is a common feature of these conditions.

DISEASE PROCESS IS EXTRINSIC TO THE BOWEL

Diarrhea results from motor or secretory dysfunction, and there are no histologic or structural changes in the bowel itself. This group includes:

(1) hyperthyroidism;
(2) diabetic enteropathy;
(3) drug-induced diarrheas (digitalis, quinidine, laxatives, and a host of others);
(4) pancreatic insufficiency (chronic pancreatitis, mucoviscidosis, and neoplasm);
(5) enzyme deficiency syndromes (lactase, etc.).

DISEASE PROCESS IS BOTH INTRINSIC AND EXTRINSIC TO THE BOWEL

Conditions included in this group vary widely in their effect upon the bowel. There may be no discernible histologic or structural changes, or the changes may be profound. In some instances it is only a matter of degree, i.e., so slight as not to be detected by ordinary methods. In other instances, the disease process is entirely outside the bowel and only secondarily involves it; for example, an ovarian tumor that initially provokes diarrhea and abdominal tenderness may lead to obstruction and ultimately even infarction of the bowel.

This group includes:

(1) specific inflammatory disorders (shigellosis, salmonellosis, amebiasis, viral gastroenteritis, and "traveler's diarrhea");
(2) mesenteric vascular insufficiency or occlusion;
(3) adjacent intra-abdominal disorders (ovarian tumor, cysts, ectopic pregnancy, lymphoma);
(4) antibiotic diarrhea (mild to full-blown pseudomembranous enterocolitis);
(5) Zollinger-Ellison syndrome;

(6) uremia;
(7) gluten enteropathy;
(8) poisoning (heavy metals, staphylococcal enterotoxin).

DIAGNOSTIC ASSESSMENT OF DIARRHEA IN THE EMERGENCY DEPARTMENT

The diagnostic parameters available in any given Emergency Department will vary greatly. It is safe to assume, however, that most will be able to accomplish a CBC, electrolytes, BUN, urinalysis, stool guaiac (or equivalent test), and a plain film of the abdomen (the older term "flatplate of the abdomen" should be discarded). Some will insist on an upright film of the abdomen as well, but it is not essential. Indeed, the above capabilities, combined with a good history and physical examination (including a rectal and proctoscopic examination) and a high index of suspicion, are more than adequate to provide an accurate diagnosis in most instances.

Most patients who present to an Emergency Department with the complaint of diarrhea will do so because it is of such frequency that it is interfering with sleep, is causing significant weakness and exhaustion, or has become associated with bleeding or abdominal pain. Confronted with a patient with all of these symptoms, we can begin to apply the previously outlined schema. The emergency physician must first make a general evaluation of the seriousness and need for supportive treatment before making further diagnostic tests (e.g., intravenous fluids, blood transfusion, electrolyte correction, etc.). These diarrhea conditions of such severity are almost all "organic" in nature. The determination of intrinsic or extrinsic (or extrinsic-causing intrinsic changes) becomes of great therapeutic importance if the extrinsic cause is rapidly treatable.

The proctoscopic examination should be decisive in excluding or including the diagnosis of ulcerative colitis, granulomatous colitis, amebiasis, or a specific bacterial colitis. Ulcerative colitis will reveal a diffusely friable and bleeding mucosa, as opposed to the ulcerating lesions of granulomatous colitis, which shows normal intervening mucosa. Multiple small punctate ulcerations will suggest amebiasis. A bacterial colitis, as with

Shigella, may be indistinguishable from a mild ulcerative colitis through the proctoscope, but the history should point the way to the correct diagnosis. If ulcerative or granulomatous colitis is seriously considered, the plain film of the abdomen should be scrutinized carefully to establish or rule out the diagnosis of toxic megacolon.

If vascular collapse and bleeding of rapid onset have been prominent features, the diagnosis of mesenteric occlusion must be considered. The syndrome of mesenteric insufficiency usually is manifested by postprandial abdominal pain, but may be associated with diarrhea. The patient generally is elderly. In acute occlusion, the presenting symptoms may be bloody diarrhea and severe abdominal pain. It rapidly progresses to atony of the bowel, vascular collapse, and death. Lesser degrees of ischemia will produce changes in the bowel mucosa characterized by shallow and linear ulceration, which usually spares the rectum. It is termed "ischemic colitis" and frequently presents with bleeding. Bleeding beyond the limits of the proctoscope should then suggest the diagnoses of colonic neoplasm, diverticulosis coli, and ischemic colitis.

In consideration of the specific inflammatory disorders, shigellosis alone, if severe enough, will produce changes in the rectal mucosa similar to mild ulcerative colitis. Salmonellosis produces no detectable changes and is more common then shigellosis. The very common "traveler's diarrhea" is thought to be due to the effects of endotoxin produced by pathogenic *E. coli.* Similarly, staphylococcal enterocolitis is the result of endotoxins, and does not involve an invasion of the mucosa. The incubation period is two to four hours, never more than six hours, and it produces explosive diarrhea and vomiting. Almost any kind of poisoning will have a similar history.

Antibiotic diarrhea occurs for the most part in patients who are postoperative and on antibiotics. The diarrhea results from altered flora in the bowel, but continuation of the pathologic process produces colitis-like changes in the mucosa. The final picture is that of pseudomembranous colitis.

The diagnosis of Zollinger-Ellison syndrome is suggested in the patient who has diarrhea and a history consistent with peptic ulcer. In 10 per cent of cases of this syndrome, diarrhea may be the only symptom. Determination of the electrolytes usually will show a hypokalemia as a result of the copious diarrhea.

A paucity of physical findings, negative laboratory data, and the appropriate history will serve to identify viral gastroenteritis.

Several of the conditions listed in the schema will rarely be diagnosed definitively in the Emergency Department. In general, conditions such as pancreatic insufficiency and gluten enteropathy will be suggested on the basis of a diligent evaluation of physical findings, corroborative laboratory data, a careful history, and a high index of suspicion. As in so many other instances, the final diagnosis for many of the conditions will depend on more elaborate in-hospital testing; however, the process of bringing the diagnosis into focus should begin in the Emergency Department, and when necessary stabilizing treatment should be initiated.

Chapter 27

DIFFICULTY IN BREATHING

Robert H. Dailey

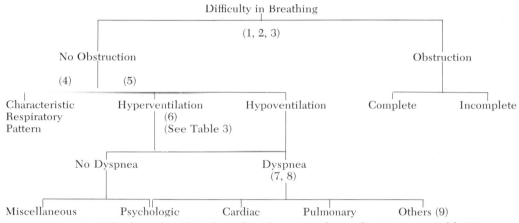

Figure 1   Difficulty in breathing logic flow sheet. (Numbers refer to items in Table 2.)

This discussion deals with the evaluation of patients presenting with the symptom or sign of difficulty in breathing. The emphasis is on approach. A lexicon of common terms is provided (Table 1) to clarify the terminology used.

INITIAL ASSESSMENT

The initial approach to the patient with respiratory distress is essentially identical to that used for any acutely ill patient, but with emphasis on adequacy of ventilation. That is, evaluation of respiration must be put in the context of the patient's general clinical state. As with all acutely ill patients, immediate threats to life must be identified with a macroscopic examination of several simultaneous components: critical observation of the patient in his most general aspects, especially respirations; fingers on the radial or carotid pulse; and several questions to obtain history and assess mental status. This macro-examination should take no more than 30 seconds to one minute, and it determines the tempo with which the remainder of the examination should unfold. If a respiratory problem is identified, a logical sequence of questions can be posed (Table 2 and Figure 1). This sequence is actually artificial: the clinician does not follow rigid formulae. It is offered, however, as a list of priorities; none should be omitted.

First, one observes the bared chest for respiratory movements. Their absence, in association with no palpable carotid pulse, immediately raises the often difficult question whether death has occurred. If the patient

527

TABLE 1. Brief Lexicon of Common Terms

1. *Respiration:* The process of gas exchange by which O_2 is gained and CO_2 lost from the body.
2. *Ventilation (alveolar):* Volume of air exchanged/min.; or vol. per breath (minus dead space) times respiratory rate.
3. *Dyspnea:* Subjective sense of shortness of breath: "air hunger."
4. *Tachypnea:* Greater than normal respiratory rate.
5. *Hyperpnea:* Greater than normal minute ventilation which just meets metabolic demands.
6. *Hyperventilation:* Ventilation which exceeds metabolic demand.
7. *Hypoventilation* (also: Respiratory Failure, Hypercapnia, Hypercarbia): Ventilation which does not meet metabolic demand.
8. *Apnea:* Cessation of breathing for indeterminate period.
9. *Respiratory arrest:* Persistent apnea.

has been observed by a nurse or ambulance attendant during the preceding five minutes, the author relies as much on their observations as on his own examination of pupils and "quick look" paddle monitor reading. Infrequently, one finds intact circulation (without shock) in the absence of respirations: the most common causes of this phenomenon are narcotic overdose, massive intracranial hemorrhage, and the apneic phase of Cheyne-Stokes respiration.

If respiratory movements are present and the circulation is intact, one must next rule out upper airway obstruction. It is rare to see complete upper airway obstruction in the Emergency Department: such patients usually are dead on arrival. However, the clinician must recognize the signs and symptoms of complete upper airway obstruction: paradoxic respirations (that is, marked chest retractions on inspiration), cyanosis, and coma; aphonia occurs if obstruction is at the vocal cords. In the absence of trauma, complete upper airway obstruction in an adult is most often due to a "café-coronary," i.e., a

TABLE 2. Breathing Difficulty

Key steps of evaluation, in sequence:

H	1. Respiratory movements present?
I	2. "Moving air"?
S	3. Upper airway obstruction?
T	4. Diagnostic respiratory pattern?
O	5. Adequacy of ventilation (= arterial PCO_2): consider rate × depth of breaths.
R	6. Dyspnea? (See Table 3)
Y	7. Objective signs on physical examination?
!	8. Laboratory, x-ray, EKG, simple pulmonary function tests.

large piece of food obstructing the glottis or trachea—frequently in a patient with dentures who has been imbibing. Under these circumstances, immediate direct laryngoscopy must be performed with bayonet forceps at the ready. If the obstructing food cannot be immediately removed, or if some other cause of upper airway obstruction is found that cannot be corrected at once, immediate tracheostomy or crycothyroidotomy must be performed. Such a patient must necessarily be managed differently in the field: the successful blind use of a plastic oropharyngeal forceps has recently been described (Eller and Haugen, 1973) as has a technique (the Heimlich maneuver) to clear the upper airway with sudden compression of the upper abdomen (Patient Care, 1976). "Restaurant cricothyroidotomy" should be performed only if the diagnosis is secure, the patient apneic, and the physician adequately equipped.

If upper airway obstruction is incomplete, stridor will be present; also, inspiration will likely be prolonged in contradistinction to the prolonged expiration seen in lower airway obstruction. These crucial findings must spark an immediate search for both the etiology and the rapidity of progression of the obstruction. In chronic upper airway obstruction without immediate life threat, simple respiratory function tests may be helpful (Sackner, 1972).

If respiratory movements are present and air is being exchanged without upper airway obstruction, the clinician should be alert to several patterns of respiration that may aid in diagnosis or necessitate immediate action (Table 4). Agonal breathing is the most important such specific respiratory pattern because it cannot sustain life. These respirations are slow, weak, shallow, and gasping, with a rapid inspiratory component. There is attendant obtundation. This pattern indicates terminal respiratory distress or the final stages of circulatory collapse. Regardless of etiology, it is an indication for *immediate* endotracheal intubation and respiratory support. One word of caution, however: in the head trauma victim one must assume that there is also a cervical fracture until x-rays prove otherwise. Under these circumstances, the head cannot safely be extended on the neck for orotracheal intubation; rather one must consider blind nasotracheal intubation, tracheostomy or cricothyroidotomy, esophageal airway, or placement of nasotracheal tube over a catheter inserted via the cricothyroid membrane. (Technique of choice in this circumstance would depend on the skills of the individual clinician.) It must be emphasized that, once a patient is being ventilated via cuffed endotracheal tube, a pneumothorax will be enlarged and/or converted to a *tension pneumothorax*. A clue to tension pneumothorax is the development of increasing pressure needed to ventilate the patient in the face of decreased chest excursions.

Several other specific respiratory patterns are either pathognomonic or helpful in diagnosis. Cheyne-Stokes respiration is phasic in nature, and frequently is misinterpreted at the bedside as hypoventilation, respiratory arrest, or hyperventilation. It is most often seen in the elderly patient with metabolic derangements and is not itself a respiratory condition necessitating treatment.

A number of characteristic breathing patterns (cluster, apneustic, ataxic, etc.) denote either anatomic or metabolic disturbances of the CNS respiratory nuclei in the pons and medulla. Although these are not often seen clinically in classic form, it is important to remember that these chaotic or irregular breathing patterns, particularly following acute rises in intracranial pressure, often immediately precede respiratory arrest. Therefore, such patients should not be left unobserved, and endotracheal intubation *must* be anticipated.

Finally, Kussmaul respirations should be mentioned. These are the deep, regular, rapid respirations classically described in patients with diabetic ketoacidosis. Such respirations represent an attempt to compensate any severe metabolic acidosis (Table 3, A–5); when accompanied by conscious respiratory effort, they may be confused with the dyspnea and/or hyperventilation of many etiologies as well as primary respiratory alkalosis.

If respirations are unobstructed and there is no characteristic respiratory pattern, an assessment of adequacy of ventilation is the next logical determination. Although such definition can be provided by an arterial PCO_2 determination, a clinical estimation must initially be relied upon. Since minute ventilation is the product of respiratory rate (8 to 16 per minute normally) and tidal volume (400-800 cc./breath normally), the importance of consciously considering rate and depth of respiration cannot be overempha-

TABLE 3. Causes of Hyperventilation°

A. Without Dyspnea
   (1) "Central" hyperventilation secondary to CVA, or Cheyne-Stokes.
   (2) Anxiety.
   (3) CNS stimulants (amphetamines, aspirin, etc.).
   (4) Early traumatic and septic shock.
   (5) Metabolic Acidosis.
      (a) Endogenous acidosis (lactic, uremic, diabetic ketoacidosis, alcoholic ketoacidosis).
      (b) Exogenous acidosis (aspirin, methanol, ethylene glycol, paraldehyde, isopropyl alcohol).
   (6) Miscellaneous: anemia, fever, hyperthyroidism.
B. With Dyspnea
   (1) Anxiety (hyperventilation syndrome).
   (2) Pulmonary.
   (3) Cardiac.
   (4) Other.

°Some of these problems represent hyperpnea more precisely than hyperventilation, i.e., ventilation does not exceed metabolic demand (e.g., fever).

sized. The depth of respiration ordinarily is more important than rate: four or five deep respirations per minute can result in adequate ventilation, whereas shallow respirations at rates of 30 or 40 are often totally inadequate. The most common causes of hypoventilation in the Emergency Department are acutely decompensated respiratory diseases, cardiovascular collapse (shock), or drug overdosages, although unusual causes may be seen, such as the "Pickwickian syndrome."

SUBJECTIVE AND OBJECTIVE FINDINGS

If ventilation is grossly adequate and the circulation is intact, a more ordered and deliberate evaluation may be made of the patient. It should be emphasized that such evaluation frequently is not done because of the patient's anxiety and obvious respiratory distress. Thus the physician is often led into a hasty and disorganized approach that misses cues and results in suboptimal care. In order best to assess the wide variety of clinical signs associated with respiratory difficulty, the patient should be examined in a semi-upright position with chest bared. During this examination, the patient must be continually assessed for worsening of his clinical condition. If such occurs, the necessity for therapeutic intervention will be in direct proportion to the rapidity and severity of clinical deterioration. Thus, the clinician

TABLE 4. *Respiratory Patterns*°

A. Agonal

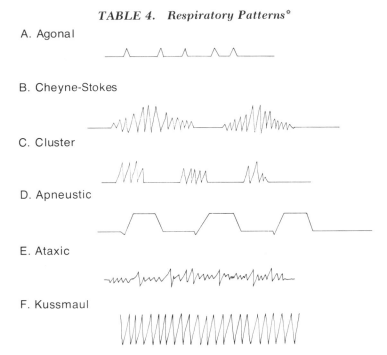

B. Cheyne-Stokes

C. Cluster

D. Apneustic

E. Ataxic

F. Kussmaul

|⟵——— 1 min. ———⟶|

°Adapted from Plum, F. and Posner, J. B.: Diagnosis of Stupor and Coma. Philadelphia, F. A. Davis Co., 1972.

should not leave the bedside until the patient is obviously either stabilized or improving.

The most important part of this evaluation is, of course, the history. This may be taken from the patient if his condition permits, or from relatives, friends, or observers. It should also involve use of the patient's old inpatient or outpatient chart, and should be detailed along conventional lines. In acute illness, it must be performed simultaneously with other examinations (Table 2). Suffice it to say that such history should be very pointed, with particular attention to elucidating positive physical findings. If the patient is acutely ill and his condition warrants immediate intervention, the history may have to be delayed, but *in no circumstances should it ever be omitted.*

Gross inspection of the patient in respiratory difficulty is the most important part of the physical examination. One should look for gross deformity of the chest wall or thoracic spine; relationship of the diaphragmatic and thoracic components of respiration; the duration and difficulty of inspiration versus expiration; presence or absence of splinting, wheezing, paradoxic chest movement, stridor, aphonia, pallor or cyanosis, etc. The neck should be observed for goiter, tracheostomy scar, tracheal deviation, and degree of neck vein distention. Unfortunately, assess-

ing central venous pressure by neck veins is often unreliable in dyspneic patients. Even if the patient is properly placed in the semi-upright position, respiratory distress produces such wide swings in intrathoracic pressure as to make central venous pressure difficult to assess by visualizing external jugular veins. But in the patient with relatively unlabored and unobstructed breathing, central venous pressure can be estimated roughly.

Cyanosis deserves special attention, as it is often misunderstood: a distinction must be made between central and peripheral (or acro-) cyanosis. Peripheral cyanosis is due primarily to circulatory failure with resultant stasis in venular and capillary beds and consequent increased oxygen extraction—thus the typical mottled cyanosis of extremities. Central cyanosis is more generalized and most readily seen in the face, especially the tongue and the tips of the nose and ears. It is due to desaturation of at least 5 gm. of hemoglobin, and is *not* directly related to adequacy of ventilation or absolute PO_2: a patient to whom oxygen is being administered will likely not be cyanotic but this fact *cannot* assure that ventilation is adequate. Also, polycythemic patients will be cyanotic at higher O_2 saturations than anemic patients.

Cough and sputum characteristics must

be recognized. Sputum should be examined both grossly and microscopically: an unstained preparation is especially useful in asthmatics to distinguish allergic from infective bronchitis (Epstein, 1972). Painful respirations, with or without splinting, are of special significance, especially in the traumatized patient. Patients with chest trauma should be evaluated especially for flail chest, pericardial tamponade, hemo- and/or pneumothorax, pulmonary contusion, and tension pneumothorax.*

Palpation is particularly helpful in patients with trauma or musculoskeletal types of chest pain. Compression in both lateral and AP diameters is useful to elicit pain of rib fractures. Fingertip pressure can identify fractures, costal muscle tears, "costochondritis," "trigger points," or subcutaneous emphysema. Percussion is most helpful to indicate either a collection of fluid in the pleural space or an elevated diaphragm. Hyper-resonance should tip one off to pneumothorax and, especially if exaggerated, tension pneumothorax. And with auscultation one must, of course, be completely familiar with the nature and significance of rales, wheezes, rhonchi, and pleural and pericardial friction rubs.

ANCILLARY TESTS

Accurate definitions of respiratory, cardiovascular, and metabolic processes are simply not possible without assays of arterial blood gases. The importance of the Pco_2 value must be emphasized, since it *defines* adequacy of alveolar ventilation: 45 mm. Hg or greater indicates hypoventilation; less than 35 mm. Hg, hyperventilation. Hypoventilation always necessitates aggressive and frequently immediate intervention. Unfortunately, because arterial blood gases take time to draw and determine, they cannot dictate clinical interventions in acutely ill patients with rapidly changing dynamic states. Rather, one must use vital signs and mental status as the most important determinants for therapeutic action, especially in airway management; and blood gases must always be interpreted in the light of clinical findings.

Maximal breathing capacity and 1- and 3-second timed vital capacity are useful bedside tests. Some degree of patient cooperation is necessary, but these tests can be used particularly well to follow a patient's objective improvement over a period of time or when comparison with previous respiratory status is desirable. Patients with acute asthma or with chronic obstructive pulmonary disease fall into these two categories, respectively.

The electrocardiogram is also very valuable in the evaluation of the patient in respiratory distress. Many pulmonary diseases have their electrocardiographic correlates, and sometimes primary cardiac disease is thus recognized as the cause for respiratory distress.

No evaluation of the dyspneic patient is complete without a *chest x-ray*. Many pathologic chest processes can be identified solely or best by x-ray. And, in the acutely ill patient, where adequate physical examination is often obscured or difficult, the chest radiograph becomes particularly valuable. If a "portable" x-ray is taken, the patient should be at least semisupine to assure a better inspiratory effort and to identify pleural fluid or subdiaphragmatic air. When a patient requires placement of a central venous pressure catheter and/or an endotracheal tube, the chest film should be taken *after* these procedures, so that proper positioning of these devices may be assessed and possible complications of the procedure detected.

One last word: An acutely ill patient must be examined and treated in an area where complete resuscitation facilities are available, where there is good lighting, and where ancillary personnel trained and experienced in handling sick people are readily at hand.

References

Eller, W. C., and Haugen, R. K.: Food asphyxiation—restaurant rescue. N. Engl. J. Med. 289:81, 1973.

Epstein, R. L.: Constitutents of sputum: a simple method. Ann. Intern. Med. 77:259, 1972.

Greenbaum, D. M., et al.: Esophageal obstruction during oxygen administration: a new method for use in resuscitation. Chest 65:188, 1974.

Levy, L. J., et al.: Ketoacidosis associated with alcoholism in non-diabetic subjects. Ann. Intern. Med. 78: 213, 1973.

Patient Care, March 15, 1976, pp. 24–39.

Plum, F., and Posner, J. B.: Diagnosis of Stupor and Coma. 2nd Ed. Philadelphia, F. A. Davis Co., 1972.

Sackner, M. A.: Physiologic features of upper airway obstruction. Chest 62:414, 1972.

Salem, M. R.: The artful intubator. Emergency Med., June 1973, p. 197.

Williams, M. H., and Shim, C. S.: Ventilatory failure. Am. J. Med. 48:477, 1970.

*See Chest Trauma, Chapter 38E.

Chapter 28

HEADACHE

Arnold P. Friedman
and Jeffrey A. Leonard

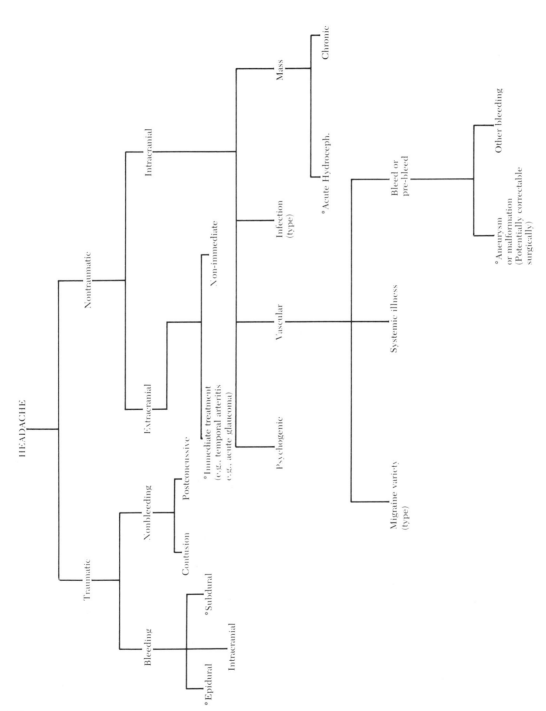

°Immediate treatment (other than pain relief) essential.

Headache occurs as a symptom in a wide variety of illnesses. Although most patients presenting to Emergency Departments with headache as a major complaint do not have significant organic disease, the minority with more serious trouble constitute an important group that needs immediate medical attention. Anyone seeking medical attention for headache should be carefully evaluated for those clues that may indicate possible intracranial disease (Table 1). This is particularly significant if severe headache develops without prior history of recurring headaches, or if a chronic headache has suddenly changed in pattern.

The diagnosis of headache associated with intracranial, systemic, and local diseases of the eye, nose, or teeth generally is based primarily on associated physical and laboratory study findings, whereas diagnosis of the major types of chronic recurring headache, migraine, and muscle contraction headache (tension), is based primarily on history.

One important first step, when possible, in establishing a diagnosis and management program is to take a comprehensive history, including a medical and family history. Particularly important questions are:

(1) When did the first attack of headache occur?

(2) Was it associated with head or neck trauma, behavioral changes, infection, neurologic symptoms, glaucoma, hypertension, or an emotional upset?

(3) What medications was the patient taking, either for the attack of headache or routinely, prior to the headache, with special attention to narcotics, tranquilizers, contraceptive pills, anticoagulants that might predispose to intracranial hemorrhage, and antibiotics that may have altered the usual clinical manifestations of meningitis?

If a mild headache relieved by salicylates is worsened by straining at the stool,

TABLE 1 *Important Symptoms to Arouse Suspicion of Serious Intracranial Disease*

1. Severe headache without prior history
2. Sudden change in chronic headache
3. Worsening with straining at stool or exertion
4. Chronic highly localized pain
5. Duration greater than one day without relief
6. Headache awakening from sleep
7. Associated convulsion
8. Memory disturbance or personality change
9. Progressive worsening

lifting, jarring, or sudden turning of the head, or if it is brought on by such exertional activities, a high index of suspicion exists for progressive intracranial disease.

The severity of the headache is an imperfect guide to the seriousness of its causes. Some of the severest headaches are due to subarachnoid hemorrhage, migraine, or emotional disorders, whereas relatively mild discomfort may be reported by patients with an intracranial tumor. The location of the pain may have some diagnostic value. Chronic unilateral or localized pain may indicate unilateral or local disease, including intracranial mass. Location of migraine tends to vary from side to side in different attacks. Headaches caused by intracranial disease may be generalized or localized in any part of the head, depending on the nature of the disease and the presence of increased intracranial pressure. The quality and character of the pain should be described as well as preheadache manifestations.

Most important in the analysis of a headache are the temporal relationships. A headache that lasts an hour, although acute and perhaps severe, is less likely to be serious than one that lasts for several hours or days. Chronic recurring headache as an isolated symptom is less alarming than a headache that constitutes a relatively new experience. Headache that awakens the patient from sleep or is present immediately upon awakening may be more serious than one that begins in midmorning when he is at work and increases during the day. The former type of headache is often seen with intracranial mass or hypertension.

Symptoms and signs associated with headache may be important guides to its underlying cause. Convulsion accompanying headache is a common symptom of organic brain disease and demands investigation, especially when of recent origin. Progressive neurologic deficits, including disturbances of recent memory and personality changes, may result from intracranial mass lesions. In the older age group, one must consider specific conditions associated with headache, such as temporal arteritis, glaucoma, vascular insufficiency syndromes, and hypertensive states. All these conditions require immediate attention and management.

Physical and neurologic examinations are essential. It is important that the pupils and optic fundi be examined. Direct attention to the cervical spine and skull should be routine. The neurologic examination should also include mental status, cranial nerves, motor system, cerebellar function, reflexes, and sensory modalities.

Laboratory Studies

Laboratory studies available in the Emergency Department that may be of value in selected headache patients include complete blood count, sedimentation rate, blood gas, electrolytes, and blood urea nitrogen and glucose. X-ray studies of the chest, sinuses, skull, and cervical spine can be of great value (see also Chapter 50).

Spinal taps in the Emergency Department are probably best reserved for those patients suspected of having meningitis or subarachnoid bleeding. All spinal fluid should be evaluated for glucose, protein, cells, and serology. If suspected meningitis was the indication for the spinal tap, the fluid should also be evaluated with a gram stain, culture, and sensitivity testing. It is frequently useful to reserve a refrigerated tube of the spinal fluid in case further studies are needed.

RECOGNITION OF BRAIN TUMOR

This is often the unmentioned fear of both examiner and patient in Emergency Departments. Yet not all brain tumors cause headache, and some tumors, especially early lesions, cause only mild intermittent headaches that may be completely relieved by aspirin. Symptoms that should alert the examiner to the possibility of intracranial tumor include the onset of a "new" or different headache pattern that has a tendency to be progressive. The headache is usually a steady, nonthrobbing, deep, dull ache which may be aggravated or produced by coughing, straining at stool, or changing posture, such as bending forward. Also frequently seen is a pattern in which headaches are worse on awakening or after being recumbent for any length of time, and gradually decrease or even disappear when the patient is upright. The mechanism for this pain is traction, either by direct local effect on pain-sensitive structures or by the effect of a mass displacing these structures. Since these pain-sensitive structures tend to be concentrated at the base of the skull, most pain generated by this mechanism tends to be poorly lateralized.

Other symptoms include "projectile vomiting," i.e., vomiting not preceded by as much nausea as would normally seem appropriate. Personality changes, which may have been noted by the patient but are appreciated more often by relatives and friends, are another nonlocalizing symptom of cerebral disease. Diagnosis of an intracranial mass cannot be made on the basis of headache characteristics alone; evaluation of other findings on neurologic examination and the results of ancillary studies are needed.

Physical findings may include nonlocalizing papilledema manifested as swelling of the optic nerve head, with engorgement of retinal veins and hemorrhages of and around the optic nerve head. A patient with specific neurologic deficits, such as hemiparesis, hemianopia, Babinski's sign, and so on, with headache, requires detailed neurologic evaluation as an inpatient.

In tumors occurring in the posterior fossa, headache referred to the occipital and nuchal region is a prominent early sign, since the inferior surfaces of the tentorium and the posterior fossa are supplied by the upper three cervical nerve roots. These tumors may make their presence known early by obstructing the fourth ventricle. In the presence of increased intracranial pressure, localization of the headache is of little value. Brain stem compression may cause somnolence and vomiting. Even though intracranial pressure may be very high in these patients, they still may not have papilledema, since it can take 24 to 72 hours to reflect the increased pressure at the optic nerve head. Acute hydrocephalus is a life-threatening emergency frequently requiring ventricular decompression.

Pseudotumor cerebri is a syndrome clinically manifested as headache, papilledema, and diminution of visual acuity. The headache is nonspecific, usually intermittent, and not a constant feature. It usually has been present for several weeks to several months before medical attention is sought. Frequently noted as part of the syndrome is the high incidence in young, obese females with menstrual irregularities. However, causes other than ovarian dysfunction are known, including Addison's disease, Cushing's disease, adrenocorticosteroid therapy or withdrawal, hypoparathyroidism, pregnancy, menarche, use of contraceptive drugs, vitamin A abuse, tetracycline use in infants, and intracranial venous sinus thrombosis. The mechanism seems to be that of cerebral swelling causing traction on pain-sensitive structures. During evaluation, visual acuity diminution is just as important a consideration as ruling out a mass lesion.

Patients who are strongly suspect for brain tumors, including "pseudotumor" patients, frequently require skull series x-rays, EEG, and brain scan. If indicated, other studies can include arteriograms, computerized axial tomography, pneumoencephalogram, or spinal tap; and a host of other studies may be necessary if the tumor is possibly a metastatic lesion.

Therapy for brain tumors should be specific for the location and histologic type, with surgery, radiation, and chemotherapy available.

INTRACRANIAL HEMORRHAGE

Head trauma is the most common cause of intracranial hemorrhage.* Spontaneous subarachnoid hemorrhage is usually caused by bleeding from pre-existing aneurysms, or a vascular malformation, but may be a manifestation of a blood dyscrasia. The clinical presentation for all spontaneous subarachnoid hemorrhage is the acute onset of severe headache. The pain is frontal or diffuse, radiating to the neck, back, and even the lower extremities. Frequently the patient

---

*See Head Trauma, Chapter 38A.

will volunteer that this is by far the worst headache he has ever had. Within minutes a variable degree of mental confusion may exist. Blood in the subarachnoid space causes a chemical meningitis, and the "meningeal signs" include a stiff neck and Kernig's sign (inability to extend the leg with the thigh flexed.) Often the patient has a mildly elevated temperature, blood pressure, and pulse.

The highly variable clinical signs and symptoms following a subarachnoid hemorrhage are in large part due to vascular spasm resulting in brain ischemia, infarct, and cerebral edema. The diagnosis of subarachnoid hemorrhage usually is strongly suggested by history and physical examination alone, but a spinal tap is diagnostic in most patients (see Table 2).

A frequent problem is differentiation between a "traumatic" spinal tap (bleeding caused by lumbar puncture) and one that truly indicates an antecedent bleed. To determine how recent a bleed has been when bloody spinal fluid is obtained requires extra observations. First, note if the spinal fluid clears as successive tubes of fluid are removed. If the last tube is not as clear as tap water, no definitive statement as to the age of the bleed can be made. If the fluid does become colorless, however, it can be assumed that the spinal tap was "traumatic." If the spinal tap does not become colorless, it is essential (a) that one of the tubes be spun in a centrifuge so that a red blood cell pellet forms at the bottom of the tube, and (b) that the supernatant fluid is clear. Any degree of xanthochromia (yellow tint) in the supernatant fluid indicates that blood has been in

TABLE 2

	RED BLOOD CELLS	MONOCYTES	PMN	PRESSURE (mm. CSF)	GLUCOSE (mg./100 ml.)	PROTEIN (mg./100 ml.)
Normal CSF	0	<5	0	<200	>40	<50
Bacterial Meningitis	N	+	+++	+	θ	+
Aseptic Meningitis	N	++	+	+	N	+
Subarachnoid Hemorrhage	+++	+	+	++	N	++
CNS Neoplasm	N	N	N	++	N	++

N = Normal
+, ++, +++ = Increased
θ = Decreased

the subarachnoid space for at least four hours before the spinal tap, and suggests an antecedent subarachnoid hemorrhage.

Further diagnosis as to the *cause* of a subarachnoid hemorrhage may be suggested by a history of progressive neurologic deficit or seizure disorder or by a cranial bruit heard through a stethoscope. All these features suggest an intracranial vascular malformation.

At times, aneurysms may be symptomatic before they hemorrhage and cause varied degrees of headache or extraocular paresis by compression of the third cranial nerve. Blood dyscrasias may be suspected if there is easy bruising or prolonged bleeding from lumbar or venipuncture sites. Further diagnostic evaluation with arteriography is often necessary. This is most commonly done after a stabilization period of several days, and only infrequently as an emergency procedure.

CRANIAL INFLAMMATION

Headache with fever should always bring to mind first the possibility of meningitis. Many agents can cause inflammation of the meninges, including blood; viral, fungal, or bacterial infection; and even metastatic disease to the meninges, such as lymphoma. The mechanism for producing pain seems to be the lowering of the pain threshold by products of inflammation to sensory nerves normally present in the pia, dura, and blood vessels at the base of the brain. The symptoms are determined by the type of structure involved, the degree of inflammation, and the location of the inflammatory process. Previously unnoticed stretching or jolting of these structures now becomes painful. This helps to explain the clinical findings of extreme pain when the patient's head is passively flexed forward, resulting in flexion of the thigh and legs (Brudzinski's sign). This sign remains present even if consciousness is altered. Meningitis headache is frequently holocranial, but tends to be worse occipitally. This may be due to the extreme reflex spasm of the cervical musculature.

In aseptic meningitis, the clinical manifestations include a more severe headache than is usually associated with simple febrile states. Virus infections are the principal causes of aseptic meningitis; however, a similar cerebrospinal fluid reaction (see Table 1) may also characterize parameningeal inflammation, such as brain abscess, encephalitis, epidural or subdural abscess, and otitis media.

Other conditions that have in common a complaint of severe headache and the presence of resistance to anterior flexion of the neck may simulate meningitis. These include subarachnoid hemorrhage, superior longitudinal sinus thrombosis, retropharyngeal abscess, and meningismus accompanying systemic infections. Furthermore, meningitis in its earliest state, with mild to moderate headache and minimal stiffness of the neck, may be mistaken for a grippelike or influenzal illness.

When meningitis is suspected, the major diagnostic procedure is lumbar puncture. Table 2 outlines some of the more frequently encountered abnormal spinal fluid values. The examiner should be aware of any recent use of antibiotics by the patient, since these may significantly modify the spinal fluid values from those seen in bacterial meningitis to those usually found in viral meningitis.

TEMPORAL ARTERITIS

Inflammation usually restricted to the temporal arteries is appropriately termed "temporal arteritis." However, the syndrome is a cranial arteritis that may involve the superficial temporal, vertebral, ophthalmic, and retinal arteries and segments of the internal carotid.

Pathologically, multinucleated giant cells are found in the media of arteries (giant cell arteritis). Symptoms include headache that is frequently localized to the temporal arteries, low-grade chronic fever, malaise, anorexia, myalgia, and weight loss. Unfortunately, temporal arteritis may present with sudden blindness, and as such is one of the more common causes of blindness in the over-50 age group that this disease frequents. On examination, the patient may have a temporal artery that is enlarged, firm, and tender to palpation. The erythrocyte sedimentation rate (ESR) is nearly always greater than 50 mm./hr. In many patients, a temporal artery biopsy may be necessary to confirm the diagnosis. If temporal arteritis is strongly suspected clinically and the ESR is elevated, the patient should be started immediately on high doses of cortisone while awaiting biopsy confirmation of the diagnosis. Many patients require corticosteroids daily for years to remain symptom-free.

SYSTEMIC ILLNESS

Headache is frequently associated with systemic infections and fever. It is usually described as dull, deep, and generalized. The headache intensity may not directly follow the patient's temperature elevations, but the mechanism of pain seems to be an excessive pial–dural artery dilatation in response to a toxic reaction caused by the presence of the foreign protein of the infecting agent. Some of those agents suspect of producing headache in this manner include viruses, bacteria, protozoa, fungi, rickettsiae, and parasites.

The clinical problem in febrile patients with headache is twofold: (1) diagnosis of the infecting agent, which may take several days with repeated cultures, x-rays, and serologic studies; and (2) the urgent problem of discovering whether meningitis is involved. Certainly those patients with meningeal "signs" require a spinal tap, but the much larger group of patients encountered in emergency practice falls into a category requiring judgment. The seriousness of untreated meningitis demands that many of these patients receive lumbar punctures.

Treatment is directed at eliminating the infecting agent whenever possible and providing symptomatic therapy for pain and fever with salicylates and mild narcotics when necessary.

Hypertension sometimes causes headaches; however, blood pressure is poorly correlated with pain. The other variable to be considered is arterial vascular tone, particularly in those arteries on the outside of the head. When for any reason arterial vascular tone is lower than usual and blood pressure is elevated, pain may be caused by excessive vascular dilatation. However, if high arterial tone is maintained the patient may have no headache, even with elevated blood pressures.

The headache most often found in a patient with hypertension is dull, throbbing, and diffuse; it may be intermittent, and typically is worse in the early morning after the patient has been recumbent for several hours.

Diagnosis usually requires little more than taking the patient's blood pressure, but in some cases of intermittent elevations of blood pressure, as is seen in pheochromocytoma, several blood pressure measurements may be necessary as early in the headache as possible.

Treatment relates to finding the cause of the blood pressure elevation, lowering the blood pressure, and symptomatic therapy of the headache with analgesics.

Other causes of vascular dilatation headaches include hypoglycemia, hypoxia, hypercapnia, and anemia. The mechanism seems to consist of local vascular responses to the metabolic abnormality.

Toxins, medications, medication withdrawal, foods, and chemical agents are recognized causes of vascular dilatation headaches. The vast numbers of agents on each list include carbon, lead tetrachloride, arsenic, insecticides, hypoglycemic agents, Apresoline, phenothiazines, alcohol, tyramine (found in aged cheese and red wine), withdrawal of caffeine, and nitrites used in most cured-meat products to keep the meat looking red (hence, "hot-dog" headaches), and monosodium glutamate, a cause of the so-called "Chinese restaurant syndrome."

VASCULAR HEADACHES OF THE MIGRAINE TYPE

There are a number of migraine variants, but certain features follow a recognizable sequence and permit classification into the types described below.

CLASSIC MIGRAINE

This occurs in approximately 10 per cent of patients with migraine. The prodromes are sharply defined contralateral neurologic manifestations, usually of a visual nature, including field defects (scintillating scotomata), but in some patients there are sensory or motor alterations, or combinations of these. The pain is unilateral and pulsatile, with anorexia, nausea, and vomiting as concomitant features. A family history of migraine is present in about 65 per cent of patients.

COMMON MIGRAINE

The prodromes of this type are not sharply defined, and they may precede the attack by several hours or days. They include psychic disturbances, gastrointestinal manifestations, and changes in fluid balance. Symptoms common to both types include local or generalized edema, irritability, pallor, dizziness, and sweating. The actual headache frequently lasts longer than in the classic type. It may last from many hours to days and may be bilateral. This is the commonest type of migraine encountered.

OPHTHALMOPLEGIC AND HEMIPLEGIC MIGRAINE

This is uncommon. Patients may have prodromal phases typical of either common or classic migraine, and then during the headache phase develop ophthalmoplegia or hemiparesis. The mechanism is felt to be actual pressure on the brain stem or cranial nerves. The deficit frequently clears in hours to days, but sometimes is permanent. Other more common causes of headache with hemiplegia include aneurysm and brain tumor, and often it is not possible to differentiate between these varied entities on a clinical level alone.

CLUSTER HEADACHE

This is characterized as a unilateral, severe headache of acute onset, usually located at the side of the face or eye. The pain recurs on the same side, is throbbing and severe, and gets its name "cluster" from its tendency to occur almost daily (frequently at night) for a few weeks, and then to disappear entirely for several months. Commonly associated with the pain are nasal congestion, lacrimation, perspiration of the face, and at times ptosis or a more complete Horner's syndrome, all occurring on the affected side. As with the other forms of migraine, the pain is believed to be related to dilatation of extracerebral cranial arteries.

Emergency treatment of migraine headaches is aimed at (a) recognition and (b) relief of pain, anxiety, and vomiting. Ergotamine tartrate is currently the most effective drug available for migraine, working as a vasoconstrictor. Definite contraindications to the use of any ergot derivative include pregnancy, vascular disease, and hypertension. If the patient is seen late in the headache phase, ergot will be less effective. Since most narcotic analgesics have marked side effects of nausea, an injectible or rectal

suppository antiemetic–sedative is often given several minutes before analgesics, and this at times may make the patient comfortable enough so that no further medications are needed.

MUSCLE CONTRACTION HEADACHE

Muscle contraction headache is also called "tension headache" because of its frequent occurrence during or following emotional stress. The pain is due in part to sustained contraction of scalp and cervical musculature. The headache usually is dull, steady, bilateral, frontal or occipital, and often described as a feeling of constriction. If examined during a headache, these patients have excessive muscular contraction of the scalp and neck with tenderness to palpation. Massage of the taut musculature can also be of further diagnostic aid as it may markedly decrease pain.

Because of the high frequency of this type of headache pattern, special attention must be paid to the differential diagnosis of upper cervical spine disease, posterior fossa lesions, and extracranial diseases of the head and neck.

Treatment with mild analgesics is usually the easiest form of therapy. Because muscle contraction headaches usually are an established method of handling emotional stress, the disadvantages of chronic use of any medication must be considered at the start, especially if narcotics or sedatives are used. Attempts to develop the patient's insight regarding the mechanism of pain formation depend on the patient-physician relationship and the degree of motivation that both exhibit.

HEADACHES FOLLOWING TRAUMA

Immediately following even minor head injury, some degree of headache is commonly present for a few hours to days. The mechanism producing pain is related to local tissue damage, sustained muscular contraction, and extracranial vascular dilatation. Brief loss of consciousness with head trauma (concussion) or prolonged loss of consciousness with possible neurologic deficits (contusion) is frequently, but not always, accompanied by headache.

Many patients seen after head trauma will require x-rays of both the skull and cervical spine for further evaluation of the causes of head pain. Fractures that traverse the groove of the middle meningeal artery are particularly serious, since laceration of this artery results in a rapid epidural accumulation of blood that can be fatal in a matter of a few hours by causing increased intracranial pressure and uncal herniation. Any patient with even a suspicion of cervical spine fracture on x-ray requires immobilization of the head and neck until neurosurgical consultation is obtained.

In patients with recent head trauma, observation with frequent vital signs is essential. Under no circumstances should these patients receive cycloplegic eye drops or sedation. Pain is usually best controlled with small amounts of codeine sulfate given intramuscularly. Because of the effect on platelets, aspirin is not recommended.

Subdural hematomas represent the accumulation of blood within the subdural space overlying the cerebral convexities, and are closely associated with trauma in the acute and subacute types. There are no characteristic symptoms that will serve to differentiate an acute subdural hematoma from cerebral contusion or laceration. The chronic variety may occur after trivial or forgotten closed head trauma. Headache is a prominent feature of subdural hematoma, although this complaint may be difficult to elicit if the patient is admitted in a confused state. In the subacute and chronic types of subdural hematoma, the clinical manifestations are those of a progressive supratentorial mass, which may be characterized by hemiparesis, focal seizures, and choked disks. Alterations in consciousness of a fluctuating nature often occur. The physician must be alert to the signs of tentorial herniation, which include a fixed dilated pupil and signs of progressive functional midbrain transection.

The diagnosis of subdural hematoma may be suspected in patients with headache following trauma who have shifts from midline greater than 2 mm. of calcified pineal glands on skull x-ray or shifts noted on sonograms. Chronic subdural hematomas are frequently demonstrable on brain scan, but as with acute subdural hematomas they may require cerebral angiography for delineation. Computerized axial tomography, when available, may be a valuable diagnostic adjunct (see Chaps. 38A and 50).

HEAD PAIN FROM EXTRACRANIAL CAUSES

Refractive error is often implicated as a cause of headache, but is only occasionally responsible. However, glaucoma causes pain and tenderness around the eye and may cause diffuse pain in the ophthalmic division of the trigeminal nerve, or a dull, poorly localized headache in addition to the local eye pain. Other symptoms include blurred vision and colored halos around lights. An acute attack of narrow-angle glaucoma can be precipitated by the physician's use of mydriatics. Regardless of the cause, diagnosis can usually be made by simple tonometry. Early treatment may frequently prevent further loss of vision or blindness.

Nasal sinus congestion, with or without infection, causes pain if there is inflammation of the mucosa and engorgement of the turbinates. This is more likely to occur with acute sinusitis than with the chronic variety. Pain may be localized to the involved sinus or referred to the teeth or other parts of the face. Diagnosis can be suspected if the sinus fails to transilluminate or if there is marked "tap tenderness." Nasal sinus x-rays are often helpful. Treatment includes decongestants and antibiotics, in addition to analgesia for the pain. Surgical drainage procedures are sometimes necessary.

Ear pain with headache is frequently a referred pain from a disease process actually in the teeth, throat, or nasal sinuses. Middle-ear infection does not often cause headache, and even when it does occur, it is usually a secondary feature to marked local pain and hearing loss.

References

Bannister, R.: Brain's Clinical Neurology, 4th ed. London, Oxford University Press, 1973.

Birkhead, N. C., Wagener, H. P., and Shiek, R. M.: Treatment of temporal arteritis with adrenal corticosteroids. J.A.M.A. 163:10, 821, 1957.

Dalessio, D. J.: Wolff's Headache and Other Head Pain, 3rd ed. New York, Oxford University Press, 1972.

Davidoff, L. M.: Pseudotumor cerebri; benign intracranial hypertension. Neurology 6:605, 1956.

Fields, W., and Sahs, A. L.: Intracranial Aneurysms and Subarachnoid Hemorrhage. Springfield, Illinois, Charles C Thomas, 1965.

Friedman, A. P.: Current concepts in the diagnosis and treatment of chronic recurring headache. Med. Clin. North Am. 56:1257, 1972.

Friedman, A. P., et al.: Classification of headache. J.A.M.A. 179:717, 1962.

Friedman, A. P., Harter, D. H., and Merritt, H. H.: Ophthalmoplegic migraine. Arch. Neurol. 7:320, 1962.

Friedman, A. P., and Merritt, H. H.: Headache; Diagnosis and Treatment. Philadelphia, F. A. Davis Co., 1959.

Haymaker, W. E.: Bing's Local Diagnosis in Neurological Diseases, 15th ed. St. Louis, C. V. Mosby Co., 1969.

Henderson, W. R., and Raskin, N. H.: "Hot-dog" headache: individual susceptibility to nitrite. Lancet 2:1162, 1972.

Laws, C. E.: Nitroglycerin head. J.A.M.A. 54:793, 1910.

Merritt, H. H.: A Textbook of Neurology, 5th ed. Philadelphia, Lea and Febiger, 1973.

Whitty, C. W. M.: Familial hemiplegic migraine. J. Neurol. Neurosurg. Psychiatry 16:172, 1953.

Chapter 29

HEMATEMESIS AND MELENA

Eddy D. Palmer

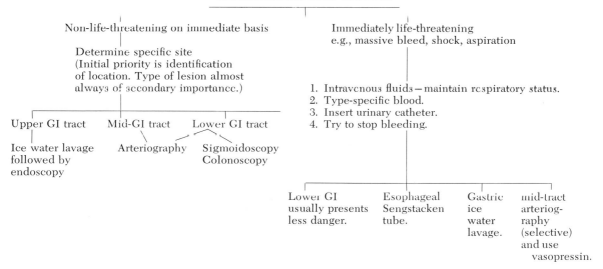

HEMATEMESIS AND MELENA

Non-life-threatening on immediate basis

Determine specific site
(Initial priority is identification
of location. Type of lesion almost
always of secondary importance.)

Upper GI tract   Mid-GI tract   Lower GI tract

Ice water lavage   Arteriography   Sigmoidoscopy
followed by   Colonoscopy
endoscopy

Immediately life-threatening
e.g., massive bleed, shock, aspiration

1. Intravenous fluids—maintain respiratory status.
2. Type-specific blood.
3. Insert urinary catheter.
4. Try to stop bleeding.

| Lower GI usually presents less danger. | Esophageal Sengstacken tube. | Gastric ice water lavage. | mid-tract arteriography (selective) and use vasopressin. |

5. If bleeding cannot be stopped, immediate operation needed.
6. If bleeding can be slowed, prepare for endoscopic and radiographic localization.

Arrival of the gastrointestinal bleeder at the Emergency Department calls for joint diagnostic and therapeutic efforts by several people; therefore a predesigned plan of action is required if confusion is to be avoided. On the other hand, no patient requires more careful individualization than does the gastrointestinal bleeder. It is therefore unrealistic to set rigid rules for managing *all* emergencies of this category. The emergency physician has some or all of these immediate responsibilities:

1. Determine whether there has been a bleed.

2. Determine whether there is active bleeding now.

3. Determine whether the bleeding source lies in the upper gastrointestinal tract (proximal to duodenojejunal junction) or more distally, or both, as the first step in identifying the responsible lesion.

4. Evaluate the patient's background medical status on which the bleed has been superimposed.

5. Judge the amount of blood lost and the patient's physiologic response.

6. Begin blood replacement.

7. Initiate efforts to stop the bleeding.

8. Initiate or arrange for immediate endoscopic and radiologic efforts to identify the bleeding source.

How far the emergency physician will go with these varied responsibilities will depend on the problem at hand. Whether he

541

will call in certain specialists—gastroenter-ologist and radiologist for emergency diag-nostic study and a surgeon to share observa-tion of the patient—will depend on his initial overview of the problem.

SUBJECTIVE

The history of hematemesis, hematoche-zia, or melena may be clear-cut and reliable, the doctor may witness them, or the patient's clothing may show the fresh stains. On the other hand, about one of five patients brought to the Emergency Department be-cause of supposed gastrointestinal bleeding is found not to have bled, the patient simply having misinterpreted something seen in the vomitus or stool as blood. Nongastro-intestinal blood that may enter and then be ejected from the gastrointestinal tract may arise from nose, tracheopulmonary tract, or, for nurslings, from the mother's nipples. Ingestion of blood for fraudulent purposes has become very rare. It is often necessary to test specimens of questioned composition for blood.

Estimation of the amount of blood lost from reports of stool and vomitus volume is likely to be wholly unreliable. It must be recalled that a person may exsanguinate into his gastrointestinal tract without any exter-nal show of blood at all. On the other hand, blood in the stomach quickly becomes di-luted and, when it stimulates rapid passage through the tract, becomes grossly diluted. A little blood goes a long way when splashed about the clothing, floor and walls, and es-timates of its volume usually are exagger-ated.

The bleeder's sudden hypovolemia, hy-potension, and anemia, plus the emotional repercussions of a sudden personal catastro-phe, must necessarily have a deleterious influence on any underlying medical prob-lem that may be present. It is essential that all information the patient or family may have about the past medical history be ob-tained early in the assessment. Unfortu-nately, shock, language problems and intox-ication often interfere with this essential communication. The background medical problems that must be of the greatest con-cern are coronary artery disease, borderline cerebroarterial disease, chronic renal dis-ease, cirrhosis, emphysema, other pulmonary insufficiency problems, and diabetes. Often, of course, the chronic disease has not pre-viously been recognized and comes to light now as a disastrous complication of the bleed.

OBJECTIVE ASSESSMENT

Assessing the severity and con-sequences of the hemorrhage at the moment of admission to the Emergency Department is an immediate responsibility of the Emergency physician. These matters, plus the principles of shock management and resuscitation, are dealt with elsewhere in this book, and only the points pertinent to the special problem at hand will be dis-cussed here.

The clinical effects of the bleed depend on both the amount of blood lost and the ra-pidity of the bleeding. In the initial stages the latter is more important than the former. A healthy adult can lose 500 ml. of blood quickly, as by blood donation, without feel-ing any adverse effects. But the sudden loss of 2000 ml. may kill. Approximately 10 per cent of unattended adults who lose half their circu-lating volume over a 12-hour period will die by the time the 50 per cent mark is reached. About one-third of people in this country who faint from gastrointestinal bleeding do so in the bathroom—and locked-in, at that. They may not receive attention for some time.

Rather often the exact duration of the bleed is not determinable, so that the first hematocrit and hemoglobin level tests may or may not reflect dilution from spontaneous efforts at volume restoration. In addition, one can seldom be sure that there was no anemia or polycythemia at the time the bleeding began. For these reasons, especial-ly, it is essential that immediate evaluation and evaluation throughout the emergency be based primarily on the vital signs and their variations. There can be little doubt that in-sufficient advantage is taken of the help the vital signs can give, owing to the inexplicable habit of relying primarily on laboratory re-ports.

The patient's general appearance on ad-mission—pallor, sweating, shock—gives es-sential information about his response to the bleed but does not permit a reliable estimate of the amount of blood lost. A helpful bedside means for judging the loss is examination of the color of the palmar creases when the fingers are forcibly extended. If there is no anemia, an intense red color is seen, even when the patient is in shock. When the circulating hemoglobin level drops below one-half of normal, the creases do not turn red upon this maneuver.

Tests of cardiovascular stability, as by the well known tilt-test, are found useful by some clinicians, but they cannot be recommended with enthusiasm because they give information only about that moment. The need is for a sign to indicate quickly a sudden rebleed or a sudden failure of the patient's homeostatic protection. The tilt-test cannot readily be repeated at frequent intervals. Recording the blood pressure, pulse rate, and respiratory rate every 15 minutes at the start and later every half-hour provides reliable information on what the bleeding is doing to the patient.

In most cases it is possible to determine whether the bleeding source is in the upper or lower gastrointestinal tract and whether the bleeding is still active when the patient is first examined, although the information may be somewhat indirect. Witnessing hematemesis answers both of these questions in a reasonable fashion. Although the stomach may retain blood for a considerable period after bleeding has actually stopped, and later eject it, this is not often the case. The rule is for the upper gastrointestinal tract to react with irritability and hyperactivity when it fills with blood, so that it quickly empties itself after bleeding has stopped.

For all patients suspected of gastro-intestinal bleeding, if hematemesis has not been witnessed or otherwise proved, a nasogastric tube should be passed for sampling of the gastric contents for blood. The ordinary nasogastric tube is much too narrow for evacuating the stomach of blood and clots; the purpose is simply to indicate whether this is upper gastrointestinal bleeding and whether any blood encountered is abundant and fresh or old and remaining only in traces.

If there has been no hematemesis and the gastric drainage contains no blood, yet melena or hematochezia is active and vital signs suggest continued bleeding, assumption of middle or lower gastrointestinal bleeding is proper. When the bleeding source is in the jejunum, ileum, or cecum it usually is difficult to know quickly when the bleeding stops and when it begins again. Changes in the vital signs are most useful.

The manner by which blood reaches the outside proves unreliable when judging its point of origin, and the clinician must be cautious not to place much diagnostic value on the appearances of vomitus and stool. One is never justified in guessing a venous source from the color of vomitus or gastric aspirate because of the rapidity with which bright red blood may turn dark in the stomach. Conversion to hematin occurs quickly in the presence of the stomach's hydrochloric acid, and black hematemesis may occur rather soon after blood has entered the stomach.

The change that blood produces in the appearance of the stool depends on the amount and rapidity of the bleeding, the location of the bleeding source, and the speed of intestinal transit. Grossly bloody stools are seen in upper gastrointestinal bleeding, when blood loss is quick and massive and transit time is rapid. Blood from the distal duodenum or jejunum must be retained in the tract at least eight hours in order to turn black. A black stool may be produced when gross bleeding arises from the ileum or below, but this is rare. Dark red is the rule. Whatever the source, in order for a black stool to be created, there must be loss of at least 100 ml. of blood and the loss must be rapid.

Gross bleeding from the right colon usually produces dark red stools. Blood from the left colon and sigmoid ordinarily is passed quickly and sometimes appears unaltered. Because it is likely to stimulate diar-

TABLE 1   Causes of Upper Gastrointestinal Hemorrhage; 1526 Adult General Hospital Patients

BLEEDING SOURCE	NO. PATIENTS	AVERAGE TRANSFUSION REQUIREMENT PER BLEED
Duodenal ulcer	402	2275
Esophageal varices	277	3530
Erosive gastritis	213	3510
Gastric ulcer	188	3200
Erosive esophagitis	96	2940
Mallory-Weiss	92	2220
Stomal ulcer	43	3210
Multiple sources	22	2240
Other lesion	82	– –
Undetermined or wrong	111	– –

rhea, it sometimes seems more thoroughly mixed with feces than one might guess it would be.

Accurate assessment of the bleed demands serial determinations of hemoglobin and hematocrit. It is a responsibility of the emergency physician to arrange for immediate determinations at the time blood is drawn for typing and cross-matching, even though he must interpret the initial report with great caution. In cases of massive bleeding there may not be sufficient time to wait for cross-match. In such cases type-specific blood is preferable.

Because of the possibility of unrecognized underlying disease, a series of screening chemical tests should be drawn at the same time. A minimum series of tests might be a glucose level, urea nitrogen, creatinine, bilirubin, calcium, potassium, sodium, chloride, and sedimentation rate.

Acute myocardial infarction is a complication in from 1 to 2 per cent of patients who have a gross gastrointestinal bleed. Therefore, electrocardiographic study is a routine requirement early in the course, with the supposition that it will be repeated in 24 hours.

During initial assessment, it is essential that the doctor keep in mind that a small proportion of gastric and duodenal ulcers that bleed perforate at the same time.

PLAN

Upon completion of emergency assessment, the plan for management concerns primarily blood replacement, efforts to stop the bleeding, and organization of the cooperative effort to identify the bleeding lesion. The rules for blood replacement for gastrointestinal hemorrhage are to risk overkill in ordering blood and to order it just as soon as the fact of hemorrhage has been established. It is the habit of many centers to ask the laboratory to cross-match six units at the start.

For most patients, whole blood will be judged the best material for intravenous resuscitation. But for patients who are elderly or have emphysema or chronic heart failure or some other cardiopulmonary threat, resuspended packed red cells prove safer and more effective than whole blood, simply because they can be infused more rapidly and in greater volume without inducing acute pulmonary edema.

In some centers central venous pressure monitoring is considered helpful or even essential for managing blood replacement, and commonly the caval catheter is placed while the patient is still in the Emergency Department. Use of this form of monitoring in gastrointestinal bleeding cannot be recommended, for three reasons. Whatever the experience of the operator, it sometimes takes a long time for him to get the catheter properly placed at a time in the emergency situation when much needs to be done for the patient. Second, there are too many complications and failures in this technique, during insertion of the catheter, and after the system is in operation. Third, interpretational errors are common in the experience of everyone who has given the technique a good trial.

When the bleeding is determined to be from the upper gastrointestinal tract, immediate ice water lavage of the stomach is recommended as the best emergency treatment, whatever the nature of the bleeding lesion, as well as an effective means for clearing the upper tract of blood in preparation for endoscopic study. This is a procedure that should be initiated in the Emergency Department soon after the patient's admission, although it often must be continued or reinitiated after the patient has reached the ward.

It is essential that the equipment and technique be correct. Ice water, not ice saline, should be used. One simply fills one basin of a double-basin cart with ice cubes and adds tap water to the top, the other basin being used for the gastric aspirate. No tube other than a French 36 Ewald tube (or larger) will do, and it is passed by mouth. If a nasogastric tube has just been passed to test the gastric contents, it must be pulled and the Ewald tube passed into the stomach. The patient is then placed in the left lateral position, and ice water is instilled by Toomey syringe or metal ear syringe. Both syringes have a large nozzle that fits the upper end of the Ewald tube well. About 200 ml. of ice water is instilled into the stomach at a time and then allowed to flow out by itself or with the help of gentlest syringe aspiration. The process is repeated until the returns indicate that bleeding has stopped. It is of primary importance that no more than mild vacuum be applied by syringe to avoid mucosal injury that might confound the interpretations of the endoscopist as he shortly tries to identify the bleeding site.

In the average case about 20 minutes of lavage are required before the gastric returns indicate that the bleeding has stopped. Bleeding cannot be controlled by this method in from 5 to 10 per cent of cases. Probably after a half-hour of continued bloody returns further lavage can be considered useless.

When the bleeding is from the mid or distal gut, there are no effective noninvasive techniques suitable for Emergency Department use for putting an end to the bleeding. Ice water enemas have been found to be ineffective.

IDENTIFICATION OF BLEEDING SOURCE

The lesion responsible for the bleed must be identified as soon as possible. The process begins during resuscitation, with differentiation of an upper tract from lower tract source and, in the case of the former, by clearing the tract of blood by ice water gastric lavage. The emergency physician has already alerted the endoscopist and radiologist to the impending necessity for an emergency diagnostic effort.

Patients with upper gastrointestinal hemorrhage require pharyngoscopy, esophagoscopy, gastroscopy, and duodenoscopy, plus barium studies of the upper gastrointestinal tract. The emergency endoscopic approach, often carried out within an hour of the patient's admission, is now accepted as essential in most centers. The procedure is done under light anesthesia with intravenous Valium and requires approximately six minutes when carried out by an experienced endoscopist.

The instrument is the end-viewing fiberoptic esophagogastroduodenoscope. The purpose of the examination is to find the smear of blood that recollects following lavage, to follow the blood back to its source, and to identify the responsible lesion. Biopsy specimens are never taken, whatever the diagnostic impression, although discovery of a tumor may well call for the taking of material for cytologic examination, provided the area is not flooded with blood.

Examination of the pharynx and esophagus is easy and rapid. The inflated stomach is vast, and most of the endoscopic time is used in the routine required to assure visualization of all mural areas. The duodenum is relatively easy to examine quickly, to its third portion, as long as the segment is relatively free of blood.

Upper gastrointestinal endoscopy in this emergent situation can be considered wholly safe in 99 per cent of cases in the hands of an experienced endoscopist. Various mechanical injuries, including perforation, are always possibilities. It can be said with confidence that endoscopy does not aggravate the bleeding.

ROENTGEN CONTRIBUTIONS

In upper gastrointestinal hemorrhage, an ordinary upper tract roentgen series ordinarily follows endoscopy to elucidate further all abnormalities of the upper tract. It, of course, cannot help with identification of the bleeding lesion.

When the bleeding is from a lower source, selective arteriography is often carried out following resuscitation. This is by far the best technique for demonstrating the level of a bleeding lesion within the small bowel and the colon short of the rectum. The arteriographer may wish to study the celiac axis, superior mesenteric and inferior mesenteric artery, or may concentrate on only one or two of the arteries.

An important advantage of arteriography is the set-up provided for intra-arterial use of vasopressin, an effective emergency therapy for certain bleeding lesions. In this approach, following cannulation of the appropriate artery, 0.3 unit of vasopressin is administered per minute, diluted in standard bottles of intravenous saline or 5 per cent glucose. The administration is precisely controlled by mechanical pump and ordinarily is continued for two to four days.

For distal colon bleeding of no more than moderate severity, sigmoidoscopic examination may answer the diagnostic question in a few minutes. Unfortunately, when lower bowel bleeding is massive, sigmoidoscopy rarely gives useful information because the field cannot be satisfactorily cleared. Whether the arteriography was diagnostic or not, emergency barium enema often follows.

DISPOSITION

When the patient presents with hematemesis or melena, a common problem for the emergency physician is simply whether the situation is severe enough to warrant hospitalization. In many cases the bleed will be judged to have been minor and to have stopped before the patient arrived. Outpatient management may well seem warranted. Ordinarily, however, conservatism must reign. Observation in a holding area for at least four hours is almost always to be considered a minimum requirement of good management.

References

Athanasoulis, C. A., et al.: Intraarterial posterior pituitary extract for acute gastric hemorrhage. N. Engl. J. Med. 290:597, 1974.

Avery Jones, F.: Hematemesis and melena: with special reference to causation and to the factors influencing the mortality from bleeding peptic ulcers. Gastroenterology 30:166, 1956.

Baum, S., et al.: Angiography in the diagnosis of gastrointestinal bleeding. Arch. Intern. Med. 119:16, 1967.

Katz, D., et al.: Sources of bleeding in upper gastrointestinal hemorrhage: a re-evaluation. Am. J. Dig. Dis. 9:447, 1964.

Palmer, E. D.: Upper Gastrointestinal Hemorrhage. Springfield, Illinois, Charles C Thomas, 1970.

Yajko, R. D., Norton, L. W., and Eiseman, B.: Current management of upper gastrointestinal bleeding. Ann. Surg. 181:474, 1975.

Chapter 30

HEMOPTYSIS

Kenneth L. Mattox

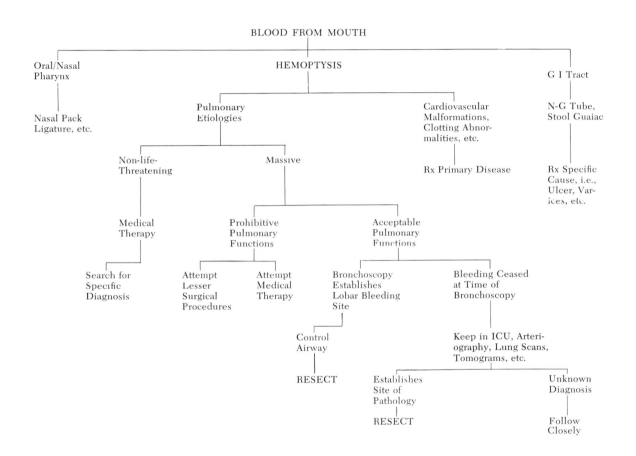

DEFINITIONS

Hemoptysis is the expectoration of blood or blood-stained sputum that originates from below the vocal cords or that has been aspirated into the tracheobronchial tree. It must be differentiated from hematemesis and epistaxis by appropriate physical examination and laboratory tests.

Massive hemoptysis is the expectoration of more than 200 ml. of blood in one coughing episode; 400 ml. of blood in any 24-hour period; 600 ml. or more within a 48-hour period; any amount of blood produced that causes airway obstruction; or chronic pro-

longed hemoptysis necessitating transfusions to maintain a stable hematocrit. Massive hemoptysis is a threat to life, not from exsanguinating hemorrhage, but from asphyxiation. As little as 150 ml. of clotted blood can form a complete cast of the tracheobronchial tree that prohibits any ventilatory effort (Mattox and Guinn, 1974). Life-threatening hemoptysis applies to the patient bleeding at such a rate as to produce exsanguination, a volume sufficient to compromise the airway, or in whom the hemoptysis is a manifestation of underlying disease that in itself is life-threatening.

ETIOLOGY

The more than 70 described etiologies of hemoptysis may be grouped into the broad general categories of: (1) trauma and foreign bodies; (2) cardiovascular lesions; (3) inflammations and infections; (4) blood dyscrasias; (5) compression syndromes; and (6) idiopathic conditions. In patients under the age of 40 years, cardiopulmonary disease, tuberculosis, foreign bodies, and bronchiectasis are the most commonly diagnosed etiologies for hemoptysis. Male patients over 40 usually have neoplasia, bronchiectasis, cardiopulmonary disease, tuberculosis, or lung abscesses as the etiology of hemoptysis. Although the most common cause of hemoptysis is infection, the distribution in terms of percentage varies depending on geographic area, ethnic concentrations, types of clinical practice, and age of the patient. Among 675 patients, Segarra (1958) found cancer in 39 per cent and bronchiectasis in 35 per cent. Smiddy, et al. (1973) found bronchitis or bronchiectasis in almost 60 per cent. Among patients with massive hemoptysis, McCollum, et al. (1975) found pulmonary tuberculosis to be the most frequent disorder. Ninety per cent of patients with hemoptysis have serious underlying disease, and in 10 per cent no cause will be found (Abbott, 1948). Other causes of hemoptysis include parasitic disease, pulmonary embolism, mitral stenosis, Goodpasture's disease, and even the presence of abnormal uterine tissue producing vicarious menstruation. In a busy thoracic clinic, 10 to 15 per cent of the patients will at some time have hemoptysis, and approximately 15 per cent of these will develop massive hemoptysis (Johnston et al., 1960).

PATHOPHYSIOLOGY

The patient with cardiovascular lesions such as mitral stenosis develops hemoptysis because of pulmonary hypertension. In the chronically ill patient with a poor gag reflex, aspiration of food or foreign bodies results in chronic infection, irritation of the bronchus, and/or lung abscesses. Among patients with cavitary disease, bleeding is usually from dilated bronchial arteries, and the bleeding site is either a rupture of Rasmussen's aneurysm or bleeding from chronic inflammation along these dilated arteries. A mycetoma may produce chronic irritation of such dilated vessels. Patients with bronchiectasis also have dilated bronchial arteries along the secondary and chronically inflamed terminal bronchioles. A patient with a pulmonary embolism or who has undergone radiotherapy to the lung may bleed directly from erosion into the pulmonary artery, pulmonary vein, or bronchial artery.

EVALUATION

Although over 90 per cent of patients with hemoptysis have a serious underlying condition, a precise diagnosis is made preoperatively in only two-thirds (Crocco, et al., 1968). Patients seek the attention of a physician because of pain or fear. A history of thrombophlebitis, exposure to pulmonary tuberculosis, previous known bronchitis, cigarette smoking, rheumatic fever, or fever and chills should be determined. It is important to note any medications a patient may have been taking, especially anticoagulants, and to ascertain the duration, character, and volume of the hemoptysis. The patient with a poor gag reflex may say that "some food went down the wrong way."

Confusion can arise when the patient has swallowed bloody sputum or has aspirated vomited blood. Hemoptysis is associated with bright, red blood and frothy sputum, whereas blood from the stomach is darker and may be mixed with food. The pH of sputum generally is alkaline; that from the stomach is acidic. Hemoptysis usually is accompanied by cough and gastrointestinal bleeding, and has an antecedent history of gastrointestinal symptoms.

On physical examination, the patient may choose to lie on his side with the pathologic lung dependent. There may be physical signs of consolidation accompanied by rales and rhonchi. Frequently, however, there is spillover of blood into both mainstem bronchi, producing confusing symptoms. An absent gag reflex may be suggestive of lipoid pneumonia and lung abscesses. Clubbing may be present in a patient with chronic lung disease. Phlebitis may be indicative of disease processes leading to pulmonary embolism. A diagnostic murmur of mitral stenosis, or a loud first heart sound, may direct attention to the cardiovascular system rather than the lungs (Table 1).

Examination of the sputum provides

TABLE 1   *Causes of Hemoptysis with Suggestive History and Findings on Examination*

ETIOLOGY	SUGGESTIVE HISTORY	PHYSICAL
Cardiovascular (e.g., CHF mitral stenosis)	Congenital heart disease Rheumatic fever Heart failure Anticoagulant therapy	Murmur, neck vein distention Pulmonary rales Peripheral signs of heart failure
Infarction	Prolonged bedrest postoperative Phlebitis Pleuritic pain Sudden onset without prodrome	Signs of thrombophlebitis Pleural effusion Tachypnea Cyanosis
Infection	Fever, weight loss, night sweats. Previous infections, nature of sputum, chronic lung disease, geographic area, family history	Cachexia, fever, pulmonary rales or consolidation
Carcinoma	Weight loss, family history, environmental factors	Evidence of metastasis Malnutrition or cachexia
Foreign bodies on aspiration	Sudden dyspnea and wheezing after coughing History of condition leading to diminished gag reflex (e.g., stroke, drug overdose, alcohol intoxication)	Diminished gag reflex Wheezing (localized) Signs of pneumonia Signs of atelectasis or hyperaeration
Vascular anomalies	Congenital malformations	Other malformations
Blood dyscrasias	Presence of chronic disease, leukemia, platelet abnormalities, anemia	Evidence of pallor, bleeding tendency (purpura)

diagnostic clues. "Rust"-colored sputum is characteristic of lobar pneumonia; frothy pink-tinged sputum characterizes pulmonary edema; and copious amounts of sputum that form layers when allowed to stand is common in bronchiectasis. The presence of frank blood is more common with infectious conditions. Microscopic examination of bloody sputum may reveal *Microbacterium tuberculosis* or specific bacterial flora. Sputum should be placed in appropriate alcohol solutions immediately upon expectoration, and submitted for cytopathologic examination.

A prothrombin time and partial thromboplastin time are the minimal clotting tests needed to screen for coagulation defects. An elevated lactic dehydrogenase with a normal serum glutamic oxylactic transaminase is suggestive of pulmonary infarction. An elevated white blood count points to infection (chronic/acute), and the hemoglobin and hematocrit reflect the extent of the hemorrhage. Among patients with Goodpasture's syndrome, an elevated blood urea nitrogen may be present. Cultures for routine fungus and acid-fast organisms are taken at the initial examination. Routine chest x-rays may reveal primary cardiovascular disease, com-

pression of the trachea or mainstem bronchi, or primary pulmonary pathology. The presence of an abscess, a tuberculous cavity, or a mycetoma suggests that the origin of the hemoptysis may be from this location seen on chest x-ray. A shadow within the pulmonary parenchyma, however, does not determine the site of pathology, since bleeding can spill into unaffected areas of the lung and cause staining or even pneumonia. In the patient with minimal hemoptysis, tomography may pinpoint specific disease processes. Congestive heart failure or wedge-shaped densities suggest specific diagnoses related to the vascular system. Radiography also is helpful in directing fiberoptic bronchoscopy biopsy forceps into specific masses for pathologic examination. Pulmonary angiography and selective bronchial artery injections are helpful, but generally are not readily available in the Emergency Department. If time permits, xenon ventilation/perfusion scans indicate differential lung function and, when combined with pulmonary function testing, serve as an extremely valuable guide when resectional therapy is considered.

Pulmonary function tests (see Chapters 3, 10, 40) are essential for determining the patient's reserve capacity and the presence of respiratory failure. Blood gas analysis provides a simple means of following the patient and detecting hypoxemia, acidosis, and hypercarbia. The patient with an FEV_1 of less than 2.0 has only a 20 per cent chance of surviving a pneumonectomy, if such is required (Boushy, et al., 1971).

In the evaluation of the patient with hemoptysis, answers should be sought to the following questions.

(1) Is the presence of hemoptysis doubtful, probable, or certain?

(2) Is there any associated upper respiratory bleeding?

(3) Is there any history of acute upper respiratory infection? smoking? related medical history?

(4) What is the volume over unit time of expectoration?

(5) Is there frank massive hemoptysis or merely blood-streaked sputum?

(6) Is this a single or repeated attack of hemoptysis?

(7) Can the patient locate the site of hemoptysis?

(8) Is there any coagulation abnormality?

The single most important consideration when contemplating resectional therapy is the localization; therefore, bronchoscopy is performed early while the patient is bleeding. Early bronchoscopy offers a 90 per cent chance of localizing the bleeding (Gourin and Garzon, 1974). Various bronchoscopic techniques have been described for clearing the airway of blood and tamponading the mainstem, lobar, and segmental bronchi of their continued oozing. When general anesthesia is utilized, the bleeding frequently has stopped at the time the bronchoscope is introduced. Therefore, topical anesthesia with general anesthetic standby and available tamponading balloons results in a higher yield of localization.

The patient presenting to the Emergency Department with massive, life-threatening hemoptysis requires rapid minimal work-up prior to therapeutic intervention. This includes an expeditious history and physical examination, complete blood count, BUN, urinalysis, prothrombin time, partial thromboplastin time, and PA and lateral x-rays of the chest, followed by bronchoscopy, control of airway, and localization of bleeding. The optimal work-up for the patient with minimal hemoptysis (time allow-ing) includes a sequential algorithm involving the aforementioned tests, in order to reach a specific diagnosis aimed toward an orderly treatment plan.

THERAPY

The approach by the Emergency Department physician should be directed toward therapy concomitant with evaluation for etiology and localization, as well as consideration of airway maintenance. If the bleeding site is known, placing the patient on the side of the pathology may help prevent spillover and preserve normal pulmonary parenchyma. Use of cough-suppressant drugs helps to decrease intrathoracic pressure. Sedation may result in decreased pulmonary artery and pulmonary bronchial artery pressures, thereby decreasing bleeding. The patient with positive acid-fast bacillus on initial stain should begin immediate antituberculous therapy. Other antimicrobial therapy directed toward treatment of bronchitis and bronchiectasis should also begin at once. Patients with penetrating injuries of the lung resulting in pneumothorax and hemoptysis commonly have cessation of bleeding with re-expansion of the lung by tube thoracostomy. Treatment of pulmonary edema with positive pressure breathing, repeated endotracheal suction, digitalization, and forced diuresis is helpful in further reducing hemoptysis. Transfusion should be administered as indicated unless pulmonary edema is present.

Immediate consultation with both pulmonary medicine internists and pulmonary surgeons is called for in the patient with life-threatening hemoptysis, and bronchoscopy should be performed in the operating room in such patients, if time allows. Indications for operation include life-threatening hemoptysis secondary to pulmonary etiologies or mitral stenosis, and situations in which the airway is compromised and asphyxia is imminent. Contraindications for pulmonary resection as a mode of surgical therapy include prohibitive pulmonary functions, a nonresectable hilar-positioned tumor of the lung, a poor general medical condition preventing general anesthesia and major surgery, grossly abnormal coagulation profile, or extensive metastatic disease. During bronchoscopy and resectional therapy, the bronchoscopist, anesthesiologist, and surgeon should take care to protect operative personnel from exposure to acid-fast organisms by wearing appropriate eye-shields and other protective equipment. The merits of both fiberoptic and rigid bronchoscopes have been widely debated, and the physician who performs bronchoscopy should be proficient in both modes.

Patients with massive hemoptysis should undergo immediate resectional therapy upon localization of bleeding site, provided, of course, there is no contraindication. Methods of airway control include the use of a double-lumen Carlen's tube, selective intubation of the right or left mainstem bronchus, and the use of tamponading balloons and packs (Heibert, 1974). In the rare patient in whom an airway cannot be maintained owing to severe hemorrhage, Mattox and Guinn (1974) have suggested the use of portable cardiopulmonary bypass during the surgical procedure. Such a device has been successfully utilized repeatedly among other moribund patients in the Emergency Department (Mattox and Beall, 1975). Intraoperatively, once amputation of the bronchial stump has been accomplished, any clot that has collected during the resection should be aspirated from the remaining bronchus or the trachea.

In the patient with prohibitive pulmonary functions, or in whom resectional therapy is contraindicated, there are lesser surgical procedures that may be useful. These include occlusion of the bronchus by permanent tamponade through the bronchoscope; ligation of the bronchus via a thoracotomy; plumbage thoracoplasty; ligation or occlusion of the pulmonary artery; and cavernostomy with packing and drainage of a bleeding cavity.

PROGNOSIS

Approximately 20 per cent of patients with minimal hemoptysis will subsequently have a second episode of bleeding from the lung (Smiddy, et al., 1973). Morbidity in minimal hemopytsis is associated with underlying disease, and the mortality usually is a complication of the underlying pathology unless the minimal hemoptysis develops into life-threatening hemoptysis (Crocco, et al., 1968). Mortality for nonoperative therapy in massive hemoptysis ranges from 50 per cent to 100 per cent. Surgical mortality fol-

lowing resection for massive hemoptysis ranges from 8 to 35 per cent. It is recommended that patients with hemoptysis be followed for at least two years.

PITFALLS

Hemoptysis poses diagnostic and therapeutic challenges to the emergency physician, the pulmonary internist, and the thoracic surgeon. A patient bleeding from the upper airway secondary to trauma or neoplasia of the trachea or larynx may have extensive hemoptysis, with spillover into one or both mainstem bronchi, and this may confuse the bronchoscopist if specific upper airway sites of bleeding have not been sought. Massive hemoptysis that ceases prior to bronchoscopy poses a problem in disposition. Such a patient may undergo prolonged bronchoscopy in an attempt to reincite the bleeding, or may be watched for several hours in the operating room or intensive care until bleeding recurs. This type of patient should be closely observed, since a number of deaths from asphyxia have occurred while the patient is in the hospital room awaiting a second bleeding episode. All reported series of hemoptysis indicate cases of idiopathic hemoptysis. Such cases should be followed closely for the presence of underlying vascular disease, Wegener's granulomatosis, or even Goodpasture's syndrome. The patient with cardiovascular disease, specifically aneurysm of the thoracic aorta and/or mitral valve disease, may present with massive hemoptysis. Therapy is directed at the correction of cardiovascular abnormalities, rather than operation on a relatively normal lung. Intrinsic disease such as liver failure and obstructive jaundice, as well as extrinsic medication, may alter the clotting profile. It is imperative that a normal clotting profile be ascertained before operative intervention.

When maximum radiotherapy to a hilar lung mass has been accomplished, hemoptysis secondary to necrosis may occur. Similar patients who have undergone successful chemotherapy for primary metastatic lung tumors may also develop hemoptysis. These central lesions may erode into a major pulmonary vein or artery, resulting in extensive, massive, exsanguinating hemoptysis. Resectional therapy in these individuals is complex and difficult, since dissection through fibrosis and neoplasia is necessary in an attempt to gain control of the hilum.

When pulmonary embolism is accompanied by infarction, with subsequent life-threatening hemoptysis, resection of that necrotic area is performed. In such a patient, pulmonary embolectomy allows for even further vascularization of a necrotic area, and will compound the volume of hemoptysis.

In the initial endoscopic evaluation, rigid bronchoscopy allows for extraction of the large clots and large volumes of blood in order to achieve control of the airway. The fiberoptic bronchoscope has a very small luminal channel for aspiration and, unless the bleeding is minimal or has first been controlled with a rigid bronchoscope, offers little, either in removing large quantities of blood or in localizing the bleeding.

Patients with pulmonary emboli, bronchiectasis, cavitary tuberculosis, penetrating lung trauma, primary pulmonary carcinoma, autoimmune disease, and cystic fibrosis each require varying approaches to the hemoptysis that is unique to each disease. The Emergency Department physician, the endoscopist, and the surgeon should be cognizant of the varying approaches based on the suspected etiology.

References

Abbott, O. A.: Clinical significance of pulmonary hemorrhage: a study of 1316 patients with chest disease. Dis. Chest 14:824, 1948.

Boushy, S. F., et al.: Clinical course related to preoperative and postoperative pulmonary function in patients with bronchogenic carcinoma. Chest 59:383, 1971.

Crocco, J. A., et al.: Massive hemoptysis. Arch. Intern. Med. 121:295, 1968.

Diamond, M. A., and Genovese, P. O.: Life-threatening hemoptysis in mitral stenosis. J.A.M.A. 215:441, 1971.

Elliott, R. C., and Smiddy, J. F.: The "territorial domain" of hemoptysis. Chest 65:703, 1974.

Garzon, A. A., et al.: Pulmonary resection for massive hemoptysis. Surgery 67:633, 1970.

Glenn, W. W. L., Liebon, A. A., and Lindskog, G. E.: Resection for Pulmonary Tuberculosis. In Thoracic and Cardiovascular Surgery with Related Pathology, 3d ed. New York, Appleton-Century-Crofts, 1975, p. 259.

Gourin, A., and Garzon, A. A.: Operative treatment of massive hemoptysis. Ann. Thorac. Surg. 18:52, 1974.

Hardy, J. D.: Pulmonary hemorrhage: causes and management. Am. Surg. 29:1, 1963.

Heibert, C. A.: Balloon catheter control of life-threatening hemoptysis. Chest 66:308, 1974.

Johnston, R. N., et al.: Haemoptysis. Br. Med. J. 1:592, 1960.

Mattox, K. L., and Beall, A. C., Jr.: Extending the art—portable cardiopulmonary bypass. J. Am. Coll. Emerg. Physicians 4:528, 1975.

Mattox, K. L., and Guinn, G. A.: Emergency resection for massive hemoptysis. Ann. Thorac. Surg. 17:377, 1974.

McCollum, W. B., et al.: Immediate operative treatment for massive hemoptysis. Chest 67:152, 1975.

Ream, C. R.: Immediate management of respiratory tract hemorrhage. Hosp. Med. 6:8, 1970.

Segarra, F. U.: Hemoptysis. N. Engl. J. Med. 258:167, 1958.

Smiddy, J. F., and Elliott, R. C.: The evaluation of hemoptysis with fiberoptic bronchoscopy. Chest 64:158, 1973.

Thoms, N. W., et al.: Life-threatening hemoptysis in primary lung abscess. Ann. Thorac. Surg. 14:347, 1972.

Tucker, G. F., et al.: The flexible fiberscope in bronchoscopic perspective. Chest 64:149, 1973.

Yater, W. M., and Oliver, W. F.: Hemoptysis. In Symptom Diagnosis, 5th ed. New York, Appleton-Century-Crofts, 1961, pp. 395–98.

Yeoh, C. B., et al.: Treatment of massive hemorrhage in pulmonary tuberculosis. J. Cardiovasc. Surg. 54:503, 1967.

Chapter 31   HYPOVOLEMIC SHOCK

Peter Rosen

TABLE 1. *Treatment of Hypovolemic Shock*

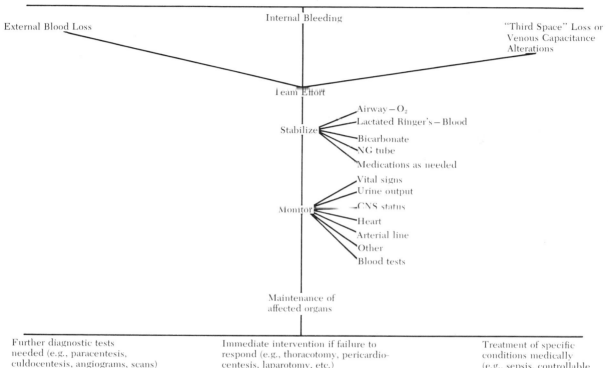

To approach management of shock rationally, it is necessary to know the pathophysiology,* but one also must rely on a preconceived plan of response. Early, organized, aggressive management is essential to salvage.

DEFINITION

Shock, like many other total body responses, has no easy definition. For all its varied etiologies, the end-result is inadequate tissue perfusion. Many of the clinical findings in shock are nothing more than reflex homeostatic efforts. Irreversible shock, like death itself, is defined as failure to respond to resuscitation. In the Emergency Department the use of any other definition can lead to premature abandonment of patients who might otherwise be saved.

Hypovolemic shock cannot be considered in complete isolation from alternative pathologic states, as it is rare to see a "pure" form of shock except in the laboratory. Frequently, in a clinical setting, no one etiology predominates. For example, the patient with a gunshot wound of the abdomen is suffering simultaneously from hypovolemia (bleeding vessels in damaged tissue), neurogenic stimuli (pain), and sepsis (lacerated bowel).

*See Chapter 4, p. 104.

A classification of the several types of shock is found in Table 1.

In this chapter we will concern ourselves only with the first of these, hypovolemic shock.

RECOGNITION

Early loss of blood produces no clinical signs or symptoms. The neurogenic component, i.e., the psychic pain surrounding the traumatic event, may predominate over the real pain or injury. It is important to realize that in young, previously healthy victims of trauma there are few recognizable clinical changes until more than 25 per cent of the blood volume has been lost. As blood loss continues, from this point on one begins to detect changes in the vital signs and appearance of the patient. The earliest clinical signs are hypotension and tachycardia. However, there may also be a brief bradycardia (Moore, 1971). As acute reduction in blood volume continues, there is progressively decreased cardiac output, the pulse weakens, and diaphoresis occurs. The patient usually is very thirsty. His mental state progresses from apathy to coma. Particularly in alcoholic patients or those with drug intoxication, psychotic behavior may develop. As pulmonary changes occur, hypoxia develops with confusion and restlessness. Acidosis occurs due to lactic acid accumulation. Respiratory compensation usually maintains pH, however, at least in the initial period.

The respiratory patterns in shock usually involve tachypnea with decreased tidal volume. There is increased work of air exchange and arteriovenous shunting. In more advanced stages of shock there is great difficulty in maintaining adequate oxygenation. The change in pulmonary compliance, which may relate to interstitial edema, is an early stage of the so-called "shock lung."

Signs in a shock patient indicating a poorer prognosis include persistently low cardiac output, higher pulmonary vascular resistance, acidosis, higher lactic acid, and *higher arterial CO_2.* Those with greater and more rapid blood loss have a worse prognosis.

RESPONSE

AT THE SCENE

The treatment undertaken at the scene depends on the capability and training of the ambulance team. External blood loss should be stopped by direct pressure after a good airway is ensured. A horizontal position should be maintained with the lower extremities elevated. If there is a question of intra-abdominal bleeding, or if blood loss has been severe, a "G" suit can be used if available. Vital signs should of course be taken, and an intravenous infusion with normal saline or lactated Ringer's should be started. Oxygen should be given and the patient kept warm and reassured.

IN THE EMERGENCY DEPARTMENT

The first obligation to the patient is triage. A small laceration of the scalp can produce a frightening, bloody appearance which cries out for attention, while the patient with a ruptured spleen may be lying unnoticed. If there is a possibility of spinal injury, the spine is protected until this question is resolved.

The resuscitation team should be summoned as a unit (a "trauma bell" that rings throughout the area can be used). The patient must then be carefully transferred to a shock cart by the Emergency physicians and nurses. Next he must be undressed. In most instances this is best performed by cutting away clothing: we have seen patients thrown into profound shock when made to sit up for removal of a T-shirt.

While the patient is being undressed, airway management should continue with high flow nasal O_2 at 15 liters/minute. Vital signs are obtained, and simultaneously the first lifelines should be placed and blood for type and cross-match (6 units) removed. The suggested initial fluid should be lactated Ringer's, although normal saline also is in frequent use. A quick history is obtained and a rapid physical examination performed. It is amazing how often the back of the patient is ignored and some important injuries missed. The evaluation of the back is performed by rolling the patient on his side, *not* by sitting him up.

Soft tissue injuries are dressed and fractures are splinted.

No diagnostic tests are performed until stabilization has been achieved.

In severe shock, blood is essential, either in the form of whole blood or as packed red cells. The use of packed red cells has been increasing owing to a lowered risk of hepatitis. Also, with whole blood there is the problem of white cell–platelet aggregates that accumulate and become trapped in the lung after transfusion. A disadvantage, however, is that infusion is slower with packed red cells. To paraphrase Walter Cannon, the patient is bleeding blood, not packed red blood cells.

Type-specific blood may be necessary, and this can be made available within minutes. This is preferable to the use of type O blood.

DIAGNOSTIC TESTS

Laboratory

There is no simple laboratory test that will determine shock or, better yet, its response to therapy. Virtually all studies are useful only as baselines, and subsequent trends in laboratory data demonstrate a response to management. The quickest and easiest studies to obtain are hematocrit (HCT), urinalysis, and central venous pressure (CVP).

The HCT is virtually meaningless except as a rough guide to volume deficit. More important is the rate of HCT change (reduction) as fluid moves into the vascular compartment. Dilution via extracellular fluid varies with the amount of blood loss. With 25 per cent or less, dilution probably occurs at about 1 cc. per minute, but with increased hemorrhage the dilution rate can increase to 20 cc. per minute. The interstitial fluid that moves into the vascular compartment causes little or no electrolyte change.

The CVP usually measures less than 10 cm. H_2O (7 to 11 cm.). An early baseline CVP is extremely helpful as it may be an early—if not the only—clue to cardiac tamponade. It also serves as a gross evaluation of fluid replacement. A Swan-Ganz type of catheter to measure pulmonary wedge pressure might be a more sensitive indicator of fluid replacement, although it is more difficult to place in an acute situation.

Urinalysis for macro- or microscopic blood and hemolysis and an indwelling catheter to measure volume of output are essential.

Studies which are useful for management, but which take longer to obtain, are: (1) blood gases; (2) electrolytes; (3) BUN and creatinine; (4) osmolality; (5) base deficit; and (6) lactate.

METABOLIC EFFECTS

1. Although eventually all shock patients suffer a metabolic acidosis, their early presentation is variable. pH is usually normal or slightly alkalotic. One must remember that the patient's pH is an unpredictable combination of respiratory alkalosis and metabolic acidosis. Too aggressive therapy with $NaHCO_3$ will produce harm by its effect on O_2–hemoglobin dissociation, by its profound resultant increase in serum osmolality, and by its paradoxic effect on the brain. As in the management of ketoacidosis, $NaHCO_3$ may produce an increase in brain acidosis with an increase in coma. This is because of its inability to cross the blood-brain barriers. As a result, peripheral alkalinization causes CO_2 to diffuse into the brain, with a subsequent drop in brain pH.

2. Most acute hemorrhages produce little or no change in serum electrolytes. The predicated increase in serum potassium is rarely seen, and in fact hypokalemia has been frequently observed. This should not be actively treated with supplemental potassium until the source of the hemorrhage has been controlled, kidney function stabilized, and persistent hypokalemia confirmed. The high serum potassium concentration of banked whole blood should also be taken into consideration.

3. Blood urea nitrogen (BUN) and creatine usually are normal early in hemorrhage unless there is underlying renal disease. This, of course, will vary with the source of the hemorrhage (e.g., with gastrointestinal hemorrhage, BUN will be elevated early; with genitourinary (GU) injuries, creatine may also be elevated early).

4. Osmolality frequently is slightly elevated to around 350 milliosmoles. This is probably due to an inability to metabolize glucose properly, with the subsequent mild hyperglycemia associated with a depressed insulin response. As a baseline and guide to future therapy, osmolality can be helpful.

5. Virtually all patients in shock have some degree of base deficit and increased serum lactate. Most of the time these will respond to resuscitation. Patients studied

with "irreversible shock" have all had persistently elevated serum lactate levels even when given massive amounts of $NaHCO_3$. Early determination of high serum lactate and base deficits may be helpful in justification of more aggressive alkalinization than is usually indicated.

X-ray

All studies are deferred until the patient has been stabilized. Even after stabilization, appropriate x-rays must be made only with great caution, as the manipulation required of the patient can again induce profound shock.

Other Studies

A full EKG is taken when all other stabilizing maneuvers have been completed.

Paracentesis or culdocentesis is performed as indicated, and only if the patient's condition permits the study.

A Foley catheter is placed in all shock patients to monitor urine output and to help define genitourinary injuries. If one cannot readily be passed (GU injury or prostatic obstruction), a percutaneous suprapubic catheter (such as the type used for peritoneal dialysis) should be passed.

THERAPY

AIRWAY MANAGEMENT

In all patients in shock, once the airway is cleared, initial airway management consists of nasal oxygen at 15 liters/minute. It is true that if pulmonary physiology is normal O_2 will not overcome the perfusion deficits present in shock, but there are enough patients in whom underlying O_2 saturation is not normal (e.g., cases of emphysema, chronic cigarette smoking, pulmonary injuries) for this routine to be beneficial. Care should be exercised in those with severe chronic respiratory disease, and for these patients assisted ventilation might be needed.

If there is any indication of compromised airway, one must immediately proceed to face-mask, mechanically assisted respirations and then to endotracheal intubation.

Post-traumatic Respiratory Insufficiency Syndrome (Shock Lung). Early in management, there is often a mildly lowered arterial PO_2. This will invariably respond to supplemental oxygen. However, there appears to be a later phase with the development of arteriovenous shunting that is less responsive. The lung is at great risk in the shock patient, and it still remains to be proved which are the exact etiologies of the dreaded insufficiency syndrome. At present the most commonly implicated factors, in addition to the underlying lung perfusion deficiency produced by the shock state, are sepsis, interstitial edema, oxygen toxicity, atelectasis, cerebral injury, microembolism of blood breakdown particles, and aspiration of gastric contents. Although electrolyte solutions had been implicated, current experimental work would seem to vindicate their use, and clinical experience indicates that the early and aggressive resuscitation of the shock victim may prevent the pulmonary sequelae.

FLUIDS

While the patient is being undressed, the airway is being managed, the initial vital signs are obtained, and the first lifeline is placed. If injuries permit, use the left arm for vital signs and the right arm for the first I.V. line. The first line should be a long, large-bore catheter CVP line. If peripheral veins are too collapsed or too distant from the site of disease, immediately place a subclavian or an internal jugular cather.* A second line is then placed: a short, large-bore catheter. If these are not producing an adequate response, further intravenous lines are added. Avoid cutting down on the ankle saphenous vein, but use the groin saphenous cut-down if there are no indications of inferior vena caval injuries.

Start therapy with lactated Ringer's solution in plastic bags. These will deliver the largest volume per minute via hand or blood pump compression and ensure maximum safety.

The fluid amounts suggested are based on adult standards. For children, quantities must be modified according to weight. As soon as 1000 cc. of fluid are infused, reevaluate the BP, CVP, pulse, urinary output, skin color, and level of consciousness. If

---

*See procedure, p. 543.

the patient has stabilized, withhold blood until the injuries can be ascertained more definitively, but continue lactated Ringer's at 500 cc./hour. If, on the other hand, the patient has made no response to a continued rapid infusion of a second 1000 cc., type-specific but not cross-matched whole blood can be started. If blood loss has been greater, type-specific blood can be started as soon as available. However, there usually is time for a trial of lactated Ringer's solution.

If the patient has made a partial response but still demonstrates a tachycardia, blood pressure deficit, and sensorium change, whole blood is started as soon as cross-match is complete.

Experimental and clinical experience indicate lactated Ringer's solution and whole blood to be a good combination of fluids. In the time required for colloids to be administered, twice the volume of lactated Ringer's can be given. Dextran should be used with caution, if at all, because of the subsequent difficulties in blood typing and the potential hazards of clotting deficiencies.

Many problems follow the administration of bank blood, and many of these would seem to be eliminated by the use of reconstituted frozen RBC. Unfortunately, most Emergency Departments do not have access to frozen blood and should be aware of certain of the risks of conventionally stored bank blood. These include: aging of RBC; hepatitis; decline in erythrocyte 2,3–diphosphoglycerate with a progressive increase in hemoglobin–oxygen affinity (left shift of O_2 dissociation curve); high serum potassium; leukocyte immunologic activations; lack of platelets; and hypothermia from administering large quantities of blood at refrigerator temperature.

Despite these risks, there is no available substitute for the combination of whole blood and balanced electrolyte solutions in the management of hemorrhagic hypovolemic shock.

RENAL MANAGEMENT

Although it is clear that the kidney is one of the organs most sensitive to the perfusion deficits of shock, it is a curiosity of clinical medicine that some patients can tolerate prolonged periods of profound shock without renal shut-down, whereas others cannot. Little can be done to protect the kidney short of overcoming the cause of shock.

Osmotic diuretics were at one time thought to protect the kidney, but recent evidence would suggest that they may actually increase renal damage. They certainly increase perfusion deficits elsewhere in the body. These diuretics should be avoided in Emergency Department management of shock. A diuretic such as furosemide has been employed and is often recommended when urine output is inadequate, but the use of diuretics is controversial in that there is evidence that clearance of substances may be reduced, while water excretion increases. The essential focus must be on restoring intravascular volume.

Later in the course of therapy, when the cause of hemorrhage has been controlled and volume restoration accomplished, a single trial dose of mannitol may be used (12.5 gm.) if the patient is anuric or oliguric. Dopamine, which acts as a renal vasodilator, may have a more beneficial effect than a diuretic; long term experience with this drug will clarify its role in maintaining renal perfusion.

All patients in shock need to be catheterized and their urine output closely monitored. Major soft tissue injuries, aged or multiple blood transfusions, and bad burns all represent special threats to the kidney because of the extra burden of major hemoglobin pigments presented to the tubules.

Complete anuria is rare even in profound shock, and suggests a traumatic disturbance of the genitourinary system. Oliguria usually responds to overall resuscitation, but if volume replacement is delayed, it may progress to anuria due to acute tubular necrosis.

CARDIAC MANAGEMENT

In the young patient cardiovascular function usually has been normal prior to injury. Shock rarely produces any observable cardiac effect other than as a preterminal event. However, in the older patient with preexisting heart disease, even a short episode of shock can induce serious dysfunction. As in patients with acute myocardial infarction, the early electrocardiogram is often nondiagnostic. Further, soft tissue and musculoskeletal injuries may make interpretation of serum enzymes inaccurate. The best cardiac management is treatment of the shock and elimination of the cause. *An aggressive approach to ventricular arrhythmias is mandatory, since cardiac arrest during hypovolemic shock is almost always fatal.*

Fluid Therapy in the Elderly Patient. The elderly patient with preinjury borderline compensation must be given fluids more cautiously, or frank pulmonary edema will ensue while there is still major volume deficit. In this group of patients it is better to use packed red blood cells, and at times one-half normal saline rather than full strength lactated Ringer's. We have also observed a paradoxic phenomenon not seen in the young patient with normal preinjury cardiac function. This is a high CVP in the face of serious hypovolemia. As volume replacement commences, the CVP drops to normal. One must be particularly careful not to overshoot on these replacements, or the CVP may rise again, signaling the beginning of serious cardiac decompensation. These patients frequently benefit from early intubation and aggressive airway management. Finally, consideration must be given to mechanical ventricular assistance devices if early response to therapy is not forthcoming.

CEREBRAL MANAGEMENT

Despite the homeostatic efforts of the organism to preserve cerebral oxygenation, cerebral function frequently is impaired. This is usually expressed by apathy, disorientation, or even frank coma. One should remember that in cases of acute or chronic alcoholism the apathy may be expressed in psychotic behavior.

A frequent source of error in the management of the multiple trauma victim is the assumption that the shock is caused by a concomitant head injury. This, in fact, is very rare except as a preterminal event or in patients with large scalp lacerations. The first priority in therapy is directed against shock and its immediate etiology. If a patient has sustained a head injury with likely trauma to the central nervous system, fluids and electrolyte solutions are ordinarily restricted to reduce cerebral edema. However, when a shock state is present such limitations must be disregarded. Cerebral edema is managed after the shock has been overcome.

Care must be exercised to prevent further damage to the cervical, thoracic, or lumbar spine. In the event of acute paraplegia some of the shock may be neurogenic, but the obligations of volume replacement are still first-order concerns.

GASTROINTESTINAL MANAGEMENT

Virtually all patients with shock will develop ileus. Furthermore, many patients may appear intoxicated. Routine placement of a nasogastric tube for intermittent suction is worthwhile.

MUSCULOSKELETAL AND SOFT TISSUE MANAGEMENT

Once the airway has been controlled and lifelines placed, soft tissue injuries must be bandaged and fractures splinted. Even while lying on a shock table, many patients will produce a significant amount of motion at a fracture site, with attendant increase in blood loss and increased chance of fat embolism.

Direct pressure to major vascular injuries is most effective. Tourniquets are rarely needed in civilian practice. Blind clamping of arteries is also to be condemned as it increases the difficulties of subsequent repair.

ANCILLARY MANAGEMENT

Severe Trendelenburg position has been shown to produce an increased stress to respiration and impairment of cerebral circulation by interference with venous return. Mild Trendelenburg is useful for increased safety in the performance of internal jugular or subclavian catheter insertions. A mild autotransfusion can be performed by elevations of both lower extremities if injuries allow. This is probably all that is necessary. If intra-abdominal bleeding is present, a "G" suit may act in a tamponade fashion as well as providing additional blood from the lower extremities.

There is some indication that regional hypothermia of the kidneys is protective against tubular necrosis. There is no easy method of achieving this in the Emergency Department. In the operating room, however, a sluice of the abdominal cavity can be carried out with iced saline.

SPECIFIC DRUG THERAPY

Tetanus Prophylaxis. All patients with traumatic injuries breaking the surface or in shock should receive 0.5 cc. of tetanus toxoid. If no complete history of immunizations can be obtained, administration of 500 units of human tetanus antitoxin at a separate site is rational. This is double the usual dose because of the possible decreased activity of the immune system during and after shock. Unless this is made a ritual management, it is easy to overlook in the rush of resuscitation—with potentially disastrous consequences to the patient.

Antibiotics. These should not be given routinely, but are indicated if there is penetration of a viscus.

Patients with open fractures and massive soft tissue injuries should also be given broad spectrum antibiotics intravenously. If antibiotics are indicated, they should be given immediately and intravenously to gain the maximum desired effect. Peripheral circulation may be so poor as to delay absorption of any medication given intramuscularly.

Analgesics and Sedatives. As a general rule not much is needed for pain relief. The supportive stabilizing maneuvers are important in the relief of pain. When particularly painful injuries are present, small doses of intravenous opiates can be used, e.g., 2 to 5 mg. morphine. Intramuscular opiates should be avoided as they will not benefit the patient while in shock, and may cause too heavy sedation subsequently when peripheral circulation improves.

An extremely important part of pain relief is verbal reassurance. Despite their apparent apathy, critically injured patients are much more aware of their surroundings than is commonly realized. Verbal preparation of the patient for common manipulative procedures such as Foley catheterization or nasogastric intubation helps greatly. Judicious and generous use of local anesthesia for cutdowns, thoracostomy, and so on, is also helpful.

In general, sedatives must be used with caution as they frequently may compound the shock state. An exception noted previously is the alcoholic patient who may respond to his hypovolemic state with development of a hyperexcited and confused state. If withdrawal is a potential hazard, this too may be an indication for some prophylactic sedation given intravenously. Once stabilization has occurred in the known alcoholic, some trauma centers infuse small amounts of alcohol intravenously to avoid an alcohol withdrawal state—which might add substantial problems to those already present. Such infusion must be done cautiously, and it is wise to err on the conservative side.

SHOCK IN NARCOTIC ADDICTS

The management of shock is difficult enough without the added problem of drug withdrawal in addicts. Narcan or Nalline should not be used unless an overdose has occurred, because they induce withdrawal during resuscitation. In any event, the target symptom in cases of overdose is respiratory depression, and small amounts of Narcan may be used to reverse this symptom without inducing a withdrawal reaction. When the time of the last "fix" is not known, and respiratory action is good, a small dose of opiate should be given I.V. Pain must be managed in the addict in the same fashion as in the nonaddict, and opiates must not be withheld merely because the addict has dosed himself prior to his injuries. Reassurance to the addict that he will not suffer withdrawal during his hospital care will make him much more manageable.

Digitalis. There rarely is indication for use of this drug in hypovolemic shock. Even when there is evidence of prior myocardial dysfunction, the first priority is restoration of volume. The electrolyte status is often unknown, and irreversible digitalis toxicity has been produced with overaggressive digitalis therapy in patients with hypokalemia.

Once volume replacement has been achieved, the use of digitalis may be considered if there is a rising CVP or high pulmonary wedge pressure. A rapid small dose should be used I.V., e.g., digoxin, 0.25 mg. No attempt at "full digitalization" should be made, and the practice of giving 1.0 or 1.5 mg. digoxin at a single dose is dangerous.

Pressors. Few shock teams would consider using vasopressors to counteract hypovolemic shock. The hypotension reflects the volume deficit, and vasopressors increase pressure but not flow. The only possible exception might be an individual with a spinal cord injury and diffuse vascular dilatation. If the patient is not responsive to blood and lactated Ringer's, consideration must be given to immediate surgical intervention.

Steroids. The use of steroids in shock is still controversial. Their use is generally warranted if there are accompanying indications (e.g., concomitant head injury or sepsis). Those who advocate steroids suggest massive doses such as methylprednisolone 30 mg./kg. I.V. The rationale for their use is that there is some beneficial effect on the microcirculation and a concomitant decrease in platelet adhesiveness. There is also vasodilatation which theoretically can improve myocardial function, as well as a modest inotropic effect on the myocardium. There is also a slight shifting effect on the O_2 dissociation curve. The postulated beneficial effects on cellular and molecular functions are still theoretical.

Diuretics. In the early phase of management, osmotic diuretics are not useful. There is no evidence that more conventional diuretics such as furosemide or the mercurials are useful either, initially. If urine flow is diminished, the best way to re-establish normal flow is with volume replacement. There is evidence that some patients will retain the salt load necessary for resuscitation and that this group of patients has a high incidence of post-traumatic pulmonary insufficiency syndrome. This group seems to benefit from furosemide therapy, but this is not a consideration for immediate resuscitation.

Electrolytes. There is no indication for supplemental potassium therapy until hemorrhage has ceased and renal function has been stabilized. A certain amount of potassium is administered obligatorily with blood transfusions, especially in the older units. Similarly, lactated Ringer's contains around 5 mEq. K/liter and penicillin about 20 mEq./million units.

Magnesium is rarely necessary unless the hemorrhage has been superimposed upon a chronic surgical illness.

Calcium also is rarely a problem in the face of the metabolic acidosis of hemorrhage. However, 1 ampule of calcium chloride should be given for every 5 units of whole blood. Rapid alkalinization may produce changes in ionized Ca^{++}, and this is another reason for care in use of this ion. Caution must be exercised in the use of calcium in the digitalized patient.

Vitamins. In the alcoholic patient multivitamins and thiamine can be of benefit, as can AquaMephyton.

Ascorbic acid is used on many surgical services, but probably can be reserved for postoperative care or for the recovery phase.

Clotting Problems. Hemorrhage may be increased owing to defects in clotting mechanics. Multiple blood transfusions also can induce a bleeding diathesis. Fresh whole blood should be used when possible. Platelet packs, antihemophiliac globulin, fibrinogen, and epsilon aminocaproic acid should all be used when there are specific indications.

Disseminated intravascular coagulation fortunately is a rare accompaniment to acute hemorrhage. It is seen most often in acute obstetric hemorrhages.

Vasodilators. One reason that advocates of steroids put forward for their use is vasodilatation. It has been suggested that vasodilators such as Dibenzyline and isoproterenol increase capillary perfusion, although there is no striking evidence of their efficacy. In cases of refractory shock, a trial of Dibenzyline therapy is warranted. Dopamine is the newest agent which may offer advantages due to vasodilatation and inotropic effects. However, the use of any pharmacologic agent *must not* blur the essential focus, which should be on restoration of circulating volume and restoration of adequate oxygen-carrying ability of the fluid in the vascular compartment (i.e., by red blood cell replacement).

EVALUATION OF THERAPY

There is no single parameter by which therapy may be monitored adequately. Pulse, blood pressure, CVP, urinary output, and cerebral functions are all helpful indications. Arterial monitoring also has been employed. The object of therapy is to stabilize the life-threatening condition until definitive management of the etiology can be accomplished. If there is early failure to respond, immediate interventions must be made when indicated, e.g., thoracostomy or pericardiocentesis. In cases of hemorrhage below the diaphragm, if all these fail, the chest should be opened and the aorta cross-clamped. On occasion a definitive repair of direct cardiac injury can be carried out. Only rarely will laparotomy be beneficial in the Emergency Department. In most instances transfer to the operating room can and should be made.

Transfer to another institution should be avoided if at all possible, but if this does become necessary the patient should be accompanied by a physician. I.V.s must be protected and fluid therapy continued. Airway management becomes even more challenging since aspiration of gastric contents during transport is always a threat. It should be emphasized that no transfer should be made until the receiving hospital or unit or operating room is prepared to accept the patient and to continue management.

EARLY CARE OF THE SHOCK PATIENT

For too many years shock units have been concerned with care of the patient only after he has arrived in hospital. Fortunately, as total emergency systems develop, more attention is being paid to the proper function of ambulance services and the care of the patient en route. New techniques are being developed to render appropriate care during extrication, as well as on site disaster management. In time this will pay high rewards in patient salvage.

References

Back, S. M., Brown, R. S., and Shoemaker, W. C.: Early prediction of acute renal failure and recovery. Am. Surg. 177(3):253, 1973.

Carey, L. L., Lowery, B. D., and Chutier, C. T.: Hemorrhagic Shock. Current Problems in Surgery. Chicago, Year Book Medical Publishers, 1971.

Lillehei, R. C., Dietzman, R. H., et al.: The pharmacologic approach to the treatment of shock. Geriatrics 27:81, 1972.

Moore, F. M.: The effects of hemorrhage on body composition. N. Engl. J. Med. 273:567, 1971.

Moss, G. S., and Saletta, J. D.: Traumatic shock in man. N. Engl. J. Med. 290:724, 1974.

Moyer, C. A., and Butcher, H. R.: Burns, Shock and Plasma Volume Regulation. St. Louis, C. V. Mosby Co., 1967.

Schumer, W., and Sperling, R.: Shock and its effect on the cell. J.A.M.A. 205:215, 1968.

Shires, G. T., and Canizaro, P. C.: Fluid resuscitation in the severely injured. Surg. Clin. North Am. 53:1341, 1973.

Shires, T. S., Camico, C. I., and Canizaro, P. C.: Shock. (Vol. XIII. Major Problems in Clinical Surgery.) Philadelphia, W. B. Saunders Company, 1973.

Shoemaker, W. G., and Monson, D. O.: The effect of whole blood and plasma expanders on volume-flow relationships in critically ill patients. Surg. Gynecol. Obstet. 137:453, 1973.

Shoemaker, W. C., Montgomery, E. S., Kaplan, E., and Elwyn, D.: Physiologic patterns in surviving and non-surviving shock patients. Arch. Surg. 106:630, 1973.

Chapter 32   PRURITUS

Howard M. Simons

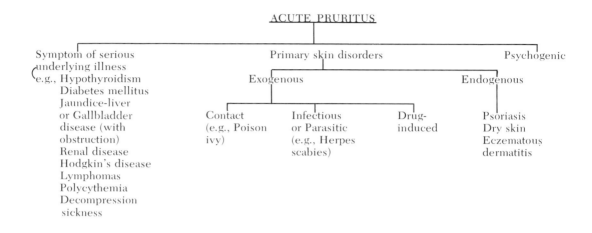

ACUTE PRURITUS

Symptom of serious underlying illness
e.g., Hypothyroidism
Diabetes mellitus
Jaundice-liver
or Gallbladder
disease (with
obstruction)
Renal disease
Hodgkin's disease
Lymphomas
Polycythemia
Decompression
sickness

Primary skin disorders

Psychogenic

Exogenous

Endogenous

Contact
(e.g., Poison
ivy)

Infectious
or Parasitic
(e.g., Herpes
scabies)

Drug-
induced

Psoriasis
Dry skin
Eczematous
dermatitis

Pruritus (itching) is the most common cutaneous symptom. It frequently is an important symptom of other skin conditions; it sometimes occurs in a generalized form without other skin disease; and it may even be the only complaint of a patient with a serious medical or surgical problem.

Pruritus in association with other cutaneous conditions usually is limited to the areas of active disease. Although this symptom may vary in severity from patient to patient with the same skin condition, the presence or absence of pruritus frequently assists recognition, as in poison ivy dermatitis in which the absence of itching makes this diagnosis very unlikely. Pruritus in relation to primary skin diseases is discussed briefly in the section on eczematous dermatitis. On the other hand, widespread or generalized pruritus in the absence of any skin disease that might produce it is a more puzzling and challenging problem for the emergency physician. It may be referred to conveniently as the "generalized pruritus syndrome."

GENERALIZED PRURITUS

Probably the most common cause of generalized or widespread pruritus is simple xerosis, or dry skin, and it seems likely that psychogenic factors can produce pruritus as well as aggravate itching from other causes. However, the emergency physician must consider various internal conditions that may produce this symptom.

Hypothyroidism, for example, may produce severe pruritus, often before other symptoms of this condition appear. However, closer examination usually discloses the dryness or fine scaling of the myxedematous patient, and the pruritus may be secondary to these changes. Although many textbooks cite uncontrolled diabetes mellitus as a cause of generalized itching, this appears to be rare, except in the severely dehydrated diabetic.

The mysterious pruritus of renal disease is characteristic of chronic renal problems. It is not related consistently to the severity of the azotemia. In liver disease, pruritus occurs only when bile flow is obstructed. It is often severe and disabling in primary biliary cirrhosis, prominent in drug-induced intrahepatic cholestasis, usually mild or transient in acute parenchymatous damage, and most variable in mechanical biliary obstruction. The degree of pruritus appears to correlate with the increase of serum bile acids.

Although pruritus is rarely found in visceral cancers, it is often the first symptom of Hodgkin's disease and mycosis fungoides, in which disorders it is sometimes intractable. It is less common in lymphomas, but reported as frequent in polycythemia. Although most cases of pruritus are aggravated by heat and hot water, the pruritus of polycythemia is especially aggravated by hot water. Pruritus is also an early unexplained symptom of decompression sickness.

RECOGNITION

Since the patient has already recognized the pruritus, the role of the emergency physician is to determine its cause(s), enabling the institution of appropriate treatment and follow-up referral. Presence or absence of a primary skin disease is the most important determination to be made and, although this is usually easy, the presence of extensive secondary lesions may cause confusion. Scaling, excoriations, erythematous areas, and small hemorrhagic crusts often result from vigorous scratching, and lichenification and pigmentary changes may occur if the process is longstanding. Patches of oozing and crusting are rare in the generalized pruritus syndrome and are more suggestive of atopic dermatitis, contact dermatitis, or secondary infection. The burrow, a fine tortuous curved ridge, is pathognomonic of scabies.

The patient's skin should be examined carefully for vesicular or bullous lesions, as these are never found in the generalized pruritus syndrome. Their presence is suggestive of *dermatitis herpetiformis*, an extremely pruritic condition in which erythematous papules and vesicles recur on the back, buttocks, and extensor aspects of the limbs. This disease is agonizingly chronic, but usually responds to sulfone therapy after the diagnosis is made.

Lichen planus is another very pruritic primary disorder in which cutaneous changes may be masked by secondary lesions. The tell-tale finding here is flat-topped, often violaceous, small papules, which are characteristically found on the wrists and ankles but may be widespread. By stretching the skin between the fingers and using a movable light source, the papules are seen to display their sharply geometric outlines and tendency to reflect more light than the adjacent normal skin. The mucosal lesions of lichen planus are white and usually in a retiform arrangement.

A thorough history may reveal renal, hepatic, lymphoreticular, or other disease which could produce generalized pruritus. In more chronic cases, the diagnoses and treatments of physicians consulted previously may be invaluable. Although medications rarely produce pruritus without a cutaneous eruption, a listing of the patient's medications may disclose a disease or symptom that the patient has forgotten.

However, *emotional stress* and *dry skin* appear to be the most common findings associated with widespread pruritus, and they occur together in the majority of cases. Xerosis is usually more pronounced on the lower legs and may result from over-use of hot water as well as from infrequent bathing. This is seen more in the elderly patient and during winter months in temperate zones, but it is not uncommon in the younger person who takes long hot baths for "relaxation." Additional factors may be the use of antibacterial or strong industrial soaps, exposure to cold winds, or living in overheated rooms. The patient may give a history of chapping very easily and of regular use of hand creams.

Dry skin is recognized initially by fine scaling and an increase in skin markings, and by cracking and increasing scale size as the process worsens. Larger areas of heavy scaling become erythematous and elevated peripherally, and assume irregularly rounded, often bizarre shapes. Sites of predilection are the lower legs, hands, and arms.

Emotional stress may be a subtle or obvious factor, denied or recognized by the patient. Since it may coexist with other causes of pruritus, it should never be regarded as the sole explanation of itchiness until other causes have been considered and evaluated. Psychogenic pruritus may be recognized by its tendency to become localized to the perianal skin or genitalia, by the patient's exaggerated descriptions of it, and by its association with stressful situations. Often it will disappear completely when the patient is working or occupied, and characteristically will flare up during the evening hours when the patient is "relaxed" or bored.

Laboratory tests are indicated to verify suspected disease, but a large battery of tests should not be ordered as a matter of routine. Blood counts and urinalyses are performed routinely in many Emergency Departments and may uncover a hematopoietic or renal abnormality that requires further investigation. If psychogenic pruritus and xerosis seem to be untenable diagnoses, blood urea nitrogen and serum bilirubin determinations are indicated.

MANAGEMENT

When underlying disease is found to explain the generalized pruritus, appropriate referral is indicated, along with some form of symptomatic therapy. However, the majority of patients with this symptom will end up with the working diagnosis of psychogenic pruritus, xerosis, or both, and the therapy should include some of the following measures, depending of course on the severity and importance of these two contributing factors.

Reassurance. The simple explanation that dry skin normally produces itching or that people normally scratch when they are under tension may be all that is needed. In a cancerphobic patient, some discussion of the negative laboratory tests might also be helpful.

Avoidance of Irritants. Hot water, over-use of soap, overbathing, and exposure to wool should be reduced or restricted. The patient usually can be persuaded to sponge bathe at the sink, where cooler water can be used "until your skin improves and can tolerate warmer water." The environmental humidity can be increased in the winter by avoiding overheated rooms and opening windows to allow the more humid outside air to enter.

Antihistamines. Although many products are effective antipruritics, diphenhydramine hydrochloride has traditional support. It is inexpensive enough to be dispensed by the emergency physician in a dosage of one or two 25-mg. capsules three or four times daily. The patient must be warned of possible drowsiness from this medica-

tion, and may also be advised to take an extra capsule at bedtime for its sedative effect.

Creams. Although corticosteroid preparations are ideal, their expense when used over large areas makes them impractical in cases of widespread pruritus. An acceptable compromise is to incorporate menthol into a weaker corticosteroid cream, as in the following:

Menthol .... 0.4 gm.
Hydrocortisone cream
    0.25 per cent..........................120 gm.

The patient should be instructed to apply the cream to the affected areas at least six times daily as an alternative to scratching. Warn the patient that menthol may be a little 'nippy" at first. Lotions often have a drying effect and should not be used where xerosis is an underlying factor.

Motivation. Treatment is almost always more effective if the patient assumes maximum responsibility for the results. A statement such as "I can tell you what to do, but *only you* can actually treat your skin" may be very helpful. If the patient understands the purpose of each therapeutic modality, he may be able to improvise, and thus improve on the therapy or adjust it to his own needs.

Tranquilizers. Only rarely is it necessary to prescribe tranquilizers for a patient with the generalized pruritus syndrome, as the other forms of therapy usually produce more rapid and reliable results. However, if the patient has discontinued a tranquilizer recently, it may be helpful for him to resume its use; if he is taking a tranquilizer "when needed," the emergency physician might suggest routine use or even a higher dose.

Systemic corticosteroids should not be used for this condition, and systemic and topical antibiotics should be reserved for specific indications. The patient must be given some insight into the nature of his condition. He must be educated as well as treated. Arrangements should be made for follow-up dermatologic care within three or four days.

SCABIES

Another cause of widespread pruritus is scabies, resulting from an infestation with the mite *Sarcoptes scabiei,* var. *hominis.* Scabies apparently is transmitted by close personal contact, e.g., from sexual partners or an overcrowded family unit.

Pruritus is the most common complaint, often very severe and usually worse at night. The primary lesion is a burrow, a thin, darkish curved tract or ridge, in which the female parasite deposits her eggs behind her as she tunnels through the skin. The most common sites for burrows are the fingers and wrists, although the genitalia, ankles, knees, and elbows are also worthwhile areas to examine. The nipples in women and the palms and soles in infants also are commonly involved. Burrows are found only rarely on the back and head. Their number may be small, often less than 10 or 12.

In most cases, and especially if the process is longstanding, secondary lesions obscure the burrows. Urticarial wheals may be seen in a wider distribution than the burrows, suggesting an allergic sensitization to the mite or its products. Papules, papulopustules, excoriations, and crusts often overlie the burrows, and inflammatory papulonodules are reported to occur on the penis and to persist for weeks or months after other scabies lesions have been eradicated. Secondary pyodermas and eczematous changes are not uncommon.

Norwegian scabies is a rare variant in which massive numbers of mites are present. Lesions are widespread, and hyperkeratosis and crusting are prominent, occasionally suggesting psoriasis.

RECOGNITION

Recognition of the burrow in its pristine form is diagnostic enough to warrant therapy, but extraction of the mite from a burrow or early papule offers the obvious advantages of definite confirmation. A scalpel blade moistened with a drop of mineral oil is used to collect scrapings from a burrow or papule, scraping vigorously enough to produce tiny flecks of blood in the oil. The oil is removed to a glass slide, and if possible the scrapings-in-oil from several other lesions are added to the same slide. Cover the slide with a coverslip (gently to avoid bubbles) and examine under low power for mites, ova, and fecal products.

In most cases, however, the burrows and early papules are hidden by secondary lesions, eczematous changes, or pyoderma, and the diagnosis must rely on the finding of multiform inflammatory lesions in characteristic locations. Interdigital or nipple lesions, consistent nocturnal pruritus, or a history of sudden onset of itching several days to weeks after sleeping in crowded conditions, all should arouse suspicions of scabies. Additionally, it is important always to ask about pruritic lesions in other family members.

MANAGEMENT

Several topical scabicides (Kwell, Eurax) are effective, and the PDR should be consulted for details of their use. A scabicide liquid—more practical than a cream as it can be spread easily over larger areas—is applied with the fingertips to all skin surfaces below the chin. Secondarily infected areas may require local and systemic antibiotics, and oral antihistamines will help to control the pruritus. Always treat close contacts who also complain of itching.

Usually itching stops and skin lesions begin to heal within a few days, although in longstanding cases with more severe secondary lesions the course will be longer. Milder cases, therefore, will be cured by the initial therapy, making follow-up care unnecessary. More severe cases, or those in which pyoderma is present, should be referred for follow-up five to seven days later. Persistence of pruritus may be due to inadequate treatment or to reinfection.

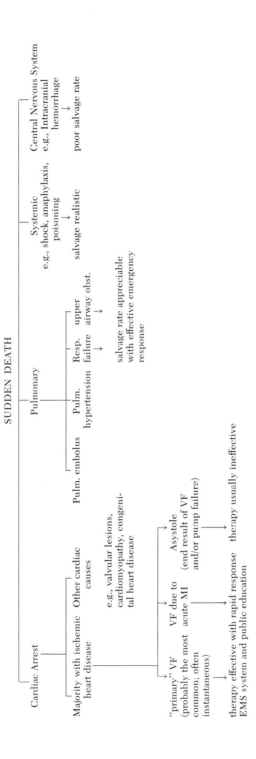

SUDDEN DEATH

Cardiac Arrest

Majority with ischemic   Other cardiac
heart disease   causes

                          e.g., valvular lesions,
                          cardiomyopathy, congeni-
                          tal heart disease

"primary" VF   VF due to   Asystole
(probably the most acute MI   (end result of VF
common; often   and/or pump failure)
instantaneous)
    ↓   ↓   ↓
therapy effective with rapid response   therapy usually ineffective
EMS system and public education

Pulmonary

Pulm. embolus

Pulm.   Resp.   upper
hypertension failure airway obst.
                ↓   ↓
              salvage rate appreciable
              with effective emergency
              response

Systemic
e.g., shock, anaphylaxis,
poisoning
        ↓
    salvage realistic

Central Nervous System
e.g., Intracranial
hemorrhage
        ↓
poor salvage rate

Chapter 33   SUDDEN DEATH

Leonard A. Cobb

INTRODUCTION

A syndrome of *sudden* death is commonly recognized when an unexpected death occurs with no premonitory symptoms or when symptoms appear minutes to several hours before the patient dies. The term *instantaneous* death has been used to describe the situation in which a patient, seemingly without symptoms, suddenly collapses from cardiac arrest and dies unless appropriate therapy is promptly administered.

The problem of sudden death is most evident in men with ischemic heart disease. Approximately 60 per cent of patients who die of ischemic heart disease experience their fatal events outside the hospital, usually precipitately (Gordon and Kannel, 1971). Furthermore, the majority of sudden deaths occur in patients who have advanced ischemic heart disease (Spain, et al., 1960; Kuller, 1969). However, it is important to recognize that other cardiac lesions also may result in sudden death, e.g., aortic and mitral valve lesions, cardiomyopathy, myocarditis, and congenital heart disease. Massive pulmonary embolism and primary pulmonary hypertension are occasional causes of this syndrome.

The frequency with which noncardiac lesions cause sudden death varies substantially depending on the criteria used and the group of patients described. Acute disorders of the central nervous system, particularly intracranial hemorrhage, may result in a rapid downhill course, with death usually due to respiratory failure and asystole. Massive bleeding and aortic dissection as well as certain infections, poisons, and anaphylaxis all may lead to a rapid death. The "cafe coronary" syndrome—upper airway obstruction due to aspiration of large chunks of food—is a dramatic, treatable cause of sudden death (Heimlich et al., 1975).

MECHANISMS OF SUDDEN CARDIAC DEATH

ELECTRICAL INSTABILITY

Ventricular fibrillation is the most common cardiac rhythm found within the first few minutes after unexpected circulatory arrest. High degrees of atrioventricular block, slow idioventricular rhythm, and cardiac arrest with straight-line EKG also may be seen, but less frequently than ventricular fibrillation (Liberthson, et al., 1974; Schaffer and Cobb, 1975). Straight-line EKGs are more commonly found in unwitnessed circulatory arrest as compared to witnessed events—presumably due to the longer delay in obtaining medical assistance. Electrical instability (represented by unifocal and multifocal premature ventricular beats, ventricular couplets and triplets, and bursts of ventricular tachycardia) is commonly present in ambulatory patients with ischemic heart disease. Although there is a statistical relationship between ventricular ectopic activity and sudden death, particularly in the post-myocardial infarction population, such electrical instability by itself is relatively non-specific as a predictor of sudden death (Coronary Drug Project, 1973; Kotler, et al., 1973). Whereas the relationship between myocardial electrical instability and sudden death may be of a causal nature, it is also possible that electrical instability and sudden death may both be secondary manifestations of underlying ischemia, prior infarction, focal areas of necrosis (Baroldi, 1975), or other processes.

In view of the prevalance of electrical instability in patients with ischemic heart disease, one might question why fatal ventricular dysrhythmias are not even more common. It is possible that the threshold for development of ventricular fibrillation varies considerably and that modulating effects of the autonomic nervous system, electrolyte disturbances, pharmacologic agents, and other factors may assume critical importance in determining whether a patient will develop ventricular fibrillation (Lown, et al., 1973).

ACUTE MYOCARDIAL INFARCTION

Acute myocardial infarction warrants special comment because of the well-recognized complication of ventricular fibrillation seen in patients with acute myocardial infarction. Experience in hospital coronary care units has shown that ventricular fibrillation complicating acute myocardial infarction is both common and treatable. Perhaps more importantly, it is preventable (Lown, et al., 1967).

"PRIMARY" VENTRICULAR FIBRILLATION

Experience with patients resuscitated from ventricular fibrillation has shown that acute myocardial infarction is by no means equivalent to the syndrome of sudden cardiac death due to ischemic heart disease. In patients resuscitated from out-of-hospital ventricular fibrillation acute *transmural* myocardial infarction appears to occur in about one-fourth of cases; and evidences of myocardial necrosis are found in fewer than one-half of surviving patients (Baum, et al., 1974; Liberthson, et al., 1974). Victims of "primary" ventricular fibrillation, i.e., ventricular fibrillation without acute myocardial infarction, commonly collapse instantaneously without prodromal symptoms. These patients have been shown to be at high risk for recurrence of fibrillation in the weeks following resuscitation (Schaffer and Cobb, 1975).

THERAPEUTIC IMPLICATIONS

MOBILE INTENSIVE CORONARY CARE UNITS

The introduction of mobile intensive coronary care units has provided a new approach for the management of out-of-hospital ventricular fibrillation. The pioneering work of Pantridge and his colleagues in Belfast has stimulated a great deal of interest and some controversy (Pantridge and Geddes, 1967). The major efforts of the Belfast group were directed toward the prevention and management of prehospital ventricular fibrillation due to acute myocardial infarction; physician participation was emphasized,

both in dispatching the mobile coronary care units and in patient management. Subsequently, rapid response *systems* were developed to assist in the management of acute myocardial infarction as well as to treat the common problem of instantaneous or near-instantaneous sudden death due to ventricular fibrillation. These systems usually are staffed by paramedical personnel and are employed to handle virtually all the common out-of-hospital medical emergencies. The organization of a prehospital emergency care system is of considerable relevance when considering the therapeutic aspects of sudden cardiac death. The sine qua non for an effective emergency care system is the ability to provide a rapid response. In several cities in the U.S. emergency care systems have been developed to provide an average three to four minute response time (the time from dispatching of the mobile intensive coronary unit until its arrival on the scene).

PUBLIC AWARENESS

Public education is an important aspect in the implementation of an emergency care system: first by providing the information necessary for patients to have appropriate access to the system, and second by involving the public in the emergency care system through widespread teaching of cardiopulmonary resuscitation (CPR). Most persons can be taught to apply CPR appropriately and effectively. The training of a large proportion of the general public, high-school age and above, probably is an attainable goal and one that holds considerable promise in improving the outcome of victims of out-of-hospital circulatory arrest.

ROLE OF PARAMEDICAL PERSONNEL

In the U.S., most emergency medical care systems are organized around emergency paramedical personnel who function under the supervision and direction of physicians responsible for emergency medical care. The capabilities of such paramedical personnel have been demonstrated in several communities, e.g., Columbus, Miami, Seattle, and Los Angeles. Fire department personnel have proved highly effective when afforded proper training and supervision; in addition, combat fire personnel often are readily available to initiate cardiopulmonary resuscitation and to provide a more rapid response than otherwise possible. Shown below are many of the behavioral objectives expected of well-trained paramedical personnel:

Expected Performance and Skills of Advanced-Level Paramedical Personnel

1. Performance of relevant history and physical examination.
2. Recognition and assessment of medical emergencies.
3. Institution of CPR and/or fluid resuscitation.
4. Appropriate airway management, including endotracheal intubation.
5. Recognition and therapy of common cardiac dysrhythmias.
6. Ability to carry out appropriate patient monitoring.
7. Knowledge of the indications for and use of defibrillator.
8. Administration of intravenous fluids and drugs under written (standing) and verbal orders.
9. Understanding and anticipation of emergency pharmacologic therapy.
10. Anticipation and institution of therapy in common medical emergencies.
11. Appreciation of psychologic problems and needs of patients and others.
12. Recording of emergency evaluation and treatment.
13. Ability to communicate succinctly by radio or telephone with supervising physicians.

RESUSCITATION

CPR has been described in Chapter 9. Although CPR is a highly effective life-sustaining procedure, it is important to recognize that this is a temporizing measure and that definitive therapy must be promptly administered. To this end, mobile intensive care has had a substantial effect in bringing the Emergency Department equipment and skills to the large numbers of patients who require therapy outside the hospital. An example of standing, written orders for paramedical personnel is summarized below. These orders have been utilized for several years in the management of over 1500 patients with ventricular fibrillation in one community (Cobb, et al., 1976).

Standing Written Orders for Paramedical Personnel Handling Cardiac Arrest

In instances of recent circulatory arrest, resuscitative efforts should be carried out as follows:
1. Verify circulatory arrest by absence of consciousness, arterial pulse, and respiration and by history from witnesses.
2. Initiate effective cardiopulmonary resuscitation. This will be the responsibility of the first unit arriving on the scene.
3. Determine the cardiac mechanism, using the oscilloscope-defibrillator electrode paddles.
4. If ventricular fibrillation is present, a 400-watt second precordial shock should be delivered and its effect on cardiac rhythm assessed.
5. An endotracheal tube is often a useful adjunct and its use is encouraged if it can be passed within 15 seconds. It is important that CPR not be interrupted for more than 15 seconds for this or other procedures. Ventilation is to be carried out with 100 per cent oxygen in patients with circulatory arrest.
6. An intravenous infusion of 5 per cent sodium bicarbonate should be initiated. (A 500-cc. flask contains a total of 300 mEq. of sodium bicarbonate, or approximately 60 mEq. of bicarbonate per each 100 ml. of solution.)

The usual total dose of sodium bicarbonate is 100 to 300 ml. of the 5 per cent solution (60-180 mEq). No more than one flask should ever be infused. After successful treatment of circulatory arrest, the sodium bicarbonate solution should be removed and a flask containing 5 per cent dextrose in water slowly infused.

7. If ventricular fibrillation persists or recurs, repeat shocks (400 watt-seconds) are indicated after infusing the initial 50 to 100 ml. of sodium bicarbonate.
8. Lidocaine, 100 mg., should be given intravenously as a single push when:

Ventricular fibrillation is refractory to two shocks or if ventricular fibrillation recurs, or when ventricular fibrillation has been successfully treated.
A total of 300 mg. of lidocaine may be administered.

9. The following drugs may also be given if resuscitation does not prove effective:
a. 0.5 mg. epinephrine (5 cc. of 1:10,000 solution) intracardiac or intravenously.
b. 5 cc. (4.5 mEq.) of calcium glucceptate directly into the intravenous needle, *not* into the I.V. tubing if sodium bicarbonate infusion is running.
10. Resuscitative efforts should not be continued indefinitely. Indications for stopping resuscitation include:
a. Straight-line EKG after the above measures have been carried out.
b. Prolonged (more than 30 minutes) arrest without any response to the above measures.
In questionable cases contact a physician by phone or radio for direction.
11. Accurate and detailed information on the appropriate forms is mandatory whenever medical decisions are made and medications administered.

12. If there is a straight-line EKG or slow idioventricular rhythm, administer intracardiac epinephrine (0.5 mg.), sodium bicarbonate as above, and calcium glucceptate.

RESULTS OF THERAPY

In a community of one-half million persons, approximately 300 instances of ventricular fibrillation were encountered annually by a fire department emergency care system. Approximately 25 per cent of patients found in ventricular fibrillation outside the hospital were resuscitated, brought to the hospital, and ultimately discharged home (Cobb, et al., 1976). Persistent major neurologic deficit in this group of patients, while occasionally encountered, only rarely prevented patients from returning to prearrest activity levels. Most instances of ventricular fibrillation occurred without obvious prodromal symptoms. Delay in the initiation of CPR was the factor most evident in unsuccessful resuscitative efforts. Patients with straight-line EKGs were rarely resuscitated.

As is the case with hospitalized patients, ventricular fibrillation which develops under surveillance outside the hospital can often be successfully managed by prompt defibrillation without CPR. However, outside the hospital this is a relatively uncommon situation, since most instances of ventricular fibrillation are not preceded by obvious alarming prodromal symptoms severe enough to alert the patient to request medical assistance (Schaffer and Cobb, 1975; Fulton, et al., 1972; Wikland, 1971).

SUMMARY

Out-of-hospital sudden death due to ventricular fibrillation is a frequently encountered major medical emergency. Resuscitative measures have proved effective if the time before initiation of CPR is less than five minutes after circulatory arrest. To this end, the training of lay persons in CPR appears to be a promising approach. Rapid institution of CPR coupled with a rapid response mobile intensive care system is probably the only effective therapeutic approach now available. In large part this is due to the infrequency of warning signs and the high frequency of near-instantaneous sudden cardiac deaths. Paramedical personnel can be trained to handle definitive resuscitation in a highly effective manner and to carry out the appropriate procedures and therapy at least as effectively as in a hospital setting where performed by physicians.

Sudden cardiac death is usually a manifestation of coronary atherosclerosis. Many, perhaps most, victims of this syndrome appear to have had a primary dysrhythmic event *not* due to typical myocardial infarction. Cardiopulmonary resuscitation with basic and advanced life support is effective in a significant number of cases if therapy is promptly administered. Patients resuscitated from out-of-hospital ventricular fibrillation show a propensity for early recurrence of ventricular fibrillation.

References

Baroldi, G.: Different types of myocardial necrosis in coronary heart disease: a pathophysiologic review of their functional significance. Am. Heart J. 89:742, 1975.

Baum, R. S., Alvarez, H., and Cobb, L. A.: Survival after resuscitation from out-of-hospital ventricular fibrillation. Circulation, 50:1231, 1974.

Cobb, L. A., and Alvarez, H.: A rapid response system for out-of-hospital cardiac emergencies. Med. Clin. North Am., 60:283, 1976.

Coronary Drug Project Research Group: The prognostic importance of premature beats following myocardial infarction. Experience in the Coronary Drug Project. J.A.M.A. 223:1116, 1973.

Fulton, M., et al.: Natural history of unstable angina. Lancet 1:860, 1972.

Gordon, T., and Kannel, W. B.: Premature mortality from coronary heart disease. J.A.M.A. 215:1617, 1971.

Heimlich, H. J., Hoffmann, K. A., and Canestri, F. R.: Food-choking and drowning deaths prevented by external subdiaphragmatic compression. Ann. Thorac. Surg. 20:188, 1975.

Kotler, M. N., et al.: Prognostic significance of ventricular ectopic beats with respect to sudden death in the late postinfarction period. Circulation 47:959, 1973.

Kuller, L.: Sudden death in arteriosclerotic heart disease. Am. J. Cardiol. 24:617, 1969.

Liberthson, R. R., et al.: Pathophysiologic Observations in Prehospital Ventricular Fibrillation and Sudden Cardiac Death. Circulation 49:790, 1974.

Lown, B., et al.: The coronary care unit—new perspectives and directions. J.A.M.A. 199:156, 1967.

Lown, B., Verrier, R., and Corbalan, R.: Psychologic stress and threshold for repetitive ventricular response. Science 182:834, 1973.

Pantridge, F., and Geddes, J. S.: A mobile intensive-care unit in the management of myocardial infarction. Lancet 2:271, 1967.

Schaffer, W. A., and Cobb, L. A.: Recurrent ventricular fibrillation and modes of death in survivors of out-of-hospital ventricular fibrillation. N. Engl. J. Med. 293:259, 1975.

Spain, D. M., Bradess, V. A., and Mohr, C.: Coronary atherosclerosis as a cause of unexpected and unexplained death. J.A.M.A. 174:384, 1960.

Standards for cardiopulmonary resuscitation (CPR) and emergency cardiac care (ECC). J.A.M.A. 227 (Supplement):834, 1974.

Wikland, B.: Medically unattended fatal cases of ischemic heart disease in a defined population. Acta. Med. Scand. (Supplement) 524:23, 1971.

Chapter 34

EVALUATION OF THE POTENTIALLY SUICIDAL PATIENT

*George R. Schwartz
and John Bulette*

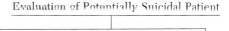

Evaluation of Potentially Suicidal Patient

Highest Risk

a. No family and friends.
b. Alcoholic.
c. Severe loss.
d. Prior attempt.
e. Organized plan including:
   1. Continual thoughts
   2. Available means
   3. Action step-preparation.
f. Chosen method of high lethal potential.

Lowest Risk

Thoughts without planning steps in individual who has suffered relatively minor loss and who does not have history of prior impulsive behavior.

Approximately two-thirds of people who go on to commit suicide have seen a physician within three months before their act (Schneideman and Faberow, 1963). When individuals attempt suicide or make a suicidal gesture they frequently are brought to an Emergency Department. But even more important, prior to an attempt, the emergency physician is in a unique position—he is often the first contact for the patient in a crisis situation, and his recognition of a patient's suicidal risk may prevent unnecessary deaths. Most individuals who are acutely suicidal are so for only a relatively short period and during this time they are extremely ambivalent about living and dying. Intervention during this period may be crucial.

Most physicians receive little training in suicidology despite the magnitude of the problem. Suicide is the tenth leading cause of death in the U.S. and the fifth leading cause between the ages of 15 and 24. The true incidence probably is higher, owing to the general abhorrence most people feel about suicide, which results in under-reporting. The philosopher Kant wrote about suicide, "It is an insult to humanity in oneself. This most individualistic of all actions disturbs society profoundly. Seeing a man who appears not to care for the things which it prizes, society is compelled to question all it has thought desirable..."

Because of the frequency of suicide and suicide attempts and the fact that such attempts are often impulsive acts related to treatable mental illness, the emergency physician should arm himself with the intellectual tools necessary to detect the patient contemplating suicide. Patients who attempt suicide usually are brought to Emergency Departments. Frequently a psychiatrist is not immediately available, and it becomes the emergency physician's responsibility to assess the likelihood of a repeat attempt.

Within the medical profession there has not been sufficient attention directed toward the problem of suicide among physicians themselves. Physicians have one of the high-

571

est suicide rates, and the number of yearly deaths from this cause exceeds the average number of graduates per year from a medical school (Schwartz, 1967). Increased communication about suicide within the medical community may enable physicians to seek psychiatric aid for themselves and thus avert tragedy.

Once a patient has made a suicide attempt and is brought to the Emergency Department, the first priority is immediate medical treatment. Knowledge of toxicology is therefore vital, since most immediately unsuccessful attempts are associated with drug ingestion. Availability of a poison control center and suitable manuals in the Emergency Department can provide information required for treatment when the substance is known. In other cases symptom analysis may point to the probable agent ingested.*

The method an individual uses cannot be used as the only factor to judge the seriousness of the attempt. For example, there may be relatively little bodily danger from 20 aspirin tablets, but if the patient believes that this is a lethal dose the lethal potential is indeed great. On the other hand, certain methods such as gunshot wounds, carbon monoxide poisoning, or hanging, in themselves, demonstrate a high potential lethality.

The greatest degree of sensitivity and sophisticated evaluation is necessary when the patient presents with depression, insomnia, or other complaints that may mask a severe depression. It is in such cases that the emergency physician's skills and knowledge of those conditions associated with suicide attempts may prevent unnecessary deaths. A key point to remember is that individuals to whom suicide seems the answer frequently will achieve a different perspective even in a matter of hours or after psychiatric treatment.

It is worthwhile to have some relevant epidemiologic information in mind. It is known that:

(a) Men complete more suicides than women, although women make more attempts.

(b) There are at least five times more attempts than actual completed suicides.

(c) The suicide rate for whites is twice that for blacks (although this may relate to differences in reporting).

(d) The incidence rises with age, although there are peaks in adolescence and in the college years.

(e) Suicide is uncommon in children; when it occurs it is almost always associated with a desire to hurt the parent.

(f) Mental illness is related to suicide and depression is of paramount importance. The highest risk is in an isolated, depressed, middle-aged alcoholic male.

There are frequent associated findings in people who attempt or actually commit suicide. First and foremost is that they have suffered a loss of some kind—loss of a loved one, job, status, health, function, or respect. Social isolation is common and includes the absence of family, friends, and strong social ties. Such social contacts provide needed support in depressed patients. Paradoxically, at the same time the depressed patient frequently seeks isolation and alienates those close to him: thus there usually is poor or decreasing social integration. People who are loosely or only slightly tied to social groups are a high risk for suicide when coping with loss.

The history and mental status examination help identify potentially suicidal patients and can help to evaluate those patients who present after an attempt. Important parts of the history include:

(a) The nature of the loss. For example, death of a person on whom the patient is dependent usually assumes more psychic importance than material loss. Loss is the sine qua non of depression and the forerunner of suicidal behavior. This includes loss of function and status, which leads to lowered self-esteem.

(b) Previous experiences coping with losses. If a person has shown marked impairment of function or suicidal thoughts after a prior loss, he is apt to repeat the same pattern.

(c) Previous depression with or without psychiatric treatment.

(d) History of impulse control, i.e., as it relates to the person's over-all stability and control. Patients with a history of drug or alcohol abuse, uneven vocational record, changing marital status, promiscuous sexual behavior, or frequent outbreaks of uncon-

---

*Specific poisons are discussed in Chapter 58B.

trolled aggression suggest poor impulse control and a higher risk of successful suicide.

(e) Family history. Certain families have a higher suicide rate. This may be important regarding the person's thoughts about alternatives. A parent who has committed suicide produces a higher risk in the offspring.

A simple mental status examination can provide the information needed to evaluate risk. The first effort is directed toward assessing the patient's higher cortical centers. If the patient is oriented in all three spheres, remembers recent and past events, and can formulate his story in an organized fashion, we can make the assumption that no organic factors are causing him to misperceive his surroundings and that there is no overt evidence of a psychotic process.

The examination should then cover the patient's mood, his affect, and his thoughts.

Mood is the patient's subjective assessment and can be found simply by asking, "How do you feel?" If the answer is "depressed" or "miserable," warning signals are being sent. The answer "fine" may be misleading, as it is a common response in some patients who are extremely distressed.

Attention should then be directed to *affect,* or the emotional response to events. Does this seem flat? Does the patient seem emotionally bare? On the other hand, is the affect somehow inappropriate to the situation? Is the patient smiling and joking while speaking of a tragic situation or a personal loss? If so, it can be a superficial defense to cover a deep sense of loss. Further questioning may penetrate a flimsy shell. A simple question such as, "Why are you laughing about something that affects you deeply?" may elicit answers relating to the patient's true feelings. If the patient has suffered a loss, his emotional response to the loss must be determined. Does he feel guilty? This may relate to a desire for self-punishment. Is there hope for improvement, or does the patient see his situation as hopeless? Often a person will avoid discussing losses and those things that make him ashamed. Frequently he will use rationalizations and an over-all glibness. Further questioning about the loss will often demonstrate the superficial nature of such defenses. The question can be asked, "Why penetrate a patient's defenses?" If they are, in fact, superficial

and easily broken, they are ineffective defenses against anxiety and depression and will certainly break down in the future under less controlled circumstances and at times when no supportive individual is present.

The way the patient expresses his *thoughts* as well as their content should be examined. Certainly a thought disorder may be detected by hearing delusional thoughts, looseness of associations, and bizarreness of expression. In the nonpsychotic patient the speed of speech may be important. Retardation of speech is characteristic of depression and is associated with frequent sighs.

The thought content may well provide the best clue. Even if the patient doesn't speak about suicide he may speak of death in general, loss of a loved person, a feeling of worthlessness, or a feeling that nobody cares about him. When such thoughts are expressed, do not at this time reassure the patient of his worth, or tell him he is wrong, but rather clarify further. The passive act of listening can be very helpful. Feelings a patient has about himself are usually not changed by facts.

Avoidance of thoughts of a serious nature can also be important. If the patient constantly avoids speaking about something you know from his history is of great importance or causing much stress, questions can be asked to attempt to bring the patient to the disturbing topic. A caveat to be observed is to beware of people who say they have recently been very depressed, but have suddenly and spontaneously recovered. The sudden recovery may indicate that the patient has found a solution to all his problems—perhaps a decision to kill himself. The physician must not avoid the question, "Have you been thinking of killing yourself?" You will certainly not give the idea to such a patient, and a straightforward question like this may allow him to speak about his thoughts. If a depressed person answers that he has not considered suicide, it is extremely useful to ask, "Why not?" What keeps him going? The answer to this sheds great light on what is really important to the individual.

If the patient has been thinking of suicide the emergency physician must then evaluate the risk. Four useful stages have been identified by Solomon (1967). These are: (1) the thought; (2) the means; (3) the action; and (4) the attempt. Evaluation should proceed carefully, asking about each of these.

The Thought. Thoughts of suicide are common. As Nietzsche wrote, "The thought of suicide is a great consolation. By means of it one gets successfully through many a bad night." Just thoughts of suicide are not a major warning flag. You must also be able to answer these questions: Are the thoughts upsetting? Are they new? Are the options finished, and is the patient emotionally drained? Does he see any hope for the future?

Means. Once the thought is present, the patient should be asked if he has decided on a means. Patients frequently will say they haven't given this aspect much thought or will say something like, "I don't know.... I guess pills or maybe I'd jump off a bridge." Of great importance is whether the person knows which pills or which bridge. Such information indicates planning, even if early. The means also give information as to the lethal potential and the point of no return. For example, when a patient shoots himself there usually is no return; ingesting pills offers much more time. Whether the means are active or passive assumes importance. For example, pills are a passive means; a gunshot is active. This also relates to the possibility of rescue. For example, a person who takes an overdose of pills outside a hospital or right before someone is scheduled to come home offers a strong possibility of rescue. Compare this with a person who goes alone to a deserted place with a gun. The setting which the patient would choose is therefore of great significance.

Action. A crucial step is taken by the person if he has initiated any action. For example, if the patient has bought a gun or has started stockpiling pills, has been walking regularly to a bridge, or has bought a rubber hose for his car. Such steps indicate a very high risk, and these patients should not be released from the hospital. It is even more serious if they have gone further and loaded the gun or attached the hose to the car. The importance of such action steps cannot be overemphasized.

Attempt. Any person who has made a previous attempt and is once again contemplating suicide falls into the highest risk category, even if he has made no action toward it. These people, once under stress, may rapidly take the action. They are frequently impulsive, and their history reveals episodes of other impulsive types of behavior.

If the emergency physician considers his patient to be at risk there is great danger in allowing the patient to leave the hospital without careful supervision. Emergency physicians rarely get follow-up on patients who commit suicide unless they follow the obituary columns in the newspaper. Any patient who indicates a method of high lethality and has taken any action step at all should not be released, even with a guardian, until psychiatric evaluation has been accomplished.

In summary, the emergency physician is frequently confronted by patients who have attempted suicide and must then assess the risk—i.e., is it a serious attempt or a gesture? Moreover, in Emergency Medicine practice there is an opportunity as well as responsibility to detect those patients who might be contemplating suicide. By looking for the loss such patients have suffered and by performing a rapid mental status examination (mood, affect, thought), it is possible to detect many such patients.

Analysis of the thoughts of suicide, the means, the action, and the attempt will enable accurate determination of risk.

References

Alvarez, A.: The Savage God—A Study of Suicide. New York, Random House, 1972.

Fedden, B.: Suicide. London Press, 1938.

Havens, L. L.: Recognition of suicidal risks through the psychologic examination. N. Engl. J. Med. 276:4, 210, 1967.

Faberow, E.: The Cry For Help. New York, McGraw-Hill, 1965.

Nietzsche, F.: The Philosophy of Nietzsche. From "On Voluntary Death" in "Thus Spake Zarathustra." New York, Modern Library 1954.

Schneidman, E.: Essays in Self Destruction. New York, Science House, 1969.

Schneidman, E., and Faberow, E.: Los Angeles suicide prevention. Am. J. Pub. Health 55:1, 1963.

Schwartz, G. R.: Loss of physicians by suicide. N. Engl. J. Med. 276:1443, 1967.

Solomon, P.: The burden of responsibility in suicide and homicide. J.A.M.A. 199:99, 1967.

Chapter 35

SYNCOPE

Milton N. Luria

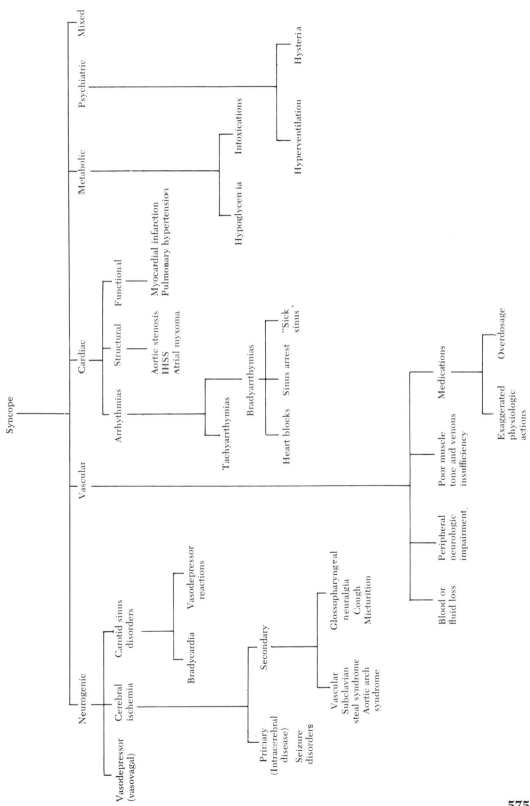

Syncope is defined as the sudden temporary loss of consciousness. In its incomplete form, it may be experienced as dizziness, vertigo, faintness, or lightheadedness. It is usually caused by a transient decrease in cerebral blood flow that results in cerebral ischemia. It has been estimated that the critical value of cerebral blood flow to maintain consciousness is 30 ml. for 100 gm. of brain tissue per minute. Syncope is an extremely common presenting complaint in the Emergency Department. It is important to understand the underlying mechanism in order to treat the symptom. Most faints are benign; some require prompt, active intervention to prevent recurrences. To recognize the patient who falls into the latter category is the challenge for the emergency physician. Some useful tests which can be done within seconds to a few hours are found in Table 1.

TABLE 1   *Useful Rapid Tests to Differentiate Type of Syncope*

---

(1) EKG and prolonged monitoring, carotid sinus pressure (monitored)
(2) Arterial blood gases
(3) Blood sugar determination, Dextrostix, response to I.V. glucose
(4) Phenothiazine test (urine) and test for other drugs (aspirin, barbiturates, etc.)
(5) Blood volume determination
(6) Hematocrit, hemoglobin
(7) Response to atropine
(8) EEG
(9) Blood pressure—reclining and with rapid standing
(10) Evocative tests (e.g., hyperventilation)

VASODEPRESSOR SYNCOPE (THE COMMON FAINT)

Vasodepressor syncope, or vasovagal syncope as it is called by some, is the most frequent cause of transient loss of consciousness. It occurs commonly in healthy individuals. The patient is usually upright—standing or sitting. The room frequently is warm or crowded. The faint may occur as a response to sudden emotional stress or after a sudden painful experience. The patient experiences a short period of nausea and profuse sweating, and develops pallor; he may hyperventilate and become weak and confused. Just before consciousness is lost, the pupils dilate; there may be a severe bradycardia at the moment it is lost. The faint is usually brief, lasting a few seconds to minutes. Consciousness returns quickly once the patient is recumbent, so that therapy consists of placing him in this position, the head lower than the rest of the body.

POSTURAL HYPOTENSION AND SYNCOPE

In postural hypotension, syncope may occur when the patient assumes the upright position. The autonomic factors compensating for the upright posture, such as reflex arteriolar and venous constriction and an increase in heart rate to compensate for pooling of vascular volume in the lower extremities, either are inadequate or fail. There is a fall in systolic and diastolic blood pressure and a variable heart rate response. The patient may develop weakness, dizziness, or syncope on sitting or standing.

Postural hypotension may be a manifestation of many disease states. It may result from loss of intravascular volume, as in severe gastrointestinal hemorrhage, marked dehydration, or massive diuresis. It may be seen in disease states with autonomic nervous system involvement, such as diabetic neuropathy, amyloidosis, and subacute combined sclerosis; in these circumstances, other symptoms referable to autonomic dysfunction may be present, such as impotence or lack of sweating. Pharmacologic agents that are ganglionic blockers may have identical effects. Postural hypotension is commonly associated with prolonged bed rest, and represents an imbalance between the hemodynamic and neurologic responses to changes in position. In old people who are relatively inactive and who have poor muscle tone and peripheral venous insufficiency, syncope may occur on standing when no other abnormality is present. Because of the lack of autonomic responses, during the presyncopal period there usually is none of the prodrome—change in heart rate, sweating, pallor, or epigastric distress—that has been noted in vasodepressor syncope.

The treatment of postural hypotension will vary, and attention must be directed to the cause. Blood transfusions or fluid replacement may be necessary. Readjustment of drug dosage may suffice. Early ambulation may help to avoid the postural hypotension of prolonged bed rest. The elderly should be advised not to get out of bed too rapidly, but instead to go from the lying to the sitting, and then after a few minutes to the standing position. For some patients, elastic stockings or elastic leotards may be necessary.

CARDIAC CAUSES FOR SYNCOPE

Because of the advances in cardiology in the past 10 to 15 years, syncope due to cardiac dysfunction must be vigorously investigated; in many cases definitive therapy is now available and effective. Fainting, when due to a cardiac cause, is a result of a sudden decrease in cardiac output. Thus, syncope may be a manifestation of a *myocardial infarction* with a markedly diminished stroke output.

In severe *valvular aortic stenosis*, syncope with effort is an ominous sign. The faint results from the fall in arterial pressure caused by vasodilatation in the muscles involved, combined with fixed cardiac output. Flow to the muscle is at the expense of that to the brain, and cerebral anoxia is the result. A transient arrhythmia or asystole may also cause syncope in the patient with obstruction of the aortic valve, and probably is responsible for syncope that occurs at rest or with minimal effort. Syncope occurring in the patient with aortic stenosis carries a grave prognosis if the latter goes uncorrected, being associated with a high incidence of sudden death. It should be considered an emergency. The patient should be hospitalized immediately and evaluated for possible early surgical aortic valve replacement.

Fainting is seen in other types of obstructive heart disease. Dizziness is common and syncope occurs in about one-third of the patients with *idiopathic hypertrophic subaortic stenosis*. Propranolol may reduce the frequency of syncopal attacks. If these are unresponsive to this drug, surgical treatment should be considered. A *left atrial myxoma* mimics mitral stenosis and should be considered in patients in whom syncope accompanies a change in position. The tumor mass shifts its position and may move down to obstruct the blood flow through the mitral valve. The tumor is often rapidly fatal if not recognized and surgically removed. In *primary pulmonary hypertension*, a syncopal episode is not infrequently the initial symptom.

A major mechanism of cardiac syncope consists of a sudden alteration in the *cardiac rhythm* or the development of *heart block*. Such a change may result in an abrupt fall in cardiac output, and the resultant decrease in cerebral blood flow may induce syncope. When the intrinsic pacemaker shifts from one site to another, there is often a transient period of asystole during which syncope may occur. With very rapid tachycardias, the diastolic filling interval may be so short that cardiac output is compromised and the patient may pass out. Likewise, a profound bradycardia may result in a markedly diminished cerebral blood flow. Syncope in older individuals should alert the physician to the possibility of heart block—either in the AV node-bundle of His or in the SA node. Adams-Stokes attacks are common in the patient who develops complete heart block with an idioventricular pacemaker. Likewise, a patient may faint with the development of a "sick sinus" syndrome, with sinus Wenckebach or sinus arrest.

Syncope due to cardiac arrhythmias or heart block usually is sudden in onset, and may occur without warning. Furthermore, when the patient regains consciousness he is usually alert. The attack may occur with the patient either standing or recumbent. Unconsciousness due to asystole occurs more quickly (4 to 8 seconds) when the patient is upright than when he is lying down.

The diagnosis of syncope caused by a rhythm disturbance or heart block has been made much easier by the use of continuous tape-recorded electrocardiographic monitoring devices. If the history seems characteristic, the patient should be monitored for several hours, even though the EKG shows a normal sinus rhythm when he is first seen. Furthermore, one cannot be certain that the premature contractions that may be seen initially in the EKG necessarily represent the mechanism for the faint. The use of the continuous tape-recorded electrocardiographic monitor may reveal a transient heart block as the more likely cause. Careful monitoring often will lead to the diagnosis. The cardiac arrhythmia can then be suppressed or prevented with appropriate drug therapy. If heart block is present, the insertion of a pacemaker may prevent further attacks. Analysis of the type of block through His-bundle electrocardiography may be of help in deciding when and if a pacemaker should be installed. For example, a combination of right bundle branch block with left posterior hemiblock can be considered a forerunner of complete heart block.

CAROTID SINUS SYNCOPE

There is a group of patients in whom the carotid sinus appears to be hyperirritable to the extent that minimal stimulation results in syncope. This syndrome is observed most commonly in elderly patients, many of whom have generalized arteriosclerosis and organic heart disease. Hyperirritability of the carotid sinus also may be seen in patients who have disease processes localized in or near the sinus area—such as a tumor or inflammatory lesion in the neck. Fainting may be caused by a tight collar, by shaving, or by turning the head to back an automobile out of a garage. As a rule there are no prodromal symptoms, and the patient is usually in the upright position before the faint.

There are three mechanisms recognized in carotid sinus syncope:

(1) In the *cardioinhibitory type*, stimulation of the carotid sinus results in slowing the heart rate due to its vagal effects on the SA and AV nodes and to the development of marked sinus bradycardia, sinoatrial block, or high degrees of atrioventricular block. Such stimulation may further result in a short period of asystole. Atropine or similar drugs may abolish this effect. Occasionally, with a hyperirritable carotid sinus, a demand pacemaker may be necessary to prevent syncope from this mechanism;

(2) In the *vasodepressor type*, impaired consciousness or fainting occurs in the absence of changes in heart rate. Peripheral vasoconstrictors are inhibited, causing vasodilatation and a fall in blood pressure. Epinephrine may prevent the development of hypotension in this case;

(3) In a rare instance, fainting may appear in a few seconds without changes either in the pulse or the blood pressure. This is known as the *cerebral type*. Symptoms may occur in any position and may be accompanied by focal neurologic manifestations. It is suggested that the syncope results from inhibition of the center for regulation of consciousness, either by a reflex mechanism or by a secondary focal circulation disturbance. The latter could occur with marked pressure on the affected carotid sinus when the other carotid artery is already thrombosed.

CEREBROVASCULAR OCCLUSIVE DISEASE AND SYNCOPE

Partial or complete occlusion of one or more of the major arteries in the neck—carotid or vertebral—may interfere with cerebral circulation and result in impaired level of consciousness and a severe case of syncope. The latter symptom is common in the *aortic arch syndrome*. With lesser involvement, lightheadedness, dizziness, weakness, and visual disturbances are present. Other focal neurologic symptoms and signs may be helpful in this diagnosis, such as hemiparesis, aphasia, or cranial nerve dysfunction. When the carotid is involved, differences in intensity of the pulse or a bruit may be present. Fainting can be caused in such patients with carotid sinus massage, and this should be performed with extreme caution and only after first listening for a bruit. Such patients may be candidates for endarterectomy. The vertebral artery system should be suspect when impairment or loss of consciousness occurs with hyperextension or lateral rotation of the head. Such attacks have been described in patients with cervical arthritis. Lastly, impaired consciousness or syncope associated with exercise of the upper extremity has been described in the *subclavian artery steal syndrome*. Again, this is surgically correctible in many instances.

COUGH SYNCOPE

Fainting may occur during a paroxysm of vigorous coughing. It is most frequently observed in men and often is associated with chronic bronchitis or chronic obstructive pulmonary disease. The duration of faint usually is brief, and there are usually no serious sequelae on regaining consciousness. Vigorous coughing and an increase in intra-abdominal pressure cause a sudden sharp rise in cerebrospinal pressure, which may "squeeze" blood from the intracranial and cerebral vessels. Thus, there is an impairment in the cerebral blood flow. Other theories that have been expressed to explain the syncope include a decrease in cardiac output due to a Valsalva effect, or a "concussive effect" caused by a rapid rise in cerebrospinal fluid pressure.

Therapy in cough syncope should be directed toward bronchitis. If the patient is a smoker, he must be urged strongly to give up this habit if he wishes to avoid further attacks.

MICTURITION SYNCOPE

Micturition syncope is seen in adult men during, or immediately after, voiding in the middle of the night. There may be no premonitory symptoms and the duration of unconsciousness is brief. Many patients give the history of drinking large quantities of alcoholic beverages, such as beer, before going to sleep. With micturition, there may be considerable deflation of the bladder. A similar type of fainting can be observed in patients with urinary retention *following* decompression of a distended bladder. It has been suggested that the fall in intra-abdominal volume may result in reflex peripheral vasodilatation. Others have attributed the faint to a Valsalva maneuver during micturition, or to the peripheral vasodilatation associated with the recent consumption of alcohol and with having been in a warm bed.

GLOSSOPHARYNGEAL NEURALGIA AND ASSOCIATED SYNCOPE

Glossopharyngeal neuralgia, like trigeminal neuralgia, is characterized by paroxysms of neuralgic pain in the throat and neck. The trigger zone is in the posterior pharynx, and the pain spreads toward the angle of the jaw and the ear. With the onset of pain the patient may develop profound bradycardia, hypotension, and, rarely, asystole. Syncope may occur as a result of the cerebral ischemia accompanying these physiologic phenomena. Atropine, or other parasympatholytic drugs, may prevent syncope by abolishing the bradycardia, presumably by preventing the vagal mediated effect. Dilantin may also be effective by raising the pain threshold, just as it does in trigeminal neuralgia.

DRUGS AND SYNCOPE

A number of commonly used drugs may be associated with syncopal attacks. *Chlorpromazine* and related *phenothiazine* drugs, used so frequently in the anxious or psychotic patient, may result in marked postural hypotension and syncope when the patient stands up. *Ganglionic blockers* and drugs that deplete catecholamines, used to treat hypertension, may result in postural hypotension and fainting. A common offender in this regard is *guanethidine.* The physician must remember that these drugs have their most profound effects when the patient is standing. If the physician, in adjusting the dosage, fails to take standing blood pressures, he may prescribe excessive amounts of guanethidine that result in dizziness or fainting when the patient rises from the lying or sitting position. *Nitroglycerin* and *Isordil* are potent peripheral vasodilators that may cause a marked fall in blood pressure, and syncope on standing. Potent *diuretics,* such as *furosemide,* may cause severe volume depletion that results in postural hypotension. *Digitalis* excess can result in complete heart block or in an arrhythmia—such as ventricular tachycardia, a slow junctional rhythm, or even ventricular bigeminy—that may result in a lowered cardiac output and subsequent insufficient cerebral blood flow. *Quinidine* in rare situations is a very unusual cause of syncope. The drug, used to prevent or reduce ventricular irritability in the form of ventricular premature contractions, may cause ventricular fibrillation. Quinidine, by prolonging the Q-T interval, may make it possible for a premature contraction to fall in the critical period of the preceding T-wave. Withholding the drug involved or adjusting the dosage should result in termination of the syncopal attacks.

HYPOGLYCEMIA

Extreme hypoglycemia is associated with weakness, sweating, confusion, and in some instances unconsciousness. Sometimes the patient, who may be elderly, appears to have had a stroke. Intravenous glucose administration causes rapid recovery. The patients usually are diabetics who are on insulin or on hypoglycemic agents. If the drugs are long-acting, it may be necessary to maintain an intravenous glucose infusion for some time to prevent the patient from again becoming unconscious.

SYNCOPE IN THE HYPERVENTILATION SYNDROME

Hyperventilation may produce a clinical syndrome in which the patient experiences "numbness and tingling of the hands, feet and face; buzzing in the head; varying degrees of reduction in the level of consciousness, described as dizziness, lightheadedness, giddiness, or fainting; blurring of vision; dryness of the mouth; stiffness of the muscles and tetany." The overbreathing, which results in hypocapnia and respiratory alkalosis, may represent an acute or chronic state and may have an organic or functional basis. It is seen as a manifestation of anoxia, encephalopathy, and salicylate toxicity. Most commonly, however, it is psychogenic in etiology. It is observed much more frequently in adolescent girls and in women than in men.

The symptoms may be focused in one or more systems and may suggest organic disease. Breathlessness is common. The patient complains of shortness of breath on performing minor tasks, the sensation of choking or gasping, a feeling of smothering, sighing, excessive yawning, or tightness in the chest. Frequently, the complaint is that the patient cannot get enough air and feels as if he is going to die. The patient may be hyperventilating while he gives his history and be totally unaware of it, and may seem to pay least attention to the respiratory symptoms. Symptoms suggesting nervous system involvement are common, e.g., dizziness, lightheadedness, blurring of vision, feelings of unreality, impairment of memory, paresthesias, and, in most severe form, occasional syncope. Chest pain is common and is usually described as a sharp fleeting twinge about the left nipple or under the left breast. Frequently there are palpitations, tachycardia, or premature beats. Musculoskeletal symptoms include myalgias, carpopedal spasm, twitching, and, rarely, tetany. The patient may complain of a dry mouth and difficulty in swallowing. Aerophagia accounts for the belching, abdominal bloating, and gas pains. Fatigue, exhaustion, weakness, and lack of ambition are common. These symptoms develop in settings of tension. The anxiety may be overt and obvious, even though the patient denies it and claims to be calm.

On hyperventilation the PCO_2 falls rapidly and the pH rises. The hypocapnia is believed to be responsible for the reduction of cerebral blood flow. This is reflected in the electroencephalogram which shows slow-wave activity. The reduction in the level of consciousness correlates well with slowing of the EEG.

The syndrome may be relieved by having the patient rebreathe into a paper bag. With proper explanation and support, the patient can understand and accept the benign nature of the symptoms. A tranquilizer is often helpful. On occasion, the symptoms are so incapacitating that psychiatric help may be needed.

HYSTERIA AND "SYNCOPE"

Hysterical fainting is important to recognize, since it may simulate vasodepressor syncope. It occurs most frequently in young girls and young women, often those with an emotional illness. The faints usually occur in the presence of others, the patient gracefully slumping to the floor or into a chair without sustaining any injury. Sometimes fluttering of the eyelids or bizarre seizure-like activity can be observed, or the patient may lie motionless for some time unresponsive to verbal commands. There usually is no abnormality in blood pressure, pulse, or skin color. Assumption of the recumbent position is not followed by recovery. The symptom represents a hysterical conversion reaction.

SUMMARY

These are the types of problem that most commonly confront the physician in the Emergency Department when a patient presents with syncope. A careful history and physical examination should be obtained and may lead to the obvious cause. It is important to assess each patient carefully in order to separate the benign faint from that of more serious consequence for which treatment now is readily available.

References

Ebert, R. V.: Syncope. Circulation 27:1148, 1963.
Engel, G. L.: Fainting. Springfield, Ill., Charles C Thomas, 1962.
Stead, E. A., Jr.: Fainting (Syncope). In MacBryde, C. M., and Blacklow, R. S.: Signs and Symptoms. Philadelphia, J. B. Lippincott Co., 1970, pp. 712–722.
Wayne, H. H.: Syncope: physiological considerations and an analysis of the clinical characteristics in 510 patients. Am. J. Med. 30:418, 1961.
Wright, K. E., Jr., and McIntosh, H. D.: Syncope: a review of pathophysiological mechanisms. Progr. Cardiovas. Dis. 13:580, 1971.

Chapter 36   VERTIGO

Robert J. Wolfson and Frank I. Marlowe

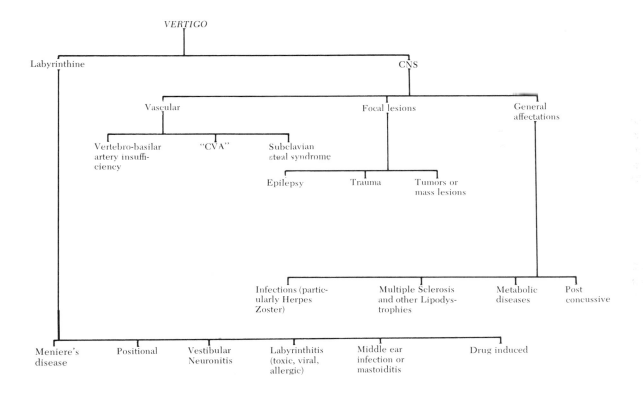

The complaint of dizziness or vertigo is commonplace in the practice of Emergency Medicine. It is a symptom which has many causes, some of which are insidiously progressive. Symptomatic therapy is necessary to control the acute manifestations of vertigo; however, every patient with this complaint deserves an investigation that is sufficiently complete to determine the likely cause, with suitable referral if tests are needed that cannot be carried out during the initial evaluation.

Vertigo may be defined as an *hallucination of motion.* In *"objective"* vertigo, the patient feels that his environment is in motion; in *"subjective"* vertigo, the patient

feels that he himself is moving. These are simply ways of describing vertigo, and have no diagnostic significance. The sensations may be rotational, or the patient may experience undulatory motion, feelings of unsteadiness, or rocking without spatial disorientation.

"Dizziness" is a term used by both patients and physicians to express a variety of sensations, including vertigo. The sensations may have differential significance, and a distinction must be made as early as possible in the examination and evaluation of the patient. Frequently, we find that the dizziness is actually a sensation of unsteadiness of gait, a period of mental confusion, faintness, giddiness, or a blurring of vision, all of which have little or no relationship to actual vertigo. Conversely, some patients use these latter terms when in fact they have experienced vertigo. Therefore, it is important to have an accurate description of the patient's complaint before proceeding with the differential diagnosis.

Vertigo as a prominent symptom has been found to occur with approximately the same frequency as one would encounter duodenal ulcer, pneumonia, rheumatoid arthritis, and appendicitis, the incidence in a general practice population being about five per 1000 patients.

Although vertigo may be caused by abnormalities within the central nervous system or the labyrinthine system, it has been shown that approximately 80 per cent of cases are due to labyrinthine involvement. In spite of its high incidence, when the cause for vertigo lies within the labyrinth the condition is rarely serious in the life-threatening sense, even though the vertigo may be overwhelming in its severity and widespread in its effects. On the other hand, causes within the central nervous system may endanger health and life. Therefore, the first thing to do when confronted with a patient suffering from vertigo is to exclude the possibility of any disorder within the

central nervous system. If this can be done, the cause will almost always be located in the inner ear.

PITFALLS TO AVOID

In order to remain on the right track, one must realize that a number of bodily functions are disturbed in a case of severe vertigo. The most misleading of all features of a vertigo attack are the accompanying nausea and vomiting. Because of this, the digestive system is frequently incriminated. However, it is not difficult to bring on nausea and vomiting by stimulating the labyrinth, as occurs in seasickness, but irritation of the stomach or gallbladder will not cause vertigo. This area of confusion can be resolved by checking for nystagmus, which always occurs during an acute vertigo attack.

One must also avoid being misdirected by the pallor, sweating, and cold, clammy appearance and weak rapid pulse that frequently accompany a vertigo attack. Not uncommonly these symptoms direct the physician's attention to the cardiovascular system rather than the labyrinth. Again, one must remember to check for nystagmus, which will be a prominent sign accompanying the vertigo attack.

The visual hallucination in which ob-

TABLE 1   *Diagnostic Tests to Aid Separation of Peripheral from Central Causes of Vertigo (in addition to careful neurologic examination)*

TEST	CENTRAL	PERIPHERAL
Electronystagmography	1. No latency 2. Persistence (nonfatigable) 3. Vertical nystagmus	1. Latency common 2. Fatigability
Caloric tests	1. Generally unimpaired except in acoustic neuroma where depressed or non-functioning on affected side	1. Impaired in vestibular neuronitis
Tuning fork	1. No diplacusis (double hearing higher pitch in involved ear)	1. Diplacusis common in Meniere's disease
Audiometry	1. Either unchanged 2. High tone loss more common in early acoustic neuroma	1. Low tones affected in early Meniere's disease
Visual fields	1. May be altered from central lesion	1. Usually normal
Angiography	1. May show mass lesion or vascular lesion	1. Usually normal
EEG	1. May show diffuse or focal abnormality	1. Usually normal
Lumbar puncture	1. Protein generally mildly elevated in neuroma	1. Normal findings expected

jects seem to be whirling around sometimes raises a suspicion that the ocular system is at fault. Severe vertigo, however, does not occur with any ocular disorder.

CAUSES OF VERTIGO WITHIN THE CENTRAL NERVOUS SYSTEM

Central vertigo can result from a variety of medical and neurologic conditions which affect the vestibular nuclei and their connections. Generally speaking, central vertigo does not have the severe rotational character experienced with a labyrinthine disorder. Nausea, vomiting and other autonomic phenomena generally are absent. Usually there are other features which indicate a lesion within the central nervous system, such as ocular palsy, unequal pupils, ptosis, facial palsy or sensory loss, dysphagia, dysarthria, long track signs (either sensory or motor), and cerebellar ataxia papilledema. Contrariwise, hearing loss and tinnitus, which are frequent accompaniments of labyrinthine and eighth nerve disorders, are rarely seen with lesions confined to the brain stem or cerebellum. The presence of vertical nystagmus (upward or downward) indicates brain stem rather than labyrinthine disease. Table 1 indicates diagnostic tests which may be indicated for differentiation; Table 2 lists the characteristics of the most common problems causing vertigo.

VERTEBRO-BASILAR ARTERY INSUFFICIENCY

This is one of the most common causes of vertigo in elderly patients. Arteriosclerosis or atherosclerosis is the most common pathologic condition leading to vertebrobasilar insufficiency, and the process may be accelerated in the presence of diabetes mellitus, hypertension, or hypercholesterolemia. The vertigo usually is momentary, and occurs with sudden changes in the position of the head. There usually are no other accompanying symptoms. The vertigo probably is produced by ischemia of the vestibular system resulting from spasm or thrombosis of the end artery.

VASCULAR ACCIDENTS

Sudden vertigo may be the earliest symptom of rupture or thrombosis of an in-tracranial blood vessel. This produces a very acute onset of severe vertigo, nausea, vomiting, and prostration, accompanied by tinnitus and deafness if the cochlear artery is involved. The symptoms may at times be indistinguishable from other types of acute labyrinthine vertigo. Usually, other neurologic signs will appear later. Hemorrhage may occur directly into the labyrinth.

MULTIPLE SCLEROSIS

Vertigo is the presenting symptom of multiple sclerosis in 7 to 10 per cent of these patients, and eventually appears during the course of the disease in up to one-third. The onset may be abrupt, with severe rotatory vertigo, nausea, vomiting, and prostration, suggesting labyrinthine disease. More often, however, the patient complains of unsteadiness and milder degrees of vertigo, usually accentuated by certain movements of the head.

Other symptoms of central nervous system involvement usually accompany this affliction. Nystagmus is almost invariably present, and a significant number of patients show vertical nystagmus. The presence of bilateral internuclear ophthalmoplegia is virtually pathognomonic of the disease. Ataxia of the eye movements on lateral gaze is also suggestive of multiple sclerosis. It should be remembered that multiple sclerosis has its onset between the ages of 20 and 40; an onset after 50 is a rarity.

EPILEPSY

Any patient who loses consciousness during a vertiginous disturbance should be suspected of having epilepsy. In about 16 per cent of epileptic patients, vertigo occurs as an aura. It may precede petit mal, grand mal, or psychomotor seizures. The diagnosis is usually easy, since the vertigo is followed by typical features of an epileptic seizure. Occasionally, a vertiginous epilepsy occurs in which vertigo is the sole manifestation of the seizure. A high index of suspicion combined with a very careful history is needed to suspect the temporal lobe as the site of origin. The presence of staring spells, rage reaction, or momentary loss of consciousness or amnesia for the entire episode may help one suspect this disorder.

TABLE 2   Differential Diagnosis of Vertigo

Disease or Conditions	Vertigo	Nystagmus	Caloric Response	Cochlear Symptoms & Signs	Associated Symptoms & Signs	Comments
1. Endolymphatic hydrops (Meniere's disease)	Severe attacks with nausea & vomiting, which last *hours* (not days or weeks)	Spontaneous during critical stage; postural in 25% of patients during first few weeks after an attack	Usually depressed in involved ear(s); progressive with recurrent episodes	Tinnitus (louder during attacks) Sensorineural hearing loss Recruitment & diplacusis usually present	Fullness in the ear during an attack; may also be noted before attack begins (as an aura)	Unilateral in 90% of patients Recurring attacks typical Interval is *variable* (days to years)
2. Benign positional vertigo	Always positional— provoked by certain head positions	Always positional— with latency, brief duration and fatigability	Normal	Absent	None	
3. Viral labyrinthitis or vestibular neuronitis	Severe 3–5 days, with nausea & vomiting Regresses over 3–6 weeks, usually	Spontaneous during severe stage; may be postural during recovery phase	Depressed in the involved ear, usually	Absent	Antecedent or concomitant acute febrile disease	Does not recur
4. Acoustic neuroma	Usually late; more often a progressive feeling of imbalance May be provoked by sudden head movements	Spontaneous type frequently present	Depressed or non-functioning labyrinth	Usually appear first Unilateral high-tone sensorineural hearing loss & tinnitus Very poor discrimination; rapid tone decay Recruitment usually absent	Decreased corneal sensitivity Facial weakness Diplopia Headache Positive x-ray findings Elevated CSF protein	Early diagnosis essential while lesion is small and may be removed with minimal sequelae
5. Vertebro-basilar insufficiency	Practically always positional—provoked by certain head positions	Usually accompanies the vertigo	Normal	Absent	Arteriosclerosis; cervical arthritis; vascular malformations	Usually seen in older age group Will invariably be other symptoms of brainstem ischemia, visual symptoms being most common

POSTERIOR FOSSA TUMORS

Acoustic neuromas account for about 80 per cent of the tumors in the cerebellopontine angle. Other tumors and lesions in this area will produce an identical clinical picture. These other lesions include meningiomas, primary cholesteatomas, metastatic tumors, and aneurysms.

Originating in the internal auditory meatus, the tumor produces its first symptoms by compression of the eighth nerve. Tinnitus occurs in 80 per cent of these patients, and is probably the most frequent initial symptom. Hearing loss usually is gradual but progressive. True vertigo occurs in only a minority of patients with acoustic neuroma. About 75 per cent complain instead of imbalance or unsteadiness. The eighth nerve symptoms increase gradually as the tumor enlarges. Occasionally, an acute attack of vertigo may occur from compression or occlusion of the internal auditory artery within the internal auditory canal. Neurologic symptoms other than those of eighth nerve origin occur when the tumor has spread beyond the confines of the internal auditory canal and compresses the adjacent brain stem, the roots of nerves five, seven, nine, and ten, or the cerebellum. A patient suspected of having an eighth nerve tumor must have an audiologic, vestibular, neurologic, and radiologic evaluation in order to confirm the diagnosis.

PERIPHERAL (LABYRINTHINE) CAUSES OF VERTIGO

MENIERE'S DISEASE

Meniere's disease is characterized by a triad of symptoms: vertigo, tinnitus, and deafness. The disease usually has its onset between the ages of 30 and 60 years, and it affects both sexes in equal proportion. It is a disorder of the inner ear, affecting both the cochlear and vestibular systems. Although the disease is primarily unilateral, bilateral Meniere's disease may be found in about 15 to 20 per cent of the cases.

In the vast majority, the initial presenting complaint is vertigo. This symptom is the most disturbing and frightening to the patient, although tinnitus and hearing loss may have preceded the vertigo by months or years. The patient may be seen during his first episode of vertigo; however, it is not unusual that several mild vertigo attacks have taken place in the past without the patient's seeking medical advice, since the episodes are often attributed by the individual to fatigue, tension, or indigestion. It is often found that only upon direct questioning will the associated symptoms of tinnitus and hearing loss be elicited.

The natural history of the disease is one of paroxysmal attacks of vertigo. The frequency and duration of each episode of vertigo follows no predictable pattern, and the severity of each attack may vary widely. The vertigo may occur suddenly and without warning, or may be preceded by a well defined aura. When an aura is present, usually a patient will first experience a feeling of fullness in the involved ear. The tinnitus then occurs, or if present prior to the attack, it will increase in loudness. Next, the ear seems blocked, because of the sudden increase in the hearing loss. Soon thereafter, the vertigo will ensue. Depending on the severity of the attack, the vertigo may last for only a few minutes; in more severe attacks it will last for several hours and will be associated with nausea, vomiting, sweating, and pallor. After the vertigo has subsided, the tinnitus usually will disappear or decrease to the level present prior to the attack. Hearing frequently recovers to its pre-attack sensitivity.

The type of vertigo experienced during a Meniere's attack usually is of a rotatory or spinning type. During this stage, the patient is unable to sit or walk because of the rotation he is experiencing. He will therefore tend to lie quietly with his head fixed in a comfortable position and to resist head movement, since this will tend to aggravate his vertigo. The degree of nausea and vomiting varies directly with the severity of the attack. Nystagmus is invariably present, and its intensity is generally proportional to the severity of the vertigo.

POSITIONAL VERTIGO

This condition is characterized by vertigo that occurs only when the head is turned in a particular manner or assumes a "critical" position. It is not to be confused with dizziness of orthostatic hypotension, which is caused by the cerebral ischemia that occurs in some patients when standing up from a sitting or recumbent position.

The vertigo may come on when the patient lies down, when he turns in bed, when the head is turned quickly to the right or left, or when he tilts his head back to look upward. Usually the vertigo is momentary, and since it is precipitated only by certain movements or positions, the patient soon learns to avoid them.

Typically, the dizziness lasts about 20 to 30 seconds and then subsides completely. The patient may feel nauseated during this time, and may even have some sweating and pallor. Turning the head in the precipitating position will cause the vertigo to recur in a similar manner.

The diagnosis is confirmed by performing a positional test. The patient sits on the table, his head turned to one side. He is then quickly lowered to a supine position, so that his head hangs over the edge of the table 30° below the horizontal. The patient's eyes are kept open, his gaze being fixed on the examiner's forehead. His eyes are watched for the appearance and duration of any nystagmus. He is asked about any subjective feeling of vertigo. The test is repeated with his head turned to the opposite side, and finally with his head brought straight back in a hanging position.

When the patient's head is placed in the critical precipitating position, there is a short latent period of a few seconds, followed by rotatory nystagmus and vertigo. The vertigo usually is severe, causing the patient to become frightened and to make an active attempt to change his head position. Nystagmus is observed beating toward the undermost ear. The nystagmus increases in rapidity of beating for a few seconds and then rapidly declines as the patient's distress subsides. Once the reaction has disappeared, the patient is allowed to sit again, at which time a recurrence of vertigo in a milder form is usually seen.

There are no other findings on the general physical examination or on neurologic and otologic evaluation. This sort of vertigo is common in the very ill-defined postconcussive syndrome. It also may be seen after exposure to very loud noise.

VESTIBULAR NEURONITIS

Vestibular neuronitis represents an acute unilateral vestibular failure whose chief symptom is vertigo. The condition differs from Meniere's disease in that there is no tinnitus or hearing loss.

The pathogenesis seems to be on a toxic or infective basis, since in a fairly high proportion of patients the onset of symptoms is associated with or occurs soon after some kind of viral illness, particularly an upper respiratory infection. Often, however, there is no clue to the possible cause. The disease is most common in the 30 to 50 age group, without preference to sex.

The vertiginous attack develops suddenly. It is a rotatory type of vertigo, frequently associated with nausea and vomiting, and the symptoms are made worse on rapid changes of position of the head. Horizontal or rotatory nystagmus usually is present and is directed toward the healthy ear.

The condition is a benign one, and recovery usually occurs within one to three months, although at times the course is more protracted. The vertigo, initially severe, usually subsides within a few hours to a few days, to be followed by a period of dysequilibrium that is aggravated by head movements of all kinds. After varying intervals, all patients become symptom-free, and no complications have been reported. Even after clinical recovery has occurred, the function of the affected labyrinth, as indicated by caloric testing, may remain permanently impaired.

The single positive test is that of vestibular function. The caloric reaction is abnormal, the diseased labyrinth showing diminished to absent sensitivity upon caloric stimulation. All other tests, including the audiometric and neurologic examination, are normal.

Conditions such as epidemic labyrinthitis, viral labyrinthitis, or acute labyrinthitis give the same symptoms and follow a similar course as vestibular neuronitis. However, in these conditions both caloric and audiometric tests are usually normal.

TOXIC AND ALLERGIC LABYRINTHITIS

An acute episode of whirling vertigo with associated nausea and vomiting may be precipitated as a direct toxic effect of certain drugs or as an allergic manifestation of the ingestion of certain foods.

Streptomycin has a specific toxic affinity to the vestibular portion of the inner ear, just as dihydrostreptomycin has a toxic affinity for the cochlear portion. In susceptible individuals, this toxicity may develop following only small doses. So predictable is this property of vestibular toxicity that streptomycin has been utilized clinically to destroy bilateral vestibular function permanently in some cases of severe Meniere's disease. Because of this toxic property, streptomycin should be administered with great care, and should be discontinued at the first sign of vestibular upset or reduction in activity as shown by caloric testing. Tobacco and alcohol will commonly produce vertigo, particularly in sensitive individuals.

Vertigo may occur as an allergic reaction to certain foods, an attack being precipitated whenever that particular food is ingested. Shellfish seem to be the most common offenders in this category.

VERTIGO SECONDARY TO MIDDLE EAR AND MASTOID INFECTION

Infections of the middle ear, whether or not involving the mastoid, may affect the labyrinth secondarily. Involvement of the labyrinth, which is separated from the middle ear only by the thin membranes of the oval and round windows, may simply be due to toxins. It may also be due to actual bacterial invasion via the emissary veins or to bone necrosis and erosion into the semicircular canal.

Because of the close anatomic relationship between the labyrinth and the intracranial structures, a suppurative labyrinthitis often will be accompanied by signs of meningeal irritation, including nuchal rigidity, opisthotonos, and Kernig's sign. The vertigo is of the irritative type, the nystagmus being directed toward the involved ear. This is increased, as is the vertigo, when the patient turns toward the affected side. In a patient with vertigo having known otitis media, one can safely assume that the vertigo is of otitic origin.

In some cases of chronic otitis media, a cholesteatoma is present and invades the mastoid. As the growth expands, it erodes surrounding tissues, including bone. This may result in the formation of a fistula into the horizontal semicircular canal. When this occurs, pressure on the tragus or the external ear canal will either cause or increase vertigo and nystagmus.

THERAPY

Although the drug treatment of vertigo itself dates back to ancient Biblical times, a good starting point is Meniere's original paper. Describing the treatment of a patient referred to him in consultation by a colleague, Meniere relates:

First of all, the intermittent character of the attacks was fought by sulphate of quinine, but the latter usually gave rise to ear noises with momentary deafness, and soon had to be abandoned, as the cure seemed to aggravate the disease. Assuming a dyspepsia as the starting point of the vertigo and vomiting, our colleague made use of all the remedies vaunted in such cases, tonics, debilitants, ferruginous medicine, bitters, carbonated waters, ice intus and extra, then the irritant and vesicatory topicals on the epigastric region, rubefacient massages, crotona oil, stibiated pomade, all with no effect. Then, in the belief that the affliction was cerebral, he bled often and copiously, he placed a large number of leeches at the temples and behind the ears, but the general debility produced by this spoliation appeared to increase the trouble and thereafter the doctor assumed that it was a cachectic state due to some errors of youth. Immediately potassium iodide was taken regularly in large doses, and for several months two grams or more of this salt were absorbed each day. The incidents continued; the patient found the noises and deafness increasing and he then thought that the alteration of the ear should be given serious consideration and he called on a wide seton at the nape of the neck, and small moxas applied to the mastoid regions, but again without success. He did not altogether forget sulphur waters and sweat baths, he used and abused everything that could be taken in whatever form, and the disease did not even yield to electricity, nor to ether instilled in the ears, so that the patient at the end of his resources, finally wanted to call on physicians specializing in diseases of the auditory apparatus.

As may be inferred from the preceding, the pharmacologic therapy of vertigo has not changed significantly in some respects over the past 100 years.

In view of the ignorance surrounding the true etiology of many forms of vertigo compounded by clinical courses which are characterized by frequent spontaneous remissions of long duration, it would seem almost impossible to formulate a rational pharmacotherapeutic program and evaluate the results thereof. In fact, Guilford in an extensive review of the literature on the medical treatment of the vertigo of Meniere's disease noted that all forms of treatment including placebos resulted in approximately two-thirds of the patients being relieved of their symptoms.

Despite these difficulties, a relatively small number of drug classes have been employed in the treatment of vertigo. Some are primarily of historic interest; others comprise the mainstay of our drug therapy. The agents currently employed are largely the same regardless of the etiology of the vertigo, whether it be central or peripheral in origin and whether it be acute or chronic.

DIETARY AND VITAMIN THERAPY

In 1934, Furstenberg, et al. outlined the dietary regimen for the treatment of the vertigo of Meniere's disease. It included a low sodium diet and administration of the acid salt, ammonium chloride. This treatment appears to have been largely abandoned at the present time. Attention has recently been focused once again on diet, based on a report (Pulec, 1972) that allergy, especially to foods, is responsible for the production of symptoms in a significant number of patients with vertigo. It has been said that the symptoms respond well to allergic management.

Almost all of the vitamins, coenzymes, and trace elements have been employed in the treatment of vertigo over the years. Nicotinic acid or niacin, which is one of the B-complex group of vitamins, has been employed since it was noted that the deficiency state, pellagra, includes within its symptom complex bouts of vertigo. The drug probably functions in the form of the amide (nicotinamide) as a weak dilator of peripheral blood vessels at the small arteriole and capillary level. This is manifested primarily as flushing of the skin and may be accompanied by some sensations of itching and burning. There is no evidence that it has any effect on cerebral blood flow, but it remains one of the most commonly advocated vasodilator substances recommended for use in the labyrinthine disorders. It is usually given orally in doses of 50 to 100 mg. four times a day or in so-called "flushing" doses in which the patient is instructed to increase the dose until he notes a flushing sensation from the medication. Its primary usefulness is in the treatment of the less acute forms of vertigo or for maintenance between acute attacks. Another nutritional element that has received wide attention in recent years has been bioflavonoids or vitamin P (lipoflavo-noid). These agents, originally isolated from such fruits as lemon, were noted to be capable of altering capillary permeability (thus the designation "P" for permeability). Subsequently these compounds were chemically identified as being derivatives of flavone, and those with biologic activity were designated as bioflavonoids. The rationale for their use in vertigo derives from the fact that one of the theories of the production of vertigo hypothesizes an increased capillary permeability as the cause of an increased production of labyrinthine fluid. Since the flavonoids have been demonstrated to have activity in diminishing capillary permeability, it was tempting to put them to the therapeutic test.

Despite several initially enthusiastic reports for the clinical efficacy of bioflavonoids in the treatment of vertigo, there remains no evidence based on well controlled studies to indicate that they are at all useful for anything other than their placebo effect.

ANTIHISTAMINIC AGENTS

The antihistamines constitute a great number of drugs representing numerous chemical categories and form the mainstay of therapy for acute and chronic forms of vertigo. The clinically useful antihistamines, as regards vertigo, fall essentially into three categories: (1) the ethanolamine group includes diphenhydramine (Benadryl) and dimenhydrinate (Dramamine); (2) the piperazine group includes cyclizine (Marezine) and meclizine (Bonine, Antivert); (3) the phenothiazine group, widely employed as psychosedatives, includes the prototype promethazine (Phenergan). The mechanism of action of the antihistamines is poorly understood, but they appear to fall into that large group of pharmacologic antagonists known as "competitive inhibitors" and are felt to act by blocking the action of histamine. Most clinically useful antihistamines also exert potent central hypnotic and anticholinergic effects. In fact, scopolamine (hyoscine) in appropriate doses is probably one of the most potent antivertiginous agents available today, although it is somewhat less well tolerated than some of the more popular antihistaminic compounds. The precise mechanism of action is not known, but the activity against motion sickness is felt to be primarily on the vestibular nuclei and vestibular central pathways.

All of the previously mentioned antihistamines and the belladonna alkaloids have been shown to be active in reducing vestibular stimulation. This rather selective central depression brought about by the above pharmacologic agents, which results in suppression of motion sickness, has made them the cornerstone of drug therapy for both the acute episode and the long term management of vertigo. These agents may be administered either parenterally for rapid onset of action or orally, as they are readily absorbed from the gastrointestinal tract, with full effectiveness apparent after about an hour and slowly diminishing activity over the ensuing three to six hours. Common treatment of an acute vertiginous attack might consist of intramuscular or intravenous dimenhydrinate (Dramamine) or diphenhydramine (Benadryl) in doses of 24 to 50 mg. every three to four hours. Supplemental treatment might well include one of the phenothiazines, especially in the face of severe nausea or vomiting. Chlorpromazine (Thorazine) may be given I.M. in doses of 25 to 50 mg. every three to four hours, and prochlorperazine (Compazine) may be given I.M. in a dose of 10 mg. every three to four hours. Scopolamine may also be used for its marked vestibular suppressant activity in doses of .6 to 1.0 mg. parenterally. Research undertaken during the military space program discovered that the most effective combination for positionally induced vertigo was scopolamine 0.6 mg. combined with dextroamphetamine 10 mg.

For treatment of the less acute forms of vertigo, oral administration of meclizine (Bonine, Antivert) in doses of 12 to 25 mg. four times daily or dimenhydrinate (Dramamine) 50 mg. four times daily is often effective. Promethazine (Phenergan) may also be employed in a dose of 25 mg. every four hours. The primary side-effect of these agents is sedation, but blurred vision, diplopia, dry mouth, hypotension, euphoria, and nervousness also have been reported. The extrapyramidal actions associated with the use of the phenothiazines in general do not appear to be a problem with promethazine in particular.

HISTAMINE AND THE HISTAMINE ANALOGUES

In view of the significant role played by the antihistamines in the therapy of vertigo it appears rather incongruous for histamine itself to have played such a large role, but it has. In a variety of diseases in which histamine is suspected of being involved in the etiology, such as allergies and various vascular headaches (cluster headache or histamine cephalalgia) in addition to Meniere's disease, attempts have been made to desensitize the patient with courses of histamine injections. There is no experimental evidence that such regimens induce significant tolerance, but they appear to have met with wide acceptance in otolaryngologic treatment. Histamine 2.75 mg. in 500 ml. of 5 per cent dextrose in water titrated over several hours appears to be widely advocated as treatment for acute exacerbations of labyrinthine vertigo despite the fact that there are no well controlled experimental or clinical trials to substantiate its effectiveness. The apparent rationale in the treatment of Meniere's vertigo appears to be postulated dilatation of cerebral blood vessels which would counteract the proposed "labyrinthine ischemia" viewed as a possible cause of vertigo. Caution must be exercised in the use of histamine in patients with a history of peptic ulcer disease or bronchial asthma as acute exacerbations might be precipitated.

Recently a histamine analogue, betahistine (Serc) had been widely promoted in the treatment of various labyrinthine disorders. It was administered orally, and its effectiveness supposedly was based on its histamine-like activity. Its effectiveness was open to serious question, and it has been withdrawn from the market.

VASODILATORS

Approximately a decade ago, several studies appeared within a short period of time tending to support the concept of angiospastic vascular change in the end arterial distribution of the labyrinthine artery as an important pathophysiologic change in labyrinthine vertigo. In response to this information interest in the clinical use of vasodilators was stimulated (Rubin and Anderson, 1958). Among these were nicotinic acid, which has previously been discussed, but the agent which appears to have had the greatest trial was nylidrin (Arlidin). This agent has previously been noted to evoke a marked increase in retinal artery blood flow, and it was felt it might exert a similar activity on labyrinthine artery blood flow. Nylidrin and similar agents (e.g., isoxsuprine) are beta-adrenergic stimulants that relax vascular smooth muscle while increasing myocardial contractility and heart rate. These actions are reported to be responsible for an increased cerebral blood flow. Nylidrin is used orally in a dose of 6 mg. three to four times a day, and isoxsuprine (Vasodilan) is used in doses of 10 to 20 mg. three to four times a day. While untoward effects with the beta-adrenergic stimulants are infrequent, the drug is contraindicated in patients with angina pectoris, acute myocardial infarction, or a history of infarction because of the risk of hypotension.

Papaverine, a non-narcotic derivative of opium, has been advocated as a cerebral vasodilator of possible value in the treatment of ischemic disorders including those of the labyrinth. Papaverine appears to act directly on smooth muscle vasculature in medium and large blood vessels, producing vasodilatation. It is used in oral doses of 100 to 300 mg. three to four times a day and is available in 150-mg. timed release capsules (Pavabid, Cerespan). Untoward side-effects encountered with papaverine are infrequent, but at least one study reported abnormal liver function in 20 per cent of patients studied while taking the drug (Ronnov-Jessen and Tjernlund, 1969).

NEWER THERAPIES

Neuroleptanalgesics. In 1965, Dowdy, et al. described their clinical experience with a mixture of drugs synthesized in the research laboratories of Janssen Pharmaceutica in Belgium. The authors described several cases in which the drug combination was able to produce immediate and dramatic relief of the subjective symptoms and objective signs of an acute attack of vertigo associated with Meniere's disease. They also reported a controlled study with normal young subjects in which administration of the drug was able to produce complete temporary suppression of vestibular reactions in eight out of nine patients. In this action, the two component drugs were significantly less effective as vestibular depressants when given alone.

Innovar is a mixture of droperidol (Inapsine), a psychotropic (tranquilizer), with a potent narcotic, fentanyl (Sublimaze) in a 50:1 ratio. It appears to be useful primarily as an ancillary agent in surgical anesthesia, producing a state of quiescence and psychic indifference to environmental stimuli referred to as "neuroleptanalgesia."

In a study of 36 patients, all of whom had pathologic spontaneous nystagmus whose origin had been clearly established as either peripheral or central, Boedts found that intravenous administration of 2 cc. of the combination of droperidol and fentanyl completely suppressed the nystagmus within one to ten minutes of administration in all patients except three with central disturbances. Clinically the injection produced immediate and complete relief of the nystagmus and other symptoms of the acute vestibular disturbance. It was further noted that a striking differential in duration of action was observed depending on whether the nystagmus was of peripheral or central origin. In cases of central origin, the nystagmus usually recurred within about 90 minutes; however, in peripheral disturbances the nystagmus did not recur within 170 minutes of the injection. This difference in duration of action would appear to be of considerable diagnostic value if it is borne out in further studies on larger numbers of patients. Innovar has been employed in doses of .5 to 2.0 cc. I.M. or I.V. for therapy of acute vertiginous attacks.

Drug-related side-effects were trivial and infrequent, consisting primarily of faintness and fatigue, with some momentary lapses into sleep. Respiratory depression, bradycardia, and extrapyramidal effects were not observed.

Hormones. Vertigo has been reported as a symptom in Addison's disease, hypothyroidism, and estrogen deficiency. In these deficiency states hormonal treatment may ameliorate vertigo, although the mechanism of action is unknown. It is unproved that these hormones have any influence in the non-deficient patient.

Perhaps in the near future a better understanding of the various basic mechanisms of vertigo will be reflected in more rational, uniform, and effective medical treatment.

References

AMA Drug Evaluation. AMA Council on Drugs, American Medical Association, Chicago, 1971, p. 20.

Boedts, D. A. A., and Vanhove, P. T. E.: Droperidol-fentanyl citrate in equilibratory disturbances. Arch. Otolaryngol. 89:715, 1969.

Dowdy, E. G., et al.: A new treatment of Meniere's disease. Arch. Otolaryngol. 82:494, 1965.

Furstenberg, A. C., Lashmet, F. H., and Lathrop, F.: Meniere's symptom complex: medical treatment. Ann. Otol. 43:1035, 1934.

Goodman, L. S., and Gilman, A.: The Pharmacologic Basis of Therapeutics, 4th ed. New York, The Macmillan Co., 1970.

Guilford, F. R.: Treatment of Meniere's disease. *In* Fields, W. S., and Alford, B. R. (eds.): Neurologic Aspects of Auditory and Vestibular Disorders. Springfield, Illinois, Charles C Thomas, 1964, p. 341.

Kubicek, W. C., and Anderson, W. D.: Blood flow changes into the dog labyrinthine arteries. Presented at Am. Acad. Opthomol. Otolaryngol., Chicago, Oct. 29–Nov. 2, 1967.

Menière, P.: Patholgie auriculaire. Gazette Medicale de Paris, pp. 29, 88, 239, 1861.

Physicians Desk Reference: Oradell, N.J., Medical Economics, Inc., 1971.

Pulec, J. W.: Medical World News, 1972, p. 41.

Ronnov-Jessen, B., and Tjernlund, A.: Hepatotoxicity due to treatment with papaverine. N. Engl. J. Med. *281*:1333, 1969.

Rubin, W. R.: Vestibular suppressant drugs. Arch. Otolaryngol. 97:135, 1973.

Rubin, W. and Anderson, J. R.: The management of circulatory disturbances of the inner ear. Angiology 9:256, 1958.

Schiff, M.: Hormones and vertigo. Arch. Otolaryngol. 97:231, 1973.

Simonton, K. M.: Meniere's disease: natural history. Otolaryngol. Clin. North Am., 1968, p. 423.

The Medical Letter: Papaverine for Cerebral and Other Vascular Disorders, *12*, No. 6:26. New York, Drugs & Therapeutic Information, Inc. (Pub.)

Section 2

Chapter 37

APPROACH TO THE TRAUMATIZED PATIENT

A. Traumatology
B. Initial Evaluation of Acutely Injured Patients

A.   TRAUMATOLOGY

C. Gene Cayten

Traumatology is the study of persons injured by external forces, the nature of the injuries, and the methods of caring for such injuries. These external forces usually are considered to involve either an object striking the human body or the human body striking an object.

Trauma has been a cause of death in every human society; homicide, accidents, and war have always taken a toll. Therefore, it is not surprising that the treatment of trauma has had a long and varied history, from primitive, homeopathic medicine (Pellegrino, 1973) to the advanced surgical procedures used in highly developed civilizations.

In Western civilization, improvements in the treatment of trauma have closely paralleled the development of surgery as a specialty. Hippocrates discussed the treatment of fractures, dislocations, and wounds in some of his initial works. Ambroise Paré, in the 16th century, was a pioneer in the management of battlefield injuries. Other pioneers in surgery, such as John Hunter, brought particular attention to the healing of wounds. Today, surgical intervention in trauma victims has become highly effective.

Although treatment of trauma has become more and more sophisticated, the incidence of trauma and its effect on society have grown. With the growth of technology since the Industrial Revolution, machines have permeated all aspects of life in industrialized nations, increasing the potential for traumatic injuries. Factories, mills, and mines, with their massive machinery; highways and roads filled with speeding vehicles; houses crammed with gadgets from power saws to lawn mowers; and farms cultivated with powerful machines are all sites for severe traumatic injury. Also, the introduction of more sophisticated weapons has had a tremendous impact on the nature and extent of trauma to the human body. Just within this century there has been a conspicuous change in the epidemiology of trauma wounds, from stabbings in the early part of the century to many more bullet injuries today. The increasing popularity of contact sports, such as football, and fast-moving sports, such as skiing, has also contributed to a rise in the incidence of trauma.

These trends toward increasing incidence of trauma have resulted in high rates of death and disability. Deaths from accidents, suicides, homicides, and other external causes of trauma have numbered over 100,000 per year for the last five years (National Safety Council, 1975). In 1971, accidents were the leading cause of working years lost. They accounted for 20.2 per cent of the total, whereas diseases of the heart accounted for 14.2 per cent (Wetzler, 1976). More than 500,000 people have been temporarily or permanently disabled each year. Accidents are the leading cause of death for Americans between the ages of 1 and 44, and they are the fourth leading cause of death for the entire population. For those 15 to 24 years of age, accidents account for more deaths than all other causes combined. In recent years, 16,000 children have died each year from trauma. Traumatic injury is also costly in economic terms. Trauma patients occupy four times as many hospital beds as cancer patients do, and account for 22 million hospital days each year—more than the total number of days for heart disease or obstetric patients. The combined costs for accidents in 1975 has been estimated at 47.1 billion dollars. This figure includes medical and hospital fees, insurance costs, and property damage. Although death rates from motor vehicle accidents have been declining in recent years, such accidents still claim a staggering total of close to 50,000 deaths each year. In 1975, motor vehicle accidents cost an estimated 21.2 billion dollars, almost half the total for all accidents.

In the 62 years from 1912 to 1974, the death rate from accidents related to work decreased by 71 per cent, from 21 per 100,000 population in 1912 to 6 per 100,000 population in 1974 (National Safety Council, 1975). In numbers, also, there was a decrease, from 18,000 deaths in 1912 to 12,600 in 1975. The number of disabling injuries related to work was still large, however, in 1972—a total of 2.3 million for all industries—and the total cost from work accidents in that year was estimated to be 15.3 billion dollars. Mining, quarrying, and construction have the highest death rates. The Occupational Safety and Health Act of 1970 mandated much more stringent precautions against occupational injuries and illnesses and required that careful records be kept of work-related injuries and illnesses.

In 1975, there were 2100 accidental work deaths in agriculture, a death rate of 54 per 100,000 workers. This rate places agriculture as the third most dangerous occupation in the United States.

The standardized death rate from accidents in the home dropped 55 per cent from 1935 to 1972. The actual number of deaths in the home in 1974 was 25,500. One out of every 53 persons in the United States was disabled one or more days by injuries received in the home in 1975.

With the increased popularity of football and other contact sports, injuries to participants have increased in recent years. Sports medicine has evolved as a major area of interest among many orthopedists and general surgeons.

THE MILITARY TRAUMA EXPERIENCE

In Vietnam and Korea, the military was able to reduce battlefield mortalities to less than 1 per cent of those injured by stabilizing trauma victims at the scene and continuing care in transit to the hospital (Harvey, 1973). This experience proved that proper integration of manpower, communication, transportation, and facilities can have a dramatic effect on trauma mortality. Attempts to apply military techniques to peacetime conditions resulted in the development of a total health care systems approach to the care of trauma victims. A monograph prepared by the National Academy of Sciences National Research Council (1966) mapped out the steps needed to establish such an approach and encouraged states and cities to apply a systems approach to the care of civilian trauma victims.

THE ILLINOIS TRAUMA PROGRAM

In Illinois, David Boyd, a trauma surgeon, was able to enlist the support of the Governor in implementing a systems approach to trauma. This approach, as it developed in Illinois, used as its basis the key concepts of (1) categorization, (2) regionalization, (3) a trauma registry, (4) manpower development, and (5) communications.

In Illinois, "a decision was made initially to proceed along the lines of categorization and designation of emergency care hospital facilities for the critically injured patient (e.g.—trauma center), and implement other essential subsystems as it appeared appropriate and became feasible. In each major community and health service district, the local health planning authority was asked to select the one hospital best suited for the care of the seriously injured (Boyd, 1974). This hospital was designated as a trauma center; eventually, there were 40 such districts or areas, each with a designated trauma center. The trauma centers were categorized as local, areawide, and regional on the basis of increasing availability of specialized personnel and care units.

A plan for hospital categorization (horizontal categorization) was developed to designate different hospitals to provide the initial care for different levels of severity of injury. Categorization governs the decision concerning where to take a patient—if there is a choice. The categorization system was planned to avoid the duplication of services in neighboring hospitals and allows staff in those hospitals which take care of the most severely injured to gain greater proficiency.

Regionalization (vertical categorization) was developed to establish special centers for the definitive care of various types of trauma, such as shock, head trauma, spinal cord injuries, and burns. In Illinois, special regional centers were established to give definitive treatment, including a regional spinal cord injury center, a nervous system trauma center, and a statewide system of burn intensive care units.

The Illinois trauma registry was developed to provide ongoing data for evaluation. The registry is a centralized record-keeping system that records "the clinical management of the injured patient . . . [and] data on demographic, epidemiologic, and health care delivery factors" (Boyd, 1974). Records are obtained from hospital-based registries. The registry thus provides essential data for planning, managing, and evaluating systematic trauma care.

Illinois also developed some new trauma and emergency medical services specialists, of which the Trauma Nurse Specialist and the Trauma-Emergency Medical Services Coordinator were particularly unique.

The "development of a comprehensive uniform . . . medical emergency communications capability, which includes simple two-way radio voice, telephone patch, and dedicated phone lines" was an objective secondary to the designation of hospitals according to a categorization and regionalization scheme. The communications system included central dispatch and "medical control of mobile elements of the system," and a "medical resource guidance system" at each regional center was planned to provide for "patient care advice, interpretation of bioelectrical data, and triage at the scene of the accident and during transportation to appropriate designated treatment facilities" (Boyd, 1974).

THE MARYLAND TRAUMA PROGRAM

In February 1973, the Governor of Maryland issued an executive order creating both the Maryland Institute for Emergency Medicine (MIEM), formerly the Center for the Study of Trauma, and the State Division of Emergency Medical Services (DEMS) within the Department of Health and Mental Hygiene. The system for the care of trauma patients was integrated into a total EMS system as Illinois had done. However, the referral of seriously ill trauma patients to a tertiary care center has progressed further than in most areas in Illinois, due partly to geography and partly to the preeminence of the University of Maryland in providing trauma care. The MIEM functions as the center of the statewide emergency medical services program, and houses the communications control center for the entire state. Approximately 900 critically ill or injured patients are transported via helicopter each year to MIEM.

THE EMS SYSTEMS ACT

Though early efforts in Illinois and Maryland focused primarily on trauma it became apparent that a systems approach to

trauma must be only one element of a systems approach to emergency medical services. Accordingly, the Emergency Medical Services Act has provided funds for the development of regionally integrated emergency care with particular emphasis on the critical patient categories of trauma, burns, cardiac emergencies, high-risk infants, poisoning, drug overdose, and alcohol intoxication, as well as psychiatric emergencies. For each critical care area, access (including appropriate transportion) must be provided to specialized critical medical care units. The regulations of the Act further require that these units be in the number and variety necessary to meet the demands of the service area. If there are no such units in the EMS region, then the system will provide access to units in neighboring areas if feasible in terms of time and distance.

The Act has served to tie trauma into a system of care that provides the appropriate manpower, training, communications, transportation, facilities, and administration for all medical emergencies.

THE PHASES OF TRAUMA CARE

Any thorough consideration of trauma and its management should account for all the phases of management discussed below.

Prevention. Students of trauma must begin with a look at ways in which trauma can be prevented. In recent years, some directions in preventing automotive trauma have become very clear. The use of seat belts and airbags has been shown to have a great influence on reducing the rates of death and disability from trauma.

The "natural experiment" of the gasoline shortage with the 55 m.p.h. speed limit probably had a major effect on diminishing highway fatalities from 55,800 in 1973 to 46,200 in 1974 (National Safety Council, 1975). Programs of better highway design, drinking-while-driving abatement, and hand-gun control have all shown potential for significantly decreasing trauma mortality and morbidity.

Pre-Hospital Care. Each war during this century has brought diminished mortality from injury. From 8 per cent in World War I, the rate fell to less than 2 per cent in the Vietnam War for victims needing medical facilities (Boyd, 1974). However, only since 1966, when the National Academy of Sciences published "Accidental Death: The Neglected

Disease of Modern Society," has emphasis been put on the pre-hospital care of trauma victims. Subsequent to this the Department of Transportation (DOT) developed the Emergency Medical Technician I (EMT-I) course and ambulance design standards, and supported pre-hospital care with funds provided under the National Highway Safety Act. During the past ten years, rapid transport ambulance services provided by funeral directors have become outmoded, and a system by which EMT's provide sophisticated medical care on the scene and en route to a trauma center in vehicles designed to allow for cardiopulmonary resuscitation has evolved.

Despite much progress, a dilemma remains as to how to provide better service to rural areas, where two out of three of motor vehicle deaths occurred in 1974.

Hospital Care. Improvements in pre-hospital care have brought several developments within hospitals. Patients who previously died before reaching Emergency Departments are now requiring expanded skills and proficiency within the Emergency Department. Emergency medicine is now the most rapidly growing specialty. There has been an increasing awareness of the need for strategically located and designated trauma centers with an increase in secondary transfers to these specialty centers. Caring for more severely injured patients has stimulated expanded research in shock and trauma units within hospitals.

The eight trauma research centers supported by the National Institute of General Medical Sciences have reduced the mortality rates for severely injured patients admitted to them from 85 to 30 per cent (HEW, 1976).

Despite such improvements, a relative lack of interest in pursuing trauma on an active, clinical, and research basis is still reflected in the paucity of governmental area involvement in such support and the relatively low successful application rate for even this existing low level of support.

Unfortunately, although death due to trauma ranks as the leading cause of death among younger people (ages 1 to 44) with the greatest number of productive years to look forward to, dollars appropriated for trauma research are very small relative to the dollars available to cancer and heart disease research. Few physicians have made a career of research or teaching of trauma, and much of the research to date has emphasized the unique features of special injuries, such as fractures and burns, and has not addressed the common denominator of trauma (NIH, 1970).

Rehabilitation. Advances in rehabilitation have paralleled the necessities of bringing military casualties back to maximal function. It has become more and more clear that prompt rehabilitation of disabled patients will greatly enhance the chance for maximal return of function. In recent years, major advances have been made in mechanical and electronic devices to improve rehabilitation. With over 500,000 people being disabled each year by trauma, the major issue is one of logistics—of getting each patient promptly into a program that can provide maximal rehabilitation.

References

Boyd, D. R.: Regionalization of Trauma Patient Care: The Illinois Experience. Illinois Med. J. *146*:33–38, July 1974.

Harvey, J. C.: Planning for career ambulance profession. Emerg. Med. Today 2(4):1, 1973.

HEW Division of EMS: A Systems Approach to the Care of Trauma Victims. 1976.

Maryland Institute for Emergency Medicine: Annual Report, 1974–1975.

National Academy of Sciences/National Research Council: Accidental Death and Disability: The Neglected Disease of Modern Society. Public Health Service Publication No 1071-A-13, 1966.

National Safety Council: Accident Facts: 1975 Edition. Chicago, National Safety Council, 1975.

Pellegrino. E. D.: Medicine, history, and the idea of man. Ann. Am. Acad. Pol. Soc. Sci. Med. Soc. *346*:9, 1973.

Surgery Training Committee of the National Institute of General Medical Sciences: Status of Research in Trauma and the Critically Injured. National Institutes of Health, Washington, D.C., 1970.

Wetzler, H. P.: Loss of working years in accidents (Letter to the Editor). N. Engl. J. Med. *294*:1348, 1976.

B. INITIAL EVALUATION OF ACUTELY INJURED PATIENTS

George R. Schwartz

During the first minutes after arrival in the Emergency Department, evaluation of the injured patient should be made at the same time that initial therapy is carried out. The airway must be cleared, hemorrhage stopped, possible fractures splinted, and suitable intravenous fluids initiated. In the severely injured, the "lifelines" must be inserted and monitors attached. Insertion of an indwelling arterial catheter can wait, but bladder catheterization, a CVP catheter, and attachment of a cardiac monitor are of high priority.

It is important to have information regarding the patient's general health as well as the presence of specific diseases, although sometimes this is not possible. Accidental injury frequently is caused by an existing medical condition. Recognition of the condition may avoid confusion and sometimes provide the key to successful treatment. For example, a person suffering an episode of hypoglycemia or syncope may be brought in still unconscious, after an automobile accident. Administration of glucose may allow full return of consciousness and prevent excessive concerns about head trauma. If the history of the accident suggests that prior loss of consciousness might have been involved, it is crucial to ensure that life-threatening conditions, apart from the trauma, are not present. For example, death can occur rapidly from a cardiac arrhythmia or an overdose of drugs, whereas the accidental injury sustained might be of little consequence.

Many serious errors in trauma evaluation occur through overconcern with the visible injuries. A laceration of the face, for example, is highly visible and might require an hour to suture. Unless there is intense concern about other possible injuries, such patients could undergo rapid deterioration from, for example, a relatively silent spleen injury while the expert facial repair is being performed. To avoid such errors and to increase diagnostic precision the evaluating physician must maintain a persistent clinical vigilance. Consideration also must be given to the type, direction, and magnitude of the forces involved in the accident, and to the physics of trauma.

BLUNT TRAUMA CONSIDERATIONS

Initially, a patient who has sustained blunt trauma to the chest or abdomen may have very few signs or symptoms. A highly emotional state often results in diminished sensory responsiveness and less awareness of pain. Also, deceleration forces can result in intestinal tears, splenic pedicle injury, and other injuries that do not result in severe pain because of limited innervation. Retroperitoneal injury may occur insidiously with enough hemorrhage to produce shock while remaining "silent" except for the symptoms caused by hypovolemia. A time-honored aphorism expresses this propensity: "Bleeding somewhere, bleeding nowhere—look in the retroperitoneum."

The history of the accident assumes importance in raising the suspicion of further injuries other than those immediately obvious. For example, if an automobile accident has occurred at 70 m.p.h. and demolished the car, an individual who was in the accident should be observed over a period of at least several hours, even if he has no symptoms. If the patient's head hit the windshield with enough force to crack the glass, there is an objective measure of the forces involved, even when a skull x-ray shows no bony injury. Parenthetically, it should be noted that a small skull fracture also is difficult to identify on x-ray, and sometimes the most serious head injury is not associated with a skull fracture.

Whether seatbelts were used can be important because of the type of injuries associated with the lap belts. For example, injury to the duodenum can occur when the individual is thrown forward against the fixed belt, resulting in compression of the intestinal segment between the belt and the vertebral column. Splenic ruptures and liver fractures also have occurred this way.

Whether the patient was thrown against the steering wheel can be important with regard to possible resultant lung and liver injuries as well as cardiac contusions and, in some instances, cardiac tamponade. Such injuries can be demonstrated by physical examination, and the chest x-ray and electrocardiogram can be confirmatory. Typical EKG findings involve nonspecific ST-T wave changes and T-wave inversions seen on the precordial leads. Later, signs of cardiac muscle injury may develop.

PRACTICAL BALLISTICS OF GUNSHOT WOUNDS

Injuries from guns are a frequent cause of death, particularly in urban areas. Many guns are available at very low prices and are sold with "no questions asked" (the so-called "Saturday Night Special"). Although such weapons are poorly balanced and relatively inaccurate, and have a greater chance of misfiring than more carefully made guns, they are still highly lethal. Police statistics show that more than one-half of all murders result from handgun injuries.

In analyzing injury resulting from bullet wounds, it is useful to know both the type of gun and type of bullet. The energy from a gun is primarily represented by the formula: $F = 1/2 \ MV^2$. "F" represents the force, "M" the mass of the bullet, and "V" the muzzle velocity. The most important determinant of the destructive potential, therefore, is the muzzle velocity. Table 1 lists some representative guns and muzzle velocities. The difference can be great with, for example, a .357 magnum having 15 times the force of a .22 caliber gun based on muzzle velocity alone, and considering the larger mass of the bullet, the difference rises to a factor of 30. Most police forces have started using the .357 magnum instead of the .38 ("police special") owing to the higher muzzle velocity.

BULLET CONSIDERATIONS

Bullets produce a shock wave in front of and lateral to their course. Where bullet velocity exceeds the speed of sound (1100 ft./sec.) there is an additional shock wave (a small "sonic boom"). When a bullet stops within a victim, all the energy is transferred, whereas a bullet that readily passes through and maintains a high velocity can produce surprisingly little damage. The development of shock waves and dissipation of missile energy are important concepts, since very severe damage frequently can occur inches away from the bullet course. For example, in injuries to the spinal cord, the bullet rarely transects the cord and, in fact, often is found lying next to the vertebra—yet total irreversible paralysis may result. Initial examination also may reveal no signs of spinal cord injury, but after several hours edema can lead to marked impairment of spinal cord functioning even to the point of total paralysis.

Police are concerned with the "stopping power" of a weapon, which means that it is desirable to have as much energy as possible dissipated within the victim. This serves literally to push him back or knock him over, regardless of where the bullet hits. As a result, bullets have been developed with special characteristics to increase "stopping power." The lead-tip bullet flattens on impact and acts like a battering ram. The entrance wound is small, but if the bullet exits the resultant wound is large. The hollow point bullet not only flattens, but tends to break up, each small fragment acting as a separate missile. The so-called "dum-dum" bullet is irregularly weighted and has more wobble, which results in extra forces owing to the rotary components. Such bullets cause a large amount of damage to surrounding tissues.

An illustration of the clinical relevance of bullet considerations occurred when a 21-year-old youth was shot through the anterior

TABLE 1   Type of Hand Gun and Approximate Muzzle Velocity

Caliber	Muzzle Velocity (ft./sec.)
.22	400
.38 special (police gun)	855
.45 automatic	850
.357 magnum	1500

thigh by a .357 magnum with a "dum-dum" bullet. The entrance wound was smaller than the exit wound. There appeared to be no injuries to the major blood vessels or nerves, distal pulses were present, and after débridement of the superficial wounds the boy was sent home on crutches. No bullet fragments were seen on x-ray. He returned the next day with a tense discolored thigh so swollen as to cause vascular and nerve compression. When the wound was explored and a fasciotomy done, extensive soft tissue injury was seen with nonviable muscle present, and pieces of clothing were discovered along the path of the missile. The femoral artery also had been transected, and vascular repair was necessary. This serves to emphasize that wounds from high energy guns and destructive bullets initially may appear minor, but require operative débridement or at least hospitalization, close observation, and the performance of suitable tests (e.g., arteriography). This example also illustrates the point that distal pulses may persist despite major proximal vessel injury.

When a bullet has passed through clothing or other substances, the presence of such foreign bodies in the wound should be suspected. The entrance wound can be enlarged under local anesthesia, debrided, and examined. The exploration need not continue into the muscle layer unless there is evidence of foreign body or nonviable tissue; these patients should be observed for any sign that more extensive exploration is required. X-ray examination usually will not demonstrate pieces of cloth. There is limited value in using prophylactic antibiotics, although they are employed widely, since problems arise from retained foreign bodies and necrosis of tissue, both of which should be removed surgically. The exception, of course, would be a case of developing cellulitis, in which systemic antibiotics can serve to limit the spread of infection.

The questioning in cases of gunshot wounds also should include consideration of the direction from which the gun was fired. One patient, for example, presented with a gunshot wound in the pelvic area, although his major complaint was shortness of breath. The knowledge that he was shot from below while climbing a fire escape directed attention to the abdomen and chest. The bullet actually had perforated the bowel in multiple areas, perforated the stomach, passed through the diaphragm, and come to rest in the chest. Subsequently, he required life-saving surgery for total repair. In the Emergency Department he needed a tube thoracotomy to drain his hemopneumothorax, as well as treatment for shock and sepsis.

SHOTGUN WOUNDS

Injuries resulting from shotguns are associated with particular problems related to the nature of the "shot" used, as well as the paper wadding that can be driven into the close-range wound. The "shot" may consist of rice or rock salt, neither of which is readily visible on x-ray. Although penetration usually is limited in such wounds, local damage to the skin can be great, and in close-range wounds there can be penetration into the abdominal or chest cavity.

KNIFE WOUNDS

Injuries resulting from knives can be deceptive. Externally they can appear to be small superficial punctures, since in the absence of large blood vessel injury the soft tissues tend to come together and seal. The history is important in assessing depth of penetration and angle of entry. If an upward motion is used, for example, a wound that seems to be over the stomach area might actually pass through the diaphragm into the chest. This sort of knife injury was commonly employed by assassins several hundred years ago. Inspection of the knife blade itself can provide information about depth of penetration.

A recent court case illustrated the need for a high level of suspicion. A young man was stabbed in the chest by a long, thin (stiletto-type) knife. He presented in no distress, but a policeman who accompanied him thought that the knife had been inserted to the hilt (five inches). A probe inserted into the external wound did not pass through the soft tissues, and the conclusion was drawn that the wound was superficial. The young man died soon after from cardiac tamponade.

The probe is a deceptive tool. Not only is it dangerous, but, because the deeper tissues rapidly seal, it will appear that the wound is superficial unless the exact path taken by the knife is followed. In cases of knife wounds of the chest, deeper injury must be considered to be present until disproved. Concern for lung, heart, esophageal, or great vessel injury requires not only an initial chest x-ray, but another taken a few hours later. One caveat is that an upright chest x-ray can appear normal even when there is up to 200 cc. of blood in the chest; a more sensitive view is provided by the lateral decubitus x-ray of the chest. A small pneumothorax also will escape detection unless a good expiratory chest film is taken. Attention to the cardiac silhouette can point to the presence of pericardial fluid. Since cardiac tamponade can be rapidly lethal, particular attention must be directed toward its diagnosis. The classic triad of hypotension, elevated CVP (neck vein distention), and a quiet heart represent a late stage at which the patient is in substantial distress. A rising CVP usually will be the early warning sign, and should be followed closely if there is any suspicion of injury to the heart. The EKG may be useful if it demonstrates diminished precordial voltage, ST-T wave changes, or signs of injury, but it is less reliable than the CVP. If cardiac tamponade is developing an immediate pericardiocentesis* should be performed, which will relieve symptoms and allow time to prepare the operating suite for a thoracotomy.

SINOGRAMS

A sinogram (injection of radiopaque contrast material along the path of the knife) can be used to determine the depth of penetration, but anyone using this test must begin by recognizing that only a positive test, showing contrast material passing into the peritoneal or chest cavity, is significant. A negative sinogram does *not* mean that the knife wound is superficial, and should not lull the physician into a false and potentially dangerous conclusion.

In cases of knife wounds, the best safeguard against error is a period of observation of the patient under conditions of suitable monitoring of vital signs.

FALLS FROM HEIGHTS

Patients who fall from buildings, ladders, cliffs, etc., experience not only the direct trauma from the fall, but also deceleration injuries that can disrupt visceral structures. Most falls result in the victim's landing on his lower extremities, and fracture of the tibia and fibula are the most common skeletal injuries. The bones of the foot are injured frequently.

Particular attention must be directed to the spine, because compression fractures, especially at the L-1 and L-2 areas, are associated with accidents in which the victim lands on his feet after falling from a height. If the os calcis is fractured, x-rays should be taken of the spine, even when clinical symptoms are relatively mild.

The presence of pelvic fractures should suggest injury to the bladder, which is, after the lung, the most common viscus injured in falls from heights. Liver and spleen injuries are somewhat less common, as are intestinal and renal trauma. However, it is not unusual to find transient hematuria, despite a normal intravenous pyelogram.

Skull fractures are less common than extremity injuries, but the coexistence of such injuries is associated with the highest mortality.

BURNS

Estimation of degree of burns and percentage of body area is important as a guide for initial treatment.* However, the type of injury frequently assumes overwhelming importance. For example, flash burns are not usually deep, whereas an electric burn might involve coagulation of all the blood in the area and extend throughout an extremity. Burns due to immersion usually are deeper than those resulting just from rapid contact. Burns from hot water or coffee occur frequently and may be the result of deliberate attack in child abuse cases.

To provide some perspective on time of immersion, it is useful to remember that, in experimental animals, a full thickness burn will result from immersion in boiling water for approximately three seconds. Hot water from a faucet rarely will exceed 140° F., and immersion in water of this temperature for approximately four to five seconds will result in second-degree burns. In treatment of burn injuries, excessive attention should not be given to the over-all percentage of burn; the more serious immediate

---

*See Procedures, page 326.

*See page 762.

problems arise from the depth and type of the initial insults. For example, sunburn frequently is a 90 per cent first- and second-degree burn from which the patient almost always survives. Therefore, an attempt should be made to determine the percentage of first, second- and third-degree burn present. A newer category, fourth-degree, involves muscle and deep connective tissue structures, as well as blood vessels and nerves. The intravascular coagulation almost invariably leads to a nonviable extremity.

TRIAGE

Triage, a French term meaning "sorting," originally was employed on a large scale in the military, the objective being to provide preferential treatment for those who could be attended readily and returned to battle, leaving aside those with more complex injuries until either they could be transferred or time became available. An "expectant" group also was separated, composed of patients whose injuries carried such a high chance of mortality or required such complex treatment that too much time would be spent by limited medical personnel.

In civilian life, barring a major disaster that causes casualties far exceeding the capabilities of available medical staff (including those within flying distance), there rarely is any need to employ the so-called "expectant" category at the scene.

Various systems of triage have been used, but the decision as to which patients are "expectant" should be made within a hospital and not on the field. All systems have in common an *"immediate"* category for those with life-threatening injuries in which a delay of a few minutes could mean life or death. Examples are a bleeding artery, airway obstruction, pneumothorax, or cardiac tamponade. Obviously, the field capability of medical personnel is crucial. If an immediate pericardiocentesis or chest tube insertion is possible, treatment at the scene may be imperative. If this cannot be done, immediate transfer is essential.

The next category involves cases in which, although patients may have severe injuries, initial examination indicates that a delay of several hours would not be harmful after simple initial treatment has been provided: for example, a person with multiple fractures but without substantial blood loss.

Once the fractures have been splinted, further immediate treatment is not essential. Many in the "immediate" category can be transferred to the "delayed" category once initial stabilization has been achieved: e.g., a probable spine fracture once the patient has been strapped securely to a spine board.

The other category includes those with no apparent injuries or only minor injuries.

EVALUATION OF THE PATIENT WITH MULTIPLE INJURIES

Table 2 illustrates the categorization of priorities necessary in a patient with multiple injuries. In such instances, it is important that there be *one* person in charge, a "trauma captain."

Initial attention must be directed at the airway, respiratory system, and cardiovascular system. Simultaneously, if cervical spine injury is suspected, a cervical collar should be placed: if the patient is bleeding, direct pressure must be applied over the bleeding sites. While this is done, life lines should be inserted for intravenous fluids, a CVP inserted, and blood for hematocrit, hemoglobin, type, and cross-matching drawn. The best initial I.V. site usually is the antecubital fossa, but it may be necessary to use a subclavian, internal jugular, or even femoral route. A cut-down is rarely needed. In cases

TABLE 2   *Summary of System of Priorities*

Basic priorities:	(1) Life; (2) Limb; (3) Function; (4) Cosmesis
Highest priority	Respiratory (facial, neck, chest) Cardiovascular Hemorrhage Neck injuries
Very high priority	Shock Retroperitoneal ⎫ bleeding Intraperitoneal ⎭
High priority	Cranial-cerebral Spinal cord Burns
Low priority	Lower G.U. injuries Peripheral nerve, vascular, skeletal Soft tissue (once bleeding controlled) Fractures (once splinted)

of severe bleeding, type-specific blood may be needed and should be available within minutes, during which time intravascular volume should be maintained by rapid infusion of lactated Ringer's solution. If equipment to retransfuse blood from the chest or peritoneal cavity is available, autotransfusion should be initiated. Oxygen should be administered at 10 liters per minute. An EKG should be taken, not only in the patient with a chest injury, but in all cases of severe injury. Medications, when given, should be intravenous. Small I.V. doses of narcotics usually are effective for analgesia. I.M. or subcutaneous injections will be absorbed variably, and therefore may be ineffective (except, of course, for tetanus toxoid).

A urinary catheter is mandatory, both to assess possible genitourinary injury and renal function and as a guide to the adequacy of fluid replacement. Approximately one-third of deaths from severe trauma result from hypovolemic shock. Therefore, without overburdening the circulation (which can be checked by CVP), the urinary output should be maintained at a rate of at least 40 cc. per hour.

Before the patient is moved further, a cross-table lateral x-ray of the neck should be taken if cervical spine injury is suspected. All suspected fractures or ligament injuries also should be splinted prior to movement.

The immediate goal is to stabilize the patient's condition and to eliminate any immediate threat to life. Once this has been achieved, further evaluation can proceed at a somewhat more leisurely pace, or the patient can be transferred to the operating suite. In some instances, however, life-sustaining surgical procedures may be necessary before the patient is transferred.

For example, if there is inadequate ventilation, intubation, tracheostomy, cricothyreotomy, thoracotomy, or ventilatory support may be essential. Similarly an immediate pericardiocentesis may be essential to preserve the life of a patient with cardiac tamponade. On occasion, immediate thoracotomy is the only way to save life—for example, when cardiac arrest and shock occur in the presence of penetrating thoracic trauma. An indwelling arterial line is a good monitoring tool that allows ready access to arterial blood for blood gas determination, and provides a direct read-out of arterial pressure.

INTRA-ABDOMINAL INJURY

Before the patient is transferred from the Emergency Department, evaluation must be carried out for intra-abdominal bleeding and visceral injury. When indicated, an upright chest x-ray or left lateral decubitus x-ray should be taken to check for free air *prior* to abdominal paracentesis or four-quadrant abdominal tap. If free blood is present, operative treatment is required. While the operating suite is being prepared, an infusion IVP, can be done, and also spleen and liver scans and angiograms, if the patient's clinical state is stable. For an effective IVP, the patient must have a near-normal blood pressure. *The most important consideration, however is maintenance of the intravascular volume and oxygen-carrying ability of the blood.*

If the patient is unconscious following a head injury and there is suspicion of intra-abdominal bleeding, an abdominal tap should be done after suitable x-rays have been taken. If a patient with abdominal injury is in shock, however, the most vital activity is to correct this state at once, and x-rays should be deferred. In such cases therapy must precede precise diagnosis, and x-ray almost always can be deferred until a more suitable time. Since intracranial bleeding will not cause hypovolemic shock, and scalp lacerations (although sometimes accompanied by excessive bleeding) rarely result in shock, an assumed diagnosis of intra-abdominal or intrathoracic bleeding should be made while the patient is being resuscitated. In this case, a peritoneal tap can be performed prior to x-ray examinations.

Use of "G" Suit

The "G" suit was derived from the military and essentially consists of an apparatus by which the lower extremities and abdomen can be compressed circumferentially.

When intra-abdominal bleeding is present, a "G" suit may provide the extra minutes of life necessary to transport the patient to the operating suite. Thoracotomy in the Emergency Department has a place, but there rarely is any benefit to be derived from emergency laparotomy.

CENTRAL NERVOUS SYSTEM INJURY

Although most cerebral injuries are not of the highest priority, careful attention to changes in neurologic condition is necessary in order to avoid missing acute subdural or epidural bleeding. The major value of skull x-rays in acute trauma is to detect midline shifts and fractures that cross the middle meningeal groove. Depressed skull fractures can be seen best on tangential x-ray views, but also should be palpable. Taping a needle or "B-B" at the site of suspected depression is helpful in evaluating the tangential x-ray.

Approximately one-half of basilar skull fractures are not detected by x-ray. However, clouding of the sphenoid sinus is a good clue, and blood behind the tympanic membrane confirms the clinical diagnosis. When computerized axial tomography is available, diagnosis of intracranial bleeding can be more rapid as well as accurate. Burr holes,* although rarely an Emergency Department procedure, are necessary if a neurosurgeon is not available and if a clinical diagnosis of acute subdural or epidural bleeding is made. Cervical spine injuries, as noted previously, are of great concern and require immediate stabilization. Nasotracheal intubation should be done if the airway is occluded. If there is evidence of spinal cord injury, attempts should be made to transfer the patient to a center for such treatment in order to obtain maximum benefit from what is at best a grim situation. At such centers, newer techniques are carried out directed at limiting cord injury, as well as older treatments such as local hypothermia.

GENITOURINARY SYSTEM INJURY

In rapid assessment, the urinalysis is the best test to check for injury to the urinary system, although it may be unreliable in complete transections of the urethra. The presence of a pelvic fracture should substantially raise the index of suspicion regarding injury to the bladder or urethra. An infusion IVP should be done on suspicion of renal injury. A urethrogram is vital if urethral laceration is suspected, and an emergency cystography should be done if bladder injury is

*See procedures page 433.

considered possible. Beware the catheter that drains frank blood: this can occur when the bladder is torn from the urethra, and the catheter, in fact, passes into the pelvis and drains a hematoma.

EXTREMITIES AND SOFT TISSUES

All suspected fractures should be splinted. Any dislocation compromising nerve or vascular function should be reduced immediately, *prior to x-ray examination.* Open fractures can be irrigated, covered with sterile dressings, and stabilized, and the patient can be made ready for surgery, unless life-threatening injuries take precedence. Where delay might occur, a large intravenous bolus of a broad spectrum antibiotic should be infused.

Whenever a fracture of thigh or pelvis is present, blood loss sufficient to cause shock may develop insidiously over a one- or two-hour period. The importance of continuous close monitoring of severely injured patients must be impressed upon every physician called upon to treat them.

OBSERVATION AREA FOR DECISION-MAKING

Any hospital that treats a large number of trauma victims should have a special area in which patients can be observed closely, with frequent assessment of vital signs and ongoing monitoring while diagnostic tests are in progress. Where such facilities are not available, far too many patients deteriorate without warning, thus providing the basis for many lawsuits.

PROBLEM CASES IN TRAUMA

A confusing situation can arise in which, despite seemingly adequate therapy, a persistent shock state remains or recurs. In this event, careful systematic review should enable detection of the cause. Beginning with the head, one can see hypotension and tachycardia from intracranial injury, but usually as a preterminal event. Injuries to the aorta can cause persistent shock, and the possibility of cardiac tamponade should not be overlooked. An acute stress in a weak heart can result in infarction, with development of cardiogenic shock superimposed on the initial hypovolemic shock. In both these cases, the CVP or pulmonary wedge pressure determination can be important tools of diagnosis.

The presence of "silent" bleeding, such as can occur from spleen injuries, injuries to the retroperitoneum, and bleeding into the pelvis, should be considered, and relatively simple tests can be performed to confirm or eliminate these possibilities if there is a high degree of clinical suspicion.

Other nontraumatic causes can rapidly develop and lead to persistent hypotension, including, for example, the development of septic shock. The possibility must be considered of drug overdose, either iatrogenic or taken by the patient prior to the accident. A nasogastric tube, with a cuffed endotracheal tube if needed, can not only decompress the stomach but, in the presence of an oral overdose, often will result in return of pill-type material many hours after ingestion. The severe injury, with resulting epinephrine release, serves to delay gastric emptying. There is certainly no harm in a trial of Narcan if an overdose of an opiate, Darvon, or similar substance is even a remote possibility.

The possibility of pre-existing conditions should not be discarded, even if rare. For example, a person with Addison's disease lacking hydrocortisone might rapidly revert to a hypotensive state. A dose of cortisone is warranted in the refractory shock patient, although the recent trend has been to give pharmacologic doses of cortisone preparations in shock states regardless. Certainly, no matter what may be the physician's philosophic outlook on the use of steroids in shock, the presence of refractory shock in circumstances in which the cause is obscure certainly warrants a trial dose of cortisone. Another condition that could occur is sudden trauma to a diseased pancreas, resulting in massive "third space" losses.

The presence of hypoxia can act as a vasodepressor and produce a shocklike state. Pulmonary status must be assessed repeatedly. For example, a pneumothorax can develop within minutes, and the subsequent hypoxia can result in hypotension and tachycardia that would not benefit from further fluid infusion; on the contrary, clinical deterioration would result.

Do not overlook the spurious finding. For example, if a blood pressure reading is taken below a brachial artery that has been punctured for arterial blood gases, the resulting arterial spasm will result in a falsely lowered blood pressure. Such a situation has occurred numerous times. In one recent instance, heroic attempts were made to bring the patient out of the shock state, including the use of fluids and vasopressors, until one of the nurses noticed that the other pulses were bounding and therefore moved the blood pressure cuff to the other arm. Such problems can be obviated with continuous arterial monitoring, although such devices are still not in widespread usage outside the university setting.

Proper evaluation of the severely injured patient requires a calm methodical approach, in order to avoid neglecting an injury or a clinical sign that might have grave consequences. A state of high sustained vigilance, together with an ability to keep many things in mind at the same time, are requirements for those who are involved in initial assessment of the injured patient.

References

Borja, A. R., Lansing, A. M., and Ransdell, H. T. Jr.: Immediate operative treatment for stab wounds of the heart. J. Thorac. Cardiovasc. Surg. 59:662, 1970.

Breen, P. C., and Rudolf, L. E.: Potential sources of error in the use of peritoneal lavage as a diagnostic tool. J. Am. Coll. Emerg. Physicians 3:401, 1974.

Chan, D., Kraus, J. F., and Riggins, R. S.: Patterns of multiple fracture in accidental injury. J. Trauma 13:1075, 1973.

Cowley, R. A., et al.: A prognostic index for severe trauma. J. Trauma 14:1029, 1974.

Dagnone, L. E.: A plan for the resuscitation of the acutely injured patient. J. Am. Coll. Emerg. Physicians 3:241, 1974.

Frey, C. F., et al.: A fifteen-year experience with automotive hepatic trauma. J. Trauma 13:1039, 1973.

Frey, C. F., Huelke, D. F., and Gikas, P. W.: Resuscitation and survival in motor vehicle accidents. J. Trauma 9:292, 1969.

Gourin, A., and Garzon, A.: Diagnostic problems in traumatic diaphragmatic hernia. J. Trauma 14:20, 1974.

Hallel, T., and Naggan, L.: Parachuting injuries: a retrospective study of 83,718 jumps. J. Trauma 15:14, 1975.

Huelke, D. F., and Snyder, R. G.: Seat belt injuries: the need for accuracy in reporting of cases. J. Trauma 15:20, 1975.

Jahadi, M. R.: Diagnostic peritoneal lavage. J. Trauma 12:936, 1972.

Kaplan, B. C., et al.: The military anti-shock trouser in civilian pre-hospital emergency care. J. Trauma 13:843, 1973.

Lewin, W.: The Management of Head Injuries. Baltimore, The Williams & Wilkins Co., 1966.

Lord, R. S., and Irani, C. N.: Assessment of arterial injury in limb trauma. J. Trauma 14:1042, 1974.

Mattox, K. L., et al.: Thoracotomy in the emergency center. J. Am. Coll. Emerg. Physicians 3:13, 1974.

Moore, F. D.: The effects of hemorrhage on body composition. J. Med. 273:567, 1965.

Naylor, R., Colyn, D., and Shires, G. T.: Morbidity and mortality from injuries to the spleen. J. Trauma 14:773, 1975.

Parmley, L. F., Mattingly, T. W., and Manion, W. C.: Penetrating wounds of the heart and aorta. Circulation 17:953, 1958.

Reynolds, B. M., Balsano, N. A., and Reynolds, F. X.: Falls from heights: a surgical experience of 200 consecutive cases. Ann. Surg. 174:304, 1974.

Reynolds, B. M., Balsano, N. A., and Reynolds, F. X.: Pelvic fractures. J. Trauma 13:1011, 1973.

Shenfeld, G.: More work for the coroner. Physician's World 1:23, 1973.

Shoemaker, W. C., et al.: Physiologic patterns in surviving and nonsurviving shock patients. Arch. Surg. 106:630, 1973.

Trollope, M. L., et al.: The mechanism of injury in blunt abdominal trauma. J. Trauma 13:962, 1973.

Van Wagoner, F. H.: A three-year study of deaths following trauma. J. Trauma 1:401, 1961.

Waller, J. A., Curran, R., and Noyes, F.: Traffic deaths: a preliminary study of urban and rural fatalities in Californians. Calif. Med. 101:272, 1964.

Whittaker, R., et al.: Earthquake disaster in Nicaragua: reflections of the initial management of mass casualties. J. Trauma 14:37, 1974.

Wise, L., et al.: Traumatic injuries to the diaphragm. J. Trauma 13:946, 1973.

Chapter 38

EMERGENCY MANAGEMENT OF TRAUMA

A. Trauma to the Head
B. Spinal Injuries
C. Trauma to the Face
D. Trauma to the Neck
E. Chest and Heart Injuries
F. Emergency Management of Trauma to the Abdomen
G. Trauma to the Extremities and Soft Tissues
H. Trauma to the Hand
I. Injuries of the Genitourinary Tract
J. Ocular Trauma
K. Trauma to the Peripheral Vascular System

A. TRAUMA TO THE HEAD

William F. Bouzarth

Automobile accidents are the number one killer in the age-group 15 to 24. Seventy-two per cent of these accident victims suffer cranial injuries. With the network of highways and byways in the United States, *no* hospital Emergency Department can escape responsibility of caring for patients with serious brain injury. The first physician called may be a general practitioner or a fully trained traumatologist. Rarely is first echelon care rendered by a neurosurgeon. Hence, this chapter is directed to the Emergency Department physician who is not a neurosurgeon.

Although cranial trauma may be classified by various methods, it is not our purpose to do so here; however, it should be stated that any open skull fracture in which the dura is lacerated or fragments are depressed is a neurosurgical problem. In closed cranial injuries, dynamic lesions are the most important. These usually represent intracranial collections of blood, such as epidural hemorrhage, subdural hemorrhage, or intracerebral hemorrhage. Cerebral edema or swelling may be equally important and is certainly more common. This latter clinical entity usually is present in every serious head injury, especially if the patient is unconscious.

Patients in the Emergency Department who are obviously unconscious constitute one-third of the admissions to hospitals for head injury; more important, 80 per cent of the total deaths from head injury come from this one-third.

THE UNCONSCIOUS PATIENT

The first principle in Emergency Department evaluation of any serious injuries is rapid assessment of the total patient, treating life-threatening injuries first (Bouzarth, 1974). This is more important in the care of the unconscious patient, for he cannot give a history or offer complaints. Priorities in the triage program may be described as A, B, C, and D: A is for airway; B is for bleeding; C for cervical spine injury; and D represents diagnostic tests.

AIRWAY

The unconscious patient who is flat on his back probably has an obstructed airway. In the supine position the muscles at the base of the tongue tend to block the upper airway, and certainly secretions will trickle down the trachea. If the patient vomits, as he is likely to do, he will aspirate the vomitus. Never be led into a false sense of security when a patient is hyperventilating. In reality, he may be doing so not because of brain injury per se, but because of a build-up of arterial carbon dioxide. It must be stressed that carbon dioxide not only stimulates respiration, but is one of most potent cerebral vascular dilating agents known. Hence, hypercarbia increases cerebral blood flow which can further exacerbate traumatic brain hemorrhage (Shenkin and Bouzarth, 1970). Also important, intracranial pressure is increased owing to this cerebrovascular dilatation, and the response is magnified if hypoxia is also present. The best way to determine respiratory efficiency is to obtain measurements of arterial PCO_2, PO_2, and pH. This is peer review of respiratory management.

If tracheal intubation is needed, one must rule out, whenever possible, a cervical spine injury. (In Chapter 10, methods of maintaining an adequate airway have been detailed.) However, no unconscious patient should be kept in the prone position for any length of time unless (1) other injuries, especially of the cervical spine, exist, or (2) some

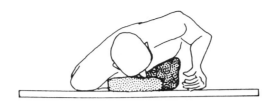

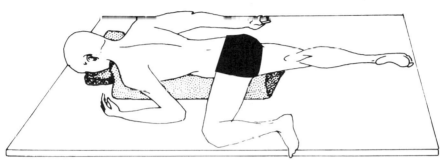

Figure 1. The head is maintained in a natural position when the patient is turned semiprone. (From Bouzarth, W. F.: The ABC's of emergency care of serious head injuries. Ind. Med. Surg. 39:21, 1970.)

type of tracheal intubation or the esophageal obstructor airway has been introduced. Otherwise, keep the unconscious patient in the semiprone position (see Fig. 1).

BLEEDING

As soon as an adequate airway has been ensured, or even while it is being established, attention should be given to control of bleeding. Except in infants with large subdural hematomas, or in brain stem injury resulting in death, one seldom sees hypotension caused by brain injury. Another neurologic cause of hypotension is spinal cord injury, usually associated with bradycardia, and it also is seen in the alcoholic patient with peripheral vasodilatation. In general, hypotension must be considered to be due to hypovolemia. All efforts should be directed toward restoring blood volume and finding the cause, such as a splenic hemorrhage. The control of scalp bleeding will be discussed later.

CERVICAL SPINE INJURY

Cervical spine injuries are, in fact, thoracic or lumbar spine fractures. First let us focus attention on those in unconscious patients. It is estimated that 5 to 10 per cent of all unconscious patients who are injured either from falling or from vehicle accidents also have spine injuries, and such patients should have cervical spine x-rays in preference to skull x-rays. A cross-table lateral cervical spine x-ray should be obtained with the shoulders depressed by pulling the arms toward the feet. It is important to see all seven vertebral bodies. Also look for widening of the posterior pharynx, which suggests spine injury.

Diagnostic indications suggesting spinal cord injury in the unconscious patient are as follows: (1) Flaccid areflexia, especially with a flaccid rectal sphincter. (2) Diaphragmatic breathing only. (3) Flexion of the forearms on the chest. (In fact, if the physician straightens the upper extremities, the forearms will flex just as soon as he lets go. This is because the injury is to the lower cervical vertebrae and the biceps muscles are not affected, so that flexion is unopposed since the triceps muscles are weak or paralyzed.) (4) By applying painful stimuli starting at the toes and working up toward the clavicle, and at the same time watching the face, you may discover that at a certain point the patient will grimace with pain—this indicates the approximate level of the spinal injury. (5) If there is hypotension without other evidence of shock, such as tachycardia, suspect a spinal cord injury. Nevertheless, do not fail to continue to search for blood loss at fracture sites, the retroperitoneal space, the spleen, and elsewhere. (6) Priapism, if present, is a characteristic sign of cord injury.

DIAGNOSTIC TESTS

The diagnostic neurologic examination should be as simple as possible and should be repeated frequently. A "mini-neurologic examination," if you will (Bouzarth, 1968). The most important part of the examination is assessment of the patient's level of consciousness. In the past, words like *stupor, semicoma,* or *coma* have been used to describe the unconscious patient. The committee that produced the glossary of terms for head injury for the Congress of Neurological Surgery notes that these words can have different meanings to various people and should *not* be used. Rather, describe the patient's reaction. For example, if he appears unconscious, will he awaken when you call his name or must you shake him? If this is unsuccessful, is light pain or strong pain required to evoke a response? For light pain use a pin stick; for strong pain pinch the skin with a hemostat.

What about the patient who is truly unconscious and does not awaken with stimulation? Does he raise his arm or try to push the painful stimulus away or does he withdraw? This is an appropriate type of response. Perhaps he just moves, but not in a defensive way. This is an inappropriate response. On the other hand, decerebrate stiffening of the extremities may result, or there may be no response at all to pain. Serial examinations may reveal that on admission a patient's response to pain was inappropriate and that 30 minutes later his response to the same stimulus was protective. This is strong evidence that he is improving, yet the examiner may still classify him as being "stuporous." Next, the pupils should be carefully checked, comparing their size and reactions to bright light. If the pupils are normal on admission, but one pupil becomes dilated and unreactive to light one hour later, this is strong evidence that an intracranial hemorrhage is producing herniation of the ipsilateral temporal lobe through the tentorium compressing the ipsilateral oculomotor nerve (see Temporal Lobe Herniation). One can record the strength in each extremity using a 0 to 4 scale. In the unconscious patient, painful stimuli may be required to compare the strength of the extremities. Using these simple techniques, it is quite possible to follow the improvement or deterioration of a patient.

A simple Neurosurgical Watch Sheet is suggested (see Fig. 2). It is basically a check-off sheet divided into units, and changes in the patient's clinical condition, good or bad, can be seen at a glance. Vital signs are obviously important in any type of trauma, and space for them is provided. It must be stressed that systolic hypertension and/or bradycardia usually indicates that intracranial pressure is increasing. Once again, hypotension is due to brain injury only infrequently, so the examiner should continue to search for other causes.

If the patient is unconscious when first seen in the Emergency Department, he is likely to remain in that state for hours to days. Baseline blood tests, especially serum electrolytes, are needed. At times, the physician is surprised to find that the head injury is minor compared to the medical reason for the unconsciousness. For example, it may not be known that the patient was a diabetic, and the blood sugar may be abnormally low or high. Alternatively, patients with chronic illness, or those who are on diuretics, may have a low serum sodium that has caused much of the unresponsiveness. Blood alcohol levels are also very valuable, even in pediatric age-groups. A serum osmolality has been found recently to be an excellent screening test, especially if it is compared to the calculated osmolality as judged by the serum electrolytes, blood sugar, and urea nitrogen. When the measured osmolality is 15 or more milliosmoles above the calculated osmolality, one has to think of alcoholism. Also, a very high osmolality indicates a poor prognosis.

There are special procedures for the evaluation of patients with serious head injuries. This usually, but not necessarily, falls into the province of a neurosurgeon. Currently, serial biplane angiography is considered to be the best method to diagnose neurosurgical traumatic lesions, but this usually requires a trained team. However, a single x-ray exposure for each injection can satisfactorily rule out subdural or epidural

UNIT		Time:						
I Vital signs	Blood pressure							
	Pulse							
	Respiration							
	Temperature							
II Conscious and	Oriented							
	Disoriented							
	Restless							
	Combative							
III Speech	Clear							
	Rambling							
	Garbled							
	None							
IV Will awaken to	Name							
	Shaking							
	Light pain							
	Strong pain							
V Non-verbal reaction to pain	Appropriate							
	Inappropriate							
	"Decerebrate"							
	None							
VI Pupils	Size on right							
	Size on left							
	Reacts on right							
	Reacts on left							
VII Ability to move	Right arm							
	Left arm							
	Right leg							
	Left leg							

Figure 2. Neurologic examination record is simple to use.

clots. This is preferable to exploratory bur-holes unless the patient is rapidly deteriorating. If arteriography is abnormal, a craniotomy is done using air-driven drills and craniotome, which requires about the same amount of time as six bur-holes. It is a good policy to use cerebral angiography if there is any doubt whether an operation is necessary.

The echoencephalogram is a safe, non-invasive technique that usually locates those midline structures, such as the third ventricle, that produce an echo. If a unilateral mass is present, these structures are displaced away from the hemorrhage and the "midline" echo will not be midline. In spite of normal readings, however, neurosurgical intervention still may be necessary, because bilateral lesions may be present that maintain the midline structures in position. The same is true for a midline pineal gland seen on a skull x-ray. On the other hand, false-positive echoencephalograms occur. Serial examinations have reduced the need for repeat cerebral angiography.

Electroencephalograms, spinal punctures, and radionuclide brain scans usually are of little help in acute cranial trauma. The only value of the EEG is in providing a baseline criterion for determining brain death in cases in which transplant surgery is in prospect.

Lumbar puncture is contraindicated in obvious head injuries. Loss of spinal fluid through a needle puncture, or through seepage from the dural hole left by the needle, can hasten brain herniation and death.

Although there are reports of brain scans demonstrating epi- or subdural hematomas, this test is not completely reliable. Brain scans have little place in the emergency situation and, in fact, may be confusing when the scalp is injured.

Computerized transaxial tomography is beginning to replace arteriography. This noninvasive technique combines the x-ray beam with computer analysis, and gives a print-out of the transverse section of the head and of the brain structures. Shifts in the ventricular system can be observed as well as the actual hematomas, which appear as high density masses. The patient must be cooperative or anesthetized. Skull roentgenograms will be discussed later. Their value in acute management has been overestimated.

Temporal Lobe Herniation

Any mass within the skull, such as epidural, subdural, or intracerebral hemorrhage and/or cerebral edema, will displace the brain. The pineal gland will shift across the midline, and echoencephalography and/or cerebral arteriography will confirm the shift. Depending on the magnitude of the shift, the medial portion of the temporal lobe, usually the uncus, also is displaced through the tentorial incisura. The oculomotor nerve and the cerebral peduncle are vulnerable at this point. The epidural hematoma that usually develops over a period of hours can produce the classic picture demonstrated in the following example.

The patient has been struck in the temporal region, and the injury may or may not have produced temporary unconsciousness. The thin temporal bone has been fractured, which caused a laceration of the middle meningeal artery. Arterial bleeding slowly dissects the dura away from the internal table and produces an enlarging hematoma. After the patient gains his senses, a headache develops that becomes increasingly more intense. He vomits and prefers to lie down, falling quickly asleep, becoming progressively more difficult to arouse and less cooperative. If the hemorrhage involves the dominant hemisphere, speech will become abnormal, and ultimately the patient will be mute. Convulsions, usually starting on the side opposite the impact site, may develop, and/or a contralateral spastic weakness may occur. At the same time, neurologic examination will reveal that the ipsilateral pupil is larger and does not react to light. The spastic weakness is due to pressure on the cerebral peduncle, which carries the crossed lateral corticospinal tract that allows voluntary movement. The dilated, fixed pupil results from compression of the oculomotor nerve that carried the fibers for pupillary constriction (Jefferson, 1938).

If surgery is performed at this point, the patient has a good chance of full recovery. Otherwise, the process continues until the uncus pushes the midbrain against the opposite tentorial edge, producing bilateral fixed and dilated pupils with bilateral spastic weakness. Decerebration occurs in which painful stimulus produces further extensor spasms. The upper limbs tend also to hyperpronate, although flexion may occur instead of extension. Soon the contralateral limbs become flaccid and motionless. The deep tendon and pathologic reflexes are absent. At this point, there is a tendency to believe the lesion is opposite the spastic limbs, giving a false localization. Later the ipsilateral limbs also become flaccid and paralyzed.

With these neurologic developments there are changes in the vital signs. In the early stages, rising blood pressure may occur, usually associated with progressive bradycardia. Respirations are slow and deep. The temperature tends to become elevated. With further brain compression, blood pressure drops, tachycardia develops, and the respirations become more shallow and slow down. Apnea occurs, and unless the patient is placed on a respirator he will soon die. A baseline EEG will be flat at this point. Cardiovascular support is necessary to prolong cardiac activity.

In such situations, if a neurosurgeon is not available, the emergency physician or staff surgeon is justified in trephining the temporal bone.* Since this syndrome can be

---

*See Chapter 17, page 432

produced by an acute subdural hemorrhage, multiple trephinations will be required. The acute subdural hemorrhage is highly lethal.

A more frequent problem is the severely injured patient who has never regained consciousness and exhibits bilateral neurologic signs, such as a dilated pupil on the same side as the more spastic extremities. This type of situation usually means a brain stem impact injury, rather than a supratentorial blood clot. These patients do not deteriorate rapidly if proper care is given. There is no doubt that high alcoholic intake and airway obstruction soon after the injury magnify the initial injury. Indeed, temporal lobe contusion, which may not cause significant brain displacement, will do so as cerebral edema and vasodilatation develop. In such cases, the treatment outlined next can offer some of these patients a meaningful survival.

Cerebral Edema and Its Treatment

Cerebral edema must be distinguished from cerebral congestion (Shenkin and Bouzarth, 1970). The first is an increase in the water content of the gray matter and/or an increase in the interstitial water of the white matter. Congestion is an increase in blood volume due to vasodilatation, and usually is due to carbon dioxide retention. Both cause the brain to swell and are made worse by anoxia. Since the swelling is limited by the skull, intracranial pressure rises.

Arterial gases usually can be adjusted using the volume-regulated respirator and varying the concentration of the inspired gases. Cerebral edema can be treated by use of adrenocortical steroids and/or diuretics. However, it must be stressed that the patient with a seriously injured brain requires careful fluid balance. In fact, the fluid management of cerebral edema is opposite to that for hypovolemic shock, but the treatment of shock takes priority. *Overhydration magnifies cerebral edema.* If there are no significant systemic injuries, the intravenous fluid intake should be limited to 600 ml./sq. m. of body surface per 24 hours (approximately 1100 ml. for a 70-kg. man). The best solution is 2.5 per cent glucose in 0.45 per cent normal saline. Serum electrolytes and urinary output are monitored. Hyponatremia is usually dilutional, but if the sodium rises above 150, if the urine output is below 500 ml./24 hours, or if the blood urea nitrogen reaches

30 mg. per cent, further fluid is needed. Usually a patient can tolerate this limited intake for five days unless he has diabetes mellitus or insipidus, a dropping blood pressure, or profuse sweating. Fluid balance is more difficult if dexamethasone and/or diuretics are used, since both tend to dehydrate the patient.

Adrenocortical steroids have had wide usage in cases of brain injury, especially dexamethasone, but there is no clinical study that statistically supports the wide clinical impression of this drug's value in acute brain trauma. If it does help combat cerebral edema, it does so by continuing action over a period of hours, and if the steroids are stopped abruptly worsening can follow. The minimal adult dose is 10 mg. of dexamethasone I.V. push and 4 mg. every four hours. With the short half-life of dexamethasone, it may be advisable to give this steroid intravenously every two hours. It is contraindicated in patients with peptic ulcer or tuberculosis. Stress bleeding in the gastrointestinal tract requires that the steroid be stopped. Finally, extra potassium may be required.

Various diuretics have been recommended, either alone or in combination. Certainly the hypertonic solutions are quick to act and can "buy" time until the neurosurgeon arrives. An indwelling urinary catheter is required. A 20 per cent mannitol solution may be given intravenously over a 15- to 20-minute period, at a dose of 6 ml./kg. of body weight (420 ml. for a 70-kg. man).

There are two side-effects that are poorly appreciated. The hypertonic agents increase cerebral blood flow as they shrink the brain. *This tends to enhance intracranial bleeding.* The second effect is rebound elevation of intracranial pressure hours later. After the diuresis, there is a readjustment of electrolytes and water. The injured brain probably gets back more water than it lost. This necessitates further hypertonic infusions or, as is being done in brain injury centers, constant monitoring of intracranial pressure and titrating the dose.

Convulsions

This complication, which can occur even after mild injury, is of great concern to the Emergency Department physician. The seizure could mean the development of an intracranial hemorrhage, but more likely it is a manifestation of direct cerebral injury. The convulsion itself can change intracranial dynamics and cause further damage, bleeding, or brain hematoma. Therefore, prevention is the goal. All traumatized unconscious patients should receive intravenous sodium diphenylhydantoin (Dilantin) (Kutt and McDowell, 1968). The total dose is two and one half times the daily oral maintenance dose for the patient's size. For the average adult, this is 1 gm. The dose is divided into four parts administered 30 minutes apart, and is complete within 90 minutes. Each dose is given at a rate of 50 mg./minute while monitoring vital signs. This does not seem to depress the level of consciousness. Patients with heart disease may be sensitive to Dilantin by this route. *Dilantin should never be given by intramuscular injection* since its absorption is unpredictable and slow. The maintenance dose is 200 mg. I. V. twice a day.

If seizures begin before the full dose is given, or start afterward, sodium amobarbital (Amytal) can be used. A 100 mg./ml. solution is injected intravenously at the rate of one ml./minute until 5 ml. have been given or the seizure stops. This can be repeated in 30 minutes. Later, intramuscular phenobarbital can be started.

In the uncommon event that the Dilantin–Amytal regimen does not control the seizures, diazepam (Valium 10 mg. at the rate of 5 mg./min.) or sodium thiopental (Pentothal) can be administered. Both tend to depress respirations, and the latter requires an anesthesiologist.

THE CONSCIOUS PATIENT

If the patient has sustained a head injury, it is important to know whether he was unconscious, for how long, and in what temporal relationship to the accident. Many times, this information can be ascertained only from the ambulance personnel.

The time-span of amnesia, especially loss of memory for events prior to impact (retrograde amnesia) is an indicator of the severity of the injury and will guide the surgeon as to the length of time that observation is necessary. A good rule-of-thumb is to observe all concussed patients for a minimum of eight hours. If, by that time, the neurologic examination is negative and the

adult patient is judged to be competent, he can be released in the care of a responsible person who is given a list of instructions outlining further observation. In the pediatric age-group, the patient should be capable of being easily aroused and not vomiting before released. In either situation, document the negative findings at time of discharge. The final neurologic examination should be detailed.

Concussion and the Postconcussion Syndrome

The diagnosis of concussion is based on the history of a mechanical force causing *temporary* neural dysfunction. The patient may have been unconscious with amnesia. In fact, there may be retrograde amnesia. On the other hand, the patient need not lose consciousness and may only complain of poor balance, visual disturbance, confusion, etc. (in 1943 a well known college football star only realized he had made the winning touchdown, a 63 yard run, when he read the Sunday paper the next day. He also had no recall of being "dazed" ten minutes prior to that, following a head-on block.) In children, vomiting is frequent, and they are more likely to have convulsions soon after injury.

What is the longest period of unconsciousness that warrants the diagnosis of concussion? There is no general agreement, but certainly ten minutes would be accepted. Further, the patient should have a normal neurologic examination one hour after injury. (Some authorities also are of the opinion that the electroencephalogram should be normal in 24 hours.) Otherwise, the diagnosis is in doubt and the patient should be admitted for further observation.

Mechanical injury to the head, with or without temporary neural dysfunction, has a tendency to produce prolonged symptoms that often are called the "postconcussion syndrome." Headaches predominate. Also, the patient is subject to episodic difficulties with the sense of balance, especially with postural change. This may be described as dizziness, lightheadedness, or a feeling as if he may black-out or faint. True rotational vertigo is uncommon. Other symptoms are lack of concentration, a tendency to be easily provoked, and a change in sleep patterns. The above are less frequent in the more serious head injury. In either group, there is a high correlation to litigation. These patients rarely seek neuro-surgical opinion after the legal aspect has been settled. Nevertheless, the postconcus-sion syndrome does occur when there is no possible compensation, which indicates that there probably is an organic basis for many of these complaints.

WHEN TO ADMIT THE CONSCIOUS PATIENT

There is considerable difference of opinion as to when to admit the conscious patient for observation. The history is impor-tant. The Emergency Department physician should estimate the magnitude of the force.* If it is so great that the physician wonders how the patient tolerated the injury, that pa-tient should be admitted. For example, a three-year-old falls out of a second story window and only bruises his head. The im-pact could have been severe enough to cause delayed cerebral edema or to tear a bridging cortical vein, yet the patient may not have lost consciousness. This patient should be admitted. On the other hand, if the same child fell off his tricycle and began vomiting hours later, it is best to admit him, although these children rarely develop neurosurgical lesions. The patient who struck his head on an open kitchen cabinet door need not be admitted, but keep in mind that delayed subdural hemorrhages have been reported following such accidents.

The physician should err toward admit-ting patients who have alcoholic intoxica-tion, for they have a tendency to reinjure themselves. Second, their sleep is deep, making it less likely that the family will arouse them every hour. Third, the chronic alcoholic with liver disease may have low prothrombin time, which increases the like-lihood of intracranial bleeding. Fourth, cere-bral atrophy is often associated with chronic alcoholism. The brain is partially suspended by bridging cortical veins near the sagittal sinus. Therefore, less commotion of the brain is needed to tear these thin-walled vessels and produce subdural bleeding.

In a retrospective study of 3500 head-in-jured patients seen in an Emergency De-partment and not admitted, a normal neuro-logic examination was found to be a reliable

factor in predicting a favorable outcome (Jones, 1974). Further, this study indicated that, if the physician considered these pa-tients to be well enough to go home, skull x-rays were "medically unnecessary." If de-sired by the emergency physician, arrange-ments can be made for skull x-rays during routine hours, provided the rare unsus-pected pathologic finding is reported to that physician or to others with knowledge of the patient. Of course, the Emergency Depart-ment records should so indicate. If the pa-tient is to be admitted, the records should demonstrate that his lack of cooperation pre-cluded adequate x-rays at that time.

In addition, there are certain "trivial" accidents that can have serious con-sequences if overlooked. Skull x-rays may indicate fractures, and therefore give reason for admission. Plastic toys with metal axles can penetrate through the thin temporal bone when propelled by a rotary lawn-mower. Pencil injuries can produce brain abscesses, and a broken point may be visual-ized on x-ray. Darts, especially the heavy lawn variety, can penetrate even the adult skull. The orbital plate is thin, so that pene-tration in the area of the globe is a potential source of delayed central nervous system in-fection. Unfortunately, skull x-rays, even a special orbital view, are usually normal in these cases. Of course, any blow from a metal tool such as a wrench, screwdriver, or rake should be considered an indication for skull x-rays.

AGITATION AND PAIN

The head-injured but conscious patient is likely to be agitated. Many times there is a correctible cause, such as a distended uri-nary bladder, tight bandage, pain, etc. On the other hand, indwelling urinary catheters, in-travenous lines, nasal oxygen tubes, physical restraints, and repeated examinations will make the patient restless. All the above are magnified by alcoholism or cerebral hypoxia.

A considerate nurse often can reduce the patient's agitation, but in the practical situation this is not always feasible. Chest restraints, encasing the hands in padded dressings, allow the patient to turn, twist, and thrash without interfering with treat-ment and observation. Nevertheless, he may get loose, pull out the I. V. and catheter, fall out of bed, and generally exasperate the Emergency Department personnel. Such pa-

---

*See Evaluation of Injury, page 598.

tients probably need some form of sedation. Chlorpromazine (Thorazine 25 mg. intramuscularly every three hours) can often quiet the patient without deepening his conscious level. In the alcoholic, fresh paraldehyde (4 to 8 ml. I. M.) administered with a glass syringe may be more effective.

In multiple trauma, the head injury may seem trivial. Strong narcotics to relieve pain from other injuries are usually contraindicated, since pupillary constriction may be produced, the level of consciousness deepens, especially for the reaction to pain, and respiratory exchange decreases, affecting blood gases. Nevertheless, pain may be so intense that narcotics are justified. Meperidine hydrocholoride (Demerol 50 to 100 mg. I. M. every three hours) may be effective, especially if supplemented with small doses of Thorazine. Stronger doses of narcotics should be used with great caution.

ANTIBIOTICS

Antibiotics generally are not required unless there is an open convexity skull or a basal skull fracture. In the latter, blood may be seen behind the drumhead, or cerebrospinal fluid drips out of the ear or nose. Many antibiotics do not penetrate the blood-brain or blood-cerebrospinal fluid barriers unless an active infection is present or the blood level of the antibiotic is high. Therefore, prophylactic antibiotics to prevent meningitis must be administered in high doses. For example, 20 million units of penicillin G by intravenous infusion is necessary on a daily basis. In the unconscious patient, beware of possible allergies. When no history is available of drug allergies and antibiotics are clearly indicated, the adult can be treated with 10 per cent chloramphenicol sodium succinate solution (50 mg./kg. of body weight I. V.). It is further recommended that bacterial cultures be obtained either of the wound, the nasopharynx, or the external auditory canal before starting treatment.

SCALP WOUNDS

Laceration cannot be evaluated properly unless bleeding is controlled. Hemostats can be clamped to the galea and reflected over the scalp to compress the vessels. This is the technique used by many neurosurgeons when doing a craniotomy. When the skull is intact, the scalp edges can be compressed

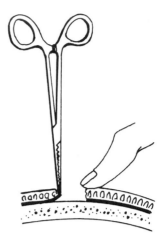

Figure 3. Hemostats clamped on the galea and reflected over the scalp, or finger pressure at the edge of the wound, stops most bleeding. (From Bouzarth, W. F.: The ABC's of emergency care of serious head injuries. Ind. Med. Surg. 39:21, 1970.)

with finger pressure to stop bleeding temporarily in order to allow proper inspection and débridement (see Fig. 3). Also, self-retaining retractors can be used to spread the wound taut. This will stop most bleeding and give a better view of the underlying pericranium and bone. If the wound cannot be adequately inspected visually, the examiner should gently palpate the bone with his index finger after putting on a sterile rubber glove. Linear fractures and depressed bone fragments are easily palpated, and these might not be seen on skull x-rays. After débridement, small scalp lacerations can be closed with through-and-through interrupted sutures about 1 cm. apart. When the galea also is lacerated and the wound gapes, this layer too should be closed with nonabsorbable sutures. The scalp sutures then are tied snugly and removed in two or three days. Also, take special note if the injury has produced a flap. If the flap has a narrow base, make sure that the flap edges bleed. If not, the flap may later become necrotic unless a plastic repair is carried out. Incidentally, there is no urgency in suturing these lacerations in the Emergency Department.

SKULL ROENTGENOGRAMS

From a medical/legal viewpoint, there is disagreement over the necessity of skull x-ray in every head injury (Bell and Loop, 1971). However, the costly over-use of skull x-rays will no doubt continue for the present. There is no doubt that skull x-rays should be of good quality and reviewed by physicians especially trained in interpretation of skull roentgenography. Unfortunately, the reverse situation is all too common, and often the uncooperative patient prevents adequate examination. In many hospitals, good quality films can be obtained only by transporting the patient to the x-ray department. This in itself diverts medical attention away from the victim. Indeed, at night and on weekends the patient may be left unattended while the films are being processed. It is recommended that an unconscious patient should not be transferred to the radiology department for skull x-rays unless: (1) he is carefully observed by a competent member of the Emergency Department staff who has immediate access to resuscitative equipment (even alert patients can have sudden seizures, vomit, aspirate, and die quickly); and (2) the films are then reviewed by a radiologist or neurosurgeon immediately—not the next morning. Otherwise, undetected abnormalities may stand as mute testimony of incompetence. If these two criteria cannot be met, skull x-rays should be delayed.

If skull films are obtained, the following findings are important: (1) a double bony density indicates a depressed bone fragment (however, for open wounds this should be evident without x-ray); (2) a linear fracture crossing the meningeal arterial groove, especially in the temporal bone or over a dural sinus, indicates a possible epidural hematoma; (3) a pineal shift suggests an intracranial hematoma, but when a calcified pineal gland would really be helpful, that is the time it will not be visualized; (4) intracranial air (pneumocephalus); (5) clouding of the sphenoid sinus indicates a basal skull fracture which will require antibiotic therapy; and (6) a foreign body, such as a bullet, can be localized.

OTHER CONSIDERATIONS

It has been demonstrated that a high percentage of adults who die from trauma have an elevated level of blood alcohol. Many enter the hospital with part of this alcohol unabsorbed in their stomachs, and their gastric contents are voluminous. Aspiration of the gastric contents should be done to remove any unabsorbed alcohol, as well as to reduce any chances of aspiration of vomitus, which is likely to occur.

In the Emergency Department, lumbar puncture is not indicated in obvious head-injured patients; indeed, it may be dangerous. However, it may be required in order to distinguish between a traumatic subarachnoid hemorrhage and meningitis.*

---

*See Chapter 17.

Figure 4. Special permit for transferring patient to neurosurgical center. (From Bouzarth, W. F.: Transferring patients with brain injury safely. Pa. Med. 77:35, 1974.)

SPECIAL PERMIT TO BE SENT WITH PATIENT

I understand that _____ is in critical condition and is being transferred to _____ Hospital for emergency neurosurgical care. I give permission, as the closest relative who is immediately available, for the _____ Hospital staff to proceed with whatever tests or treatment they consider necessary, including emergency brain or spine surgery.

I also agree to come to _____ Hospital or to help get other relatives (who may be closer to the patient) there as soon as possible.

I realize that the patient is in critical condition and may not live to reach _____ Hospital, or that when he or she arrives, the medical findings may be such that emergency surgery is not in the patient's best interests.

Date _____

Signature _____

Witness _____

Relationship _____

INTERHOSPITAL TRANSFER

Nearly one-half of the hospitals in the United States have fewer than 200 beds, and many do not have neurosurgeons on the active staff. With the development of trauma centers and, more recently, head injury treatment centers, interhospital transfer is a reality (Craig and Hunt, 1959; Bouzarth, 1974). The A, B, C, and D of acute care, as previously outlined, must be maintained during transportation. Since vomiting is more likely to occur, gastric aspiration should be done unless a cuffed endotracheal tube or esophageal obstructor airway has been inserted. Further, if there is any possibility of shock, it is a good idea to carry one unit (500 ml.) of blood for every 15 minutes of travel time.

The relatives should be informed that transfer is needed even though death can occur en route, and that the neurosurgeon may not recommend surgery (see Fig. 4). Send a copy of the watch sheet and caution the ambulance driver about safety.

Special Pediatric Problems

In mild injuries, the younger the patient, the more likely he will have a seizure and/or vomit. Also, he will be more difficult to arouse, just as a normal child is more difficult to awaken in the middle of the night. On the other hand, the pediatric patient tends to make a better recovery from serious brain injury. If lumbar puncture is to be performed, the needle should be placed near the L5 spinous process.*

Infants with subdural hematoma or effusion can develop a massive increase in intracranial pressure. The anterior fontanelle bulges and is tense. Immediate subdural taps may be indicated.* The infant may need a transfusion.

---

*See Chapter 17.

References

Bell, R. S., and Loop, J. W.: The utility and futility of radiographic skull examination for trauma. N. Engl. J. Med. *284*:237, 1971.

Bouzarth, W. F.: Neurosurgical watch sheet for craniocerebral trauma. J. Trauma 8:29, 1968.

Bouzarth, W. F.: Transferring patients with brain injury safely. Pa. Med. 77:35, 1974.

Bouzarth, W. F., et al.: A guide to evaluate serious head injuries. Bull. Am. Coll. Surg. *59*:21, 1974.

Craig, T., and Hunt, W.: Emergency care of extradural hematoma. J.A.M.A. *171*:405, 1959.

Jefferson, G.: The tentorial pressure cone. Arch. Neurol. Psychiatr. *40*:857, 1938.

Jones, R. K.: Assessment of minimal head injuries: indications for in-hospital care. Surg. Neurol. 2:101, 1974.

Kutt, H., and McDowell, F.: Management of epilepsy with diphenylhydantoin sodium. J.A.M.A. *203*:969, 1968.

Shenkin, H. A., and Bouzarth, W. F.: Clinical methods of reducing intracranial pressure. N. Engl. J. Med. *182*:1465, 1970.

B. SPINAL INJURIES

William F. Bouzarth

INTRODUCTION

Spinal cord injury is catastrophic and devastating. It is estimated that the average annual rate of incidence is about 50 persons per million population, and one-half of these victims die within a year of their injury. Further, the cost of acute care in hospitals, of care in rehabilitation centers, and of chronic care is staggering. According to Young (1970), the life-long cost for care of one paraplegic is $400,000, which in the entire United States would amount to 2 billion dollars per year. Although efforts are being made to prevent spinal cord injury, to offer the injured "preventive" extrication and transportation to a hospital Emergency Department, and to treat the victim properly in hospitals, results are still notoriously poor. With ongoing research, and with federally-supported spinal cord injury centers, there is considerable hope for the many victims yet to come.

The Emergency Department physician can train ambulance attendants to recognize spinal injury, to perform safe extrication, to immobilize the patient during transportation, and to start medical and supportive treatment. A report of 300 proved cervical spine injuries indicates that 57 per cent had some type of motor loss, yet the diagnosis was not made in the first 24 hours of hospital admission in 37 per cent of cases, and was delayed for one month in 25 per cent (Bohlman, 1972). Ten patients (3 per cent) developed paralysis after unguarded, unintentional manipulation while in the hospital. The emergency physician can assist the many other specialists—neurosurgeons, orthopedists, neurologists, and psychiatrists—by providing each patient with proper professional services in the first few hours after injury. This chapter will focus upon serious spinal cord injury per se, and will place secondary emphasis on subluxations, fractures, and/or dislocations.

ETIOLOGY AND PATHOPHYSIOLOGY

Open injuries are caused by missiles, knife blades, ice picks, and massive forces that literally tear the patient apart. Closed injuries, which are more common, can occur from: (1) a fall, regardless of how a patient lands; (2) diving accidents; (3) a blow on the top of the head; (4) forced flexion or hyperextension of the neck or body; (5) electric shock (in which paralysis may be delayed); or (6) even after a twist or lift that results in an extruded disk fragment. Spinal cord injury was found most frequently among male auto drivers of 18 to 35 years of age, either unmarried or in some marital difficulties, who were involved in a vehicular accident.

Bony elements including the intravertebral disk also may be fractured and/or displaced, and such injuries may or may not produce secondary damage to the cord. A recent analysis of diving accidents indicates that cervical cord injury occurred after the impact, suggesting improper water rescue in victims with unstable spine injuries (Kewelramani and Taylor, 1975).

It is well known that the spinal cord can be damaged without producing x-ray evidence of structural abnormalities of the bone. This is especially true in patients with rheumatoid arthritis who have a tendency toward profuse bleeding, and in the elderly with cervical spondylosis. In the latter, forcible flexion or extension of the neck compresses the intraspinal neural elements between the anterior arthritic ridges and the hypertrophic ligamentum flavum, thereby damaging the cord. This usually produces central cord necrosis. Recent experimental

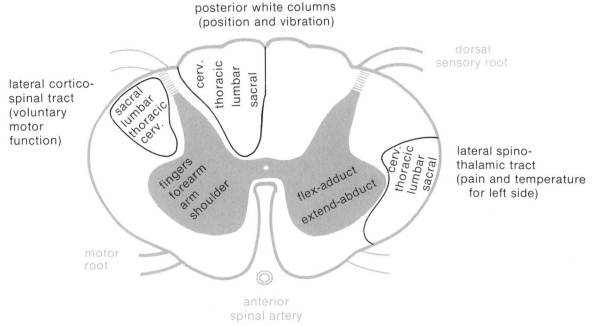

Figure 1. Cross section of spinal cord.

work indicates that the central gray matter stores and releases various catecholamines that are formed in brain cells and migrate down into the spinal cord by way of the long neural tracts of the white matter. With central cord injury, these molecules are released and cause local vasomotor changes that in time destroy the central tissue and, with severe injury, the white matter also. Thus, the cord may be destroyed biochemically. For this reason, local spinal hypothermia, dexamethasone, and other drugs show some promise.

The spinal cord has been compared to a telephone cable, with the vertebral bodies as poles. This analogy is not exact if one considers that: (1) electrical impulses to and from the brain are carried in the white matter and synapse in the gray matter on a segmental basis; (2) there is a layered arrangement of the long tracts in the white matter (see Fig. 1); (3) neural cells of the gray matter can generate their own "calls;" (4) the arterial and venous blood supplies, when traumatized, tend to damage the cord differentially; (5) a lesion may appear clinically to be higher or lower than it actually is; (6) the spinal cord is a segmental organ with the 31 segments close to their vertebral counterpart cephalad, but less so caudad (all the sacral segments are opposite the L1 vertebra); and (7) there are no private lines for the sense of touch.

EXAMINATION OF A PATIENT WITH SPINAL INJURIES

In cases of spinal injury, a detailed examination must be recorded in contradistinction to the "mini-examination" recommended for cases of serious brain injury. The initial examination is one of the most crucial factors in arriving at the decision to recommend surgery and in determining prognosis. For example, the observation of a feeble movement of the toe, a small area of perianal hypalgesia, a muscle twitch when the deep tendon reflex is tested, or even the presence of a Babinski sign indicates an incomplete lesion with a better prognosis. Localized back or neck pain and tenderness is an important clue to spinal injury, especially if there is radiation into one or more limbs.

In the description of spinal injury syndromes, the following definitions are important:

(1) *Arm* designates that part of the upper limb located between the elbow and shoulder.

(2) *Leg* designates that part of the lower extremity between the knee and ankle.

(3) The suffix–*esthesia* refers to all sensation, according to some authorities, and only to tactile sensation according to others. To avoid confusion, absence of sensation will be called *anesthesia;* diminished touch sensation, *hypesthesia;* hypersensitivity to touch, *hyperesthesia;* abnormal sensation without stimulation, *paresthesia;* and perverted response to stimuli, *dysesthesia.* (Position and vibration senses travel in the ipsilateral posterior columns.) (Fig. 1.)

(4) The suffix–*algesia* refers only to sense of pain. *Analgesia* denotes no sense of pain; *hypalgesia* denotes diminished pain; and *hyperalgesia* refers to increased perception of pain. This sensation and temperature sense travel in the contralateral anterolateral spinothalamic tract (Fig. 1).

(5) The suffix–*plegia* indicates total paralysis of a limb or limbs; *monoplegia* means paralysis of one limb; *hemiplegia,* paralysis of upper and lower limb on the same side; *crossed hemiplegia* refers to involvement of the ipsilateral upper limb and contralateral lower limb; *diplegia* means affliction of both upper extremities; *paraplegia,* of lower extremities; and *quadra-* or *tetraplegia* involves all four limbs.

(6) The suffix–*paresis* means that some movement is present (an incomplete lesion).

(7) *Spinal shock* indicates complete loss of function below the level of the lesion. The patient has an areflexic flaccid paralysis of the limbs including the rectal sphincter, with anesthesia up to that level. Because of loss of sweating and shivering, there is a tendency toward poikilothermia. In spite of paralysis of the bowel and bladder, priapism occurs in many cases. A tendency toward hypotension may be exhibited without the other findings of circulatory shock; in fact, bradycardia is common. This state may be completely reversible within minutes to days, especially in cases of concussion of the cord; alternatively, there may be a permanent loss of function, or only partial return. It is said that, if there is no improvement within 24 hours, there will be no return. Within a few weeks, however, spasticity, hyperreflexia, and mass-reflex state may develop.

There still is considerable confusion about the meaning of the term "quadriplegia." In the true sense, this is a complete paralysis of all limbs and indicates a lesion at C5 or above. But what term is to be used when the patient cannot move the lower extremities or extend the forearms, but can flex them—or, in other words, when the lower limbs are plegic and the upper limbs are paretic? Perhaps the term should be "para-

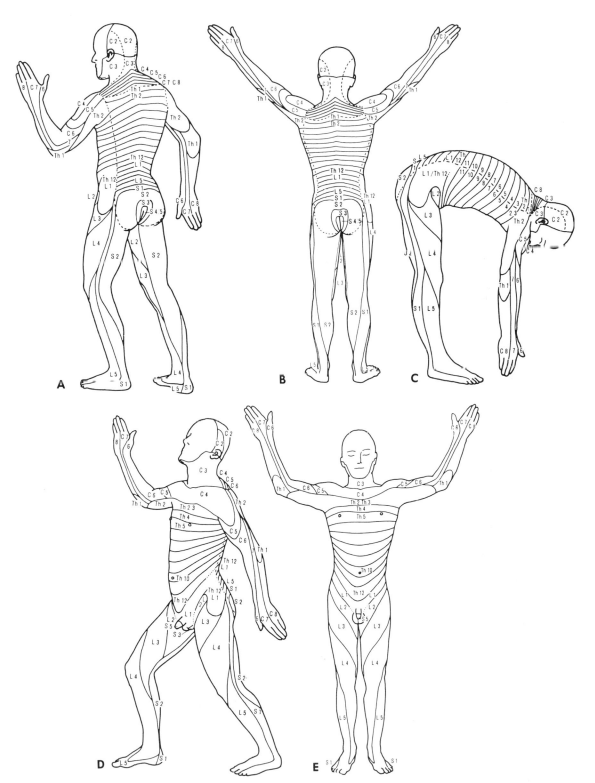

Figure 2. Dermatomal distribution. The representation on the face is for pain sensation only (see onion-skin syndrome).

plegic-diparetic" or a C6 quadriplegia. On the other hand, if there is movement in one or both lower limbs, this would be a C6 quadriparesis. What is being stressed in this terminology is the location of the cord lesion by motor examination. None of the above describes sensation. Therefore, terms are needed to distinguish a total (complete) loss of function from a partial (incomplete) loss. The term "complete" quadriplegia or paraplegia means no movement, with anesthesia below the level of the lesion. Thus, a complete C6 quadriplegia has a different clinical connotation from an incomplete C6 quadriplegia (some sensation present) or from a C6 quadriparesis. The sensory distribution by dermatomes can be confusing (see Fig. 2, A–E).

COMPLETE NEUROLOGIC SYNDROMES BY CORD SEGMENTS

Patients with upper cervical lesions (C1, 2, and 3) used to die either on the scene or soon after admission to the hospital, but, with modern resuscitative techniques, life can be sustained for months; in fact, the patient may be able to sustain his own life for a time inasmuch as the trapezius, sternocleidomastoid, and platysma muscles contract for this vital function. Anesthesia includes the neck and posterior scalp (C2) with hypalgesia or analgesia of the face (onion-skin pattern, to be described). In the C4 lesion there is some diaphragmatic movement and neck movement, with normal neck sensation. In lesion C5, when the patient is prone the scapula can be moved toward the midline and the shoulders can be elevated slightly. Otherwise, the upper limbs are immobile. Sensation is present in the shoulders and lateral arm. At cord segment C6 there is a tendency for the upper limbs to be held in the "hold-up" position, with the hands half closed, and at times, the forearms are flexed across the chest when the deltoid function is diminished. It is also characteristic that when the limbs are straightened by the examiner, and then released, the flexed position of the forearm is resumed. Sensation is present in the lateral forearm. Involvement of the C7 segment is not so easily recognized, since the triceps may have some function, radial deviation of the hand is now possible, and sensation is

present in the thumb. When the lesion occurs at the C8 segment, triceps function is good but intrinsic hand muscles are paralyzed. The patient has sensation in the middle finger, however.

Injury in the first thoracic segment is demonstrated in the hand by paralysis of the abductor pollicis brevis, but with normal triceps function. There is sensation in the fifth finger but not in the medial forearm. At the next segment (T2), motor function in the upper extremity is normal, but sensory loss is exhibited in the medial aspect of the arm and part of the axilla. At T4 there is anesthesia to the nipples. It should be stressed that C3-4 sensory supply by way of the supraclavicular nerves meets the T4 dermatome. Unless a careful check is made in the axilla and medial arm, the level may be incorrectly diagnosed. A cord lesion at the T10 segment produces anesthesia to the umbilicus. When the patient lifts his head off the bed, the umbilicus rises due to paralysis of the inferior recti muscles (Bevor's sign).

The five lumbar cord segments are located under the T11-L1 vertebral bodies. When injury occurs at the L1 segment, the cremasteric reflex is absent and anesthesia extends to the top of an imaginary bikini bathing suit. Paraplegia is still present. With the lesion at L2, slight hip flexion is possible and the condition may be described as a paraparesis. The cremasteric reflexes are present. Sensation is noted in the upper anterior thigh. Localization of injury at L3 is demonstrated by definite hip flexion, with some adduction of the thigh. Sensation is present in the lower part of the anterior thigh. With an L4 transsection it is possible for the patient to extend the leg, and the knee jerk may be present but usually is depressed or absent. Sensation extends to the medial knee and leg. A lesion at L5 produces weakness of the extensor hallucis longus and paralysis of the peroneal muscles. Sensation is present in the medial ankle.

Since the sacral and coccygeal spinal segments that make up the conus medullarus are small, it is unusual to get a clear-cut division between segments. However, when the S1 root is injured, the ankle jerk is depressed or absent, the biceps femoris muscles are weak, there is no sensation in the great toe, posterior thigh, or saddle area, and the rectal sphincter flaccid (Fig. 2,A, B).

INCOMPLETE SYNDROMES

The Brown-Séquard syndrome or hemisection of the cord is usually produced by a knife blade. There is ipsilateral paralysis with loss of position and vibratory sense, and contralateral loss of pain and of temperature sensation. Touch is only slightly impaired, if at all. *Acute anterior spinal cord injury (anterior spinal artery syndrome)* results in immediate paralysis, with hypesthesia and hypalgesia to the level of the lesion and preservation of position and vibratory senses. The patient with *acute central cervical spinal cord injury* manifests greater loss of motor power in the upper limbs as compared to the lower extremities, usually with retention of urine and varying degrees of sensory loss below the lesion. Paresthesias and/or dysesthesias often are present in the upper limbs.

The next four syndromes may result from: (1) vertebral artery occlusion due to fracture/dislocation of the lower cervical spine; or from (2) direct injury to the cervicomedullary junction and upper cervical segments. The *Déjérine onion-skin pattern* is a hypalgesia or analgesia of the face caused by involvement of the spinal tract of the trigeminal nerve. *Horner's syndrome* is represented by ptosis, miosis, and anhidrosis. *Posterior-inferior cerebellar artery syndrome* produces one or more of the following: dysphasia; dysphonia; hiccups; nausea; vomiting; vertigo; and cerebellar dysfunction. On examination, the patient demonstrates an ipsilateral paralysis of the soft palate, Horner's syndrome, cerebellar asynergy, and analgesia of the face, with a contralateral analgesia of the limbs and trunk. Nystagmus and/or forced eye deviation may be present. *Crossed hemiparesis or plegia* indicates brain stem localization. There is ipsilateral loss of function in arm and contralateral loss in the leg.

Usually, *incomplete spinal cord injury* represents any combination of the above, especially with spasticity, hyperreflexia, and pathologic reflexes. There is great variability of sensation and motor function, especially from one side to the other, and cord localization may be difficult. Injuries of the L1 vertebra may produce both upper and lower neuron signs, and those below which affect the cauda equina produce lower motor-neuron-type weakness.

The blood supply to the cord comes from branches off the vertebral arteries and the aorta. Studies of human anatomic specimens have indicated that there are three areas (C1, T4, and L1) where collateral circulation is sparse. Hence, a C5-6 dislocation that partially compresses the vertebral arteries as they travel within the bony spinal elements can produce a C1 lesion, due to decreased blood flow through the midline anterior spinal artery that originates from both vertebrals. The great radicular artery of Adamkiewicz originates from the aorta, usually enters the bony spinal canal at L1, and sends branches up to T4, another watershed area. Therefore, a lumbar fracture can produce a T4 localization.

EXTRADURAL SPINAL HEMATOMA

Another vascular syndrome that can occur even after minor injury, especially in patients under anticoagulation therapy or with rheumatoid arthritis, is the *extradural spinal hematoma*. The cord or cauda equina can be compressed within minutes to hours, producing a total neurologic lesion. Progressively severe neck or back pain is a prominent symptom, and there is a tendency for the segmental localization to rise (cephalad march) as the hematoma dissects and compresses in both directions.

EMERGENCY DEPARTMENT MANAGEMENT

As soon as a cord injury is suspected, immobilization is required with immediate attention to airway management. A properly trained ambulance crew should deliver the accident victim securely strapped to a spine board, but if they fail to do so this should be done promptly on arrival at Emergency, the patient being moved en bloc. In neck injuries, sandbags should be placed next to the patient's head. Halter traction (10 lb.) has been recommended by some authorities, but there are some disadvantages in that the airway may be further compromised, and 10 lb. (a weight difficult to tolerate for any prolonged period) may not provide adequate immobilization. Since the spine board does not interfere with x-ray, a cross-table lateral and an anteroposterior x-ray should be obtained of the suspected area. For neck injuries, the shoulders must be depressed by

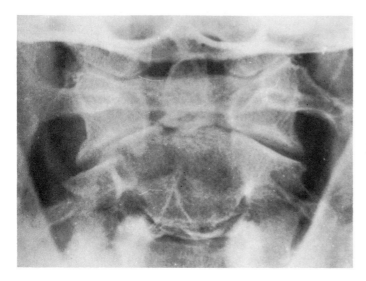

Figure 3. Open-mouth anteroposterior view which demonstrates an odontoid fracture.

pulling the hands toward the feet so that the seventh cervical vertebra is visualized. It must be stressed that the more difficult it is to see this vertebra, the more likely is there to be a cervical fracture and/or dislocation, since there is paralysis of the muscles that depress the shoulders while the elevators such as the trapezius are unaffected. At times, "swimmers'" views, or tomography, may be required to visualize the lower cervical spine. In addition, an open-mouth view for the odontoid process is required (see Fig. 3). *Flexion and extension views, which may be a part of the routine cervical spine examination, are contraindicated.*

Always inspect the posterior pharyngeal soft tissue for hemorrhage and/or edema that widens the soft tissue shadow, indicating cervical spine injury. Once a fracture and/or dislocation is confirmed, skull tongs should be applied. The Gardner-Wells tongs are recommended.*

Respiratory insufficiency may be expected with cord lesions, especially in the high cervical area. Mechanical ventilation is usually required for a C4 transection lesion, and almost always for C1, 2, and 3 lesions. In the urgent situation, an endotracheal tube is inserted by a "blind nasal" technique or passed over a flexible fiberoptic bronchoscope, since neither requires hyperextension as does the laryngoscope. The esophageal obturator airway or simple bag-to-mouth ventilation of the paralyzed patient can bridge the gap until tracheostomy can be performed. Arterial PCO_2, PO_2, and pH must be obtained periodically and the gases corrected by adjusting the volume-regulated respirator and concentration of the inspired gases.†

Another frequent problem is paralytic ileus, which further decreases respiratory efficiency. The diaphragms are elevated, thus reducing respiratory exchange. The work of respiration becomes more difficult and the patient rapidly fatigues. Gastric dilatation can result in regurgitation and pulmonary aspiration. Bowel sounds may be absent and, with lesions above the T8 segment, rigidity and tenderness of the anterior abdominal wall also is absent. Therefore, it is extremely difficult to diagnose intra-abdominal surgical lesions. It is advisable that the circumference of the body be measured daily at the level of the umbilicus. An increasing circumference is a direct measure of the magnitude of the paralytic ileus. Base-line abdominal x-rays aid in future evaluation of gastrointestinal complication. Passing a nasogastric tube for continuous suction for two to five days is recommended to prevent abdominal distention. During this period, intravenous fluids are administered, monitoring the serum electrolytes and osmolality. The patient usually will not defecate for at least a week. Enemas are usually retained, have no value, and in fact may give trouble. When the patient begins to have bowel sounds and can take

*See page 436.   †See Chapter 10.

food by mouth, rectal suppositories can be given every second day before breakfast.

Even in partial lesions, the urinary bladder is paralyzed. Early catheterization is required, therefore, and this requires meticulous technique. Current practice is for the bladder to be emptied every four to eight hours by intermittent catheterization. The frequency of catheterization is determined by the volume of urine, 500 to 700 ml. being attempted between each catheterization. This program reduces the complications that occur with long term indwelling catheters.

Bedsore precautions should be started early. The skin should be kept dry, powdered with talc, and massaged periodically. Sheets should be kept unwrinkled. Since the spine-injured patient may also have extremity fractures, special care must be given to the skin under a cast. If the bony lesion requires immobilization and/or traction, the patient must be placed on a turning device (Stryker frame or Foster bed) and turned every two hours. This places a great deal of stress on the nursing staff, but is an absolute necessity. With cervical spine injuries, the physician should supervise the first turning for each shift of nurses, not only to make sure it is done correctly but to ensure that the patient has not been made worse in the face-down position. Turning frames provide only two positions, whereas the patient in bed can also be placed on his side, which has definite advantages. Flotation pads, alternating air mattress, or a water bed can be used with a diligent nursing staff, and obviates the need for a turning frame which is universally uncomfortable to most patients (and nurses!).

DIFFERENTIATION BETWEEN SPINAL SHOCK AND TRAUMATIC SHOCK

There has been some confusion about spinal shock and traumatic shock. Both produce hypotension, but spinal shock, although not responsive to transfusion, will improve with 1 per cent solution of Neosynephrine intravenously. Spinal shock is likely to slow the pulse. Because of this tendency to hypotension, the patient cannot be placed in the sitting or erect position without difficulty.

CORTICOSTEROIDS

Dexamethasone has been used widely in treatment of trauma to the central nervous system. Its exact mechanism of action is not known and, in fact, there is no good clinical proof that spine injuries are aided by this steroid. Nevertheless, following current practice, it should be administered first in the Emergency Department, giving 10 mg. I.V. push and then 5 mg. every three hours. This can be tapered off after five days. One problem with this steroid is stress ulcers. G.I. bleeding can occur, so it is not recommended for patients with a history of peptic ulcer. Active tuberculosis can be worsened and is also a contraindication to steroid use.

ANTIBIOTICS AND ANALGESICS

Antibiotics seem to be used universally in early management of spinal injury. Pulmonary complications lead to infection, and catheterization makes the urinary tract very susceptible. There may be some wisdom in holding off antibiotics until an infection actually arises, and then treating the infection with the appropriate antibiotic. Otherwise, the flora may be changed so that infection may be due to an antibiotic-resistant organism. Urinary prophylaxis with Mandelamine is indicated when the patient can take medicine orally.

Relief of pain, paresthesias, and/or dyesthesias in acute phase is difficult. Often these symptoms are magnified by the patient's own anxiety. Since blood flow to the muscles is diminished, intramuscular medication may not be absorbed in the expected fashion. If heavy sedation or narcotics are given, whatever voluntary respiration is present may be further depressed, leading to cerebral anoxia. However, if the patient is on assisted respiration, the better part of valor is to give adequate tranquilizers and narcotics to keep him comfortable in the acute phase. Morphine tends to slow respirations. Drug addiction is a frequent complication in such patients, and this should be kept in mind. However, the disturbing sensory symptoms begin to resolve within a week. Later, other annoying pain and dysesthesias develop.

SURGICAL INDICATIONS AND CONTRAINDICATIONS

The neurosurgeon, often with orthopedic consultation, has a major responsibility for surgical intervention. The following brief discussion is offered so that the emergency physician can better understand the complexities of such decisions.

Most discussions concerning surgical procedures mention lumbar puncture and/or myelography. Although lumbar puncture is a procedure that the emergency physician should be able to perform, it is difficult in the paraplegic and very hazardous in the quadriplegic; consequently, *both become neurosurgical procedures in the patient with cord injury,* and, in fact, lumbar puncture may be contraindicated. Pantopaque myelography can be performed without moving the patient from the supine position by inserting a spinal needle at the C1-2 level.

There is considerable difference of opinion as to the operative management of spinal cord lesions. Schneider (1962) lists nine indications, whereas Guttmann (1973) is much more conservative. Also there is considerable diversity concerning what type of operation to recommend; that is, posterior laminectomy versus anterior body fusion with diskectomy. Experts vary widely on the timing of each type of operation. In Bohlman's series (1972), 10 per cent of the patients worsened or developed paralysis after surgery. Bohlman feels laminectomy to be indicated only in patients with massive epidural hemorrhage, since laminectomy is associated with high mortality and loss of motor function.

Most authorities agree that progressive deterioration of neurologic function is a definite indication for immediate surgical intervention. This can be manifested by increasing weakness and/or decreasing sensory perception, as well as by progressive "cephalad march," as seen in acute epidural hemorrhage. Thus, recorded baseline and serial examinations provide the main clue. Another indication is the presence of open fractures or penetrating wounds that require débridement to prevent abscess formation or meningitis. Penetration of the bowel prior to spinal injury makes débridement more imperative. Bone fragments in the spinal canal, especially depressed laminae, constitute another indication. Intraspinal bullet fragments also have been listed. Schneider (1962) considers the syndrome of the acute anterior spinal cord injury to be a firm indication. The anterolateral approach in the cervical region has gained more favor, especially when the lower vertebral bodies are involved.

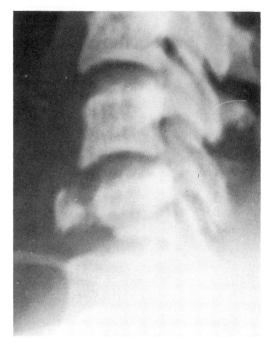

Figure 4. "Tear drop" fracture of C6 wedge compression of the vertebral body (postlaminectomy film).

Nerve root injuries, as they enter the intravertebral foramina, and including the intraspinal cauda equina, represent a different problem from spinal cord injuries. Decompressive lumbar laminectomy seems to offer a better prognosis than conservative treatment without surgery. In cervical lesions, decompression of the highest nerve root may change a complete C6 quadriplegia to a C7 level and greatly improve rehabilitation. Thus, nerve root decompression has been recommended by some authorities, even in cases involving complete spinal lesions.

Certain bony abnormalities, with or without neural dysfunction, have a clear indication for surgical correction. The acute "tear drop" cervical fracture/dislocation (see Fig. 4) should be reduced with skull traction and fused early. If a significant fracture or dislocation cannot be reduced by traction, open reduction is then essential.

Surgery is contraindicated for the patient with a complete lesion when first examined, unless there is a block demonstrated by myelography or by jugular compression test, and no bony structural changes are noted. However, this is still in dispute. Certainly if there is no improvement after 24

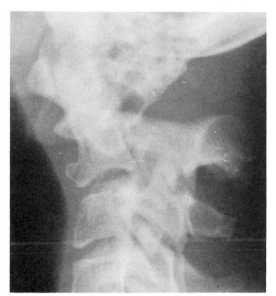

Figure 5. "Hangman's" fracture with the axes being dislocated in the C3 vertebral body and an axial avulsion fracture of the neural arch.

hours, there is very little likelihood of surgery proving beneficial. The syndrome of acute central spinal cervical cord injury has also been listed as a contraindication. "*Hangman's*" fracture (see Fig. 5) usually responds better to a brace, cast, or halo cast for six to eight weeks. Cervical lesions, C4 or above, may lose any remaining diaphragmatic function, thus making surgery dangerous, and it is not recommended unless the lesion is progressive. Obviously, treatment of traumatic shock or other death-producing systemic injury should take priority over spinal surgery. Finally, if proper facilities and qualified surgeons are not available, cervical cord neurosurgery is contraindicated.

The decision for definitive treatment of patients with spinal cord lesions should be a neurosurgical one. A decision to fuse the spine is often shared with the orthopedist. There is a high chance that any decision will appear to be wrong to a colleague, to the patient, to his family, or to 12 jurors. Indeed, a decision not to operate may appear wrong to the responsible neurosurgeon if, next morning, he finds the patient now has a complete lesion. It is even worse to operate on an incomplete lesion and have the same result. Both conditions occur in the best of hands. However, the attitude of society today is that the treatment was wrong if the patient doesn't get better. Indeed, the patient himself often tends to blame the neurosurgeon for his infirmity.

Without a doubt, the serious spinal cord and/or brain injury can be tragic to the patient, his family, the well-meaning neurosurgeon, and society at large. Only society and medical research can improve the situation in the future. Continuing education is recommended so that the Emergency Department physician can do his share in properly treating today's victim according to the standards of today's knowledge, and in stimulating the development of adequate prehospital care.

References

Bohlman, H. H.: The results of cervical spine trauma: general and specific. American Academy of Orthopedic Surgeons Instructional Course No. 17, Jan. 30, 1972.

Guttmann, L.: Spinal cord injuries. Oxford, Blackwell, 1973.

Kewalramani, L. S., and Taylor, R. G.: Injuries to the cervical spine from diving accidents. J. Trauma *15*:130, 1975.

Schneider, R. C.: Surgical indication and contraindication in spine and spinal cord trauma. Clin. Neurosurg. 8:157, 1962.

Young, J.: Development of systems of spinal cord injury management with a correlation to the development of other isoteric health care systems. Ariz. Med. *27*:1, 1970.

C. TRAUMA TO THE FACE

Errikos Constant

INTRODUCTION

Facial trauma constitutes one of the most common injuries seen in Emergency Departments. In the U.S. the main cause is vehicular accidents. In a study of over 1000 facial injuries, it was found that 54 per cent occurred while the patient was riding in a motor vehicle, 17 per cent happened in the home, 11 per cent occurred during the pursuit of athletic activities, and 6 per cent were the result of animal bites. In motor vehicle accidents, the face is the anatomic region that most often sustains injury (Brooks, Nahum, and Siegel, 1970).

Facial injuries may involve the facial skeleton, the soft tissues, and certain vital structures of the face, such as the seventh cranial nerve, the parotid gland and its duct, and the lacrimal apparatus. Restoration of both function and appearance is the primary goal of treatment. Prompt recognition and skillful management of these injuries usually give excellent results and facilitate the subsequent physical and psychologic rehabilitation in the patient (Converse, 1963).

Although a facial injury may be the most obvious and dramatic wound in an injured person, it may be the least important in terms of patient survival. A complete history and physical examination of the injured person should be performed, and injuries to the cervical spine, central nervous system, abdomen, chest, and extremities must be recognized and treated first.

Some of these patients become involved in personal injury litigations with which the emergency physician also may find himself associated, even years later (Schultz, 1967 and 1977). Accurate description of the injury and the method of treatment is of inestimable value. Photographs are most helpful, but, if not taken, a sketch by the physician indicating the injuries sustained (including measurements of lacerations) will refresh the memory in later years.

RECOGNITION AND MANAGEMENT OF LIFE-THREATENING SITUATIONS IN PATIENTS WITH MAXILLOFACIAL INJURIES

Facial trauma, unaccompanied by other injuries, seldom threatens the patient's life. In those few instances in which it does, it is due either to (a) airway obstruction or (b) blood loss.

Airway Obstruction. Brisk bleeding from the oral cavity and nose may obstruct the airway, especially with the patient in the supine position. Prompt suctioning of the oropharynx is mandatory to remove all clots and foreign bodies (broken teeth, denture fragments, etc.). If the patient is able, he should be encouraged to sit up and clear his mouth and airway. If he must lie down, the prone position is preferable. The "post-tonsillectomy position" (patient on his side, head down, neck extended) is usually the safest method to transport a patient with a maxillofacial injury.

Posterior displacement of the tongue causes airway obstruction and frequently is seen in association with bilateral condylar or parasymphyseal fractures of the mandible. Allowing the patient to bend forward or pulling the tongue forward with a suture gives immediate relief.

Massive edema of the tongue, floor of the mouth, and oropharyngeal tissues may occlude the airway. Endotracheal intubation is a swift and safe method to relieve the obstruction and, in most instances, is preferable to tracheostomy. If the patient is unconscious, it is best that he be intubated immediately. Tracheostomy, best performed in an operating room (Eiseman and Spencer, 1963), may become necessary if intubation is needed for periods longer than a few days.

Blood Loss. Shock is seldom the result of blood loss from extensive facial injuries. Its presence should alert one to the possibility of an intrathoracic, intra-abdominal, or extremity injury.

Pressure dressings, with sterile gauze held firmly in place by an elastic bandage, will temporarily arrest most of the bleeding seen about the face. If a large artery is severed (e.g., the external facial), careful clamping of the vessel with a hemostat is necessary. A few well-placed sutures will control the bleeding of most tongue lacerations.

Bleeding from lacerations of the gingiva, floor of the mouth, and buccal mucosa may be controlled temporarily by rolling a sterile gauze, placing it over the wound, and having the patient bite down on it.

Nasal bleeding may be brisk, and may require both a postnasal pack and an anterior pack for control.*

The treatment of shock from blood loss should be prompt and vigorous.†

---

*See page 417.
†See page 553.

SOFT TISSUE INJURIES OF THE FACE

RECOGNITION OF SOFT TISSUE INJURIES

Recognition of the common types of facial soft tissue injuries and an understanding of their characteristics is essential in treatment planning.

Contusion. Blunt trauma results in a crushing injury to the soft tissues, with the overlying skin remaining intact. Extensive edema, or a large hematoma, may be seen in a contused area. In severe contusions, gradual necrosis of the skin may occur, requiring débridement. The underlying nerves may be crushed and the patient may experience anesthesia. The integrity of the underlying facial skeleton should be determined by careful clinical and roentgenographic examination.

Abrasions. These may be superficial or may extend deeply into the dermis. When grossly contaminated with foreign particles (e.g., gravel, gun powder), they may "tattoo" the skin if not treated properly.

Lacerations. These may have clean-cut edges when inflicted by a sharp object, or the edges may be ragged and contused. They may penetrate deeply, severing important muscles, nerves, or ducts. Stellate lacerations are often caused by blunt trauma and commonly have irregular and contused wound margins.

Avulsion Flaps. These are lacerations with extensive undermining. The rich vascular supply of the face insures the survival of most of these flaps. However, a very narrow base in relation to length may result in necrosis of its distal portion. Similarly, a thick flap, one that is severely contused, or one that has been twisted for a long time, may fail to survive.

Avulsion of Soft Tissue. This results in complete loss of skin. Immediate coverage with a skin graft may be necessary to avoid infection. Granulating wounds should be avoided in the face.

Burns of the Face. See Chapter 39A.

Soft tissue injuries of the face that are easily overlooked are as follows:

(1) Contusions and lacerations in the scalp, postauricular area, and eyebrow.

(2) Transverse eyelid lacerations. These seal promptly due to lack of skin tension.

(3) Lacerations and hematomas of the nasal septum.

(4) Lacerations of the oral commissure, floor of the mouth, or palate.

THE MANAGEMENT OF SOFT TISSUE INJURIES

General Considerations. Most soft tissue injuries may be repaired in the Emergency Department. If they are extensive, however, or if vital structures (e.g., the facial nerve) are involved, repair should be performed in the operating room where adequate lighting, instruments, and assistance are available and the distractions of a busy Emergency Department are absent.

Timing of Repair. The surgical adage states that primary repair of soft tissue wounds should be carried out within eight hours from the time of injury, but a rational approach is to evaluate each wound individually. Three factors must be considered: (a) the type and degree of contamination; (b) the resistance of the host; and (c) signs of inflammation. Thus, a forehead laceration, caused by a relatively clean shattered windshield, may be free of any signs of inflammation 24 hours later and can be repaired primarily. A similar laceration caused by a dirty instrument on a farm may already be infected in three to four hours and a primary repair would be inadvisable.

If during the initial evaluation the decision is to delay primary repair because of other life-threatening injuries, the wounds should be cleansed gently with saline and soap, saline soaks should be initiated, and a broad spectrum antibiotic administered. Under these circumstances, a facial wound may be closed as late as 48 hours after the injury.

In instances where a facial wound has not received attention for 36 to 48 hours, the wounds should be cleansed, and saline soaks initiated. In about five days, in the absence of any inflammatory signs, this wound usually can be closed. Antibiotics may be started in cases of contaminated wounds, although with adequate local care there are differences of opinion as to their efficacy.

Anesthesia. Most soft tissue injuries may be repaired using local anesthesia. Adequate premedication is recommended to help allay apprehension, avoid restlessness, and achieve a measure of analgesia. Meperidine (Demerol) and diazepam (Valium) in appropriate doses are often helpful. Caution is essential, however, if there is a concomitant head injury.

Lidocaine (Xylocaine) 1 per cent with 1:100,000 epinephrine is an excellent local anesthetic that provides hemostasis within five to ten minutes. Toxic reactions are rare and are related to inadvertent intravascular injections or overdosage. In extensive facial lacerations in which a large volume may be required, Xylocaine 0.5 per cent with 1:200,000 epinephrine may be used. Allergic reactions are exceedingly rare, but a positive history should be heeded and a different anesthetic used. Whatever local anesthetic the surgeon chooses, he must know its pharmacologic effects and be prepared to treat its toxic and allergic reactions.

Anesthesia may be achieved with minimal discomfort to the patient if the solution is injected slowly, preferably under the wound margins. A sharp disposable 27-gauge needle is used. The face lends itself nicely to block anesthesia, which may be supplemented by infiltration anesthesia (Fig. 1).

In children, small lacerations may be repaired under local anesthesia. Bundling, gentle restraint, compassion, and patience are required. Extensive soft tissue injuries in children are best repaired under general anesthesia.

Local anesthesia should be administered before the patient's face is scrubbed.

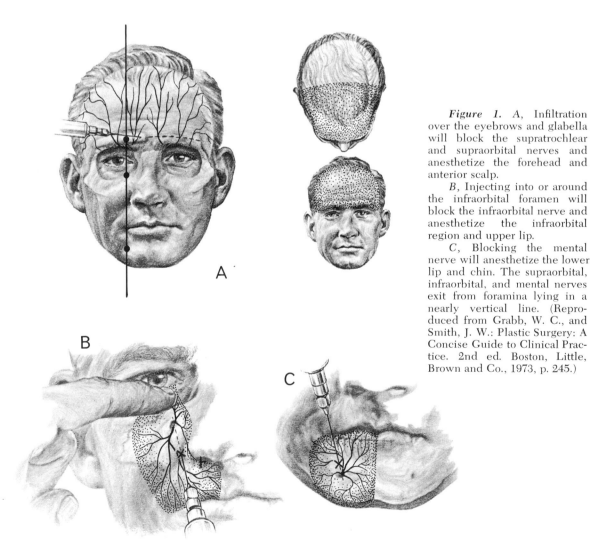

Figure 1. A, Infiltration over the eyebrows and glabella will block the supratrochlear and supraorbital nerves and anesthetize the forehead and anterior scalp.

B, Injecting into or around the infraorbital foramen will block the infraorbital nerve and anesthetize the infraorbital region and upper lip.

C, Blocking the mental nerve will anesthetize the lower lip and chin. The supraorbital, infraorbital, and mental nerves exit from foramina lying in a nearly vertical line. (Reproduced from Grabb, W. C., and Smith, J. W.: Plastic Surgery: A Concise Guide to Clinical Practice. 2nd ed. Boston, Little, Brown and Co., 1973, p. 245.)

The face can then be cleansed thoroughly without any discomfort to the patient. The function of the facial nerve and all areas of sensory loss should be recorded accurately prior to the administration of local anesthesia.

Treatment of Soft Tissue Injuries of the Face. The following fundamental principles of wound care should be observed in treating soft tissue injuries of the face:

(*a*) After the administration of anesthesia, wash the face and neck with a bland soap and copious amounts of saline. Shaving is unnecessary unless the patient has a beard or mustache. Do not shave the eyebrows.

(*b*) Sterile drape the face and neck (Fig. 2). Avoid operating through a keyhole in a towel.

(*c*) Obtain perfect hemostasis. Bleeding vessels should be clamped accurately and tied with fine ligatures. Small bleeding points may be electrocoagulated.

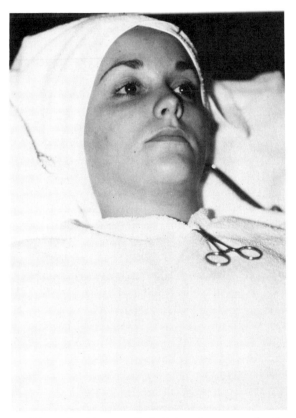

Figure 2. Four sterile bath towels — one under the head and shoulders, another wrapped around the forehead to exclude the hair, and two lying diagonally across the chest — give excellent exposure for repair of facial lacerations. The ears, when injured, may be left exposed. *Do not work through a keyhole in a towel.*

(*d*) Excise crushed and devitalized tissue conservatively. Remember that facial skin and its specialized structures (lips, eyelids, eyebrows, alae of the nose and ears) are difficult to reconstruct and should never be sacrificed unnecessarily. If in doubt about the viability of a tissue, preserve it.

(*e*) Explore all wounds gently, systematically, and completely. Remove blood clots and foreign material. Palpate carefully to ascertain the integrity of the underlying facial skeleton.

(*f*) Irrigate the wound copiously with saline to remove all blood clots and foreign material. Continue irrigation with each layer of closure.

(*g*) Atraumatic technique is essential. Handle tissues gently with skin hooks and avoid grasping the skin edges with forceps. Forceps, when required, should be finetoothed.

(*h*) Suture wounds meticulously. Muscles responsible for facial expression and mastication should be approximated carefully with absorbable suture to restore their function. Subcutaneous tissue is then approximated with 5–0 absorbable suture, and an inverted subdermal suture will relieve tension on the skin edges. Fine approximation of the wound margin is then achieved by atraumatic 6–0 nylon interrupted sutures (Fig. 3). These may be removed safely in four to five days. Although absorbable sutures generally are employed, some physicians advocate the use of fine colorless or white synthetic nonabsorbable suture material for the deep tissues. Excellent illustrations of many suturing techniques applicable to facial injuries also may be found in several textbooks (see Selected Reading List: 1,2,5).

(*i*) Appropriate tetanus immunization should be given.

Treatment of Common Types of Soft Tissue Injury. CONTUSIONS. The contused area should be washed gently with soap and water. Judicious application of cold during the first 12 hours and heat thereafter may help to decrease the edema. The efficacy of proteolytic agents (e.g., chymotrypsin) in reducing edema has not been substantiated (Rosenthal et al., 1970). If employed, they should be administered immediately after the injury has been sustained. Hematomas should be aspirated under aseptic technique and a pressure dressing applied. At times, blood clots may

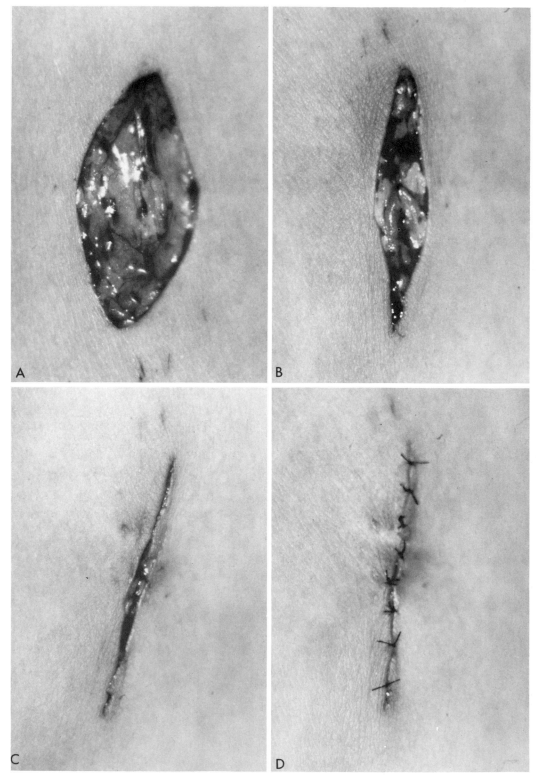

Figure 3.   *A*, After hemostasis and irrigation, the wound is ready for closure.
B, Subcutaneous sutures close the dead space.
C, Sturing the deep dermal layer brings the wound margins together.
D, 6–0 nylon sutures placed through the epithelium 1 mm. on either side of the wound will even up the margins.

be evacuated through a small, well-placed incision. Severely contused tissues may eventually necrose, requiring excision.

ABRASIONS. All superficial abrasions should be washed with soap and saline. If infection is avoided they should heal with minimal, if any, scarring. Application of antibiotic or bacteriocidal ointment two to three times daily until epithelialization is complete may be helpful. If gross contamination is present, a brush should be used to remove all foreign material.

Abrasions that extend deeply into the dermis heal with some scarring. Gross contamination (e.g., if the face has been dragged along the road, or if gun powder particles are imbedded in the tissue) should be treated vigorously while the wounds of entry are still open. If a brush fails to remove these "tattoos," painstaking removal of each particle with the point of a No. 11 Bard Parker blade is essential. Dermabrasion with a rotary disk in the operating room may be necessary if the "tattooing" is extensive. Grease can be removed using a small amount of ether on a sponge, followed by irrigation.

LACERATIONS. Meticulous, atraumatic closure of a laceration will result in a scar that seldom requires revision (Fig. 4). If the edges are ragged or severely contused, conservative trimming will improve the final result. Lacerations may run across normal crease lines. Attempts to change their direction by means of Z-plasty at the time of primary closure usually are inadvisable.

Stellate lacerations frequently result in unsightly scars. These lacerations consist of several small flaps whose contused apices may not survive. If they are small and located where the surrounding tissue may be mobilized, excision in the direction of the skin lines may prove to be the ideal solution.

AVULSION FLAPS. Tiny epidermal or dermal flaps, such as those seen when the forehead has struck a windshield, should be irrigated profusely; glass fragments should be removed, the flaps smoothed gently into their beds, and a pressure dressing applied. Revision and dermabrasion usually are necessary in six months' time to improve the cosmetic effect.

In large horseshoe flaps, the viability of

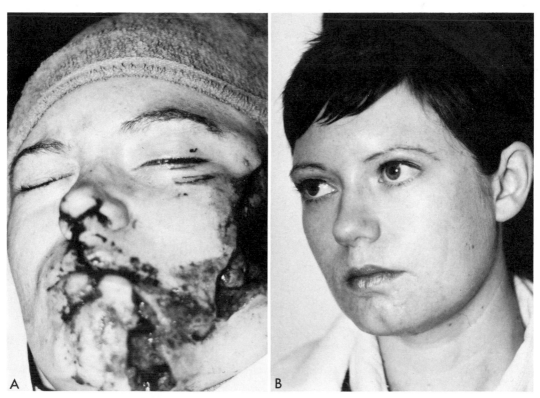

Figure 4. A, Facial lacerations repaired a few hours following injury.
B, Nine months later. The scars are acceptable and revision is unnecessary.

their distal end may be questionable. It is best to replace these in their beds and to suture them carefully. Usually a greater length survives than expected, and excision of the necrotic segment may be carried out later. These flaps often heal with a "trap door scar," an unsightly puckering above the surrounding tissues. The subsequent use of Z-plasties to correct this deformity may never be entirely satisfactory. If feasible with a small flap, an ideal solution is to convert a horseshoe flap into a linear scar by an elliptic excision placed in the direction of the skin lines. This may be done either at the initial repair or several months later (Converse, 1974).

AVULSION OF SOFT TISSUE. If the area of full thickness skin loss is small and located where undermining and primary closure can be done without distorting the surrounding facial features, this is often the best treatment. If this is not convenient, skin grafting or well-designed regional flaps may be necessary (Converse, 1974; Schultz, 1977). If the avulsed skin is brought in with the patient, it may be replaced, provided it is not severely contused and contamination is minimal. The tissue should be washed thoroughly and kept in saline. Its chances of survival are enhanced if it is defatted and sutured back within two hours from the time of injury (Grabb and Dingman, 1972).

Treatment of Injuries of Specific Soft Tissue Structures of the Face. The repair of certain soft tissue structures of the face deserves special consideration.

GINGIVA AND ORAL CAVITY MUCOSA. Oral mucosal lacerations should be sutured, the incidence of infection being no greater than if they are left open. Four-0 silk usually is employed since it is comfortable for the patient. Absorbable suture is used in children to avoid the task of suture removal. When the gingiva has been stripped from the alveolar ridge and necks of the teeth, it should be secured in place with a suture through the papilla, and around the tooth through the interdental space. If the wound is the result of contusion, suturing should be loose. Some physicians avoid closure of mucosa unless the wound is gaping, and they claim satisfactory results thereby.

TONGUE. Tongue lacerations must be sutured carefully to insure hemostasis and proper healing. Four-0 silk mattress sutures serve well with deep bites, and are best left in place for at least ten days. In children, 3–0 absorbable suture may be used.

LIP. Ideally, through-and-through lip lacerations should be repaired in three layers: mucous membrane is approximated with 5–0 absorbable suture, orbicularis oris muscle and subcutaneous tissue with 4–0 absorbable suture, and skin with 6–0 nylon. Approximating the muscle layer is necessary in order to reconstitute the oral sphincter. Proper alignment of the mucocutaneous junction is essential for a good cosmetic

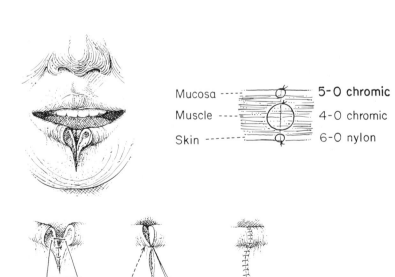

Figure 5. Stages in repairing a through-and-through lip laceration. Accurate approximation of the mucocutaneous junction early in the repair is essential to avoid notching. (Reproduced from Curtin, J. W.: Basic plastic surgical techniques in repair of facial lacerations. Surg. Clin. North Am. 53:44, 1973.)

result (Fig. 5). In cases of forceful contusion or tooth puncture, the nonvisible mucous membrane may be left unsutured and irrigated daily.

NOSE. Through-and-through lacerations require meticulous repair of the nasal mucosa with 5–0 absorbable suture, and of the skin with 6–0 nylon. Proper alignment of the alar rim and columella is necessary to obtain a good cosmetic result. Suturing back an amputated portion of the nose is almost always doomed to failure. Although reconstruction of this structure is difficult, the attempt is nevertheless worthwhile, since successful cases have been reported (Grabb and Dingman, 1972).

EAR. The excellent blood supply of the ear frequently insures its survival even after severe contusions and lacerations. Because ear reconstruction is difficult and often unsatisfactory, no part of it should be excised unless definitely necrotic. In cases of severe injury, the various parts should be unraveled and sutured, using 5–0 absorbable suture for the cartilaginous framework and 6–0 nylon for the skin. Hemostasis should be perfect to avoid hematomas (Fig. 6).

Dressing an injured ear is equally as important as careful repair, if a seroma or hematoma is to be prevented. Moist cotton pledgets should be packed into the convolutions of the auricle to achieve equal pressure throughout, using gauze and Kling to apply proper pressure. After 48 to 72 hours the ear should be inspected to determine its viability and for drainage of any seroma or hematoma that may have accumulated.

Seromas or hematomas following blunt trauma to the ear should be evacuated (aspirated or drained) and dressed carefully to prevent a "cauliflower" ear.

Although suturing back an ear that has been torn off completely is usually a futile exercise, successful replantation has been reported in the literature (McDowell, 1971; Mladick et al., 1971). The management of these cases is complex.

EYELIDS. Through-and-through lacerations of the eyelids should be sutured in three layers: tarsal plate and conjunctiva, orbicularis oculi muscle, and skin. Suture material and knots should be placed in such a manner that they do not lie against the globe, in order to prevent corneal abrasions

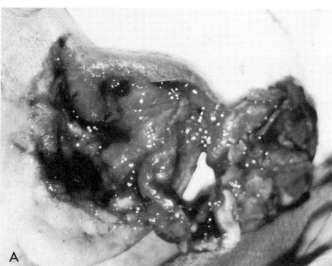

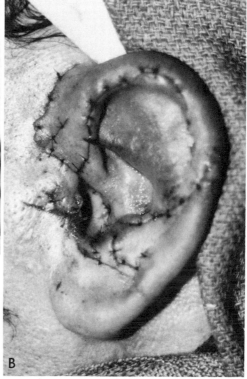

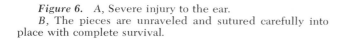

Figure 6. *A,* Severe injury to the ear.
B, The pieces are unraveled and sutured carefully into place with complete survival.

or ulcerations. Injuries to the levator palpebrae muscle must be recognized and treated promptly if ptosis of the eyelid is to be avoided (Converse, 1974).

Loss of part of the eyelid with exposure of the cornea should be recognized, and the services of a physician versed in ophthalmic plastic surgery should be sought (see Selected Reading List, No. 3).

COMPLICATIONS

Most complications of immediate treatment of soft tissue injuries are related to the development of hematomas, infections, and unsightly scars.

Hematomas. These contribute to wound pain, delay primary wound healing, and predispose to infection. Meticulous hemostasis will prevent their formation, but once they develop they should be evacuated and appropriate measures taken to prevent their recurrence.

Hematomas of the auricle and nasal septum are especially disastrous. Large hematomas in the oropharynx may cause an airway obstruction requiring tracheostomy.

Infections. These seldom develop in facial wounds caused by vehicular accidents. Animal and human bites or grossly dirty wounds are more likely to become infected, and a broad spectrum antibiotic should be given, in addition to thorough débridement of the wound.

Prompt recognition and vigorous treatment of all facial infections is essential. Midface infections may progress along the angular and ophthalmic veins into the cavernous sinus, causing thrombosis. This disastrous complication is manifested by fever, eyelid edema, chemosis, ophthalmoplegia, and delirium, and can result in death.

Infections of the auricular or nasal septal cartilages (often the result of untreated hematomas) are rare, but produce characteristic deformities ("cauliflower" ear, "saddle" nose) (Converse, 1974).

Scars. Disregarding the principles of soft tissue repair may result in unsightly scars that are sometimes difficult if not impossible to correct (Fig. 7) and that may have a profound psychologic effect on the patient for the rest of his life. Judicious revision of scars should not be carried out earlier than four to six months from the time of injury.

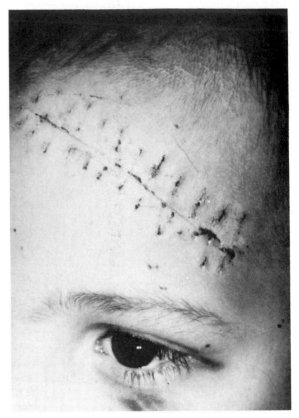

Figure 7. Revision of this wound to eliminate the cross-hatched suture marks is almost impossible. If left alone, this wound would have healed by contraction and epithelization, leaving a scar less objectionable and easier to revise.

The vagaries of these procedures should be explained to the patient as well as the course of scar formation. A scar that appears unsightly during the red/purple phase may be barely noticeable in the final white stage.

FRACTURES OF THE FACIAL SKELETON

A careful clinical examination combined with an adequate roentgenographic evaluation will establish the correct diagnosis of most facial fractures.

ROENTGENOGRAPHIC EVALUATION

A "facial bone fracture series" should be obtained in all patients with maxillofacial injuries. These should include: (*a*) Waters view; (*b*) posteroanterior view of the face; (*c*) lateral view of the face; (*d*) posteroanterior view of the mandible; (*e*) right and left oblique of the mandible; and (*f*) Towne view. A host of other views are available to clarify special problems, and the advice of a roentgenologist should be sought.

Dental films may be of inestimable value. Periapical films of the teeth and occlusal films of the maxilla or mandible show these structures in detail. "Panorex" views show the teeth, rami, and body of the mandible with clarity.

Maxillofacial injuries often are associated with skull and cervical spine injuries. Skull and cervical spine x-rays must be obtained before definitive therapy is initiated in these patients.

CLINICAL EXAMINATION

Frontal Sinus, Naso-orbital, and Frontoethmoidal Region. A depression above the glabellar area often indicates a depressed fracture of the anterior wall of the frontal sinus. Edema and supraorbital anesthesia may be present. The integrity of the posterior wall of the sinus should be determined by appropriate roentgenograms. Displaced fractures of the posterior wall involving dural tears that lead to cerebrospinal fluid (CSF) rhinorrhea, or injury to the frontal lobe, demand immediate neurosurgical consultation (Newman and Travis, 1973; Schultz, 1977).

Patients with fractures of the naso-orbital and frontoethmoidal area present with marked periorbital ecchymosis, subconjunctival hemorrhage, and a depressed nasal bridge. The medial canthal ligaments are disrupted, leading to an increased intercanthal distance (telecanthus, traumatic hypertelorism) (Converse, 1963, and 1974).

CSF rhinorrhea should be suspected in these patients, but its recognition may be difficult when it is mixed with blood or nasal secretions. The flow of a clear, nonviscous, salty-tasting fluid, which increases when the patient sits up or coughs, is suggestive of CSF rhinorrhea. The fluid can be tested for glucose, which is absent in nasal secretions, and for protein, whose content is less than that seen in serum.

The Middle Third of the Face. The zygoma, maxilla, and nasal bones comprise the middle third of the face. Of these, fractures of the zygoma and maxilla often go

unrecognized, but injuries to the nasal bones are easily recognized and are the most common fractures of the facial skeleton (Schultz, 1977).

NOSE. Clinical examination is far more important than roentgenography. Lateral deviation or depression of a patient's usual nasal contour often indicates a fracture or dislocation of the nasal bones or lateral cartilages. If the deformity is subtle, it may be obscured by edema, and it may be necessary to defer final diagnosis for several days. Crepitation may be present; in its absence, the patient must be relied upon to help determine whether the deformity is old or new. Speculum examination may reveal lacerations or fracture dislocations of the septum. A septal hematoma must be recognized and treated promptly (Converse, 1974); failure to do so may result in a septal abscess, destruction of the septal cartilage, and a "saddle" nose deformity.

MAXILLA. In contrast to nasal fractures, which often are seen independently, maxillary fractures are frequently seen in conjunction with nasal and zygomatic fractures. Again, clinical examination is more valuable then roentgenography (Fig. 8). If the maxilla can be moved back and forth, it is likely that the whole palatal segment is fractured. Fracture of one-half of the palate results in lateral flaring of the involved seg-

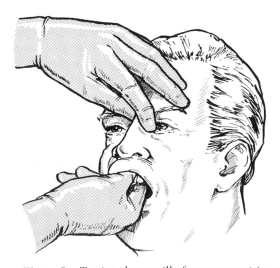

Figure 8. Testing the maxilla for movement is an excellent method to determine its integrity. Roentgenograms often are misleading. (Reproduced from McGregor, I. C.: Fundamental Techniques of Plastic Surgery and Their Surgical Applications, 6th ed. Edinburgh, Churchill Livingstone, 1975.)

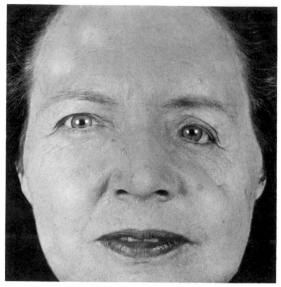

Figure 9. A flat left cheek and inferior displacement of the globe and the lateral canthus in a malar bone fracture. These changes may be obscured by edema during the early post injury period. (Reproduced from Converse, J. M.: Reconstructive Plastic Surgery, Vol. II. Philadelphia, W. B. Saunders Co., 1964.)

ment with a laceration frequently seen in the midline of the palate. If the maxilla and the nose as a unit can be rocked back and forth, a fracture of the whole maxillary complex is obvious. Malocclusion is invariably seen in displaced maxillary fractures.

ZYGOMA (MALAR) BONE AND ZYGOMATIC ARCH. Periorbital edema and ecchymosis, subconjunctival hemorrhage, and anesthesia of the upper lip, maxillary teeth, gingiva, and cheek should lead the physician to suspect a fracture of the body of the zygoma. In displaced fractures, the cheek prominence is flattened when compared to the other side, and palpation of the lower orbital rim may show a separation of the zygomaticomaxillary suture line. An inferior displacement of the globe and its lateral canthus may be present (Fig. 9). Subcutaneous emphysema in the cheek indicates that the integrity of the paranasal sinuses has

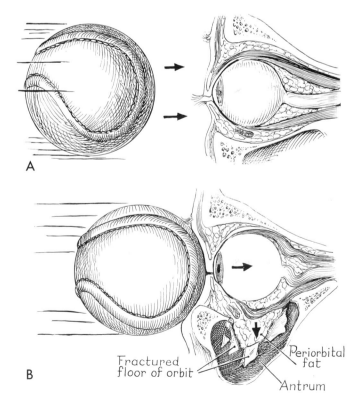

A

B

Fractured floor of orbit

Periorbital fat

Antrum

Figure 10. Blow-out fracture of the orbital floor. The periorbital fat and the inferior oblique and inferior rectus muscles are herniated into the antrum. (Reproduced from Converse, J. M.: Reconstructive Plastic Surgery, Vol. II. Philadelphia, W. B. Saunders Co., 1964.)

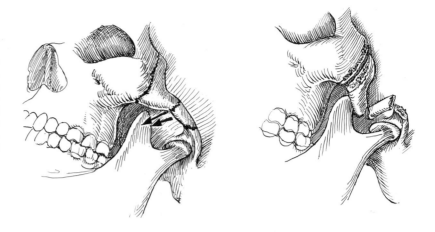

Figure 11. The medially displaced zygomatic arch fragments may impinge on the coronoid process, limiting mandibular excursions. (Reproduced from Converse, J. M.: Reconstructive Plastic Surgery, Vol. II. Philadelphia, W. B. Saunders Co., 1964.)

been violated. The patient should be warned against blowing his nose, which will increase the emphysema. Antibiotics should be given to prevent a midface soft tissue infection.

A "blow-out" fracture occurs when the floor and medial walls of the orbit are fractured, allowing herniation of the orbital contents (fat, inferior oblique, and inferior rectus muscles) into the maxillary sinus. In addition to diplopia, there is enophthalmos and limitation of upward gaze (Fig. 10) (Converse et al., 1967).

Zygomatic arch fractures should be suspected when there is an indentation over the arch. There may be trismus and limitation of mandibular excursion, as the medially displaced fragments impinge on the coronoid process (Fig. 11).

MANDIBLE, ALVEOLAR PROCESS AND TEETH. The key to the diagnosis and treatment of these structures is occlusion. Occlusion is the position in which a patient's teeth meet comfortably when he bites, and the physician should become acquainted with this anatomic relationship. The patient's statement, "My teeth don't meet right," ordinarily is a sign that the mandible, alveolar process and teeth, or the maxillae have sustained an injury with displacement.

Inspection and palpation, both intraorally and extraorally, will reveal most fractures of these structures (Fig. 12). The patient may complain of pain and tenderness over the fracture site. Anesthesia of the lower lip is present if the inferior dental nerve has been damaged. Tenderness over the temporomandibular joint and deviation of the jaw toward one side on opening may suggest a condylar fracture.

THE EYE. In all fractures of the middle third of the face, a complete eye examination is necessary.* Considering the severity of many midface fractures, injuries to the globe are remarkably few.

---

*See Chapter 15

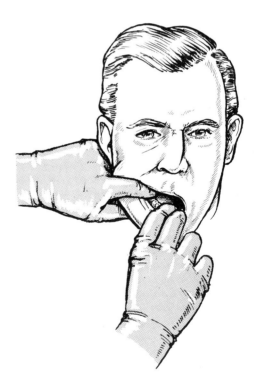

Figure 12. Careful intraoral and extraoral inspection of the mandible will detect many mandibular fractures. Forceful demonstration of crepitation at the fracture site, causing additional injury to the neurovascular bundle in the mandibular canal, is unnecessary. (Reproduced from McGregor, I. A.: Fundamental Techniques of Plastic Surgery and Their Surgical Applications, 6th ed. Edinburgh, Churchill Livingstone, 1975.)

Management

GENERAL CONSIDERATIONS

Many facial fractures are treated in the operating room. Certain procedures, however, may be carried out in the Emergency Department under local anesthesia. These are: (a) closed reduction of simple nasal fracture; (b) reduction of alveolar process fracture; (c) replantation of an avulsed tooth; (d) closed reduction of a simple mandibular fracture; and (e) reduction of a dislocated temporomandibular joint.

Undisplaced fractures of the facial skeleton need no treatment. If the fracture involves the maxilla or mandible, a high calorie, high protein liquid diet should be prescribed for four weeks until bony union occurs. It is wise to check the patient's occlusion periodically to confirm that the fragments have not been displaced.

TIMING OF REPAIR

If a patient has sustained an isolated injury (e.g., a nasal fracture), prompt closed reduction under local anesthesia may be carried out safely. Maxillofacial trauma, however, is often associated with other life-threatening injuries that require immediate treatment. If a general anesthetic is given, repair of the soft tissue injuries should be carried out at the same time, and treatment of facial fractures may be delayed until the patient's condition stabilizes. On occasion, if a patient's condition allows it, reduction of facial fractures may be carried out simultaneously.

Since alcohol ingestion frequently is associated with vehicular accidents and altercations, many patients with facial injuries arrive in the Emergency Department with stomachs filled with food and alcohol, in addition to blood, rendering them poor candidates for general anesthesia. A nasogastric tube should be used to empty the stomach, especially if a general anesthetic must be used because of associated life-threatening injuries.

Facial fractures may be reduced with good results as late as two weeks following injury. Consequently, focusing attention on the immediate treatment of these injuries, and neglecting—or overlooking—other life-threatening or potentially serious conditions should be avoided.

ANESTHESIA

General anesthesia is used in the treatment of most displaced facial fractures. However, local anesthesia can be used in the procedures described below.

NASAL FRACTURES. A simple, clinically displaced nasal fracture may be reduced either immediately after the injury, before the onset of edema, or several days later when the edema subsides. Premedication with Valium and Demerol is helpful. Three-inch rolled cotton pledgets are soaked in a solution of 5 per cent cocaine containing several drops of 1:1000 Adrenalin, and

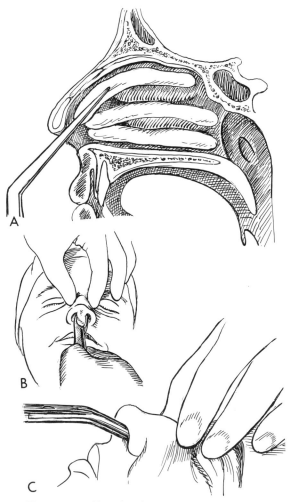

Figure 13. Closed reduction of nasal fracture.

A, Anesthesia is accomplished by cocaine-soaked cotton packs.

B and C, The nasal bones and septum are manipulated into position by means of an Asche forceps and the fingers of the left hand. (Reproduced from Converse, J. M.: Reconstructive Plastic Surgery, Vol. II. Philadelphia, W. B. Saunders Co., 1964.)

thoroughly squeezed out to remove excess solution. Under direct visualization one pack is placed along the floor of the nose, another along the roof, and the third along the middle turbinate. Using Xylocaine 1 per cent with 1:1000,000 epinephrine, the external nose is anesthesized by bilateral infraorbital nerve blocks and by infiltrating the root of the nose (Dingman, 1961). It is important to wait 15 to 20 minutes to achieve complete anesthesia.

An Asche or Walshom type forceps is inserted under the displaced nasal pyramid, which is manipulated along with the septum into proper position (Converse, 1974; Schultz, 1977). A depressed nasal bone on one side only may be elevated by a flat No. 3 knife handle (Fig. 13).

When the operator is satisfied, both by palpation and careful observation, that the nasal pyramid and septum are at the midline, nasal packs are inserted to support the fractured bones and to prevent hematomas. These are removed in two to three days. A nasal splint made of plaster of Paris, or one commercially available, is held over the nose for five to seven days for protection.

If the septum is injured, the patient should be warned that a deformity may appear gradually, often months later, and that further septal and nasal reconstruction may be necessary (Fry, 1967).

Injuries to Teeth. Fracture of a crown of a tooth, exposing its dentin or pulp, is a most painful situation. A commercially available celluloid crown form, held in place with zinc oxide eugenol paste, gives good relief until a dental consultation can be obtained.

A subluxated tooth should not be extracted, but manipulated gently into its proper position and then immobilized.

An avulsed tooth should not be discarded, especially in a youngster. It should be placed in cold saline, and the services of an oral surgeon experienced in replantation should be obtained. Teeth replanted within one-half hour of the accident may remain vital with gingival and periodontal reattachment. Later replants may become devitalized, and root resorption is frequently seen (Lu, 1973; Massler, 1974).

Alveolar Process Fractures. These occur more frequently in the maxilla than in the mandible. Adequate anesthesia may be achieved by injecting Xylocaine 1 per cent with 1:100,000 epinephrine into the buccal or labial sulcus and in the palatal area. The displaced alveolar plate is manipulated into position and immobilized by an arch bar attached to the intact teeth on either side. A liquid diet is prescribed for three to four weeks.

Fractures of the Mandible. Closed reduction of simple, minimally displaced fractures of the mandible may be achieved by a wide variety of techniques. One method involves the application of commercially available arch bars to the maxilla and mandible, after which rubber bands are applied to pull the teeth together into occlusion (Fig. 14). When normal occlusion is established, the rubber bands are replaced by loops of wire to immobilize the jaws for four to six weeks.

Fractures of one or both condyles often are treated by interdental fixation for four weeks. Fractures of the coronoid require no treatment. Most other fractures of the mandible require evaluation and treatment by a specialist.

Temporomandibular Joint Dislocation. This may occur from a blow to the lower jaw, a wide yawn, or simply opening the mouth too wide. The patient discovers that he is unable to close his mouth. Roentgenograms will demonstrate the condyle at, or anterior to, the articular eminence.

The administration of Valium and Demerol, at times with a muscle relaxant, frequently will result in spontaneous reduction of the dislocation. Injection of a local anesthetic into the masseter and internal pterygoid muscles to relieve spasms may aid in the reduction.

Manual reduction is accomplished by applying downward and posterior pressure with the index finger in the buccal sulci, while the thumbs push the chin upward. If this fails, the administration of general anesthesia or an open reduction becomes necessary (Fig. 15).

Following manual reduction of the dislocation, the patient is given analgesics and advised to remain on soft foods and to avoid opening the mouth wide for approximately three weeks. Recurrent dislocations result in temporomandibular joint arthropathy (Dingman and Constant, 1969).

FRACTURES OF THE FRONTAL SINUS, NASO-ORBITAL, AND FRONTOETHMOIDAL

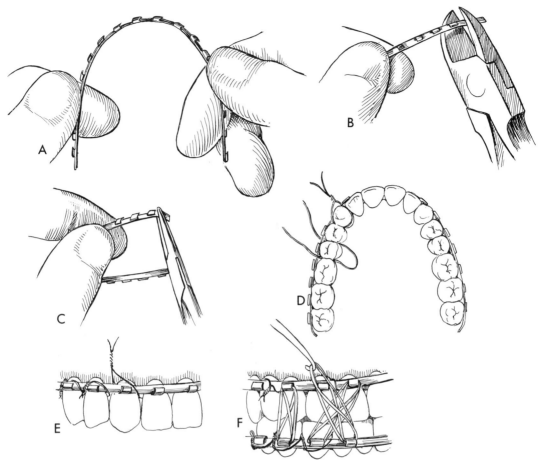

Figure 14.   *A, B,* and *C,* A commercially available arch bar is shaped to fit the maxillary and mandibular arches. *D* and *E,* Stainless steel wire secures the bar to the necks of the teeth.

    F, The maxilla and mandible are brought into occlusion and held in place with rubber bands. (Reproduced from Converse, J. M.: Reconstructive Plastic Surgery, Vol. II. Philadelphia, W. B. Saunders Co., 1964.)

REGION. Open reduction of the anterior table of the frontal sinus usually restores the forehead contour (Schultz, 1977). If the nasofrontal duct is injured and cannot be reconstructed, some authors recommend the occlusion of the duct, removal of the mucous membrane, and obliteration of the sinus cavity to prevent a mucopyocele (Newman and Travis, 1973). This complication is rare. If the posterior table is injured, resulting in a dural tear and cerebrospinal rhinorrhea, antibiotics should be administered and a neurosurgical consultation obtained promptly.

    In fractures of the naso-orbital and frontoethmoidal area, the fragments telescoped in the orbital or ethmoidal areas must be brought forward and the medial canthal ligaments reattached to correct the telecanthus. Nasolacrimal injuries should be repaired (Converse, 1974; Converse and Smith, 1966).

    MAXILLA. The goal of treatment of maxillary fractures is the establishment of normal occlusion. This is achieved by the application of arch bars, interdental fixation, and suspension of this unit to the zygomas or frontal bone (craniofacial suspension) (Converse, 1974).

    ZYGOMA AND ZYGOMATIC ARCH. Open reduction and interosseous wiring of the malar bone restores the cheek contour adequately. In "blow-out" fractures, the emphasis on the complications of enophthalmos and diplopia led to a policy of routine exploration of the orbital floor. This notion has been challenged recently, and operative intervention is reserved for a very few selected cases (Crikelair et al., 1972; Putterman, Stevens, and Urist, 1974).

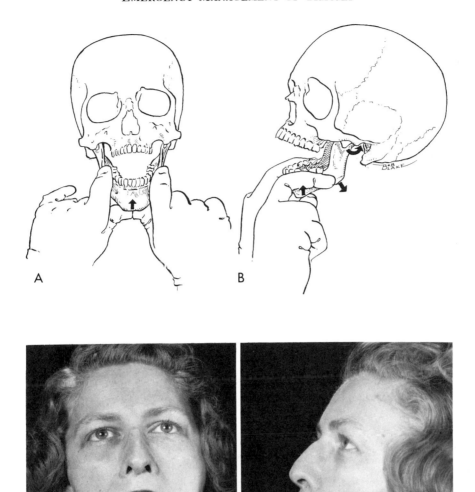

Figure 15. Method of reducing a dislocated temporomandibular joint. First the fingers in the buccal sulci apply pressure downward, then the thumbs push the chin upward and backward. (Reproduced from Converse, J. M.: Reconstructive Plastic Surgery, Vol. II. Philadelphia, W. B. Saunders Co., 1964.)

Depressed fractures of the zygomatic arch are elevated to restore the facial contour. On occasion, a severely depressed fracture may impinge on the coronoid process and interfere with lateral excursions of the mandible (Fig. 11). This must be corrected by elevating the fragments to their proper position.

Complications

The most common complication of nasal fracture treatment is the improper positioning of the nasal pyramid through inability to maintain the position of the nasal bones or lateral cartilages. This, along with the drifting of the nasal septum mentioned earlier,

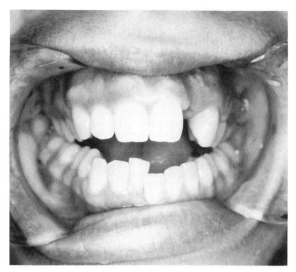

Figure 16. An open bite with only the molar teeth meeting. This is the result of bilateral condylar fracture.

may result in a poor cosmetic result and airway obstruction, requiring additional operations for correction.

Inadequate immobilization, local infection, and (rarely) osteomyelitis may lead to nonunion of fractures of the mandible. Malocclusion, occasionally with severe open bite, may be seen if the occlusal relationships of the teeth are not maintained. This is also noted in inadequate reduction of condylar fractures (Fig. 16).

RECOGNITION AND MANAGEMENT OF INJURIES TO THE VITAL STRUCTURES OF THE FACE

Three structures of vital importance may be involved in facial trauma. The prompt recognition and management of these injuries is very important.

FACIAL NERVE

Penetrating lacerations in the parotidomasseteric area may injure the main trunk of the facial nerve or one or more of its five main branches (forehead, eye, upper lip, lower lip, and—least important—cervical). The function of each should be tested and recorded prior to the administration of local or general anesthesia. Intelligent evaluation

and expert repair will free the patient from the burden of lifelong facial disfigurement.

If feasible, neurorrhaphy should be performed at the time of the initial soft tissue repair under general anesthesia. If the repair cannot be carried out during the first three days following injury, during which time the distal ends can be identified with the help of a nerve stimulator, the ends should be tagged with a clip or a black silk thread and a neurorrhaphy performed shortly after the 21st day (McCabe, 1972; Miehlke, 1974). If the branches of the facial nerve have been severed distal to a line dropped from the lateral canthus of the eye, neurorrhaphy is unnecessary (Fig. 17). Careful approximation of the muscles and soft tissues in this location results in significant return of facial expression within six months.

Facial paralysis may be seen in the absence of penetrating lacerations. Severe contusions (axonotmesis, neurapraxia) may be the cause. In addition, some 30 to 50 per

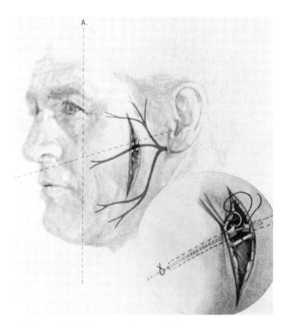

Figure 17. Repair of severed branches of the facial nerve in lacerations lying anterior to line A are unnecessary. Wound closure usually will result in good facial function within six months. Stensen's duct is found just below a line drawn between the tragus of the ear and the upper lip. A polyethylene tube threaded through the papilla will appear in the wound if the duct is severed. It also serves to splint the site of repair. (Reproduced from Grabb, W. C. and Smith, J. W.: Plastic Surgery: A Concise Guide to Clinical Practice, 2nd ed. Boston, Little, Brown and Co., 1973.)

cent of transverse fractures of the temporal bone may be associated with facial paralysis (Miehlke, 1974).

PAROTID GLAND AND DUCT—SUBMAXILLARY GLAND AND DUCT

A laceration of the capsule or substance or the parotid gland should be closed with a small rubber drain in place. Any salivary fistula that forms invariably ceases to drain as the wound scars down.

Recognition of injury to Stensen's duct, and its proper management, is essential to avoid the vexing problems of a salivary pseudocyst and a parotid duct fistula. The papilla of Stensen's duct, located next to the maxillary second molar tooth, should be visualized to determine if saliva can be expressed from it. If not, a polyethylene catheter should be inserted into the papilla and advanced until it presents itself into the wound. Repair should be carried out over the tube, which is left in place for two weeks (Fig. 17) (Abramson, 1974; Pallin and Trail, 1970).

The buccal and/or zygomatic branch of the facial nerve frequently is involved when Stensen's duct is severed, and a neurorrhaphy should be carried out at the same time. Lacerations of the submaxillary gland are infrequent, and any salivary fistula that forms ceases to drain shortly. Lacerations of Wharton's duct need not be repaired, as the new fistula drains into the mouth.

THE LACRIMAL SYSTEM

Naso-orbital fractures and, less frequently, lacerations of the medial canthus of the eye will injure the lacrimal excretory system (punctum, canaliculus, lacrimal sac, and nasolacrimal duct). Prompt recognition and treatment of these cases is essential to avoid the complications of epiphora and dacryocystitis (Converse, 1974).

Probing the duct system or injecting a dye into the sac to see it appear in the inferior meatus of the nose will help establish the diagnosis. These diagnostic maneuvers may need to be delayed until the edema subsides. Repair is done in the operating room at the time of injury, or days later when the swelling subsides. Good results have been reported in late repairs (Converse, 1974).

CONCLUSION*

Victims of maxillofacial injuries may be facially disfigured for life. Since the face is probably the most important portion of one's body image, the psychologic impact of such a disfigurement may be devastating. A long period of rehabilitation, both psychologic and physical, may be required to return these victims, often young when injured, to their careers and to a normal life. Prompt recognition and intelligent, skillful management of these injuries during the first few hours after the injury usually will give satisfactory results and hasten the return of these victims to their families, jobs, and society.

SELECTED READING LIST

1. Converse, J. M.: Kajanjian and Converse's Surgical Treatment of Facial Injuries. 3d ed. Baltimore, The Williams and Wilkins Co., 1974.

   The life work of two outstanding leaders of modern plastic surgery, Doctors Kajanjian and Converse, is contained within these two volumes. The early management and subsequent rehabilitation of facial trauma victims are described authoritatively and within a historical perspective. A classic in its field.

2. Dingman, R. O., and Natvig, R.: Surgery of Facial Fractures. Philadelphia, W. B. Saunders Co., 1964.

   An outstanding monograph describing the diagnosis and treatment of fractures of the facial skeleton with great clarity. Excellent illustrations.

3. Grabb, W. C., and Smith, J. W.: Plastic Surgery: A Concise Guide to Clinical Practice. 2d ed. Boston, Little Brown & Co., 1973.

   Fifty-three contributors cover all aspects of plastic and reconstructive surgery in this current, concise text. Well written with excellent bibliography.

4. Guralinck, W. C.: Textbook of Oral Surgery. Boston, Little Brown & Co., 1968.

   The body of knowledge that comprises modern oral surgery is covered in this concise text.

5. McGregor, I. A.: Fundamental Techniques of Plastic Surgery and Their Surgical Applications, 6th ed. Edinburgh, London, and New York, Churchill Livingstone, 1975.

*Acknowledgment: I am indebted to Drs. John Wiegenstein and Don G. Davis for their many helpful suggestions in the preparation of this manuscript.

A delightfully written brief text that conveys to the reader eloquently the magic, versatility, and challenge of modern plastic surgery.

6. Mustardé, J. D.: Repair and Reconstruction in the Orbital Region. Baltimore, The Williams and Wilkins Co., 1966.

A superb and unique book written by the surgeon who originated or perfected many of the techniques described. The authoritative text on reconstructive plastic surgery of the orbital region.

7. Rowe, N. L., and Killey, H. C.: Fractures of the Facial Skeleton. 2d ed. Edinburgh, Churchill Livingstone, 1968.

A comprehensive textbook on the management of facial injuries written by two outstanding British oral surgeons. Written clearly and authoritatively, it is a book of reference for all interested in facial trauma.

8. Schultz, R. C., Facial Injuries, Chicago. Year Book Medical Publishers, Inc. 1977.

A fine account of one surgeon's extensive experience in this field. A concise and clearly written text with excellent diagrams and illustrations.

References

Abramson, M.: Treatment of parotid duct injuries. Laryngoscope 183:1764, 1974.

Brooks, S. H., Nahum, A. M., and Siegel, A. W.: Causes of injury in motor vehicle accidents. Surg. Gynecol. Obstet. 131:185, 1970.

Converse, J. M.: Kajanjian and Converse's Surgical Treatment of Facial Injuries. 3rd ed. Baltimore, Williams & Wilkins Co., 1974.

Converse, J. M.: Facial disfigurement in automobile accidents. J.A.M.A. 185:354, 1963.

Converse, J. M., and Smith, B.: Naso-orbital fractures and traumatic deformities of the medial canthus. Plast. Reconstr. Surg., 38:147, 1966.

Converse, J. M., Smith, B., Obear, M. F., and Wood-

Smith, D.: Orbital blow-out fractures: a ten-year survey. Plast. Reconstr. Surg. 39:20, 1967.

Crikelair, G. F., Rein, J. M., Potter, G. D., and Cosman, B.: A critical look at the "blow-out" fracture. Plast. Reconstr. Surg. 49:374, 1972.

Dingman, R. O.: Local anesthesia for rhinoplasty and the nasal septum in rhinoplastic surgery. Plast. Reconstr. Surg. 28:251, 1961.

Dingman, R. O.: Correction of nasal deformities due to defects of the septum. Plast. Reconstr. Surg. 18:291, 1956.

Dingman, R. O., and Constant, E.: A fifteen-year experience with temporomandibular joint disorders. Plast. Reconstr. Surg. 44:119, 1969.

Eiseman, B., and Spencer, F. C.: Tracheostomy: an underrated surgical procedure. J.A.M.A. 184:684, 1963.

Fry, H.: Nasal skeletal trauma and the interlocked stresses of the nasal septal cartilage. Br. J. Plast. Surg. 20:146, 1967.

Grabb, W. C., and Dingman, R. O.: The fate of amputated tissues of the head and neck following replacement. Plast. Reconstr. Surg. 49:28, 1972.

Lu, M.: Replantation of avulsed anterior teeth in patients with jaw fractures. Plast. Reconstr. Surg. 51:377, 1973.

Massler, M.: Tooth replantation. Dent. Clin. North Am. 18:445, 1974.

McCabe, B.: Injuries to the facial nerve. Laryngoscope 82:1891, 1972.

McDowell, F.: Successful replantation of a severed half ear. Plast. Reconstr. Surg. 48:281, 1971.

Miehlke, A.: Extratemporal injury and repair of the facial nerve. Otolaryngol. Clin. North Am. 7:467, 1974.

Mladick, R. A., Horton, C. E., Adamson, J. E., and Cohen, B. I.: The pocket principle: a new technique for the reattachment of a severed ear part. Plast. Reconstr. Surg. 48:219, 1971.

Newman, H., and Travis, L. W.: Frontal sinus fractures. Laryngoscope 83:1281, 1973.

Pallin, J. L., and Trail, M. L.: Trauma to the parotid region. South. Med. J. 63:1389, 1970.

Putterman, A. M., Stevens, T., and Urist, M. J.: Nonsurgical management of blow-out fractures of the orbital floor. Am. J. Ophthalmol. 77:232, 1974.

Rosenthal, S. G., Song, C. J., Bromberg, B. E., and Adamson, R. J.: Chymotrypsin—effects on water content and strength of healing wounds. Plast. Reconstr. Surg. 46:287, 1970.

Schultz, R. C.: Facial Injuries. Chicago, Year Book Medical Publishers Inc., 1977.

D. TRAUMA TO THE NECK

William E. DeMuth, Jr., and Gary G. Nicholas

INTRODUCTION

The neck is a compact area that contains major components of three life support systems: the respiratory system, the central nervous system, and the cardiovascular system. Thus, the initial evaluation and management of blunt and penetrating neck injuries must be well planned and executed.

Emergency care of the patient with neck

injury should be undertaken at the scene of the accident if qualified personnel are in attendance. First priority must be given to the establishment of a satisfactory airway. Aspiration of the upper airway, orotracheal intubation or cricothyroidotomy may be required. Secondly, or concomitantly, the control of hemorrhage is best accomplished by direct pressure applied to the wound. Third, two large caliber intravenous lines should be placed. Blood should be drawn for type and cross-match of at least four units of whole blood. For transportation, the patient should be in the supine position in order to decrease the risk of air embolism. In evaluating the airway and the vascular structures, one must be mindful of the possibility of doing more damage to existing cervical spine or cord lesions. The latter are discussed in another chapter, but basic precautionary measures must be mentioned here. If the head is held in a deviated position, it must not be corrected by manipulation, lest the cord be damaged by vertebral misalignment. Pain and rigidity of the cervical muscles likewise should be respected, for underlying spine injury may be present. A cervical collar or other support should be applied at the scene.

The cross-table lateral roentgenogram, which must include all seven cervical vertebrae, is the most important x-ray to be taken in patients with head and neck injuries.

Exploration of a penetrating neck wound in the Emergency Department is contraindicated. Hemorrhage may be exacerbated and blind clamping may cause serious damage to underlying vital structures. All penetrating neck wounds that disrupt the platysma muscle require formal exploration by a qualified surgeon in a well equipped operating room. Although there is some minor controversy on the dogma to explore all penetrating wounds deep to the platysma, the vast majority of authors favor compulsory exploration (Fogelman and Stewart, 1956; Jones, Terrell, and Salyer, 1967; Knightly, Swaminathan, and Rush, 1973). Fogelman reported a series of 100 cases of penetrating neck wounds, and noted a mortality of 35 per cent in those that were not explored. Patients in his series who had immediate exploration had a mortality of 5 per cent. The urgency of formal exploration also has been well documented. There is a fivefold increase in the mortality rate for patients in whom exploration is delayed beyond six hours (Fogelman and Stewart, 1956). Blunt neck injury likewise may require formal exploration.

Mechanism of Injury — Anatomic and Ballistic Considerations

Classically, injuries have been categorized as blunt or penetrating. Although useful, this classification falls short when missiles are considered. Perforations caused by knives, ice picks, and similar instruments damage by destroying tissue in the direct path taken by the penetrating object. The intimate anatomic relationships found in the neck predispose to multiple structural injuries.

On the other hand, the remarkable compactness and mobility of the neck are great assets. Posteriorly, heavy muscles and the cervical skeleton afford great protection of the anterior visceral compartments, and the mandible shields the throat anteriorly. Well developed visual and auditory reflexes cause cervical flexion and extension of the arms that act to protect the anterior neck in times of danger.

The larynx and trachea are the most anterior of the vital cervical structures, and therefore are prone to be damaged by blunt or sharp objects. Although vulnerable to injury, these structures are accessible for establishing an airway if obstruction is present. The thyroid cartilage is easily identified by palpation, as is the trachea in most patients. A finger placed at the upper end of the thyroid cartilage reveals the prominent notch. Two to three centimeters down is the clear interval between the thyroid and cricoid cartilage, the cricothyroid membrane.

For practical purposes, low velocity bullets such as the .22 caliber rimfire inflict injuries only within the wound track. Although structures directly hit may be extensively damaged, the devastating temporary cavity with wide tissue destruction characteristic of high-velocity missiles is not seen.

PENETRATING BULLET INJURIES

In civilian life, few patients sustaining high velocity bullet wounds of the neck reach the Emergency Department alive. Indeed, survival after a direct hit is rare even in military situations. Expanding bullets used in hunting firearms are so destructive that only victims with tangential wounds have a chance of surviving. The full-jacketed bullet demanded by the Geneva Convention in the military is somewhat less destructive, but still deadly in the neck. Even with tangential wounds, cavitation may result in damage to deep structures that may not be recognized because of the absence of obvious tissue damage. Even when high-velocity bullets do not strike a vital structure, the temporary cavity formed is enormous and is proportional to the velocity of the missile. Expressed mathematically, kinetic energy, the determinant of wounding capacity, is: $KE = mass \times velocity^2$. Obviously, small increments in velocity result in marked increases in wounding capacity.

What applies in the neck also pertains to other anatomic locations. Tissues richly endowed with elastic tissue, such as skin and lung, are very resistant to the effects of high-velocity missiles, whereas structures having high specific gravity, such as bone and liver, are especially prone to such damage. Vessels demonstrate substantial resistance but, as in other situations in which vascular injuries may occur, intimal disruption may be present without gross damage to the vessel exterior.

BLUNT INJURIES

Just as penetrating wounds may seem deceptively innocent, apparently innocuous blunt injuries can cause severe life-threatening injuries. Cyanosis, dyspnea, and subcutaneous emphysema suggest cricoid fracture with tracheal avulsion. Blunt trauma may be more subtle, but extensive vascular, CNS, and visceral injury may be produced (Chodosh, 1968; Mant, 1972; Simeone and Goldberg, 1968; Towne, Neis, and Smith, 1972). Vascular injury secondary to blunt trauma usually is produced by intimal disruption with subsequent thrombosis, with or without embolization. Central nervous system injury may involve secondary intracranial hemorrhage or direct trauma of the spinal cord in association with cervical spine fractures and dislocations. Visceral injuries may include disruption of the trachea or esophagus by the sudden compression of air trapped in

their lumina. Hemorrhage into the thyroid may lead to respiratory distress.

Whereas a superficial knowledge of ballistics affords some understanding of the magnitude of injury expected, blunt forces for the most part are poorly quantitated and cannot even be estimated in most deceleration injuries, in which an extraordinary number of variables act to modify the forces.

AIRWAY INJURY

Despite the well-recognized necessity for early establishment of an adequate airway in instances of facial, cervical, and thoracic injuries, lives are still lost for lack of clear understanding of the problems and the correct actions to take to deal with them. Most important is resuscitation and the preparation for definitive care.

Airway injury may manifest itself by obstruction, subcutaneous emphysema, coughing up blood, change of voice, or signs of hypoxia. The presence of stertorous breathing in association with restlessness, cyanosis, and increased use of accessory respiratory muscles makes the diagnosis of airway obstruction and hypoxia obvious. Noisy respiration or the complete absence of ingress and egress of air is an obvious sign. Snoring or stertorous breathing in the comatose patient often is dismissed as something seen in normal sleep, a dangerous supposition in the injured. Blood, mucus, vomitus, loose teeth, and dentures found in the mouth are obstructing agents that should be looked for and removed. Retraction of the suprasternal space and sternum gives additional clues to upper airway obstruction.

Since obstruction of the airway caused by aspirated blood, vomitus, or foreign bodies is frequent, aspiration of the oropharynx and trachea should be the first maneuver performed in the establishment of the airway. If manipulation of the upper airway is inadequate (and it should be successful in over 90 per cent of instances), endotracheal intubation should be undertaken. If this is not possible, cricothyroidotomy should be performed. In the hypoxic, hemorrhaging patient this is a much easier procedure than standard tracheotomy. (The method to perform a cricothyroidotomy is illustrated on page 420.)

As a less desirable alternative, transtracheal catheter ventilation has been employed. Needles or small cannulae are inserted through the cricothyroid membrane or trachea. In general, air movement through these small devices is inadequate to sustain life. If a single skilled attendant is faced with a need for cardiopulmonary resuscitation, the method may be useful if gas under pressure is applied to the airway. A No. 14 catheter can be inserted into the airway in a few seconds and, if oxygen at 60 psi and a 6-liter flow rate is passed into the catheter intermittently, adequate aeration will result. The pressurized tank valve should be opened and closed to provide inspiration and expiration on a 1:2 ratio. The adequacy of the airway is determined by the presence of ventilation indicated by chest expansion; the absence of those findings suggests airway obstruction. If it is not immediately apparent that ventilation has been improved, associated thoracic injuries such as tension pneumothorax or hemothorax should be sought.

ASSOCIATED THORACIC INJURIES IN NECK TRAUMA

Complete evaluation of the airway includes examination of the thorax for evidence of pneumothorax, tension pneumothorax, or hemopneumothorax. Cyanosis and respiratory distress will persist after the upper airway has been cleared if tension pneumothorax is present.

Physical examination of the involved hemithorax will reveal hyper-resonance with decreased breath sounds. Shock may persist, after what appears to be adequate correction of hypovolemia, as a result of concomitant hemorrhage. Tension pneumothorax demands immediate aspiration with a large bore needle, or the insertion of a chest tube that can be placed to water-seal drainage. A similar picture of persistent shock and respiratory distress can be seen in patients with massive hemothorax. However, dullness to percussion with an absence of breath sounds will be noted on the involved side. Needle aspiration or placement of a chest tube will confirm the diagnosis.

Persistent bleeding after initial decompression may demand immediate thoracotomy, particularly if injury to the great vessels is suspected.

Radiographic confirmation of intrathoracic injury should be obtained, but not at the expense of jeopardizing the resuscitation of a critically ill patient. If any suspicion of such injury is present, tube thoracostomy is immediately indicated. The aphorism that the treatment of a pneumothorax is a chest tube, not a chest x-ray, holds considerable validity.

LARYNGEAL FRACTURE

Compression of the larynx against the cervical vertebral bodies by a direct blow to the neck, as from an automobile steering wheel, may produce a laryngeal fracture with associated airway obstruction. Besides the previously described symptoms of airway obstruction, the three most common symptoms of laryngeal fracture are: subcutaneous emphysema; aphonia; and severe facial pain (Shumrick, 1973). Coughing may extrude air through a small mucosal tear in the larynx and produce massive subcutaneous emphysema. Aphonia is the result of deformation of the larynx that follows fractures with subsequent overriding of the fragments. Massive hematomas located in the glottic area also may produce aphonia. Facial pain may be exacerbated by swallowing or coughing.

The best diagnostic sign of a fractured larynx is the loss of normal anatomic landmarks produced by the laryngeal cartilages. Flattening of the anterior neck is noted, with loss of prominence of the thyroid cartilage. Closed blunt injury of the airway has been reported to result in complete disruption of the trachea from the larynx (Chodosh, 1968). The trachea retracts into the superior mediastinum, and an inability to palpate the trachea in the neck should alert one to the possibility of this diagnosis.

The diagnosis of laryngeal injury may be facilitated by soft tissue x-rays of the cervical region. Laryngograms utilizing water soluble contrast media are also valuable. Direct laryngoscopy is a useful technique.

Prior to manipulation of the fractured larynx, tracheostomy should be performed, since the partially compromised airway may be totally occluded in the attempted examination.

Open reduction and fixation with internal stents and wiring to produce stabilization constitutes the definitive treatment.

COMBINED AIRWAY AND VASCULAR INJURY

The presence of bubbling, frothing blood in the wound or airway suggests a combined tracheal and vascular injury. When concomitant airway and vascular injury is suspected, the passage of an endotracheal tube, the cuff of which, if possible, should be inflated below the tracheal or laryngeal injury, is the best means of controlling the airway. Once the cuff is inflated, digital pressure applied to the bleeding wound will control most bleeding vessels in the neck.

Hemorrhage from a penetrating neck wound should be controlled by external pressure. Circumferential bandaging, wrapping or taping is absolutely contraindicated. Major vessel injury in association with disruption of the trachea may produce airway obstruction from aspiration of blood. In these patients, as well as in those with closed space hematoma compressing the trachea, immediate intubation or cricothyroidotomy is necessary. Hemorrhage in the neck produces unique problems, but the likelihood of hypovolemic shock must not be overlooked. Insertion of two large-bore intravenous lines and immediate crossmatching of whole blood is mandatory. A healthy adult suffering trauma will be able to tolerate at least 2 liters of balanced salt solution in the course of the initial resuscitation.

COMPLICATIONS OF AIRWAY INJURY

Complications of treatment of airway injury may be either immediate or delayed. Immediate problems may arise if the pharyngeal or laryngeal mucosa is torn in the course of inept endotracheal intubation. Hemorrhage may occur if the thyroid gland or the contents of the carotid sheath are injured in the course of cricothyroidotomy or tracheostomy. Late complications include laryngeal or tracheal stenosis. Phonation may be impaired if the recurrent laryngeal nerve has been injured.

VASCULAR INJURY

Types. Next to airway obstruction, bleeding is the most common cause of death in cervical injuries. Penetrating wounds of the neck may easily extend into the superior mediastinum with injuries of the great vessels. The carotid and vertebral arteries, as well as the jugular veins, may be the source of major bleeding from cervical injuries.

The large external jugular veins are very superficial and prone to injury by lacerations and stab wounds. Suicide attempts notoriously involve these vessels. Injuries of the large veins may give rise to torrential external bleeding. Despite its being a low pressure system, venous bleeding within the fascial compartments of the neck also may result in airway compromise and cerebral edema due to the obstructed venous outlet. This dreaded complication of thyroidectomy is well known to all surgeons. Added to this is the possibility of air embolism resulting from air being sucked into open cervical veins.

Air Embolism. When injury has occurred to a large vein, such as the internal jugular, air embolism must be considered. This is best avoided by transporting the patient supine and applying pressure to the wound. If there is a suspicion that air embolism has taken place, the patient should be placed on his left side.

Control of Bleeding. Most external bleeding can be controlled by direct digital pressure over the wound. Carotid artery injuries may be more difficult to control, but in no instance should circumferential neck dressings be applied. When the wounding instrument (knife, ice pick, or other object) is found protruding from a neck wound, it should not be removed or otherwise manipulated in the Emergency Department. These objects frequently penetrate major vessels and afford a tamponade effect which, if removed, may result in fatal hemorrhage. They should be removed in the operating room during cervical exploration or thoracotomy, where vessel control is possible.

Probing or attempted clamping of vessels in bleeding wounds of the neck is absolutely contraindicated in the emergency room. Serious injuries of major vessels, the thoracic duct, the brachial plexus, or the recurrent laryngeal nerve have followed such efforts.

Definitive treatment of vascular injuries is carried out in the operating room. In general, major arteries are reconstructed and venous injury can be treated by ligation.

Cerebral Blood Flow Considerations. The circulation to the brain is entirely dependent on the carotid and vertebral blood flow. In addition to the rapid blood loss that follows major arterial injuries in the neck, attempts to stop this loss may result in cerebral hypoxia. Digital pressure may control external bleeding, only to result in retention of blood within the fascial compartments of the neck, thus adding a strangling pressure effect upon the airway. Since continued bleeding will result in death from loss of blood volume, this chance must sometimes be taken.

Major vessel injury in the neck is unique in several respects. Cerebral infarction may result from disruption of one of the major cervical vessels, or later as a result of a failed vascular reconstruction. Vascular injury may be manifest by hemorrhage, thrombosis, or formation of an arteriovenous fistula. Late sequelae include the formation of traumatic aneurysms (Teal et al., 1972).

Hemorrhage may occur externally, or it may be contained within the fascial compartments of the neck. These contained hematomas may cause compression of the trachea, with subsequent airway obstruction. Pulsation of a hematoma suggests major underlying vascular injury. The absence of pulsation either in the upper extremity or in the temporal artery suggests a major vessel thrombosis. Ischemia of the upper extremity or brain is likewise indicative of vascular compromise. A continuous bruit or thrill in the area of injury is diagnostic of an arteriovenous fistula. Central nervous system symptoms may provide evidence of vascular compromise. The "lucid interval" so typical of epidural hemorrhage may be seen following blunt trauma to the carotid artery, with intimal disruption and subsequent propagation of thrombosis (Caldwell and Hadden, 1948; Towne, Neis, and Smith, 1972). Thrombosis of the vertebral artery may be manifest as brain stem ischemia and cerebellar signs such as cranial nerve deficits, ataxia, and long tract signs. This usually occurs in association with fractures of the transverse processes or partial subluxation of the upper cervical spine (Simeone and Goldberg, 1968). Subarachnoid hemorrhage may occur with disruption of the vertebral artery at the base of the skull (Mant, 1972).

Angiography probably is indicated only for those patients in whom there is no obvious need for exploration of the neck (Smith et al., 1974). Ashworth reported that one-third of the patients with major vascular injury in his survey showed no clinical evidence of this injury (Ashworth, Williams, and Byrne, 1971).

INJURIES TO PHARYNX AND ESOPHAGUS

Injuries of the pharynx and esophagus do not pose a threat to life in the few hours following injury. The esophagus lies deep and just anterior to cervical vertebrae, and deep penetration usually is required to perforate it. Unrecognized, these wounds may lead to fatal infections of the mediastinum, sometimes causing infection that dissects upward to the hyoid bone and results in upper airway obstruction.

Injury to the esophagus frequently is manifest by dysphagia or spitting up blood. However, early in the postinjury period there may be no symptoms that can be attributed to the esophagus or pharynx. If a satisfactory airway has been established and hemorrhage is controlled, a PA and lateral film of the neck and chest, combined with an esophagogram utilizing water-soluble radiopaque contrast material, is very useful in establishing the diagnosis of esophageal injury. Esophagoscopy also is a useful maneuver in this regard.

If the recognition of esophageal injury is delayed because of associated injuries or overlooked at the time of initial evaluation, mediastinitis with abscess formation and sepsis is likely to occur. Swelling due to inflammation in the visceral fascial compartment of the neck may produce late airway compromise. The finding of pneumomediastinum may not be evident for several hours, so a repeat x-ray may be necessary.

The treatment of esophageal injuries is carried out at the time of neck exploration in the operating room. Closure of the disruption and drainage is the preferred method of management. If seen after the development of abscess and infection, drainage of the area may be all that is possible. Antibiotics should be started as soon as the diagnosis of food passage perforation is made. Broad spectrum antibiotic coverage is essential owing to the variety of bacteria found in the oropharynx and esophagus. Treatment should be directed at both aerobic and anaerobic organisms.

NEUROLOGIC INJURY

Spinal cord injury may occur in conjunction with penetrating or blunt neck injuries.

It is essential that unstable cervical spine fractures be recognized in order to avoid possible damage to the spinal cord. Any evidence of neurologic deficit in the extremities should alert the physician to this possibility. Cross-table lateral radiographs should be obtained if there is any suspicion of spine injury. The neck should be splinted until it is demonstrated that no cervical spine injury has occurred.

Other neurologic injuries occurring in association with neck trauma are not life-threatening; however, their recognition is important to the subsequent care of the patient. Brachial plexus injury may be caused by external pressure of hematomas or from fractures of the clavicle. A preliminary neurologic examination is of great importance medicolegally. Functional integrity of the brachial plexus is easily ascertained by testing sensory and motor function of the hand and arm. Direct laceration or avulsion of the components of the plexus is also possible. Injury to the phrenic nerve may be diagnosed if a high, immobile diaphragm is noted on physical examination. Fluoroscopy of the diaphragm can provide future documentation of this injury.

Injury to the stellate ganglion may result in a Horner's syndrome. The resulting pupillary inequality may on occasion be misinterpreted to indicate intracranial injury.

Stridor or alteration in phonation may be seen with injury to the vagus nerve, or, specifically, the recurrent laryngeal branch. Airway obstruction can occur when bilateral damage has taken place. Weakness of the trapezius muscle will indicate damage to the spinal accessory nerve as it courses through the posterior cervical triangle. Deviation of the tongue toward the injured hypoglossal nerve will be seen if this cranial nerve is damaged in the upper portion of the anterior cervical triangle.

The definitive management of nerve injury in the neck consists of relief of any external pressure, as in the patient with a hematoma compressing an adjacent nerve, or primary repair of the nerve if possible. Results of primary repair probably are as good as, or better than, delayed repair, except in the case of massive tissue loss or gross contamination.

THORACIC DUCT

Injury to the thoracic duct poses no immediate threat to life. Failure to recognize this injury at the time of exploration of the neck wound may lead to a fistula that will require a secondary procedure for closure. Suspicion of this injury should be raised when a penetrating injury has occurred in the left supraclavicular region. Thoracic duct fistulization can produce significant fluid and protein loss. Treatment consists of ligation of the duct proximal and distal to the point of injury.

SELECTED READINGS

1. Fogelman, M. J., and Stewart, R. D.: Penetrating wounds of the neck. Am. J. Surg. 91:581, 1956.

   This is a review of 100 cases that documents the value of early exploration of all penetrating neck wounds.

2. Jones, R. F., Terrell, J. C., and Salyer, K. E.: Penetrating wounds of the neck: an analysis of 274 cases. J. Trauma 7:228, 1967.

   The authors review 274 cases of penetrating neck injuries and outline the initial method of management.

3. Fitchett, V. H., Pomerantz, M., Butsch, D. W., Simon, R., and Eiseman, B.: Penetrating wounds of the neck. Arch. Surg. 99:307, 1969.

   This is a review of the authors' experience with neck wounds seen in Vietnam.

References

Ashworth, C., Williams, L. F., and Byrne, J. J.: Penetrating wounds of the neck. Am. J. Surg. 121:387, 1971.

Caldwell, H. W., and Hadden, F. C.: Carotid artery thrombosis: report of eight cases due to trauma. Ann. Intern. Med. 28:1132, 1948.

Chodosh, P. L.: Cricoid fracture with tracheal avulsion. Arch. Otolaryngol. 87:461, 1968.

Committee on Trauma, American College of Surgeons. Early Care of the Injured Patient. 1st ed. Philadelphia, W. B. Saunders Company, 1972.

Fogelman, M. J., and Stewart, R. D.: Penetrating wounds of the neck. Am. J. Surg. 91:581, 1956.

Jones, R. F., Terrell, J. C., and Salyer, K. E.: Penetrating wounds of the neck: an analysis of 274 cases. J. Trauma 7:228, 1967.

Knightly, J. J., Swaminathan, A. P., and Rush, B. F.: Management of penetrating wounds of the neck. Am. J. Surg. 126:575, 1973.

Mant, A. K.: Traumatic subarachnoid haemorrhage following blows to the neck. J. Forensic Sci. Soc. 12:567, 1972.

Oppenheimer, R. P.: Airway...instantly. J.A.M.A. 230:76, 1974.

Shumrick, D. A.: Trauma of the larynx and lower airway. Otolaryngology 3:609, 1973.

Simeone, F. A., and Goldberg, H. I.: Thromboses of the

vertebral artery from hyperextension injury to the neck. J. Neurosurg. 29:540, 1968.

Smith, R. F., Elliott, J. P., Hageman, J. H., Szilagyi, D. E., and Xavier, A. O.: Acute penetrating arterial injuries of the neck and limbs. Arch. Surg. 109:198, 1974.

Teal, J. A., Bergeron, R. T., Rumbaugh, C. L., and

Segall, H. D.: Aneurysms of the cervical portion of the internal carotid artery associated with nonpenetrating neck trauma. Radiology 105:353, 1972.

Towne, J. B., Neis, D. D., and Smith, J. W.: Thrombosis of the internal carotid artery following blunt cervical trauma. Arch. Surg. 104:565, 1972.

E. CHEST AND HEART INJURIES

Panagiotis N. Symbas

The third leading cause of death in the U.S. is trauma, and a significant number of these fatalities are due to chest injuries. The availability of high speed travel and the considerable violence in our society have resulted in this great increase in thoracic trauma.

The magnitude of injury to the intrathoracic organs cannot be determined by external appearances alone. Blunt trauma may have left only a few external marks of injury and yet may have caused extensive internal damage. The extent of an injury from a bullet also cannot be determined accurately from the wound; internal damage depends on the velocity of the bullet, its size, the distance traveled, and its pathway in the thorax (see *Evaluation of Trauma*, p. 598, for ballistic considerations).

The thoracic injury can be due to nonpenetrating trauma, commonly as the result of a vehicle accident, or to penetrating trauma, frequently due to missle or knife wounds. Depending on the cause of the thoracic injury, some special injuries of the thorax may result. Blunt trauma may result in a fracture of the ribs, with or without flail chest wall segment; hemothorax; pneumothorax; subcutaneous emphysema; contusion of the lung; rupture of a bronchus; rupture of the aorta, contusion of the heart or, rarely, rupture of the interventricular septum, and rupture of the aortic or atrioventricular valves or the free cardiac wall. Penetrating trauma, on the other hand, may cause only subcutaneous emphysema; hemothorax, pneumothorax or both; sucking wound of the chest; laceration of the lung, trachea, or bronchus; contusion of the lung; penetrating wound of the esophagus or diaphragm; and penetrating wound of the heart or great vessels (Symbas, 1972).

The initial management of any of these thoracic injuries is the same as in any other form of major injury and consists of restoration of adequate function of the respiratory and cardiovascular systems. After the initial resuscitation, each type of injury is specifically managed according to the outlines given later in this chapter. The physical examination should be repeated after initial patient management so that less obvious but equally or more detrimental coexisting injuries will be detected.

CHEST WALL

RIB FRACTURE

Fracture of the ribs is the most common chest injury, occurring in approximately 85 per cent of cases of nonpenetrating trauma. It is usually the result of some form of blunt trauma to the thoracic cage, although missile injury can result in fracture of one or more ribs. Owing to the inward displacement of the fractured ribs during external blunt injury, laceration of the parietal and visceral pleura and lung may occur, resulting in an escape of air from the lung into the pleural space or the subcutaneous tissue.

The chief clinical manifestation of rib fracture is chest wall pain, which usually is accentuated at the site of the fracture by deep inspiration, by movement of the chest wall, or by pressure over the fractured rib. Also, crepitus of subcutaneous tissue at the site of the fracture, at the ipsilateral chest wall, or at the neck or the whole trunk due to subcutaneous emphysema, and signs and symptoms of pneumothorax or hemopneumothorax frequently are present (Fig. 1). The diagnosis of rib fracture should be suspected in a patient with the above clinical findings, particularly when subcutaneous emphysema

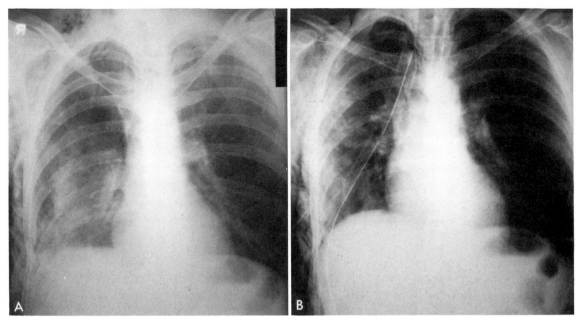

Figure 1.   Fracture of the right eighth rib with loculated pneumothorax, pneumomediastinum, and subcutaneous emphysema. *A,* Before insertion of chest tube. *B,* After insertion.

is present following blunt trauma. The diagnosis can be confirmed by chest x-ray, particularly an overexposed film that shows rib detail. Lack of evidence of rib fracture on a routine chest x-ray does not exclude its presence.

The treatment of simple, uncomplicated rib fractures should be directed toward the relief of pain and the prevention of its perils—particularly marked splinting of the injured side with lack of expansion of the lung, retention of secretions, pneumonitis, and various degrees of respiratory insufficiency. The pain can be relieved either with an intercostal nerve block, the duration of which is unpredictable and which may vary from a few minutes to several hours, or by the administration of narcotics, usually for the first three or four days, to be replaced later with other analgesics. Judicious administration of narcotics is mandatory so that the patient will be comfortable and yet not be oversedated with supression of the cough reflex and decreased respiratory excursions. After an analgesic is provided, most patients with uncomplicated fracture of the ribs can be discharged and followed the next day and thereafter in the outpatient clinic or office. However, children and elderly patients should be admitted to the hospital; the first for observation of coexistent intrathoracic

injuries, which could be present and not initially evident (Bickford, 1962), and the latter for provision of optimal relief of symptoms, for pulmonary toilet, and for the prevention of pulmonary complications, all of which are quite likely to occur when the elderly are treated on an outpatient basis (Hardy, 1963).

For many years in the past, strapping of the chest with adhesive tape was frequently used for treatment of rib fracture. However, because of its disadvantages, e.g., decrease of respiratory excursion, retention of secretions, pulmonary infection, and respiratory insufficiency, this treatment has generally been abandoned. The chest pain subsides a few days after the injury, and delayed pneumothorax and hemopneumothorax, which may be expected in the presence of the sharp edges of fractured ribs, seldom occur.

SUBCUTANEOUS EMPHYSEMA

Subcutaneous emphysema may be due to either blunt or penetrating injuries of the chest. Its localization at the site of a penetrating wound may result from the entry of atmospheric air through the skin wound into the subcutaneous tissue or, more often, from air escaping through a wound of the lung into the pleural space, leading to pneumothorax, and from there (through the wound of the parietal pleura) into the subcutaneous tissue. Rarely, subcutaneous emphysema due to laceration of the lung may be present without pneumothorax. A plausible explanation for this phenomenon is a history of previous pulmonary or pleural inflammatory processes with fusion of the visceral and parietal pleura. Because of the symphysis, escaping air from the injured lung, having no access to the pleural space, passes directly into the subcutaneous tissue. In some cases, however, the pleural symphysis may be tenuous, and some time after the injury separation of the pleural surfaces may occur, permitting air from the lacerated lung to enter the chest cavity, resulting in a delayed pneumothorax. Therefore, observation and repeat x-rays are necessary. Subcutaneous emphysema at the site of injury from blunt trauma is almost invariably associated with rib fracture and laceration of the lung. Subcutaneous emphysema in the neck only, following penetrating or blunt injury to the thorax, may be the earliest sign of an undetected major intrathoracic injury to the esophagus or the major airways.

Subcutaneous emphysema can be diagnosed easily by observation, by palpation, or by chest x-ray (Fig. 1). It usually is asymptomatic, but when very extensive may create discomfort. Treatment is required only to relive discomfort, as when the emphysema extends rapidly to obliterate vision or causes painful pressure on the external genitalia. Then, a few skin incisions parallel to the skin creases are sufficient to decompress the subcutaneous space. In the absence of pneumothorax, a chest tube should not be inserted. Rather, the patient should be observed and followed with serial chest x-rays, with the institution of closed thoracostomy drainage if and when pneumothorax or hemopneumothorax occur.

TRAUMATIC ASPHYXIA

This clinical entity is a rare sequela of blunt trauma to the chest. An injury of this type forces the anterior chest wall backward, compressing the heart against the vertebral column. This sudden compression of the heart, especially of the thin-walled right atrium, forces the blood to flow back into the valveless veins of the upper chest, neck, and head. The retrograde force is so great that multiple petechial hemorrhages and stasis occur in the minute veins of the skin and mucous membranes, resulting in a characteristic bluish-purple mottling of the skin of the head, neck, and upper thorax, as well as small hemorrhages in the subconjunctival tissues. Although the appearance of patients with traumatic asphyxia is quite alarming, usually this clinical entity is free of symptoms and requires no special therapy, except for assuring the patient that it is self-limiting process, usually lasting two weeks.

HEMOTHORAX

Accumulation of blood in the pleural space may be due to blunt or penetrating injuries of the intrathoracic organs or chest wall vessels. Depending on the state of the pleural space, the blood may be free or loculated. The amount and the rate of intrathoracic bleeding depends on the source and the duration of the hemorrhage. The state of the accumulated hemothorax, whether it is clotted or nonclotted, appears to depend on the rapidity of the bleeding and the time elapsed from hemorrhage to drainage. Slow bleeding in the presence of good function of the heart and lungs allows sufficient time for depletion of some of the coagulation factors and prevention of clotting (Symbas, 1969). Accumulation of blood in the pleural space results in compression of the ipsilateral lung. Massive hemorrhage may cause displacement of the mediastinum with compression of the contralateral lung. The patient may be asymptomatic or may have symptoms and signs of respiratory or circulatory insufficiency.

The diagnosis of hemothorax can be strongly suspected when physical findings of free or loculated fluid or air and fluid accumulation in the thoracic cavity are present (absent breath sounds, dullness to percussion, etc.). When the patient's condition permits, the diagnosis should be confirmed by chest x-ray, which will show diffuse opacification of the involved hemithorax when radiographs are made with the patient in a supine position, opacification of the lower chest with or without air fluid level if films are taken with the patient erect, or a localized density at the site of injury if the pleural space is partially obliterated (Fig. 2).

The best treatment of hemothorax in most cases is continuous drainage with a closed thoracostomy tube. As a rule, the fifth intercostal space at the midaxillary line is the ideal site for insertion of the tube in pa-

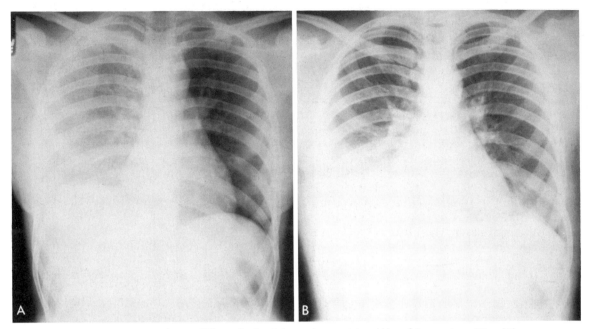

Figure 2.   Hemothorax. Films obtained in supine position (*A*) and in erect position (*B*).

tients with nonloculated hemothorax or hemopneumothorax. The fourth or fifth space at the anterior axillary line is also used. The chest bottle is connected to a conventional 14–20-cm. H_2O suction, and the amount of drainage should be recorded frequently. Continuous massive drainage indicating bleeding of arterial origin is unlikely to be self-limiting, and emergency thoracotomy should be performed. Progressively decreasing drainage, on the other hand, provided that the chest tube is functioning, indicates that the intrathoracic bleeding will be self-limiting. Therefore, closed thoracostomy serves two important functions: the evacuation of blood and air from the thoracic cavity, and as an excellent indicator for the need for thoracotomy. In addition, blood collected in a sterile chest bottle containing sterile normal saline can be autotransfused, a routine practice in our institution for the past seven years (Symbas, 1969, 1972).

Occasionally, evacuation of a hemothorax is incomplete owing to malposition of the chest tube or clotting of intrathoracic blood. Retained blood resulting in radiographic opacification of less than one-half of the involved hemithorax will be resolved and absorbed within four weeks after injury in the majority of patients. If this does not occur, as is the case in a few patients, surgical evacuation of the hemothorax and decor-

tication of the lung should be performed electively. A larger undrained hemothorax, on the other hand, should be surgically evacuated within the first few days after the patient's injury. The probability of spontaneous resolution in this case is remote (Maloney, et al., 1961; Samson, et al., 1946). An undrained hemothorax may become infected or organized to produce fibrothorax, which will prevent free expansion of the involved lung, resulting in the so-called "trapped lung." The latter will result in repeated respiratory infections and, eventually, in bronchiectasis.

PNEUMOTHORAX

Traumatic pneumothorax is the result of blunt or penetrating injury to the lung, the tracheobronchial tree, the esophagus, or the chest wall. Depending on the rate and the amount of the accumulated air in the pleural cavity and the integrity of the pleural space, simple, tension, or open pneumothorax ("sucking" chest wall wound) may develop.

SIMPLE PNEUMOTHORAX

A pneumothorax is considered to be *simple* when the accumulated air in the pleura results only in prevention of expansion of the ipsilateral lung, without displace-

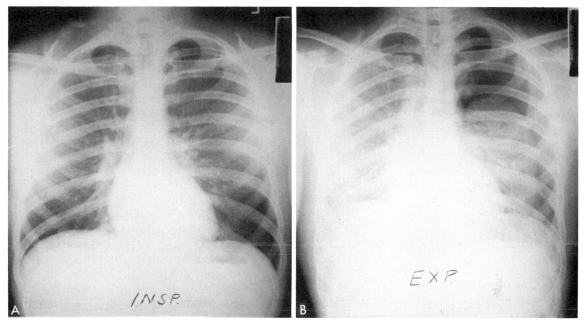

Figure 3. X-ray films obtained during inspiration (A), and expiration (B). Note that the small pneumothorax is clearly seen in B.

ment of the mediastinum and/or the ipsilateral hemidiaphragm, and without communication with the atmosphere.

Depending on the degree of lung compression, the extent of pulmonary injury, and the status of pretraumatic pulmonary function, the patient's clinical picture may vary from complete absence of symptoms to severe dyspnea. In addition to signs of air present in the pleural space, physical examination may reveal subcutaneous emphysema either restricted to the site of the chest injury or extending to other areas of the body. The diagnosis is confirmed by chest x-ray, particularly when significant pneumothorax is present, but when there is only a small amount of air in the pleural space the condition may not be evident in the conventional inspiratory film (Fig. 3, A). A small pneumothorax is easily seen when an expiratory chest x-ray is obtained (Fig. 3, B). A pneumothorax involving less than 15 per cent of lung area may be treated by close observation if the patient does not require assisted ventilation or general anesthesia. If either of the latter two situations exists, or if the pneumothorax is greater than 15 per cent, closed tube thoracostomy should be performed. In the patient with free pneumothorax, the tube is inserted through the fifth intercostal space at the midaxillary line,

whereas in loculated pneumothorax the tube should be placed in the air pocket. The thoracostomy tube is removed 24 hours after it has stopped functioning. Confirmation of complete lung re-expansion should be obtained by repeat chest x-ray 12 to 24 hours after removal of the thoracostomy tube.

TENSION PNEUMOTHORAX

Accumulation of air in the pleural space under pressure, resulting not only in the collapse of the ipsilateral lung, but also in the displacement of the mediastinum toward the contralateral side is called tension pneumothorax. This phenomenon occurs when there is no free communication of the pleural space with the atmosphere and when the site of injury of the lung acts as a one-way valve, allowing air to escape into the pleural space during inspiration and inhibiting its return to the lung during expiration. The resulting collapse of the lung, and particularly the displacement of the heart to the contralateral pleural space, precipitates severe cardiorespiratory embarrassment. The diagnosis of this most lethal—but fortunately rarely seen—clinical entity should be suspected in a patient with thoracic trauma, pneumothorax, and displacement of the point of maximum cardiac impulse away

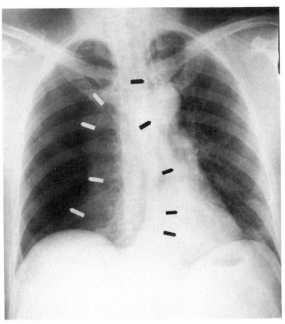

Figure 4. Tension pneumothorax on the right side with displacement of mediastinal structures away from it.

asymptomatic or severely dyspneic. Small sucking wounds of the chest in patients with relatively normal lung can be tolerated quite well for a considerable length of time. This, of course, is not true when the diameter of the stoma of the chest wall defect is greater than the diameter of the patient's trachea, because air will then move preferentially in and out of the chest through the wound rather than through the trachea and lung. The diagnosis of this entity can easily be suspected from the noise made by the air entering and leaving the pleural space during respiration and by the obvious disruption of the continuity of the chest wall. Closure of the sucking wound should be performed as soon as possible by surgical repair or with application of Vaseline gauze, and a thoracostomy tube should be inserted through a separate incision in all patients with a sucking wound before the wound is closed in order to prevent the conversion of a sucking wound of the chest with open pneumothorax to a more lethal condition, tension pneumothorax.

SUCKING WOUND OF THE CHEST

from the side of the pneumothorax, particularly if the patient manifests severe respiratory insufficiency. The diagnosis of tension pneumothorax is easily confirmed, when the patient's condition permits, by a chest x-ray which demonstrates pneumothorax with displacement of the mediastinal structures away from it (Fig. 4). When the patient's symptoms are severe, however, and the physical findings of tension pneumothorax are present, a No. 15 gauge needle or a thoracostomy tube should be immediately inserted into the pleural space. This will relieve the symptoms promptly, and the diagnosis will be confirmed by the exit of air under pressure from the pleural space. Following the initial decompression of the pleural space, the pneumothorax is handled with a conventional thoracostomy tube connected to a waterseal bottle.

SUCKING WOUND OF THE CHEST

When the pleural space is not obliterated by adhesions, disruption of the continuity of the chest wall following trauma will result in a sucking wound and extensive pneumothorax. Depending on the size of the opening on the chest wall and the condition of the lung, the patient may be completely

FLAIL CHEST

Fracture of more than two ribs in continuity in more than one place each results in an instability of the chest wall segment that is supported by the fractured ribs. This segment moves paradoxically during respiration, inward during inspiration, and outward during expiration (Fig. 5). This paradoxic movement, however, is not present in all parts of the chest wall. Multiple fractured ribs posteriorly underneath the scapula or beneath a well-developed latissimus dorsi muscle usually do not result in an unstable chest wall segment thanks to splinting by these structures. The patient with a flail chest may be exchanging air effectively or may be severely dyspneic. This depends on the size of the unstable chest wall segment and especially on the magnitude of the concomitant insult to the lung.

Flail chest can be readily diagnosed by observing the movement of the chest wall during respiration, particularly during deep inspiration. The asymptomatic young patient with flail chest should be followed closely both clinically and by blood gas determinations so that if and when respiratory embarrassment occurs assisted ventilation may be instituted. Progressive hypoxemia and hypercapnia indicate the need for ventilatory

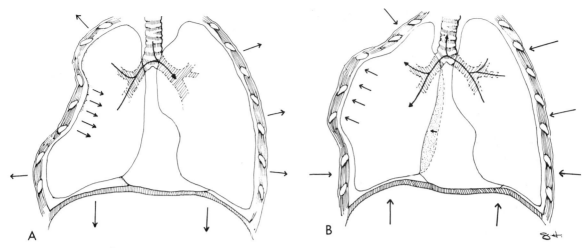

Figure 5. Paradoxic movement of the unstable "flail" segment of the chest wall. *A*, During inspiration; *B*, during expiration.

support. In the dyspneic patient, on the other hand, tracheal intubation initially—and a tracheostomy later, if needed—should be performed and assisted ventilation instituted.

Periodic blood gas determinations should be performed to regulate both the percentage of oxygen administered and the tidal volume and to maintain a normal range of blood gases. After the third postinjury day and recovery of the lung from the traumatic insult, some of these patients may be able to ventilate sufficiently with an oxygen mask alone, even though the chest wall segment is still unstable. For this reason, they should be evaluated every day for the possibility of weaning them from the respirator by determining blood gases and tidal volume after the respirator has been substituted by a "T"-piece for 20 to 30 minutes. If these values are found satisfactory, the tracheal tube should be removed and assisted ventilation discontinued, even though the unstable chest wall segment may persist. In the past, various methods of traction were used with Kirschner wires or towel clips for external fixation of the flail chest wall segment. Because they do not assure adequate ventilation and are cumbersome, inefficient, and potentially dangerous, these modes of therapy have been abandoned.

PENETRATING OR BLUNT INJURY TO THE LUNG

Injury to the lung from penetrating trauma is commonly due to knife or bullet wounds and always results in disruption of the continuity of the visceral pleura with various degrees of laceration and contusion of the lung. Leakage of air and blood through the visceral pleural wound results in diffuse or localized pneumothorax or hemopneumothorax. Depending on the amount of air or blood leak into the pleural space, the patient may be relatively asymptomatic or may have various degrees of respiratory or circulatory insufficiency. Patients with a lung wound—particularly those caused by bullets—usually have hemoptysis shortly after injury or several days later. After the hemothorax or hemopneumothorax is evacuated, most penetrating wounds of the lung heal slowly with concomitant decrease in the leakage of air and blood. However, injury to a major branch of the tracheobronchial tree or pulmonary vessels sometimes will require surgical intervention. Occasionally, due to hepatization of the injured lung, particularly when the wound was caused by a high velocity missile or close-range shotgun injury, bleeding from the lung continues and thoracotomy will be required to control the blood loss. Emergency thoracotomy for control of bleeding usually involves oversewing the wound or wounds of the lung, but occasionally this is not sufficient and resection of the injured lung will be necessary.

Penetrating injury of the lung rarely may result in infection or lung abscess formation, particularly when the missile injury is accompanied by foreign material such as

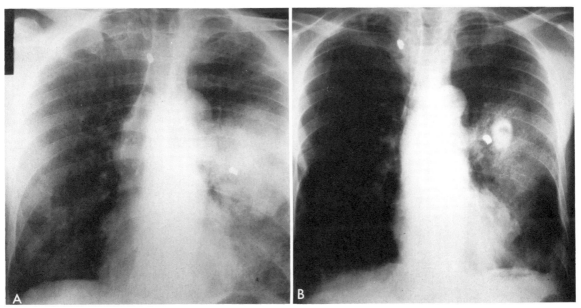

Figure 6. A, Contusion of the lung from bullet wound. B, Cavitation of the contused lung one day after the injury.

clothing or shotgun wadding. Also, the contused area of high velocity missile wounds may cavitate (Fig. 6) or become organized into a fibrous solitary mass.

Blunt injury of the lung frequently results in contusion of the ipsilateral or even the contralateral lung sometimes with laceration of visceral pleura and the lung. The force transmitted to the lung from blunt trauma results in extravasation of blood into the interstitial and alveolar spaces, precipitating consolidation of the lung. Depending on the extent of the injury and the preinjury status of pulmonary function, a patient with pulmonary contusion may be totally asymptomatic or may complain of dyspnea. Frequently, immediate or delayed hemoptysis may last for several days. The diagnosis of contusion is established by chest x-rays, particularly those obtained several hours after the injury. Therefore, a negative chest x-ray shortly after the injury does not exclude the presence of lung contusion, since the radiographic manifestations of insult to the lung frequently appear 12 to 24 hours after the clinical manifestations. The chest x-rays of a bluntly contused lung may demonstrate a localized or, more frequently, a diffuse infiltrate of the ipsilateral or even the contralateral lung—in addition, of course, to other roentgenographic manifestations of blunt thoracic injury.

The treatment usually is supportive, with good pulmonary toilet, avoidance of fluid overload, and ventilatory support, as required. Several days of this form of therapy usually result in clearing of the consolidation or infiltrate, with restoration of the lung to its preinjury status, although infection, pneumonitis, or, very rarely, lung abscess may develop.

PENETRATING OR BLUNT INJURY OF THE MAJOR AIRWAYS

Penetrating wounds of the lower neck or upper chest may involve the trachea or the major bronchi. Owing to lack of protection of the cervical trachea by bony structure, this tracheal segment is most frequently injured from penetrating wounds.

Severe blunt trauma to the thorax may result in a partial or complete tear of the trachea or major bronchi (Eastridge, et al., 1970). The patient's clinical condition following injury of the airway depends on the size of the wound in the tracheobronchial tree, the level of the injury, the magnitude of the injury to the other lung, and also whether the flow of air from the tracheobronchial lumen to the pleural space is bidirectional, unidirectional, or stopped because of obliteration of the traumatic defect.

Patients with major unidirectional air

flow are most likely to be severely symptomatic, with dyspnea and hypotension because of the frequent development of tension pneumothorax. The symptoms in patients with bidirectional flow are directly related to the size of the hole and the level of the injured tracheobronchial tree. Patients with a defect of the airway sealed by adjacent tissue usually are relatively asymptomatic unless the injured area of the trachea has resulted in an unstable segment which collapses, particularly during expiration. The clinical picture in patients with injury of the tracheobronchial tree may vary from the very grave—severe dyspnea, cyanosis, hypotension with or without massive subcutaneous emphysema—to the asymptomatic, except for mild hemoptysis or perhaps minimal subcutaneous emphysema.

Injury to the tracheobronchial tree should be suspected in patients who experience severe blunt trauma to the chest with the above clinical manifestations, especially the very ill patient with massive air leak in whom the insertion of one or two chest tubes does not result in improvement and expansion of the involved lung, or in the patient who has persistent lobar atelectasis, despite a good clinical appearance. Penetrating wounds of the lower neck or upper chest should always raise suspicion of tracheal injury, particularly when associated with a massive air leak, subcutaneous emphysema, or hemoptysis (Symbas, 1975).

Once the diagnosis of rupture of the tracheobronchial tree is suspected, bronchoscopy should be performed to establish the diagnosis by direct visualization of the site of injury. Repair of the traumatic defect should be performed as soon as possible.

TRAUMATIC PERFORATION OF THE ESOPHAGUS

Traumatic perforation of the esophagus, except for that due to esophageal instrumentation, which will not be considered here, is associated with missile or knife wounds of the neck, chest, or upper abdomen or, less frequently, with blunt trauma to the abdo-

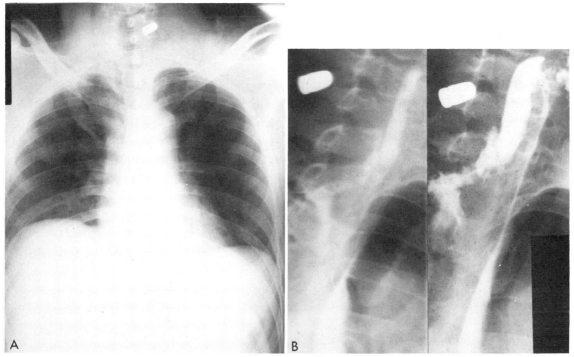

Figure 7. A, Chest x-ray showing swelling subcutaneous emphysema and a missile in the lower neck region in a patient with a bullet wound of the lower neck.

B, Admission esophagogram shows extravasation of the radiopaque material. (Reproduced with permission from Symbas, P. N., Tyras, D. H., Hatcher, C. R., Jr., and Perry, B.: Penetrating wounds of the esophagus. Ann. Thorac. Surg. *13*:552, 1972 and from the publisher, Little, Brown and Co., Boston.)

men or chest and rarely with accidental insufflation or pressurized air into the patient's mouth.

Pain is the most common symptom of perforation of the esophagus, its location depending on the site of the perforation. The pain may be located in the epigastrium when the lower esophageal segment and particularly when its intraperitoneal portion is injured. Chest pain may be the predominant symptom when the intrathoracic esophagus is perforated or the pain may be in the neck if the cervical esophageal portion is injured (Symbas, 1972). The patient usually is febrile and may be hoarse or have dysphagia or respiratory distress. When the perforation involves the cervical esophagus, it is accompanied by local tenderness, subcutaneous emphysema, and some resistance of the neck to passive motion (Fig. 7, A). Perforation of the intrathoracic esophagus causing mediastinal emphysema and mediastinitis may manifest with subcutaneous emphysema in the neck, mediastinal "crunch," splinting of the chest wall, and respiratory distress or shock. Abdominal tenderness and rigidity are the most common signs of perforation of the intra-abdominal, and not infrequently of the lower thoracic esophageal segment. Chest and neck x-rays, in the presence of cervical esophageal perforation, may demonstrate widening of the superior mediastinal shadow, subcutaneous emphysema in the neck (Fig. 7, A), and increased distance between the trachea and vertebrae (prevertebral shadow). When the thoracic esophagus is perforated, x-rays may reveal widening of the entire mediastinal shadow, mediastinal or subcutaneous emphysema of the neck, and hydrothorax or pneumothorax (Fig. 8, A).

The diagnosis of esophageal perforation is suspected when some or all of the above clinical and x-ray manifestations are present, although some of these clinical features may easily be attributed to coexisting injuries of other organs. For this reason, esophagography should be performed in all patients with penetrating wounds close to the esophagus or in those where the bullet or weapon may have traversed the mediastinum.

Esophagography may be performed with either absorbable or nonabsorbable radiopaque material as soon as the patient's condition is stable. The films should be taken from both frontal and lateral views, both during and after swallowing the radiopaque material. With perforation, contrast media may be seen to extravasate from the esophageal lumen during swallowing, or radiopaque material may be noted at or near the region of the esophagus after swallowing is completed (Figs. 7, B and 8, B).

Treatment of esophageal perforation should be instituted as soon as the diagnosis is suspected, and consists of suspenison of oral alimentation, constant gastric suction through a nasogastric tube, and administration of broad spectrum antibiotics and, if needed, blood volume expanders.

After the diagnosis is established, the patient should be operated on as soon as feasible. At operation, the esophageal wound should be sutured, if possible, and the adjacent area widely drained. For intrathoracic or intraperitoneal esophageal perforation, gastrostomy and feeding jejunostomy also should be performed. The results of this form of therapy are excellent for cervical esophageal perforation, whereas intrathoracic esophageal wounds carry a high risk.

Injury of the Diaphragm

Traumatic injury of the diaphragm is due to penetrating injury and/or blunt trauma. These two types of diaphragmatic injury differ considerably in their clinical manifestations and management.

PENETRATING INJURY OF THE DIAPHRAGM

This form of injury is the most commonly encountered diaphragmatic trauma. It is frequently due to a bullet or stab wound of the lower chest and upper abdomen, although such wounds in other areas of the body may reach the diaphragm. Penetrating diaphragmatic injuries usually do not manifest by a special clinical picture; rather the clinical manifestations are those of any of the concomitantly injured intrathoracic or intraperitoneal organs. In general, the patients frequently have symptoms and signs of intraperitoneal bleeding or peritonitis or signs and symptoms of hemothorax or pneumothorax. In some cases, particularly those with chronic diaphragmatic injury, symptoms and signs of abdominal visceral obstruction or strangulation may be present. The diagnosis of penetrating injury of the diaphragm should be suspected when proximity of the

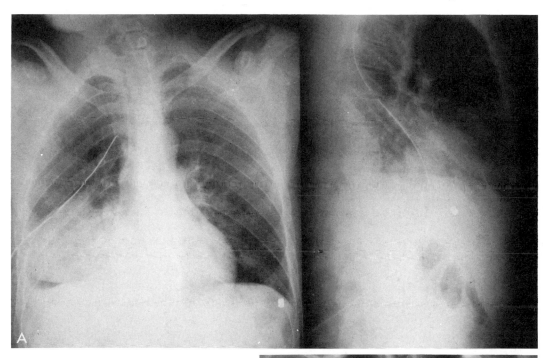

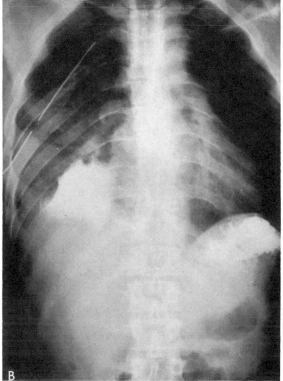

Figure 8. A, Chest x-ray in a patient with bullet wound of the right side of the chest. The bullet is located in the left side of the chest.

B, Admission esophagogram shows extravasation of radiopaque material into the right chest. (Reproduced with permission from Symbas, P. N., Tyras, D. H., Hatcher, C. R., Jr., and Perry, B.: Penetrating wounds of the esophagus. Ann. Thorac. Surg. *13*:552, 1972; and from the publisher, Little, Brown and Co., Boston.)

external wound indicates that the missile or knife possibly has traversed the diaphragm, particularly when it appears to be abnormal on chest x-ray. Nevertheless, the diagnosis usually is established at the time of exploratory laparotomy or thoracotomy for the repair of coexisting intraperitoneal or intrathoracic injury. As a general rule, preoperative management consists of general resuscitative measures for intraperitoneal and/or intrathoracic injury, the diagnosis of this injury, and its surgical repair, if indicated. Repair of small penetrating injuries usually is performed incidentally during exploratory laparotomy for major intra-abdominal injuries.

NONPENETRATING INJURY OF THE DIAPHRAGM

Rupture of the diaphragm usually is the result of a severe blunt injury of the abdomen or upper abdomen and lower chest. It commonly involves the membranous portion of the left hemidiaphragm, usually in a radial direction. Thanks to protection by the liver, rupture of the right diaphragm occurs less frequently. Following the rupture of the left diaphragm, a diaphragmatic hernia is usually formed without a sac. Absence of a hernia sac and the differential pressure between the left pleural and peritoneal cavities cause herniation of intraperitoneal organs. Initial compression of the ipsilateral lung soon may be followed by displacement of the mediastinum away from the involved side. Owing to these anatomic changes, the patient may develop symptoms and signs of respiratory and cardiac embarrassment, and, because of the compromise of the gastrointestinal lumen and the blood supply of the herniated viscera, he may present with symptoms of gastric or intestinal obstruction or visceral ischemia and gangrene. Depending on the magnitude of the herniation of various organs and the degree of the compromise of the herniated viscera, the patient may become severely symptomatic immediately after the injury, or after a dormant period of varying lengths. On physical examination, in addition to the signs of visceral obstruction or gangrene that may be present, the breath sounds are absent, and bowel sounds may be heard in the left thorax. The diagnosis of rupture of the diaphragm should be suspected in all instances of severe blunt trauma, particularly when accompanied by any of the above signs shortly after the in-

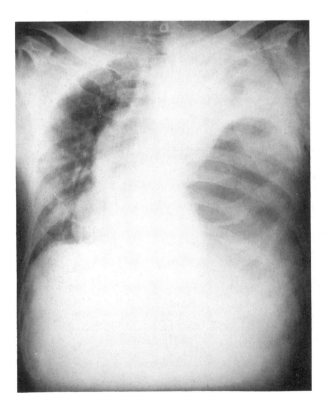

Figure 9. Chest x-ray of a patient who had sustained blunt injury to the abdomen four months earlier.

jury—or days, weeks, or even months after the injury.

Clinical suspicion of the diagnosis should be enhanced when the chest x-ray shows absence of the normal contour of the diaphragm with compression of the left lung (with or without displacement of the mediastinum) and radiolucency in the left chest compatible with loculated pneumothorax or air in a distended herniated stomach or bowel (Fig. 9). Once the diagnosis is suspected, in addition to routine resuscitative measures, a nasogastric tube should be inserted as soon as possible and connected to constant suction. Chest x-ray may locate the tube in the chest If the stomach has herniated into the left pleural space, confirming the suspected diagnosis. In addition, the applied suction will decompress the gastrointestinal tract and improve the patient's clinical picture. The diagnosis usually is confirmed by a barium contrast study of the gastrointestinal tract which demonstrates viscera containing contrast material in the chest. Once the diagnosis is established, the patient should be operated on as soon as possible to prevent necrosis of the herniated viscera and severe cardiorespiratory embarrassment.

Penetrating Wounds of Great Vessels

Penetrating wounds of great vessels commonly are due to missile or stab wound injury and usually are associated with a penetrating wound of the chest, upper abdomen, or lower neck. The true incidence of these wounds is not known, since many of these patients succumb shortly after injury, and autopsy examinations are not performed on all patients dying from trauma.

Penetrating injuries of the great vessels usually manifest by massive hemothorax with or without hemorrhagic shock. When an intrapericardial segment of the great vessels is injured, cardiac tamponade with or without hemothorax is commonly the presenting clinical syndrome (Symbas, 1974). Carotid or subclavian artery injury may present with an absent or weak pulse distal to the wound. The patient may be hemiplegic or comatose, or a progressively enlarging hematoma may be observed. Massive hematoma formation may cause symptoms and signs of compression of the superior vena cava, trachea, or esophagus. Arteriovenous, aortocardiac, or aortopulmonary fistulas also may be present.

The diagnosis of great vessel injury is

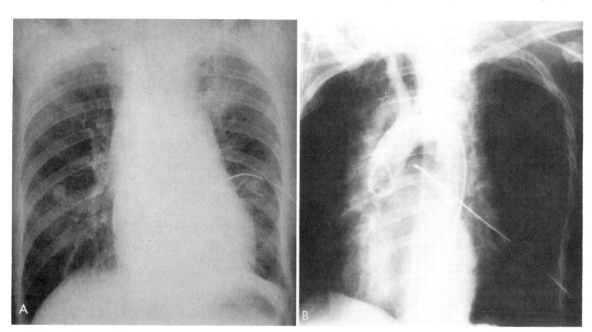

Figure 10. A, Admission chest x-ray in a patient who had sustained a bullet wound of the right supraclavicular fossa. The bullet was imbedded to the left of the spine at T7 level. She had no more bleeding after 500 ml. of blood was drained immediately after the chest tube was inserted.

B, Aortography of the same patient done shortly after admission, showing a false aneurysm of the aortic arch, an aortic arch to left brachiocephalic vein fistula and poor filling of the descending aorta. (Reproduced with permission from Symbas, P. N.: *Traumatic Injuries of the Heart and Great Vessels*, 1972; and from the publisher, Charles C Thomas, Springfield, Ill.)

suspected when bleeding into the pleural space is massive and/or continuous, or when a missile has traversed the mediastinum, especially when accompanied by widening of the mediastinal shadow (Fig. 10, A). When the bleeding is self-limited, the diagnosis is also suspected in the presence of a new murmur or aneurysm formation.

The suspected diagnosis of great vessel injury in patients with massive intrathoracic bleeding is established at the time of emergency surgery. When emergency thoracotomy for bleeding is not required, the suspected diagnosis of great vessel injury should be confirmed with arteriography to define the type and site of the injury so that a proper surgical approach can be planned. The arteriographic picture of great vessel injury may vary from a false aneurysm to arteriovenous aortocardiac or aortopulmonary fistula to a small irregularity of the arterial wall (Fig. 10, B).

The initial treatment of patients with great vessel injury depends on the clinical manifestations, but usually involves restoration of circulating blood volume, relief of cardiac tamponade (see *Procedure*, p. 326), and provision of adequate ventilation. The first of these resuscitative measures can be accomplished to a great extent, as we have done over the past seven years, by autotransfusing the blood drained from the hemothorax.

When continuous bleeding is the clinical manifestation of a penetrating wound of great vessels, the patient should be operated on as soon as possible. When the diagnosis is suspected from other manifestations of such a wound, repair of the wound should be carried out after the diagnosis is confirmed by arteriography. At the time of surgery, the chest and neck should be prepared and draped widely so that the initial thoracotomy incision may be extended if needed. Emergency thoracotomy for intrathoracic bleeding usually is performed via an anterolateral incision through the fourth intercostal space, which is extended, if needed, posteriorly or anteriorly to the opposite pleural space, or to the neck and supraclavicular fossa (Fig. 11). Repair is accomplished using either partial tangential occlusion of the injured vessel or after cross clamping it proximal and distal to the wound. Cardiopulmonary bypass is used if the ascending aorta is clamped, or temporary external shunting is used when the innominate artery or descending aorta is clamped. Only clamping proximal and distal to the wound is needed if the subclavian artery is injured.

RUPTURE OF THE AORTA

Rupture of the aorta is one of the most lethal cardiovascular injuries resulting from

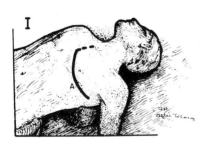

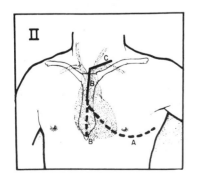

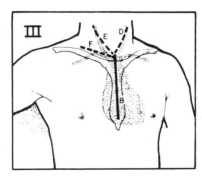

Figure 11. Diagrammatic illustration of the incisions utilized for the management and repair of penetrating wounds of the aorta and great vessels. (Reproduced with permission from Symbas, P. N.: Traumatic Injuries of the Heart and Great Vessels, 1972; and from the publisher, Charles C Thomas, Springfield, Ill.)

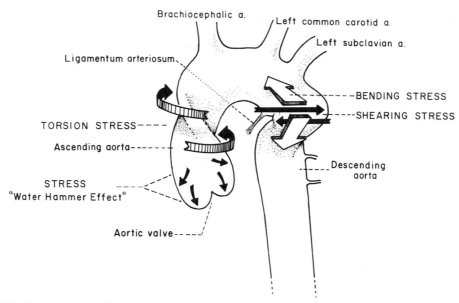

Figure 12.   Diagrammatic illustration of the forces responsible for the aortic rupture from blunt trauma. (Reproduced with permission from Symbas, P. N.: Traumatic Injuries of the Heart and Great Vessels, 1972; and from the publisher, Charles C Thomas, Springfield, Ill.)

blunt trauma. It is estimated that the vast majority of patients with aortic rupture succumb at the scene of the injury or during transportation to a medical facility, with only 10 to 20 per cent living long enough for emergency hospitalization (Parmley, et al., 1958; Spencer, et al., 1961). They can be treated successfully if the diagnosis is made early and treatment is instituted promptly. The usual sites of aortic rupture are the aortic isthmus (immediately distal to the origin of the left subclavian artery) and the ascending aorta, although rupture may rarely occur in the distal descending or abdominal aorta. However, the overwhelming majority of patients surviving long enough for surgical treatment have rupture of the aortic isthmus.

Rupture of the aorta occurs as a result of compressive or decelerating trauma and is the result of a variety of forces acting on the aortic wall (Fig. 12). The patient with aortic rupture usually is desperately ill from other coexisting injuries (musculoskeletal, abdominal, or heart) but may be asymptomatic with no evidence of external injury. Coexisting injuries may mask the signs of aortic rupture. Therefore, a high index of suspicion is required in order to establish the diagnosis of aortic rupture.

The symptoms of chest pain, dyspnea, back pain, or inability to move the lower extremities, of which the patient with rupture of the aorta usually complains, are not specific and may be due to another injury. On the other hand, the signs of aortic rupture are more specific. Our experience, and that gained from reviews of the literature, reveals the frequent occurrence of a triad of signs which appears to be of significant diagnostic value in the early postinjury period (Symbas, 1973). This triad consists of (1) increased pulse amplitude and blood pressure of the upper extremities, (2) decreased pulse amplitude and blood pressure of the lower extremities, and (3) roentgenographic evidence of widening of the mediastinum (Fig. 13, A). However, it must be remembered that widening of the mediastinal shadow may be the only finding. Less frequently, increased blood pressure and pulse amplitude of the upper extremities without widening of the mediastinal shadow may be the only manifestation. For this reason, when the above triad is present in a patient who has sustained severe blunt trauma, the diagnosis of rupture of the aorta is fairly certain. The diagnosis should be confirmed by aortography (Fig. 13, B), which should, therefore, be performed as soon as possible in all patients with blunt trauma and the above triad, with widening of the mediastinal shadow alone, or new unexplained increased pulse amplitude and blood pressure of the upper extremities.

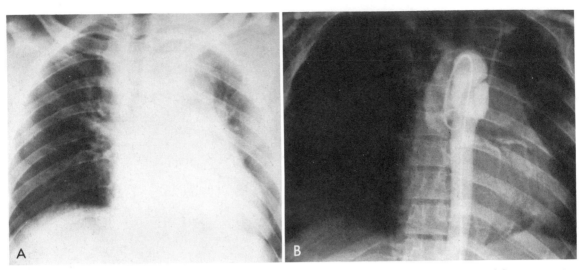

Figure 13. A, Widening of the mediastinum shortly after a vehicle accident. B, Aortogram of the same patient shortly after his admission showing a false aneurysm just distal to the left subclavian artery.

The danger of exsanguination is constantly present in patients with rupture of the aorta, and for this reason repair of the rupture should be performed as soon as possible after the diagnosis is confirmed angiographically. The repair can be done with the use of femoral vein to femoral artery partial bypass or with temporary external local shunt. The results of surgical treatment are usually most gratifying.

Occasionally, if facilities for immediate surgical repair of the lesion are not available, or when other injuries or coincidental infection dictate delay of corrective surgery, treatment with an antihypertensive drug, as in patients with dissecting aneurysm of the aorta, might be an excellent adjunct in the management of these patients. Transfer to a hospital with appropriate facilities for elective repair of the lesion should be effected as soon as the patient's condition permits.

HEART

Penetrating Wounds of the Heart

Penetrating wounds of the heart usually are due to bullet or stab wounds frequently inflicted to the chest and upper abdomen. Over 50 per cent of the victims with penetrating cardiac trauma succumb shortly after the injury (Blalock and Ravitch, 1962; Suggs, et al., 1968) from exsanguination or cardiac tamponade, and those remaining survive for various periods of time so that many of them, if treated immediately and properly, may recover completely from their cardiac wound. The clinical manifestations of penetrating wounds of the heart usually are dependent on the site and size of the cardiac wound and the state of the pericardial wound. When the pericardial wound remains open and allows free drainage of the intrapericardial blood, the cardiac wound manifests with symptoms and signs of hemorrhage and hemothorax, whereas when the pericardial wound is obliterated with blood clot and adjacent lung or prepericardial fat the escaping blood from the cardiac chamber cannot drain into the pleural space, and cardiac tamponade ensues.

The patient with tamponade may be restless, complaining of air hunger, or may be in shock. His skin may be cold and moist and his lips and digits mildly cyanotic. Visible superficial neck veins may be distended and have paradoxic filling during inspiration (Kussmaul's sign). The blood pressure may be unobtainable, or the systolic pressure below normal level with a decrease during inspiration of 10 mm. Hg or more ("paradoxical pulse"). The pulse pressure is narrow, and the pulse is rapid and hypodynamic. The heart sounds may or may not be distant and muffled, and the central venous pressure is elevated.

The diagnosis of penetrating cardiac wound should be suspected in a wounded patient with cardiac tamponade or with sig-

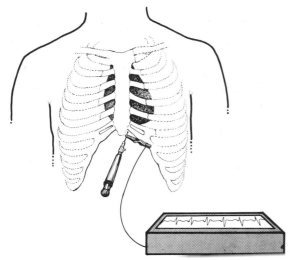

Figure 14. Pericardiocentesis through the paraxiphoid route. (Reproduced with permission from Symbas, P. N.: Traumatic Injuries of the Heart and Great Vessels, 1972; and from the publisher, Charles C Thomas, Springfield, Ill.)

nificant intrathoracic bleeding. When the clinical manifestation of the suspected cardiac wound is that of tamponade, immediate pericardiocentesis with a thin-wall metal needle or, preferably, a plastic #17 or #18 gauge catheter or needle should be performed through the left substernal paraxyphoid route with the patient in a semierect position, 35 to 40 degrees, and the needle pointing toward the left shoulder (Fig. 14). During pericardiocentesis, continuous monitoring with an electrocardiogram is desirable, but should not be done at the expense of delaying prompt pericardial decompression. If nonclotting blood is obtained, the diagnosis of cardiac injury and cardiac tamponade is certain, and the pericardial space should be decompressed as much as possible. If a plastic catheter or needle is used for the pericardiocentesis, it should be left in place for continuous drainage of the intrapericardial blood until the cardiac wound is surgically repaired.

When the clinical manifestations of penetrating wounds of the heart are hemothorax and signs and symptoms of blood loss, the pleural space should be drained with a closed thoracostomy tube. Blood drained from the pleural space may be autotransfused, if needed, with the administration of other blood volume expanders. The expansion of the circulating blood volume benefits not only the patients with cardiac wounds

and a clinical picture of blood loss, but also those with a clinical picture of cardiac tamponade. However, in patients with tamponade, the hemodynamic improvement following the administration of blood volume expanders is of short duration. Therefore, definitive treatment of these patients, as well as those with continuous blood loss, should be provided as soon as possible.

The definitive treatment for patients with cardiac wounds and massive unrelenting blood loss is exploratory thoracotomy and cardiorrhaphy. However, the definitive treatment for the patients with cardiac wounds and cardiac tamponade was not uniform in the past. After the historic introduction of cardiorrhaphy for cardiac wounds by Rhen in 1896 and pericardiocentesis by Dupuytren in 1826, the treatment of traumatic cardiac tamponade has varied. Presently, multiple pericardiocentesis as a definitive mode of therapy is of historic interest only. Although surgical repair, only in the face of recurrence of tamponade after one or two pericardiocenteses, has compared quite favorably with immediate surgical repair alone, it should be discouraged.

The progressive improvement of means of transportation has resulted in prompt arrival at hospitals of patients with more severe cardiac wounds which can be handled successfully only by immediate surgery. In addition, the unpredictable course of traumatic pericardial tamponade following an initial favorable response to pericardiocentesis, coupled with the remarkable advancement in the fields of resuscitation, anesthesia, and cardiac surgery, strongly supports the policy of immediate surgery for all patients with penetrating wounds of the heart (Symbas, 1975).

While light general anesthesia is administered and the entire anterior chest is prepped and draped, the operating team should be ready for rapid thoracotomy and decompression of the pericardium in case of rapid deterioration of the patient's condition. An anterolateral submammary incision performed on the involved side may be expanded as needed to the opposite side or to the neck (Fig. 15). After the pericardial space is rapidly decompressed, bleeding through the cardiac wound is controlled digitally, and the cardiac wound is repaired, usually with ease. Injured sizable branches of the coronary arteries are repaired under cardiopulmonary bypass, either primarily or

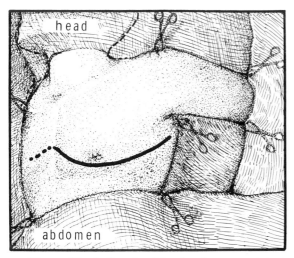

Figure 15. Left anterolateral submammary incision. (Reproduced with permission from Symbas, P. N.: Traumatic Injuries of the Heart and Great Vessels, 1972; and from the publisher, Charles C Thomas, Springfield, Ill.)

with the use of a reversed saphenous vein graft, whereas small severed branches are simply ligated. During hospitalization and after discharge, the patient with a penetrating wound of the heart should be observed closely for symptoms and signs of residual post-traumatic cardiac lesions, e.g., shunt, valvular lesions, myocardial aneurysm, or retained projectiles. These defects may be repaired electively when needed.

BLUNT INJURY TO THE HEART

Various types of blunt trauma to the chest, ranging from contact sports to compression of the thorax between two objects, have resulted in cardiac injury. Presently, the commonest of all is the "steering wheel injury" from automobile accidents. These blunt injuries damage the heart: (*a*) by sudden accelerations or decelerations of the chest, causing the heart to be thrust against the chest wall; (*b*) by compression of the heart between the sternum and the vertebral column when the former is suddenly driven in by a forceful blow; and (*c*) by sudden and violent increases in the intrathoracic or intra-abdominal pressure which may produce subendocardial hemorrhages or even rupture of the heart.

Blunt trauma to the heart may cause a variety of cardiac lesions: (*a*) myocardial contusion; (*b*) rupture of the free cardiac wall, the interventricular spetum, or the aortic, mitral, and tricuspid valves.

CONTUSION OF THE HEART

The pathologic lesions of myocardial contusion vary in extent and nature from small areas of petechiae or ecchymosis to contusion of the full thickness of the cardiac wall which may result in immediate or late rupture.

The most common symptom of myocardial contusion is pain, which usually is identical to that of myocardial infarction or ischemia but usually is not relieved by coronary vasodilating drugs (DeMuth, et al., 1967). Asymptomatic myocardial contusion has been reported, but it is likely that the history of chest pain was not obtained in these patients because of the presence of severe pain from injuries to the other parts of the body. The chest pain starts immediately or within a few hours after the trauma. The patient may also complain of palpitations or tachycardia, or he may be dyspneic or hypotensive. Virtually all dysrhythmias have been observed in patients and in experimental animals with myocardial contusion (Louhimo, 1967). Premature atrial or ventricular contractions are the most frequent types of irregularity noted, with paroxysmal ventricular tachycardia, fibrillation, and idioventricular rhythm being frequent causes of death following cardiac contusion. Myocardial contusion may coexist with hemopericardium manifested by symptoms and signs of cardiac tamponade, as well as early or late post-traumatic pericarditis.

Presently the most readily available diagnostic test for myocardial contusion is the 12-lead electrocardiogram, which should be obtained in all patients who sustain blunt injury, particularly those involving the precordium. Electrocardiographic abnormalities precipitated by contusion of the heart range from transient to long lasting disturbances of rhythm, to evidence of pericarditis or focal muscular damage, to changes typical of myocardial infarction. These abnormalities return to normal in a much shorter time than those produced by frank myocardial infarction, are frequently present shortly after the trauma, or may not appear until 24 to 48 hours later. Therefore, serial electrocardiograms should be done in patients who sustain blunt trauma to the thorax to detect the early- and late-appearing electrocardiographic changes. Unfortunately, electrocardiographic abnormalities other than those indicating muscle damage from cardiac contusion are relatively nonspecific since they can be precipitated by other conditions not infrequently present in traumatized patients (hypoxia, hypovolemia, shock, etc.). Despite the error in specificity, the 12-lead electrocardiogram has proved to be the most reliable diagnostic tool offering a practical, relatively accurate, and dependable means of evaluating the injured patient.

Other laboratory studies have not been found to be of great diagnostic value. Serum enzymes are so frequently elevated in concomitant liver, lung, and skeletal muscle injuries or in hemorrhagic shock that they are not very useful in establishing this diagnosis. However, the specific enzymes from myocardial damage (e.g., CPK) may be useful, although not indicative of degree or location of damage.

The treatment of myocardial contusion is similar to that of myocardial infarction. Digitalis should be used cautiously and only in the presence of cardiac failure or atrial fibrillation with a rapid ventricular response; antiarrhythmic drugs, lidocaine, procainamide, or quinidine, can be given for control of arrhythmias and especially of ectopic beats. Anticoagulants should not be administered because they might precipitate myocardial or intrapericardial bleeding, and coronary dilators should not be prescribed because they have little or no effect on the pain and may cause harmful systemic vasodilatation.

RUPTURE OF THE HEART

Forceful compression against the vertebral column may cause rupture of the heart at the time of injury. Immediate myocardial discontinuity also may be caused by laceration from a sharp rib or sternal bone fragment, or delayed rupture may occur at the site of a myocardial contusion as late as two weeks following the initial blunt trauma. Very rarely the heart may be ruptured by violent compression applied to the abdomen and legs. Cardiac rupture may involve the free wall, with clinical manifestations of hemopericardium and cardiac tamponade, or may involve the interventricular septum or the aortic, mitral, or tricuspid valves, manifesting with symptoms and signs of congestive heart failure.

The diagnosis of rupture of the heart should be suspected when a patient experiences severe blunt injury and has a clinical picture of cardiac tamponade or congestive heart failure. However, in the face of symptoms and signs of cardiac tamponade, massive myocardial contusion must be considered, as the clinical manifestations may be identical to those of cardiac rupture. In such cases, pericardiocentesis should be performed immediately to relieve possible cardiac tamponade, but the diagnosis should be confirmed at emergency thoracotomy and followed by closure of the cardiac defect.

The diagnosis of rupture of the cardiac valves or interventricular septum should be suspected in patients who sustain severe blunt trauma and develop congestive heart failure. The symptoms of cardiac decompensation in these patients may appear immediately after the injury or following a relatively asymptomatic period of days or even years. The diagnosis of rupture of the cardiac valves or ventricular septum should be strongly suspected in patients who develop a valvular regurgitant murmur, or murmur of ventricular septal defect (with or without symptoms of cardiac decompensation) following severe blunt trauma.

In the symptomatic patient with rupture of the cardiac valves or interventricular septum, treatment should be supportive both before and after the diagnosis is established. Common measures used include assisted ventilation, good pulmonary toilet, and careful administration of digitalis and diuretics. If the patient fails to respond to this treatment, cardiac catheterization should be performed as soon as possible. Clinical deterioration combined with the specific data of cardiac catheterization will serve as indicators for emergency surgical repair. In patients with compensated congestive heart failure, cardiac catheterization and angiography should be performed following recovery from the initial trauma. If the cardiac lesion is found to be hemodynamically significant, elective repair should be performed.

AUTOTRANSFUSION FROM HEMOTHORAX

A major factor in the successful resuscitation of patients suffering severe trauma with massive blood loss is the prompt availability of blood for transfusion. The blood commonly used in such patients is the ho-

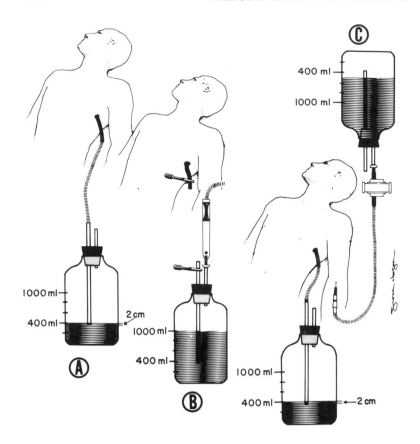

Figure 16. Autotransfusion from traumatic hemothorax. (Reproduced with permission from Symbas, P. N.: Autotransfusion from hemothorax: experimental and clinical studies. J. Trauma *12*:689, 1972; and from the publisher, The Williams & Wilkins Company, Baltimore.)

mologous banked blood which carries the attendant risks of serum hepatitis and transfusion reactions. These risks are accentuated by the not infrequent necessity of transfusion "type–specific" (uncrossmatched) blood in life-and-death situations. The ideal blood for transfusion is that which is promptly available and is free of these familiar complications. The blood which meets these criteria is that contained by a massive hemothorax in cases of major intrathoracic trauma not involving diaphragmatic penetration. Following the experimental (Symbas, 1969) and clinical (Symbas, 1969, 1973) demonstration of the alterations of the blood components contained in a hemothorax and the safety of autotransfusion of blood from traumatic hemothorax, almost all patients with massive hemothorax at our institution have been autotransfused.

In patients with traumatic hemothorax, an Argyle No. 34 or 36 French plastic tube is inserted into the involved pleural space and connected to a chest bottle containing 400 ml. sterile normal (0.9 per cent) saline solution and maintained under suction of approximately 15 cm. of H_2O (Fig. 16, A). If repletion of lost blood is required, autotrans-

fusion is performed in one of two ways: (*a*) the mixture of blood and saline in the chest bottle is passed through a blood administration set, filtering particles greater than 40 μ, and is infused into the patient (Fig. 16, *C*). While this is being infused, a second sterile chest bottle with saline is connected to the chest tube to continue the drainage and (*b*) the conventional vacuum blood transfusion plastic bag is first filled from the chest bottle and then, from it, conventional transfusion is carried out. To date, at out institution more than 200 patients have been autotransfused with one of these two techniques and none of them manifested any side-effects which could be attributed to the autotransfusion.

References

Avery, E. E., Mörch, E. T., and Benson, D. W.: Critically crushed chests. A new method of treatment with continuous mechanical hyperventilation to produce alkalotic apnea and internal pneumatic stabilization. J. Thorac. Surg. 32:291, 1956.

Bickford, B. J.: Chest injuries in childhood and adolescence. Thorax 17:240, 1962.

Blades, B.: Ruptured diaphragm. Am. J. Surg., *105*:501, 1963.

Blalock, A., and Ravitch, M. M.: A consideration of the

nonoperative treatment of cardiac tamponade resulting from wounds of the heart. Surgery *52*:330, 1962.

Cooper, F. W., Jr., Stead, E. A., Jr., and Warren, J. V.: The beneficial effect of intravenous infusions in acute pericardial tamponade. Ann. Surg. *120*:822, 1944.

Culiner, M. M., Roe, B. B., and Grimes, O. F.: The early elective surgical approach to the treatment of traumatic hemothorax. J. Thorac. Cardiovasc. Surg. *38*:780, 1959.

DeMuth, W. E., Baue, A. E., and Odom, J. A.: Contusion of the heart. J. Trauma, *7*:443, 1967.

Drews, J. A., Mercer, E. C., and Benfield, J. R.: Acute diaphragmatic injuries. Ann. Thorac. Surg. *16*:69, 1973.

Dupuytren: Cited in Cazan, G. M., Jr.: Multiple laceration of the auricle. U.S. Armed Forces Med. J. *3*:253, 1952.

Eastridge, C. E., et al.: Tracheobronchial injury caused by blunt trauma. Am. Rev. Resp. Dis. *101*:230, 1970.

Haller, A., and Donahoo, J. S.: Traumatic asphyxia in children: pathophysiology and management. J. Trauma *11*:453, 1971.

Hardy, J. D.: Thoracic emergencies in the aged. Am. J. Surg. *105*:543, 1963.

Herbert, W. M., et al.: A regimen for the early care of the patient with crushed chest. J. Trauma *4*:325, 1964.

Louhimo, I.: Heart injury after blunt trauma. Acta Chir. Scand. (Suppl. 380)*134*:1967.

Maloney, J. V., Jr., Schmutzer, K. J., and Raschke, E.: Paradoxical respiration and "pendelluft." J. Thorac. Cardiovasc. Surg. *41*:291, 1961.

Parmley, L. F., et al.: Nonpenetrating traumatic injury of the aorta. Circulation *17*:1086, 1958.

Ren, L.: Über penetirende Herzwunden und Herznaht. Arch. Klin. Chir. *55*:315, 1897.

Samson, P. C., et al.: The management of war wounds of the chest in a base center. The role of early pulmonary decortication. J. Thorac. Surg. *15*:1, 1946.

Seybold, W. D., Johnson, M. A., III, and Leary, W. V.: Perforation of the esophagus. Surg. Clin. North Am. *30*:1155, 1950.

Spencer, F. C., et al.: A report of fifteen patients with traumatic rupture of the thoracic aorta. J. Thorac. Cardiovasc. Surg. *41*:1, 1961.

Symbas, P. N.: Autotransfusion from hemothorax J. Trauma *12*:689, 1972.

Symbas, P. N.: Traumatic Injuries of the Heart and Great Vessels. Springfield, Illinois, Charles C Thomas, 1972.

Symbas, P. N.: Great vessel injury from penetrating trauma. J. Cardiovasc. Surg. (11th World Congress, International Cardiovascular Society, Barcelona, Sept. 1973), pp. 620–625, 1975.

Symbas, P. N., et al.: Penetrating cardiac wounds: A comparison of different therapeutic methods. Ann. Surg. *83*(4): 377–381, April, 1976.

Symbas, P. N., et al.: Autotransfusion and its effects upon the blood components and the recipient. *In* Zuidema, G. D., and Skinner, D. B. (eds): Current Topics in Surgical Research, Vol. 1. New York and London, Academic Press, 1969, pp. 387–398.

Symbas, P. N., et al.: Penetrating cardiac wounds: A comparison of different therapeutic methods. Ann. Surg. (in press).

Symbas, P. N., et al.: A study of autotransfusion from hemothorax. Southern Med. J. *62*:671, 1969.

Symbas, P. N., et al.: Penetrating wounds of the esophagus. Ann. Thorac. Surg. *13*:552, 1972.

Symbas, P. N., et al.: Penetrating cardiac wounds. Significant residual and delayed sequelae. J. Thorac. Cardiovasc. Surg. *66*:526, 1973.

Symbas, P. N., et al.: Rupture of the aorta: a diagnostic triad. Ann. Thorac. Surg. *15*:405, 1973.

Symbas, P. N., et al.: Traumatic rupture of the aorta. Ann. Surg. *178*:6, 1973.

Symbas, P. N., et al.: Penetrating wounds of the great vessels. Ann. Surg. *179*:757, 1974.

Sugg, W. L., et al.: Penetrating wounds of the heart: An analysis of 459 cases. J. Thorac. Cardiovasc. Surg. *56*:531, 1968.

Watson, J. H., and Bartholomae, W. M.: Cardiac injury due to nonpenetrating chest trauma. Ann. Intern. Med. *52*:871, 1960.

F. EMERGENCY MANAGEMENT OF TRAUMA TO THE ABDOMEN

James R. Mackenzie

INTRODUCTION

This chapter is concerned with the immediate management in the Emergency Department of a patient who has suffered an accidental, deliberate, or iatrogenic application of force (which is usually mechanical but may be thermal or chemical) to the abdominal cage or its viscera. The applied force may be diffuse, such as a blow causing a blunt abdominal trauma, or concentrated, such as a missile causing penetrating or perforating abdominal trauma. The resultant damage may be inconsequential, life-threatening, or complicated by associated injuries or conditions that either mask the seriousness of the abdominal injury or themselves cause death or permanent disability.

Three themes are constant throughout this chapter:

1. The unity of the chest and abdomen (the truncal cage and its viscera) — injury to one part of the trunk invariably involves or affects the function of the other.

2. The essential unity between pre-hospital, Emergency Department, and definitive care — recognition and resuscitation from physiologic deficits caused by abdominal injuries are the essential roles of the emergency medical technician (EMT) and the emergency physician (EP). The recognition and confirmation of the abdominal injury are the combined responsibility of the EP and the trauma leader; the decision to observe or repair suspected abdominal injuries is the sole responsibility of the trauma leader.

3. Survival and the quality of survival depend on saving time between the appearance and correction of physiologic or anatomic deficits produced by abdominal injuries.

Management of patients with abdominal trauma beyond the Emergency Department will be considered only as it adds perspective to the themes of this chapter.

HISTORICAL BACKGROUND

The history related to the diagnosis and treatment of abdominal wounds is bound up in the history of warfare. Blunt abdominal trauma was limited to those who rode in the cavalry or in chariots, or were pushed off fortress walls, thrown off cliffs, or stoned as a means of execution. Such injuries usually were musculoskeletal or cranial, and the few internal injuries encountered probably were due to rupture of swollen and fragile malarial spleens.

The diagnosis of most penetrating or perforating abdominal injuries was obvious, and those who survived the battlefield were treated. The Egyptians washed the wounds, removed spears and arrows, applied oil, wine, or root juices as local antiseptics, and used stimulants and drugs such as mandragora and opium for pain relief. The Greeks inherited Egyptian medicine and the Romans improved upon their legacy. Celsus sutured the large intestine, peritoneum, and skin but noted that it was useless to suture the small bowel. The Arabs devised cataplasms for local anesthesia. Roger of Palermo worked at Salerno in the 12th century and reintroduced the intestinal suture, which he performed over a hollow tube, and stopped hemorrhage by digital compression, torsion, ligature, and styptics.

The decision to perform an exploratory laparotomy for evidence of visceral injuries in abdominal trauma did not pose the dilemma for the ancient physician that it does for his modern counterpart. Then, as now, wounds from sharp instruments missed vital organs in many; however, operative mortality approached 100 per cent. Indeed, triage on the field of battle often removed the decision-making power from the surgeon, since those considered to be mortally wounded were left to die or to be slain by the enemy or were sometimes killed by their comrads as an act of mercy as mentioned in the first and second books of Samuel of the Old Testament.

CONTROVERSY CONCERNING LAPAROTOMY

The controversy concerning laparotomy for the diagnosis and operative management of abdominal wounds became a serious and practical concern in 1836, when Baudens reported that only half of his operative cases from the French-Algerian War in 1830 had survived. Sims advocated laparotomy, but Walter in 1859 and Kinlock in 1863 were the first to perform abdominal operations in the United States for blunt and gunshot wounds, respectively. Reclus found that 66 of 88 dogs with abdominal bullet wounds survived without surgery and therefore continued the practice of nonoperative treatment of gunshot wounds. The British in the Boer War in 1899 advocated operative intervention in gunshot wounds to the abdomen, but fewer survived wounding with surgery than wounding without surgery, and this mode of treatment was again abandoned.

Laparotomy became mandatory for the treatment of all suspected missile wounds to the abdomen during World War I because the new high-velocity missiles caused both greater visceral damage and a higher mortality rate (85 per cent). Surgical exploration of the abdomen had become safer with the introduction of endotracheal anesthesia and better understanding of the management of sepsis and shock, and improved surgical techniques had been developed. As a result of this policy, mortality rates improved with each new conflict: 56 per cent by the end of World War I, 25 per cent during World War II, 12 per cent during the Korean conflict, and 8.5 per cent during the Vietnam War (Heaton et al., 1966). The mortality rate from civilian injuries approached 55 per cent during the period 1927–1942 but is less than 5 per cent today (Nance et al., 1974).

The success of mandatory exploration of all penetrating abdominal wounds in wartime led to the general acceptance and adoption of this mode of treatment for similar civilian injuries by 1945. However, Shaftan (1960) and Nance et al. (1974) have shown that selected laparotomy for cases with the indications listed in Figure 4 lowered morbidity and mortality. The reason for the improvement is that few civilian stab or missile wounds penetrate the coelom or cause significant visceral injuries. Therefore, in a great number of civilian patients with penetrating abdominal trauma, mandatory laparotomy is meddlesome and leads to complications. Thus, the management of penetrating abdominal wounds has come full circle since Bauden first advocated operative intervention in some penetrating wounds of the abdomen.

The recognition of the essential unity between resuscitation and operative correction of the wound was the final great advance in the care of the treatment of abdominal wounds. Prince Gedroity showed that rapid operation before deterioration of the patient saved lives in the Russia-Japanese War. Blood and fluid replacement were shown to delay deterioration from shock and peritonitis during World War I and the Spanish Civil War. But it was only late in World War II, according to Beecher (1955), that prompt operative repair was considered merely a continuation of the resuscitative treatment begun at the time the injured man was located.

CLASSIFICATION

The emergency physician must be programmed like a computer to rapidly diagnose and initially treat the patient with abdominal injuries *before* he is first faced with the problem. A set of classifications will help the physician to rapidly obtain a clinical picture of the patient through the use of the history, physical examination, routine or special laboratory data, or special diagnostic procedures; to rapidly diagnose life-threatening conditions and to reverse them; to determine the urgency with which the patient must be treated by operative intervention; or to pro-

ceed with further resuscitative procedures in a more sophisticated unit (intensive care unit) or conduct further laboratory tests or diagnostic procedures in the Emergency Department or suitable observation area. (One such unit, termed "Emergency Decision-making Unit" was described in Chapter 1.)

The classification of abdominal injuries will therefore include: (1) the anatomic sites involved; (2) resulting physiologic deficits; (3) etiology of the injury; (4) predisposing conditions that led to or complicated the injury; and (5) other injuries caused by the accident. These classifications stress that it is the *trunk* that is injured and that a blow to the chest or abdomen may structurally and functionally alter the other.

ANATOMIC CLASSIFICATION
(Fig. 1)

Injuries to the trunk may involve the truncal cage mechanism, which includes the cage itself and its controlling mechanisms (brain, spinal cord, and peripheral nerves), and or its viscera. The viscera are in turn divided by the diaphragm into those that lie predominantly in an area of negative pressure, the thoracic cavity, and those that lie predominantly in an area of positive pressure, the abdominal cavity. When this common wall is disrupted, the pressure difference will often force the mobile abdominal viscera into the thoracic cavity.

The thoracic viscera are divided into *lateral* (lungs) and *medial* (mediastinal) *structures*, since evidence of anatomic or functional disruption of these sites will depend upon the physical or radiologic examination of the lateral or medial aspects of the chest, respectively. The abdominal viscera are divided into *solid organs*, which bleed profusely when injured and lead to early signs of hypovolemic shock but late signs of peritonitis, and *hollow organs*, which tend to lead to early signs and symptoms of peritonitis but late signs of hypovolemic shock due to third space fluid sequestration.

Each item of information gathered about the patient should be tested by the emergency physician against this anatomic classification or program. He should ask the following questions: "Does this mean truncal cage or visceral injury? Is the latter above or below the diaphragm? If below the dia-

Truncal cage mechanism
1. Control mechanisms—central nervous system, spinal cord, peripheral nerves
2. Truncal cage
   a. Soft tissue—skin, subcutaneous fat, muscle, fascia, diaphragm
   b. Hard tissue—bones (ribs, sternum, spine, pelvis), cartilage (costal cartilage, intravertebral disc, and symphysis pubis)

Viscera below the diaphragm
1. Solid organs
   a. Intraperitoneal—spleen and liver
   b. Extraperitoneal—kidneys, pancreas, aorta, and inferior vena cava and their large branches
2. Hollow organs
   a. Gastrointestinal tract
   b. Genitourinary tract

Viscera above the diaphragm
1. Lateral—lungs
2. Medial—mediastinum
   a. Respiratory—tracheobronchial tree
   b. Cardiovascular-lymphatic—heart, arteries and veins (pulmonary and systemic) and lymphatics
   c. Gastrointestinal—esophagus

Figure 1   Anatomical classification of truncal trauma.

phragm, is it solid or hollow? What new information is needed to fit the diagnosis into one or more anatomic sites?" The information from these questions superimposed upon anatomic classification will lead the emergency physician to the most precise diagnosis of the sites of injury.

The physical examination—i.e., what is visualized (inspection), felt (palpation), heard (percussion or ausculation), smelled, and sometimes even tasted—usually will define involvement of the truncal cage mechanism by the injuring agent. On the other hand, visceral injuries usually are *suggested* when a physiologic deficit is defined or suspected (i.e., failure to ventilate, distribute, diffuse, or perfuse), by the history related to the traumatic event (blunt abdominal trauma and high-velocity missiles often cause visceral injury), or by a change in the initial condition of the patient with time (especially development of peritonitis). Visceral injury usually is *proved* by the use of laboratory investigations or by special diagnostic procedures, e.g., x-ray, central venous pressure (CVP), peritoneal lavage, ultrasound, or angiography. The *absence* of visceral injuries is often suspected by the rapid response and stabilization of the patient to the initial resuscitative measures.

In conclusion, the physician who has been programmed with an anatomic classification of what *could* be injured is equipped to gather information that can be rapidly formulated into a precise diagnosis of the injury and therefore a plan for its management. If information is insufficient for a precise diagnosis, then the program will help the physician to formulate a plan for further investigation.

PHYSIOLOGIC DEFICITS (Fig. 2)

Injury to the truncal cage mechanisms or its viscera may cause one of four basic physiologic deficits—errors in (1) ventilation, (2) distribution of inspired air, (3) diffusion, or (4) perfusion—which may kill the victim, cause prolonged disability, or maim the patient for life. The emergency physician must be programmed to suspect, promptly recognize, and manage these deficits, for this is his raison d'être.

Prompt recognition of physiologic deficits and their immediate successful reversal depends initially upon clinical rather than laboratory observations repeated frequently at regular intervals and applied in a routine manner. Included are observations of the cardiovascular respiratory system, measurements of the pulse and respiratory rate and rhythm, blood pressure, urinary output and specific gravity, CVP, and response to therapy—especially response to clearing of the airway, ventilation, and bolus replacement of suspected fluid and blood losses. Organization of data may be aided by a trauma "tote board" (see Fig. 13). However, laboratory tests are useful to establish baseline values, to help confirm a suspected diagnosis, and to indicate response to therapy, e.g., changes in blood gases in response to ventilation.

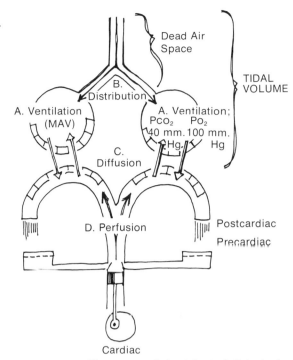

Cardiac

Figure 2. The causes of physiologic deficits in the trauma patient.

Errors in ventilation
1. Upper airway Obstruction
2. Damage to the truncal cage mechanism

Errors in distribution
1. Lower airway obstruction
2. Decreased tidal volume
3. Decreased functional residual capacity

Errors in diffusion (see Fig. 3)

Errors in perfusion
1. Low cardiac output shock
   a. Precardiac—hypovolemia, increased capacitance
   b. Cardiac—pericardial (tamponade), myocardial (prolonged anoxia, arrhythmias), endocardial (ruptured valves)
   c. Postcardiac—use of vasoconstrictors in shock
2. High cardiac output shock—not usually seen in the Emergency Department

The emergency physician who treats abdominal injuries and therefore potential thoracic and other multiple injuries must be aware of the most frequent causes, clinical diagnoses, and means of immediate reversal of common physiologic deficits (Fig. 2). (For more detailed discussion, see Chapter 3.)

1. Errors in ventilation (Fig. 2) are caused by upper airway obstruction and damage to the truncal cage mechanism.

(*a*) Upper airway obstruction above the carina causes stridor, indrawing of the lower rib cage, intercostal spaces, and tracheal tug. Treatment consists of removal of the obstruction.

(*b*) Damage to the truncal cage mechanism including the central nervous system can cause an alteration in rate of respiration or size of the tidal volume (TV). Failure of the lower rib cage to flair indicates a decrease of 150 cc. or more in the TV. To correct hypoventilation, ventilate the patient. Administering oxygen without a mechanism for ventilation will not correct this deficit, as the oxygen cannot reach the unventilated alveoli. A decreased TV also leads to regional hypoventilation (see errors of distribution), since the area of the lung will not expand if the rib cage over it does not expand.

2. Errors in distribution (Fig. 2) indicate that inspired air does not reach the alveoli of all parts of the lung, leading to regional hypoventilation. Therefore, some parts of the lung will be perfused but not ventilated, causing shifting of unoxygenated blood into the systemic circulatory system ($\dot{V}/\dot{Q}$ deficits). Significant errors are always accompanied by cyanosis and decreased oxygen content of arterial blood. Errors in distribution are caused by obstruction of the bronchial tree below the carina, decreased TV, or decreased functional residual capacity (FRC).

(*a*) Obstruction of the bronchial tree below the carina is frequently due to aspiration of gastric contents in the patient with abdominal trauma. It can be prevented by the routine use of a nasogastric tube, placing the patient in a prone position, or by oropharyngeal suction and placement of a cuffed endotracheal tube. The routine use of a nasogastric tube also will help to determine the presence or absence of upper gastrointestinal bleeding, correct a decreased FRC caused by gastric distention, and prevent troublesome distention of the abdominal viscera during the preoperative period. Diagnosis and treatment of obstruction to the airway below the carina are discussed in Chapter 3.

(*b*) Decrease in tidal volume is discussed under hypoventilation. Correction of this deficit consists of ventilating the patient.

(*c*) Decrease in functional residual capacity is caused by abdominal—especially gastric—distention due to swallowed air or air forced into the stomach during positive pressure ventilation via a face mask. It leads to decreased mobility of the diaphragm and lower rib cage and is the most common cause for decreased residual air in the lungs after a normal expiration. Routine placement of a nasogastric tube may be life-saving. Pneumothorax also frequently causes decreased FRC.

3. Errors in diffusion. Contused lung, aspiration, and massive replacement of blood loss by crystalloid fluids are the most common causes for pulmonary edema in the patient with abdominal trauma. In such situations, a high index of suspicion and the findings of an increasing re-

spiratory rate (accurately measured), appearance of rales in the bases of one or both lungs, and changes in the P_{O_2} over baseline blood gases are the most sensitive indices available for diagnosis of the condition. The use of a nasogastric tube and a cuffed endotracheal tube will prevent aspiration.

4. Errors in perfusion (Fig. 2). Blood loss leading to poor venous return is the most common cause of low cardiac output shock (i.e. precardiac or pre-load shock) in abdominal trauma. It must be remembered, however, that there are cardiac and postcardiac causes of low cardiac output shock (mentioned in Fig. 2).

In suspected abdominal trauma remember the following considerations:

(*a*) Signs of shock, including a urine output of less than 2 ml./minute, *and* a rise in the specific gravity without obvious reason indicate occult bleeding, usually abdominal or less often retroperitoneal or mediastinal.

(*b*) Raised neck veins or an increased CVP with clinical or urinary signs of shock must be considered as due to cardiac tamponade until proved otherwise.

(*c*) Correction of hypovolemic shock after a rapid (5 to 10 minutes) infusion of 10 ml./kg. of Ringer's lactate, saline, or blood implies a mild blood loss; 20 ml./kg. implies a major blood loss; and 40 ml./kg. implies a life-threatening blood loss. This formula can be used for infants, children, and adults (Morse, 1976).

(*d*) Evidence of a decreased cardiac output after an initial response to the rapid infusion of 10 to 20 ml./kg. of fluid implies continued occult bleeding; after the rapid infusion of 40 ml./kg., it implies exsanguination.

(*e*) In the latter instance, further investigative procedures must cease, and the patient must be transferred immediately to the operating room for surgical intervention.

(*f*) A significant decrease in blood pressure, rise in pulse rate, or drop in urinary output after the institution of continuous positive pressure breathing indicates hypovolemia or tension pneumothorax *until proved otherwise.*

In conclusion, the emergency physician must immediately recognize and reverse errors in ventilation, distribution, diffusion, and perfusion if the patient is to survive the initial, insult-causing abdominal injury.

ETIOLOGY (Fig. 3)

The causal agent and the circumstances in which it was applied must be considered when treating a patient with abdominal trauma. A significant number of patients with knife wounds or blunt injuries will need

Penetrating
1. Stab wounds
2. Gunshot wounds
3. Shotgun wounds
4. Fragmentation missles
5. Flying objects (e.g., lawnmower blades)
6. Falls on sharp objects (e.g., picket fences)

Non-penetrating (blunt)
1. Non-specific (motor vehicle accidents, sports injuries, home, industrial)
2. Seatbelt injuries
3. Blast and crush injuries

Iatrogenic
1. Endoscopies (with or without biopsies)
   a. Upper and lower gastrointestinal tract
   b. Peritoneoscopy
   c. Culdoscopy
2. Paracentesis or low thoracocentesis (especially trocar)
3. Liver biopsy or percutaneous transhepatic cholangiography or angiography
4. Endoesophageal placement of nasotracheal oxygen catheter
5. Barium enema

Ingestion injuries
1. Corrosives
2. Foreign bodies

Perversion injuries
1. Enemas
2. Foreign bodies
3. High pressure hose

Figure 3 Etiologic agents causing abdominal injury.

observation only, since they will not have significant visceral injuries (Nance et al., 1974; Shaftan, 1960). In contrast, virtually all high-velocity missile wounds must be explored—even though no visceral injury is demonstrated—since most of these agents will cause a great deal of tissue damage, especially to solid organs (Demuth, 1966). Injuries have been divided into penetrating, nonpenetrating (blunt), iatrogenic, ingestion, and perversion.

PENETRATING ABDOMINAL TRAUMA (PAT)

STAB WOUNDS

Knives, scissors, screwdrivers, pencils, glass bottles, automobile radio antennae, bicycle spokes, and numerous other instruments may be used to inflict stab wounds to the abdomen. It must be remembered that stab wounds to the chest up to the area of the fourth rib also can produce trauma to the abdominal viscera. The size, shape, and depth of the wound are important in determining what viscera, if any, are involved.

Shaftan and later Nance popularized the approach of selective rather than mandatory celiotomy of stab wounds to the abdomen. This policy was established because they found a 25 to 75 per cent incidence of negative laparotomies; one-half of the so-called "positive" laparotomies were performed for insignificant visceral injuries that would have healed without operative intervention. They also found a 8 to 11 per cent morbidity rate in those cases with negative explorations or unnecessary positive explorations, and delay until indications for mandatory celiotomy appeared did not seem to increase mortality or morbidity. The 50 to 75 per cent who avoided celiotomy usually could be discharged three to four days later.

Therefore, the emergency physician performs three functions in managing stab wounds to the abdomen in the Emergency Department: (1) resuscitation of the patient with physiologic deficits; (2) recording baseline information, including stability and changes with time and treatment so that the trauma surgeon can determine whether the indications for mandatory laparotomy listed in Figure 4 are present; and (3) initiation of investigations to determine the presence or absence of significant visceral injuries.

GUNSHOT WOUNDS*

Tissue damage due to bullets or other missiles is proportional to the loss of kinetic energy (KE) between entry and exit of the missile from the body (DeMuth, 1966). The loss of KE is expressed as tissue displacement radial to the trajectory of the bullet. Missiles with high KE produce a large cavity and consequently much damage during passage, while collapse of the tissue obliterates the cavity after passage and gives a false impression of tissue normality. The rest of the loss of KE is due to friction and is expressed as coagulative heat. Damage done by missiles is greatest in solid organs, muscle, skin, and bone and least in subcutaneous tissue and lung.

---

*See also Evaluation of Trauma for missile considerations.

Etiologic agents
1. High-velocity gunshot wounds
2. Type III shotgun wounds
3. High-velocity mines or other fragmentation missiles
4. Agents left behind—for example, stakes, glass bottles

Presenting or delayed signs
1. Peritoneal injury, i.e., peritonitis (especially tenderness, rebound tenderness, guarding, or rigidity)
2. Loss of bowel sounds
3. Evisceration of viscus or massive wounding to the truncal cage
4. Unexplained shock
5. Positive diagnostic studies
   a. Visible blood from the stomach or rectum
   b. Massive hematuria with confirmation of injury by rectal examination, IVP, cystogram, or cystoscopy
   c. Needle aspiration or peritoneal lavage for blood, bile, or intestinal contents
   d. Plain films (displacement, fluid, or air)
   e. Arteriogram
   f. Unexplained increasing abdominal girth
   g. Injuries noted on peritoneoscopy, sigmoidoscopy, panendoscopy, or culdoscopy

Stability—unstable, deteriorating, or irreversible

Figure 4 Protocol for mandatory exploration of the abdomen.

KE at the muzzle (muzzle velocity) is expressed in foot-pounds and is equal to the mass of the missile in grains times the square of the velocity in feet per second, divided by twice the gravitational acceleration in feet per second; that is,

$$KE = mv^2 \div 7000 \times 32.2 \times 2,$$

or

$$KE = mv^2/4,508,000$$

In the preceding formula, 7000 is a conversion factor

Most handguns have a muzzle velocity of 500 to 1500 feet per second; military rifles have a velocity of 2000 to 3000 feet per second. Impact velocity will depend on the characteristics of the missile (ballistic coefficient) and the distance of the target from the muzzle. The missiles with the best coefficients (e.g., M-16) will lose 6 per cent, and round-nose bullets (.22) will lose 16 per cent of their muzzle velocity per 100 yards (DeMuth, 1969). Some bullets are soft-nosed or drilled and are designed to expand, tumble, or shatter upon impact, thus imparting all or most of their KE to the tissue before exit. Therefore, an M-16 bullet with a velocity of 3250 feet per second could have at least 14 to 16 times more impact energy at

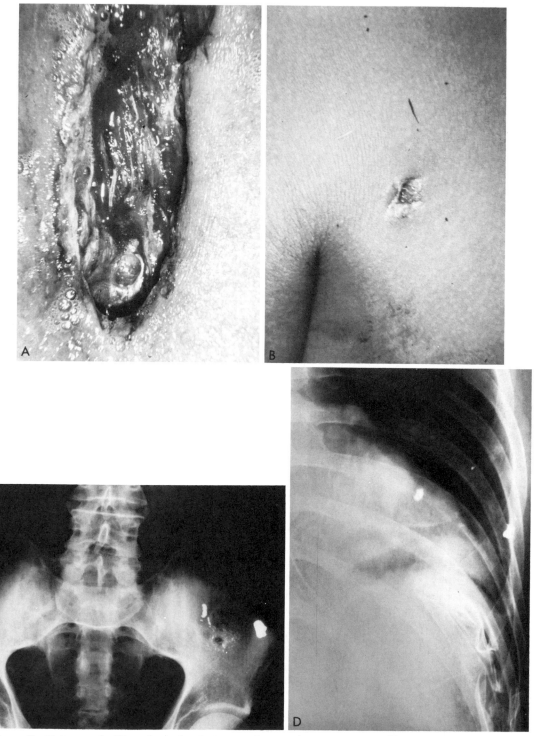

Figure 5. Exit wounds. Wounds can be obvious, as the one shown in *A*, created by an M-16 bullet as it left the abdominal wall; or they may be occult, as the one shown in *B*, which was near the intergluteal cleft. If no exit wound exists, then the bullet must still be in the truncal cavity. *C*, An x-ray of a patient who was shot in the left pelvic region. The bullet hit the left iliac bone, then part of it ricocheted into the left side of the chest, damaging the spleen and diaphragm during its course (*D*).

point-blank range and 25 yards respectively than a .22 calibre handgun. It will impart most of its energy to the tissue in its trajectory, and tissue damage including exit wounds will obviously vary accordingly. Fragmented missiles will have several trajectories, causing even more damage (Fig. 5, A, B, C).

The lighter bullet has less inertia (I = mv) and tends to be deflected by tissue planes of the truncal cage and therefore may be deflected away from the abdominal cavity. The smaller, low-velocity missile may penetrate the abdominal cavity and separate rather than damage the mobile viscera, since it will have lost most of its KE on impact with the solid tissues of the truncal cage (tissue drag). As a consequence, Nance et al. (1974) have suggested expectant treatment of patients with wounds caused by low-velocity bullets with a small mass. The same criteria listed for mandatory laparotomy in stab wounds are used for patients with gunshot wounds (GSW) to the abdomen. Shaftan suggests that this form of treatment will significantly lower morbidity and hospital stay, since 25 to 50 per cent of an increasing number of homicides in the U.S. are due to handguns. There is still substantial controversy among surgeons, however, particularly with regard to gunshot wounds.

The function of the emergency physician in treating GSW to the abdomen is fundamentally the same as for stab wounds. However, he must remember that patients with wounds caused by high-velocity missiles are unstable and that laparotomy is mandatory, in spite of the clinical appearance of the wound or apparent state of health of the victim.

SHOTGUN INJURIES

This term implies a pellet load, although it may be slugs. The powder, size of pellets, choke of gun, and distance to target all determine the KE at impact and, therefore, destructive effect. The *pattern* is the area over which the pellets are dispersed. A close pattern having a diameter of 15 cm. or less concentrates KE and produces wide and deep tissue destruction. In addition to the pellets, the wad, plastic cups, and clothing are usually buried deep in these close pattern wounds.

There are numerous combinations of pellets, powder, and choke, but the most frequently used is 12-gauge with shells containing No. 6 pellets or larger. Full choke fired at 10 yards will concentrate 95 per cent of the pellets within a circle 22 cm. in diameter and within a 44 cm. diameter circle when fired from a cylinder bore. Doubling the distance doubles the diameter of the pattern and quadruples the area. At 20 yards, one-quarter of the muzzle velocity of 1300 feet per second is lost.

Sherman and Parrish describe three types of injuries: Type I, or long-range (over 7 yards), injuries seldom penetrate the truncal cavity; Type II (3 to 4 yards) may perforate a large number of visceral structures in the truncal cavity, making location of all perforations impossible. The mucosa of the intestines usually do not part in these wounds and heal unaided, while operative handling spills intestinal contents and contaminates the cavities. Therefore, Type I and II wounds may be treated expectantly. The emergency physician can institute the same type of management for these wounds as for stab and low-velocity gunshot wounds.

Type III wounds are sustained at point-blank range, causing massive tissue destruction and shock and have a 50 to 65 per cent mortality (Bell, 1971). These patients, if they survive the initial injury, need immediate operative intervention. The role of the emergency physician is to start resuscitation and to send the patient *immediately* to the surgical service. Operative intervention is mandatory and time is of the essence.

All shotgun wounds to the abdomen have twice the mortality rate (27.6 per cent in Bell's 1971 series) of other gunshot wounds (12.5 per cent in Nance's series). Those involving the chest have an even greater mortality rate.

OTHER PENETRATING WOUNDS

Fragmentation missile wounds are becoming more frequent with the advent of urban conflict and should be treated like shotgun wounds because of their KE characteristics and patterns.

Impalement wounds and flying missiles from lawnmowers are like stab wounds except that they are larger, dirtier, and more likely to require wide debridement of the wound and operative correction of visceral injuries. As in stab wounds, the impaling object, if still present in the wound, should be removed only by the attending surgical team, and then usually in the operating room under anesthesia.

IATROGENIC INJURIES

Inadvertent perforation of the gastrointestinal tract may follow endoscopic procedures. Abdominal sites include the lower end of the esophagus and stomach during panendoscopy or one of its variations; colonic perforation following sigmoidoscopy and colonoscopy, especially with biopsy; and small bowel damage following peritoneoscopy, especially with tubal cauterization for sterilization. Paracentesis and low thoracentesis, liver biopsy, splenoportography, percutaneous transhepatic cholangiography, or percutaneous transhepatic portal venography may also cause bile peritonitis and intraperitoneal bleeding, or small or large bowel perforations with peritonitis. These injuries may go unrecognized, or the symptoms of injury may be delayed for one to three days or even several months for subphrenic collections of bile or pus (Zollinger, 1972). Therefore, it is important for the emergency physician to keep this type of injury in mind when patients arrive in the Emergency Department with unexplained fever, peritonitis, or evidence of intraperitoneal bleeding. Barium enemas can also cause colonic perforations, but these are usually recognized at the time. If not, they are readily diagnosed on a flat plate of the abdomen.

Improper placement of a nasopharyngeal oxygen catheter or an endotracheal tube connected to positive pressure ventilation or inadvertent connection of the nasogastric tube to an oxygen outlet instead of suction while resuscitating a patient in the emergency department can cause severe damage to the esophagus and stomach within minutes. The usual injury to the esophagus is laceration and bleeding, but there may be perforation of the intra-abdominal lower end with escape of free air into the peritoneal cavity. The usual injury to the stomach is severe distention with lacerations and/or perforation along the lesser curvature. The distended stomach causes respiratory distress. The acute rise in intragastric and therefore intra-abdominal pressure may compress the inferior vena cava, leading to

interrupted venous return to the heart and preload shock. Perforation of the stomach and escape of oxygen into the intraperitoneal cavity may also lead to an acute rise in the intra-abdominal pressure and obstruction of the inferior vena cava.

Recognition of this complication is made on clinical grounds with the appearance of blood in vomitus or in the nasogastric tube, rapid abdominal distention, and cardiorespiratory distress. Immediate treatment rather than confirmation of this complication is imperative if death is to be avoided. Oxygen is stopped, and the nasopharyngeal catheter or endotracheal tube is removed from the esophagus. If the oxygen was inadvertently administered through the nasogastric tube, it is left in place and immediately connected to gentle suction. If a nasogastric tube is not in place, it should be cautiously but rapidly introduced while being careful to avoid further lacerations to the esophagus or the lesser curvature of the overdistended stomach. Often the distention cannot be relieved by this method, since the distended stomach also distorts and blocks the gastroesophageal junction, or the distention may be limited to the antrum by a transverse fold at or near the incisura. The distention, and hence the obstruction, to the passage to the nasogastric tube may be relieved by positioning the patient prone or on the right side. If these methods of relief fail and the patient is in cardiorespiratory distress, then a No. 14 needle or cannula should be passed percutaneously into the distended stomach, or if this fails, a minor laparotomy should be performed through the linea alba. Time, as usual, plays its part in survival.

PERVERSION INJURIES

Anything goes! The injuring agents may include anything from enemas to foreign bodies to high-pressure hoses used to "goose" the victim. Perforation can occur below or above the peritoneal reflection. Those related to the anal sphincter and levator ani may cause necrosis and gas gangrene. Other injuries perforate the bladder, generally just above the neck in the area of the trigone. Those above the peritoneal reflection lead to peritonitis.

Diagnosis should be suspected in patients with rectal, urinary tract, or vaginal bleeding or with signs and symptoms of peritonitis or unexplained shock (see Fig. 4). Confirmation depends upon the history, which is often inaccurate because of the embarrassment of the situation; rectal and vaginal examination for foreign bodies, blood, or abscesses; urinalysis for blood; physical examination of the abdomen; and three radiographic views of the abdomen for evidence of perforation. Further diagnostic procedures should be left to the treating surgeon.

BLUNT ABDOMINAL TRAUMA

Blunt abdominal trauma (BAT) accounts for 0.1 per cent of hospital admissions but 1 per cent of all trauma admissions to hospital. It includes percussion injuries from pedestrian–motor vehicle accidents, seatbelts, and sports, home, and industrial accidents. Automobile accidents account for 50 per cent of all blunt injuries, but 70 to 75 per cent of all BAT (Ballinger, 1973).

BAT is associated with a 10 to 30 per cent mortality rate. Di Vincenti et al. (1968) reviewed 518 patients treated for BAT at Charity Hospital, New Orleans between 1951 and 1966: 10 per cent died before treatment; 5 to 6 per cent died following nonoperative treatment (3 to 4 per cent due to error in diagnosis and 1 to 2 per cent from other severe injuries), and 9 per cent died following operative intervention for an overall mortality rate of 24 to 25 per cent. Davis (1976), reporting from the same institution for the period of 1967–1973, treated 437 cases of BAT: 3.4 per cent died before treatment was instituted; 0.7 per cent following nonoperative treatment; none from misdiagnosis of abdominal injuries; and 9.2 per cent following operation. *It is important for the emergency physician to note* that the improved results between the two series depended upon prehospital and emergency department diagnosis and care, and better selection of patients for expectant management. There was no improvement in mortality figures for those who ultimately were chosen for surgery.

Injury to liver, diaphragm, kidney, combined pancreas and duodenum, or retroperitoneal areas carries a higher mortality than injury to the spleen and urinary bladder. Isolated pancreatic and hollow organ injuries have the lowest mortality. The high mortality

rate with the first group seems to be due to associated injuries, especially to the head, as well as to the abdominal injury.

Occupant survival from blunt abdominal trauma due to motor vehicle accidents may rise in the next few years with the introduction of lower speed limits in both Canada and the United States and the wider use of seat belts. Ontario introduced a 60 m.p.h. speed limit (it had been 70 m.p.h.) and compulsory use of restraint systems on January 1, 1976. The death rate and serious injury rate immediately dropped by 30 per cent even though collision rates had risen 3 per cent. Australia and other countries have shown that much of the reason for lowered death and serious injury rates was due to the decrease in head and spinal injuries (Henderson and Wood, 1973). Thus, survival from abdominal trauma in the future may be due to a decreased incidence of associated injuries.

The percentage of those with abdominal injuries who reach the hospital alive may even increase owing to a higher survival rate per accident, as noted above. They may also temporarily increase because abdominal injuries are traded for the more serious cranial–upper spinal injuries with the redistribution of forces by the seat belt. Kolowski and Rost first described injuries due to the wearing of seat belts in 1956. Williams and Kirkpatrick showed that lap belts produce more serious visceral injuries than the three-point restraining system, which causes more injuries to the truncal cage. The three-point restraining system is superior in preventing injuries to the pregnant uterus (Crosby and Costello, 1971). Therefore, the mandatory installation of comfortable three-point restraining systems in new cars should ultimately result in an absolute decrease in abdominal injuries.

The mechanism of injury in trauma to the abdominal cage is either a percussion blow to the hard and soft tissue or a crushing effect between the forward inertia of the abdominal contents or posterior abdominal wall and the external restraint. If the restraint is narrow, such as the rim of a steering wheel or a narrow lap belt displaced above the anterior superior iliac spines, the rectus muscle and subcutaneous tissue may be cut in half even though the skin is intact. Either mechanism, percussion or crushing, tends to produce external bruising, while crushing can also produce a defect in the muscles.

Abdominal viscera are damaged by

crushing the organ against the posterior abdominal wall, especially the spine. Pancreatic injuries from falling on the handlebars of a bicycle in children is an example. Shearing forces between mobile and fixed organs also cause damage. Finally, an increased intra-abdominal pressure may rupture the hollow viscera.

Blunt trauma, as its name describes, is indiscriminate. There usually are no entry or exit wounds to guide the physician to the area of damage. The care of the patient with blunt abdominal trauma, therefore, concerns the patient who has potential multiple areas of the body involved by trauma, as opposed to the care of the patient with penetrating abdominal trauma, who, at worse, has multiple organs of the trunk involved by the injury. The major role of the emergency physician in blunt abdominal trauma, therefore, is resuscitation. However, it is also important to initiate studies that will identify major visceral injuries, since mandatory laparotomy usually takes precedence over other mandatory explorations.

DEGREE OF STABILITY

The life of the trauma victim is in jeopardy from the moment instability or mandatory indications for operation first appear (Fig. 4) until the disruption produced by the injury is corrected. The emergency physician (in consultation with the trauma team) must therefore be programmed to repeatedly consider whether to continue with resuscitation and diagnosis or to rapidly transfer the patient to the operating room for correction of the injuries. The patient with truncal injuries can be categorized for this purpose as *stable* (before or after resuscitation), *unstable, deteriorating,* or *irreversible.*

Stable implies the absence of physiologic deficits at the time of examination, or if present, the deficits are easily reversible without continued effort. Exceptions to this definition are wounding by medium- or high-velocity missiles; Type II shotgun wounds; high-velocity fragments from mines, grenades, etc.; and wounds that produce moderate or major bleeding. Those exceptions place the patient in the *unstable* category, since the very nature of the wound or deficit demands mandatory exploration.

Unstable implies the continued need for resuscitative measures even though vital signs and physiologic deficits have been restored. The patient's life must be considered in jeopardy from the moment instability appears until the wound has been repaired.

Deteriorating implies that signs of physiologic deficits are still present in spite of resuscitative measures. This patient must be moved to the operating room without delay, even though further diagnostic tests or resuscitation are mandatory, so that thoracotomy or laparotomy may be instituted at the instant it is deemed necessary. Delay in the transfer of the deteriorating patient often means unnecessary death between the Emergency Department and the operating room table.

Irreversible implies that the injury or its complications will kill the patient in spite of treatment. Irreversible lesions usually involve the head and the spine but include massive loss of viscera or tissue from the truncal cage.

ASSOCIATED CONDITIONS

Morbidity and mortality increase in both penetrating and blunt abdominal trauma in the presence of multiple abdominal organ injury; with extra-abdominal injuries, especially to the head and chest; and with central nervous system depression due to ingestion of drugs or alcohol. Morbidity and mortality also increase with preinjury disabilities such as diabetes, heart attacks, or psychosis. The associated conditions increase morbidity and mortality directly; and indirectly by distracting attention from the abdominal injury or by obscuring the signs and symptoms of abdominal injury. The emergency physician must recognize morbid conditions associated with abdominal trauma and understand and combat their lethal effects. Blunt abdominal trauma associated with a heart attack is an example of a possible dilemma facing the emergency physician. Shock may be due to precardiac causes (hypovolemic or vasodilation drugs), cardiac (tamponade, myocardial infarction, beta-blocking effects of antihypertensive drugs, or traumatic valvular disruption), postcardiac (rupture of the aorta), or a combination of all three types of shock. (Figure 6 diagrams some possibilities in the context of a "cascade of triage.")

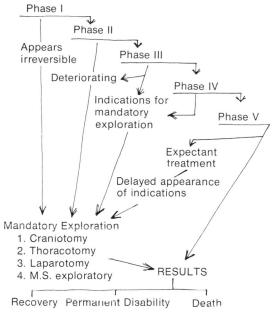

Phase I

Phase II

Appears
irreversible

Phase III

Deteriorating

Phase IV

Indications for
mandatory
exploration

Phase V

Expectant
treatment

Delayed appearance
of indications

Mandatory Exploration
1. Craniotomy
2. Thoracotomy
3. Laparotomy
4. M.S. exploratory

RESULTS

Recovery   Permanent Disability   Death

Figure 6. Cascade of Emergency Department triage (see text).

DIAGNOSIS OF ABDOMINAL TRAUMA

SIGNS AND SYMPTOMS OF BLUNT ABDOMINAL TRAUMA

The signs and symptoms of blunt abdominal trauma cover a wide clinical spectrum. The victim may present with signs and symptoms of injury to the abdominal cage mechanism only; with cage injury plus occult injury to the viscera; or with obvious severe injury to the viscera with signs and symptoms of cardiovascular and respiratory collapse. Indeed, the usual signs and symptoms of abdominal visceral injury may be overshadowed in the patient obtunded by head, spine, or chest injuries, or by ingested drugs; or by intrinsic metabolic defects such as diabetes. Delay in the diagnosis of visceral injuries in these patients may lead to a higher morbidity and mortality than is necessary.

Injury to the control mechanism of the abdominal cage (head, dorsicervical spine) produces signs and symptoms discussed in Chaps. 38A and B and will not be repeated. Injury to the soft tissues of the abdominal cage may produce severe pain, especially with movement, which may result in decreased tidal volume breathing. Indeed, deep breathing may be used to unmask occult pain due to truncal injury. The skin, subcutaneous and musculofascial tissues may be obviously bruised, welted, or lacerated from the external blow or from a compound fracture. Steering wheel or seatbelt injuries may cause separation of the tissue beneath an intact skin, and the separation may be readily seen or palpated beneath the area of the blow. Tenderness originating from the abdominal wall can be differentiated from tenderness originating from the peritoneum by tensing the muscles of the abdominal wall by straight leg elevation 2 inches off the bed. If tenderness to direct palpation disappears with tension, then the pain originates from a deeper plane than the muscles; if present but less, both the wall and the deeper structures may be involved; if flexion produces the pain, then, of course, it originates from the wall.

Injury to the cartilaginous and bony abdominal cage produces pain and tenderness directly over the area and often obvious deformities and crepitus with movement. The signs and symptoms have been discussed under the chapters dealing with the chest, spine, and bony pelvis. It is important to point out that tenderness or crepitus to remote palpation, as shown in Figure 7, or directly over the fracture is a much more reliable method of demonstrating the presence of hard tissue injury than is the use of x-rays, which might initially appear to be negative. Rectal and vaginal examination by palpation must be considered part of the search for bone or joint injury to the pelvis, as well as part of the search for rectal, prostatic, bladder, and vaginal injury (Fig. 7D).

The victim's sides and back must be examined in the same manner as the anterior abdominal cage. The patient is turned like a log, and the cervical spine is protected by traction or by a collar unit until spinal injury has been ruled out. Otherwise, the diligent search for other injuries may lead to inadvertent spinal cord damage, especially in the unconscious patient. This part of the examination could be deferred in the unconscious patient until lateral neck (cervical spine) x-rays are taken.

Intra-abdominal injury should be suspected in anyone who presents with severe injury to the soft or hard tissues of the truncal cage, shock, peritonitis, loss of liver dullness on the right side, or obliteration of Traube's space on the left. Davis et al. (1976) found that 187 (43 per cent) of 437 cases of BAT

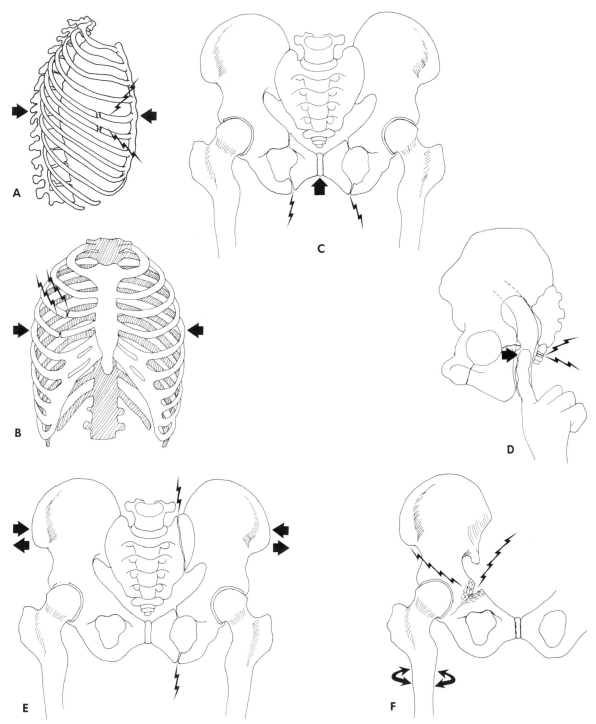

Figure 7. The diagnosis of fractures of the truncal cage mechanism. A rapid way to elicit pain at the site of fractured ribs is to produce anteroposterior compression over the sternum, which will elicit pain at the site of fractures of the lateral portion of the ribs (*A*) while lateral compression of the rib cage elicits pain over the costochondral joint and the posterior aspect of the ribs (*B*). The exact site of the fractured ribs and the number is then elicited by palpation directly over the site indicated by the pain.

Anteroposterior compression over the symphysis pubis causes pain in the pubic bones of itself (*C*). Confirmation of fractures includes direct palpation externally or by rectal or vaginal examination and x-ray (*D*). Lateral compression or distraction causes pain over injured sacroiliac joints or pubic symphysis or fractured iliac bones (*E*). Rotation or flexion of the hip bone causes pain in the injured acetabulum or sacroiliac joint (*F*). Although x-ray will confirm the diagnosis of a fractured pelvis or ribs, a negative x-ray must be viewed with suspicion if there are signs of tenderness in the above situation.

were asymptomatic on arrival in the Emergency Department; 84 of the 187 (45 per cent) ultimately developed signs and symptoms requiring laparotomy, and 64 (76 per cent) had significant injuries. *Therefore, the emergency physician must ensure that all patients with blows to the trunk or deceleration injuries (falls or motor vehicle accidents) who initially present without signs and symptoms are treated as though they actually had intra-abdominal injuries.* These patients must be examined repeatedly in the Emergency Department or admitted to a team who will carry out this function.

ASSOCIATIONS OF INJURIES

Fractures of the lower ribs suggest possible laceration of the liver on the right, or of the spleen on the left, especially if the patient has pain in the respective shoulder tip. This pain may be enhanced by the Trendelenburg position or by deep breathing and is accompanied by evidence of blood loss. Indeed, the patients often complain that they cannot sit up because they feel faint and they cannot lie down because of the shoulder pain. Other signs of intraperitoneal blood loss include shifting dullness in the flank to percussion and abdominal distention, which is usually due to the accompanying ileus. Fractures of the bony pelvis indicate possible rectal or genitourinary disruption. Blood on the palpating finger, prostatic mobility, or bulging of the anterior rectal wall provides conclusive evidence of pelvic visceral injury. Bruises or welts over the epigastric area from a steering wheel, handlebars of a bicycle, or kick by a horse may indicate pancreaticoduodenal injuries. These same signs due to a misplaced seat belt over the lower abdomen may mean a crushed terminal ileum or a lacerated pregnant uterus. Acute flexion over the belt will also produce injury to the dorsolumbar spine often accompanied by liver and diaphragmatic injury.

Shock due to occult blood loss on admission to the Emergency Department or developing soon afterward indicates damage to intraperitoneal solid viscera, fractured pelvis or femur; or laceration of the great vessels of the mediastinum. The amount of blood and other fluids necessary to restore urine flow and the CVP indicates the severity of the initial bleeding, while a continued need for fluid after the initial rapid replacement indicates further fluid loss most likely due to bleeding (Morse, 1976).

Obliteration of Traube's space indicates a subscapular hematoma or a tear of the spleen, especially if other signs and symptoms of splenic trauma are present. Obliteration of the space may also be caused by an enlarged liver, a stomach full of fluid (no air bubble), or a chronically enlarged spleen.

Disruption of a hollow viscus due to BAT may be accompanied by loss of air and fluid contents into the general peritoneal cavity, the lesser sac, or the retroperitoneal space. Gas escaping into the intraperitoneal space leads to loss of liver dullness to percussion over the area of the liver bed below the sixth rib laterally and the fifth rib anteriorly when the patient lies in the semi-erect position or on the left side. This is usually the earliest sign of rupture of a hollow viscus and may be confirmed by x-ray. Escape of air into the retroperitoneal space or lesser sac will only be detected on x-ray films of the abdomen (Fig. 10D).

Other signs of perforation such as tenderness, rebound tenderness, rigidity, rectal and vaginal tenderness, and absence of bowel sounds, i.e., signs of peritonitis, are usually absent on admission but appear within two hours. *Therefore, accurate observations of these signs must be recorded on admission and at frequent intervals.* Bowel sounds may be absent on admission owing to reflex ileus rather than to peritonitis. Therefore, this sign is only of use if bowel sounds are initially present and then subsequently disappear. Finally, the signs and symptoms of peritonitis may appear several hours or even days later due to loculation of the intestinal contents in the retroperitoneal space or lesser sac (Walt and Wilson, 1975). Similarly, peritonitis due to intraperitoneal bleeding is usually delayed. Of course, both solid and hollow organs may be disrupted by BAT in which case the clinical picture may include the signs and symptoms of both.

SIGNS AND SYMPTOMS OF PENETRATING ABDOMINAL TRAUMA

Like BAT, penetrating abdominal trauma (PAT) produces a wide clinical spectrum. The wounding instrument may penetrate only the truncal cage; or it may penetrate the abdominal cavity without injury to the viscera, it may cause insignificant injury to the viscera (example, an ice pick wound to the right lobe of the liver is no more significant to the ultimate survival of the patient than a liver biopsy), or it may cause devastating injury to most of the viscera of the truncal cage (example, a fragmented M-16 bullet).

The fundamental job of the emergency physician, apart from resuscitation, is to determine the nature of the penetrating instrument and the circumstances under which it produced the wound; the trajectory of the stabbing instrument or missile and therefore the likelihood of causing significant visceral injury; and finally, the presence or absence of visceral injury.

Nature of the Penetrating Instrument (Fig. 3). All wounds produced by military rifles, high-velocity mines, and Type III shotgun wounds demand mandatory exploration with or without evidence of visceral injury because their high KE at impact will most likely cause visceral damage. Once the emergency physician determines that the patient has been wounded by these instruments, he should proceed with routine, but judicious, use of laboratory tests listed below.

Trajectory. The trajectory of the wounding instrument will usually indicate the possibility of visceral damage. The instrument may penetrate any part of the truncal cage or the truncal cage mechanism but—except for head, spinal, or pleural injuries—the entry produces few, if any, physiologic deficits. On the other hand, the exit wound may be large and interfere with physiologic function in the same manner as blunt abdominal trauma. A line drawn between these two wounds will usually indicate the viscera damaged by the trajectory of the bullet (Fig. 5 *C* and *D*). It must again be emphasized that wounds entering or exiting as high as the fourth rib on the right and the fourth interspace on the left may produce damage to the abdominal viscera, while wounds as low as the 11th rib may produce visceral injuries to the chest. The entry wounds to the abdominal or thoracic viscera may be hidden in three circumstances: iatrogenic (endoscopies); perversion (rectal, vaginal, urethral, or bladder); and missile wounds entering a skin crease (mines, perverted attempts at murder; Fig. 8) or into the thigh, buttock, or shoulder.

Visceral Injury. The signs and symptoms of visceral injury, occult or obvious, are the same for PAT as they are for BAT and will not be reiterated. The big advantage that the emergency physician has in diagnosing visceral injury due to PAT as opposed to BAT is that establishment of the trajectory of the wound by clinical and radiologic examination indicates the possible viscera involved. It is important to remember that if an exit wound is not found, the missile must still be present somewhere in the abdomen, as shown in Figure 5C.

LABORATORY TESTS

Laboratory tests are used as baseline studies for future comparison or as aides to

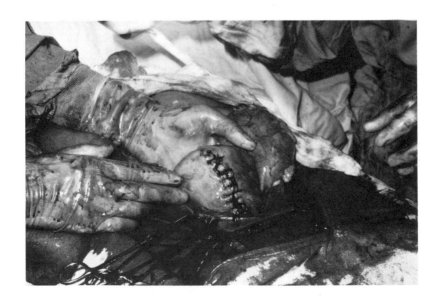

Figure 8. Hidden entrance wounds. A pregnant Vietnamese lady was charged with fraternizing with U.S. soldiers by the Viet Cong. They placed a rifle into her vagina and pulled the trigger. The bullet perforated the anterior fornix, opened the pregnant uterus, killing the fetus, lacerated the bladder, and exited through the anterior abdominal wall, but did not kill the victim.

confirming a clinical diagnosis. *Laboratory tests should never be used as a substitute for clinical judgment in the acute situation,* either as a diagnostic tool or as an indication for treatment since the patient may expire before the results are obtained.

ROUTINE RADIOLOGIC EXAMINATIONS

Radiologic examination of the trunk is an important aid in the precise location and diagnosis of an abdominal injury and is an adjunct to, but not a replacement for, the clinical examination. Judgment must be exercised in its use, since it must not interefere with resuscitation or delay laparotomy in the unstable patient. Potentially useful x-ray examinations used in the following sequence include:

1. Supine anteroposterior views of chest and abdomen; if warranted, inspiratory and expiratory and Pennel views for suspected peridiaphragmatic and pelvic injuries, respectively.

2. Semi-upright, semi-erect exposures of chest and abdomen.

3. Right lateral decubitus of the abdomen and, if warranted, of the chest and a lateral view of the dorsolumbar spine. If the patient has a suspected spinal fracture or is unconscious, a cervical collar or traction must be applied, and the patient turned like a log to avoid spinal cord damage. The physical examination of the back may be completed at this time.

4. IVP, when indicated, is performed at the time of the supine films unless angiography is contemplated, which will also produce an IVP.

5. Stereo x-rays and magnification radiography aid the physician into interpreting chest and abdominal injuries, especially of the spine, ribs, sternum, and pelvis. *Lateral films of the spine are unnecessary with stereo.*

A standard methodical approach should be used in viewing and interpreting x-rays. Essentially, the purpose for the x-rays is to determine whether the truncal cage, the viscera, or both are involved by trauma. Therefore, the anatomic classification of truncal trauma should be used as a guide to the sequence in which the x-rays should be read and interpreted (Fig. 1). The soft and hard tissue of the trunk, including retroperi-

toneal areas, are viewed first, then the area around the diaphragm, the mediastinal structures of the chest followed by the lungs, and finally the solid and hollow organs of the abdomen. The following rules are useful:

1. The interpretation of abnormalities should be left until the standard reading of the films is complete. Otherwise the obvious abnormalities may distract the physician's attention from the subtle changes.

2. Fractures of truncal bones indicate possible visceral damage immediately beneath them (spleen, liver, bladder, urethra).

3. A foreign body or displaced fractured rib lying as high as the fourth rib on the right and the fourth interspace on the left may involve abdominal viscera, while those as low as the eleventh rib on both sides may involve the thoracic viscera.

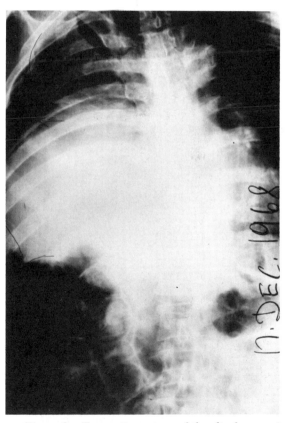

Figure 9. Traumatic rupture of the diaphragm. A "raised diaphragm" on the right may actually be liver protruding through a ruptured hemidiaphragm. The diagnosis was confirmed by instillation of a small volume of CO_2 (100 cc.) into the peritoneal cavity, which produced a small pneumothorax. The dome of the liver may be damaged, and therefore, angiography should be performed preoperatively if the patient is stable.

4. Missiles tend to fragment: therefore, look for more than the obvious fragment. The absence of a missile on x-ray when no exit wound is visible indicates embolization or penetration beyond the trunk into an arm or a leg.

5. An "elevated diaphragm" on the right may be liver protruding into the chest through a ruptured diaphragm. It may indicate a ruptured dome of the liver as well (Fig. 9).

6. Air originating from rupture of the stomach, duodenum, or colon is found in one of three places in the abdomen: (a) free in the peritoneal cavity settling in the most inde-pendent position, i.e., under the diaphragm in the upright, the flank in the decubitus, and outlining the falciform ligament (the double wall sign) in the supine; (b) limited to the lesser sac with perforation of the stomach (there may be an air-fluid level present); and (c) stippling the area behind the duodenum when this structure is injured (Fig. 10A to F).

7. The spleen, kidneys, or liver may be enlarged or distended, indicating subcutaneous hematoma or hemorrhage limited to that area. The stomach is often displaced medially with indentations along the greater curvature due to hemorrhage of a ruptured spleen into the gastrosplenic ligament. This sign may be

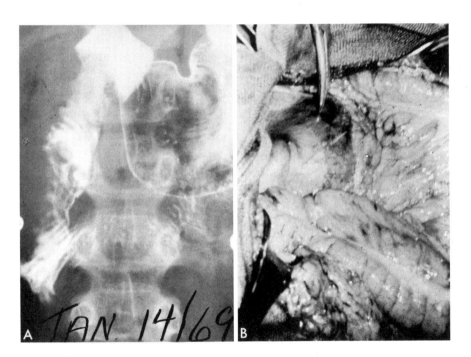

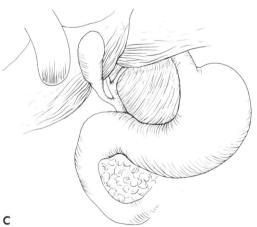

Figure 10. Pancreaticoduodenal injuries. There are two types of duodenal injuries. The least injury is a bleed between the submucosa and the muscularis which accentuates the natural transverse duodenal folds of Kerck-ring, and appears as "stacked coins" or a "coiled spring" on air- or water-soluble con-trast x-rays (A). Bleeding may dissect between the fibers of the muscularis mucosa and ap-pear at operation as a subserosal hematoma (B) or even a retroperitoneal hematoma(C).

enhanced by installation of 200 cc. of air into the stomach through the nasogastric tube. However, if rupture of the stomach or duodenum is present, air will escape into the spaces indicated in item 6. Care must be taken to avoid respiratory embarrassment or vomiting and aspiration with this technique.

8. Loss of the psoas shadows indicates retroperitoneal bleeding.

9. Separation of the gas-filled colon from the preperitoneal fat line indicates blood or fluid in the flank. Flotation of the small bowel toward the center of the abdomen and an enlarged opaque space between their walls also indicate free fluid in the abdominal cavity.

McCort (1966) has written a pertinent, well-illustrated book on the radiologic diagnosis of trauma for those who wish more details than are included here.

SPECIAL DIAGNOSTIC PROCEDURES

Four-Quadrant Peritoneal Tap or Lavage. This will indicate the presence of blood, bile, pancreatic juice, or intestinal contents in the abdominal cavity. Suggested indications for tap or lavage are outlined in Figure 11. A four-quadrant tap often can precede lavage, since it is easy to do, requires only a Potter needle and syringe, and will be positive in 88 per cent of the cases (Davis et al., 1976). Truncal radiology should precede the tap or lavage, since air introduced by these procedures can be confused with air from a perforated viscus.

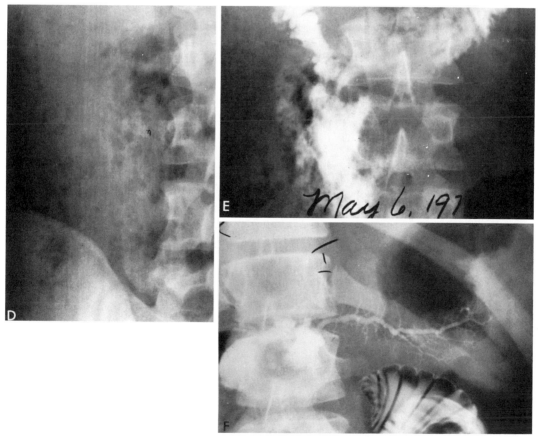

Figure 10. Continued. The second type of injury is perforation of the duodenal wall with escape of air, bile, pancreatic juice, and duodenal succus entericus into the retroperitoneal tissues, causing inflammation, infection, and death if not promptly recognized and treated. Preoperative diagnosis depends upon demonstration of air in the retroperitoneal space around T12 and L1 (*D*). Water-soluble contrast medium will often delineate or confirm the perforation (*E*). ERCP will delineate pancreatic and biliary injuries preoperatively. *F* shows one performed on a patient who developed a pseudocyst three weeks after being crushed between two cars. The main duct was not transected, and therefore the patient was treated expectantly. The pseudocyst resolved.

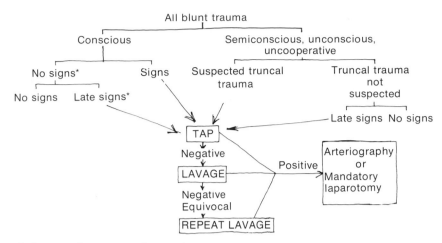

Figure 11.   Indications for peritoneal tap or lavage.

All patients with suspected blunt abdominal trauma are considered for lavage at the Hamilton General Hospital, Hamilton, Ontario. Conscious patients however, are only tapped if they develop early or late indications for mandatory laparotomy (Fig. 5). All patients who are obtunded, unconscious, or uncooperative are submitted to tap. Exceptions are those with known isolated systems injury, such as an isolated blow to the skull.

If the tap is negative, peritoneal lavage is performed. If the return is equivocal, i.e., newsprint can be read through the return tubing, the lavage catheter is left in place. The test is negative if the return remains equivocal after repeated lavages during a 12-hour period. Stable patients with positive taps proceed to three-vessel abdominal arteriography. Unstable patients proceed directly to laparotomy.

Returns which contain bile, pancreatic juice, intestinal contents, feces, and inflammatory fluids are considered positive.

Angiography (Fig. 12). Patients who have PAT or BAT and who have had minor bleeding and are stable at the time of tap or lavage may not need laparotomy. These people can undergo three-vessel angiography (celiac, superior, and inferior mesenteric arteries). The findings are peculiar to each individual organ and include extravasation of dye into the peritoneal cavity or viscera when bleeding is still active; radiolucent defects due to hematomas; and evidence of arteriovenous shunting (Lim et al., 1972).

The interpretation of angiographic findings must be very carefully considered and must match the clinical picture, since false

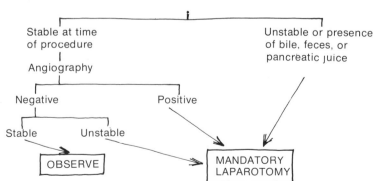

Figure 12.   Indications for abdominal angiography. Arteriography is used to confirm the presence of significant organ injury in stable patients who have: BAT with a positive peritoneal tap or lavage; or PAT due to stab wounds, low velocity GSW, or Type I and Type II SGW. Mandatory laparotomy is indicated by the arrows in the diagram. Patients with bile, feces, or pancreatic juice in the tap or lavage, or patients with moderate or major bleeding, usually proceed directly to mandatory laparotomy.

positive and negative results are common. Arteriography of the aortic arch should always be performed in conjunction with abdominal arteriography in order to locate occult injuries to the great vessels of the thorax.

Ultrasound. Ultrasound detects abnormal enlargement of solid organs and collections of fluid. This diagnostic aid is mobile and could be used more often to aid the diagnosis of abdominal and thoracic injuries, especially with the development of the new gray scale model.

Sinograms. Sinograms have been used to delineate penetration of the abdominal cavity. However, frequent false negative results, and positive tests that led to laparotomies for insignificant injuries (15.9 per cent in one series) (Streichon, 1909) have led to greatly decreased use. Clinical observation, peritoneal lavage, and angiography have largely replaced this mode of investigation.

Endoscopy. The peritoneoscope can be introduced through the abdominal stab wound after the peritoneal lavage. Air must be introduced into the cavity first. Its use is limited to observation of bleeding, liver trauma, and damage to pelvic organs. Positive identification of traumatized organs is important, but negative findings should be treated as though the procedure had not been done.

Panendoscopy may supplement other diagnostic procedures in the future to delineate gastric and duodenal trauma as well as trauma to the esophagus and could be used to detect hematomas and perforation of these organs. The diagnostic accuracy of panendoscopy could be enhanced if an erect film of the abdomen were taken following the procedure in order to detect free air that may have been introduced into the intraperitoneal cavity, behind the duodenum, or into the lesser sac. Air instilled into the duodenum may also outline the stacked-coin appearance of a duodenal hematoma (Fig. 10 A).

Endoscopic Retrograde Choledochopancreatogram (ERCP). ERCP has been used to detect rupture of the pancreatic duct and could be used to detect rupture of the extrahepatic biliary tree. It could be used both preoperatively and intraoperatively in order to diagnose injuries to the duodenum or retroperitoneal area around the pancreas without opening the duodenum or performing a Kocher maneuver (Fig. 10F). Sigmoidoscopy can likewise be used both pre- and intraoperatively to detect trauma to the rectum and rectosigmoid area.

MANAGEMENT

THE SURVIVAL EQUATION

Survival (S) is directly proportional to the ability of the trauma system to respond to the accident with adequate and appropriate care (AAC) and is inversely proportional to the severity of the initial injury (I) and to the square of the time lapse between the injury and stabilization of the unstable patient (T^2); that is, $S = KAAC/IT^2$, where K is a constant for any trauma system and relates to the coordination or meshing of the plans for survival of the various echelons of trauma care (first aid at the scene; ambulance services; Emergency Department care; and definitive care by the trauma team and its back-up services); and to the number of opportunities for testing and coordinating the plans.

The survival equation is imprecise, but is defined in mathematical terms in order to dramatize the importance of the trauma components of the emergency medical services system which affects outcome. The severity of the injury is the only independent variable in the equation. The other variables depend upon the organization of personnel, space, equipment, and back-up facilities to carry out a plan for survival. Each echelon of care will have its own plan of action, but the equation assures that the plans of the lower echelon will mesh with the plans of the next higher one (K). Since the trauma team is ultimately responsible for all trauma patients, the plans for care of this type of patient by all echelons, including care in the Emergency Department, will be subservient to it. It is the responsibility of the Emergency Department, however, to coordinate the plans of action for emergency medical care of several tertiary care services for efficient use of its facilities (Mackenzie et al., 1976).

The decision to mesh the plans of action for trauma care at the different echelons is political and involves crossing boundaries of influence. It is, therefore, important to negotiate and record in writing the formula for meshing the plans. It is only when the meshing is completed and the system has been tested under fire and modified as necessary that K will be maximized for any given community or trauma system.

The preceding section of this chapter discussed the methods used to diagnose abdominal injury in the patient with suspected multiple trauma. An effective plan to maximize K in the Emergency Department can be instituted based upon the rational use of diagnostic procedures, resuscitation, and the first appearance of signs and symptoms of deterioration or of other criteria for mandatory exploration.

THE EMERGENCY DEPARTMENT PLAN FOR SURVIVAL

The objectives of the emergency department plan for survival are simple: to recognize and reverse pulmonary deficits; to stop major bleeding and restore perfusion; to determine the presence of thoracic, abdominal, spinal craniocerebral, and musculoskeletal injuries and to assign priorities of treatment in that order (resuscitative or definitive); and to transfer the patient to the next echelon of care (trauma service) whenever instability cannot be corrected or the diagnosis of the extent of the injuries has been completed. The objectives are instituted in five phases: Phase I, rapid assessment for priorities of treatment; Phase II, resuscitation; Phase III, the second (repeated) assessment; Phase IV, diagnosis of occult injury; Phase V, disposal. This plan of action is called the cascade of Emergency Department triage (Fig. 6).

Sometimes, the phases are instituted concurrently in the unstable or deteriorating patient, but sequentially in the patient with subtle injuries. Deteriorating patients are culled from each phase of this plan for mandatory treatment by the trauma team (usually exploration) and each patient is treated as a spinal injury until proved otherwise. Figure 13 indicates a time and treatment "tote board" to organize care, particularly when multiple procedures are being done.

Phase I—Rapid Assessment. Care starts when information about a trauma patient is radioed to the Emergency Department by the ambulance service; continues during the transportation of the patient in the Emergency Department from the ambulance entrance to the resuscitation area for life-threatened patients; and ends with the

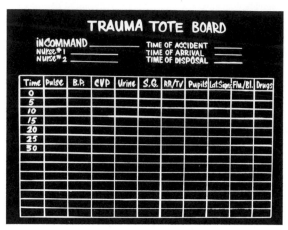

Figure 13. Time and treatment tote board. The tote board is designed to identify the treating team and its commander; and patient progress and response to treatment matched against elapsed time (five minute intervals). The board and a large stopwatch are located near the head of the patient so that T^2 of the survival equation is always visible to the team. One member of the team is assigned to obtain and record the information on the tote board.

routine institution of measures designed to gain cardiovascular-respiratory control and obtain blood for routine laboratory data and cross-matching.

The emergency physician and his staff should immediately prepare space, equipment, and personnel to receive the patient(s) upon communication from the ambulance service. A resuscitation team with a physician captain is assigned to each patient as he arrives. If this is not possible, the institution of the Disaster Plan should be considered. The staff should alert the necessary back-up facilities, especially the trauma service, laboratory services, x-ray, intensive care unit, and the operating room about the nature of the incoming cases.

The emergency physician should meet the victim at the ambulance entrance and accompany the patient to the space set aside and prepared for the care of life-threatening illnesses or injuries. If there is more than one patient arriving at the same time, then the head of the resuscitation team assigned to the patient by the emergency physician will perform this duty. (In the latter instance, the emergency physician becomes the triage officer rather than head of the resuscitation team.) On the way to the resuscitation area, the leader should look for signs of life; evidence of external bleeding (which he or one of the stretcher bearers should stop immediately); obvious evidence of head injury; and obvious evidence of musculoskeletal fractures.

Each member of the resuscitation team will have been assigned specific duties in the resuscitation room. One member will observe and record the time of accident, time of arrival, vital signs, previously ingested drugs, and will attach an EKG monitor. A second member of the team will start and regulate the intravenous infusion and take blood for routine laboratory tests and cross-matching. A third member will care for the airway and ventilation, including endotracheal intubation, and will assess and treat the patient as though he had a cervical spinal injury. The fourth member of the team, usually the leader, will institute cardiac massage if necessary. This duty allows the leader to continue Phase I assessment while utilizing his abilities.

The cascade of care passes to Phase II when the foregoing plan has been instituted unless the patient has had cardiorespiratory arrest or an irreversible craniocerebral, truncal, or musculoskeletal injury, in which case mandatory exploration in the operating room must supervene.

Phase II—Resuscitation. Phase II begins during Phase I if vital signs are absent, since the diagnosis of cardiorespiratory arrest demands immediate action. It continues concurrently during other phases in the cascade and ends with definitive care (operative or expectant) of the patient. This phase of management is devoted to reversing the physiologic deficits mentioned in Figure 2 and to the prevention of further injuries. The emergency physician must therefore decide within moments of arrival if death, cardiac arrest, or physiologic deficits exist and then institute appropriate management.

Deterioration during resuscitation demands transfer of the patient from the Emergency Department to the operating room where resuscitation, including mandatory exploration of that part of the anatomy causing the deterioration, continues. The priority for exploration is instability due to craniocerebral, truncal, and bleeding musculoskeletal injuries. In some instances all three systems must be explored concurrently, but the area with uncontrollable hemorrhage leading to deterioration (usually the abdomen) will be explored first. If deterioration is not present, then the treatment progresses to Phase III.

Phase III—The Second (Repeated) Assessment. Phase III begins when the patient responds to the resuscitation measures instituted in Phases I and II and continues until the patient has been definitively treated. Data gathered from previous phases (assessment, management, and response to management), together with a detailed physical examination and results from laboratory and radiologic examinations, will in most instances define the injuries received by the patient; the physiologic deficits caused by them; further diagnostic procedures necessary to precisely define the extent of the injuries and physiologic deficits; and the method(s) to be used to definitively treat the patient.

The history, physical examination, and response to treatment should accurately identify the extent of injuries to the skull, truncal cage mechanism, and the musculoskeletal system as well as stability of the patient and should suggest the extent of damages to the contained viscera. These results then indicate the need for further investigations, including urine output and specific gravity; central venous pressure, complete blood count, and blood gases for confirmation of bleeding or shock; and blood gases, tidal volume, and minute volume for confirmation of occult respiratory distress.

Approximately half of the avoidable deaths in the Emergency Department happen during Phase III and are related to the inappropriate use of radiologic examinations. The patient with BAT faces this risk because more time is spent on the radiologic examination than any other phase of management; other investigations and even resuscitation is halted owing to the fear of radiation exposure to the *team;* the attention of the team shifts from patient to management to interpretation of x-rays; and the rapid movement of the deteriorated patient from the x-ray table to the operating room is logistically impossible. *Therefore, the radiologic examination must be aborted, bypassed, or continued in the operating room in any patient who is suspected of deterioration.*

The indications for mandatory exploration (Fig. 4) are usually apparent, and resuscitation is complete at the end of Phase III. These patients should be explored immediately, since they are at risk from death or severe disability until definitive care is given (T^2 in the equation). The rest pass to Phase IV or directly to Phase V.

Phase IV—Diagnosis of Occult Injuries. Phase IV begins with the realization that some patients are unstable at the end of Phase III, but the cause of the instability is obscure. It ends when the cause of the instability has been identified (it is usually due to occult bleeding into the peritoneal, retroperitoneal, mediastinal, or cranial spaces) and mandatory exploration of the affected area has been instituted or when the instability has been disproved (Fig. 6). The diagnosis is usually confirmed when the emergency physician and trauma surgeon use the special diagnostic procedures in the manner indicated previously. The usual sequence is tap, lavage, endoscopy, and finally angiography. It should be remembered that bilateral carotid, aortic arch and three-vessel abdominal angiography should be done each time arteriography is contemplated, since the additional time spent on the other two areas is short and occult injuries to the head and chest are frequently associated with BAT.

Phase V—Disposal. Most of the suspected multiple injured patients fall into Phase V; that is, they remain stable either before or after resuscitation and they lack indications for mandatory exploration. These patients are treated expectantly (see under the etiologic headings) and sent to the intensive care unit or an observation ward. Some will develop delayed indications for mandatory exploration, usually laparotomy or instability. These patients must be then treated in the same manner as those whose instability and indications for mandatory exploration appeared in one of the preceding phases of the cascade. However, it must be emphasized that this form of expectant treatment can only be performed if the patient is constantly monitored by the intensive care unit staff and regularly reviewed by the leader of the trauma team.

In summary, if time (T^2), instability, and indications for mandatory laparotomy are always kept uppermost in the minds of the Emergency Department team while treating suspected abdominal trauma, the cascade of Emergency Department care should lead to low death and permanent disability rates with a low complication rate due to a reduction of unnecessary exploration of visceral cavities.

ORGANIZATION

The successful Emergency Department must be organized to carry out the survival plan for abdominal trauma. The plan relates to the survival plans for all life-threatening illnesses as well as the management plans for other care provided in the Emergency Department for economical and organization reasons. Organization involves space, equipment, personnel, and back-up facilities.

Space. All life-threatening emergencies should be treated in the same area of the Emergency Department. The skills and equipment and back-up facilities necessary for the resuscitation of a patient with cardiorespiratory distress from multiple trauma is virtually the same as that necessary for resuscitation from a cardiac arrest or severe overdose. The number of interchangeable rooms necessary to provide for support of the patient with a life-threatening condition will depend upon the peak average load of this type of patient in the Emergency Department and the policies governing the length of stay in the Emergency Department before disposal to a definitive care facility. These rooms should be located away from the receiving area of the Emergency Department and as close to the inhospital diagnostic facilities as possible. Space for other Emergency Department functions such as minor operating rooms and observation facilities should also be located in this area, since the number of life-threatening emergencies in the average Emergency Department would not keep the resuscitation team occupied. The skills necessary to perform these latter functions are also akin to those necessary for the resuscitation rooms.

Most Emergency Departments are organized to accommodate the single victim, which is a common occurrence, and disasters, which rarely happen. However, although multiple victim emergencies (MVE) descend upon most Emergency Departments several times each year, the organization and space available for their care are usually lacking. Therefore, the area set aside for life-threatening emergencies should have at least two rooms capable of comfortably handling two victims each. This allows the same resuscitation team to care for two victims at one time, thus sparing personnel when multiple victims arrive. The minimum area for the rooms and their relationship to other Emergency Department space is discussed elsewhere (Mackenzie et al., 1976).

Equipment. GENERAL. The trauma room must have (1) adequate background white light, which will facilitate complete examination of the patient, including his true color; (2) operating-room lights suspended from the ceiling at each patient location for adequate visualization of orifices and for performance of diagnostic procedures; (3) a sufficient number of electrical outlets to run the myriad machines used in resuscitation and monitoring; and (4) outlets for an unlimited supply of air, oxygen, and suction. The electrical, gas, and suction outlets should be suspended from the ceiling on mobile carriers to allow for adequate movement of the resuscitation and trauma teams around the patient.

The stretcher at each station should be high enough to allow the team to work comfortably; sturdy enough to perform closed chest cardiac massage; capable of tilting; interchangeable with special care unit beds, especially ICU; and designed for quick radiologic examination without further injury to the patient. The former functions of the stretcher are usually compromised if the latter radiologic function is built into it, or vice versa, although many complicated and expensive stretchers have been designed.

Open shelves at eye level should contain all the equipment necessary for the Emergency Department diagnosis and resuscitation of the trauma patient. Some form of color-coding that is standard and recognizable for Emergency Equipment throughout the hospital should be used for the equipment stored on the shelves, e.g., green for respiratory equipment, red for cardiovascular equipment, and yellow for drugs. Packaged trays for "prepping" and draping the patient, performing diagnostic and resuscitative procedures on the trunk, insertion of catheters, or stopping bleeding should be similarly color-coded. Interchangeable equipment carts could be used instead of shelves, but they must be designed to store the equipment at eye level.

A large trauma tote board and stopwatch prominently placed near the head of the patient are used to record the resuscitation events; to force the team captain to continuously review all aspects of patient management; to keep time prominent in the minds of the team; and to review the effectiveness of Emergency Department management after the emergency has passed (Fig. 13).

SPECIFIC. The equipment necessary to diagnose and resuscitate the patient with abdominal trauma is the same as that necessary to diagnose and treat other life-threatening situations. Equipment that ranges in size,

such as endotracheal and chest tubes and needles, should be stored together with their connectors in such a way that the person using them can easily identify and pick out the size and shape necessary for the situation.

Equipment necessary for the diagnosis and management of the patient with abdominal trauma includes a basic prep and drape tray with scalpel, clamps, etc., to which can be added a Potter needle for abdominal paracentesis and peritoneal dialysis catheter with trochar for peritoneal lavage; a proctosigmoidoscopy tray of the fiberoptic variety; nasogastric suction equipment (Salem, 50 cc. syringe, and intermittent suction machine), and endoscopy equipment (usually kept in a central place, because of expense). A laparotomy tray with basic equipment to expose the viscera in order to clamp the large vessels, is mandatory for the rare salvageable case who is exsanguinating as he reaches the Emergency Department. However, most patients who suddenly need operative intervention have been slowly deteriorating in the Emergency Department for some time, usually while being x-rayed, and should have been moved previously to the operating room under terms outlined in the cascade plan for Emergency Department care of the trauma patient.

THE EMERGENCY DEPARTMENT DIAGNOSIS AND MANAGEMENT OF SPECIFIC INJURIES TO THE ABDOMEN

The Emergency Department diagnosis and management of most cases of abdominal trauma present few problems in management if the Emergency Department plan for survival is followed (Fig. 6). However, injuries to the structures in the hepatoduodenal ligament (extrahepatic biliary tree, hepatic artery, and portal vein) the diaphragm, the pancreaticoduodenal area, and the rectum may produce changes so subtle as to be missed, and the patient may be discharged from hospital. The person with delayed rupture of the spleen may also be discharged from the Emergency Department as having suffered insignificant injuries. *Beware*, therefore, of the Emergency Department patient who appears to have "insignificant injuries" following BAT or "superficial PAT," especially if the patient is under the influence of drugs or alcohol or is in any other way obtunded.

INJURIES TO THE DIAPHRAGM

A ruptured diaphragm may be undetected for years. Often the first indication of this injury is intestinal obstruction caused by strangulated herniated abdominal viscus through the rent of the left diaphragm, or recurrent pneumonitis due to a paralyzed diaphragm. Often it is found incidentally on chest x-ray.

Suspicions should be aroused in cases of suspected raised intra-abdominal pressure against a closed glottis, such as a blow to the abdomen or flexion injury pivoting around the lower lumbar spine; PAT in the upper abdomen or thorax; bowel sounds in the chest on the left; the appearance of a "raised diaphragm" to percussion on the right; shoulder-tip pain on the affected side increased by deep breathing or Trendelenburg position (Kehr's sign); air-fluid levels above the left diaphragm or an "elevated" right hemidiaphragm on chest x-ray; or when pneumoperitoneum and pneumothorax coexist. Emergency Department confirmation of a ruptured diaphragm includes paradoxical motion of the diaphragm on fluoroscopy, since the phrenic nerve is damaged in 75 per cent of the cases. However, once the suspicion is raised, the trauma team should be called to handle the patient.

INJURIES TO THE STRUCTURE IN THE HEPATODUODENAL LIGAMENT

Injuries to the structures in this ligament are usually due to PAT, especially high-velocity gunshot and shotgun wounds to the upper abdomen. Three clinical situations exist:

(1) Penetrating wounds, or rarely BAT, causing damage to all structures present as shock due to blood loss, especially from the portal vein. Most of these patients die before admission to to Emergency Department or shortly thereafter. The survivors are obvious candidates for immediate laparotomy.

(2) In an isolated blunt injury to the common bile duct or main hepatic duct or its branches, with no other abdominal injury, bile slowly collects in the subhepatic space but, unlike infected bile associated with a ruptured gallbladder, does not produce immediate severe peritonitis. Instead the peritonitis is mild, the signs and symptoms are insidious, and the diagnosis is often delayed for nine days to five weeks (Zollinger, 1972). The patient may complain of right upper quadrant pain but is usually released after a period of observation. A quiescent interval of days or weeks then ensues before abdominal distention with pain, tenderness, and spasm, followed by nausea, vomiting, fever, jaundice, and white stools appear or abdominal paracentesis yields bile. The emergency physician will be hard pressed to identify these patients and may send some home. A high index of suspicion because of the nature of the accident may lead the physician to perform a peritoneal lavage, but this may be negative for bile at first.

(3) Some patients have other intra-abdominal trauma and are explored, but the rupture of the extrahepatic biliary tree is missed. The rupture is usually diagnosed by the trauma surgeon when bile pours out a drain site, but even some postoperative cases may be discharged only to return to the Emergency Department with the above symptoms. Therefore, emergency physicians should be aware of the delayed appearance of signs and symptoms of rupture of the extrahepatic biliary tree whenever a case of unexplained abdominal distention or jaundice appears in the Emergency Department. Although bile peritonitis is supposed to have an 85 per cent mortality rate, Zollinger reported only 1 death in 16 patients who had rupture of the hepatic duct or its radicles.

PANCREATICODUODENAL INJURIES

These injuries fall into four classes: Class I, duodenal hematoma, contusion, or incomplete perforation of the duodenum; Class II, complete perforation of the duodenum, usually retroperitoneal, without pancreatic injury; Class III, duodenal injury with hematoma, complete or incomplete perforation with minor injury to the pancreas without laceration of the main pancreatic duct; and Class IV, duodenal injury and major pancreatic injury such as laceration of the main pancreatic duct, massive contusion, or multiple lacerations. These injuries present a major challenge to the emergency physician. Diagnosis was delayed for more than 24 hours in 10 of 36 patients (28 per cent) in one series in which 4 of them had Class IV injuries (Lucas et al., 1975). Treatment delayed for less than 24 hours does not affect mortality, but it increases precipitously to 40 to 65 per cent after that time. Delayed diagnosis does not cause an increase in morbidity, hospital stay, or number of operations in Class I injuries, but these factors increase three- to sixfold in Class IV injuries (Walt and Wilson, 1975).

Admission findings are often subtle: minimal tenderness of the abdominal wall which progresses to rebound tenderness, guarding, and rigidity; more abdominal signs appear as the patient becomes sober; and radiologic evidence of stippling of the retroperitoneal area around the pancreaticoduodenal area and the transverse mesocolon which increases on subsequent films especially after instillation of air into the stomach with a nasogastric tube. The emergency physician will only make the diagnosis if he is suspicious of it in all patients with blunt abdominal trauma and gunshot, shotgun, and stab wounds to the right upper quadrant, no matter how trivial, and performs repeated physical and radiologic examinations in these patients until they are sober. Confirmaton of the diagnosis consists of panendoscopy, ERCP, and contrast studies (Fig. 10).

RECTAL INJURIES

These injuries are the easiest of the intra-abdominal injuries to diagnose but are so often missed because rectal examinations are not routinely done on all trauma patients. Some injuries are obvious, especially perversion injuries, while the rest will be suspected with blood on the palpating finger. The diagnosis is confirmed by sigmoidoscopy, pelvic views showing gas in the extraperitoneal pelvic tissue, and instillation of Gastrografin dye diluted four times by saline into the rectum.

SUMMARY

Abdominal wounds present a challenge to the emergency physician. A few injuries will be fulminating, usually as a result of hemorrhage, and the patient's life depends upon the orchestration of the skills of many professionals in a compact period of time. Other abdominal injuries represent a

diagnostic challenge. Some will initially have the obvious signs and symptoms leading to mandatory laparotomy, while others will need diagnostic tests to confirm the need for laparotomy. *Mortality and morbidity will be minimal in the difficult cases if an Emergency Department plan for survival is developed which applies to all patients.* This plan usually revolves around a cascade of events that identifies certain patients for mandatory laparotomy based upon signs and symptoms of instability or the other indications for laparotomy.

Unfortunately, there are a few injuries, usually associated with retroperitoneal structures, that have few signs or symptoms of visceral disruption. Such patients are often sent home, or diagnosis is otherwise delayed. They return to die when their injuries are obvious to everyone.

Organization of the Emergency Department for the care of the patient with abdominal trauma, together with a plan for survival, and repeated testing and improvement of the system will keep the latter group a small part of the total Emergency Department experience. This strategy has and will improve survival and quality of life for those who suffer from such injuries.

References

Adams, F.: The Genuine Works of Hippocrates (translated from the Greek). New York, William Wood, 1886.

Balligner, W. F.: Splenectomy. Current Prob. Surg. 1:51, February 1965.

Balligner, W. F., Rutherford, R. B., and Zuidema, G. D.: The Management of Trauma, 2nd ed. Philadelphia, W. B. Saunders Co., 1973, Chapter 11 (Abdominal Injuries), pp. 396–455.

Bell, M. J.: The management of shotgun wounds. J. Trauma 11:522, 1971.

Castiglioni, A.: A History of Medicine, 2nd ed. (translated from the Italian and edited by E. B. Krumbhaar). New York, Knopf, 1947, pp. 209–210.

Committee on Automotive Safety: Automobile safety belts during pregnancy (editorial). J.A.M.A. 221:20, 1972.

Crosby, W. M., and Costello, J. P.: Safety of lap belt restraints for pregnant victims of automobile collisions. N. Engl. J. Med. 284:632, 1971.

Davis, J. J., Cohn, I., and Nance, F. C.: Diagnosis and management of blunt abdominal trauma. Ann. Surg. 183:672, 1976.

De Muth, W. E.: Bullet velocity and design as determinants of wounding capability; an experimental study. J. Trauma 6:222, 1966.

De Muth, W. E.: Bullet velocity as applied to military rifle wounding capacity. J. Trauma 9:27, 1969.

De Muth, W. E., Jr.: The mechanism of shotgun wounds. J. Trauma 11:219, 1971.

Di Vincenti, F. C., Rives, J. D., and Laborde, E. J.: Blunt abdominal trauma. J. Trauma 8:1004, 1968.

Fitzgerald, J. B., Crawford, E. S., and De Bakey, M. E.: Surgical considerations of nonpenetrating abdominal injuries. Am. J. Surg., 100:22, 1960.

Garrison, F. H.: History of Medicine. Rev. ed. Philadelphia, W. B. Saunders Co., 1960.

Heaton, L. D., Hughes, C. W., Rosegay, H., Fischer, G. W., and Feighny, R. E.: Military practices of the United States Army in Viet Nam. Curr. Probl. Surg., 1:59, November 1966.

Henderson, M., and Wood, R.: Compulsory wearing of seatbelts in New South Wales, Australia: An evaluation of its effects on vehicle occupant deaths in the first year. Med. J. Austr. vol. 2, 1973.

Lim, R. C., Jr., Glickman, M. G., and Hunt, T. K.: Angiography in patients with blunt trauma to the chest and abdomen. Surg. Clin. North Am. 52:551, 1972.

Loria, F. L.: Historical Aspects of Abdominal Injuries. Springfield, Ill., Charles C Thomas, Publisher, 1968.

Lucas, C. E., and Ledgerwood, A. M.: Factors influencing outcome after blunt duodenal injury. J. Trauma 15:839, 1975.

Mackenzie, J. R., Harvey, J., Horton, R., Johnson, P., and Strickler, A. C.: A Method For Auditing Ambulance Services In A Specific Area. Proceedings of Seventeenth Conference of the American Association for Automotive Medicine, Oklahoma City, Oklahoma, November 1973, pp. 418–431.

Mackenzie, J. R., Jelenko, C., III, James, P., and Frey, C.: A guideline for the organization of an emergency department in the university setting. J. Am Coll. Emerg. Physicians 5:364, 1976.

McCort, J. J.: Radiographic Examination in Blunt Abdominal Trauma. Philadelphia, W. B. Saunders Co., 1966.

McNally, N. H.: The Ontario Ambulance Service Program: Bridging gaps in our medical care system. Ontario Med. Rev., May 1970 (Part I) and June 1970 (Part II).

Means, R. L.: Bile peritonitis. Am. Surg. 30:583, 1964.

Morse, T. S.: Teaching Initial Management of Shock in Children. Proceedings of the Sixth Annual Meeting of the University Association for Emergency Medical Services. Philadelphia, May 1976.

Nance, F. C., Wennar, M. H., Johnson, L. W., Ingram, J. C., Jr., and Cohn, I., Jr.: Surgical judgement in the management of penetrating wounds of the abdomen: Experience with 2212 patients. Ann. Surg. 179:639, 1974.

Ryzoff, R. I., Shaftan, G. W., and Herbsman, H.: Selective conservatism in penetrating abdominal trauma. Surgery 59:650, 1966.

Shaftan, G. W.: Indications for operation in abdominal trauma. J. Surg. 99:657, 1960.

Sherman, R. T., and Parrish, R. A.: Management of shotgun injuries. J. Trauma 3:76, 1963.

Streichen, F. M., Efron, G., Pearlman, D. M., and Weil, P. H.: Radiographic diagnosis versus selective management in penetrating wounds of the abdomen. Ann. Surg. 170:978, 1969.

Surgery in WW II. In General Surgery, published by the Medical Department, United States Army, 1955, Vol. 2, pp. 5–7.

Vance, B. M.: Traumatic lesions of the intestines caused by non-penetrating blunt force. Arch. Surg. (Chicago) 7:197, 1923.

Walt, A. J., and Wilson, R. F.: Management of Trauma: Pitfalls and Practice. Philadelphia, Lea & Febiger, 1975.

Williams, J. S., and Kirkpatrick, J. R.: The nature of seat belt injuries. J. Trauma 11:207, 1971.

Zollinger, R. M., Jr., Keller, R. T. and Hubay, C. A.: Traumatic rupture of the right and left hepatic ducts. J. Trauma 12:563, 1972.

G. TRAUMA TO THE EXTREMITIES AND SOFT TISSUES

David P. Simmons and William R. MacAusland, Jr.

RECOGNITION

Optimal management depends on prompt recognition.

(1) A *history* of the mechanism will help predict the probable injury if it is interpreted in light of the regional anatomy. For example, a knee striking the dashboard of a car should suggest possible patellar fracture and hip dislocation.

(2) The *physical examination* may merely confirm the suspected diagnosis, but it is critical to establish the baseline status of the skin and neural and vascular structures. The depth and extent of skin injury should be estimated. The vascular state can be assessed by noting the presence of capillary filling and palpating the radial, dorsalis pedis, and posterior tibial pulsations. Finally, testing of both motor and sensory function of the major peripheral nerves is absolutely necessary for the neurologic examination.*

---

*See procedure 10.

(3) *Immobilization* through splinting is the next essential step to prevent further skin, neural, or vascular complications, to provide relief of pain, and to decrease bleeding.*

(4) Last, *x-rays* will further help finalize the orthopedic diagnosis, and definitive treatment then may follow this vital sequence.

MANAGEMENT

Any major skin, nerve, or vessel injury usually calls for consultation services. In the absence of these, proper orthopedic management requires immobilization of any fracture or ligament injury, even if only suspected. The type of immobilization selected depends on the anticipated timing of the next phase of treatment. Orthopedic Procedure Section 1 illustrates splinting techniques suitable for several days of protection. Where swelling is extreme or other injuries predominate, it may be reasonable to splint, ice, and elevate a part for later reduction and/or casting.

All open wounds should be irrigated immediately with sterile saline. The surrounding intact skin should be swabbed with an antiseptic solution. The wounds should be covered with dry sterile dressings, which should not be disturbed again until definitive wound care is undertaken. Most extremity hemorrhage can be controlled readily by simple, *sustained* compression. Tourniquet application or hemostatic clamping within wounds is rarely necessary.

All open fractures and dislocations are treated as true emergencies in order to prevent infection. *Closed* fractures and dislocations are only relative emergencies, depending on the degree of displacement, the anticipated difficulty of reduction, and the associated nerve or vessel injuries. Fractures and dislocations with associated ischemic deficits, locally or distally, are true emergencies. Immediate manipulative reduction should be performed by the emergency physician if the ischemia is severe. Fractures and dislocations with neural deficits may be true emergencies in which prompt reduction is imperative if neurologic function is deteriorating. Lacerations of joints, tendons, and vessels must be recognized and considered for primary repair. No skin laceration should be closed without careful examination for deep injury to vital structures.

COMPLICATIONS

The major complications of trauma to the bony extremities are skin, soft tissue, neural, and vascular. Most, if not all, that did not exist at the time of injury can be prevented by proper initial care. Early splinting in proper alignment with compressive, but not constrictive, bandaging will decrease bleeding, swelling, and pain. Instruction on self-observation, with prompt reporting of any change, guards against early, rapid deterioration of the outpatient. Physician follow-up within 24 to 48 hours will insure recognition and treatment of delayed complications.

A common, often underestimated, difficulty relates to bruising or crushing of muscle with hematoma formation. These injuries may be extremely painful and may require a prolonged time before normal function is regained. Local ischemic necrosis within fascial compartments and heterotopic bone formation (myositis ossificans) are less common, but potentially serious, complications. The former usually occurs with the forearm or calf muscles; the latter in the thigh. The degrees of pain, swelling, induration, and loss of adjacent joint motion are indicators of the potential severity of these injuries.

Proper management of severe contusions includes the same principles advanced for fractures and dislocations. Application of local ice in the first 48 hours is beneficial in decreasing bleeding and relieving pain, whereas heat will have the opposite effect. Later in the course, heat may promote resorption of blood and faster healing through vasodilatation. Systemic or local proteolytic enzymes may offer some theoretic advantages, but probably are ineffective. Where ischemia threatens, surgical release of fascial compartments may be necessary as an emergent operative procedure.

Specific Management

The details of management must be approached by considering the problem

---

*See procedure 1.

"regions" as they present for diagnosis, treatment, and prevention of complications. A major separation of orthopedic problems is possible according to the x-ray findings.

(1) *X-rays positive.*
   (a) fracture.
   (b) dislocation.
(2) *X-rays negative.*
   (a) strain and rupture.
   (b) laceration.

THE NECK[*]

Major forces are required to fracture or dislocate the cervical spine, but even minor forces can result in neurologic injury. An early, thorough neurologic examination is most important, because the discovery of progressive changes may necessitate prompt surgical treatment. Scalp lacerations and abrasions may signal the direction of applied forces. The physical examination is otherwise of little use in separating the various lesions.

X-RAYS POSITIVE

Fracture. All should be immobilized with a four-poster cervical brace, and the patient should be kept recumbent (Procedure 1). A complete neurologic examination should be recorded promptly. Fracture reduction is the decision of the consultant. The main complication is cord or nerve root injury; if this is not present with the original injury, it may be prevented entirely by the surgeon.

Dislocation. See Fracture.

X-RAYS NEGATIVE

Strain and Rupture. If the neurologic examination is negative, immobilization with a soft collar, plus symptomatic treatment, is adequate. Beware of incomplete or "negative" x-ray studies, as spontaneous reduction of neck dislocations is common. When in doubt, immobilize in a four-poster cervical brace and obtain specialist consultation.

Laceration. Neural injury will rarely occur, but major bleeding can result from arteries and veins that may require primary repair. Penetrating wounds usually merit ex-

[*]See also Chapter 38B.

ploration under optimum surgical conditions.

THE BACK

Major forces are required to fracture or dislocate the dorsolumbar spine. Minor forces, in contrast, may herniate discs and strain ligaments or muscles. The initial neurologic examination is most important in order to document progressive deficits. Radiating leg pain with passive straight leg raising helps identify individual nerve root compression associated with disc herniation.

X-RAYS POSITIVE

Fracture. The patient should be kept recumbent and supine, but log rolling may be done for essential examinations and x-rays. A complete neurologic examination should be recorded promptly. Reduction is the decision of the consultant. The main complication is cord or nerve root injury. If it is not present with the original injury, it may be entirely prevented by the emergency physician.

Dislocation. See Fracture.

X-RAYS NEGATIVE

Strain and Rupture. These injuries usually are ligamentous or muscular, but they may be related to the intervertebral disc, particularly if neurologic signs and symptoms are present. Analgesics, muscle relaxants, heat, and external support may help, but bed-rest is the most beneficial treatment. Complications will result from premature mobilization without muscular rehabilitation. If acute loss of bladder, bowel, or motor function develops, prompt surgical decompression may be indicated.

Laceration. These are rarely accompanied by neural injury, but penetrating wounds (e.g., gunshot) may require surgical exploration.

UPPER EXTREMITY: SHOULDER-ARM

Leverage through the arm may cause major proximal injury with seemingly minor trauma. Moreover, the splinting effects of gravity against the trunk may mask serious injury.

X-RAYS POSITIVE

Fracture. **CLAVICLE.** Most displacement is acceptable, and application of a clavicular strap (Procedure 1) is protective and comforting. However, serious neural or vascular difficulties may arise in either upper extremity if not observed serially. Immobilization is useful for approximately three weeks in children, and for six weeks in adults.

SCAPULA AND PROXIMAL HUMERUS. As even considerable displacement is acceptable, a sling and swathe (Procedure 1) usually is sufficient treatment. In adults, this should be followed by early (one to two weeks) active motion exercises. When reduction is indicated, general anesthesia frequently is necessary owing to the proximal location. Skin, neural, and vascular injuries are not associated commonly, but humeral head dislocations often occur. Satisfactory lateral x-rays must be obtained to insure their recognition and treatment.

HUMERAL SHAFT. These fractures usually are displaced, but often are self-reducing by gravity. Sling and swathe immobilization is sufficient (Procedure 1) but coaptation splints may be more comfortable (Procedure 9). Skin puncturing is very common, but arterial injury is rare. Although the radial nerve frequently is injured, exploration almost never is necessary because of the high incidence of spontaneous recovery.

Dislocation. **HUMERAL HEAD.** These injuries are very common. The humeral head usually lies anteriorly. The injury presents as a subacromial depression and a painful, immobile shoulder. Reduction should be obtained promptly (Procedure 8). Since relaxation is necessary to prevent fracture or neurovascular injury during reduction, anesthesia may be indicated (Procedure 4). After reduction, sling and swathe immobilization for six weeks is necessary to prevent recurrence. However, in patients over 50 years of age, active motion exercises should be begun after one week to prevent stiffness. Immobilization for anything other than symptoms is not necessary in recurrent dislocations. The skin and vessels usually are intact, but the axillary nerve frequently is compressed. This deficit presents as locally decreased sensation (Fig. 1) and loss of deltoid muscle function. Fortunately, spontaneous recovery after reduction is usual.

ACROMIOCLAVICULAR. These injuries are very common and often are not recognized. If displaced, they are easily noted upon examination. Otherwise, standing AP x-rays of both shoulders with weights in the hands may be necessary to demonstrate the lesion. Early repair may be indicated if displacement is full in a young person, but sling treatment is satisfactory for most injuries. Skin, neural, and vascular complications are rare, unless restrictive strapping is used as a method of treatment.

STERNOCLAVICULAR. Although this is rare, a retrosternal position may affect the airway and require emergent reduction. Surgery often is necessary to accomplish this.

X-RAYS NEGATIVE

Strain and Rupture. **ROTATOR CUFF TEAR.** This is an injury of middle age, pre-

Figure 1. Sensory distribution of axillary nerve. (Adapted from DePalma, A. F.: Management of Fractures and Dislocations, 2nd ed. Philadelphia, W. B. Saunders Co., 1970, p. 605.)

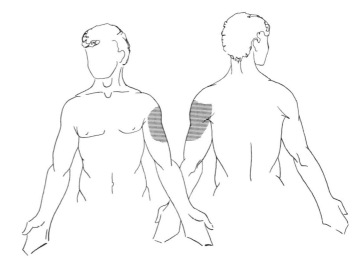

senting as apical shoulder pain. There is weakness or loss of active abduction and loss of ability to hold against gravity when passively abducted. A diagnostic injection of local anesthetic may be useful to test strength without pain inhibition (Procedure 6). Treatment is sling support, but surgical repair may be indicated for complete ruptures in active young people. Skin, neural, and vascular injuries are not associated.

BICEPS RUPTURE. This is an injury of middle age. There is acute loss of biceps strength with distal movement of the biceps mass upon active contraction. Surgical repair may be indicated in the young; otherwise, sling support is sufficient. Skin, neural, and vascular injuries are not associated.

TENDINITIS/BURSITIS. Acute shoulder pain without injury is the presenting complaint. The symptoms frequently are precipitated by strenuous or repetitive use. Point tenderness at the shoulder is typical. A calcific deposit adjacent to the greater tuberosity may be seen on the x-ray, but is not essential for the diagnosis. Local injection with steroid is the most effective treatment (Procedure 6). Oral anti-inflammatory agents are a useful secondary measure. A sling, ice, and analgesics should also be considered.

MISCELLANEOUS. Beware of the rare, but commonly missed, lesions with "negative" x-rays such as posterior humeral head dislocation, sternoclavicular dislocation, Pancoast's syndrome, and cervical root lesions.

Lacerations. Significant deep structures rarely are involved, but all adjacent musculotendinous, neural, and vascular structures should be checked for function (Procedure 10).

ELBOW

X-RAYS POSITIVE

Fracture. **SUPRACONDYLAR HUMERUS.** This is a common pediatric injury. Reduction should be prompt and exact, with adequate anesthesia to avoid the frequent neurovascular complications. A single failed reduction attempt should result in hospital admission for traction treatment (Procedure 2). If the fracture is undisplaced, a posterior splint in flexion and a sling are sufficient (Procedure 1). As ischemic contracture of the forearm musculature is insidious and disas-

trous, with or without reduction, nerve and vessel function must be followed carefully (Procedure 10).

JOINT FRACTURES, PEDIATRIC. These are difficult to diagnose by x-ray alone. A careful physical examination, and comparison x-rays of both elbows, are essential. Each epiphysis should be checked for appearance and position (Fig. 2). If the fracture is undisplaced, a posterior splint and a sling are sufficient (Procedure 1). Displacement usually requires reduction, frequently by surgical methods. Ischemic contracture of the forearm musculature may occur here, as with supracondylar fractures (Procedure 10).

JOINT FRACTURES, ADULT. The common types involve the olecranon and the radial head. Frequently, surgery is necessary to replace or remove displaced fragments. If the fracture is undisplaced, a posterior splint and a sling are sufficient (Procedure 1), but active elbow motion should begin early. Neurovascular complications are less frequent than in children, but nevertheless are serious (Procedure 10).

Dislocation. **OLECRANON AND RADIAL HEAD.** These occur at all ages and in all directions, but usually are posterior. They are easily reduced if treated early, but anesthesia may be necessary (Procedures 4 and 8). Commonly overlooked complications are associated avulsion fractures, which may have to be reduced separately or even replaced surgically. Comparison x-rays of the other elbow are necessary in children (Fig. 2). The neurovascular risks are similar to those of the supracondylar fracture (Procedure 10).

RADIAL HEAD DISLOCATION. This is rare without an associated ulnar fracture, which is displaced and may be distal (Monteggia fracture). It is easily missed if the fracture is noted first. Both need prompt reduction, often surgically. The skin commonly is punctured by the ulnar fracture fragments.

X-RAYS NEGATIVE

Strain and Rupture. **LATERAL EPICONDYLITIS (TENNIS ELBOW).** This usually occurs after strenuous use of the extremity. There is point tenderness over the lateral epicondyle (Fig. 2). The pain is reproduced by giving resistance to active finger and wrist extension. Elbow motion usually is full and painless passively. The initial treatment should be rest and splinting

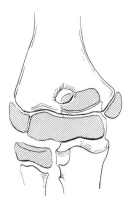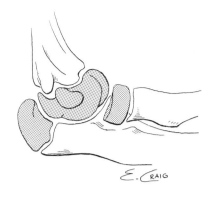

Figure 2. Elbow epiphyses. (Adapted from Blount, W. P.: Fractures in Children. Baltimore, The Williams & Wilkins Co., 1955, p. 4.)

(Procedure 1), but a local steroid injection may be helpful (Procedure 6).

MEDIAL EPICONDYLITIS (LITTLE LEAGUE ELBOW). This occurs in young pitchers, who become tender over the medial apophysis (Fig. 2). Treatment always is cessation of throwing, with a splint if symptoms are acute (Procedure 1). Local steroid injection is never indicated. The apophysis may be displaced and may require operative replacement. There may be evidence for ulnar nerve irritation chronically (Procedure 10).

OLECRANON BURSITIS (HYDROPS). A large, soft, fluid-filled mass presents and persists over the olecranon, caused by direct trauma or chronic irritation. Treatment is to aspirate and immobilize. These masses may be infected, so fluid analysis is useful; they may become infected after the most careful aspiration. Recurrent bursitis usually responds to local instillation of steroid (Procedure 6).

RADIAL HEAD SUBLUXATION (NURSE-MAID'S ELBOW). This occurs in very young children after a longitudinal pull on the arm. It presents as an irritable child with an immobile elbow. The cartilaginous radial head will not be seen on the x-rays. The subluxation is reduced by forceful supination and extension; anesthesia usually is not necessary. The complication is recurrence if the elbow is not immobilized with a posterior splint for three weeks (Procedure 1).

LACERATION. The ulnar nerve is the most accessible structure. It commonly is injured by a fall on the flexed elbow (Procedure 10). Primary repair usually is not indicated, but should be considered.

WRIST

X-RAYS POSITIVE

Fracture. **DISTAL RADIUS (COLLES).** There is a characteristic deformity of dorsal displacement and radial shortening. Restoration of the normal relationships promotes normal function, but may not be necessary in the very elderly. Reduction usually is easily obtained by longitudinal traction and manipulation (Procedure 9). The choice of a splint or cast depends on the ease of follow-up (Procedure 3). The fracture may be open owing to an inconspicuous puncture of the skin by the ulna. The median nerve may be injured, and needs careful initial assessment with serial observation (Procedure 10). Swelling and vascular compromise present a real danger to the hand as well, and loosening of the splint (splitting the cast) may be necessary in addition to mere elevation of the part. The inherent instability of these fractures necessitates frequent x-rays until healing has occurred. For these reasons, careful, frequent follow-up is imperative.

EPIPHYSEAL SEPARATION. This is a pediatric injury that presents exactly like a Colles' fracture. Reduction must be gentle, with adequate anesthesia to avoid further epiphyseal plate injury (Procedures 4 and 9). A long arm cast is indicated initially (Procedure 3). These injuries rarely are open, but again the median nerve is at risk (Procedure 10). Fortunately, secondary growth disturbance is rare.

NAVICULAR. This common injury of all ages often is missed. Local tenderness (in the snuff-box) is a cardinal sign even if the x-ray is negative. The bones rarely are displaced. Immobilization with a long arm cast incorporating the thumb is the most complete form of treatment (Procedure 3). These fractures are prolonged in healing, and some may result in avascular necrosis—particularly if the fracture is more proximal and if immobilization is inconsistent. Skin, nerve, and vessel injuries are rare.

BOTH BONES OF THE FOREARM. These fractures occur at all ages. The worst may have little physical deformity as they are completely displaced and shortened. The reduction usually is difficult and requires adequate anesthesia (Procedures 4 and 9). The cast or splint chosen must go above the elbow to control the rotational instability (Procedure 3). Adult reductions must be exact, and surgery usually is required. There is more leeway in children's fractures, but there must be no rotational deformity. These commonly are open injuries, especially over the ulna, but nerve and vessel injury is not usual. Post-injury swelling may be extreme, and close follow-up is essential (Procedure 10). A displaced single bone fracture means a possible elbow or wrist dislocation; x-rays of the entire forearm from wrist to elbow are a necessity. A greenstick (incomplete) fracture in a child should be broken completely through at the time of reduction to prevent recurrent angulation during healing.

Dislocation. **LUNATE, PERILUNATE, TRANSNAVICULAR.** These injuries are uncommon, but usually missed initially. There should be wrist deformity and limitation of motion. The lateral x-ray is invaluable to detect these lesions (Fig. 3). Closed reduction should be attempted promptly, but open reduction often is needed. Major trauma is necessary to cause these injuries, so that skin, nerve, and vessel injury frequently is seen (Procedure 10).

X-RAYS NEGATIVE

Strain and Rupture. All wrist "sprains" are navicular fractures until proved otherwise by x-ray and examination two weeks after injury. Therefore, they should all be splinted. The complications are late and serious (e.g., non-union, avascular necrosis, and degenerative arthritis) if the original lesion is not recognized and treated.

Laceration. The superficial, volar position of major tendons, nerves, and vessels

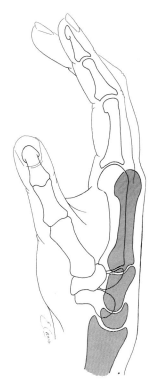

Figure 3. Lateral x-ray of wrist. (Adapted from DePalma, A. F.: The Management of Fractures and Dislocations, 2nd ed. Philadelphia, W. B. Saunders Co., 1970, p. 985.)

means that serious multiple injuries are common. Primary repair of all or most of these structures usually is indicated. The carpal joints are rarely entered. The complication is prolonged or permanent loss of function if not recognized and treated acutely (Procedure 10).

HAND*

X-RAYS POSITIVE

Fracture. **METACARPAL NECK (BOXER'S FRACTURE).** This fracture presents as a "dropped knuckle" with good finger function after a fist fight. The fingers should be compared for any rotational deformity. The fracture should be reduced (Procedure 9) if angulation is severe (greater than 45°), or if there is any rotation. Splinting should be in flexion for three weeks (Fig. 4). The com-

---

*See also Chapter 38H.

monest complications are stiffness after long immobilization, and skin injury from too much pressure by the cast or splint.

METACARPAL SHAFT. These fractures often are multiple. The more radial in the hand is the bone, the more critical is the displacement. The oblique type of fracture is very unstable. Rotational deformity cannot be accepted. Reduction is accomplished by traction, and splinting should be done in flexion (Fig. 4), with care to prevent rotation. Swelling often is great, but skin, nerve, and vessel injuries are rare.

METACARPAL BASE (BENNETT'S AT THE THUMB). These are articular fractures that often involve dislocation, so that anatomic reduction is necessary. Surgery frequently is required. Undisplaced fractures should be held in a short arm cast with the thumb included (Procedure 3).

PHALANGEAL SHAFTS. (1) *Proximal Phalanges.* These fractures need to be perfectly reduced. Children's fractures usually are epiphyseal. They generally can be reduced by longitudinal traction and splinting in the functional position of flexion (Fig. 4 and Procedure 9). Oblique, comminuted, and articular fractures usually require surgery. Swelling may be a problem, but skin, nerve, and vessel difficulties are uncommon unless immobilization devices are too tight.

(2) *Middle Phalanges.* See Proximal Phalanges.

(3) *Distal Phalanges.* These fractures usually are the result of a crushing injury. They are very painful and may have a subungual hematoma to release (by a heated paper clip pushed through the nail). The nail itself serves as a splint and a dressing, so removal should be avoided. The hand should be elevated and treated symptomatically. The fracture does not require specific treatment.

(3) *Joint Fractures.* These fractures commonly are underestimated (e.g., "chip" fractures that actually represent avulsion injuries). If displaced, they need reduction, frequently by surgery. Undisplaced fractures should be splinted in the functional position (Fig. 4). Early follow-up x-rays are important in order that recurrent displacement may be recognized. Early (two weeks) active motion is important to preserve finger function. The common complications are progressive dis-

location if they are not reduced and splinted, and stiffness if they are not mobilized early.

Dislocation. **INTERPHALANGEAL.** This is a very common injury, readily reduced by longitudinal traction (Procedure 8). Anesthesia usually is not needed if reduction is performed promptly. Splinting should be in the functional position (Fig. 4). A search should be made for a volar fragment on x-ray, which must be reduced or late instability will result. If active motion is begun early (ten days) permanent stiffness will be resisted.

METACARPOPHALANGEAL. The most common site of dislocation is at the thumb. The flexor tendons entrap the metacarpal head. This is a difficult reduction (Procedure 8), usually requiring anesthesia (Procedure 4), and frequently surgery. Splinting should be in flexion; active motion should begin early (ten days).

X-RAYS NEGATIVE

Strain and Rupture. **MALLET FINGER (BASEBALL FINGER).** This is the very common result of direct trauma to the tip of a finger. It presents as a drooping finger tip that represents an avulsion of the extensor tendon from the base of the distal phalanx. A "chip" or avulsion fracture may be seen on x-ray. Splinting in comfortable extension is necessary for six weeks. The skin should be observed closely for pressure necrosis caused by the splint or hyperextension of the joint.

ULNAR COLLATERAL LIGAMENT METACARPOPHALANGEAL JOINT OF THUMB (GAMEKEEPER'S THUMB). This is very common and very easily missed. The x-ray may show a "chip" or avulsion fracture at the ulnar aspect of the base of the proximal phalanx. The joint will be unstable to stress testing (Procedure 7). It may be treated by a cast in adduction (Procedure 3) or by primary surgical repair. Late instability is the complication.

INTERPHALANGEAL COLLATERAL LIGAMENT. This infrequent injury usually is missed, but may be detected by stress testing (Procedure 7). It should be splinted in flexion (Fig. 4), but mobilized by early active exercise (ten days).

FLEXOR PROFUNDUS TENDON RUPTURE. This is infrequent but easily missed. The

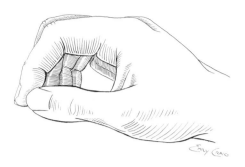

Figure 4. Position of function. (From Blount, W. P.: Fractures in Children. Baltimore, The Williams & Wilkins Co., 1955, p. 114.)

tendon avulses from the base of the distal phalanx. The injured finger rests in extension, and the others lie flexed. Surgical repair is required or there eventually will be no function of the tendon.

Laceration. The superficial position of tendon, nerve, and vessel results in easy and frequent injury. Injury to any of these structures requires primary surgical repair.

LOWER EXTREMITY: HIP

X-RAYS POSITIVE

Fracture. **PELVIC.** This is common after falls and automobile accidents. Injuries often are fatal and should not be underrated. Local palpation and pelvic compression should elicit pain and crepitation. The fractures, even if widely displaced, rarely require other than symptomatic treatment. This includes bed-rest. A close study is essential for severe bleeding and possible genitourinary injury. The antigravity suit (the "G-suit") may support circulation temporarily while volume is being replaced.

ACETABULAR. These are common with automobile accidents. Displacement usually is not acceptable in joint fractures. Reduction generally necessitates skeletal traction (Procedure 2) or surgery. The complications are the same as with any pelvic fracture initially, and degenerative arthritis of the hip appears later.

HIP. These are most common in the elderly, but children also are affected. Since undisplaced fractures are hard to see on x-ray, hip pain on passive rotation may be most diagnostic. With displacement, the leg will be shortened and externally rotated. Skin traction (Procedure 2) is useful initially for pain relief, but most fractures need reduction and internal fixation to prevent poor healing, loss of function, and the complications of bed-rest. Skin, neural, and vascular difficulties in the limbs are rare, but general systemic complications are frequent and often lethal.

TROCHANTERS. These are avulsion injuries. The patient may walk in, but treatment with crutches and rest to decrease symptoms is useful. There should be no complications unless the pain is incapacitating or the displacement is extreme.

FEMORAL SHAFT. This is a common major injury. The leg will be shortened and externally rotated. It can always be treated with traction initially (Procedure 2), with surgical treatment a later option. A skin opening is common. There often is a serious associated vascular injury that may require primary surgical repair (Procedure 10).

Dislocation. **HIP.** Major trauma is necessary to cause this injury. The displacement usually is posterior, but may be anterior (Fig. 5). It constitutes a true emergency and requires prompt reduction (Procedure 8). General or spinal anesthesia usually is necessary, but I.V. sedation (Pro-

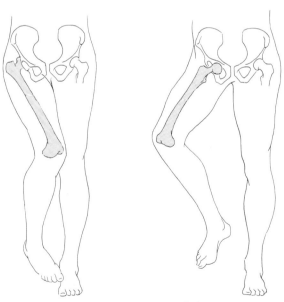

Figure 5. Positions of hip dislocations. (From Nardi, G. L.: Surgery, 3rd ed. Boston, Little, Brown and Co., 1972, pp. 971 and 972.)

cedure 4) may be sufficient if treatment is immediate. There may be an associated acetabular fracture preventing reduction or causing instability. The sciatic nerve is vulnerable posteriorly (Procedure 10). A patellar fracture commonly accompanies posterior dislocation. The late complication is avascular necrosis of the femoral head if reduction is delayed more than several hours.

X-RAYS NEGATIVE

Strain and Rupture. Pain on hip examination, with "negative" x-rays, usually means an undisplaced hip or pelvic fracture in the adult and a slipped capital femoral epiphysis in the child. Legg-Perthes' disease (avascular necrosis) and sepsis are other major considerations in the child. Children commonly report only knee pain with hip diseases and injuries. Skin traction is effective to decrease pain (Procedure 2). All cases that are merely "suspicious" should be protected with rest and crutches, and provided with early follow-up to prevent complications arising from missed diagnosis. A slipped epiphysis or an undisplaced hip fracture may require prompt surgical fixation to prevent progressive displacement.

Laceration. Rarely, the sciatic nerve may be injured posteriorly and the femoral artery, vein, and nerve anteriorly. Early recognition (Procedure 10) is essential. Primary surgical repair may be indicated.

KNEE

X-RAYS POSITIVE

Fracture. JOINT. Intercondylar and plateau fractures will present with blood in the joint. Aspiration may yield fat mixed in blood, a valuable diagnostic sign (Procedure 5). Treatment usually is by traction, most commonly skeletal through the proximal or distal tibia (Procedure 2). If the fracture is displaced, operation often is necessary to reduce and stabilize internally. Skin injury usually is not a problem, but peroneal nerve and/or popliteal artery injuries commonly go unrecognized (and thus untreated), with serious long term effects (Procedure 10).

PATELLA. This common injury may be difficult to see on x-rays. If the fracture is undisplaced, treatment by immobilization in a cylinder cast or posterior splint is sufficient (Procedures 1 and 3). If the fracture is displaced, surgical repair or removal is necessary. A skin abrasion or laceration into the joint is common, but neural and vascular injuries are rare. The joint lacerations require immediate surgery.

AVULSIONS. Small "chips" seen on knee x-rays may represent major ligamentous injuries. These should be treated with immobilization in a cylinder cast and crutches for approximately six weeks. If the fractures are displaced, surgical repair of the injured ligaments may be indicated. A stress examination may be useful in determining significance or severity (Procedure 7).

Dislocation. PATELLA. This is a very common injury, especially in young girls and women. They are always laterally displaced, but may reduce spontaneously and elude diagnosis. Reduction is easily accomplished with knee extension and lateral patellar pressure. Anesthesia usually is not necessary (Procedure 4). A check x-ray, for possible osteochondral fracture and loose body, is important before and after reduction. A cylinder cast is necessary for treatment of the first episode, but recurrent dislocations need only symptomatic treatment acutely. The complication is recurrent dislocation if the injury is not immobilized until the torn soft tissues are healed; this takes a minumum of six weeks.

KNEE. Major trauma is necessary to cause this dislocation. Reduction by manual traction should be immediate, and followed by posterior splint or cylinder cast immobilization (Procedures 1 and 3). Peroneal nerve and popliteal vessel injuries are the rule, so that careful baseline and serial observations are necessary (Procedure 10). Surgical treatment often is necessary for the vessel, nerve, and ligament injuries.

FIBULAR HEAD. This injury is very rare. It should present as a visible and palpable prominence. Treatment usually is by closed reduction and immobilization in a long leg cast (Procedure 3). The peroneal nerve function must be noted and followed carefully (Procedure 10).

X-RAYS NEGATIVE

Strain and Rupture. LIGAMENTS. These are extremely common injuries that often are underestimated. The medial ligaments are involved most frequently. A rapid, large joint effusion (blood) usually develops.

Aspiration may assist in diagnosis and relief of pain (Procedure 5). Stress testing is important to establish the diagnosis (Procedure 7). In a child, instability on stress examination indicates that there has been an epiphyseal separation. Knee pain in a child very often results from hip pathology. A spontaneously reducing patellar dislocation may mimic medial strain. The treatment is cylinder cast immobilization (Procedure 3). Major disruptions may require surgical repair. Neurovascular and skin injuries are rare.

MENISCUS. This very common injury usually is medial. The history may show that the knee may snap, lock, or buckle. There commonly is local medial joint line tenderness. The knee should be protected with crutches until the acute symptoms resolve. Early surgical treatment is only indicated when knee motion is fixed ("locked").

QUADRICEPS RUPTURE. This occurs in the elderly. The patient cannot actively extend the knee or hold against gravity. Surgical repair is necessary, but the knee should be splinted acutely to avoid further disruption (Procedure 1).

PATELLAR TENDON RUPTURE. This is a rare injury. The patient cannot actively extend the knee or hold against gravity. Surgical repair is necessary.

Laceration. Even "superficial" lacerations commonly involve the joint. Puncture wounds are especially hazardous. X-rays should be checked for possible intra-articular gas or foreign body. Surgical exploration is required to prevent infection. Nerve and vessel injuries may occur with posterior trauma, and may need surgical repair (Procedure 10).

LEG AND FOOT

X-RAYS POSITIVE

Fracture. **TIBIAL SHAFT.** These injuries are very common at all ages. The leg usually is shortened and externally rotated if the fracture is displaced. Reduction by longitudinal traction (Procedure 9) after sedation (Procedure 4) normally is successful. Immobilization in a long leg cast (Procedure 3) is necessary to control rotation of the fracture. Post-injury swelling can be a major problem that, like nerve and vessel function, must be followed carefully (Procedure 10). Elevation will prevent most of the difficul-

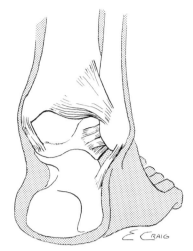

Figure 6. Ankle anatomy. (Adapted from DePalma, A. F.: The Management of Fractures and Dislocations, 2nd ed. Philadelphia, W. B. Saunders Co., 1970, p. 155.)

ties, but splitting of the cast may be necessary.

FIBULAR SHAFT. These fractures usually are due to direct trauma. If they are isolated injuries (that is, not related to ankle fractures or ligamentous strains), they rarely require other than crutch protection.

MALLEOLAR. This common ankle injury is extremely variable in type and often is open (Fig. 6). It always is a joint fracture that requires exact reduction, often surgical. Anesthesia is necessary for reduction (Procedures 4 and 9). A long leg cast is necessary for immobilization (Procedure 3). Swelling is a problem, but neural and vascular injury is rare. Ischemic skin injury related to persistent displacement is common, and thus prompt reduction is important. Elevation will prevent most soft tissue difficulty, but splitting of the cast may become necessary.

METATARSAL. These fractures are very common and frequently multiple. Swelling occurs quickly, so that there is little apparent deformity. The fractures rarely need reduction. Treatment is by protected weight bearing and/or a short leg walking cast (Procedure 3). Foot elevation is important in order to avoid soft tissue complications.

PHALANGES. The mechanism of these injuries usually is stubbing or crushing. If deformity is apparent on physical examination, reduction can be accomplished by longitudinal traction and manipulation. Immobilization for three to six weeks is achieved by taping the injured toe loosely to an adjacent toe. The great toe may be splinted effectively with plaster (Procedure 1). Crutch protection may be helpful to relieve symptoms and promote prompt healing.

Dislocation. **TALAR, SUBTALAR, MIDFOOT.** These rare injuries are often skin and vascular emergencies arising from the displacement. Prompt reduction by longitudinal traction and manipulation is essential. A splint is sufficient to immobilize and decrease soft tissue complications (Procedure 1). Delay in reduction may result in loss of the foot. Elevation after reduction is extremely important in order to decrease swelling.

TOE. Metatarsal-phalangeal and interphalangeal dislocations are rare, but usually are easily reduced by longitudinal traction. Splinting is accomplished by taping the injured toe to an adjacent toe. Splinting for two to three weeks generally is sufficient.

X-RAYS NEGATIVE

Strain and Rupture. **GASTROCNEMIUS FASCIA ("PLANTARIS RUPTURE").** This is an injury of middle age. It is caused by a sudden, violent muscular strain, with resulting sudden pain in the calf. There is local tenderness, with good active plantar flexion of the ankle. It is important to differentiate this from heel cord rupture. The treatment is symptomatic. Crutch protection, followed by a ½-inch heel lift, is useful.

HEEL CORD RUPTURE. The presentation of this injury may be the same as that of gastrocnemius fascia rupture, except that the patient cannot stand on his toes, and squeezing the calf will not plantar flex the ankle, thus proving a complete rupture (Fig. 7). Treatment can consist of immobilization in a short leg cast (Procedure 3), with the foot in a gravity position of equinus, or surgical repair.

DELTOID LIGAMENT RUPTURE. This is an eversion injury, with resulting medial ankle tenderness and swelling (Fig. 6). X rays may show lateral displacement of the talus or a fibular fracture. Stress testing may demonstrate the rupture if the x-ray is negative (Procedure 7). The talus position must be restored to normal. A long leg cast (Procedure 3) and crutch protection is necessary for six weeks to achieve optimum healing. An all too common complication is late instability of the ankle. In children, the tibial epiphysis may displace, requiring reduction and a long leg cast for approximately three weeks (Procedure 3). The foot should be elevated after these injuries to prevent soft tissue complications.

LATERAL COLLATERAL LIGAMENT. This is the most common ankle injury. In-

Figure 7. Squeeze test for ruptured heel cord. (From MacAusland, W. R., Jr.: Orthopedics. Boston, Little, Brown and Co., 1965, p. 283.)

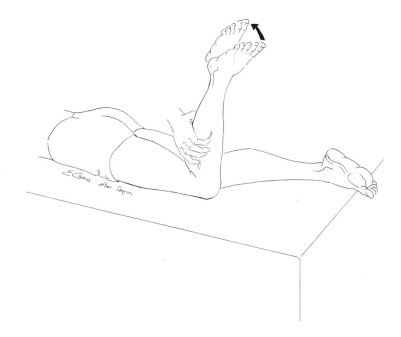

version is the mechanism of injury. Lateral ankle swelling and tenderness will be found (Fig. 6). Stress testing will define the extent of the tear (Procedure 7). A short leg cast (which may be the walking type) for six weeks is minimum treatment for severe tears (Procedure 3). The all too common complication is late instability of the ankle. In children, the distal fibular epiphysis may avulse; this requires a short leg cast for approximately three weeks. The foot should be elevated after these injuries to prevent soft tissue complications.

Laceration. There are superficial neural, vascular, and tendinous structures that are susceptible to laceration near the ankle. They may require primary repair. A plantar laceration of the foot threatens important nerves; repair should be considered (Procedure 10).

H. TRAUMA TO THE HAND

E. Jeff Justis

INTRODUCTION

The hand is a specialized organ that requires sensibility, mobility, and active musculotendinous units for normal function. Anything that interferes with these modalities can seriously impair a patient's manual dexterity and affect his employability and life style, often irretrievably. Physicians responsible for initial care of the injured hand have the unique opportunity to recognize potential problems and specific injuries early. Delay in evaluation and institution of effective planned management can lead to an unnecessarily poor result.

Hand injuries often are seen in the Emergency Department as separate entities, a concept that enables the physician to concentrate on the pathologic anatomy before him. When hand injuries are associated with other more serious injuries, those that threaten life must, of course, take precedence, although every effort should be made to prevent disability that may arise through inadequate examination or follow-up.

INITIAL EVALUATION

Regardless of the innocent appearance of a minor injury or the obvious damage in a serious injury, each patient presenting in the Emergency Department with an injured hand should receive as a minimum the following assessment and initial care.

OBSERVATION

Observe the hand for obvious open injury, severe arterial or venous bleeding, or devitalized parts. Most bleeding can be controlled by sustained local pressure and elevation, although ligature of an arterial bleeder occasionally may be required. Do not blindly grasp tissue in the depths of a wound with a hemostat, however, as damage to nerves, tendons, and other structures may result. Rather, try to isolate the offending vessel, even if a tourniquet must be used temporarily.

Observe for altered posture. This is especially useful in children. The diagnosis of a severed tendon can be made merely by noticing an alteration in the normal resting position of the hand (Figs. 1, 2, 3, *A–D*).

X-RAY EXAMINATION

At least two views should be taken. Not only is this necessary for completeness in a full evaluation, but specific fractures, dislocations, foreign bodies, and other pathologic conditions may be recognizable only on roentgenograms. Special views (e.g., navicular) should be specified when needed.

TETANUS PROPHYLAXIS

Toxoid booster, toxoid initial immunizing dose, or tetanus immune globulin (Hyper-Tet) should be given, depending on the patient's previous immunization history

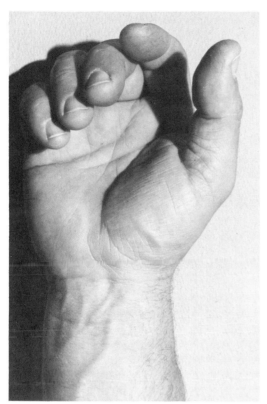

An initial irrigation may be possible without anesthesia. However, the use of a digital block or of local infiltration anesthesia will facilitate thorough inspection and cleansing of the wound. As a means of decreasing the patient's pain, Xylocaine or another local anesthetic agent may be used as an initial topical irrigant prior to injecting gently through the wound into undisturbed tissue. For more than the simplest wound, or when deep probing is anticipated, nerve block is preferred.

DIGITAL NERVE BLOCK AND WRIST BLOCK ANESTHESIA

Satisfactory anesthesia either for thorough inspection of the wound or for definitive treatment can be obtained readily and safely in hand injuries through good digital nerve block or wrist block anesthesia. A small bore needle (25 to 27 gauge) is used

Figure 1. Normal resting posture of hand, anteior view. Note the increase in flexion of the fingers from the index to the fifth finger due to differences in relative resting tension of the flexors.

and the type of wound. Use caution in giving equine antitoxin, as an allergic idiosyncrasy may lead to anaphylactic shock, even with skin testing. Hyper-Tet is much preferred if previous immunization has been inadequate—250 units is an adequate dosage in most circumstances.

Simple Wounds

The first principle in the management of any wound to the hand is, of course, *thorough cleansing.* However, the hand *should not be soaked* in pHisoHex or any other antibacterial solution. Rather, *wash* the hand with pHisoHex, Betadine, or plain soap and water to remove the superficial dirt from the *undamaged* skin. The wound itself should be irrigated *only* with normal saline. (Antiseptics damage cells, and pHisoHex contains a preservative producing a tissue reaction that will interfere with wound healing.)

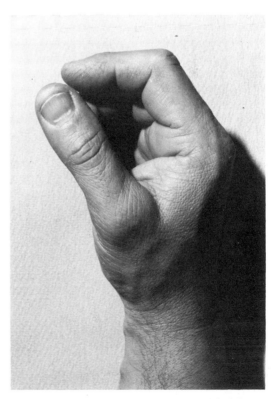

Figure 2. Normal resting posture of hand, radial view.

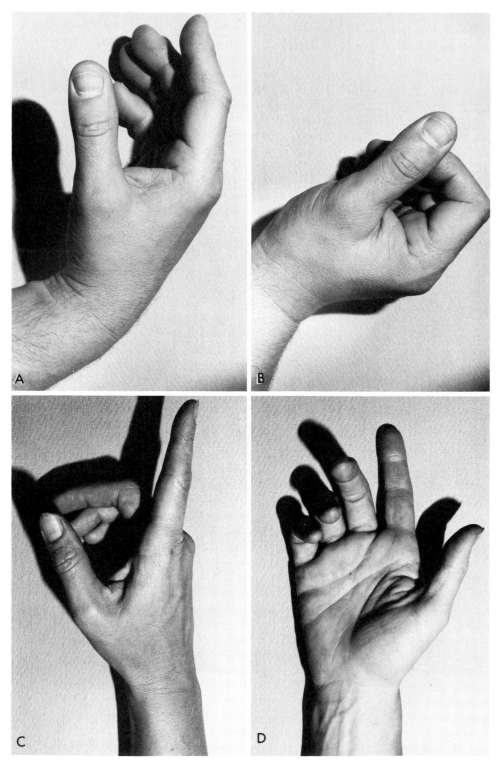

Figure 3. A, Extension of the fingers and the thumb is increased when the wrist is allowed to flex passively.
B, Flexion of the fingers is increased as the wrist is allowed to passively extend. *C* and *D* show abnormal posture of
a hand in which both flexor tendons to the index finger have been severed. Variations from this posture would be
present if only one flexor tendon had been severed. Each of the remaining fingers would be affected similarly by
abnormalities of the tendinous structures.

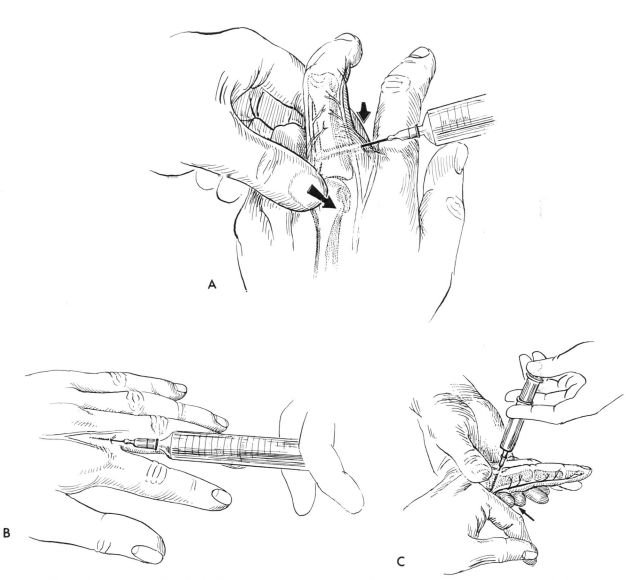

Figure 4. A, Raising dorsal wheal by transverse injection in subcutaneous tissue across metacarpophalangeal joint area. B, Small bore needle passed toward the palm to side of metacarpal neck. C, Anesthesia of digital nerve by injection of approximately 1 cc. of 1 per cent Xylocaine. (From Chase, R. A.: Atlas of Hand Surgery. Philadelphia, W. B. Saunders Co., 1973, p. 31.)

and 1 per cent Xylocaine or other appropriate anesthetic solution *without epinephrine* is injected as follows:

For digital nerve block, minimal pain is produced by raising a dorsal wheal at the region of the metacarpophalangeal joint, and injecting transversally in the subcutaneous tissue across the dorsum of the metacarpal neck to anesthetize the dorsal digital branches of the radial and ulnar dorsal branches (Fig. 4*A*), and then by injecting toward the palm to each side of the metacarpal neck (Fig. 4*B*). The volar or proper digital nerves are anesthetized by injecting approximately 1 cc. in their region as shown in Figure 4*C*.

For a complete wrist block, subcutaneous injection of the dorsal branch of the ulnar nerve just distal to the ulnar styloid and of the superficial branch of the radial nerve in the region of the anatomic snuff-box will provide good anesthesia to the dorsum of the hand. The palmar cutaneous branches of the radial nerve, the median nerve, and the ulnar nerve may be anesthetized by raising a subcutaneous wheal across the volar surface of the wrist. The median and ulnar nerves must be anesthetized by injecting deeper, but the injection should be proximal to the distal flexor crease of the wrist so as to avoid injecting with pressure in the carpal tunnel itself. The median nerve is found just to the radial side of the palmaris longus tendon or midline of the wrist. When injecting, one should avoid injection directly into the median or ulnar nerve. If a parathesia is produced, either insert the needle further or withdraw it slightly so as to avoid intraneural injection. The ulnar nerve is injected just proximal to the pisiform and along the radial border of the flexor carpal ulnaris. Care should be taken to avoid injection directly into the ulnar artery, which lies just to the radial side of the ulnar nerve at the wrist.

DETAILED EXAMINATION

The single most important factor in the successful management of superficial wounds is a working knowledge of the anatomy. After initial observation and x-ray examination, a more detailed evaluation is required.

Complete sensory evaluation is often impossible in children. One may test the autonomous zones of sensibility (Fig. 5) in cooperative patients by asking them to describe the difference in sensibility between one area and another. Dryness in these areas, secondary to loss of autonomic nerve supply, is also a reliable indication of nerve deficit, even in children.

Motor evaluation may require only observation of the posture of the hand (Figs. 1 to 3); however, not only severed tendons, but dislocations and fractures also may alter the

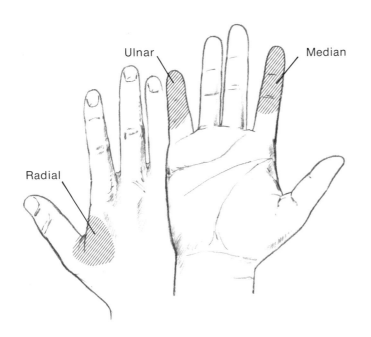

Figure 5. Autonomous zones of sensibility (areas supplied by single innervation).

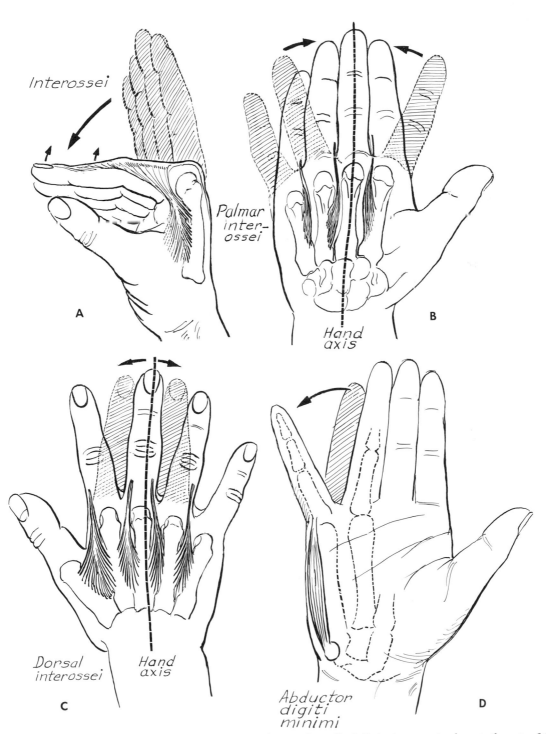

Figure 6 *A–D:* Evaluation of the interosseous muscles. *A,* The pull of all the interossei palmar to the axis of the metacarpophalangeal (MP) joints and dorsal to the interphalangeal (IP) joint axis acts to flex the MP joints and extend the IP joints. *B,* The palmar interossei adduct the fingers to the hand axis. *C,* The dorsal interossei act as abductors from the hand axis which falls in the middle of the long finger. *D,* The abductor digiti minimi is the dorsal interosseous equivalent of the little finger.

normal resting posture. Each *extrinsic* muscle may be evaluated separately by demonstrating to the cooperative patient the movement desired. *Intrinsic muscle* function may be difficult to assess in the injured hand, although one may be able to palpate contraction in the first dorsal interosseous muscle, indicating the presence of function in the motor branch of the ulnar nerve (Fig. 6). Function of the thenar muscles does not always mean an intact median nerve, since the deep portion of the flexor pollicis brevis is ulnar innervated, and the other thenar muscles similarly may receive all or part of their innervation through the ulnar nerve.

TREATMENT

Always suspect deep injury and remember the closeness of important structures. If you are certain after thorough evaluation that the wound is, in fact, superficial and uncomplicated, perform an irrigation and mechanical cleansing under an anesthetic. An arm tourniquet may be used for 10 to 15 minutes without causing significant pain when observation of deep structures is required in the Emergency Department. After elevation of the arm for three to five minutes, a blood pressure cuff may be elevated to 250 mm. Hg for a bloodless field.

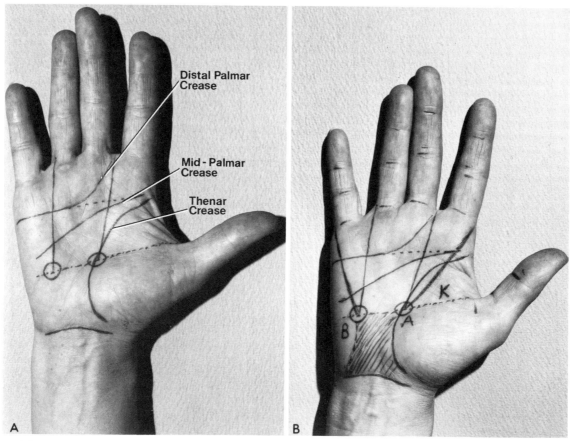

Figure 7. Surface anatomy. *A,* Important landmarks: distal; palmar crease; midpalmar crease; thenar crease. *B,* Kaplan's line (k) parallel to a line connecting extremes of the distal palmar crease and midpalmar crease. Point *A,* where Kaplan's line crosses the previously described thenar crease, is the most important point of emergence of the motor branch of the median nerve. This also is the area of take-off of the sensory nerves to the thumb and of the radial digital nerve to the index finger, which passes rather superficially diagonally to the radial border at the base of the index finger. The point where Kaplan's line crosses the line extending from the ulnar border of the ring finger marks the hook of the hamate, where the motor branch of the ulnar nerve curves radially, crossing the palm to supply the intrinsic muscles of the hand. This also marks the point of emergence of the ulnar digital nerve to the little finger as it courses diagonally to the ulnar border of the base of the little finger. Notice the shaded area extending distal to the flexor crease of the wrist, which represents the area of the carpal tunnel that contains the median nerve, the flexus pollicis longus, the four flexor sublimi, and four flexor profundi to the fingers.

Superficial flaps of skin should be replaced unless grossly damaged. Skin sutures should be nonabsorbable to minimize reaction, and catgut generally should not be used in suturing lacerations. Many small finger wounds can be dressed adequately with a Band-Aid. More extensive wounds should be immobilized with a wrist splint and/or a bulky dressing, maintaining the wrist and fingers in a functional position. The patient should be instructed to maintain the elevated position (above heart level) in the postoperative period until there is no further swelling and normal function is restored.

Complicated Wounds

TENDON AND NERVE INJURIES

The innocent appearance of many hand wounds may hide a major problem. The severance of a *tendon*, even to the fifth finger, or of a digital nerve can lead to significant impairment of function if unrecognized. Caution must be exercised in deciding that a tendon is *not* severed, since a patient can actively flex or move a digit with a tendon that is partially severed. One clue to any damage is that pain usually is produced during motion, and blood may be present within the sheath. Tendons that are partially severed can rupture two to three weeks later if unrepaired and unprotected. Nerve function can overlap to the extent that the patient will not notice the difference in sensibility between two sides of a digit, for example, and one definitely can be mistaken as to the loss of sensibility. For this reason it is most important to know what to expect in the way of anatomy in the region of the laceration (Fig. 7, *A*, *B*). To overlook a severed nerve is not at all uncommon, and the burden of proof is on the examiner. Thus, operating room exploration of major hand wounds often is necessary on referral from the Emergency Department.

Examination of Tendons. In examining the flexor tendons of the fingers, stabilization at the distal interphalangeal joint will demonstrate profundus action (Fig. 8). Holding the other fingers in extension will allow demonstration of the flexor sublimis that flexes the proximal interphalangeal joint (Fig. 9).

Treatment. In general, do not attempt tendon or nerve repair in the Emergency Department. Occasionally, a surgeon who has had some experience in hand surgery will perform a limited repair of, for example, extensor tendons in the Emergency Department, under certain ideal circumstances. *Primary repair* of flexor tendons may be attempted if a surgeon skilled in this type of work is available and if operating room facil-

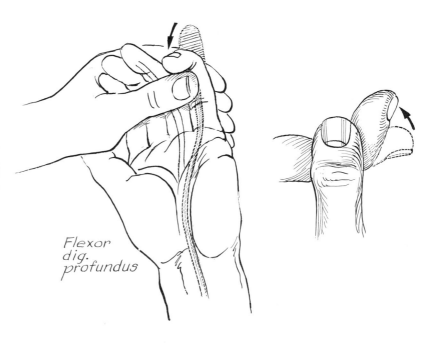

Figure 8. Testing the function of the profundus tendon. (From Chase, R. A.: Atlas of Hand Surgery. Philadelphia, W. B. Saunders Co., 1973.)

Flexor dig. profundus

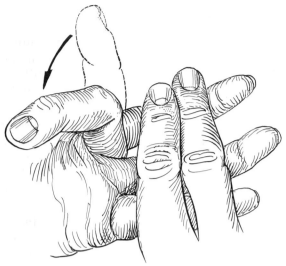

Figure 9. Testing the sublimis tendon. (From Chase, R. A.: Atlas of Hand Surgery. Philadelphia, W. B. Saunders Co., 1973.)

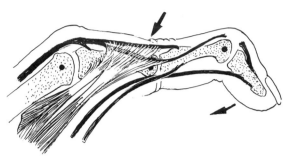

Figure 10. Rupture of the extensor tendon at insertion into the distal phalanx, the "baseball" or "mallet" finger. (From Chase, R. A.: Atlas of Hand Surgery. Philadelphia, W. B. Saunders Co., 1973.)

ities are adequate. If in doubt, merely close the skin loosely and refer the patient to someone knowledgeable in hand surgery. *Delayed primary repair* may offer a good result under select circumstances. The important principle to remember is that delay in repair of nerves and tendons *is not harmful* (and may be beneficial) if careful cleansing and skin closure are accomplished initially.

Common Tendon Injuries. Closed tendon injuries involving the extensor mechanism, such as "mallet (baseball)" finger (Fig. 10) and "boutonnière" deformity (Fig. 11), usually can be successfully managed conservatively. "Mallet" finger deformity, in which there is an avulsion of the distal extensor attachment resulting in a flexion deformity, can be treated by applying a simple metal splint that places the *distal interphalangeal joint only* in a neutral or slightly extended position. Hyperextension of this joint is not necessary and may be detrimental, since the blood supply to the skin may be compromised during forced hyperextension of this joint. Fixed flexion of the *proximal* interphalangeal joint (as in the older method of treatment of "mallet" finger by application of a finger cast, maintaining flexion of the proximal joint and extension of the distal joint) is both unnecessary and definitely harmful to this joint. The extended position of the distal joint must be maintained consistently for six to eight

weeks in adults, four to six weeks in children. Similarly, treatment of a "boutonnière" deformity is by application of a straight splint to immobilize the proximal interphalangeal joint in extension. The metacarpophalangeal joint and the distal interphalangeal joint should not be immobilized.

Extensor tendons occasionally can be repaired in the Emergency Department if the facilities and the experience of the treating physician are adequate. For the very common lacerations of the extensor hood over the metacarpophalangeal joint, a pull-out "roll stitch" may be utilized to provide firm closure; the MP joint should be splinted in full extension for about four to five weeks. One should use caution, however, in dealing with wounds that may be caused by another person's teeth (human bite wounds). Such wounds notoriously are contaminated with serious pathogens. In general, no human bite should be sutured primarily. The wound should be left open for adequate drainage; secondary closure may be performed if there is no evidence of infection in

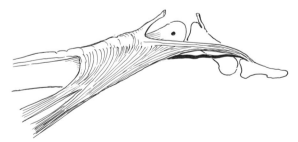

Figure 11. Rupture of the central slip of the long extensor tendon near its insertion into the middle phalanx, the "boutonnière" deformity. (From Chase, R. A.: Atlas of Hand Surgery. Philadelphia, W. B. Saunders Co., 1973.)

five to seven days. Antibiotics should be used. With dog bites there is less chance of infection, but even with adequate débridement and irrigation the safest approach is a secondary closure.

"No Man's Land." It is my feeling that a "no man's land" exists for any tendon injury in the distal forearm, wrist, or hand under the following circumstances:

1. Inadequate facilities: for example, poor lighting; poor equipment in the Emergency Department; absence of a pneumatic tourniquet; inadequate assistance; large, clumsy, or malfunctioning instruments; or an inadequate suture selection.

2. A physician who is inexperienced in tendon repair work or unfamiliar with the local anatomy—or an experienced surgeon who is fatigued.

3. Any situation in which there is doubt on the part of the physician providing initial treatment that adequate repair of the severed tendon can be performed and that proper follow-up can be continued.

The reason that the classic *"no man's land"* has become so much of a part of our vocabulary in dealing with hand injuries is that, occasionally, clumsy or large sutured repair of a flexor or extensor tendon at *other* locations in the hand will work satisfactorily and provide a good result. However, this same type of repair performed in "no man's land" (the area of the fibrous flexor sheath of the flexor tendons of the fingers and thumb, approximately from the distal palmar crease to the proximal interphalangeal joint) will inevitably fail. Given proper conditions, as described above, flexor tendon repair done as a primary or delayed primary procedure, even in "no man's land," can be expected to provide a satisfactory result in most cases. A half-severed tendon should be treated in basically the same way as one completely severed, for a smooth repair is essential for adequate function. If it remains unrepaired, late rupture is a distinct possibility.

WRINGER INJURIES

Wounds sustained by severe compression of the hand and forearm, usually between rubber or steel rollers, are classified generally as "wringer injuries." Often there is no outward suggestion of the degree of injury, and massive edema, and even Volkmann's ischemic contracture, are the sequelae if this injury is inadequately treated.

"Bursting wounds" of the fingers and in the thenar and hypothenar areas, may look like lacerations, but in fact are due to increased internal pressure and should not be closed. Avulsion of skin is common, and occasionally the most obvious damage is at the elbow or shoulder where the roller spins as it is blocked in progression up the extremity.

Treatment. Initial treatment consists of thorough cleansing of the skin (even if no lacerations are present), tetanus prophylaxis, and application of a compressive dressing with elevation of the extremity well above the heart level. The dressing consists of a single layer of nonadhesive gauze (Adaptic, Zeroform, etc.), fluffs and gauze separating each finger, Webril or other cast padding, and Kerlex. *No circular cast should be used.* A stockinette may be applied over the entire dressing, but Ace or other elastic bandages usually are *too* constrictive and should be used with *extreme caution.* The patient should be admitted for observation.

IMPENDING ISCHEMIA AND VASCULAR INJURIES

In compressing injuries as noted above, *Volkmann's ischemia* is a serious complication. Supracondylar fractures of the elbow or damage to the brachial, radial, or ulnar arteries from other cause, also may result in ischemia to the muscles of the forearm and/or hand that eventually causes fibrosis, contracture, and permanent disability. The earliest and most important sign of impending ischemia is *pain on passive stretch* of the involved muscles—usually the flexor group of forearm muscles. Sensory changes are variable, as is the presence or absence of a pulse.

With Volkmann's ischemia, the radial pulse usually is not palpable and delayed capillary filling is evident. *Early fasciotomy* is indicated, and for many wringer or crush injuries this may be done prophylactically in view of the severity of this complication and the likelihood of its development in this type of injury.

Traumatic Arterial Thrombosis. With laceration or traumatic thrombosis of the major arterial supply, the hand will exhibit pallor and distal pulses will not be palpable. With this type of injury, salvage of an extremity or hand is possible through vascular anastomosis at any level performed by a skilled surgeon. (Surgeons expert in microvascular techniques have successfully anastomosed digital arteries at the distal interphalangeal joint level.) If the time of ischemia exceeds four to six hours, some permanent muscle damage will have occurred. Some surgeons recommend radial or ulnar arterial repair even when only one artery is severed, but, if the total blood supply to the hand or part is adequate clinically through collaterals, one must exercise judgment in considering the necessity for such repair.

Fractures and Dislocations

Obvious deformity may indicate a fracture or dislocation. X-rays should *always* be obtained. This is important not only in order accurately to determine the method of reduction, but also for obvious medicolegal reasons.

SPRAINED OR "JAMMED" FINGERS

These are frequently seen in the Emergency Department. Unfortunately, when no abnormality is seen on x-ray these injuries often are inadequately treated. If a ligament is completely torn, as demonstrated clinically by lateral instability, immobilization or, occasionally, surgical treatment will be required—especially if the *ulnar collateral ligament of the thumb* is involved.

Initial treatment must include protective splinting in the functional or curved position (not on a straight splint or tongue blade) and taping to an adjacent finger. The patient should be followed as an outpatient so that *mobilization* can begin as soon as the acute pain lessens, and so that conditions occasionally unrecognized, such as "mallet" finger and "boutonnière" deformity, can be adequately treated.

PROXIMAL INTERPHALANGEAL JOINT DISLOCATIONS

Dislocations of this joint are common (Fig. 12). These usually can be reduced by a gentle pull in the direction of the deformity under digital block anesthesia. One should check for lateral instability after reduction. Immobilize by taping the affected finger to its neighbor with a little cotton pad between the fingers and applying a dorsal splint *(curved aluminum)* to prevent hyperextension of the finger, but so as to *allow* full active flexion as tolerated. The splint can be discontinued after a week or so and the patient can be permitted to continue protective, full flexion of the finger, which should

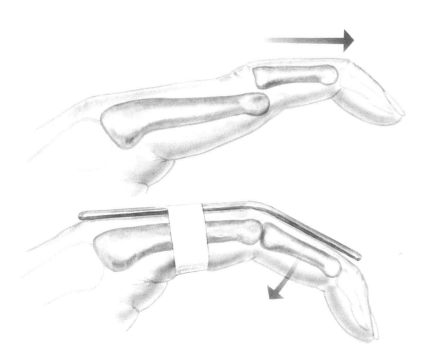

Figure 12. Proximal interphalangeal joint dislocation and reduction with dorsal blocking splint.

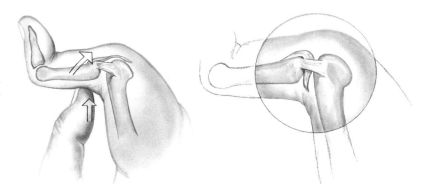

Figure 13. Dislocation of metacarpophalangeal joint of the thumb.

be taped to its neighbor. Thus, severe limitation of motion can be averted.

METACARPOPHALANGEAL JOINT DISLOCATIONS

These dislocations, particularly of the thumb, may resist closed reduction. This is because of a locking of the metacarpal head anterior to the volar plate, which is displaced with the dislocation. There is no objection to attempting closed reduction in the Emergency Department. MP joint dislocations of the thumb are reduced by *pushing* the proximal phalanx distally (on the proximal dorsal aspect) until it can be flexed forward easily over the metacarpal head (Fig. 13). No attempt should be made to pull the finger back into place, as this will only tighten the structures on each side of the metacarpal head, effectively blocking relocation. If closed reduction is unsuccessful, one should be prepared to perform an open reduction as soon as practical.

FRACTURES OF THE PROXIMAL PHALANX

These fractures (Fig. 14, *A*, *B*) often are volarly angulated owing to the intrinsic tendinous pull across the fracture; thus, these fractures often are stable in full flexion of the MP joint. This serves to relax the intrinsics and to allow the reduction to be maintained. Occasionally, particularly with multiple fractures, Kirschner wire internal fixation is necessary.

Be cautious in treating *spiral nondisplaced fractures* of the metacarpals or phalanges, as these often will have a *rotary* component, so that the finger will rotate under or on top of an adjacent finger during flexion of the finger, thus disabling the entire hand. Accordingly, be sure to check rotation with the finger in slight flexion. This rotary component often can be corrected by taping to an adjacent finger and maintaining the finger in slight flexion on a curved metal splint.

AVULSION FRACTURES

Avulsion fractures (Fig. 15) often appear to be quite innocent, and only an x-ray obtained by stressing the joint in the opposite direction can demonstrate its instability. These fractures often require open reduction and internal fixation for adequate stabilization. Similarly, condylar fractures of the phalanges are unstable and often must be treated with internal fixation.

In dealing with fractures of the hand or fingers, as a general rule, *no extreme position of a finger should be maintained for longer than ten days*, and, except for certain unstable fractures, most metacarpal and phalangeal fractures may be adequately controlled in the functional position (Figs. 1 and 2). Do not depend on radiographs to determine adequate healing. Most hand fractures should not be immobilized for over *three weeks*. Early motion will prevent permanent disabling stiffness.

The Mangled Hand

The severity of mangling hand injuries is quite obvious, since this open wounding involves skin, nerve, tendon, and bone. Bleeding may be quite severe, but usually can be controlled through elevation and an adequate pressure dressing, with the fingers molded into a somewhat functional position.

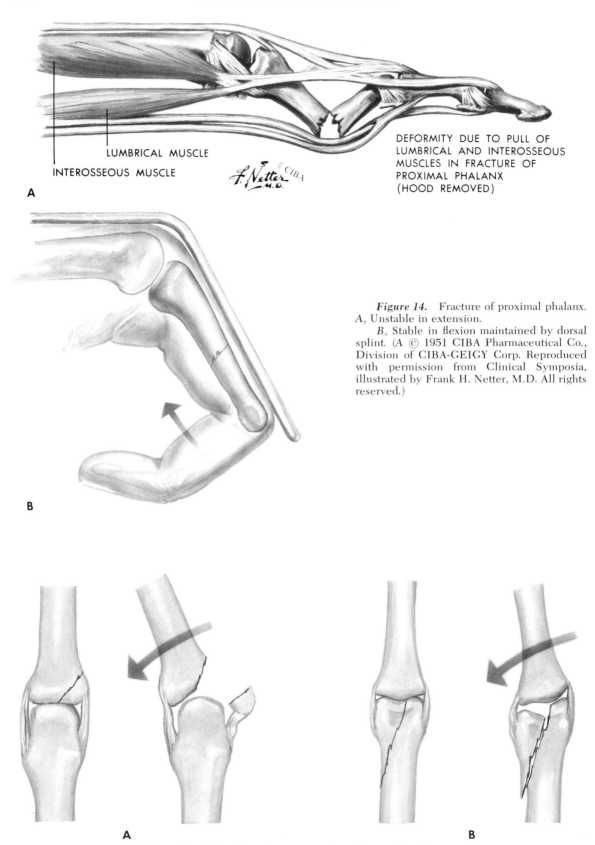

A

INTEROSSEOUS MUSCLE   LUMBRICAL MUSCLE

DEFORMITY DUE TO PULL OF
LUMBRICAL AND INTEROSSEOUS
MUSCLES IN FRACTURE OF
PROXIMAL PHALANX
(HOOD REMOVED)

B

Figure 14. Fracture of proximal phalanx.
A, Unstable in extension.

B, Stable in flexion maintained by dorsal
splint. (*A* © 1951 CIBA Pharmaceutical Co.,
Division of CIBA-GEIGY Corp. Reproduced
with permission from Clinical Symposia,
illustrated by Frank H. Netter, M.D. All rights
reserved.)

A   **B**

Figure 15.   *A,* Avulsion fracture. *B,* Unstable condylar fracture.

If definitive care is readily available, a bulky protective dressing can be utilized as temporary splintage until the patient can be transferred to the operating room. Occasionally, it may be necessary to elevate the extremity and apply a tourniquet to control bleeding, so that the injury can be evaluated more accurately.

TREATMENT

The first principle of treatment is thorough irrigation and débridement of all devitalized tissue and all foreign material. This is followed by stabilization of the skeleton (with Kirschner wires) and limited closure. If in doubt, one should apply a nonadhesive dressing and leave the wound open in preparation for a *delayed primary closure* (up to seven to ten days postinjury) or *secondary closure* (after ten days). A primary repair is one carried out during the first six hours following wounding. A delayed primary closure includes the repair of structures before significant granulation tissue develops — in this case, the wound usually can be separated bluntly. Secondary repairs are made after granulation has matured and there is fibrous tissue ingrowth. One usually should not attempt definitive suture of a nerve or tendon in such a severely mangled hand injury, although these structures may be loosely approximated to facilitate later identification and repair. Occasionally, damaged parts of the hand are brought in separately. These should be saved, as one occasionally may utilize the skin of amputated parts for full thickness or split thickness skin grafting.

Amputations

In general, amputations should not be treated as Emergency Department procedures unless an adequate operating area is present. For the best long term results in finger amputations, one should:

1. Identify and resect nerves as far proximally as possible.
2. Identify and ligate (or cauterize) the digital arteries.
3. Perform adequate irrigation and débridement to prevent infection, since the period of morbidity and the time that the patient is away from work may be lengthened greatly if an infection develops.

TIP AMPUTATIONS

These are considered separately here, since damage to the pulp is the critical factor. Tight closure over the exposed distal phalanx is contraindicated, and some form of local flap (Kutler, Klienert, etc.) may be necessary. Split or full thickness free grafts may be satisfactory if there is sufficient pulp pad remaining (Fig. 16). A Stent dressing should be applied (Fig. 17). If in doubt, tip amputations may be left open and delayed primary repair carried out as an elective procedure. Some studies indicate that allowing tip amputations to heal by secondary intention produces satisfactory results in most patients, although the time for complete healing may be excessive. If the avulsed fingertip is brought in with the patient, there is a temptation to replace it. This usually fails to take. In children, however, it may be worth trying. Remove the fatty layer from the inside and trim off the outer cornified layer prior to replacement.

Reimplantation. Selected patients may deserve consideration for possible reimplantation. Considerations that must be made and conditions that must be present include:

1. Clean amputations and minimally damaged distal parts.
2. Because of vessel size, reimplantation of a finger may not be successful in a child. It may be technically easier to reimplant an entire extremity.
3. A team of surgeons capable of performing microvascular surgery for distal amputations or standard vascular and nerve anastomoses for proximal amputations.
4. Patients or parents must have a complete understanding of all the facts relating to management and the complications that may follow reimplantation.

Even if a surgical team is not geographically close, if the emergency physician feels that a patient presenting with an amputation is an otherwise ideal candidate for reimplantation, arrangements can be made for transfer of the patient to a reimplantation center, preferably within four hours. Chartered aircraft often are available to provide rapid transport from smaller communities.

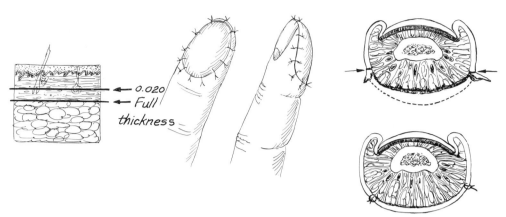

Figure 16. Finger tip amputation; repair with full thickness graft. (From Chase, R. A.: Atlas of Hand Surgery. Philadelphia, W. B. Saunders Co., 1973.)

The amputated parts should be placed in Ringer's solution in a plastic bag, and the bag should be placed in ice water for preservation and transportation. *Do not freeze* the part or place it in antiseptic solution, soapy water, or distilled water.

Foreign Bodies

A seemingly superficial foreign body can be exceedingly difficult to locate and remove, especially in an Emergency Department situation, and deep foreign bodies should be left for definitive surgical exploration. All patients should be x-rayed, since even nonmetallic foreign bodies, such as glass or painted wood, may be visible. Xeroradiography may aid in localization if the foreign body is not visible using standard x-ray techniques. Tetanus immunization is a *must*, since the depths of a puncture wound may harbor an ideal anaerobic medium for the growth of clostridia.

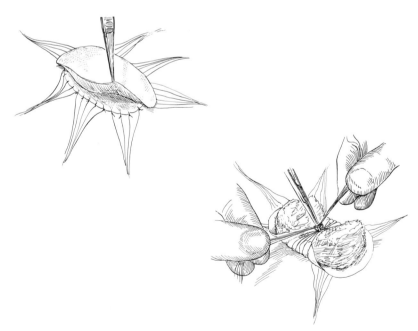

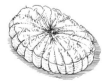

Figure 17. The Stent dressing; uniform pressure applied by tie-over dressing. (From Chase, R. A.: Atlas of Hand Surgery. Philadelphia, W. B. Saunders Co., 1973.)

Removing a large piece of wood, metal, or fish fin can lead to a false sense of security, since a portion of the foreign body may remain to cause chronic pain and infection. It is far better to perform a complete surgical exploration under ideal conditions than to leave a foreign body imbedded in a hand, merely because of a lack of facilities for adequate exploration in the Emergency Department.

INJECTION INJURIES

An innocent appearing puncture in the skin of the thumb or a finger (usually the index) may be the site of entrance of grease, paint, or solvents injected under pressure of 3000 to 7000 lb. per square inch. (Such pressures commonly are used in the application of commercial materials. By comparison, home or hobby spray compressors produce a rather harmless 40 to 60 lb. per square inch of pressure.) The high pressure of industrial compressors is sufficient to force the material along the tendon sheaths and neurovascular bundles and into the potential spaces of the hand. Damage is not only mechanical but chemical, and the distinguishing feature of this type of foreign body penetration is the excruciating pain that develops within two to three hours of the injection.

Treatment. Local incision and drainage is totally inadequate. Definitive treatment includes extensive débridement and removal of all foreign material. Even with adequate and immediate treatment, amputation or numerous reconstructive procedures eventually may be required, but loss of function can be minimized with early recognition of this occult problem. Remember the classic signs:

1. A small puncture wound oozing paint, grease, or other material.
2. Excruciating pain developing over a two- to three-hour period.
3. Swelling and pain on passive motion of the digit.

SNAKE BITE*

Although deaths from envenomation by the three poisonous viperids (rattler, copper-

head, moccasin) and the one elapid (coral snake) indigenous to the United States are uncommon, the morbidity is significant, especially in the upper extremity. At least a part of the disability resulting from snake bite may be iatrogenic, and is therefore preventable. The natural fear and panic accompanying snake bite may lead to overvigorous incision, tourniquet application, and ice application, with resultant secondary damage. The classic signs of envenomation must be present before treatment is begun: (1) Fang marks; (2) *immediate* pain; (3) rapid swelling.

Other variable findings include: petechiae, bullae, and hemorrhagic transudate from fang punctures. Later, paresthesias, necrosis, and tissue slough will develop. Initial symptoms should appear within one hour; if they are not then present, the wound should be cleansed, tetanus prophylaxis given, and the patient reassured. The bite may have been inflicted by a nonpoisonous snake, and in any case envenomation varies with the size of the poisonous snake and other factors. Thus, treatment should be individualized, depending on the degree of apparent toxicity.

Treatment. LOCAL TREATMENT. Do not incise the wound unless the degree of local pain and swelling is indicative of a serious bite. In the latter case, make an incision through the skin only, connecting the fang marks. If the wound is critical, both fang marks and intervening skin should be *excised* with a ¼- to ½-inch margin. Cool the extremity with padded ice packs, but do not immerse in ice water or allow to freeze. Immobilize the hand and arm in the functional position and at heart level.

SYSTEMIC TREATMENT. General supportive measures should be instituted. The venom must be neutralized by antivenom (Wyeth's polyvalent antivenom). This is produced from horse serum to which many patients may be highly allergic, necessitating desensitization or the use of hyperimmune serum. Skin testing is essential and, if a patient is allergic, the risk of giving polyvalent antiserum must be weighed. Local infiltration of the bite area may be worthwhile in the arm or forearm, but not in the hand or fingers, since more fluid would be pumped into an already swollen tight area to produce even more damage. Intravenous or intra-arterial infusion with an arm tourniquet in

*See also page 822.

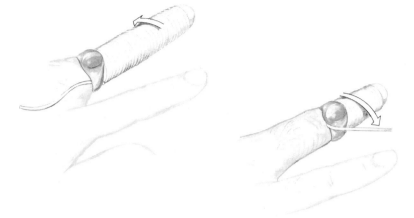

Figure 18.　Ring removal.

place is preferred. The antivenom is mixed with 100 ml. isotonic saline and 100 mg. of Solu-Cortef and injected over a 20-minute period. Ancillary medication is given, including analgesics, antibiotics, and tetanus prophylaxis, and the patient is admitted for observation.

Early fasciotomy of the forearm may be necessary if swelling is significant and there is any indication of an impending ischemia.

RING REMOVAL

With most patients who present with a swollen finger from an insect bite, edema, sprain, or fracture, rings can be removed by wrapping the finger with string from the tip down to the ring, and then inserting the string under the ring. The string is unwound as the ring is pulled distally (Fig. 18). This cannot be done, of course, with lacerations or crush injuries. In this case, cutting the ring either with diagonal cutters or a special ring cutter is the procedure of choice.

FISH HOOKS

If a fish hook is caught in the soft fleshy part of the skin, and the point of the fish hook is tenting up the skin, the area first should be anesthetized; then the hook can be pushed gently through the skin and the barb cut off, so that the unbarbed portion can be backed out (Fig. 19). There invariably is an element of contamination, and one certainly should place these patients on antibi-

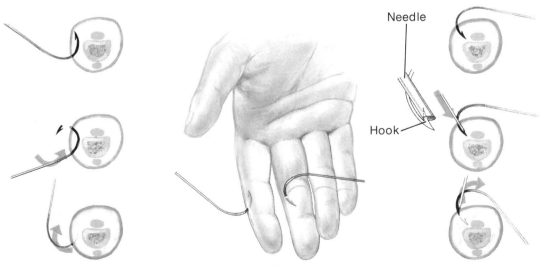

Figure 19.　Fish-hook removal.

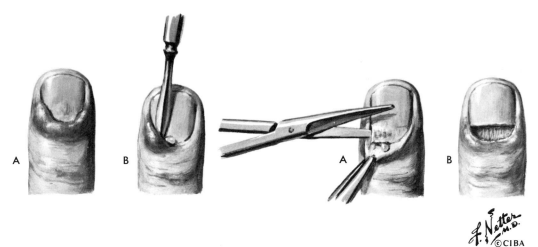

otics and observe the part carefully for inflammatory signs over the next several days. If the fish hook has penetrated and is pointing toward or into deeper structures, the procedure, after adequate anesthesia, is to insert a No. 18 needle adjacent to the barbed portion of the hook so that the beveled open end of the needle fits over the barb. The needle and the hook are then backed out together. This is particularly applicable if the hook actually lies against the bone of the finger so that it cannot be pushed through without excessive damage to the tissue.

INFECTIONS

The most common infection seen in the hand is a *paronychia*, usually caused by *Staphylococcus aureus*. Occasionally, local drainage can be established by raising a corner of the nail and retracting the eponychium (Fig. 20). Some infections require proximal incision (under digital block anesthesia) with a dressing placed under the raised eponychium for drainage.

The *"Felon"* or distal pulp space infection, usually caused by staphylococci or streptococci, results in an extremely painful tense distal pulp that requires incision and drainage. A midlateral incision is made on the side of the pulp exhibiting maximal swelling and tenderness (Fig. 21). Do not "fishmouth" the end of the finger; usually it is unnecessary to make an incision in the opposite side of the pulp. However, if the infection is obviously "pointing," even on the volar surface of the finger, the incision for drainage should be made directly over the center of the abscess.

Tenosynovitis (Fig. 22A). Infection of

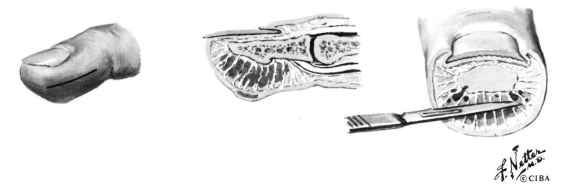

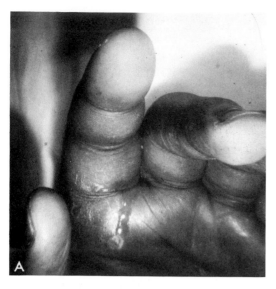

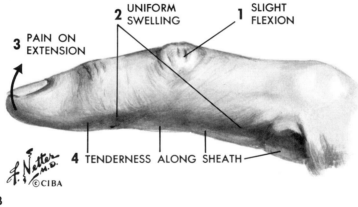

Figure 22. A, Tenosynovitis. B, Four findings in tenosynovitis (Kanavel's four cardinal points). (*B,* © 1951 CIBA Pharmaceutical Co., Div. of CIBA-GEIGY Corp. Reproduced with permission from Clinical Symposia, illustrated by Frank H. Netter, M.D. All rights reserved.)

a flexor tendon sheath may follow a puncture wound or occasionally may develop spontaneously (hematogenous origin). The classic signs of this serious infection are (from Kanavel) (Fig. 22, *B*):

1. Mild flexion contracture of the affected finger.

2. Uniform swelling of the entire volar surface of the finger.

3. Pain on passive extension.

4. Tenderness all along the flexor sheath.

TREATMENT. Early incision and drainage is required to prevent severe scarring and subsequent loss of function. This should not be done in the Emergency Department; the extensive exposure, dissection, and postoperative management required generally makes it vital that a surgeon experienced in the hand be consulted as soon as possible.

"Collar-button" abscess is a synovial sheath infection that extends proximally to the palmar subcutaneous tissue. The infection may then go through to the dorsal soft tissues. Incision must be made on both palmar and dorsal surfaces for adequate drainage (Fig. 23).

Hand Infections and Antibiotics

In dealing with patients with hand infections it is helpful to classify them tentatively on the initial examination as either "medical" or "surgical" hand infections.

SURGICAL HAND INFECTIONS

This term implies those in which there is localization of the infectious process to a closed space, such as in the "felon" or pulp abscess, the subungual abscess or paronychia, flexor tenosynovitis, dorsal subcutaneous space infection, thenar space infection,

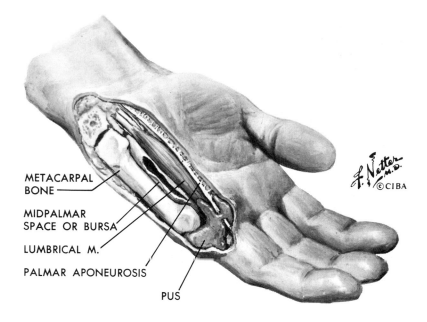

Figure 23. Collar button abscess. (© 1951 CIBA Pharmaceutical Co., Div. of CIBA-GEIGY Corp. Reproduced with permission from Clinical Symposia, illustrated by Frank H. Netter, M.D. All rights reserved.)

METACARPAL BONE

MIDPALMAR SPACE OR BURSA

LUMBRICAL M.

PALMAR APONEUROSIS

PUS

or infections in any closed or semiclosed space in the hand or wrist. These infections, in which there is actual accumulation of fluid under pressure (for example, synovial fluid, suppuration, or a foreign body such as paint, etc.), will not be benefited per se by antibiotic treatment. Antibiotics in these cases should be utilized to prevent generalized spread of the infection and to control lymphangitis or septicemia. The primary treatment, however, remains surgical, and until the pressure in the closed space is relieved by surgical means the infection cannot be controlled. Occasionally, acute symptoms subside with antibiotics alone, but significant local damage may occur.

"MEDICAL" INFECTIONS

This, on the other hand, implies infections such as cellulitis, inflammatory reactions following foreign body penetration, or questionable cases in which one cannot be sure whether localized abscess or fluid formation has occurred. These infections generally can be controlled through the use of antibiotics, elevation of the extremity, immobilization, and occasional warm compresses to increase the local blood supply. Most purulent hand infections involve *Staphylococcus aureus*, and some staph-sensitive antibiotic such as penicillin generally should be utilized. In severe infections, it is wise to begin with methicillin or cephalothin. If culturable material is available for specific identification, the antibiotic sensitivity of the organism can be obtained. In cellulitis, injection of a small amount of nonbacteriostatic saline into the area, followed by aspiration and culture, will give positive results in about 50 per cent of cases.

Gunshot Wounds

Close range low-velocity bullet wounds usually are incurred in the hand by patients cleaning small handguns. These low energy wounds generally require less extensive débridement than do high-velocity bullet wounds. Primary treatment consists of a thorough cleansing and superficial débridement followed by elevation of the hand, splinting in a functional position, and close observation. There may be a "blast" injury to adjacent nerves with sensory or motor deficit, but early exploration is not indicated. Exploration and repair of nerves or tendons can be done after the initial swelling has subsided, if necessary. Tendons may become adherent in deep scar tissue and require tenolysis. Neurolysis may be necessary after two or three months. With low-velocity bullet wounds, fractures often are nondisplaced, though comminuted, and definitive treatment may require only that the hand be splinted in a functional position.

High-velocity bullet wounds and *shotgun wounds* are much more destructive and require considerable débridement at the time of initial treatment. Shotgun wounds damage primarily through the bulk of the material exploded into the hand, whereas high-velocity missiles damage by the tremendous energy that must be absorbed by the surrounding tissues. Thus, with the latter, damage may extend well beyond the bullet tract itself. *Treatment* again must include cleansing the surrounding skin, copious irrigation, and débridement of all obviously devitalized tissue. Tendons or nerves should not be repaired, but the skeleton may be stabilized with K-wires. Closure should not be attempted, but the hand should be dressed and splinted in a functional position and elevated; a second look under anesthesia is taken 36 to 48 hours later, at which time closure may be possible, either locally or through flaps or grafts.

Thermal Injuries

BURNS

Of all wounds of the hand, burns can present the greatest problem. If there is full thickness loss of skin, the function of underlying structures is adversely affected and the development of postburn cicatrix can lead to marked deformity of fingers, even though there may have been no direct involvement of joints. Initial treatment of localized burns should consist of ice, followed by gentle cleansing and application of some nonadhesive and antibacterial dressings. If the burn is well circumscribed, one might consider *primary excision* and *grafting.*

However, some time usually must pass before demarcation is obvious and the exact extent of the burn can be determined. The single most important factor in preventing deformity is the position in which the hand must be placed. *In contrast to the splinting recommended for other hand injuries, the burned hand should be splinted so that the metacarpophalangeal joints are in flexion and the proximal and distal interphalangeal joints are in extension.* The wrist should be extended and the thumb abducted.

ELECTRIC BURNS

In electric burns, the initial appearance of the extremity may not indicate accurately the degree of damage. From the point of en-

trance of a high voltage current to the point of exit, whole muscle groups literally may be cooked through the passage of the electric current. An entire segment of the median or ulnar nerve may be completely coagulated by the internal heat produced by current flow through the tissues. Early decompression of the affected parts of the hand and forearm is indicated, and may require *extensive fasciotomy* and débridement to prevent secondary muscle necrosis through vascular compression. Electric "flashburns" or "arc" burns usually are more superficial and should be treated as thermal burns.

FROSTBITE*

Cold injured tissue may present with degrees of hyperemia, blistering, and necrosis of skin and subcutaneous tissue. Cellular death due to direct freezing is responsible for some of the damage, but progressive infarction secondary to thrombosis of vessels results in deep necrosis and loss of digits. Adequate treatment must be begun immediately.

Treatment. Rapid rewarming at 40° C. has been established as the most efficient means of preventing further damage. The extremity should be elevated to lessen edema. Low molecular weight dextran should be given to decrease blood viscosity and promote capillary flow. Of course, tetanus prophylaxis and antibiotics should be given. Sympathetic block may be indicated 24 to 48 hours after injury. Admission to the hospital for observation and subsequent treatment is necessary.

Prophylactic Antibiotics in Hand Injuries

In any hand injury in which there is no devitalized tissue, no foreign material, a normal blood supply, no accompanying debilitating medical condition, diabetes mellitus, or immunologic abnormality, adequate per primam healing is the rule; antibacterial agents are not necessary, since the patient's own immunologic response should control the minimal degree of contamination inevitable in any open injury. The treating physician, then, should perform a thorough surgical débridement and cleansing so that any

---

*See also page 770.

wounds satisfy these ideal conditions. Obviously, with crushing injuries, foreign body penetration, or devitalizing injuries one cannot, during the initial examination and treatment, be sure that all the factors likely to lead to an infectious process have been eliminated; it is for this reason that prophylactic antibiotics are utilized. At one end of the scale of injuries there may be patients with minor lacerations and minimal contamination who do not need to be placed on prophylactic antibiotics; they should be observed in the postoperative period for any evidence of inflammatory reaction or early infection. At the opposite end of the scale, of course, are those patients with rather massive crush injuries and obviously untidy or dirty wounds who should be placed on prophylactic antibiotics. If antibiotics are used prophylactically they should be started, preferably intravenously, prior to any surgical procedure. This is particularly true if a tourniquet is used, so that the extremity will be perfused with the antibiotic solution prior to closure of the wound and prior to the accumulation of blood in dead spaces. The degree to which the treating physician utilizes prophylactic antibiotics depends in large measure on his experience and on the degree to which he will be able to follow the patient. There is no harm in failing to place a patient on antibiotics if one can observe him closely for the development of infection, so that adequate treatment (such as removal of the sutures and beginning antibiotics) can be initiated. The harm, rather, lies in allowing a patient to develop an infection that is untreated for a period of several weeks; irreparable and significant damage can be the result.

Steroids and Hand Injuries

Many hand surgeons utilize steroids locally in the management of tendon repairs and tendon grafts and in other elective surgical procedures. There is no clear evidence that steroids offer any advantage in the management of acute hand injuries and certainly not in the emergency situation. Similarly, there is no evidence that systemic or topical steroids offer any particular advantage in the emergency management of hand burns.

References

American College of Surgeons: Prophylaxis Against Tetanus in Wound Management. Bull. Am. Coll. Surg. September, October 1967.

Beal, J. M.: Frostbite. Ill. Med. J. 136:592, 1969.

Beck, A. Robert, Jewett, T. C., Jr., and Allen, J. E.: Emergency room treatment of wringer injuries in children. Hosp. Top. 45:85, 1967.

Bingham, D. L. C.: Acute infections of the hand. Surg. Clin. North Am. 40:1285, 1960.

Boswick, J. A., Jr.: Initial care of hand injuries. Postgrad. Med. 48:179, 1970.

Boyes, J.: Bunnell's Surgery of the Hand. 5th ed. Philadelphia, J. B. Lippincott Co., 1970.

Brower, T. D.: Volkmann's ischemic paralysis. Surg. Clin. North Am. 40:491, 1960.

Brown, H. G.: Electrical and cold injuries of the hand. Orthop. Clin. North Am. 1:321, 1970.

Burkhalter, W. E., et al.: Experiences with delayed primary closure of war wounds of the hand in Vietnam. J. Bone Joint Surg. 50-A:945, 1968.

Eaton, R. G., and Butsch, D. P.: Antibiotic guidelines for hand infections. Surg. Gynecol. Obstet. 130:119, 1970.

Entin, M. A.: Infections of the hand. Surg. Clin. North Am. 44:981, 1964.

Entin, M. A.: Crushing and avulsing injuries of the hand. Surg. Clin. North Am. 44:1009, 1964.

Flatt, A. E.: Minor hand injuries. J. Bone Joint Surg. 37-B:117, 1955.

Granberry, M. W.: Gunshot wounds of the hand. Hand 5:220, 1973.

Green, W. L.: Results of primary and secondary flexor tendon repairs in no man's land. J. Bone Joint Surg. 56:1216, 1974.

Heycock, M. H.: On the management of hand injuries caused by woodworking tools. Br. J. Plast. Surg. 19:58, 1966.

Kleinert, H. E.: Finger tip injuries and their management. Am. Surg. 25:41, 1959.

Kleinert, H. E., et al.: Reimplantation of amputated digits and hands. Orth. Clin. North Am. 4:957, 1973.

Mann, R. J.: Paint and grease gun injuries of the hand. J.A.M.A. 231:933, 1975.

Matev, I.: Wringer injuries of the hand. J. Bone Joint Surg. 49:722, 1967.

Milford, L.: Shotgun wounds of the hand and wrist. South. Med. J. 52:403, 1959.

Milford, L.: The Hand. Campbell's Operative Orthopedics. 5th ed. St. Louis, The C. V. Mosby Co., 1971.

Moberg, E.: Evaluation of sensibility in the hand. Surg. Clin. North Am. 40:357, 1960.

Moberg, E.: The treatment of mutilating injuries of the upper limb. Surg. Clin. North Am. 44:1107, 1964.

Parks, B. J., and Horner, R. L.: Electrical burns of the hand. J. Occup. Med. 15:967, 1973.

Ramos, H., Posch, J. L., and Lie, K. K.: High pressure injection injuries of the hand. Plast. Reconst. Surg. 45:221, 1970.

Riordan, D. C.: The primary treatment of acute hand injuries. N.O. Med. Surg. J. 103:365, 1951.

Salisbury, R. E., et al.: Management of electrical burns of the upper extremity. Plast. Reconst. Surg. 61:648, 1973.

Smith, E. B.: Acute hand trauma. J. Nat. Med. Assoc. 60:304–306, July 1968.

Snyder, C. C., Straight, R., and Glenn, J.: The snakebitten hand. Plast. Reconst. Surg. 49:275, 1972.

Spinner, M., et al.: Impending ischemic contracture of the hand. Plast. Reconst. Surg. 50:341, 1972.

Stark, H. H., Wilson, J. N., and Boyles, J. H.: Grease-gun injuries of the hand. J. Bone Joint Surg. 43-A:485, 1961.

Whitson, T. C., and Allen, B. D.: Management of the burned hand. J. Trauma 11:606, 1971.

Williams, C. S.: Initial treatment of acute hand injuries. J. La. State Med. Soc. 124:205, 1972.

I. INJURIES OF THE GENITOURINARY TRACT

A. Richard Kendall and Lester Karafin

RENAL TRAUMA

Introduction

The incidence of renal trauma appears to increase each year as our motor vehicles achieve higher speeds and the Friday evening knife and gun clubs change areas of our major cities into battlefields. Waterhouse and Gross (1969) reported 116 cases of renal trauma in over 9500 patients admitted to the King's County Trauma service over a five-year period. The greatest number of injuries occur in men during the early years of adult life, although children also are prone to renal injury, probably owing to the absence of significant perirenal adipose tissue. The kidneys are ideally located to avoid injury, being protected by the lumbar spine and rib cage. However, injuries to these bony structures often affect the kidneys secondarily. It is important to stress that a diseased kidney (e.g., hydronephrotic, tumor-bearing, etc.) may be more prone to injury than a normal kidney, and this must always be given consideration at the time of emergency investigation.

CATEGORIES

Renal injuries in the past have been categorized by cause, e.g., blunt or penetrating, or by type, e.g., contusion, laceration, or pedicle injury. Blunt or nonpenetrating injuries still exceed penetrating injuries by a four-to-one margin, although Scott et al. (1969) reported a 7 per cent incidence of injuries to the kidney in a total of 2500 penetrating wounds of the abdomen.

Recognition

All patients with trauma to the upper abdomen and/or flank areas, as well as to the lower rib cage, should be considered as potential candidates for renal trauma. This applies, for example, to the patient being evaluated for possible hepatic or splenic injury following fracture of the lower rib cage. Individuals who have fallen from heights and landed on their buttocks have been found to have injuries of the kidney and the renal vasculature.

Following assessment of the vital signs, abdominal examination is imperative to elicit tenderness or a mass in the flank or upper abdominal area or the presence of muscle guarding. Because of the likelihood of other associated serious intra-abdominal injuries, the nature of the renal injury may

TABLE 1   *Renal Trauma*

EVALUATION	FINDINGS
Urinalysis	Hematuria
Abdominal x-rays	Obliteration of psoas shadow, alteration of renal outline
Augmented excretory urography	Visualization of kidneys, assessment of contralateral kidney
	Assessment of function or disruption
Renal angiography	Disruption of blood vessels assessing severity of injury, parenchymal disruption, extravasation
Renal scan	Assess degree renal trauma
Retrograde urography	Little use in renal trauma evaluation unless kidney does not visualize with augmented excretory urography and angiogram should precede

be obscured. In addition, bleeding in the retroperitoneal area may give few initial symptoms. Table 1 indicates general tests in use for evaluation of renal injury.

In every abdominal injury, *early* urinalysis is mandatory. Most patients, except the extremely ill, can void spontaneously on demand, and routine catheterization simply to obtain a urine specimen in the patient with an upper abdominal or flank injury is to be avoided when possible. Depending on the degree of injury, one may expect to have gross or microscopic hematuria, but unfortunately, as demonstrated by Scott et al. (1969), 29 per cent of patients with penetrating renal injury did not have significant hematuria. If the patient is catheterized, one cannot be sure if the microscopic hematuria is due to instrumentation or, indeed, to primary trauma.

Only in the rare situation of massive bleeding with uncontrollable hypotension should an individual with suspected renal trauma enter the operating room before x-ray studies are obtained. Augmented excretory urography (large dose of contrast material) with tomography should be performed immediately after stabilization of the vital signs. Not only should some indication of the degree of injury thus be obtained, but (of equal importance) the presence and function of the contralateral kidney can be determined. The preliminary film of the abdomen may demonstrate obliteration of the psoas shadow, possibly by a retroperitoneal hematoma, and the renal outline should be scrutinized for evidence of disruption. Following administration of contrast material, there may be delay in visualization of the injured kidney due to poor perfusion, possibly secondary to reflex arterial spasm. The nephrogram may demonstrate disruption of the cortex, and urinary extravasation may be noted as contrast is excreted (Fig. 1).

In earlier years retrograde urography was utilized more widely, but today it has only a small role in the evaluation and recognition of renal trauma. Although there still may be an indication for this procedure when the kidney cannot be visualized by other means, renal angiography is a more productive procedure. Certain centers are extremely enthusiastic over angiography, but it should not be utilized routinely and each case must be individualized. However, if there is nonvisualization, significant uri-

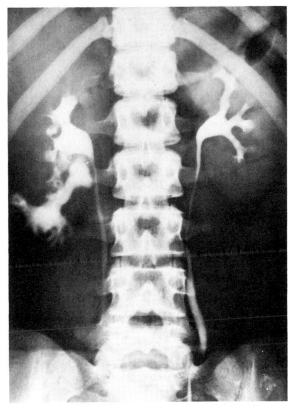

Figure 1. Disruption of cortex of right kidney on IVP with urinary extravasation.

nary extravasation, or evidence of continued blood loss, renal arteriography should be performed prior to contemplated operative exploration (Fig. 2, *A*).

The renal scan also is useful in determining the presence and degree of renal trauma (Fig. 2, *B*).

Treatment

The vast majority of patients with renal trauma can be handled conservatively without the need for operation. Following blunt trauma in which satisfactory visualization of the kidney is obtained on excretory urography, and in which there is evidence of little or no extravasation, the patient should be admitted to the hospital for close follow-up evaluation. Hemoglobin and hematocrit values are determined at least every 12 hours — or more frequently, as dictated by the condition of the patient. The same per-

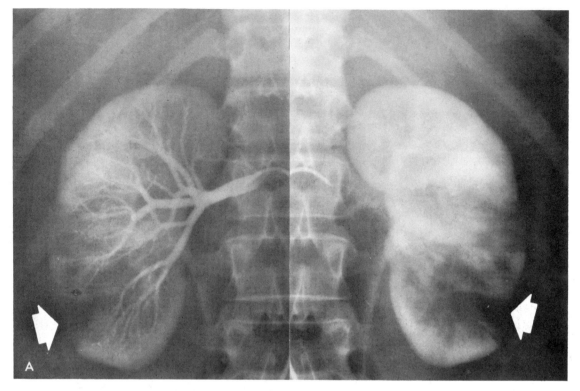

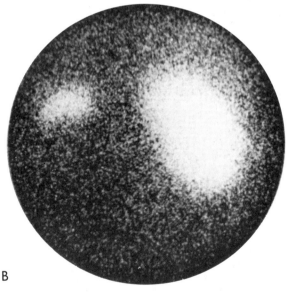

Figure 2. *A,* Angiogram demonstrating disruption of cortex of lower pole. *B,* Renal nuclear scan demonstrating injury to right lower pole.

son who examined the patient on admission should repeat his observations every few hours thereafter to detect any changes in abdominal signs. The presence of increased muscle guarding, an enlarging mass, or a progressively falling hemoglobin count and hematocrit may be an indication for angiography and possible exploration. The only absolute indication for emergency intervention in renal injuries is potential exsanguination, as seen in pedicle injuries, severe lacerations with massive extravasation or hemorrhage, or disruption of the ureteropelvic junction (Fig. 3). There is some debate regarding surgical exploration. Some urologists advocate surgical exploration of all kidneys demonstrating even minor extravasation. We and others assume a more conser-

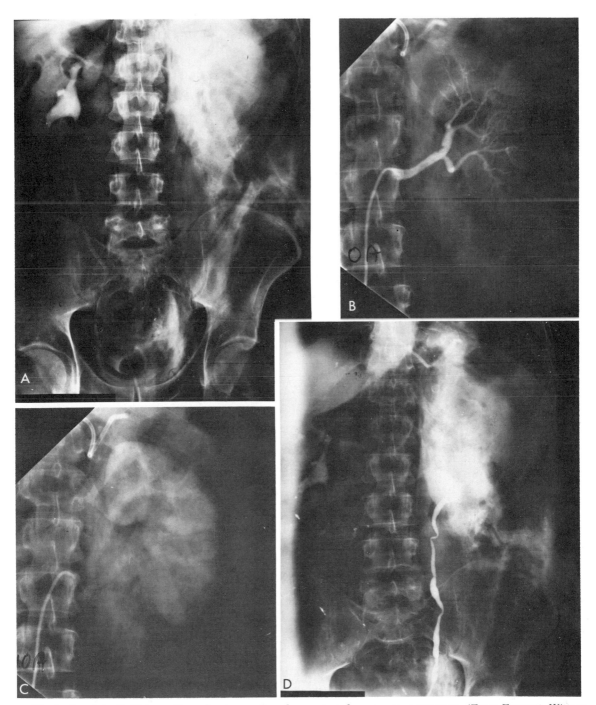

Figure 3. A to D, Extraperitoneal extravasation demonstrated on gravity cystogram. (From Emmett, Witten: Clinical Urography, Philadelphia, W. B. Saunders Co., 1977.)

vative, nonoperative approach in these "minor injuries." The controversy arises from the fact that the average patient will respond favorably to bed rest, intravenous fluid administration (due to secondary ileus), and analgesics.

PROPHYLACTIC ANTIBIOTICS

At the present time there is diversity of opinion over the value of "prophylactic" antibiotics. Although there is no convincing evidence that they reduce morbidity, the traumatized kidney may be more prone to infection via the hematogenous or ascending routes, and therefore their use is justified in the seriously injured patient.

Further Hospital Evaluation

The patient is kept at strict bed rest until gross hematuria resolves, and daily urinalysis is performed. Once there is evidence of subsiding hematuria with diminution in microscopic hematuria, gradual increased ambulation is permitted. Following full ambulation, the patient may be discharged for at least another week of convalescence at home. The time of return to "full activity" is dictated by the severity of the injury and the clinical course of the patient.

Although patients with penetrating injuries of the kidney also may be handled conservatively in a similar fashion, it is obvious that the vast majority of these undergo operative exploration because of the possibility of injury to another organ. If the excretory urogram demonstrates no evidence of extravasation and normal renal architecture, the kidney may be palpated at the time of operation, but definitive exploration and mobilization are best deferred. Even if there is a small nonexpanding hematoma in the perirenal space, opening of Gerota's fascia probably is not warranted. However, in the presence of significant extravasation, or if during the course of abdominal exploration the perirenal hematoma demonstrates expansion in size, the renal vasculature should be primarily secured and the kidney definitively explored and repaired as indicated. In general, nephrectomy is to be avoided, and more conservative procedures should be attempted, such as primary hemostasis and suture repair or partial nephrectomy. A preoperative renal angiogram is a great help in determining just how an injured kidney can best be salvaged.

Sequelae

Although the true incidence of complications following renal trauma cannot be determined because of failure of detection or inadequate follow-up in asymptomatic individuals, numerous potential sequelae are possible.

(1) Delayed bleeding. Following discharge from the hospital, the patient should be instructed to avoid strenuous exercise for at least two months. Not infrequently a patient is discharged following the disappearance of microscopic hematuria only to have recurrent bleeding several weeks thereafter. On occasion this secondary bleeding has required operative intervention and resulted in loss of a kidney.

(2) Renal hypertension occasionally may occur as a result of localized ischemia or unsuspected vascular injury.

(3) Hydronephrosis, secondary to either the formation of a urinoma or extrinsic scarring about the ureteropelvic junction, has been encountered on several occasions.

(4) Perinephric abscess.

(5) Renal artery aneurysm.

(6) Arteriovenous fistulae. These are being reported in greater numbers since the advent of angiography, and certainly may become symptomatic and require operative consideration.

Follow-up excretory urograms are necessary to detect possible sequelae.

URETERAL TRAUMA

INTRODUCTION

Ureteral injury secondary to external trauma occurs far less often than in the kidney, but appears to be more frequent following penetrating, rather than blunt, injuries. The most common ureteral injury is iatrogenic, being secondary to abdominal operations, ureteral instrumentation, or radiation therapy.

RECOGNITION OF URETERAL INJURY

Following blunt or penetrating abdominal injury, the physician must have a high index of suspicion. An augmented excretory urogram is mandatory. In the presence of serious ureteral injury, detailed films should demonstrate extravasation of urine caused by loss of continuity or obstruction at a specific level.

TREATMENT

Immediately upon demonstration of loss of continuity of the ureter, cystoscopy and the passage of a ureteral catheter should be attempted. If there has been incomplete disruption, and if the catheter can be passed into the renal pelvis, this alone may be satisfactory therapy in cases of minimal extravasation. However, the patient must be watched carefully for evidence of any expanding flank mass or sepsis. In the presence of significant extravasation, the most conservative therapy is ureteral exploration, drainage of extravasated urine, and primary ureteral repair. One of the more difficult problems is the patient with ureteral injury secondary to gunshot wounds. In these cases, there usually is devitalization of the ureter both proximal and distal to the area of injury, and it is necessary to trim the ureter until it bleeds in order to assure viability of the anastomotic site.

Injuries to the lower ureter may best be handled by reimplantation into the bladder, rather than by uretero-ureterostomy. Occasionally, when large areas of ureter have been destroyed, a diverting nephrostomy is necessary, ureteral reconstitution being carried out usually at a later date. Numerous techniques are available for ureteral replacement. A bladder flap may bridge the defect to the lower ureter, or a segment of ileum occasionally may be interposed between the ureter and bladder. The kidney may be mobilized downward so as to achieve added ureteral length and to permit a uretero-ureteral anastomosis, and on a very rare occasion autotransplantation into the true pelvis has been performed. At the present time transuretero-ureterostomy (anastomosis to the contralateral ureter) has gained in popularity.

SEQUELAE

The following sequelae may occur after ureteral injury:
(1) Ureteral stricture with hydronephrosis.
(2) Periureteral urinoma with hydronephrosis.
(3) Retroperitoneal abscess.
(4) Uretero-intestinal fistula.

A postoperative or postinjury urogram is essential to detect potential complications that may remain clinically silent.

VESICAL TRAUMA

INTRODUCTION

The bladder is unique, inasmuch as it is one of the few organs of the body subject to trauma that continually changes its shape and capacity. In the child the bladder is more of an intraperitoneal organ, whereas in the adult it is located rather deep in the pelvis behind the symphysis pubis. Only in the case of strategically placed missiles or a fracture of the pelvis is the empty bladder easily injured. However, when the bladder is distended it extends higher in the abdomen, raising the reflection of the peritoneum. In this location it is more prone to both penetrating and blunt injury. Three major types of injury to the bladder may occur.

(1) Blunt trauma to the lower abdomen may result in a simple bladder contusion or actual vesical rupture, with the perforation frequently occurring in the dome (the portion covered by peritoneum), and subsequent intraperitoneal extravasation of urine.

(2) Crush injuries to the pelvis may cause the bladder to be penetrated by spicules of bone, with extravasation of urine into the extraperitoneal, perivesical space.

(3) Penetrating injuries to the bladder from without are usually due to knife or gunshot wounds and, although any form of extravasation can occur, it also is important to consider other surrounding viscera and major blood vessels.

Another form of vesical injury is iatrogenic following pelvic operations or endoscopic instrumentation.

A simple contusion is an injury to one or more layers of the vesical wall in which there is no demonstrable extravasation of urine. Extraperitoneal rupture usually occurs with fractures of the bony pelvis, and indicates a rupture of the bladder wall below the area covered by peritoneum. Intraperitoneal rupture most commonly follows trauma to the lower abdomen with the bladder distended. The dome of the bladder covered by peritoneum is the weakest, most unsupported area, and thus is prone to rupture with extravasation of urine intraperitoneally. A combination of intra- and extraperitoneal rupture may result from penetrating injuries.

RECOGNITION

With any injury to the lower abdomen, and certainly whenever there is a fracture of the bony pelvis, bladder injury should be suspected. Fractures of the bony pelvis result in a significant degree of hemorrhage, and the marked bleeding and hematoma formation with instability of blood pressure, etc., may obscure the diagnosis.

Classically, the patient has quite severe lower abdominal pain with tenderness to palpation, although pain is surprisingly minimal in some patients. Dullness to percussion may represent either hematoma formation or a distended bladder that cannot be evacuated. As will be discussed under injuries to the membranous urethra, injuries are possible to both structures, and injury to one does not preclude injury to the other. The presence of hematuria following injury to the lower abdomen should focus attention on the bladder, although potential injury to the lower ureter or, as in the case of diffuse abdominal injury, the kidney, should never be discounted.

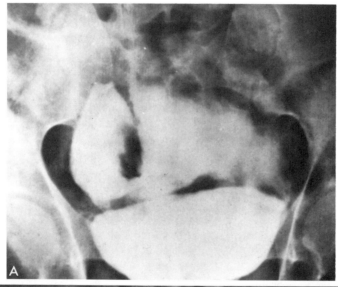

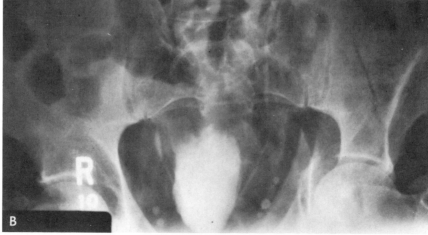

Figure 4. *A,* Intraperitoneal extravasation demonstrated on gravity cystogram. *B,* "Tear drop" bladder secondary to compression by perivesical hematoma.

Depending on the nature of the injury, diagnostic studies should be delayed only long enough to begin appropriate intravenous fluid and stabilization of blood pressure. Practically speaking, the patient should be moved immediately to an x-ray facility where a No. 18 Foley catheter is passed under aseptic conditions. If the catheter does not pass easily into the bladder, further attempts should be avoided and a retrograde urethrogram performed to evaluate possible injury to the membranous urethra. If the catheter is passed into the bladder and sanguinous urine is obtained, the bladder should be evacuated and approximately 150 ml. of contrast media instilled by gravity. Films are taken with the bladder distended in the AP and both oblique projections, and again after drainage of the contrast material to delineate possible extravasation obscured by the contrast-filled bladder. Based on the cystogram, one can usually determine whether there has been intra- or extraperitoneal rupture of the bladder (Figs. 3 and 4, A). However, in the case of an extensive pelvic hematoma, the bladder may be compressed into the so-called "tear drop" bladder with the hematoma sealing the bladder and preventing extravasation (Fig. 4, B). Prompt and properly performed cystourethrography should permit the proper diagnosis, and cystoscopic examination is rarely, if ever, warranted. Diagnosis by instilling a measured volume of fluid into the bladder, and then determining the volume drained, is misleading, and there is no longer any reason for this unscientific and error-prone method of investigation.

In extensive abdominal injuries, intravenous urography may be necessary to rule out possible injury of the kidney and/or ureter. In a well-coordinated x-ray department, a cystourethrogram and intravenous urogram can be performed quite rapidly without danger to the patient.

TREATMENT

Basic teaching must be that rupture of the bladder with extravasation of urine demands immediate operation. With newer antibiotics, minor extraperitoneal rupture of the bladder has been treated simply by urethral catheter drainage. However, this increases the danger of pelvic accumulations, and, for safety's sake, vesical exploration should be performed in all intraperitoneal ruptures as soon as the condition of the patient allows. Operative therapy includes the following stages.

(1) Thorough drainage of the perivesical space with evacuation of extravasated urine.

(2) Suprapubic cystostomy with at least a No. 32 de Pezzer catheter.

(3) Wherever possible, the rent in the bladder is closed and hemostasis obtained.

(4) In the presence of an intraperitoneal rupture, the peritoneal cavity is inspected and extravasated urine evacuated.

(5) The ureteral orifices should be observed; this procedure is enhanced by the intravenous administration of methylene blue. If the injury is in the area of the ureteral orifices, the surgeon must satisfy himself as to their patency before terminating the operation.

SEQUELAE

Complications following injury and rupture of the urinary bladder most often are due to delay in definitive diagnosis and operative therapy. Potential sequelae include: (1) Perivesical abscess and systemic sepsis; (2) rare obstruction of the vesical neck from perivesical hematoma or cicatrix formation; (3) occasional osteomyelitis of the pelvis; (4) vesical calculus formation secondary to prolonged catheter drainage; and (5) persistent vesicocutaneous fistula.

INJURIES OF THE MEMBRANOUS URETHRA

INTRODUCTION

Inasmuch as injuries to this structure may have serious complications, including impassable urethral stricture, urinary incontinence, or impotence, they represent the greatest potential morbidity of all injuries of the genitourinary tract. Although the membranous urethra itself is rarely injured except by urethral instrumentation, in the male complete or partial tear at its junction with the prostate gland is not uncommon. This most frequently occurs following automobile accidents in which the somewhat distended bladder and attached prostate gland are sheared from the membranous urethra, which is fixed by its attachments to the pelvic bones. This type of injury is associated most commonly with multiple pelvic fractures, and usually is a complete, not partial, tear.

RECOGNITION

A high index of suspicion is necessary in an individual with a fracture of the pubic rami who has hematuria or any difficulty in voiding. This injury occurs above the urogenital diaphragm, so that all bleeding and/or urinary extravasation occurs within the pelvis, and very little abnormality may be found on examination of the perineum and genitalia (Fig. 5). Pain in the suprapubic area, with tenderness to palpation and dullness to percussion, as found in vesical rupture, are quite common. Rectal examination may reveal the prostate gland to be high-riding or, as is quite frequent, a large pelvic hematoma may be palpable. Quite frequently during rectal palpation one may encounter fragments of the fractured pelvis.

When an avulsion injury of the posterior urethra is suspected, a retrograde urethrogram is preferable to the passage of a urethral catheter. Injudicious use of the catheter may convert a partial tear into a complete one, and render reconstitution of the urinary tract more difficult. In this type of injury, as contrast material is injected aseptically per urethra, extravasation into the pelvis is obvious when the contrast media are mixed with the perivesical blood. In a complete tear, no contrast material enters the urinary bladder; in a partial tear, one may see extravasation as well as contrast in the bladder. An intravenous urogram should demonstrate the high-riding bladder filled with contrast material without any extravasation, inasmuch as the sphincteric mechanism of the posterior urethra is operational.

TREATMENT

At the present time, treatment of this type of injury is undergoing critical reevaluation. In the past, therapy of choice was suprapubic exploration, drainage of the perivesical space, insertion of a cystostomy tube, and passage of a urethral catheter per meatus, which was then advanced and manipulated until it entered the bladder. Light traction was maintained on the Foley catheter to approximate the severed urethra, and the catheter was maintained for at least three weeks.

This type of operation, with blind approximation of the membranous urethra, involves a great deal of morbidity owing to urethral stricture formation, and is not now considered advisable.

Urologists seem to be split into two major camps. The first advises exploration with evacuation of the hematoma and direct suture approximation, or simple repositioning of the prostatic to membranous urethra. Subsequent stricture formation, if it develops, can be cared for at a later date. The second, more conservative view advocates immediate simple cystostomy without exploration of the retropubic space or evacuation of the pelvic hematoma. Within three to four months, the prostate gland rides low in the pelvis and closely approximates the area of the membranous urethra, and the very short fibrous tissue stricture responds well to urethroplasty. This technique avoids any urethral instrumentation, which may convert a partial tear into a complete one.

SEQUELAE

Following all types of repair, a membranous urethral stricture is most common, often requiring secondary urethroplasty. A significant degree of incontinence has been encountered, although recent reports following cystostomy with delayed elective urethroplasty indicate a much decreased incidence. It must be recognized that injury to the pelvic nerves may result in the significant sequela of impotence. Besides these later complications, postoperative pelvic infection and abscess formation are a distinct possibility that may be prevented by not opening the perivesical hematoma. Occasional cases of osteomyelitis may develop.

INJURIES OF THE DISTAL OR ANTERIOR URETHRA

Introduction

The urethra can be considered to be divided into the posterior urethra, which includes the prostatic and membranous portions, and the anterior urethra, which includes the bulbous and pendulous segments. Injuries can occur secondary to in-

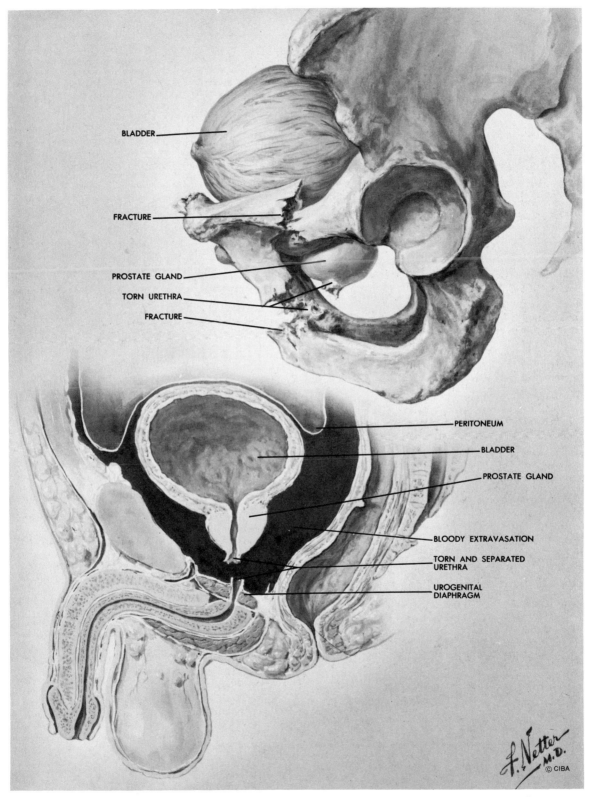

BLADDER

FRACTURE

PROSTATE GLAND

TORN URETHRA

FRACTURE

PERITONEUM

BLADDER

PROSTATE GLAND

BLOODY EXTRAVASATION

TORN AND SEPARATED URETHRA

UROGENITAL DIAPHRAGM

Figure 5. Disruption of membranous urethra with extensive perivesical hematoma. (© 1954, Ciba Pharmaceutical Company Division of Ciba-Geigy Corp. Reproduced with permission from the Ciba Collection of Medical Illustrations by Frank H. Netter, M.D.)

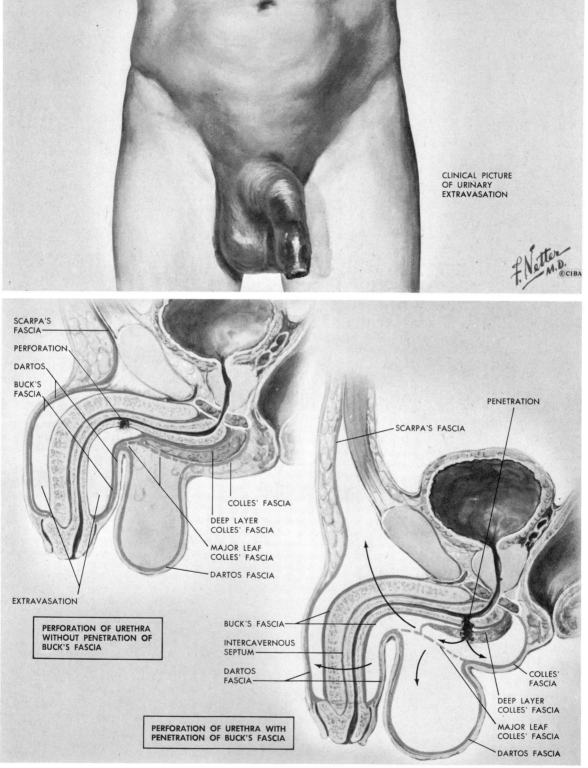

Figure 6. Pathways of urinary extravasation following injury of the urethra below the urogenital diaphragm. (© 1954, 1965 Ciba Pharmaceutical Company, Division of Ciba-Geigy Corp. Reproduced with permission from the Ciba Collection of Medical Illustrations by Frank H. Netter, M.D.)

strumentation, either by the physician or through the introduction of foreign bodies into the urethra by the patient himself. Injuries to the anterior urethra usually are a result of being struck in the perineum, and often are referred to as a "straddle" injury. With rupture of the urethra and extravasation of urine and blood through Buck's fascia, progressive extravasation may occur into the scrotum, into the perineum back to the central tendon, and even up the anterior abdominal wall under Scarpa's fascia (Fig. 6). This is in direct contrast to injuries to the posterior urethra, which result in pelvic extravasation and hemorrhage.

RECOGNITION

Following the injury, which usually can be pinpointed by a check on the patient's history, there is swelling and tenderness in the perineum, the degree depending on the extent of injury: for example, there may be only a urethral contusion without rupture, or frank rupture of the urethra itself with extravasation. The classic finding is dripping of blood from the urethral meatus. Inasmuch as the injury is distal to the urethral sphincter, there may be a constant ooze of blood, not only the hematuria seen with bladder and posterior urethral injuries. If recognition has been delayed, extensive perineal and scrotal swelling secondary to extravasation may occur.

Confirmatory diagnosis rests on the retrograde urethrogram, which in the case of frank rupture will demonstrate extravasation of contrast material (Fig. 7).

TREATMENT

Spontaneous voiding is to be avoided until the extent of injury has been determined. If there is no evidence of extravasation and only minimal perineal ecchymosis or induration, a urethral catheter can be passed and maintained for three to four days. If there is evidence of considerable extravasation or perineal hematoma, after passage of the urethral catheter, exploration of the injured urethra is warranted. The extravasated urine and hematoma are evacuated, the area debrided, and the incision either closed with a drain in place or packed loosely open. Following complete healing of the perineum, the urethral catheter usually may be

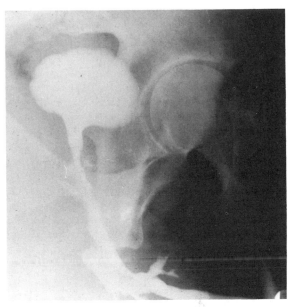

Figure 7. Retrograde urethrogram demonstrating extravasation from the bulbous urethra.

removed by the eighth to tenth postoperative day. If there has been extensive urethral injury, suprapubic cystostomy and perineal drainage may be necessary. On the rare occasion when a urethral catheter cannot be passed, suprapubic cystostomy should be performed and the urethra exposed perineally. At this time, only drainage may be carried out, but if there has been complete disruption of the urethra, reanastomosis occasionally may be performed. Again depending on the degree of injury, a urethral catheter may or may not be used as a stent. Whenever suprapubic cystostomy is indicated, the catheter should not be removed postoperatively until normal voiding occurs following clamping of the catheter, or preferably not until a voiding cystourethrogram demonstrates absence of extravasation and obstruction.

COMPLICATIONS

Complications of injuries to the anterior urethra include: (1) Perineal phlegmon with possible extensive loss of tissue and skin; (2) urinary tract infection secondary to the indwelling catheter; (3) localized urethritis secondary to the indwelling catheter; and (4) urethral stricture secondary to No. 3, the injury itself, or periurethral extravasation. Urethral stricture formation may be avoided somewhat by earlier drainage of the perineum, preventing periurethral fibrosis, and judicious use of nonreactive urethral catheters. Resulting strictures can be treated by the conservative methods of urethral dilatation or internal urethrotomy; a refractory stricture may warrant definitive urethroplasty in the future.

INJURIES OF THE GENITALIA

Introduction

Injuries of the scrotal and penile skin should be treated in the same manner as cutaneous injuries elsewhere in the body. A particularly common injury results from penile skin being caught in a zipper. Under local anesthesia, the zipper can be removed and the skin sutured primarily.

ANTERIOR URETHRA

Because the urethra traverses the penis, all the information imparted in the previous section may pertain if the anterior pendulous urethra is injured. Strangulation of the penis due to either rubber bands, rings, or clamps should be treated very conservatively. Following removal of the cause, amputation should never be performed initially, even if the penis appears frankly gangrenous. The vascularity of this organ is truly amazing, and what appears initially to be gangrenous may become revitalized. At a later date, when the area of devitalized tissue is well demarcated, débridement or even partial amputation may be indicated. At this time a longer segment of penis usually will be salvagable than would have been the situation if immediate amputation had been carried out. After severe injuries to the penis with involvement of the urethra, urinary diversion may be indicated, either by suprapubic cystostomy or by perineal urethrostomy.

Occasionally, blunt trauma to the penis results in a rupture of Buck's fascia with considerable bleeding. Although this usually responds to conservative treatment, exploration and hemostasis sometimes may be warranted.

On rare occasions a patient has attempted emasculation with complete transection of the penis. Although in the past this has been treated as for an amputation for carcinoma, with diversion of urine by way of a perineal urethrostomy and hemostasis of the penile stump, the imagination of some urologists has been stimulated. In recent years there have been reports of reanastomosis of the severed penis, but we believe that success will continue to be very limited.

Human bites of the penis often are not admitted by the patient, but if these are not treated with irrigation, débridement, and antibiotics, a severe and rapidly progressing cellulitis may develop.

AVULSION OF THE SKIN OF THE PENIS AND SCROTUM

Loss of skin from the penis and/or scrotum is an uncommon but urgent situation resulting from numerous causes. In this mechanized age, one of the most common causes of such denudation is the "power take-off injury." The moving elements of factory or farm machinery engage a trouser leg and twist upward to the genital area. Here the thin, elastic, redundant skin of the penis and scrotum is grasped and avulsed, often in one piece. The skin of the penis usually tears loose just behind the coronal sulcus, and the glans is thus spared any injury (Fig. 8). This type of injury rarely involves the corpora or the spermatic cord as the overlying skin is loosely attached. The plane of cleavage in the scrotum usually is along the dartos fascia superficial to the cremasteric muscle. The cremasteric reflex may be the reason for testicular sparing.

Complete denudation of the skin of the penis and the scrotum creates an acute emergency in which resurfacing should not be delayed. Repair of the denuded penis may be performed utilizing pedicle flaps from the scrotum to cover partial defects, or scrotal skin also may be utilized by burying the denuded penis in a subcutaneous scrotal tunnel, and freeing it at the time of a second operation. The remaining scrotal skin almost always is adequate for covering the testes and, if available, also should be utilized to resurface the penis, as already stated. The elasticity and great viability of scrotal tissues should always be borne in mind. In the absence of adequate scrotal skin to resurface the penis, a split thickness skin graft (Fig. 8, B) from either the inner aspect of the thigh or the lower abdomen may be utilized. In the absence of satisfactory amounts of scrotal

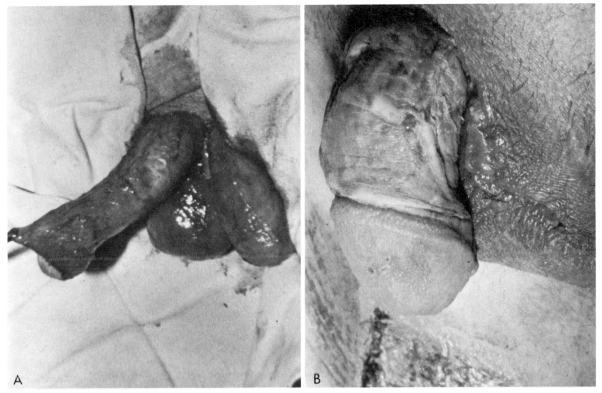

Figure 8. A, Avulsion of the skin of the penis and scrotum. B, Resurfacing of the penis by a split thickness skin graft.

skin to cover the testes, the latter may be buried in the superficial tissues of the thigh just under the skin, where the temperature is similar to that of the normal scrotum, or the testis and spermatic cord may be covered by a split thickness skin graft.

INJURY OF THE TESTICLE

Direct injury to the testicle itself is rather unusual, thanks to the active cremasteric reflex that causes retraction of the testicle when danger threatens. Most injuries of the testicle are nonpenetrating, and conservative therapy including bed rest, local ice compresses, and elevation of the scrotum has been advocated in the past.

However, it is now recognized that, when the tunica albuginea is ruptured, extensive bleeding may occur with replacement of the seminiferous tubules by hematoma. When there is progressive scrotal distention in these cases, surgical intervention is warranted, with drainage of the blood from the scrotum and early repair of the rup-

tured tunica. It has been amply demonstrated that, if early drainage and repair are not carried out, atrophy of the testicle occurs in a significant number of cases. Even minor trauma to the male genitalia may focus attention on an abnormal testicle previously asymptomatic: for example, neoplasms may be unmasked by minimal testicular trauma.

FOREIGN BODIES

Most frequently, foreign bodies are self-inserted into the urethra. In some instances they migrate into the bladder and require cystoscopic or operative removal. If the end of the object is visible, removal can be accomplished with the use of a fine hemostat and lubricant. If foreign bodies cannot be visualized, they may be passed spontaneously during voiding or may require operative extraction. Care must be taken not to injure the urethra by attempts at extraction. The trauma arising from an unsuccessful extraction attempt can result in added difficulty as a result of edema.

J. OCULAR TRAUMA

John Purcell and George L. Spaeth

RECOGNITION AND MANAGEMENT

BLUNT TRAUMA

Blunt trauma to the eye and its adnexa can cause extensive ocular damage that may not be evident on casual examination.

(a) Periorbital edema and *ecchymosis* (the "black eye"): Edema and ecchymosis are the result of damage to blood vessels about the orbit. They extend across the bridge of the nose to involve the nontraumatized eye. The ethmoid sinus may be ruptured, allowing air to enter the orbital tissues with consequent crepitus; this may become worse when the nose is blown.

(b) Blow-out fracture of the orbit (Figure 1): When an object, often larger than the orbital rim inlet (fist, ball, rock), strikes the eye, the eye and the orbital tissues are compressed. This increased intraorbital pressure may blow-out the weakest point of the orbit, which is usually the floor. Fat, fascia and the inferior oblique and inferior rectus muscles prolapse into this fracture site, and may occasionally be trapped. Diplopia on upward or downward gaze (usually up) owing to limitation of the motion of the eye from incarcerated tissues may occur. Damage to the infraorbital nerve causes anesthesia or hypesthesia of skin over the medial one-third

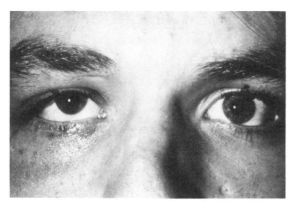

Figure 1. A fracture of the orbital floor ("blow-out fracture") may be present in the absence of obvious signs of trauma. Limitation of eye movement can be a valuable sign, as it is here, where there is limitation of upward gaze in the left eye due to trapping of the inferior oblique muscle.

of the lower lid, extending onto the maxilla, and "numb" upper teeth on the alveolar ridge beneath this area. Crepitus may be palpable along the orbital rims or within the orbit from communication with the maxillary sinus air or ethmoid.

When a blow-out fracture is suspected, the patient should promptly have a thorough eye evaluation and an x-ray examination of the orbit. Treatment may be cold compresses for 24 hours followed by warm compresses, a broad spectrum oral antibiotic, and a warning not to blow the nose lest air be forced from the sinus into the orbit. Referral to an ophthalmologist for a complete evaluation and any necessary treatment within the next few days should always be made. During this period the visual acuity should be carefully and repeatedly monitored. Orbital swelling following trauma can cause delayed loss of vision due to ischemia or direct compression of the optic nerve. Should such occur treatment must immediately be given to correct the situation or permanent loss of vision may result.

In most instances of blow-out fracture surgical repair is *not* required or advisable. Diplopia can be transient. Improper surgery, on the other hand, has caused unnecessary loss of vision.

(c) Hyphema (settled blood in the anterior chamber, Figure 2): Bleeding from the iris blood vessels, which may result from any type of trauma, is the most frequent cause for hyphema. The patient may have serious associated signs, such as somnolence and vomiting; in such cases a severe glaucoma usually is present. On the other hand, the patient may be almost asymptomatic, except for blurred vision, even when the hyphema is extensive. Hyphemas are ocular emergencies. They are a certain sign that the eye has received a severe blow and that its health is in jeopardy. No drops, manipulation, or further ocular examination should be performed. A shield should be placed over the eye and the patient immediately placed under an ophthalmologist's care. The patient's head should be kept in an upright position to prevent the blood from occluding the entire angle recess, which could occur in

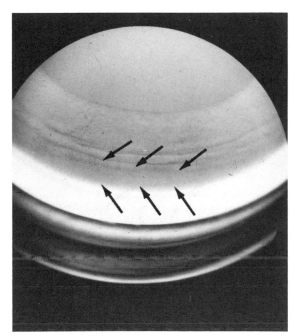

Figure 2. Hyphema may be easily visible following direct trauma to the globe. In other cases it can be detected only by slit lamp examination or gonioscopy, as illustrated here.

placed into the anterior chamber the lens may cause an acute rise of the intraocular pressure, with consequent cloudy cornea, blurred vision, and pain. This is an ocular emergency. An ophthalmologist should be consulted, who may attempt to reposit the lens by placing the patient in a supine position and dilating the pupil.

If a lens dislocates posteriorly into the vitreous the chief symptom is blurred vision. A "shadow" may float across the field of vision. This is a less emergent situation, but referral to an ophthalmologist should be made. In most instances the lens dislocates only partially, remaining close to its normal position but slipping anteriorly, causing the anterior chamber to become shallower. This may induce a secondary angle-closure glaucoma, which is a true medical emergency; the pressure in the eye may exceed the retinal arterial pressure and so cause rapid and permanent blindness. Prompt lowering of the intraocular pressure is mandatory. This is best accomplished by administration of intravenous acetazolamide (500 mg. per 70 kg. of body weight) or oral glycerol (1 cc. per kg. body weight), or both. Commercially available preparations of glycerol are more palatable than the plain product. Acetazolamide has a sulfa base and therefore the patient should be questioned regarding allergy prior to its use. If vitreous is trapped in the pupil, pupillary-block glaucoma may lead to a secondary angle-closure glaucoma. Treatment, again, is acetazolamide or glycerol. Miotics (pilocarpine) usually should not be used as they increase the degree of pupillary block. Prompt referral to an ophthalmologist is proper.

Dislocation of the lens may not be easily seen. Tremulousness of the iris or, more definitely, tremulousness of the lens should be looked for with the slit lamp. Uneven shallowing of the anterior chamber is another clue.

(f) Rupture of the globe: Blunt trauma can rupture the globe with surprising ease. As the scar is often hidden under the conjunctiva, the correct diagnosis will occasionally be missed unless the possibility of scleral rupture is specifically eliminated. Vision is usually markedly reduced and the eye is soft.

In questionable cases surgical exploration usually should be carried out. The patient should be given antibiotic drops, tetanus toxoid, systemic antibiotics, a protective

the supine position. If an ophthalmologist is not immediately available, the patient's eyes should be patched and after sedation (the purpose of which is to decrease rapid movement of the eyes) the patient should be kept in a darkened room. Aspirin should not be given because of its effects upon platelet function. The question of whether to use myotics or mydriatics is one best left for the ophthalmologist.

(d) Traumatic iridocyclitis: Iritis, manifested as an outpouring of inflammatory cells and exudate into the anterior chamber, is usually present following blunt trauma. The patient's eye is red (predominantly over the ciliary body), and the pupil miotic. Photophobia and pain are the chief complaints; their intensity varies with the degree of intraocular inflammations. Treatment, often cycloplegic and corticosteroid drops, should usually be managed by an ophthalmologist. Corticosteroids must be used with special caution as such eyes are predisposed to steroid-induced glaucoma.

(e) Dislocation of the lens: The most common cause for lens dislocation is trauma. Dislocation may be partial or complete (Figure 3). When partially or completely dis-

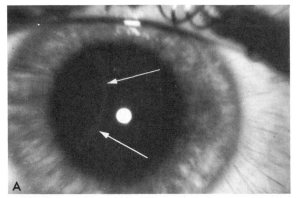

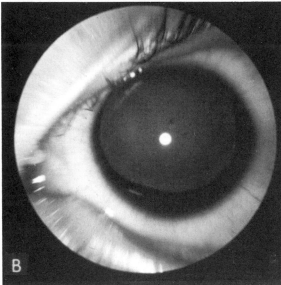

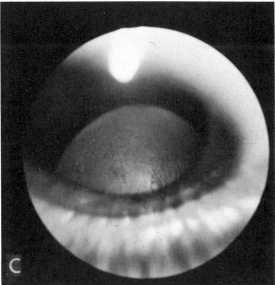

Figure 3. Partial or complete dislocation of the lens is most readily noted when the pupil is dilated (*A*). When the lens is only minimally dislocated, diagnosis is difficult; the most reliable sign is tremulousness of the lens itself. Usually a sign of trauma, it may also be seen in localized ocular or more generalized systemic disease, such as aniridia (*B*) and homocystinuria (*C*).

eye shield and be instructed not to eat or drink anything before the necessary surgical repair.

(*g*) *Contusion injuries:* At the time of the initial examination the pupil should be dilated (see Table 2 for contraindications) and the fundus examined. Hemorrhages of the retina or vitreous warn of possible retinal tears and demand further evaluation. A peculiar white sheen due to edema of Henle's fiber layer in the retina is known as "commotio retinae." In the macular region this may lead to permanent damage to vision. There is no specific treatment.

All patients with blunt trauma to the eye should have a fundus examination by an ophthalmologist, although this need not be performed immediately, especially in cases where the ocular media are not clear. It usually should take place within three to four days.

LACERATING INJURIES

(*a*) Lids:

Superficial lacerations of the skin, lids, and brow that do not involve the lid margins, the lacrimal apparatus, or the deep tissues may be closed primarily with interrupted 6–0 silk or synthetic sutures by the emergency physician.

Avulsions of the lid (Figure 4), lacerations of the lid margins, and lacerations involving the canalicular apparatus need to be repaired by one familiar with the specialized structures involved. Improper approximation of the lid margins will cause notching that is unsightly and may result in exposure of the eye. Improperly repaired canalicular lacerations may result in excessive tearing, with maceration of the skin and blurring of

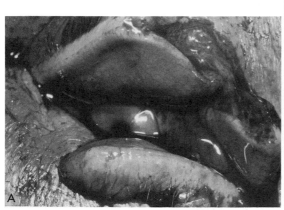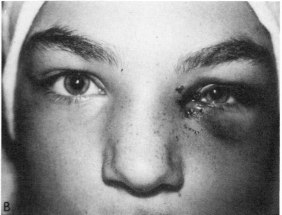

Figure 4. Trauma to the lid causing a tear of the lid margin (A) or involving the canaliculus (B) needs special surgical repair.

vision. The canaliculi should not be probed.

(*b*) Conjunctival lacerations smaller than 1 cm. may be left open; larger ones should be sutured with an absorbable suture (such as 7–0 gut) *after determining that there is no underlying ocular damage.*

(*c*) Lacerations to the cornea and sclera are ocular emergencies. A topical antibiotic drop should be instilled, systemic antibiotics started (see Appendix), the lid covered with a shield and light patch, tetanus toxoid given, and the patient prepared for surgery under general anesthesia.

(*d*) Intraocular foreign bodies: Any injury to the eye should raise the suspicion of an intraocular foreign body. This may enter the eye without clinically apparent external ocular damage, although usually fluorescein stain will demonstrate a point of entry. Specialized radiologic examination of the eye should be performed where such a possibility arises, and is highly sensitive in indicating the presence of a radiopaque foreign body (Figure 5). Metal (especially copper) is toxic to the eye and needs to be removed. Cases with intraocular foreign bodies should be managed in a fashion similar to that prescribed for cases with a ruptured globe. Removal may be difficult, especially if the object is nonmagnetic, and the prognosis should be considered guarded at best. Referral to an ophthalmic center is necessary.

CHEMICAL OR THERMAL TRAUMA

(*a*) Alkali and acid burns are true emergencies that require the *highest priori-*ty. Alkaline materials are potentially more disastrous than acid because of rapid penetration of the material into the cornea. The nature and concentration of the agent, and the time in contact with the eye all influence the extent of the permanent injury.

Irrigation of the eyes should, of course, be done as soon as possible. Never should treatment await arrival at the Emergency Department. Water, or where this is not immediately available, beer, urine, or any other reasonably safe fluid should be used. On arrival in the Emergency Department the usual routine should be abandoned and the patient's eyes irrigated *as soon as possible.* Any source of water may be used. It is helpful to have a reservoir of 1000 cc. of normal saline with I.V. tubing attached for prompt use. The eyes should be opened manually, using a lid speculum, topical anesthetic (proparacaine, tetracaine) applied, and irrigation with at least 2000 cc. normal saline for each affected eye performed. Particulate matter should be removed with cotton-tipped applicators or forceps. Systemic analgesia may be needed.

The extent of injury can be gauged by the opaqueness of the cornea and the blanched or white appearance of the conjunctiva. Severity increases as these are more pronounced. An ophthalmologist should be consulted promptly to continue treatment and decide whether hospitalization is necessary.

(*b*) The chief sources of ultraviolet radiation injuries are "sun lamps," welding arcs, and carbon arcs. There is generally an interval period of six to 12 hours before the onset of symptoms, which begin with irritation

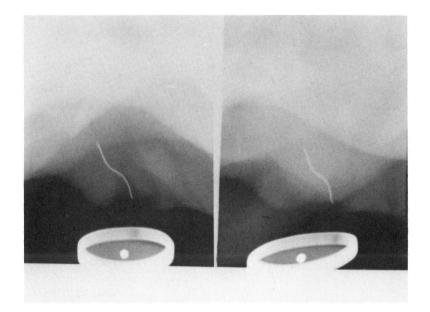

Figure 5. A history suggesting possible intraocular foreign body or the observation of a penetrating injury usually indicates the need for radiologic studies designed to demonstrate radiopaque intraocular foreign bodies such as that seen here.

and redness and continue on to severe photophobia and blepharospasm. The ultraviolet rays cause an irritation of the superficial corneal epithelium which can be detected by applying fluorescein topically and observing this with a blue light; involved areas will stain green. Diffuse involvement with punctate staining often will be noted.

These patients are very uncomfortable, but have a brief, self-limiting eye injury that may be safely handled by the emergency physician. A topical anesthetic (proparacaine) affords immediate relief and facilitates examination. The pupils are then dilated with tropicamide (Mydriacil) 1 per cent. This short-acting cycloplegic will relieve the pain of reflex ciliary spasm. Both eyes may be patched with semipressure dressings, and the patient instructed to see an ophthalmologist in 24 hours if still uncomfortable. Systemic analgesics may be prescribed.

The patient should *not* be given continued topical anesthetic drops for relief of pain as this may lead to retarded epithelial healing and serious ocular damage.

CORNEAL ABRASIONS AND CORNEAL FOREIGN BODIES

Corneal abrasions occur from many sources. The patients usually experience pain, photophobia, injection, and tearing. Topically applied fluorescein (after topical anesthetic to facilitate the examination) delineates the area of abraded corneal epithe-

lium. These patients may be helped by short-acting cycloplegics (tropicamide 1 per cent or cyclopentolate 1 per cent), which give relief from the ciliary spasm and iritis that usually accompany these injuries. Such mydriasis is not always needed or desirable. Stronger agents such as atropine and scopolamine usually are not employed. A topical antibiotic drop may be applied. If the injury is severe or deep, a pressure dressing should be applied to the involved eye and the patient instructed to see an ophthalmologist within 24 hours. A frequent occurrence is bilateral corneal abrasions resulting from prolonged wearing of hard contact lenses. The lenses should not be used again until healing is complete.

Corneal foreign bodies are such a frequent occurrence that the physician in the Emergency Department should be thoroughly familiar with them. These occur from hammering, grinding, working under cars, motorcycling without goggles, and from any source conceivable. The important considerations are: (1) to make sure that there is no intraocular penetration of a foreign body, (2) to be sure there is not more than one foreign body, and (3) to make certain that the treatment is not worse than the illness. After topical anesthetic drops are applied the patient should have a thorough search for other debris in both cul-de-sacs. If any are present these should be carefully removed with cotton-tipped applicators or forceps.

Foreign bodies actually embedded in the cornea are removed at the slit lamp with a "spud," an 18-gauge needle or jeweler's forceps. First the depth of the injury should be established; if superficial, the foreign body may be removed safely by lifting it off with one of these instruments. If deep within the stroma, the patient is probably best referred to an ophthalmologist. Rust surrounding the foreign body should be removed as completely as possible at the initial treatment. The patient may benefit from a short-acting cycloplegic (tropicamide 1 per cent), and antibiotic drops should be instilled every four hours. A patch is generally not necessary. The patient should be instructed that the foreign body sensation will return after the anesthetic wears off and will persist for 12 to 24 hours. If there is any doubt as to the full extent of a foreign body injury consultation should be obtained.

CONJUNCTIVAL FOREIGN BODIES

Foreign bodies lying on the surface of the conjunctiva are usually best removed without prior administration of anesthetic drops. Such is true even when on the undersurface of the lid. In such cases removal of the object should be associated with almost immediate disappearance of symptoms.*

---

*Thanks are given to Doctor W. Annesley and the Retina Service, Doctor G. Shannon and the Oculoplastic Service and Doctor P. Laibson and the Cornea Service of Wills Eye Hospital, who supplied many of the photographs illustrating Chapters 38 and 51.

References

Asch, M. J., et al.: Ocular complications associated with burns: review of a five-year experience including 104 patients. J. Trauma 11:857, 1971.

Blecker, G., and Keith, L.: Fractures of the Orbit. Baltimore, The William & Wilkins Co., 1970.

Edwards, W. C., and Layden, W. E.: Monocular versus binocular patching in traumatic hyphema. Am. J. Ophthal. 76:359, 1973.

Ferguson, C.: Deep, wooden foreign bodies of the orbit. Trans. Am. Acad. Ophthal. Otolaryngol. 74:778, 1970.

Frueh, B.: Transient blindness following blunt trauma to the eye. Am. J. Ophthal. 71:1034, 1971.

Goldman, R. J., and Hessbury, P. C.: Appraisal of surgical correction in 130 cases of orbital floor fracture. Am. J. Ophthal. 76:152, 1973.

Griffith, J. D.: Transient blindness following seemingly trivial head injury in children. N. Engl. J. Med. 278:648, 1968.

Laibson, P., and Oconor, J.: Explosive tear gas injuries of the eye. Trans. Am. Acad. Ophthal. Otolaryngol. 74:811, 1970.

K. TRAUMA TO THE PERIPHERAL VASCULAR SYSTEM

Robert B. Rutherford

BACKGROUND AND PERSPECTIVE

The management of peripheral vascular injuries has greatly improved over the last two decades as advances in the definitive surgical approach to occlusive arterial disease in civilian practice have been applied to large numbers of vascular injuries incurred on the battlefields of Korea and South Vietnam.

The first crude vascular repair was performed over two centuries ago, and the basic suture techniques as we know them today, including even the use of autografts and homografts, were well worked out by the end of the first decade of this century, thanks mainly to the classic works of Carrell (1907) and Guthrie (1907). Therefore the stage was set for the application of these techniques to vascular injuries by the outbreak of World War I. Yet it was not until the Korean conflict was well under way over 40 years later that this came to pass. The development and use of high velocity missiles and high explosives during World War I, the treatment priorities imposed by mass casualty situations, and the inordinately long evacuation times from the embattled trench to the operating theater all combined to perpetuate a discouragingly high failure rate and to establish the attitude that there was no place for primary vascular repair in military medicine. Even under the more optimal conditions of civilian practice, treatment rarely went much beyond hemostasis, and not only was the injured artery usually ligated at the expense of its patency but so was the accompanying vein—whether injured or not. For inexplicable reasons, this attitude was perpetuated through World War II (DeBakey and Simeone, 1954), when direct repair was attempted in only slightly over 3 per cent of arterial injuries and end-to-end anastomoses were performed in only eight instances. The over-all amputation rate was 49 per cent.

The Korean conflict shared a period of very rapid advancement with cardiovascular surgery, when bold innovative approaches seemed commonplace. Rapid evacuation of casualties, ample blood replacement, antibiotics, improved vascular instruments, and a more stable fighting front with trained surgeons at forward (MASH) hospitals set the stage for the complete reversal of the previously conservative military attitude toward vascular injuries. Immediate repair was attempted in 88 per cent of arterial injuries. In these cases the amputation rate was only 13 per cent; of those in whom ligation of the injured vessel was carried out, 51 per cent suffered amputation.

The present-day approach to vascular injuries can be said to stem from this experience, although important refinements have been added by subsequent developments in civilian practice and in Vietnam. However, today's relatively optimistic outlook toward peripheral vascular injuries cannot be solely ascribed simply to adopting a policy of immediate operative repair. Rapid transportation, availability of blood and antibiotics, abandonment of mass tourniquet techniques, a better appreciation of the true nature of certain forms of arterial injury (particularly those due to high velocity and blunt trauma), the increased use of arteriography, the recognition of the importance of fracture stabilization, proper débridement of the traumatized arterial segment, liberal use of fasciotomy, repair of concomitant venous injuries, the success of saphenous vein grafts in bridging major vascular defects in the face of gross contamination and extensive tissue destruction, heparin anticoagulation, the introduction of Fogarty balloon catheters, and improved suture material and instruments—all have contributed greatly to the steady improvement in our results in the management of peripheral vascular injuries over the last two decades.

When we consider peripheral vascular injuries, the emphasis is naturally on arterial injuries. Peripheral venous injuries rarely present as an isolated clinical problem in the Emergency Department. An isolated venous injury, even to a major peripheral vein, usually will present as no more than a hematoma, although secondary thrombosis of the vein can and occasionally does occur, and can lead to all of the usual postphlebitic sequelae. Even beyond the Emergency Department, in the operating room the surgeon usually encounters venous injuries only in relation to injury to the adjacent artery. The best known consequence of concomitant venous injury is the formation of an arteriovenous fistula, but another important consequence, one that has been fully appreciated only recently, is the effect of venous occlusion, when the injured vein is not repaired, on blood flow through the repaired artery. In fact, acute deep venous occlusion may reduce arterial flow by as much as 33 to 50 per cent (Shires and Patman, 1966).

Nevertheless it is the arterial injury that attracts most attention, both in the Emergency Department and in the operating room. A wide spectrum of arterial injuries may be encountered, depending on the mechanism of the injury. Examples of these are shown in Figure 1. Penetrating wounds may take the form of a small puncture, a lateral or through-and-through knife wound, or a low velocity bullet hole. An artery will be cleanly destroyed if directly hit by a high velocity bullet, but even on a near miss it may be literally torn apart by the explosive energy released in the temporary cavity that develops in the bullet's wake.* Blunt trauma may result in contusion and segmental spasm of the artery, but more commonly it will cause segmental thrombosis because of intramural hematomas, flaplike intimal tears, or circumferential intimal disruption. Furthermore, even though for the purposes of this discussion arterial injuries are considered as a separate entity, they are rarely an isolated consideration clinically. Associated injuries to the accompanying veins and nerves, concomitant fractures or dislocations, varying degrees of muscle or other soft tissue destruction, and contamination of the wound with bacteria and foreign material frequently compound the problem.

---

*See also Evaluation of Trauma, p. 599.

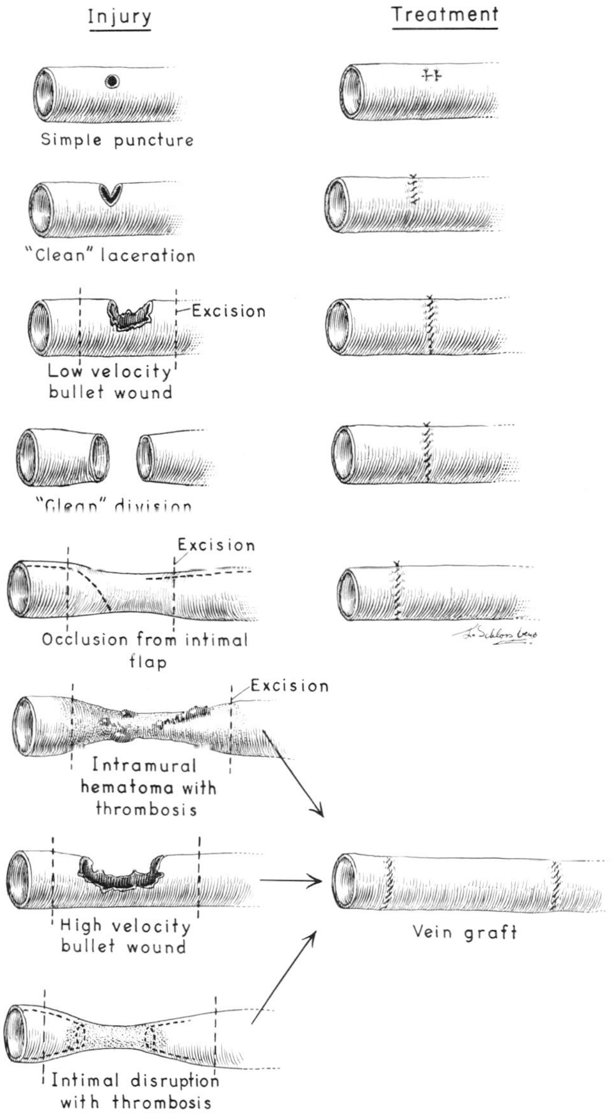

Injury   Treatment

Figure 1. Common forms of arterial injury with the likely method of repair. (From Ballinger, W. F., et al.: The Management of Trauma, 2nd ed. Philadelphia, W. B. Saunders Co., 1973.)

Simple puncture

"Clean" laceration

Low velocity bullet wound — Excision

"Clean" division

Occlusion from intimal flap — Excision

Intramural hematoma with thrombosis — Excision

High velocity bullet wound

Vein graft

Intimal disruption with thrombosis

Besides the nature of the arterial injury itself, other factors that play a role in the degree of arterial insufficiency produced are the level or site of injury, the collateral circulation, and, occasionally, in the older patients seen in civilian practice, underlying chronic occlusive arterial disease. A good example of the importance of the location of the injury and the collateral circulation is the popliteal artery, which not infrequently is injured by displaced fractures above or below the knee joint or by dislocation of the joint itself, in addition to penetrating trauma. The popliteal artery is the only major artery traversing the midsection of the lower extremity, unlike the superficial and deep femoral arteries above and the three main infrapopliteal branches below. Most of its geniculate collaterals leave it over a relatively short distance, so that they are often also occluded, either directly by the initial trauma or secondarily by segmental thrombosis of the main artery. The high amputation rate associated with ligation of an injured popliteal artery was first documented in World War I, when it was reported by Makins (1919) to be 60 per cent. Even today popliteal artery injury carries an amputation rate of approximately 30 per cent, almost twice that of the next most serious site of peripheral arterial injury, the common femoral. Of course, higher amputation rates are to be expected as a natural consequence of an acute traumatic occlusion than with the acute thrombotic occlusion of an already arteriosclerotic artery, in which the the gradual narrowing of the artery prior to occlusion provided both the stimulus and time for the development of collateral channels.

RECOGNITION

The key to successful management of acute arterial injuries in the Emergency Department is prompt and accurate diagnosis. The possibility of an arterial injury should be entertained whenever a penetrating wound is found along the course of a major vessel, particularly if there is excessive bleeding from the wound or a rapidly expanding hematoma. However, if the artery has been completely severed and its ends have contracted and become occluded by thrombus, the wound itself may not arouse suspicion. Nonpenetrating injuries are a less obvious and therefore more treacherous cause of arterial injury. In particular, the existence of a displaced fracture, a dislocation, or extensive soft tissue damage should arouse suspicion of concomitant arterial injury. Thus, a high index of suspicion is essential when examining injured extremities. This is particularly true of patients with multiple injuries or those who are unconscious. The unconscious patient or the patient whose other injuries are causing a great deal of pain or distress may not call attention to the extremity even when there has been a traumatic arterial occlusion.

The physician in the Emergency Department should check peripheral pulses on all extremities as a *routine* in evaluating trauma victims, not just those with obvious extremity wounds and skeletal injuries. Examination of the extremity distal to a wound or fracture usually will indicate an arterial injury by the absence of pulses and by changes in temperature and color. The five P's of acute arterial occlusion—pain, pulselessness, pallor, paralysis, and parasthesias—are featured in most medical school texts and lectures. Unfortunately, a diagnosis of an arterial injury by physical examination is not always that easy. Even something as seemingly objective as the presence or absence of peripheral pulses may be misleading. For example, in 271 documented arterial injuries reported by Shires et al. (1966) from Parkland Memorial Hospital, distal pulses were present on admission to the hos-

pital in 25 per cent, and in 15 per cent these pulsations were considered to be normal in amplitude. In a later review from the same institution, normal pulses on admission were recorded in approximately 10 per cent of arterial injuries. Therefore, it must be realized that in approximately 10 to 15 per cent of significant arterial injuries, distal pulses may initially be normal to palpation.

Confusion may result when examining extremities in the presence of shock. Shock may not only mask or mimic the classic signs of arterial insufficiency, but, in association with minor or subclinical degrees of arteriosclerosis, may lead to confusing differences between compared extremities. Conversely, it may be difficult to decide, in older patients, if absent peripheral pulses are due to injury or to pre-existing disease. A history of claudication or the presence of trophic skin changes (absent hair growth, thickened nails, shiny, atrophic skin, and loss of subcutaneous fat) should be sought to clarify this situation. It is also important to examine the injured extremity serially for the disappearing pulses that signal delayed occlusion, the pulsating hematoma of a false aneurysm, or the bruit of an arteriovenous fistula. It is not uncommon, particularly in blunt trauma, for there to be intramural hematomas or an intimal tear. These do not immediately cause occlusion but, because of associated vasospasm or subintimal dissection, eventually will lead to thrombosis.

Capillary filling should be noted, not only as an aid to diagnosis but as one index of viability. However, *one common mistake is that the viability of the limb—and therefore the degree of urgency for repair—is estimated entirely upon the apparent viability of the skin, without realizing that the viability of ischemic nerves and muscles is much more limited than that of skin.* The work of Milan and Tattoni (1963) showed that myelin degeneration and axon retraction began in nerves as early as four to six hours after the onset of ischemia and that discoid degeneration with progressive loss of contractility affected up to 90 per cent of muscle fibers by 12 hours. Once this change has occurred, only partial recovery is possible. Thus, failure to recognize that the skin is not the best gauge of viability may lead to serious leg disability from nerve deficits or ischemic muscle contractures.

The extremity should be carefully tested for sensory and motor function. Major areas of complete anesthesia or obvious digital paralysis or footdrop should be considered *late* signs of ischemia. It is particularly important to examine carefully those patients who complain of persistent pain in the distal forefoot or toes or who feel weakness, numbness, or tingling in their feet. For unknown reasons, the earliest signs of ischemic neuropathy usually appear in the distribution of the peroneal nerve. The sensory distribution of this nerve on the foot is often limited to the dorsum of the base of the first and second toes. This small area may easily be overlooked in checking for sensation. In addition, pain sensation is one of the last modalities to be involved; therefore the patient must not be merely checked with a pin for pain sensation but must also be tested for light touch. In addition to light touch, proprioception often disappears early; therefore, one should ask the patient to identify which toe the examiner is moving and the direction in which he is moving it while this activity is shielded from his view. The first muscles to become involved are usually the extensor hallucis longus and anterior tibial. Thus, weakness in dorsiflexion of the great toe or ankle may appear before other motor loss is evident. Not only should the patient be asked to dorsiflex his foot and wiggle his toes, but the strength of these motor functions should be compared with that of the opposite extremity.

The Doppler ultrasound probe can be extremely valuable in evaluating patients in the Emergency Department with peripheral vascular disease—particularly in peripheral arterial injuries—and it should be standard equipment in every major Emergency Department. Experience is required in the use of the probe, e.g., in distinguishing the characteristics of unobstructed and postobstructive flow, but this skill can be readily acquired. By listening with the Doppler probe over the known anatomic course of the arterial tree, one usually can determine the level and extent of arterial obstruction and the patency of the arteries below the obstruction. It is even possible to measure the perfusion pressure reaching the distal tissues (Strandness and Sumner, 1972). In this regard, Lavenson and his associates in Vietnam (1970) found a reliable correlation between audible flow through nonpalpable distal (e.g., posterior tibial) arteries and limb viability. Audible flow in the distal artery usually indicates a perfusion pressure of at least 30 mm. Hg, which often is sufficient to maintain viability. However, this pressure can be determined with accuracy using an ankle pressure cuff.

Finally, the value of arteriography in evaluating arterial injuries cannot be overemphasized. It is useful: (1) in dissociating arterial spasm from mechanical obstruction; (2) in providing earlier diagnosis when the clinical evidence is not conclusive; (3) in identifying the level of the occlusion for more precise surgical exploration; (4) in assessing the condition of the collateral circulation; and (5) in detecting unsuspected incomplete occlusions, false aneurysms, and A-V fistulas. It is unnecessary *only* in penetrating wounds when the existence and location of the arterial injury are obvious. Therefore, although arteriography is not advised in the simpler penetrating wounds, particularly when the arterial tree has been surveyed with the Doppler ultrasound probe, it usually should be obtained in the more extensive penetrating wounds and in cases of arterial occlusion secondary to blunt trauma. However, it is not necessary to obtain arteriography preoperatively in these circumstances. In most cases, when the existence of an arterial injury is known, it is more expedient to obtain an intraoperative arteriogram at the beginning of the procedure than to take the time to obtain it in the Department of Radiology before proceeding to the operating room. On the other hand, arteriography should be obtained before taking the patient to the operating room in cases where there is a question of whether a peripheral arterial injury exists. Most trauma centers are using arteriography with increasing frequency in serious penetrating wounds, major fractures and dislocations, or extensive soft tissue damage of the extremity—even when there is no clear evidence of arterial injury—before proceeding with operative repair. One thing this increasing use of arteriography has taught us is that what is often diagnosed as "arterial spasm in association with a major fracture or soft tissue injury" is not spasm at all but an intrinsic arterial lesion causing partial or even complete obstruction of the arterial lumen. It would be wise for physicians in Emergency Departments to operate under the premise that traumatic arterial spasm does not exist, even though, in fact, it occasionally does. Table 1 indicates the diagnostic tests important in evaluating peripheral vascular injuries.

TABLE 1   *Special Diagnostic Tests of Aid in Evaluating Vascular Injuries (In addition to meticulous physical examination)*

1. Doppler ultrasonic probe.
2. Limb blood pressure measurements.
3. Arteriography.
4. Radiography to determine associated injuries.

MANAGEMENT

The most pressing indication for treatment of arterial injuries and the first order of business in the Emergency Department is, of course, exsanguinating hemorrhage. Unfortunately, and all too commonly, the inexperienced physician will be found frantically and blindly clamping in the depths of a wound filled with blood. This not only allows additional blood loss at a time when it can least well be tolerated, but, unless vascular clamps are available and used, the injury to the artery and other tissues may be compounded, necessitating a more extensive débridement and possibly the need for a segmental vascular graft when a simple reapproximation would have otherwise sufficed. Control by clamping is permissible in open, superficial wounds, particularly if the physician is experienced and if sterile vascular clamps are available, as they should be in every Emergency Department. However, persisting with blind attempts at clamping, with poor exposure in a pool of blood and in the face of continuing rapid blood loss, is inexcusable.

The use of tourniquets is also to be condemned, except under the most trying circumstances, because, if improperly applied, they occlude collateral circulation as well as the injured vessel. Furthermore, because their application is rarely correct, they usually occlude the venous outflow without controlling arterial inflow, thereby increasing the bleeding from the wound and the risk of postischemic muscle compartment swelling.

Direct pressure over the wound or over the course of the artery proximal to the wound will control almost any bleeding. Injured patients are usually hypercoagulable, and five to ten minutes of continuous pressure often will produce hemostasis even in the face of a major arterial injury. If this fails, pressure should be reapplied and the patient

taken to the operating room, where this pressure can be maintained with a sterile gloved hand while the patient is anesthetized, the extremity prepared and draped for surgery, and control obtained by the surgeon through a short proximal incision over the course of the artery.

Once the diagnosis of a peripheral arterial injury has been established, its relative priority in the over-all management of the patient must be established. Such a decision obviously depends on the seriousness of the associated injuries as well as on the immediate threat presented by the arterial injury itself. Although it is axiomatic that arterial repair should be performed as soon as possible, it is equally true that, once the possibility of exsanguinating hemorrhage has been controlled, there may be no immediate threat to life or limb from this injury. Trauma to the other vital systems may deserve prior or at least concomitant attention.

Nevertheless, the consequences of delay in restoring arterial circulation to the extremity must be recognized in making such a decision. Although the oft-quoted six- to 12-hour "golden period" is only relative, the results of treatment do correlate well with this. Edwards and Lyons (1954) noted that gangrene was rare following successful repairs undertaken within six hours of injury, but that it occurred in over 50 per cent beyond 12 hours. In Jahnke's experience (1953) with 77 consecutive arterial repairs during the Korean conflict, no amputations were required when the delay was 12 hours or less but were required in 29 per cent after this lapse of time. The results are even worse with blunt trauma. Makin (1966) found that when the repair of arterial injuries associated with a fracture or dislocation was delayed more than 12 hours, 80 per cent required amputation and the remaining 20 per cent suffered permanent disability. When the delay was under 12 hours, the amputation rate was 16 per cent.

Obviously, establishing that the patient has a viable extremity does not mean that the arterial injury should not be repaired. There is no assurance that further propagation of the thrombus that is occluding the artery will not cut off additional collaterals and change the situation from that of a viable extremity to that of a nonviable one. The guiding philosophy should be to *repair all arterial injuries as soon as possible.*

However, under certain circumstances

one is justified in electing not to follow this dictate. For example, with an obviously viable extremity and in the face of extensive, badly contaminated wounds, one might elect simply to debride the wounds and leave the arterial repair until later, when the problems of infection and tissue coverage of the graft will not be so great. Second, in a patient involved in a serious accident in whom multiple system injuries are suspected but not manifest, it might be wise to allow a few additional hours for these injuries to make themselves apparent, rather than to rush the patient to the operating room for repairs of an arterial injury, particularly if the extremity appears viable. Third, if the threat to life due to associated injuries is great and might be increased by undertaking arterial repair, one might be willing to accept the consequences of delayed repair if the extremity appeared viable, and even if the limb would not be expected to survive without early repair. The priority of life over limb obviously must be observed. Fourth, arterial repair should not be undertaken if associated skeletal or neuromuscular damage in that extremity precludes the restoration of useful limb function. Finally, it must be recognized that it may be wise to delay or even not undertake the repair of arteries which are minor and not essential to limb survival or function. As Eiseman (1970) pointed out, in reporting on complications which arose from repairing minor or noncritical arteries in the Vietnam conflict, it is not ordinarily essential to limb survival, in the young at least, to repair (a) the brachial artery between the profunda and the elbow collaterals, (b) the ulnar or radial artery alone at any level, (c) the profunda femoris artery, (d) the superficial femoral artery proximal to the geniculate collaterals, and (e) the anterior tibial, the posterior tibial, or peroneal artery alone at any level.

On the other hand, in a more favorable environment, and particularly when not restricted by priorities dictated by other injuries, it probably is wise at least to explore all potential injuries to "name" arteries, regardless of how inconsequential they may seem, even if viability is not an issue. Late aneurysm formation and arteriovenous fistulae may thus be avoided, and it is always possible that those successfully repaired arteries may serve an unexpected later purpose.

Once hemostasis is no longer a problem and the diagnosis has been established, Emergency Department staff should proceed with the preparation of the patient for surgery, inserting at least two large-bore intravenous cannulas, restoring blood volume, typing and cross matching the patient for 2 to 4 units of blood, and administering tetanus prophylaxis. Broad spectrum antibiotic coverage should be administered intravenously in large doses in the Emergency Department prior to operation if these agents are to have a "prophylactic" effect. The indications for antibiotics are not only the usual ones of shock, tissue ischemia, and gross contamination, but also the possibility of having to place a prosthetic graft during the arterial reconstruction. If the viability of the extremity is marginal it is particularly important to maintain the patient's blood pressure and to keep the involved extremity in a dependent position relative to the heart to maximize the perfusion pressure distally in the limb. This is particularly important if delay is anticipated before repair can be performed. Vasodilators should not be given. Anticoagulants should be withheld until the wound has been thoroughly explored and debrided and arterial reconstruction is about to take place. Occasionally in simpler arterial injuries, anticoagulants will not be used even intraoperatively. Neither heat nor cold should be applied, normal body temperature being ideal. Finally, since it is important not to use the superficial vein in the same extremity in grafting, because of the risk of concomitant deep venous injury, the contralateral leg or ipsilateral upper extremity should be shaved as well as the injured extremity. Although many of the above functions will be taken over by the surgical team that undertakes the patient's vascular reconstruction, the emergency physician should proceed with these routine preoperative preparations until he has been relieved of responsibility for his patient.

REPLANTATION

The reattachment of an amputated part of an extremity—the ultimate in the management of peripheral vascular injuries—is a matter that requires preparation and forethought. The subject has been thoroughly covered by Malt (1974). In general, only upper extremities are replanted, and then only when there are no other serious injuries. This procedure should not be undertaken unless there is available an experienced team with vascular surgical, neurosurgical, and orthopedic skills. It usually is performed only when there is a lack of extensive tissue disruption and contamination (i.e., a "clean" amputation) and when the patient is well motivated, emotionally stable, and young. Each Emergency Department should develop its own policies and procedures for such an undertaking in collaboration with the appropriate staff surgeons so that the indications are clear and the method of handling the severed extremity is clearly detailed. Ordinarily the artery to the severed extremity is cannulated as atraumatically as possible and cold heparinized saline is perfused by gravity until the venous effluent is clear; then the limb is wrapped in a sterile dressing.

COMPLICATIONS OF INITIAL MANAGEMENT

The *specific complications* of the initial or Emergency Department management of peripheral vascular injuries are mainly related to three aspects: *failure to achieve hemostasis properly; failure to diagnose the vascular injury early; and failure to observe the urgency for vascular reconstruction and minimize the ischemic period.* These pitfalls have been described above, and failure to avoid them will be measured in terms of nerve palsies, ischemic neuritis, and occasionally reflex sympathetic dystrophy—as well as compartmental swelling, with resul-

tant myonecrosis or ischemic contractures and, finally, amputation for gangrene.

References

Abbott, W., Mione, P. J., and Austen, W. G.: Effect of venous interruption on arterial circulation. Surg. Forum 25:246, 1974.

Brisbin, R. L., Geib, P. O., and Eiseman, B.: Secondary disruption of vascular repair following war wounds. Arch. Surg. 120:522, 1970.

Carrel, A.: The surgery of blood vessels. Johns Hopkins Bull. 18:18, 1907.

DeBakey, M. E., and Simeone, F. A.: Battle injuries of the arteries in World War II. Ann. Surg. 140:318, 1954.

Edwards, W. S., and Lyons, C.: Traumatic arterial spasm and thrombosis. Ann. Surg. 140:318, 1954.

Guthrie, G. C.: Heterotransplantation of blood vessels. Am. J. Physiol. 19:482, 1907.

Harris, W., and Malt, R.: Late results of human limb replantation. J. Trauma. 14:44, 1974.

Jahnke, E. J., Jr., and Seeley, S. F.: Acute vascular injuries in the Korean war: An analysis of 77 consecutive cases. Ann. Surg. 138:158, 1953.

Lavenson, G. S., Rich, N. M., and Baugh, J. H.: Value of ultrasonic flow detector in the management of peripheral vascular disease. Am. J. Surg. 120:522, 1970.

Makin, G. S., Howard, J. M., and Green, R. L.: Arterial injuries complicating fractures or dislocations: the necessity for a more aggressive approach. Surgery 59:203, 1966.

Makins, G. W.: Gunshot injuries to the blood vessels. Bristol, England, John Wright & Sons, Ltd., 1919.

Malan, E., and Tattoni, G.: Physio- and anato-pathology of acute ischemia of the extremities. J. Cardiovasc. Surg. 4:2, 1963.

Nolan, B.: Vascular injuries. J. Roy. Coll. Surg. 13:72, 1968.

Shires, G. T., and Patman, R. D.: Vascular injuries in the care of the trauma patient. New York, McGraw-Hill Book Co., Inc., 1966.

Strandness, D. E., and Sumner, D. S.: Non-invasive methods of studying peripheral arterial function. J. Surg. Res. 12:419, 1972.

Chapter 39

SPECIAL PROBLEMS IN TRAUMA

A. BURNS
John A. Moncrief

PREHOSPITAL CARE

Frequently the first people at the scene of burn injuries are firemen and policemen. Shortly thereafter ambulances arrive. Burn treatment should be begun immediately by those first to arrive.

The patient's airway should be checked first, and in cases where smoke inhalation is evident, oxygen by mask should be started. The presence of perioral or intraoral burns is a strong indication that significant smoke inhalation has occurred. Stridor and retractions suggest burns of the glottis or vocal cords.

At the scene attempts to classify burns in terms of degree are fruitless. Instead, the patient's hot clothing should be removed and ice or cool water applied to the burned areas for 10 to 15 minutes. Overzealous use of ice should be avoided because of its potential for lowering total body temperature.

If time permits, simple washing of the burned areas with soap and water followed by coverage with a sterile dressing would be helpful, particularly if the hospital is more than 15 minutes from the scene.

If the ambulance team has the capability to begin intravenous infusions, one should be started with normal saline or lactated Ringer's solution. This should be done for all but the obviously minor burn.

Topical creams or ointments should not be employed in prehospital treatment.

MANAGEMENT IN THE EMERGENCY DEPARTMENT

INITIAL CONSIDERATIONS AND ASSESSMENT

As with any patient first seen in the Emergency Department or in the initial treatment area, an over-all assessment of the patient's status must first be made. If not already done, an airway should be established

and oxygen started if smoke inhalation is likely. All covering material and clothing should be removed, and the patient inspected closely from head to toe, front and back, with an eye toward discovering unsuspected injury. In addition, as detailed a history as possible must be obtained from the

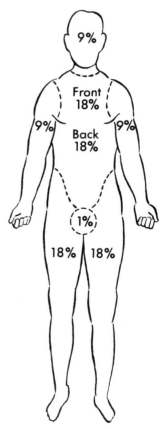

Figure 1. "Rule of Nines." Use of this type of body surface description allows for rapid estimate of the area of burn. Each segment should be examined separately and the total arrived at by simple addition. Errors in estimate of area of burn due to variations of body contour with weight and age are of no clinical significance in establishing initial fluid requirements. The ease of use through the years has firmly established the practicality and validity of this system.

patient or his relatives or companions. This should deal primarily with the specific injury, but also should provide important contributory information about the patient's past medical or social history. The circumstances of the accident are to be reconstructed as closely as possible, as damage to deeper tissues or organs may be anticipated, depending on the circumstances of the injury. For example, exposure to high voltage electric current as opposed to household current, inhalation of toxic combustion products resulting from the burning of synthetic material, or knowledge that the accident occurred within a closed space—all are important in patient evaluation. Associated injuries or contact with toxic caustic or corrosive chemicals may be discovered. Once this general information has been obtained and a general view of the patient accomplished, more specific attention directed toward the burn injury itself can be undertaken.

For purposes of discussion, initial burn care can be divided into several convenient groups. These are not necessarily presented here in the order of their temporal impor-

tance, as indeed one aspect of resuscitative therapy may be much more urgent in a given patient than in another, and only experience and clinical judgment will determine the order of priority. In actual practice all the steps usually are being accomplished simultaneously, with appropriate emphasis being directed more forcefully in one direction or another.

ESTABLISHING AN ADEQUATE AIRWAY

The most urgent requirement in any trauma patient is an adequate airway. In the absence of facial burns with their attendant extensive edema, or the inhalation of toxic combustion products, airway problems in the burn patient ordinarily are not of great immediate importance. Ventilation problems may develop later in the postburn period, but generally do not require prompt emergency treatment in the immediate postburn period. The most dramatic occurrence of airway problems is in the patient suffering

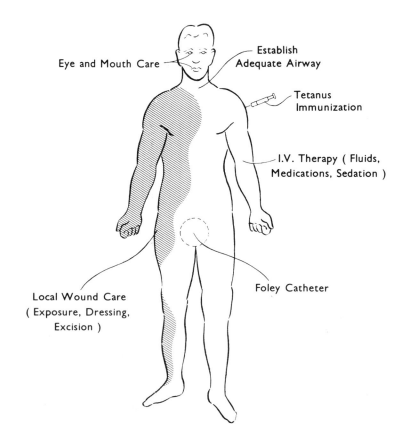

Figure 2. Assurance of an adequate airway is the first priority, with intravenous fluid resuscitation in close succession. Wound care should be delayed until the other aspects of treatment are firmly under way or established. In practice, all the procedures are accomplished in essentially a simultaneous fashion with emphasis placed where the clinical situation dictates.

Eye and Mouth Care

Establish Adequate Airway

Tetanus Immunization

I.V. Therapy (Fluids, Medications, Sedation)

Foley Catheter

Local Wound Care (Exposure, Dressing, Excision)

from overwhelming inhalation of toxic combustion products. Frequently such a patient does not show significant burn injury to the body surface. This is typical of the inhalation injuries seen in firemen and in those burned in industrial accidents, where the patient is "overcome with smoke"—in reality a combination of carbon monoxide poisoning and a severe, fulminant, rapidly progressive and extensive tracheobronchitis. Under these circumstances respiratory exchange is markedly impaired and the oxygen-carrying capacity of the red cells severely diminished.

When burn injury occurs about the face and neck, edema of these structures develops with varying rapidity, in part in response to the fluid resuscitation therapy undertaken. Although the appearance of edema is most dramatic in second degree burns, the greatest impairment of the airway and greatest danger to the patient occur in those whose burns are deeper. The third degree burn tissue is dry, inelastic, and indeed is shrunken somewhat from its original contour. The obligatory edema that occurs beneath it causes an encroachment on the softer tissues of the neck, resulting in constriction of the pharyngeal airway, fixation of the mandible, often in a retracted position, and marked edema and eversion of the lips, causing difficulty in evacuation of oral contents. As so many of these patients are nauseated at this early stage, the risk of aspiration of gastric contents is high because of an inability to evacuate the oral cavity. A nasogastric tube may be necessary to decompress the stomach. No food should be given by mouth in major burns during the immediate postburn period.

It is best to provide an adequate airway in these patients by the most expeditious means available. Although in the past tracheostomy has been advocated, experience indicates that this procedure is difficult to accomplish in the Emergency Department, in the recovery room, or during the initial phase of resuscitation. Indeed, it may add unwarranted hazards. Consequently, it is recommended that an airway be established, if possible, by utilizing either a nasotracheal or endotracheal tube inserted through the nose or mouth with the aid of direct laryngoscopy. Whether the patient requiring respiratory support can be managed without an inflated cuff or danger of aspiration of the gastric contents will determine primarily the need for having the cuff about the endotracheal tube inflated at all times. If support can be managed without inflating the cuff, so much the better; but if it is necessary to inflate the cuff it should be deflated periodically in the hope of avoiding tracheal erosion. In general, the endotracheal tube should be removed after four to five days, unless there is some overriding need for its retention, and then the cuff should be deflated if at all possible. In some instances tracheostomy may be essential, particularly if there is associated severe facial injury.

There are, of course, occasions when a cuff must be left inflated for long periods of time and the patient must be carried on progressively higher concentrations of inspired oxygen as well as increasing respiratory pressures (PEEP). This is usually necessary only in cases of significant damage to the tracheobronchial tree from irritating products of combustion. The main problem is determining in advance when such respiratory support is necessary. When the patient is first seen in the Emergency facility, it may not be obvious that pulmonary complications are going to supervene. A history of exposure to toxic combustion products or of having sustained injury within a closed space that forced inhalation of such products should lead to a high index of suspicion, and prophylactic therapy should be strongly considered. The carboxyhemoglobin determination can indicate to some extent the degree of smoke inhalation. In addition to the endotracheal tube and respiratory support, the patient with obvious or strongly suspected respiratory damage should receive methylprednisolone, 20 mg. per kg. in a single bolus intravenous administration daily for three to five days in an attempt to prevent pulmonary edema. Clinical experience would indicate that this is helpful under these circumstances, but strong statistical evidence is not yet available. The use of bronchial lavage is controversial and not recommended at this time.

SEDATION AND ANALGESIA

Many patients who have sustained thermal injury require analgesia and/or sedation to relieve pain. One must differentiate between the restlessness and irritability of hypoxia and those due to pain. If there is any question, arterial blood gases should be measured immediately. Application of cool compresses to the burn wound will assuage the local pain to a considerable degree. It is not necessary to immerse the patient in ice water or to use ice compresses. Simple cool compresses from water are sufficient. Application should be continued until the patient is essentially free of pain. Then the compresses are removed. This may take 30 to 60 minutes.

Medication administered as a sedative or analgesic to the burn patient must be given intravenously in the immediate postburn period. Because of the derangements of circulatory dynamics, any medication given intramuscularly or subcutaneously during this time will be absorbed in such an erratic fashion that an unpredictable dose response will occur. For this reason administration of anything by routes other than the intravenous may result in late pick-up of the medication and oversedation. The type of intravenous medication utilized should be individualized to the patient. The most commonly used are morphine and meperidine, which can be given intravenously in appropriate doses every two to four hours as necessary. It is best to begin with the smallest doses possible (e.g., 1 to 3 mg. morphine I.V.) to avoid hypotension and respiratory depression. Barbiturates should not be used, as they often act more as a stimulant than as a sedative or analgesic. Such agents as diazepam or hydroxyzine offer sedation without significant respiratory depression — although episodes of apnea have occurred with intravenous diazepam and should be anticipated.

TETANUS PROPHYLAXIS

The risk of tetanus is significant in the burn patient population. For this reason, immunization should be carried out promptly. If the patient has been actively immunized within the past five years, only a tetanus toxoid booster shot is necessary. Although it may be possible to avoid booster administration if the patient was immunized within the year prior to the burn, it is not certain in this patient population whether such protection is sufficient. Contrary to some popular beliefs, the burn patient is quite capable of an anamnestic response to a tetanus toxoid booster, and indeed antitoxin levels frequently are higher in the burn patient population following tetanus toxoid booster injec-

tions than they are in the normal unburned population.

If the patient has never received any active tetanus immunization, it is worthwhile to protect him with hyperimmune human antitetanus gammaglobulin. This is commercially available and should initially be administered in a dose of 250 units. The injection should provide protection for a period of four to six weeks, at which time the dose should be repeated. At the same time the patient should be started on active immunization utilizing alum-precipitated toxoid. Although the evidence is unclear at the moment, previous experience with simultaneous administration of antitoxin and toxoid would indicate that alum-precipitated toxoid is to be preferred to fluid toxoid under these circumstances.

ANTIBIOTIC COVERAGE

In general, prophylactic systemic antibiotic therapy is contraindicated in the treatment of thermal injury. For the small burn wounds it is not necessary, and for the patient who has sustained extensive thermal injury administration must be continued over such a protracted period that the only significant result is the emergence of bacterial flora resistant to the antibiotic being administered. In addition, systemic antibiotics cannot be delivered in sufficient quantity to the singularly avascular burn wound where the bacteria reside in such large numbers. Historically penicillin was employed during the earliest phase of burn treatment in an attempt primarily to treat streptococcal burn sepsis and provide prophylaxis. Some centers continue to use penicillin or an antibiotic with activity against gram-positive cocci, although firm evidence of benefit from such treatment has not been demonstrated.

Should there be associated injuries, such as open fractures or open head wounds, or pre-existing illness, such as upper respiratory infection, that in themselves dictate the use of antibiotic therapy, such administration with amounts and dosage schedules usual for the basic disease can be accomplished. Later in the postburn course systemic antibacterial therapy may be indicated, but not in the immediate postburn period. Suitable cultures direct specific therapy.

INTRAVENOUS RESUSCITATION

As the result of the thermal injury there is a marked derangement of the cardiocirculatory dynamics. The magnitude of this alteration is in general proportional to the extent and depth of the thermal injury and involves not only the central pumping mechanism (the heart), but also the peripheral vasculature. Such changes do not occur in minor burns and in this classification we would consider any partial thickness burn of less than 20 per cent of the body surface or any full thickness burn of less than 10 per cent of the body surface. Electric injuries usually require volumes of fluid far out of proportion to the extent of surface injury.

Following thermal injury there is a loss of capillary integrity, which in burns of 30 per cent of the body surface or less is limited to the burn area and in a larger burn is present throughout the body, but most marked within the burn area. This loss of capillary integrity is such that substances of a molecular size as great as 150,000 Å pass freely through the capillary membrane. This complete capillary permeability to the principal colloids within the vascular compartment negates their colloid oncotic effect, and thus Starling's law is not an effective force under these circumstances. Both clinical and laboratory experimental evidence clearly show that intravenous fluids administered during this period produce expansion of the plasma volume only as the result of high rates of fluid administration, and this is completely independent of the type of fluid administered. In other words, *salt solutions are as effective as colloidal solutions during this period of altered capillary permeability.* Indeed, in large burns, unless one exceeds 4.5 ml. per kg. per hour in the rate of administration of fluid, there is no significant increase in plasma volume. Again, this is regardless of the type of fluid administered.

At some time between 18 and 36 hours postburn this altered capillary permeability is reversed. By some unknown mechanism the body regains its ability to retain colloidal substances within the vascular compartment. The change is undetected by any clinical observation, but experimental studies clearly show this to be the case. Thus, during the second 24 hours postburn one would anticipate that the administration of colloid would be effective in maintaining plasma volume, and indeed such is the case.

With the above information in mind, one can utilize any of the various fluid formulae that have been advocated for the resuscitation of the burn patient. Realize that any fluid formula used is simply a means of initiating fluid resuscitation therapy and that the rate and type of fluid administration must be altered according to the patient's clinical response to that therapy. The primary guides to adequacy of fluid therapy are clearness of the sensorium, adequacy of the peripheral capillary flow, presence or absence of signs of pulmonary edema indicating fluid overload, rate and quality of the peripheral pulse, and adequacy of urinary output. The CVP, while a late indicator, may be useful. Early changes may be detected through measurement of the pulmonary wedge pressure by means of a Swan-Ganz catheter which can detect early signs of fluid overload. All the factors should be carefully evaluated periodically; however, hourly urinary output is used as the prime guide in the evaluation of the efficacy of resuscitation, and in general an adequate urinary output is considered to be evidence of adequate fluid resuscitation therapy.

Table 1 outlines the more popular of the various fluid resuscitation formulas available. One should familiarize himself thoroughly with any one of these formulas and use the one with which he feels most comfortable and from which he gets optimal results. Clinical experience indicates that proper utilization of any of these resuscitation formulas will result in effective resuscitation of the patient by all the clinical parameters available to us.

It must be emphasized that in all the formulas utilized fluid resuscitation therapy is calculated on the basis of extent of burn. Depth of burn is not considered in calculating the initial fluid dosage. However, clinical experience would indicate that the deeper burns require larger amounts of fluid and that the range of fluid requirement for a given extent of burn is quite large. In addition, initiation of fluid resuscitation therapy is calculated from the time of onset of injury, not from the time the patient is first seen in the treatment facility. Ordinarily one-half the calculated daily requirement is administered in the first eight hours postburn, with the remainder being administered in the subsequent 16 hours. Thus a delay in initiation of therapy requires vigorous fluid infusion.

TABLE 1 Fluid Administration

Selection of a specific fluid resuscitation formula should be dictated primarily by the attending physician's familiarity with the given technique. Clinical response indicates little in favor of any one formula and, indeed, as the table indicates, total sodium and total fluids in the first 48 hours are almost identical.

Formula		First 24 Hours	Second 24 Hours	Total
Brooke	°Colloid °°Electrolyte G/W	1.5 ml./kg./% burn 0.5 ml./kg./% burn 2000 ml.	0.75 ml/kg./% burn 0.25 ml./kg./% burn 2000 ml.	(70 kg − 40% burn) 12,400 ml. fluid 1694 mEq. Na
Evans	Colloid Electrolyte G/W	1.0 ml./kg./% burn 1.0 ml./kg./% burn 2,000 ml.	0.5 ml./kg./% burn 0.5 ml./kg./% burn 2000 ml.	12,400 ml. fluid 1736 mEq. Na
Parkland	Colloid Electrolyte G/W	None 4 ml./kg./% burn None	°°°None or 500 ml as needed None Ad lib (Sufficient to maintain urine output)	13,200 ml. fluid 1716 mEq. Na

°Colloid = Plasmanate, plasma, dextran.
°°Electrolyte = Ringer's lactate.
°°°If urine output cannot be maintained with G/W alone, give 500 ml. colloid as necessary.

The main differences in the fluid formulas have to do more with the constituent quantities administered than with the total quantity given. If one calculates the total quantity of fluid and the total mEq. of sodium administered in the Brooke formula or the Parkland formula or the Evans formula, there is only about 5 per cent variation in the three. In the Brooke formula and in the Evans formula, colloid, electrolyte solution, and glucose and water are administered throughout both the first and second postburn day, with smaller quantities being administered in the second 24-hour period. In the Parkland formula, resuscitation during the first 24 hours is with electrolyte solution alone (Ringer's lactate), and in the second 24 hours no salt water is administered as a tremendous salt load is already on board. If one finds, with this therapy, that urinary output cannot be maintained with glucose and water alone, during the period subsequent to the first 24 hours, small quantities of colloid (500 ml.) can be administered, usually with a prompt response.

USE OF BLOOD

Unless there are associated injuries such as hemothorax or loss of blood from the body from some other source, the administration of whole blood is not to be considered during this initial period of treatment. Although a loss of red cell mass can be clearly demonstrated as a result of thermal injury, the loss of noncellular elements from the vascular compartment so far exceeds this loss of red cell mass that there is a resulting progressive hemoconcentration, which usually does not begin to correct itself until the middle of the second postburn day. It is not until the third to the fifth postburn day, when mobilization of the edema fluid occurs, that the true level of hemoglobin or hematocrit can be readily appreciated. Thus, during the immediate postburn period (first five days) the administration of whole blood is contraindicated for the treatment of the burn injury itself, as it merely aggravates the already increased blood viscosity and diminishes oxygen delivery to peripheral tissues.

In utilizing urine output to monitor adequacy of the fluid resuscitation one is guided by both the rate and character of urine production. A flow of 30 to 50 ml./hr. usually is considered sufficient in adults, but when the Parkland formula is used volumes of 50 to 100 ml./hr. are advocated. Such rates are not produced in a steady manner, but characteristically wide fluctuations of flow occur, requiring close monitoring and rapid adjustments in fluid administration. In children (20 to 30 ml./hr.) and in infants (10 to 20 ml./hr.) proportionately lower rates are accepted.

RENAL CONSIDERATIONS

Large amounts of microscopic sediment are seen in the urine following thermal injury, but the gross appearance usually is clear. Should pigment (hemoglobin and/or myoglobin) appear, this is evidence of deeper burn injury. Unless cleared from the urine by increased urine flow, an obstructive nephropathy and acute tubular necrosis may supervene. Under such circumstances one should abandon the calculated rates of fluid administration and significantly increase the rate of the intravenous fluid therapy to promote a brisk diuresis. If such cannot be accomplished by increasing fluid load alone, use of a diuretic is indicated. Mannitol (50 gm.) or furosemide (80 to 120 mg.) is effective in helping to clear the urine.

One must be aware that during the administration of a diuretic the rate of urine flow is no longer a guide to the adequacy of fluid resuscitation; therefore, other parameters must be more heavily relied upon.

LOCAL CARE OF THE BURN WOUND

Small burns of the trunk and extremities that do not require grafting can readily be treated on an outpatient basis. The wound should be cleansed thoroughly with soap and water, the hair shaved around it, and a dry, sterile dressing applied. Five to seven days later the dressing can be changed down to lower layers of the dressing that are firmly adherent. If there is no obvious evidence of gross infection, another clean dressing can be placed over this; again, after another five to seven days, the dressing is removed, at which time the burn wound should be freshly healed, allowing complete removal of the dressing.

Burns of the face or perineum, unless of extremely limited extent, cannot be adequately treated on an outpatient basis. At least for the initial two to five days these should be treated in the hospital, with the wound exposed to the air. Thorough cleaning with soap and water and shaving of the perineum is necessary. It is not necessary to shave the head in the presence of a facial burn unless the burn is deep and extensive, but certainly the hair should be kept away from the burn wound. Because of the tendency for the development of a purulent conjunctivitis with the attendant risk of corneal erosion and perforation, the eyes must be irrigated at least once every shift with saline and a bland ointment instilled (sulfacetamide or methylcellulose), with meticulous care being taken to maintain good hygiene. The mouth should be cleaned and the teeth brushed at least twice daily to prevent the development of stomatitis. This can be most readily accomplished with an electric toothbrush, particularly if the patient is unable to help himself.

In more extensive and deeper burns, local care of the burn wound is accomplished in a fashion similar to that used in smaller wounds, but on a grander scale. The wounds are cleansed thoroughly with soap and water and irrigated with saline, and all hairy surfaces are shaved. Any loose epidermis is debrided away, but any firmly adherent skin is allowed to remain in place, as experience indicates that this facilitates the healing of the burn wound beneath it. Large blisters and bullae may be infected even though intact. After evacuation of fluid, the loose epidermis overlying the blisters and bullae can be reapproximated to the burn surface and held in place with a light dressing for 24 hours until a firm fibrin coagulant binds it to the underlying wound.

It should be emphasized that the burn wound itself should take last priority in the treatment of the acutely burned patient, except in the case of very minor wounds. The main risk to the burn patient from the standpoint of the burn surface itself is that of infection, which does not ordinarily supervene in a significant degree for 72 to 96 hours postburn. Resuscitation efforts must take priority over local care of the wound.

In general, patients managed on an outpatient basis are best treated with an occlusive dressing changed every five to seven days until the wound beneath is healed. Topical and local antibiotic therapy are not advocated for these small wounds. Larger wounds are best treated by the exposure method and application of topical antibacterial therapy. This type of therapy should be dictated by what is available and by which substances the attending physician knows best as well as by what may be indicated by the type and location of the burn wound itself. There has been no clear-cut demonstration of advantage of one type of therapy over another, and each has its proponents. It should be noted that Sulfamylon causes pain on application and requires daily or more frequent changes; therefore it should be used primarily in hospitalized patients.

Under some circumstances the wounds may be immediately excised and grafted either at the same time or 24 hours later. This is particularly advantageous in small, circumscribed, full thickness burn wounds, such as contact burns or steam press burns in which the depth of burn is obvious, the outlines are sharply circumscribed, and the patient's general condition permits this immediate approach to the burn wound. Usually recovery is rapid and the patient can be discharged from the hospital within ten days. He usually returns to light work within three weeks.

ASSOCIATED INJURIES

Associated injuries in the burn patient should be cared for at the same time that the burn resuscitation is being accomplished. Blunt abdominal or thoracic injuries that require operative intervention should be approached promptly once resuscitation is well under way. Associated fractures can be immobilized by skeletal traction but it is unwise to immobilize a burned extremity in plaster or to attempt any type of internal fixation in the presence of a high risk of fulminant infection. Skeletal traction can be utilized quite effectively for alignment of fractured fragments, and even though the pins may be placed through areas of full thickness burn, osseous complications are minimal. A small ring sequestrum occasionally may form.

Where there has been a circumferential burn of third degree, symptoms of compression, whether in an extremity, the abdomen, or the chest, may require escharotomy. The clinical symptoms should guide the selection of this therapy.

Severe burns are best treated in a specialized burn center because of the high risk of mortality.*

---

*For hand burns, see p. 732.

SUNBURN

Although usually of minor long term consequence, severe sunburn can provide substantial distress to a patient. Moreover chronic exposure to the sun (ultraviolet rays, 290 to 320 nm) is associated with the development of skin cancer. Theoretically, sunburn is the only burn which can affect 90 per cent of the body with full survival; however, severe sunburn may indeed require intravenous fluid therapy. Topically, the most important consideration is thorough washing and avoidance of breaking small blisters. Topical creams may be soothing, particularly if they contain one of the "caine" local anesthetics. Caution should be employed because of the possibility of allergic reaction. Cool compresses offer substantial relief.

The best plan is protection. Although most of the commercial "sunscreen" preparations are effective in the laboratory, they readily wash off or leave with sweat, making frequent application essential. The best sunscreen preparations are: (a) 5 percent para-aminobenzoic acid in 70 to 95 percent ethyl alcohol; (b) Escalol (506) (2.5 percent 150 amyl p-N, N-dimethyl amino benzoate) in 65 to 95 percent alcohol. These preparations can protect fair-skinned people for at least four hours after one application, even with sweating. They are cosmetically acceptable as well. Most commercial preparations have limited effectiveness.

References

Alexander, J. W., Dionigi, R., and Meakins, J. L.: Periodic variation in the antibacterial function of human neutrophils and its relationship to sepsis. Ann. Surg. *173*:206, 1971.

Arturson, G.: Pathophysiological aspects of the burn syndrome: with special reference to liver injury and alterations of capillary permeability. Acta Chir. Scand. (Suppl.) *274*:1, 1961.

Baxter, C. R.: Crystalloid Resuscitation of Burn Shock. In Polk, H. C., Jr., and Stone, H. H. (eds.): Contemporary Burn Management. Boston, Little, Brown & Co., 1971, pp. 7–32.

Baxter, C. R.: Topical Use of 1.0% Silver Sulfadiazine. In Polk, H. C., Jr., and Stone, H. H. (eds.): Contemporary Burn Management. Boston, Little, Brown & Co., 1971, pp. 217–225.

Baxter, C. R. et al.: A circulating myocardial depressant factor in burn shock. Transactions of Third International Congress on Research in Burns. Bern, Hans Huber Publishers, 1971, pp. 499–503.

Birke, G., et al.: Studies on burns. IX. The distribution and losses through the wound of I-albumin measured by whole-body counting. Acta Chir. Scand. *134*:27, 1968.

Foley, F. D.: The burn autopsy: fatal complications of burns. Am. J. Clin. Pathol. 52:1, 1969.

Foley, F. D., and Shuck, J. M.: Burn-wound infection with phycomycetes requiring amputation of hand. J.A.M.A. 203:596, 1968.

Gump, F. E., Price, J. B., Jr., and Kinney, J. M.: Blood flow and oxygen consumption in patients with severe burns. Surg. Gynecol. Obstet. 130:23, 1970.

Harrison, H. N., Bales, H., and Jacoby, F.: The behavior of mafenide acetate as a basis for its clinical use. Arch. Surg. 103:449. 1971.

Harrison, H. N., et al.: The relationship between energy metabolism and water loss from vaporization in severely burned patients. Surgery 56:203, 1964.

Jelenko, C. III, and Ginsburg, J. M.: Water-holding lipid and water transmission through homeothermic and poikilothermic skins. Proc. Soc. Exp. Biol. Med. 136:1059, 1971.

Krause, W., Matheis, H., and Wulf, K.: Fungaemia and funguria after oral administration of Candida albicans. Lancet 1:598, 1969.

Moncrief, J. A.: The status of topical antibacterial therapy in the treatment of burns. Surgery 63:862, 1968.

Moncrief, J. A.: Effect of various fluid regimens and pharmacologic agents on the circulatory hemodynamics of the immediate postburn period. Ann. Surg. 164:723, 1966.

Moncrief, J. A., and Teplitz, C.: Changing concepts in burn sepsis. J. Trauma 4:233, 1964.

Moyer, C. A., Margraf, H. W., and Monafo, W. W., Jr.: Burn shock and extravascular sodium deficiency-treatment with Ringer's solution with lactate. Arch. Surg. 90:799–811, 1965.

Order, S. E., and Moncrief, J. A.: The Burn Wound. Springfield, Illinois, Charles C Thomas, 1965.

Shuck, J. M., and Moncrief, J. A.: The management of burns. Part I. General considerations and the Sulfamylon method. Curr. Probl. Surg., February, 1969, pp. 1–52.

Shuck, J. M., Pruitt, B. A., Jr., and Moncrief, J. A.: Homograft skin for wound coverage: a study in versatility. Arch. Surg. 98:472, 1969.

Stone, H. H.: Wound Care with Topical Gentamicin. In Polk, H. C., Jr., and Stone, H. H. (eds.): Contemporary Burn Management. Boston, Little, Brown & Co., 1971, pp. 203–216.

Teplitz, C.: Pathology of Burns. In Artz, C. P., and Moncrief, J. A.: The Treatment of Burns. Second edition. Philadelphia, W. B. Saunders Co., 1969, pp. 22–88.

Teplitz, C., et al.: Pseudomonas burn wound sepsis. I. Pathogenesis of experimental Pseudomonas burn wound sepsis. J. Surg. Res. 4:200, 1964.

Wilmore, D. W., et al.: Supranormal dietary intake in thermally injured hypermetabolic patients. Surg. Gynecol. Obstet. 132:881, 1971.

Wilson, J. S., and Moncrief, J. A.: Vapor pressure of normal and burned skin. Ann. Surg. 162:130, 1965.

B.   DISORDERS DUE TO COLD

Loren A. Johnson

TYPICAL PRESENTATIONS

A policeman discovers a 25-year-old alcoholic in an alley. The patient has stiff distal movements and a cold abdomen. The nurse takes a rectal temperature below the limits of the ordinary clinical thermometer. A weather thermometer reads 84° F.

A child gets lost overnight in a light squall without his jacket. What are his chances?

A skier has a stiffly frozen foot under a boot-top fracture.

A mountain climbing party is stranded. Do the conditions warrant helicopter evacuation?

A farmer experiences purplish discoloration of his nose, hands, and feet outdoors in wintertime.

HISTORY AND INCIDENCE

Overwhelming cold stress may be generalized, causing accidental hypothermia, or localized, causing frostbite, immersion injury, or chilblains. These disorders can occur independently or together, usually in cold climates, and especially during war.

In his retreat from Moscow in 1812, Napoleon lost most of his Grande Armée of 80,000 to the cold, prompting the first scientific observation by his staff surgeon, Baron Larrey, of the phenomenon of the "white death" of hypothermia that followed heavy sleetfalls, and the gangrene of frozen tissue exposed to fire. Modern warfare has given us no fewer casualties from frostbite, among aviators in World War II and infantrymen in Korea; hypothermia, among victims of ship sinkings in the North Atlantic; and trench foot, among the armies of Europe. Some advances in prevention and therapy have been made from these experiences, but hypothermia and cold injury continue to pose a significant threat to all cold-exposed peoples around the world and a considerable treatment challenge in the Emergency Department.

BASIC CONSIDERATIONS

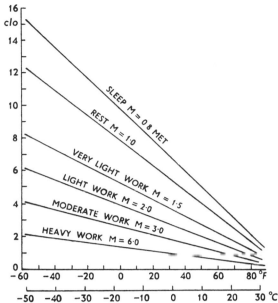

Figure 1. Total insulation of clothing needed for different metabolic rates. (From Burton, A. C., and Edholm, O. G.: Man in a Cold Environment. London, Edward Arnold, Ltd., 1955, with permission.)

As expressed by the law of Arrhenius, the logarithm of chemical reactions in the physiologic range varies directly with the absolute temperature. This results in about a 10 per cent change in biochemical activity for each Centigrade degree of temperature change. By adjusting rates of heat production and heat loss, homeotherms maintain a stable deep body temperature range for optimal enzyme functioning. In man, this range is 97.5 to 99.5° F., or 36.4° to 37.5° C., and is maintained by the use of clothing and by adjustments in sweating, vasomotor tone, exercise, shivering, and basal thermogenesis, under the control of the hypothalamus (Figs. 1 and 2).

Heat may be convected, conducted, irradiated, and released by evaporation from the body. Clothing reflects heat and retains a warm air envelope, known as the private climate. Its insulating value has been de-

COOLING POWER OF WIND EXPRESSED AS "EQUIVALENT CHILL TEMPERATURE"																						
WIND SPEED		TEMPERATURE (°F)																				
CALM	CALM	40	35	30	25	20	15	10	5	0	−5	−10	−15	−20	−25	−30	−35	−40	−45	−50	−55	−60
KNOTS	MPH	EQUIVALENT CHILL TEMPERATURE																				
3 - 6	5	35	30	25	20	15	10	5	0	−5	−10	−15	−20	−25	−30	−35	−40	−45	−50	−55	−65	−70
7 - 10	10	30	20	15	10	5	0	−10	−15	−20	−25	−35	−40	−45	−50	−60	−65	−70	−75	−80	−90	−95
11 - 15	15	25	15	10	0	−5	−10	−20	−25	−30	−40	−45	−50	−60	−65	−70	−80	−85	−90	−100	−105	−110
16 - 19	20	20	10	5	0	−10	−15	−25	−30	−35	−45	−50	−60	−65	−75	−80	−85	−95	−100	−110	−115	−120
20 - 23	25	15	10	0	−5	−15	−20	−30	−35	−45	−50	−60	−65	−75	−80	−90	−95	−105	−110	−120	−125	−135
24 - 28	30	10	5	0	−10	−20	−25	−30	−40	−50	−55	−65	−70	−80	−85	−95	−100	−110	−115	−125	−130	−140
29 - 32	35	10	5	−5	−10	−20	−30	−35	−40	−50	−60	−65	−75	−80	−90	−100	−105	−115	−120	−130	−135	−145
33 - 36	40	10	0	−5	−15	−20	−30	−35	−45	−55	−60	−70	−75	−85	−95	−100	−110	−115	−125	−130	−140	−150
WINDS ABOVE 40 HAVE LITTLE ADDITIONAL EFFECT.		LITTLE DANGER			INCREASING DANGER (Flesh may freeze within 1 minute)					GREAT DANGER (Flesh may freeze within 30 seconds)											
		DANGER OF FREEZING EXPOSED FLESH FOR PROPERLY CLOTHED PERSONS																				

Figure 2. The effect of wind on temperature. (From Air Force Survival Manual 64-3. Courtesy of the U. S. Air Force.)

fined in the unit known as the clo, which is equal to that of a standard suit that keeps the average man warm at 60° F. Unfortunately, standard clothing provides little protection from wind and wetness. So, for all-weather purposes, clothing is worn in closely-fitting layers with outer garments that shed wind and water, but allow egress for body moisture; wool garments that retain insulative value when wet; and inner garments that keep warm air close to the body. Footgear is insulative, moisture-wicking, and nonconstrictive, and the hands are covered with a mitten shell that reduces the surface area for radiant heat loss. Above all, the highly vascular head and neck are covered by a hood that can conserve up to 50 per cent of the heat produced by the body at temperatures below 40° F.

Shivering creates heat through phasic contractions of truncal muscles. However, intense shivering during overnight exposure can exhaust glycogen stores at four to five times the basal metabolic rate, and lead to metabolic acidosis, with only a 50 per cent net heat gain due to impairment of peripheral vasomotor tone.

Blood flow in the capillary beds of fingertips can be reduced as much as 99 per cent by deep vasoconstriction, which creates a distinct insulating temperature gradient between the body periphery and the body core. Additional heat conservation derives from the counter current heat exchange mechanism in the limbs, wherein warm arterial blood is cooled gradually by the surrounding venae comitantes.

From the standpoint of localized cold stress, the only protective mechanism for the distal extremity is the hunting phenomenon, a periodic vasodilatation that occurs after a few minutes of limb immersion at 59° F. (15° C.). Much of the flow is through arteriovenous anastomoses, and it becomes insufficient in the presence of hypothermia. Thus, the limb is sacrificed in favor of life, unless internal body warmth is restored.

Good conditioning, a large body mass, a thick subcutaneous fat pad, and acclimatization to cold are all protective against hypothermia and cold injury. Fat has one-third of the thermal conductivity of muscle; however, despite a greater body fat percentage, women are subjectively less tolerant to cold than are men. Certain chronically cold exposed peoples are said to possess brown fat, which protects the nape of the neck and is capable of thermogenesis. Most racial groups from temperate latitudes can acclimatize to cold, showing improved vasomotor control, more adequate periodic vasodilation in the extremities, and superior heat conservation in the body core, after a few weeks of chronic exposure. On the other hand, ethnic groups of warm weather origin have trouble acclimatizing. For example, Negro military personnel in Korean and Alaskan operations have been shown to be six times more vulnerable to frostbite than their Caucasian counterparts (Orr and Fainer, 1952). In addition, certain persons may have specific hypersensitivity or vulnerability to the cold, in the form of recurrent respiratory infections, vasomotor rhinitis, Raynaud's phenomenon, and cold hypersensitivity diseases.

ACCIDENTAL HYPOTHERMIA

Occurrence and Diagnosis

Accidental hypothermia is the pathologic state of a reduction in the deep body temperature to below 95° F. (35° C.), due to accidental cold stress. With continuing stress, this condition may be progressive and fatal unless body warmth is restored and concomitant metabolic aberrations are corrected.

In most cases, the etiology of hypothermia can be ascribed to one of three sets of accidental circumstances, from which one can better determine therapy and prognosis. First, there is the hypothermia of cold water immersion, which is the principal cause of death following boating accidents, and usually amounts to the brief but overwhelming exposure of an otherwise healthy victim. Second, there is the hypothermia of cold weather exposure; in this too, most victims are healthy, but they may be exposed for longer periods of time, in a marginal heat balance situation. Third, there is the hypothermia of cold stress among the aged, intoxicated, or debilitated, wherein the victim's condition impairs thermogenesis and heat retention, even under modest stress.

The diagnosis of hypothermia usually is made by taking the rectal temperature with a low reading thermometer. Few Emergency Departments have such a device on hand, so it frequently is necessary to use the thermoprobe device with the hypothermia blanket, which must be obtained from the operating room and calibrated with a standard control temperature before use. A weather thermometer is less precise, but can be used if a low-reading medical thermometer is unavailable.

Clinical Features

As the deep body temperature begins to fall, the healthy nonintoxicated individual undergoes an increase in shivering and vasoconstriction, and a general increase in sympathetic tone, with an elevated blood pressure, heart rate, and respiratory rate. Below 95° F. (35.0° C.), the shivering and vasoconstriction become even more intense, and fine manual dexterity for self-protective behavior, such as fire-starting, is lost. The victim appears well oriented and is able to maintain a normal posture, but begins to show apathy, poor judgment, memory lapses, dysphasia, dysarthria, and ataxia. Up to this point, the hypothermia is said to be mild and entirely reversible if the victim is insulated from further heat loss.

Below 90° F. (32.2° C.), the hypothermia can be said to be moderately severe. Full-scale shivering is replaced by marked muscular rigidity and stiff distal movements. There may be a glassy stare with marked obtundation, progressing to stupor. The blood pressure may not be detectable with a sphygmomanometer, but a strong carotid pulse usually is present. Breathing becomes shallow and irregular. The heart rate begins to slow and fails to respond to atropine, although a tachycardia may persist, and supraventricular arrhythmias, ventricular extrasystoles, and T wave inversion may appear on the electrocardiogram.

Below 82° F. (27.8° C.), the hypothermia is profound, with deep coma and rigidity. The EKG may show the classic J wave or Osborne wave notching at the end of the QRS complex (Fig. 3). Pulmonary edema with white frothy expectoration can occur, and there is great risk of ventricular fibrillation resistant to cardioversion, and of asystole and apnea. The lethal temperature can be highly variable, with survival recorded at deep body temperatures as low as 68° F. (20° C.). Among the aged, the intoxicated and debilitated, and also newborn infants, impairment of thermogenesis and decreased heat retention ability can result in death, even when the cold stress is modest.

As a cause of coma, hypothermia might be overlooked, in the absence of shivering. The presence of skeletal muscle artifact on the EKG and a cold feeling to the abdominal skin provide useful clues in the initial evaluation. In addition, the profoundly hypothermic state could be mistaken for death, since a rigid posture, bluish discoloration, and the absence of a stable cardiac rhythm may present an appearance not unlike rigor mortis. Under these circumstances, tissue oxygen requirements are greatly reduced and the central nervous system may remain viable over prolonged periods, despite poor perfusion, so that the only criterion for hypothermic death is failure to revive after continuous resuscitation and rewarming.

The rewarming phase of severe hypothermia is not just a mirror image of the cooling phase; it introduces the additional haz-

Figure 3. Serial lead II electrocardiograms taken during the rewarming process, showing bradycardia, skeletal muscle tremor, and the prominent J or Osborne waves, which are pathognomonic of hypothermia. With rewarming, there is a gradual emergence of P waves and a gradual increase in the heart rate. (From Fernandez, J. P., et al.: Accidental hypothermia. J.A.M.A. *212:*153, 1970.)

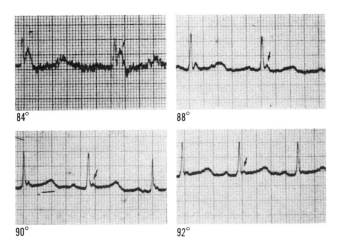

ard of circulatory collapse, or "rewarming shock," which probably is due to the combination of lactic acidosis, hypoxemia, dehydration, and an increased functional demand on the heart, in the face of myocardial glycogen depletion. Rapid active external rewarming exacerbates this phenomenon by causing premature perfusion of the cold periphery, leading to a central temperature afterdrop, with chilled venous blood returning to the heart. Passive rewarming sometimes can be accomplished by merely insulating the patient from further heat loss, supporting ventilation, and correcting fluid and electrolyte abnormalities; however, several hours are required, which further compound the stress and add to the risk period. Methods for rewarming the body internally, therefore, have proved safest and most effective.

Pathogenesis

With the hypothermia of cold water immersion, most people can maintain a normal body temperature in water above 60° F., and some individuals, such as long-distance swimmers, can tolerate much colder water. For victims of ship sinkings during World War II, immersion at 29 to 30° F. for more than 90 seconds was uniformly fatal, whereas immersion at 40° F. for up to one hour was fatal to only 50 per cent of victims (McCance, 1956; Molnar, 1946). More recently, it has been suggested that hypothermia, rather than drowning, is the more common mode of death after cold water boating and canoeing accidents; also that survival time might be enhanced by using the life vest and maintaining a flexed posture, if rescue is imminent, rather than trying to swim to safety. A cover for the back of the neck is thought to protect the hypothalamus from conductive heat loss.

With the hypothermia of cold weather exposure, collapse usually occurs about one hour after the victim first shows signs of exhaustion or obtundation, and death may follow as soon as one hour thereafter. In most cases, the victim's heat balance will have been marginal for some time prior to the collapse, and the exhaustion can be ascribed to prolonged stress, intense shivering, dehydration, and lactic acidosis. Predisposing factors include poor physical conditioning, fatigue, inadequate water and carbohydrate intake, poor judgment, poor survival skills, and inadequate preparation for wilderness outings. Consequently, this condition has been called "the killer of the unprepared."

With the hypothermia of cold stress among the aged, the intoxicated or debilitated, and neonates, exposure usually is relatively prolonged, and metabolic aberrations and complications may be quite severe. Although the great importance of temperature control for the neonate has been acknowledged, it has been recognized only recently that hypothermia is a common mode of death in the elderly who live in poorly-heated homes (Fox, et al., 1973). Besides the primary condition, causal factors may include trauma, cerebrovascular accident, sepsis, hypoxia, hypothyroidism, hypoadrenalism, poor nutrition, malabsorption syndrome, hypoglycemia, severe dermatoses, methanol poisoning, and overdosage of drugs that impair shivering and vasomotor tone, such as barbiturates, phenothiazines, and ethanol. This complexity of pathologic circumstances may make it almost impossible to determine if the hypothermia is the cause or the consequence of the coma, and this probably is the reason why the mortality rate for severely hypothermic patients in this category was 60 per cent, prior to the use of internal rewarming techniques. Even now, survival still may depend more on the underlying health of the patient, and on the nature and duration of the cold stress, than on any particular therapeutic modality.

Many investigators, beginning with Claude Bernard in 1855, have recognized a relationship between hypothermia and hypoglycemia, and it has long been known that intense shivering causes rapid depletion of glycogen in the liver, skeletal muscles, and myocardium. Shivering can be abolished by lowering the blood sugar with insulin, and can be restored by giving glucose, however, previous fasting and the withholding of glucose enhance the survivability of deeply hypothermic rats, possibly through influences on the end-stage serum potassium and pH levels. Consequently, glucose and insulin probably are best withheld from the deeply hypothermic patient until the body is warm enough to have a metabolic demand, and until the serum potassium level is found to be safe.

Thyroid hormone and catecholamines

are calorigenic, and cold exposure is a potent stimulus for the release of both; however, hypothermia and acidosis impair their biologic potency. Consequently, the presence of hypothermia poses grave problems for the hypopituitary, hypoadrenal, or myxedematous patient, during and after rewarming. Some clinicians routinely give thyroid hormone and corticosteroids to all comatose hypothermia victims, presuming that there may be a hormonal deficiency state caused by stress; however, assays of these hormones usually are normal. Of some historical interest however is the development of hypoadrenalism in the late President John F. Kennedy, attributed to prolonged cold water immersion.

Initial increases in the rate and depth of respiration during the cooling phase of hypothermia reflect an increase in aerobic metabolism, which may be as high as 3.59 times the basal metabolic rate. As cooling commences, the oxyhemoglobin dissociation curve shifts to the left, representing a marked decrease in the oxygen-carrying capacity; however, there is an increased solubility of oxygen in cooled plasma, so that the Po_2 may be relatively normal. With further cooling, the respiratory quotient may drop to as low as .32, carbon dioxide level falls, and hypoxia becomes the predominant stimulus to respiratory function. Consequently, oxygen should be administered to the deeply hypothermic patient only after ventilatory control has been established.

For a variety of reasons, prolonged hypothermia causes dehydration, electrolyte depletion, and prerenal azotemia. In most cases, there is a lack of thirst and no water intake. As cooling commences, fluid shifts from the plasma to the tissues, and there is a hypo-osmotic diuresis and electrolyte wasting, despite reduced glomerular filtration. After rewarming, there may be excessive potassium excretion, possibly due to adrenal hypersecretion.

Other postrewarming sequelae of hypothermia may include persistence for several days of the hypotension and J wave aberration on the EKG; the development of alkalosis and dyserythropoiesis, with a steady fall of the hemoglobin over three weeks; silent myocardial infarction; pancreatitis; septicemia; and neurologic syndromes, including peripheral neuropathy, amnesia, and exaggerated emotional responses. Some of these may be related to microinfarcts (Duguid, et al., 1961; Mant, 1964). Bronchopneumonia, with growth of adventitious organisms, occurs almost invariably with deep hypothermia, presumably as a result of injury to the respiratory tract. Early broad-spectrum antibiotic therapy and vigorous tracheobronchial toilet are indicated.

Treatment

As soon as hypothermia is recognized in the field, action must be taken to prevent further heat loss. Wet clothing is removed, the victim is placed in a dry sleeping bag, and external heat sources, such as the bodies of warm companions, are applied. If the victim is alert, hot drinks can be given, and isometric exercises should be encouraged. Frequent sweet meals are helpful, particularly when there is intense shivering, but alcoholic beverages in depressant amounts are avoided. If the victim is unconscious, litter evacuation is sought as soon as possible, and special attention is given to airway maintenance, ventilation, and resuscitation. Oxygen is given only in the presence of constant external ventilatory control (bag-valve or endotracheal intubation).

Two devices now in use by some mountain reserve groups assist rewarming in the field. The hydraulic sarong is a portable hypothermia blanket that provides ample external heat for the maintenance of body temperature during evacuation. The applied heat is controlled just above the external body temperature, so as to minimize the risk of rewarming shock. The heated oxygen breathing device uses an exothermic chemical reaction to heat inspired oxygen, and has the advantage of a central rewarming effect, but the amount of heat that can be returned via the respiratory route is small.

Internal Rewarming

Of the several techniques for internal rewarming, heated extracorporeal circulation probably is the most physiologic but least practical for Emergency Department use. On occasion, open cardiac massage and pericardial lavage with warmed saline have been necessary in cases of cardiac standstill or ventricular fibrillation that proved refractory to cardioversion.

Among methods more practical for the

Emergency Department, peritoneal lavage is safe and can be initiated promptly to effect critical phase rewarming, usually within four hours. In addition, there is the added benefit of the elimination of hydrogen ion through dialysis. Isotonic peritoneal dialysate is heated through a polyethylene blood warming coil at 100°F., and exchanged 2 liters at a time, every 20 to 30 minutes, with the object of raising the rectal temperature above 86°F. (30°C.) as soon as possible, to obviate the danger of refractory ventricular fibrillation. Care must be taken that the endotracheal cuff is inflated, as vomiting may ensue. Theoretically, central rewarming also could be effected with warm isotonic enemas in the field and in the Emergency Department; however, the rectal temperature would not be available for monitoring. Gastric lavage also might be effective, but neither of these techniques has been popularized as adjuncts to therapy.

Once the rectal temperature exceeds 86°F. (30°C.), a hydraulic hypothermia pad or warm water bath can be used to raise the deep body temperature at a rate not in excess of 2°F. or 1°C. per hour, at the same time maintaining control of the metabolic acidosis and electrolyte abnormalities. Ideally, the applied temperature is controlled about 5 to 10°F. above the rectal temperature, and the limbs are insulated or suspended out of the water so that a more central rewarming effect is accomplished. During this phase of rewarming, there may be persistent bradycardia, atrial arrhythmias, hypotension, and oliguria, which are appropriate to the metabolic state of the patient at low body temperatures, and frequently will correct spontaneously with full rewarming. The temptation for those inexperienced in the management of hypothermia to rewarm the patient faster, or to give vasoactive, antiarrhythmic, diuretic, or endocrine drugs, must be avoided, in as much as (1) rapid external rewarming may cause sudden shifts in electrolytes and acid metabolites, and (2) drug effectiveness depends on correction of the temperature depression and acidosis. In uncomplicated cases, a gradual regaining of consciousness and orientation, as the deep body temperature approaches normal, provides the best index to good therapy.

During stabilization and convalescence, the risk of rewarming shock gradually diminishes over the first 24 hours, and careful monitoring is continued with the patient at strict bedrest. The need for fluid, electrolytes, corticosteroids, thyroid hormone, insulin and glucose, vasopressors, and digitalization must be considered on an individual basis. Antibiotics usually are indicated early after a sputum sample, or the tip of the endotracheal tube is obtained for culture and sensitivity. Special attention is given to the treatment of impending withdrawal syndromes, since alcoholics or drug abusers might be more likely to develop hypothermia. With adequate insulation, rest, nutrition, and respiratory care, a considerable (if not complete) recovery from the pulmonary, erythropoietic and neurologic lesions can be expected.

COLD INJURY TO PERIPHERAL AREAS

Occurrence

Cold-exposed peripheral tissue may be injured by one of three processes. *Frostbite* is a refrigerating and ischemic insult to the tissue, from atmospheric or contact exposure at below freezing temperatures. *Immersion* or *trench foot* injuries occur less often, from the ischemia and impaired local energy metabolism attendant to immersion in water less than 50°F. (10°C.) for more than 12 hours, or from exposure to moisture at similar temperatures for more than 24 hours. *Chilblains* occur infrequently, as a chronic nodular subcutaneous vasculitis, usually about the pretibial area, from chronic or recurrent cold exposure. Of the three, frostbite deserves principal consideration as an acute traumatic event, most amenable to emergency treatment.

Clinical Features

Frostbite begins insidiously with paresthesias and numbness, as an extremity or exposed area of tissue begins to freeze from its distal and outer surfaces. Freezing that reaches just into the epidermis usually appears as a shallow blanched wheal formation of the nose or ears, known as frostnip or incipient frostbite, and disappears with contact rewarming, leaving only mild erythema. Freezing that penetrates more deeply into skin and underlying structures results in one of four degrees of injury, from which one can determine the prognosis and therapy.

Superficial frostbite is a part or full-thickness injury to the skin of an extremity, with additional damage to sensitive underlying structures such as nerves, muscles, and vasculature. It appears as a pale waxy area, with a doughy consistency to the touch. The injury is non-necrotizing, and the deep neurovascular dysfunction is for the most part reversible, so that edema, itching, burning, deep pain, and coarse tactile sensation return on rewarming, leaving a characteristic appearance from which one can assess the depth of injury. If the edema remains mild and the mottled cyanotic appearance changes to rubor without vesicle formation, the injury is first-degree, and only desquamation and transient swelling, erythema, and cold-sensitivity will be expected over the next few weeks.

The formation of thick, clear, or pink vesicles extending dorsally down to the tips of the digits indicates that the frostbite is second-degree; the edema gradually resolves and the vesicles contract and dry within two to three weeks, forming a dark eschar. The area looks necrotic, but the germinative layer of dermis is intact, so that sloughing of the eschar after four weeks reveals poorly keratinized skin, which is easily traumatized. Eventually, there is complete healing with partial regeneration of toenails or fingernails. Late sequelae usually include paresthesias, hyperhidrosis, and transient or persistent cold sensitivity, with reactive vasodilatation, tingling pain, and edema, to even the most mild cold exposure. Occasionally, edema of an urticarial type and systemic allergic-type sensitivity can occur.

Deep frostbite is a necrotizing injury to skin and soft tissues, which may involve the more resistant connective tissue and bone, in the full thickness of an extremity. The injured part appears pale and lifeless, and feels hard or woody in texture, devoid of movement or sensation. Deep neurovascular function is severely damaged or lost, so that on rewarming the mottled cyanotic appearance persists, bordered by the clear vesicle formation of second-degree injury. Deep swelling and pain develop over the next several hours, and small dark vesicles form over the next few days. As the swelling resolves, the formation of a thick gangrenous eschar within two weeks, and the occurrence of deep aching and burning pain in two to five weeks, indicate that the injury is *third-degree*, and some functional regeneration and healing can be expected. The eschar or carapace protects the underlying fibrous healing, granulation, and epithelialization processes, which usually require two to three months for completion. Pain, hyperhidrosis, and risk of moist gangrene are significant during this period. Trophic ulcerations, severe cold sensitivity, and arthritis may appear as late sequelae.

In *fourth-degree* frostbite, the entire thickness of the distal portions of the digits or extremity are devitalized and relatively painless after rewarming. There is mild-to-moderate edema, and gangrene is slow to develop once the edema resolves. Demarcation between living and dead tissue takes about one month, and spontaneous amputation takes at least another month.

Immersion injuries tend to be more diffuse than frostbite injuries, with ischemia involving the entire thickness of the limb. When severe, the prognosis is similar to deep frostbite, and the likelihood of amputation is high.

Pathogenesis

Freezing can damage tissue by disrupting enzyme function, by denaturing proteins, and by desiccating the cell through ice crystal formation in the extracellular fluid, which becomes hyperosmotic with respect to the intracellular fluid. However, it is a well-known fact that less specialized tissues can survive unquestionable freezing. Indeed, human extremities immersed in iced saline undergo skin freezing as the deep limb temperature drops below 50° F. (10° C.). After a few minutes, there is cell wall damage in nerves, muscles, and arteries, and the serum creatinine phosphokinase level rises. Nonetheless, the skin may recover unharmed as long as its neurovascular supply remains intact. By contrast, freezing below −5° C. (−21° F.) damages skin irreparably (Keatings and Cannon, 1960).

To counteract the desiccating effect of freezing, dimethyl sulfoxide, an experimental freely diffusing osmotic buffer, has been somewhat effective when applied topically to superficial frostbite lesions; however, this substance is exothermic when mixed with water, and its therapeutic benefit may derive from earlier rewarming (Wood, 1970).

Prolonged cooling, with or without freezing, also can cause ischemic injury as a result of arteriospasm and microvascular stasis. Numerous animal studies have shown that there is sequential arterial and arteriolar constriction; venular and capillary dilatation; capillary leakage; arteriovenous shunting; platelet, fat, and red blood cell aggregation; and thrombosis in small veins. When external warmth is applied, perfusion from deep vessels tends to return slowly in relation to the accelerated oxygen demand, exacerbating the ischemic insult. Rapid rewarming minimizes this discrepancy, and has been shown to be a highly effective measure for saving tissue and promoting recoverability. As such, it is the proved keystone for successful therapy, but the circumstantial delays usually encountered with the evacuation of frostbite victims often make rapid rewarming hard to achieve in the ideal.

Sympathectomy relieves arteriospasm, closes arteriovenous shunts, and promotes collateralization into the area of frostbite, but is a major surgical procedure that is contraindicated during the acute phase of therapy, because blood flow may be diverted preferentially to uninjured tissues. The intra-arterial injection of sympatholytic drugs obviates these problems, since it can be performed easily and selectively, and appears nearly as effective in saving tissue and promoting recoverability as rapid rewarming, in the rabbit's foot model (Snider et al., 1974). An immediate alpha-blocker, tolazoline hydrochloride, is mixed with a long-acting alpha-blocking substance, reserpine, in saline, and is given by bolus. The reserpine effect begins in three to 24 hours, and persists for two to four weeks. This technique has yet to be evaluated clinically in a controlled study.

Several other measures have been employed to enhance microvascular perfusion, but most, including intravenous heparin administration, systemic vasodilators, ethanol, enzymes, steroids, and flavenoids, have not proved useful. Antisludging agents, such as low molecular-weight dextran and experimental non-ionic sulfactants, may prove helpful with more clinical experience. Other measures to be evaluated include hyperbaric oxygen therapy and the use of aspirin.

Factors that predispose a victim to local cold injury include constrictive clothing; use of vasoconstrictive drugs such as nicotine; obstructive vascular disease; and an ectomorphic habitus. Mountain climbers face the additional stresses of evaporative heat loss, dehydration, and hypoxemia, and their injuries may be particularly severe, as are those suffered by victims of contact with supercooled metal or liquids, those who have superimposed burns or fractures, and those who experience rough handling of injured tissue.

Refreezing poses a great hazard to an extremity, once thawed, and almost certainly results in total tissue destruction. Indeed, many victims of frostbite have been able to walk to safety on frozen feet that remained usable and salvageable because premature rewarming was avoided.

Treatment

For frostnip or incipient frostbite, simple contact rewarming, such as the application of cupped hands to the affected nose or ears, is sufficient.

For superficial or deep frostbite, the yet-unrewarmed part should be immersed gently in a well-agitated water bath at 104 to 108° F. (40 to 42° C.) for 20 minutes, or until there is erythematous flushing. Pain may be excruciating at this time, and analgesia and sedation may be required. Ethyl alcohol may be the only sedative available in the field, and is useful for this purpose. Smoking is prohibited because of its peripheral vasoconstrictive effects, and constrictive clothing is loosened while general body warmth is restored.

The technique of rapid rewarming is feasible for prehospital use, if rescue personnel are properly trained and equipped to control the immersion temperature, treat the pain, and evacuate the victim gently by litter. This is particularly advisable as an alternative to prolonged spontaneous rewarming during evacuation. For field use, preheated water can be poured on to a wrapping of towels; however, special care must be taken to avoid overheating, repeated cold exposure, or mechanical trauma to tissues.

In the Emergency Department, thorough history-taking and examination will reveal the nature and duration of the cold stress. Rapid rewarming is completed, but the injured part is never subjected to repeated rewarming, even if it has become cold again. Early measures that might be undertaken include the administration of low molecular weight dextran, and the selective intra-arterial injection of sympatholytic drugs with radiologic and vascular surgical consultation—necessary for optimal treatment of this severe threat to limb.

The injured surface then is bathed in an antiseptic solution and cradled very gently in an open fashion, with sterile cotton between the fingers and toes. Care is taken not to rupture any vesicles, but those ruptured should be debrided. Gentle whirlpool treatments, with a dilute lukewarm antiseptic solution, are begun early and continued twice daily. These reduce the risk of infection, aid débridement, give the patient a sense of progress in therapy, and soften the eschar for physiotherapy; this should begin early, with frequent active mobilization of each involved joint, otherwise passive mobilization is required. Constricting eschars are bivalved, and the extremity is elevated frequently to minimize swelling. The patient is immunized against tetanus. Any blebs with the appearance of infection are opened, drained, and cultured, and antibiotics are used expectantly, awaiting culture and sensitivity. An immediate gram stain may be helpful.

Amputations, revisions, and dermatoplasties almost always should be delayed until there is complete demarcation and separation of gangrenous tissue. In this way, large amounts of underlying tissue may be conserved, except when early liquefaction or the development of moist gangrene or infection necessitate early amputation.

For the late sequelae of edema, hyperhidrosis, and pain associated with vasospasm, sympathectomy may be of value when symptoms are intractable. It also reduces moisture and speeds gangrenous demarcation, thus reducing the likelihood of infection during convalescence. However, the result may be impotence, excessive regional dryness, and failure to relieve that portion of the pain that is purely neuropathic. Temporary ganglionic blockade or sympatholytic agents may help in evaluating its effectiveness, and also provide an alternative to surgery.

The patient's diet should be high in protein and ascorbic acid. Alcohol is permissible, but cigarette smoking should be avoided. Occupational therapy is helpful in boosting morale and diverting attention from the injury during the prolonged convalescence.

COLD HYPERSENSITIVITY

Cold urticaria, cold agglutinin syndrome, and paradoxical cold hemoglobinuria are conditions associated with immunologic hypersensitivity to cold exposure.

With cold urticaria, wheals and generalized urticaria can occur in response to localized or generalized skin chilling, probably because of a skin-sensitizing serum factor. The symptom pattern may be familial, sporadic, or in association with multiple myeloma, cryoglobulinemia, or syphilis. Similar symptoms can arise from previous local cold injury.

With cold agglutinin hypersensitivity, intravascular erythrocyte agglutination results from cold-reacting antibody-erythrocyte attachment, and hemolysis results from the agglutination and the attachment of complement. A purplish discoloration occurs in cold-exposed peripheral parts, such as the hands, feet, nose, and ears, without the initial blanching phase that distinguishes Raynaud's phenomenon. Pain may occur with cold air or food intake. The anemia is worse during the winter, and general chilling with a sensitive antibody response can lead to sudden bouts of hemolysis, sometimes requiring transfusion. The spleen may or may not be enlarged, and spherocytosis usually is not seen. The condition may be idiopathic, possibly developing into a chronic disease in later life, or it may be induced by lymphoma or infections such as Mycoplasma pneumonia or mononucleosis. Diagnosis is based upon in vitro tests for agglutination, and management consists mostly of helping the patient avoid cold stress.

With paroxysmal cold hemoglobinuria, severe hemolysis can be effected by antibodies of the IgG type, which can occur with syphilis, autoimmune diseases, and postviral states. Treatment consists of antibody suppression, corticosteroid administration, and protection from the cold.

References

General

Burton, A. C., and Edholm, O. G.: Man in a Cold Environment. London, Edward Arnold, Ltd., 1955.

Carlson, L. D., and Hsieh, A. C. L.: Cold. *In* Edholm, O. G., and Bacharach, A. L. (eds.): The Physiology of Human Survival. London, Academic Press, Inc., 1965, pp. 15–31.

Gates, D. M.: Man and His Environment: Climate. New York, Harper & Row, 1972.

Kantor, F. S.: Urticaria; and Rosse, W. F.: Hemolysis Due to Cold-Reacting Antibodies. *In* Beeson, P. B., and McDermott, W. (eds.): Textbook of Medicine. Philadelphia, W. B. Saunders Co., 1975, pp. 117–9 and pp. 1444–5.

Accidental Hypothermia

Fuhrman, F. A., and Crismon, J. M.: The influence of acute hypothermia on the rate of oxygen consumption and glycogen content of the liver and on the blood glucose. Am. J. Physiol. *149*:552, 1947.

Gregory, R. T., and Doolittle, W. H.: Accidental hypothermia. Part II. Clinical implications of experimental studies. Alaska Med. *15*:48, 1973.

Grossheim, R. L.: Hypothermia and frostbite treated with peritoneal dialysis. Alaska Med. *15*:53, 1973.

Horvath, S. M., and Spurr, G. B.: Effects of Hypothermia on the General Metabolism. *In* Dripps, R. D. (ed.): Proceedings of Symposium on the Physiology of Induced Hypothermia. Washington, National Research Council, 1956, pp. 8–25.

Hudson, L. D., and Conn, R. D.: Accidental hypothermia, associated diagnosis and prognosis in a common problem. J.A.M.A. *227*:37, 1974.

Maclean, D., et al.: Metabolic aspects of spontaneous rewarming in accidental hypothermia and hypothermic myxoedema. Q. J. Med. *48*:371, 1974.

Mant, A. K.: Some post-mortem studies in accidental hypothermia. Med. Sci. Law *4*:44, 1964.

Matthews, J. A.: Accidental hypothermia. Postgrad. Med. J. *43*:662, 1967.

McCance, R. A.: The Hazards to Men in Ships Lost at Sea, 1940–1944. Medical Research Council, Special Report Series 291, London, 1956.

McNichol, M. W.: Respiratory failure and acid-base status in hypothermia. Postgrad Med. J. *43*:674, 1967.

Pugh, L. G.: Accidental hypothermia in walkers, climbers, campers: report to the Medical Commission on Accident Prevention. Br. Med. J. *1*:123, 1966.

Weyman, A. E.: Accidental hypothermia in an alcoholic population. Am. J. Med. *56*:13, 1974.

Zingg, W.: Accidental hypothermia. Can. Med. Assoc. J. *96*:214, 1967.

Cold Injury to Peripheral Areas

Busby, D. E.: Cold Injury and Hypothermia. Clinical Space Medicine, NASA CR 856. Albuquerque, Lovelace Foundation for Medical Education and Research, 1967, pp. 128–149.

Carpenter, H. M., et al.: Vascular injury due to cold. Arch. Pathol. *92*:153, 1971.

Duguid, H., Simpson, R. G., and Stowers, J. M.: Accidental hypothermia. Lancet *2*:1213, 1961.

Fox, R. H., et al.: Body temperatures in the elderly: a national study of physiological, social and environmental conditions. Br. Med. J. *1*:200, 1973.

Keatinge, W. R., and Cannon, P.: Freezing point of human skin. Lancet *1*:11, 1960.

Kimmo Kyösola, D. M.: Clinical experiences in the management of cold injuries: a study of 110 cases. J. Trauma *14*:32, 1974.

Knize, D. M., et al.: Use of antisludging agents in experimental cold injuries. Surg. Gynecol. Obstet., *129*:1019, 1969.

Lapp, N. L., and Juergens, J. L.: Frostbite. Mayo Clin. Proc. *40*:932, 1965.

Mills, W. J., Jr.: Frostbite, a discussion of the problem and a review of the Alaskan experience. Alaska Med. *15*:27, 1973.

Molnar, G. W.: Survival of hypothermia by men immersed in the ocean. J.A.M.A. *131*:1046, 1946.

Orr, K. D., and Fainer, D. C.: Cold injuries in Korea during the winter of 1950–51. Medicine *31*:177, 1952.

Snider, R. L., et al.: Intra-arterial sympathetic blockade in treatment of frostbite. Surg. Forum *9*:237, 1974.

Ward, M.: Frostbite. Br. Med. J. *1*:67, 1974.

Washburn, B.: Frostbite. N. Engl. Med. J. *266*:974, 1962.

Wood, D. C., et al.: Some experimental studies with dimethyl sulfoxide (DMSO) in cold injury. Curr. Ther. Res. *12*:97, 1970

C.   RADIATION INJURY

George L. Voelz

Management of ionizing radiation cases have been infrequent—virtually nonexistent in most hospital Emergency Departments. This is in stark contrast to the high public interest and concern over radiation as an environmental hazard. However, the likelihood of such injuries undoubtedly is increasing as the use of radiation sources and machines continues to proliferate.

Ionizing radiation is any radiation, either particles or electromagnetic energy, with sufficient energy to produce ions in matter. If the radiation passes through tissue, ioniza-

tion of molecules within cells produces immediate biochemical changes that may lead to more visible biologic effects later, such as the acute radiation syndrome, chromosomal aberrations, cell death, cellular repair, or malignant transformation. Ionizing radiations may be separated into two general classes: (1) *penetrating radiations* (x-rays, gamma rays, or neutrons); (2) *nonpenetrating radiations* (alpha or beta particles).

Penetrating radiations can produce damage through the entire portions of the body exposed, either whole-body or localized exposures. Such exposures occur from sources outside the body, such as x-ray machines, accelerators, or gamma sources. These are termed *external* radiation and have produced the majority of serious radiation cases. The nonpenetrating radiations produce their damage by either immediate contact with or contamination of the skin (beta burns) or by internal deposition through inhalation, skin absorption, wounds, or ingestion. Alpha particles do not have sufficient penetrating power to cause external damage, even skin damage, but are serious internal contaminants. *Internal* contamination is an important concern in health protection of radiation workers, but has resulted in emergency medical problems only in a few instances of maladministration of radiopharmaceuticals.

RECOGNITION OF IONIZING RADIATION INJURY

HISTORY

Radiation injury problems will almost always present with a known history of exposure. The patient usually will know that he was exposed to a radiation-producing machine or a radioactive source. Thus the estimate of damage and need for treatment is likely to be a more difficult problem than the initial identification of the diagnosis or the nature of the insult.

There is always an exceptional case to disprove the rule. Here the presenting symptoms and course must ultimately raise the question of radiation as a potential agent. Presenting complaints of flu (nausea, vomiting), mumps (swollen parotid glands), skin ulcerations, burns, or bone marrow depression have been noted when a history of radiation exposure was not known or suspected immediately.

ACUTE RADIATION SYNDROME

The acute exposure of the whole body or a major portion to a large amount (over 100 rem) of penetrating radiation results in a progressive series of signs and symptoms known as the *acute radiation syndrome*. A summary of the principal characteristics of the acute radiation syndrome after exposures of various magnitudes is shown in Table 1. Time relationships of the principal signs, symptoms, and hematologic changes are shown in Figure 1.

Initial symptoms of anorexia, nausea, vomiting, and fatigue occur within two to six hours after exposure. The severity of symptoms is variable, so that their intensity is not very meaningful. Absence of nausea and vomiting suggests a relatively low dose. The presence of fever, diarrhea, delirium, or hypotension initially suggests the possibility of a supralethal dose. Prodromal symptoms subside within a few hours to several days if

TABLE 1 *Dose-Effect Relationships Following Acute Whole Body Irradiation (X- or Gamma)*

WHOLE BODY[°] DOSE (RAD)	CLINICAL AND LABORATORY FINDINGS
5–25	Asymptomatic. Conventional blood studies are normal. Chromosome aberrations detectable.
50–75	Asymptomatic. Minor depressions of white cells and platelets detectable in a few persons, especially if baseline values established.
75–125	Minimal acute doses that produce prodromal symptoms (anorexia, nausea, vomiting, fatigue) in about 10–20% of persons within 2 days. Mild depressions of white cells and platelets in some persons.
125–200	Symptomatic course with transient disability and clear hematological changes in a majority of exposed persons. Lymphocyte depression of about 50% within 48 hours.
240–340	Serious, disabling illness in most persons with about 50% mortality, if untreated. Lymphocyte depression of about 75 + % within 48 hours.
500+	Accelerated version of acute radiation syndrome with gastrointestinal complications within two weeks, bleeding, and death in most exposed persons.
5000+	Fulminating course with cardiovascular, gastrointestinal and CNS complications resulting in death within 24–72 hours.

[°]Conversion of rad (midline) dose to radiation measurements in R can be made roughly by multiplying rad times 1.5. For example, 200 rad (midline) is equal to about 300 R (200 × 1.5).

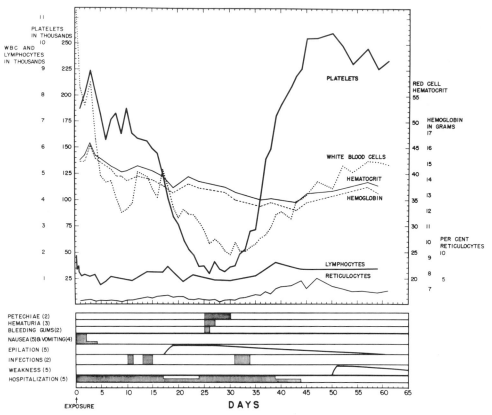

Figure 1. Average hematologic values, clinical signs, and symptoms of five patients exposed to 236 to 365 rad in the Y-12 criticality accident. (Courtesy of Dr. Gould Andrews, Oak Ridge Associated Universities, Oak Ridge, Tennessee.)

supralethal doses are not involved. There follows a relatively symptom-free latent period for a week or more; shorter latent periods are present after higher doses.

Skin erythema may appear within minutes to hours following a single large exposure, but it is not a very reliable sign in evaluating exposure severity because of variations with the energy (penetration power) of the radiation. If produced by penetrating radiation, serious systemic injury is certain.

An early and important clinical indicator of damage is the response of the peripheral lymphocyte count. If there are 1200 or more lymphocytes per cu. mm. at 48 hours after exposure, the likelihood of survival is very good. Lesser counts at this time suggest more serious exposures; less than 500 lymphocytes per cu. mm. at 48 hours suggests a poor prognosis. A fluctuating leukocytosis is present for the first few days after exposure.

LOCALIZED RADIATION SKIN BURNS

Radiation burns may occur in a localized area of skin as a result of direct contact with a high dose radiation source or exposure to an intense radiation beam. The possibility of a radiation burn may be recognized after an exposure, but in the absence of such history the presence of an area of burning pain without known cause is the presenting complaint. There may or may not be noticeable erythema in the area. The physical findings at the burn area are deceptively minor compared to the possible future injury.

Radiation burns develop much more slowly than do thermal burns. The severity of the burn may not be evident for several weeks. Erythema comes in waves during the first two to three weeks. Damage to the blood supply becomes evident over this same period, and after high exposures may proceed to ulceration, necrosis, and gangrene.

RADIOACTIVE CONTAMINATION

Radioactive material may be present on the skin or in wounds if the exposure occurs around radioactive sources, transportation casks, or industrial plant process equipment which are damaged at the time of the accident. If there is any question about the possible presence of radioactive contamination on the patient, a survey with beta-gamma and alpha survey instruments should be made.

Many radioactive contaminants are in particulate (insoluble) form which will not pass through intact skin. They continue to irradiate the skin (and body) until removed. Some liquid forms of contaminants may pass through the skin. Wounds or burns are a potential source of entry to the body for all types of contaminants. Inhalation and ingestion of radioactive contaminants are common modes of exposure. All loose contamination will transfer to other people, clothing, or instruments on contact.

The most important initial action when radioactive contamination has occurred is simply to recognize its presence before the patient or attending medical personnel begin to move around the hospital and "track" the contamination to other parts of the building. Even if the levels are not harmful, such movements make the subsequent radiologic surveys and clean-up procedures unnecessarily difficult and expensive.

MANAGEMENT OF IONIZING RADIATION CASES

INITIAL CONSIDERATIONS

The evaluation of radiation (alleged or real) injury requires an immediate assessment of the type of potential radiation injuries or complications—external (whole-body, non-uniform, or local), radioactive skin contamination, internal emitters, and associated physical injuries. This information is gathered by history initially. If associated physical injuries are life threatening, these should be treated first by conventional means. During these proceedings, information should also be gathered by both history and physical measurements to identify any significant radioactive contamination.

An important planned emergency procedure is to identify resources within the hospital and the community that can aid in radiologic assessments. The hospital list should include all individuals licensed to handle radioactive materials—pathologists, radiologists, and nuclear medical specialists. External resources would include local health physicists, medical physicists, or other specialists with training in radiologic health. The U.S. Energy Research and Development Administration (formerly U.S. Atomic Energy Commission) can be contacted to activate their regional radiologic assistance teams that are available for advice both by telephone and by professional radiologic assistance at the scene.

SKIN CONTAMINATION

Radioactive contamination on the skin usually will not be high enough to present a direct radiation hazard of any seriousness to the attending personnel. Attempts should be made to isolate the room and area so that personnel do not track radioactive material to other rooms. The containment and clean up will be markedly assisted by use of paper (kraft or newspaper) on the floor and radiologic monitoring of all personnel and equipment before leaving the room (area). Attending persons should wear scrub suits, surgical gown, gloves, and shoe covers. The latter are removed to prevent tracking when leaving the area. In a few exceptional cases, the use of respirators may be advisable to prevent inhalation of radioactive particles during the initial assessment and decontamination efforts.

The patient clean-up is usually fairly simple: removal of contaminated clothing, showering (if ambulatory), or washing skin surfaces with detergent and water. After each washing, the skin is monitored with survey instruments to evaluate the progress. If washing does not remove contaminants satisfactorily in areas that are covered with hair, clipping may be helpful.

Skin wounds require some special attention. Wash the contaminants away from the wound, if possible. Débridement of the wound surfaces may be necessary if particles are embedded. If the contaminant is an alpha-emitting isotope, measurements should be made by experienced health physicists since alpha particles have such poor penetration power that they are masked by any moisture, blood, or tissue. Special radiologic instrumentation may be used to advantage in these cases.

INITIAL MANAGEMENT OF ACUTE RADIATION INJURY

The most difficult part of medical management of radiation exposure is probably the evaluation of the degree of exposure and the distribution of the dose over the body. During the first few days up to several weeks, diagnostic evaluation and preparation for later therapeutic measures are the main activities, unless the exposure has been excessively high (supralethal—1000 rad or more). In the latter case, a constellation of immediate symptoms including nausea, vomiting, diarrhea, and shock will require symptomatic, supportive, and palliative treatment during what will probably prove to be a relatively short course—perhaps two to ten days. Treatment will generally require antiemesis, sedation, vasopressor agents, and fluid replacement.

No special therapy has been successful for local skin burns due to ionizing radiation. These should be treated in a manner similar to that used in thermal burns with bland ointments and protective dressings. In case of beta burns, surgical excision and fullthickness skin grafting is advisable as soon as the area can be delineated because of the prolonged, painful nature of the burn and the poor healing quality of this lesion.

The mild exposure case (less than about 125 rad whole body exposure) will require evaluation to confirm the dose, but will generally require only reassurance that no serious effects are anticipated and that treatment is not needed. If there is any concern that a higher dose might have occurred, the patient should be followed weekly on an outpatient basis for diagnostic hematologic changes during the first month after exposure. The individual can be advised that any slight statistical increases in risk of late effects, such as cancer or leukemia, that may be identified in large population studies are really very small incremental risks for any given individual case. On the other hand, it is prudent to advise males that initiation of birth control methods for several months is advisable in order to avoid any potential congenital defects in conceptions during this period. After several months, this potential risk is essentially back to normal and further precautions are not needed.

Those cases in the intermediate dose ranges (200 to 1000 rad whole-body dose) will require close medical observation and probably active treatment during the period of peak bone marrow depression at about 20 to 30 days after exposure. Because of the delay of these hematologic effects, the only initial treatment is symptomatic treatment of nausea and vomiting. There is need for prompt planning for future therapeutic measures that may be required. The problem, quite simply, is one of keeping the patient alive for five or six weeks until his bone marrow function begins to recover.

The therapeutic requirements will fall into the following areas:(1) control of infections—protection from exogenous infection by reverse isolation techniques or preferably "clean" room environments, use of antimicrobial drugs, transfused leukocytes, and immune globulin; (2) control of bleeding—use of platelet transfusions or fresh whole blood and protection from trauma; (3) rest, psychologic support, and other supportive therapy as needed. Heroic efforts to save the patient's life in suspected lethal exposures (over 500 rad) might include the use of bone marrow transplantation within ten days of the exposure, which is about two weeks prior to the period of anticipated maximal bone marrow depression. Cross circulation with a patient having a more nearly normal hematopoietic system has also been entertained as a measure that might be considered during the period of maximal marrow suppression.

Fortunately, there is a period of a week or more available to arrange for special consultation and advice on the necessary hospital services as well as time to move the patient to a hospital staffed to provide the necessary laboratory, bacteriologic, and hematologic services.

TREATMENT FOR INTERNAL CONTAMINATION

The treatment of internal assimilation of radioactive isotopes is similar to that followed when other toxic substances have been absorbed. The response will vary depending on the mode of exposure—skin absorption of wounds, ingestion, or inhalation. Irrigation of the nose, mouth, and pharynx; removal of gastric contents; and the use of purgatives can produce gastrointestinal absorption.

The exposure to certain ingested radioisotopes can be reduced by the use of chemical antidotes, blocking agents, and isotopic dilution techniques. Agents to consider for specific isotopes are: Cesium-137—1 gm. of Prussian blue (ferric ferrocyanide) orally (this compound is not approved for drug use, but has been used safely in humans); Iodine-131—3 to 5 drops of saturated solution of potassium iodide in water; Phosphorus-32—1 gm. stable phosphate; Radium-226—$MgSO_4$ (Epsom salts), 10 gm. in 100 ml. of water; Strontium isotopes—aluminum phosphate gel, 100 ml.; Tritium—force fluids to patient tolerance. All of these antidotes are most effective if started immediately after exposure.

There are no prophylactic methods for use after inhalation of insoluble particulates. Lavage of the bronchopulmonary tree has been successful in removing 25 to 50 per cent of inhaled insoluble radioactive particulates in dogs if initiated in the first week. This technique should be used only after careful consideration of the long-term risk of the exposure hazard against the immediate risk of a procedure. It must be performed by a team of specialists experienced in bronchopulmonary lavage.

The excretion of some radioisotopes can be enhanced (thus the radiation dose is reduced) by the use of a chelating agent that binds the nuclide into a soluble complex. The principal agent used clinically is the calcium salt of diethylene-triamine-pentaacetic acid (Na_3Ca-DTPA). The physician must apply for permission to obtain and to use it under an investigational new drug permit through the Division of Biomedical and Environmental Research, U.S. Energy Research and Development Administration, Washington, D.C. It has been useful for several transuranic elements—plutonium, americium, californium, and neptunium; rare earths—cerium, yttrium, lanthanum, and scandium; and zinc. A typical treatment regimen is to give 0.5 to 1 gm. of Na_3Ca-DTPA intravenously in 250 cc. of isotonic saline or 5 per cent glucose as soon after exposure as the treatment decision can be made. Aerosol administration of the drug has also been used experimentally and found to be convenient and effective. There have been no serious side-effects to this drug, although kidney irritation and increased zinc excretion are potential hazards. Routine clinical urinalyses should be used to recognize development of kidney tubule damage. This effect is reversible by reducing the dosage or stopping drug administration. This drug has produced teratogenic effects in mice and should not be administered to females when pregnancy is possible.

References

Cronkite, E. P., and Bond, V. P.: Radiation Injury In Man, Its Chemical and Biological Basis, Pathogenesis, and Therapy. Springfield, Illinois, Charles C Thomas, 1960.

International Atomic Energy Agency: Diagnosis and Treatment of Radioactive Poisoning. Proceedings of WHO and IAEA Scientific Meeting, October 15–18, 1962, Vienna, 1963. (For sale in U.S. through UNIPUB, Inc., P.O. Box 433, New York, N.Y. 10016.)

International Atomic Energy Agency: Manual on Radiation Haematology. Technical Reports Series No. 123, IAEA, Vienna, 1971. (UNIPUB, Inc., P.O. Box 433, New York, N.Y. 10016.)

International Atomic Energy Agency: Planning for the Handling of Radiation Accidents. Safety Series No. 32, Vienna, 1969. (UNIPUB, Inc., P.O. Box 433, New York, N.Y. 10016.)

International Atomic Energy Agency: Symposium on the Handling of Radiation Accidents. Proceedings Series ST1/PUB/229, Vienna, 1969. (UNIPUB, Inc., P.O. Box 433, New York, N.Y. 10016.)

Kornberg, H. A., and Norwood, W. D. (ed.): Diagnosis and Treatment of Deposited Radionuclide. New York, Excerpta Medica Foundation, 1968.

National Academy of Sciences, National Research Council: The Treatment of Radiation Injury. Publication 1134, Report of the Committee on Pathologic Effects of Atomic Radiation. Washington, D.C., 1963.

Saenger, E. L. (ed.): Medical Aspects of Radiation Accidents. Washington, D.C., U.S. Government Printing Office, 1963.

Thoma, G. E., and Wald, N.: Diagnosis and management of accidental radiation injury. J. Occup. Med. 1:421, 1959.

World Health Organization: Diagnosis and Treatment of Acute Radiation Injury. Proceedings of a Scientific Meeting Jointly Sponsored by the International Atomic Energy Agency and the World Health Organization. Geneva, 1961.

Andrews, G. A., et al.: Criticality Accident at the Y-12 Plant. Ibid., pp. 27–48.

D. FAT EMBOLISM

Leonard F. Peltier

GENERAL CONSIDERATIONS AND PATHOPHYSIOLOGY

Fat embolism is important because it is the most frequent cause of death following skeletal injuries and the fourth most frequent cause of death following vehicular accidents (Garden, 1972). Fat embolism is a pulmonary complication of injury to bone and soft tissue (Weisz, 1971). It usually is a self-limited disease that should end in complete recovery. In this condition, fat appears in the circulating blood, not in the fine emulsion of a metabolic lipemia, but in droplets large enough to occlude capillaries and arterioles. These fat droplets arise from ruptured fat cells at the local sites of injury, enter the vascular system by the process of intravasation, and are carried to the lungs where they lodge in the pulmonary vessels as emboli. Although fat droplets can be demonstrated easily in the circulating blood, the number of fat emboli in the systemic circulation, e.g., brain, kidney, etc., is very small compared to the number in the lung. The processes of intravasation and embolization begin immediately after injury and continue intermittently for several days. The extent of these processes is influenced by the amount of motion or manipulation of the injured tissue and by the degree of hypovolemia or hypovolemic shock. Therefore, careful splinting, smooth transport, and gentle handling, along with prompt and adequate correction of hypovolemia, are important steps in prophylaxis.

The mechanical blockage of a portion of the pulmonary vascular bed by fat emboli increases the resistance to flow, increases the pressure in the pulmonary artery and increases the work of the right ventricle. Engorgement of the pulmonary vascular bed decreases the compliance of the lung and increases the work of breathing. A change in the ventilation–perfusion ratio may occur. These changes begin as soon as emboli appear in the lung, shortly after injury. Hypovolemia or hypovolemic shock occurring concurrently reduces the effectiveness of the heart's response to a demand for an increased cardiac output.

The lung parenchyma produces lipase to remove the emboli. As hydrolysis of the triglycerides to glycerol and fatty acids occurs, a chemical pneumonitis results. There is an increase in the permeability of the capillary and alveolar cell junctions, with leakage of fluid and protein into the alveolar walls and into the alveoli themselves. Lung surfactant activity is decreased. Functional residual capacity is reduced, and there is a diffusion barrier. All these changes — (1) decreasing compliance; (2) increasing work of breathing; (3) changes in ventilation–perfusion ratios; (4) diminishing functional residual capacity; and (5) a diffusion barrier — promote poor oxygenation of venous blood and result in arterial hypoxemia.

CLINICAL PRESENTATIONS

Clinically fat embolism is a particular form of post-traumatic pulmonary insufficiency (Horovitz et al., 1974). It is seen particularly in patients with fractures, especially fractures of the pelvis, femur, tibia, and ribs. It occurs most frequently in patients with multiple fractures and crushing injuries and can be separated clinically from the other causes of post-traumatic pulmonary insufficiency by its classic petechial hemorrhages (Pazell and Peltier, 1972). It occurs more frequently in patients who have been hypovolemic or who have had hypovolemic shock. Patients with fat embolism usually have thrombocytopenia (< 150,000 per cu. ml.) and electrocardiographic abnormalities. Occasionally a chest x-ray will show widespread changes.

Of greatest importance, however, are the changes in the arterial blood gas concentrations. Hypoxemia (< 60 torr) is very characteristic.

Table 1 shows the problem list of a 27-year-old man admitted to the hospital two hours after the motorcycle he was riding was struck by another vehicle. Problems 1 to 4 can be identified by physical examination and confirmed by x-ray without difficulty. Since none of the fractures are open fractures there will not be visible blood loss, but swelling and hemorrhage in the areas of the fractures over the next 48 hours will seques-

TABLE 1   Problem List: 27-year-old Male

1. Fractures pelvis (3 rami).
2. Fracture femur, shaft, right.
3. Fracture tibia, shaft right.
4. Multiple abrasions and contusions.
5. Shock (BP 70/ − on admission), hypovolemia.
6. Hypoxemia (PaO_2 45, 24 hours after admission) inapparent.

ter at least 3000 ml. of fluid and blood. Depending on the severity and extent of the abrasions and contusions (Problem 4), a significant amount of blood and fluid may be lost into these tissues also. This helps to explain Problem 5, shock. In injured patients shock is almost always due to hypovolemia associated with blood loss, either externally, into the body cavities, or into the soft tissues. It is important to consider the extent of fluid and blood loss into soft tissues around areas of fracture, crushing, or contusion, since these losses frequently are underestimated or ignored entirely. The identification of Problem 6 requires measurement of the arterial blood gases. This procedure should be done regularly and frequently in every severely injured patient.

A review of this problem list 24 hours after the admission of the patient should strongly suggest that another problem, fat embolism, may be added soon.

DIAGNOSIS

Fat embolism occurs in patients of all ages (Weisz et al., 1973). It is not a rare or unusual condition. The diagnosis should not be made by exclusion or as a last resort; rather, it should be anticipated (Table 2).

Fat embolism occurs in association with fractures, usually multiple, of the pelvis, femur, tibia, and ribs. The significance of multiple rib fractures should not be overlooked because, in addition to furnishing fatty marrow for emboli, they cannot be immobilized effectively and may make respiration much more difficult.

Hypovolemia and shock accompanying multiple skeletal and soft tissue injuries in the absence of external bleeding are caused by the sequestration of blood and fluid in the sites of local injury. The extent to which this occurs is almost always underestimated.

There is a synergistic relationship between shock and fat embolism (Derks and Peters, 1973; Pazell and Peltier, 1972). Fat embolism is more likely to occur in patients who have had hypovolemia and shock for a period of more than six hours. The sharp drop in hemoglobin often associated with the onset of clinical fat embolism is a reflection of this untreated blood loss.

Since fat embolism is essentially a pulmonary complication, respiratory distress, i.e., tachypnea and dyspnea, is frequent. While its significance is difficult to evaluate at the bedside, it occurrence is an absolute indication for the measurement of the blood gases. We have not found changes in temperature (i.e., fever) to be a useful indicator for either the diagnosis or prognosis of fat embolism, although it is one of the parameters usually followed.

Disturbances of consciousness, e.g., confusion, disorientation, coma, and neurologic disturbances, are frequent in patients with fat embolism. In seriously injured patients it may be difficult to separate those changes due to fat embolism from those due to head injury. In general, changes due to fat embolism are diffuse, without localization, and may change quickly. Echoencephalographic and angiographic studies are normal. A frequent misdiagnosis is delirium tremens. The duration and severity of the neurologic disturbances is directly related to the degree and duration of hypoxemia. There appears to be no relationship between the severity of the neurologic signs and the prognosis for recovery. Any suggestion of a disturbance of consciousness in a severely injured patient is an absolute indication for the measurement of the blood gases.

TABLE 2   The Diagnosis of Fat Embolism

Clinical
   Skeletal injuries:
      Pelvis, femur, tibia, ribs
   Hypovolemia − shock
   Respiratory distress:
      Tachypnea, dyspnea
   Disturbances of consciousness:
      Confusion, disorientation, coma
   Petechial hemorrhages

Laboratory
   Measurement of arterial blood gases
   Platelet count
   EKG
   Chest x-ray

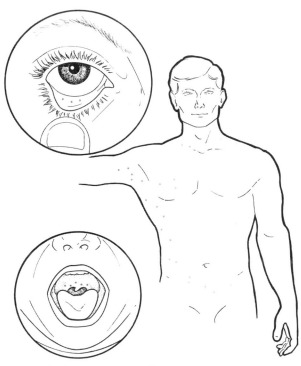

Figure 1. Diagram illustrating the usual distribution of the petechial rash seen in fat embolism. (From Peltier, L. F.: Fat embolism. Orthoped. Clin. N. Am. *1*: 13, 1970.)

The classic clinical finding in patients with fat embolism is petechial hemorrhages. These may appear as early as 12 hours after injury or as late as three or four days. They can be seen most easily in the axillae and along the flanks, although they occur over the entire trunk and occasionally on the face and extremities (Fig. 1). They can be seen in the subconjunctiva and over the sclera. They

may be accompanied by hemorrhages in the eye grounds. The petechiae come in crops and fade after 48 hours. The presence of six to 12 classic petechiae firmly establishes the clinical diagnosis of fat embolism. The petechial rash is not an embolic phenomenon but an indication of a general increased capillary fragility. This can be demonstrated by a capillary fragility test (Fig. 2).

The measurement of the arterial blood gases is essential for the diagnosis as well as the treatment of fat embolism. The end-result of the embolic process in the lung is arterial hypoxemia. This appears soon after injury and may progress or persist for five to seven days. In any patient with multiple skeletal injuries it is advisable to measure the arterial blood gases initially and at intervals of 12 hours for at least the first 48 hours.

Thrombocytopenia ($<150,000$ cu. mm.) is characteristic of fat embolism (Bradford et al., 1970; Pazell and Peltier, 1972). Although a portion of the decline in the platelet count may be due to the consumption of platelets in the normal clotting of the multiple hematomata and to the lack of platelets in old bank blood which the patient may receive by transfusion, the major cause of this thrombocytopenia is the consumption of platelets by aggregation around the embolic fat droplets. The platelet count may decline early after injury and reach levels of 50,000/cu. mm. Five to seven days after injury, there is a rebound phenomenon, and the platelet count becomes greater than normal. There is some evidence that the degree of thrombocytopenia parallels the degree of arterial hypoxia.

There is a high incidence (80 per cent)

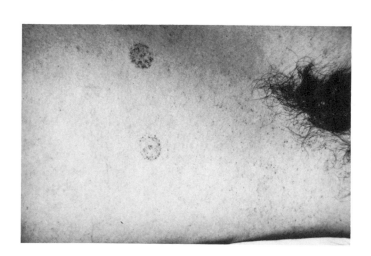

Figure 2. Typical petechiae seen in the axilla and on the chest wall. Notice especially how the application of the suction cup of the EKG lead has resulted in a shower of petechiae. This demonstrates the increase in capillary fragility associated with fat embolism.

of electrocardiographic abnormalities in patients with fat embolism. These are primarily changes indicative of right heart strain and are best appreciated in vector cardiograms.

A chest x-ray on admission is important because it may show pulmonary contusions. Changes in the chest x-rays due to fat embolism occur in only about one-third of the patients. They are characterized by a diffuse fine pattern of densities and are nonspecific. There is no correlation between the appearance of the chest x-ray and the arterial blood gases.

In patients with skeletal injuries: (1) fat droplets can be demonstrated in the circulating blood directly by staining methods and indirectly with a Doppler flow meter; (2) similar fat droplets can be found in the urine; and (3) an elevation of the serum lipase activity can be found three or four days after injury. All of these findings occur in more than 50 per cent of patients with fractures, indicating the ubiquity of the phenomenon of fat embolism. Unfortunately, they are of no prognostic value and do not give any indication regarding which patients will be significantly affected. Although interesting and useful for research purposes, these tests are not helpful in early diagnosis and management.

TREATMENT

The prophylactic treatment of fat embolism (Table 3) begins at the accident scene

TABLE 3   *Treatment of Fat Embolism*

Prophylaxis
  Prevention of shock:
    Proper splinting, careful transport, gentle handling
    Early and adequate volume replacement of fluids and blood
  Prevention of hypoxemia:
    Early administration of O_2 (40%) by mask or nasal prongs

Treatment
  Mechanical support of respiration with a volume respirator:
    Intubation, tracheostomy, PEEP
  Corticosteroid hormones in pharmacologic doses

---

with proper splinting of the fractures; continues with gentle transport to the hospital; and relies on careful handling of the patient in the Emergency Department during the clinical and x-ray examinations. These are important in limiting the amount of fat intravasating and in decreasing the extent of the hypovolemia and shock. Early and adequate replacement of lost fluid and blood is essential.

Since hypoxemia is the fundamental physiologic defect, its prevention by the early administration of O_2 would appear to be reasonable. We have observed that patients never allowed to become hypoxemic are less likely to develop serious pulmonary insufficiency, and for this reason suggest O_2 administration, 40 per cent, by mask or nasal prongs in the Emergency Department in patients with serious skeletal injuries.

If it becomes impossible to maintain a $PaO_2 > 60$ torr with 40 per cent O_2 inhalation, consideration must be given to intubation or tracheostomy and the use of a fixed volume ventilator. These should be operated with a tidal volume slightly greater than normal. The use of PEEP (positive end expiratory pressure) is sometimes quite helpful. There is no benefit in raising the PaO_2 above 100 torr.

In the seriously ill patient, when the PaO_2 cannot be maintained above 60 torr by means of a mechanical respirator and O_2 concentrations of 60 per cent, we would advise the intravenous administration of corticosteroid hormones in pharmacologic doses for a period of three to five days (Ashbaugh and Petty, 1966; Fischer et al., 1971).

While the intravenous administration of ethanol (5 per cent ethanol–5 per cent dextrose) for the treatment of fat embolism has been advocated in the past, this method of treatment has become outmoded. Ethanol is still used by some in the humidifying chamber of the respirator. The use of digitalis and rapid digitalization may be indicated in the treatment of those patients exhibiting signs of incipient heart failure and EKG signs of right heart strain. Its use is predicated on the support of the right ventricle which is working against a sudden increased load. There are no indications for the use of heparin or low molecular weight dextran in the treatment of fat embolism (Peltier et al., 1974).

References

Ashbaugh, D. G., and Petty, T. L.: The use of corticosteroids in the treatment of respiratory failure associated with massive fat embolism. Surg. Gynecol. Obstet. 123:493, 1966.

Benoit, P. R., Hampson, L. G., and Burgess, J. H.: The value of arterial hypoxia in the diagnosis of pulmonary fat embolism. Ann. Surg. 175:128, 1970.

Bradford, D. S., Foster, R. R., and Nossel, H. L.: Coagulation alterations, hypoxemia and fat embolism in fracture patients. J. Trauma 10:307, 1970.

Derks, C. M., and Peters, R. M.: The role of shock and fat embolism in leakage from pulmonary capillaries. Surg. Gynecol. Obstet. 137:945, 1973.

Fischer, J. F., et al.: Massive steroid therapy in severe fat embolism. Surg. Gynecol. Obstet. 132:667, 1971.

Garden, R. S.: The war of the roads. Injury 4:109, 1972.

Horovitz, J. H., Carrico, D. J., and Shires, G. T.: Pulmonary response to major injury. Arch. Surg. 108:349, 1974.

McCarthy, B., et al.: Subclinical fat embolism: a prospective study of 50 patients with extremity fractures. J. Trauma 13:9, 1973.

Pazell, J. A., and Peltier, L. F.: Experience with sixty-three patients with fat embolism. Surg. Gynecol. Obstet. 135:77, 1972.

Peltier, L. F., et al.: A panel discussion of fat embolism. Arch. Surg. 109:12, 1974.

Sproule, B. T., Brady, T. L., and Gilbert, T. A. L.: Studies on the syndrome of fat embolism. Canad. Med. Assoc. J. 90:1243, 1964.

Weisz, G. M.: The cause of death in fat embolism. Chest 59:511, 1971.

Weisz, G. M., Rang, M., and Salter, R. B.: Posttraumatic fat embolism in children. J. Trauma 13:529, 1973.

Wertzberger, J. J., and Peltier, L. F.: Fat embolism: the importance of arterial hypoxia. Surgery 63:626, 1968.

Wilson, R. F., et al.: Respiratory and coagulation changes after uncomplicated fractures. Arch. Surg. 106:395, 1973.

Wrobel, L. J., Virgilio, R. W., and Trimble, C.: Inapparent hypoxemia associated with skeletal injuries. J. Bone Joint Surg. 56A:346, 1974.

E. LASER AND MICROWAVE INJURIES

Leon Goldman

APPLICATIONS OF THE LASER

Lasers are used extensively in industry for metalworking of many types, for information handling in many diverse fields including computer technology and video disk communications, and also for monitoring of construction. In the military, lasers are used for ranging, communications, radar, and weaponry. An important use of lasers is the laser-induced thermonuclear fusion advanced as a partial answer (some years hence) to the energy crisis and also for use in weaponry. Related to this is the recent development of uranium enrichment by lasers.

These several applications mean increasing use of high- and higher-output laser systems or many types of lasers ranging from the x-ray region of the spectrum to far into the infrared zone. Increasing concern about exposure to operating personnel is therefore necessary as is, in some instances, exposure of the general public.

Fortunately, there is an awareness of the need for concern on the part of both industry and government. An example of excellent cooperative work is the recent American National Standards Institute Manual on the Safe Use of Lasers.

DIAGNOSIS AND TREATMENT IN MEDICINE

For diagnosis, laser radiation is used for transillumination of tissue, acoustical holography (where the laser is combined with ultrasonics), in the examination of infants and of the fetus in utero, and for the diagnosis of breast cancer. Lasers are also used for microemission spectroscopy, even at the organelle and cellular level, as well as for examination of blood and tissues for cations. In addition, laser communications and laser computer technology are used to provide better medical care through patient examination, information collection, storage, and retrieval.

In therapeutics, laser surgery is used extensively for eye surgery for diabetic retinopathy, detached retina, etc., and for investigative laser surgery. Laser surgery with high-output systems is still in an investigative stage, but is used in dermatology for resistant portwine birthmarks, tattoos, and various accessible cancers. Laser surgery is also used for the removal of burn eschar and immediate graft replacement, vulvectomies for cancer, in liver trauma, and in other conditions. It is expected that with the development flexible high-output laser systems there will be even more extensive uses for laser surgery.

LASER REACTION IN TISSUE

The laser reaction in tissue is, in brief, a nonspecific coagulation necrosis similar to that of an electric burn. In more than 14 years of research and clinical applications of the laser, there has been no evidence of carcinogenesis.

OUTLINE OF THE TREATMENT OF LASER INJURIES

ACUTE EYE TRAUMA

1. Consultation with an ophthalmologist is necessary in laser injuries.
2. Topical and systemic steroids, including Blephamide ophthalmic suspension.
3. Fundus picture and detailed description of the current injuries, if these occur in a large laser facility.
4. Repeat examination at least within 24 hours since most laser eye injuries usually will not be severe.
5. Chronic eye hazards.
   a. Possibly may occur from continued exposure to low intensity impacts; detection possible by frequent eye examinations.

SKIN INJURIES FROM ACCIDENTAL OR INTENTIONAL EXPOSURES

1. Acute. Treat as for electrical burn—in general most will be mild.
   a. Topical corticosteroids if mild.
   b. Topical antibiotics if indicated.
   c. Débridement, excision, and graft replacement if injury is severe.
   d. For contaminated wounds (infections from materials processed; radioactive compounds), debride locally and irrigate with saline. If radioactive contamination has occurred, suitable steps should be instituted.
2. Chronic.
   a. Bland creams to avoid dryness; no evidence of carcinoma, as yet, from chronic laser radiation exposure (no data yet on U.V. lasers).

RESPIRATORY SYSTEM

1. Acute.
   Evaluate the hazards of material processing as regards substances, industrial hygiene, etc. Therapy, local and systemic, should be directed toward the toxicity of substances inhaled.
2. Chronic exposure.
   Evaluate the hazards with laboratory tests and analyses of materials, pulmonary function, hematology, etc.

PREVENTION OF LASER INJURIES

1. A definite program of laser safety.
2. Protection.
   a. Area control.
   b. Personnel.
      (1) Specific laser-protective glasses for eyes.
      (2) Skin protection.
      (3) Environmental protection in material processing.

As indicated for material processing, eye protection should be considered for open processes and consideration also given to the production of pulmonary irritant or toxic materials such as phosgene from laser impacts on certain types of firebrick, beryllium from some alloys, etc. Treatment should be given for inhalation of toxic substances. In addition to the acute treatment, the patient should continue to be watched for chronic changes. Pulmonary edema may occur in hours depending on the nature of the substances inhaled.

If the injuries from laser occur in an establishment where there is an extensive laser facility, special forms must be used to record complete data in the emergency treatment. For example, in eye injuries the exact location and description of the lesions must be given. Here, a fundus picture will help considerably. For the skin also, if necessary, pretreatment and post-treatment photographs also should be taken to evaluate the type and location of the burn. In air pollution from laser processing it is necessary, again, that the patient be examined repeatedly to determine any late effects of such atmospheric exposures.

Patients should always be reassured that the laser is not carcinogenic.

MICROWAVE EXPOSURES

GENERAL CONSIDERATIONS

The immediate concern with an injury from microwave is eye exposure. Lens damage probably has not occurred in humans from cumulative exposure to low levels of microwave energy. Lens damage could not occur in a human from acute exposure microwave energy without severe facial burns.

The other area of concern with microwave injury is the exposure of the testes.

Harmful effects of microwave therapeutic diathermy develop from exceeding the recommended doses for such therapy. This may occur through error, may be intentional, or may develop in a treated area with reduced pain sensitivity. It is necessary that rings, pins, metal, and dentures be removed before these treatments are given. This precaution also includes metallic orthopedic prostheses. Microwave ovens, a spin-off from radar research and predicted to have a rosy future, will have few hazards if radiation is below the government standard of 10 mW./cm.² (to have 1 mW./cm.² 5 cm. from the oven when new and 5 mW./cm.² after use). Eye injuries and secondary virus infections may develop, chiefly through misuse. Some microwave ovens have been implicated in pacemaker malfunctions.

TREATMENT OF MICROWAVE INJURIES

EYE

Again, the same precautions are used for immediate treatment and follow-up care as with the laser, described previously. Be-cause of the danger of possible cataract formation from severe or unusual microwave exposure, the patient should be examined for a long period following exposure or accident, and the power density of exposure determined definitely. This subject of eye involvement, as indicated, is still controversial, especially with respect to occupational exposures.

TESTES

If there has been some concern about exposure to high-output microwave, even without discomfort to the scrotal area, it is well that, after a period of some three to four weeks, detailed examinations of the sperm be performed to reveal any late sequelae. Burns may develop from metal contacts on the skin by absorption of microwave radiation.

BODY BURNS

The treatment is that of an electrical burn.

References

American National Standards Institute: Safe Use of Lasers. 1973.

Appleton, B.: Microwave cataracts. J.A.M.A. 229:407, 1974.

Appleton, B.: Results of Clinic and Surveys for Microwave Ocular Effects. DHEW Publication No. (FDA) 73–8031, BRH/DBE73–3.

Goldman, L., and Rockwell, R. J., Jr.: Lasers in Medicine. New York, Gordon and Breach Science Publishers, 1972.

Goldman, L.: Applications of The Laser. Cleveland, CRC Press, 1973.

Moore, W., Jr.: Biological Aspects of Microwave Radiation. HEW National Center for Radiological Health TSB4, July, 1968.

F.   NEAR-DROWNING

James E. Gerace

GENERAL CONSIDERATIONS

DEFINITIONS

Webster defines *drown* as to "die by suffocation in water or other liquid." The terms "drown," "drowning," and "drowned" thus all have a lethal connotation. Near-drowning is the term used for a submersion from which an individual survives at least temporarily. In clinical usage, the terms "drowning" and "near-drowning" are modified, depending on whether aspiration occurred and on the type of fluid aspirated. Delayed drowning (secondary drowning; post-immersion syndrome) is defined as near-drowning with recovery followed by a recurrence of respiratory symptoms.

INCIDENCE

Drowning ranks as the third leading cause of accidental death in the United States, accounting for about 8000 deaths annually. Though all ages are affected, the greatest incidence is in the second decade. Drowning occurs most frequently in rivers and canals, with lakes ranking second and beaches third. The incidence of near-drowning is unknown but is thought to be greater than that of drowning.

PATHOPHYSIOLOGY

Hypoxemia is the single most important consequence of near-drowning. Its degree and duration depend on the duration of submersion and whether fluid was aspirated. Approximately 10 to 20 per cent of victims do not aspirate water because of laryngospasm and/or breath-holding. Although the PO_2 can rapidly decrease to tensions incompatible with life, early resuscitation can result in rapid and complete recovery. With aspiration of fluid, hypoxemia occurs almost immediately, is more severe, and more difficult to treat. Hypoxemia occurs because of shunting of blood through perfused but nonventilated alveoli. The major underlying mechanism of nonventilation of alveoli following fresh water aspiration is thought to be alteration of the normal surface tension properties of surfactant, with collapse of the alveoli. With sea water aspiration, hypoxemia results from fluid in the alveoli preventing ventilation. Reflex airway closure and a decrease in compliance occur in both fresh and sea water aspiration, and may contribute to hypoxemia.

During recovery from near-drowning, hypoxemia may remain while the patient breathes room air, even after the alveolar–arterial gradient on 100 per cent oxygen returns to normal. This suggests that areas of non-uniform ventilation or diffusion problems cause hypoxemia even after the absolute intrapulmonary shunt is no longer of clinical significance. This may result from aspiration pneumonitis, organization of proteinaceous exudate, alteration of the alveolar capillary membrane, or infection.

Acidosis is common following near-drowning, and may be respiratory, metabolic, or a combination. The PCO_2 can rise rapidly during periods of apnea or hypoventilation, and the hypoxemia that frequently occurs may result in the excess production of lactate. Usually the patient has been resuscitated and is either breathing spontaneously or being ventilated when blood gases are first drawn. Thus, the PCO_2 is often normal or low, while the pH remains low since the metabolic component persists longer.

Pulmonary edema is common in near-drowning, being reported in up to 75 per cent of cases with either fresh or sea water aspiration.

With sea water aspiration, pulmonary edema is thought to be due to hypertonicity, which results in a movement of fluid or plasma from the vascular system into the alveoli. Following fresh water aspiration, pulmonary edema appears to be due to injury of the alveolar capillary membrane and alteration of surfactant, both of which allow exudation of protein-rich plasma.

Although blood volume changes have seldom been measured in human near-drowning victims, clinical experience as well as laboratory observations indicate that sea water near-drowning can produce hypovolemia and even shock as fluid passes from the vascular system into the alveoli. Although fresh water near-drowning can produce hypervolemia, this is usually transient owing to a redistribution of fluid into other body compartments, including the lungs. Thus, either type of near-drowning can cause hypovolemia and may lead to hypotension or shock.

Cardiac function in near-drowning is influenced by hypoxemia, changes in blood volume and serum electrolytes, and acidosis. Atrial fibrillation and premature ventricular contractions are the most frequently observed arrhythmias. Ventricular fibrillation is a probable cause of death in some victims who die shortly after submersion, but is uncommon in subjects who reach a hospital.

Electrolyte changes are seldom of a magnitude to be of clinical significance. Although profound changes may occur acutely, spontaneous recovery usually is so rapid that by the time the patient reaches the hospital the derangements are mild or nonexistent. However, more caution should be exercised in patients with renal impairments.

Hematocrit and hemoglobin values

usually are normal in both fresh and sea water near-drowning victims, suggesting that most victims do not aspirate large quantities of fluid. Hemolysis, resulting in hemoglobinuria and hemoglobinemia, can occur following either type of aspiration, although it is more common with fresh water.

Renal abnormalities have been observed in both fresh and sea water near-drownings. These most commonly consist of proteinuria and/or cylindruria; however, transient azotemia and acute renal failure have been reported. It appears most likely that hypoxemia, hypotension, and lactic acidosis are the major factors producing renal abnormalities; however, hemoglobinuria and myoglobinuria should always be considered and treated if present.

CLINICAL MANIFESTATIONS

The predominant clinical features are related to the lungs and the nervous system. Respiratory signs and symptoms vary considerably in type and severity and include apnea, shallow rapid breathing, a substernal burning sensation, pleuritic chest pain, inability to take a deep breath, rasping cough, expectoration of pink frothy sputum, dyspnea, cyanosis, rales, rhonchi, and dullness of the lung fields. Pyrexia and leukocytosis are common and do not necessarily indicate the presence of infection. The chest roentgenogram is frequently abnormal, often correlating poorly with signs and symptoms, ranging in severity from patchy infiltrates to extensive pulmonary edema.

The most common neurologic findings are restlessness and lethargy, which usually are transient. Seizures occasionally occur shortly after the acute insult. Unconsciousness is fairly common although usually of brief duration, responding to initial resuscitative measures and improvement of oxygenation. In those with mild hypoxia, recovery usually is rapid and complete. With severe hypoxia prolonged residual neurologic deficits may result.

LABORATORY

Arterial blood gases constitute the most important tests following near-drowning and should be performed in all victims as soon as possible. The chest roentgenogram is a valuable method of following the course of the patient. It usually returns to normal in 12 hours to six days, and a worsening of the roentgenogram or the persistence of infiltration for ten days or longer may indicate the presence of a bacterial pneumonia superimposed on the aspiration. The electrocardiogram, serum electrolytes, CBC, plasma hemoglobin, creatinine, BUN, urinalysis, and sputum for smears and cultures should be obtained as early as possible and repeated as indicated.

TREATMENT

CONSIDERATIONS

Near-drowning victims require prompt and vigorous therapy. The physiologic derangements present and the type of therapy required are remarkably similar in fresh and sea water near-drowning victims. The most significant include lack of spontaneous respiration, hypoxemia, acidosis, and pulmonary edema.

AT THE SCENE

The single most important immediate requirement of all near-drowning victims is the restoration of effective ventilation. A delay in initiating resuscitation of only a few seconds may mean the difference between recovery and death. Mouth-to-mouth resuscitation should begin as soon as possible—i.e., in the water for those rescuers who are able to do so, and on shore for those who are not. Elaborate lung-draining procedures are contraindicated as they waste valuable time, are ineffective, and may induce vomiting. The mouth and upper airway, however, must be patent; thus, dentures, secretions and debris should be rapidly removed.

If there is evidence of cardiac arrest, closed cardiac massage must be given in addition to mouth-to-mouth resuscitation. Oxygen by mask should be administered as soon as it is available and in as high a concentration as possible. Mechanical devices, preferably hand-operated or controlled, can be utilized as soon as they are available. If the victim has been submerged or unconscious for more than a few seconds it is likely that acidosis is present, and intravenous sodium bicarbonate, 0.3 to 0.4 mEq/lb., may be safely administered.

EN ROUTE TO HOSPITAL

Therapy must be continued until the victim recovers or it is certain that he has expired. The return of consciousness and of spontaneous respiration should not lull one into a false sense of security. Although ventilatory assistance may no longer be required, it is likely that hypoxemia is present. Thus, all patients who have lost consciousness or aspirated water should be treated with oxygen and transported to an emergency department where a more complete evaluation can be performed.

IN THE EMERGENCY DEPARTMENT

Initial evaluation and therapy should be aimed at intensive respiratory care. The requirement for ventilatory assistance and oxygen will be governed by the clinical status of the patient and by the results of arterial blood gas analysis. Ventilatory assistance is generally required if the patient is not breathing, if the P_{CO_2} is greater than 50 mm. Hg, or if the P_{O_2} is less than 50 mm. Hg while on maximum concentrations of oxygen. This should be accomplished initially via mask: prolonged ventilation, however, will require endotracheal intubation.

Following resuscitation, hypoxia usually becomes the most pressing clinical problem. Oxygen should be administered to raise the P_{O_2} to 60 to 80 mm. Hg. This may require only a simple nasal cannula or a nonrebreathing mask or, possibly, a volume respirator and positive end-expiratory pressure (PEEP).

Respiratory acidosis is treated by ventilation. When metabolic acidosis is severe (i.e., pH below 7.20), bicarbonate (44 to 88 mEq.) should be administered intravenously. One should be careful in the administration of bicarbonate, however, because once proper oxygenation is achieved lactic acid is rapidly metabolized and the acidosis reversed.

Cardiac arrhythmias usually respond to correction of hypoxemia and acidosis: if not, they should be treated by standard methods. If shock is present, therapy with vasor pressors and volume expanders may be needed.

Pulmonary edema usually responds well to bed rest, oxygen, and diuretics. In the presence of hypovolemia the effect of diuretics may be limited. Nebulized 20 to 30 per cent ethyl alcohol may be used in order to change the surface tension of pulmonary edema bubbles. In the presence of profound pulmonary edema with severe respiratory embarrassment it may be necessary to apply positive pressure ventilation and PEEP.

The combination of pulmonary edema and shock presents a difficult clinical problem. In this situation treatment with colloids such as albumin or plasma is recommended in order to increase the intravascular osmotic pressure and draw fluid into the vascular system from the lungs. This therapy, however, is not without hazard, as in the presence of injury to the alveolar capillary membrane this material may pass from the pulmonary capillaries into the alveoli.

Electrolyte abnormalities are seldom of clinical significance, and the routine administration of saline to all fresh water near-drownings and the use of water solutions in all sea water near-drownings is not recommended. Treatment should be given only when significant derangements exist.

Convulsions and restlessness usually respond to reoxygenation of the patient. Should that prove ineffective, 5 to 10 mg. diazepam intravenously or barbiturates can be used as required. Cerebral edema can occur and may be treated with dexamethasone, 10 to 20 mg. I.V. followed by a maintenance dosage of 4 to 6 mg. every six hours, or by infusion of 20 per cent mannitol in a dosage of 1.5 mg./kg. body weight over 30 to 60 minutes.

Mild azotemia and proteinuria do not require treatment. Acute tubular necrosis is managed by standard means. Hemoglobinuria is best treated by maintaining an adequate urine flow.

Extensive hemolysis, though rare, may lead to severe anemia and is best treated with packed cells.

Bronchospasm, if present, may be treated with a bronchodilator such as nebulized isoproterenol or intravenous aminophylline, 250 to 500 mg. given over five to 15 minutes.

Bacterial pneumonia occasionally may occur in near-drowning victims, especially if heavily polluted water is aspirated. Although transient fever and leukocytosis are common, bacterial pneumonia is not. Thus the routine use of broad spectrum antibiotics in all near-drowning victims is not recommended. Antibiotic therapy should be withheld until there is definite indication, such as persistent fever and leukocytosis, the presence of a predominant organism on smear and culture, or clinical deterioration.

Although corticosteroids have been used in the treatment of near-drowning because of the inflammatory reaction that may be present in the lungs and because some victims aspirate gastric contents, to date there is no evidence that these hormones are of value in the treatment of water aspiration. Thus, in the absence of gastric aspiration, there is not clear indication for the administration of corticosteroids.

Intermittent positive pressure breathing (IPPB) may be of value in improving oxygenation and in preventing atelectasis.

In instances where large amounts of water have been swallowed, the stomach should be decompressed via a nasogastric tube.

COMPLICATIONS

POST-IMMERSION SYNDROME

The major complication of near-drowning is secondary drowning or the post-immersion syndrome. This has been reported in individuals who appear to recover from the acute insult and are allowed to go home. Respiratory symptoms usually begin within a few hours and are profound. The syndrome is most likely to occur following near-drowning in sea water or in heavily polluted water and is commonly associated with secondary infections. This is usually prevented by admitting all near-drowning victims who have aspirated water or lost consciousness to the hospital for at least 24 hours' observation, with monitoring of vital signs, arterial blood gases, and the chest roentgenogram, and by prompt treatment as previously outlined. When this syndrome occurs, the patients are usually sicker and have a lower survival rate than those who are immediately admitted to the hospital. With this syndrome vigorous therapy with all the modalities mentioned above, including antibiotics, is recommended.

References

Fuller, R. H.: Drowning and the post-immersion syndrome. A clinicopathologic study. Milit. Med. *128*:22, 1963.

Giammona, S. T., and Modell, J. H.: Drowning by total immersion: effects on pulmonary surfactant of distilled H_2O, isotonic saline, sea water. Am. J. Dis. Child. *114*:612, 1967.

Grausz, H., et al.: Autorenal failure complicating submersion in sea water. J.A.M.A. *217*:207, 1971.

Griffin, G. E.: Near-drowning: its pathophysiology and treatment in man. Milit. Med. *131*:12, 1966.

Martin, C. M., Barrett, O. N.: Drowning and near-drowning: a review of ten years' experience in a large army hospital. Milit. Med. *136*:439, 1971.

Modell, J. H., et al.: Blood gas and electrolyte changes in human near-drowning victims. J.A.M.A. *203*:337, 1968.

Modell, J. H.: The pathophysiology and Treatment of Drowning and Near-Drowning. Springfield, Charles C Thomas, 1971.

Moser, R. H.: Drowning: a seasonal disease. J.A.M.A. *229*:563, 1974.

Rivers, J. E. et al.: Drowning. Its clinical sequelae and management. Br. Med. J. *2*:157, 1970.

Rutledge, R. R., and Flor, R. J.: The use of mechanical ventilation with positive end-expiratory pressure in the treatment of near drowning. Anesthesiology 38: 794, 1973.

G. TRAUMA FROM ENVIRONMENTAL PRESSURE ALTERATIONS

George R. Schwartz

DECOMPRESSION DISEASES

Nitrogen-Related Disease States

PATHOPHYSIOLOGY

Humans exposed to gaseous environments containing physiologically inert gases (i.e., air containing approximately 80 per cent nitrogen) distribute these gases through the body in proportions that depend on the partial pressure of the inert gas and its solubility in water, body solutions, and fat. Generally, we are concerned with nitrogen, but in some artificial environments helium is used to replace nitrogen.

If environmental pressure suddenly decreases, nitrogen tends to come out of solution. If the pressure is much lower and the change is rapid, bubble formation occurs. Pain in the joints is an early symptom, owing to their sensitivity to internal pressure changes. Nitrogen bubbles may occlude the blood vessels of the lungs or brain. Bubbles within fat cells can cause bursting and release of fat into the circulation, compounding the problem with fat embolism. Air embolism (discussed subsequently) also may occur if the pressure changes cause disruption of the lung, and in such instances the nitrogen bubbles are of much less consequence than the lung damage and resulting air embolism, which may be rapidly fatal.

The degree of "bends" symptoms depends predominantly on the rapidity of decompression, the number and size of the bubbles, and the areas in which they lodge. A small amount of bubble development can occur with no symptoms. Physical activity increases the symptoms both in severity and speed of onset. This probably is related to increasing vascular turbulence and formation of vacuum cavities by muscle and joint movement. Individual susceptibility depends primarily on body build. Poorly perfused fatty tissues in which nitrogen has a higher solubility support bubble growth well. Therefore, individuals with more fat are more susceptible and develop more severe symptoms.

PREDISPOSING SITUATIONS

(a) Scuba diving with too rapid ascent.
(b) Flying in aircraft after scuba diving.
(c) Rapid ascent or decompression in an airplane.
(d) High altitude flying with inadequate pressurization of cabin and inadequate denitrogenation.
(e) Tunnel workers with too rapid ascent (caisson disease).

TIME COURSE OF SYMPTOMS OF BENDS

Most symptoms will appear within one hour, with onset in some cases within minutes and in others more delayed (Table 1). After three hours, very few people will get new symptoms or develop initial symptoms. However, if exposure to depth is followed by exposure to reduced atmospheric pressure, symptoms may develop as late as 12 hours after the dive. If symptoms are seen after 24 hours, the condition almost certainly is not decompression sickness.

TABLE 1 Time Course of Symptom Development in Bends

MINUTES	PERCENTAGE WITH SYMPTOMS
30	50
60	85
180	95
360	99

(*From* U.S. Navy Diving Manual 8:32–1, Navy Department, Washington, D.C., Sept., 1973.)

SYMPTOMS IN DIVERS COMPARED TO THOSE IN AVIATORS

In divers, the symptoms are somewhat different from those developing in aviators, owing to the increased dissolved nitrogen in the diver's blood and tissues in relation to the greatly increased pressure under water, as well as to the greater physical work usually being performed by divers. Decompression sickness thus is generally more severe in divers, and permanent sequelae are more common. In divers the latent period before clinical symptoms develop is dependent primarily on depth of dive, rate of ascent, and physical activity. Other factors also are important: for example, whether earlier dives had occcured that day and the amount of "surface time" between dives. Divers' manuals contain tables that coordinate the various factors and indicate safety limits. Particularly useful is *The New Science of Skin and Scuba Diving* (Association Press, 1975) and the U.S. Navy Divers' Manuals.

Bends. The characteristic symptoms (Table 2) involve pain in joints and bones,

TABLE 2 Type of Symptoms (Bends)

TYPE	PERCENTAGE MANIFESTING
Local pain—legs or joints	90
Dizziness (staggers)	5
Paralysis	2
Chokes (shortness of breath)	2
Collapse	0.5–1

worsening with movement, and usually not confined to a single site. The pain usually is described as deep and gnawing. Exposure to cold increases the symptoms. The pains disappear rapidly on descent, and return on immediate reascent.

PROTECTION

In situations of known predicted rapid ascent, protection against bends can come from denitrogenation prior to diving or flying. For example, exposure to 100 per cent oxygen for periods of 16 hours or more will reduce the incidence of bends to zero. However, even prebreathing with oxygen for one hour can reduce the chance of symptoms by almost 50 per cent.

DIAGNOSTIC TESTS

The history is of greatest importance in diagnosis. However, there may be some x-ray findings including bubbles in joints, bursae, tendon sheaths, or muscles. If there has been increased pulmonary pressure during ascent, mediastinal emphysema may be present and pneumothorax may occur. Ultrasound apparatus may detect bubbles in the vascular system. If rupture of the lung occurs, air embolism may result, with possible disastrous consequences as large amounts of air are released into the vascular space.

Chokes. Chest pain, cough, and variable degree of dyspnea are seen. The cough may be paroxysmal and is nonproductive. The pain may be pleuritic in nature, or sometimes is described as burning substernal pain. In advanced stages, cyanosis and syncope may occur. An additional finding is that of a fiery red pharynx. These symptoms are believed to reflect nitrogen "bubble" pulmonary emboli with pulmonary irritation and reflex cough responses. The possibility of fat embolization contributing to the clinical picture has been suspected on histologic grounds (Clay, 1963). If there is no evidence of lung damage (e.g., pneumothorax), air embolism is not a factor.

Chest x-ray, EKG, and auscultation are inconsistent aids. Rales may be heard and right heart dilatation may occur, although even with severe symptoms these findings may not be present. Chest x-rays during an acute episode have demonstrated right heart enlargement. Arterial blood gases may demonstrate hypoxia and hypocarbia with mild acidosis.

Skin Lesions. A pruritic, warm, painful, blotchy red rash may occur, usually on the torso, resulting from nitrogen bubble emboli in the distal vessels of the skin. During descent the lesions will disappear. However, once present, the areas again may become tender and edematous five to six hours after ascent. Small skin blebs that produce a burning sensation are a slightly different manifestation. These are thought to be due to nitrogen gas trapped in the glands of the skin. Pruritus may be an early symptom. The skin manifestations are themselves harmless, but if widespread may be a sign of impending chokes, CNS involvement, or cardiovascular irregularity.

Central Nervous System Manifestations. The CNS symptoms may range from mild headache to "staggers," delirium, and coma. Convulsions and transient loss of vision may occur, as well as signs of spinal cord impairment. The type of symptoms produced depends on the site of embolization and any reflex spasm that occurs. Some neurologic symptoms may take days or weeks to disappear. Permanent sequelae are not common in aviators, but they occur more frequently in divers.

On the EEG, irregular slowing has been seen when focal deficits from cerebral gas embolization are present.

Cardiovascular Symptoms. Cardiovascular symptoms include hypotension, bradycardia, syncope, arrhythmias, and even coronary occlusion. The presence of cardiac symptoms or signs requires continuous monitoring. *When death occurs in decompression sickness, it almost always is from cardiovascular disturbances.*

Delayed Shock Syndrome. Hypotension may occur, and in one to three hours circulatory collapse and pulmonary edema can develop. This is believed to be associated with loss of intravascular volume and secondary hypovolemic shock, coupled with increased pulmonary endothelial permeability and pulmonary hypertension. The proposed mechanism involves widespread nitrogen gas and fat emboli causing ischemia and increased capillary permeability. Local hypoxia causes release of kinins, histamine, and other vasoactive substances. The result is loss of fluid from the vascular compartment into the lung parenchyma and systemic vascular "pooling."

EMERGENCY TREATMENT OF DECOMPRESSION SICKNESS

The best treatment is immediately to transport the patient to a decompression chamber, where the total decompression regimen may take 24 to 28 hours.* The patient should be kept at total rest with 100 per cent oxygen by mask, at 5 liters per minute, in a slight Trendelenburg position, lying on his left side to reduce chances of gas bubbles forming a "lock" in the heart, which if present can seriously reduce cardiac output. Some authorities recommend the use of an inert gas such as helium with the oxygen to avoid oxygen toxicity, although some experiments have suggested that the nitrogen bubbles may enlarge during the breathing of the oxygen-helium mixture (Strauss and Kunkle, 1974).

Supportive treatment includes intravenous fluids monitored by CVP if a shock state is present. A vasopressor can be used to correct the hypotension resulting from widespread vasodilatation, but replacement of fluids is essential in view of "third space losses." Urine flow, blood pressure, and pulse should be monitored. IPPB should be used if pulmonary edema is present. Morphine and diuresis offer little effectiveness in this form of pulmonary edema. If transportation is by plane, it should fly as low as possible and continuous oxygen should be supplied. A cardiac monitor should be used during transport to detect potentially lethal arrhythmias.

If a decompression chamber is not available, the patient should be kept at complete bed rest, breathing oxygen by nasal cannula, and should remain in slight Trendelenburg position on his left side. Sedation usually is necessary. Unless symptoms are confined to joints and are mild, a cardiac monitor is advisable and respiratory function should be monitored by serial arterial blood gas determinations.

Each Emergency Department should have the 24-hour telephone number of the nearest decompression chamber. If questions arise, the Air Force School of Aerospace Medicine in San Antonio will provide 24-hour consultation.

---

*See U.S. Navy Divers' Manual.

Nitrogen Narcosis

Owing to the high pressure with underwater descent, increased nitrogen is dissolved in the blood. The effects of the nitrogen have been termed "rapture of the depths," descriptive of the development of an apathetic, slightly euphoric mental state. Mild effects may be seen at depths as shallow as 50 feet, and below 200 feet most people will experience significant impairment of logical thought. The phenomenon of nitrogen narcosis led to the growth of helium-oxygen environments for prolonged sojourns underwater, since a similar effect is not found with helium.

Where nitrogen narcosis is present, suitable action should include direct assistance of the diver by his companion, and the return of both to the surface using suitable decompression schedules. If possible, a fresh diver should be sent to assist.

Diving Accidents

There are two major types of diving units in use: the "open-circuit" and the "closed-circuit." The latter employs 100 per cent oxygen, and the exhaled gas goes through a canister where carbon dioxide is absorbed. It is dangerous because of the inefficient carbon dioxide removal with aging of the material in the canister, and the limitations on depth due to high concentration oxygen under pressure, which can result in lung damage.

The "open-circuit" uses a tank of compressed air, a valve, and a regulator which can be inspiration-triggered or of a forced-air type. These units need routine inspection and should be used only by those familiar with their limitations.

Although great fear is voiced about equipment failure, almost all catastrophes in fact result from human error, e.g., inattention to well known safety procedures, fatigue, lack of attention to time, and inadequate familiarity with the equipment. The most serious problems in diving arise from air embolism.

Air Embolism

When "skin diving," a lungful of air is inhaled and the diver heads for the bottom or as far as he can go. The increasing pressure on descent will decrease the volume of air within the lungs, and the volume will increase upon ascent. However, the volume will not at any time be greater than the original inspired volume. As a result, air embolism is not a danger in skin diving.

However, when diving with a scuba tank, a lungful of air can be taken well beneath the surface, and with volume increase upon ascent rupture of the lungs can occur, resulting in rapidly fatal air embolism. A quantity of air at 100 feet underwater will occupy four times the volume at the surface. Thus, when a diver ascends it is essential that he exhale continuously. The actual rate of volume expansion becomes more rapid as the surface is approached. Once the lungs are at full expansion, an additional volume change from only an additional 4-foot ascent is sufficient to rupture a portion of the lung. The exact damage can vary from a minimal pneumothorax and mediastinal emphysema to a total pneumothorax, with air in the arterial tree leading to cerebral air embolism and rapid loss of consciousness.

Treatment involves prompt recompression, as well as the other methods mentioned for air in the vascular compartment. A tension pneumothorax may develop and require immediate thoracostomy, or at least insertion of a needle to release the trapped gas. However, a simple, nonprogressive pneumothorax will respond well to needle aspiration. The needle can be inserted into the second intercostal space at the midclavicular line. However, a tube thoracostomy is the safest procedure in all cases and eliminates the need for repeat chest x-rays at frequent intervals.

EBULLISM

This is a syndrome of air embolism caused by exposure to altitude where the total ambient pressure approaches 47 mm. Hg (63,000 feet) or less. The result is not only acute hypoxia, but "evaporation" or "boiling" of body fluids, with widespread air bubble formation. Animal studies demonstrate vaporization at the entrance of the great veins into the heart, which causes blockage of venous return and a fall in cardiac output. Bubbles are widespread throughout the heart and arterial system (Dunn, et al., 1965). This is rapidly fatal,

owing primarily to cardiac and cerebral hypoxia. Lung rupture may not occur if the airway is open.

The ebullism syndrome is essentially untreatable at the present time, unless it happens accidentally in a vacuum test environment and treatment is instituted within one to two minutes. The treatment includes rapid recompression to hyperbaric levels. The body position, as for any air in the intravascular compartment, should be slight Trendelenburg, left lateral position. Artificial ventilation may be necessary, and chest tubes must be inserted if pneumothorax has occurred. Aspiration of gas is feasible from the right heart and can be done through a CVP catheter.

EXPLOSIVE DECOMPRESSION INJURIES

This sort of injury will occur almost exclusively in conditions of very high altitude flight or space flight, where the change in pressure is extremely large and rapid. Time of useful consciousness is less than 10 seconds.

TYPE OF INJURY

Explosive decompression can cause internal injuries to those gas-containing organs, owing to rapid expansion. Pulmonary damage, with hemorrhage and air emboli, can result. Tympanic membranes may rupture, and sinus pressure can cause extreme pain. The G.I. tract probably would not be damaged significantly, however, since severe lesions are very difficult to produce experimentally. There also is danger of injury from flying objects in this sort of decompression, and people have even been pulled out of aircraft through small portholes when a window was lost.

Blast Injury

High pressure blast injuries are produced by explosions or rapid decompression. The effects are primarily those of direct trauma related to the intensity of the blast wave.

Death results chiefly from disruption of the vascular structures of the lungs, with hemorrhage, hemoptysis, air embolism, and respiratory failure. Nonlethal blast injury will result in damage to the tympanic membrane and pressure damage to the hearing apparatus, producing hearing loss that may be permanent.

Injuries to abdominal viscera have been reported. Hypoxia and cardiac contusion can result in arrhythmias.

Brain injuries secondary to blasts have been reported with hemorrhage into the brain substance. Air embolism from the lung also may be involved in CNS abnormalities.

Injuries to the bony skeleton from blast waves through air or water are rare, unless contact is made through solid structures transmitting the blast pressure.

TREATMENT

Treatment of blast injuries should focus on the lungs and heart. Blood pressure and oxygenation should be supported. Chest tubes frequently are required because of hemopneumothorax. Hemorrhage into the G.I. tract should be expected on the basis of animal experiments, and CNS hemorrhage may occur depending on the degree of blast pressure.

PRESSURE DISORDERS OF THE EAR

AEROTITIS MEDIA (BAROTITIS MEDIA)

This is a noninfectious condition caused by a pressure differential between the air in the tympanic cavity (middle ear) and that of the surrounding atmosphere.

Ordinarily, the pressure is equalized in the middle ear through the eustachian tube. With altitude increase of approximately 500 feet, the air in the middle ear expands, and sufficient pressure develops to open the eustachian tube and allow exit of air. On descent, air must pass into this cavity through the eustachian tube. If there is edema of the tube, as may occur with upper respiratory infections or a mechanical obstruction, the air may not be able to pass back through the eustachian tube on descent. The problem almost always occurs on descent, as the positive pressure from the expanding gas in the middle ear generally can push through even an edematous eustachian tube. The anatomy

of the eustachian tube is such that air passage from the nasopharynx into the middle ear cavity is opposed in the resting anatomic position. Contraction of the dilator muscles occurs with swallowing, yawning, or a Valsalva maneuver, allowing opening of the normal eustachian tube. However, if this tube is obstructed, negative pressure occurs, and with altitude change symptoms of pain, vertigo, and tinnitus develop. If the altitude change without equalization is 2000 to 3000 feet, the tympanic membrane may rupture.

As a result of the relative negative pressure produced by deficiencies in middle ear ventilation on descent, negative pressure trauma to the tissues occurs with hyperemia, mucosal edema, and petechiae. There is outpouring of fluid transudate within the middle ear, which may be mixed with blood.

Acute barotitis media may occur when an individual has a respiratory infection, if altitude change is very rapid, or occasionally if he is asleep during descent. Once a substantial negative pressure has developed within the middle ear, the usual procedures (yawning, Valsalva, swallowing) are ineffective in opening the eustachian tube.

DELAYED OTITIS MEDIA

This usually occurs after breathing oxygen, which fills the middle ear cavity. As the oxygen is absorbed, negative pressure is produced and fluid accumulates in the middle ear. This normally occurs after sleep, and is felt to be related to decreased swallowing during sleep and a consequent reduced tendency to equalize pressure.

Clinical Symptoms—Acute Barotitis Media. One or both ears may be affected. Symptoms begin during or immediately after descent from altitude, and pain can be mild or intense. If the tympanic membrane ruptures, a sharp pain occurs, often accompanied by a loud noise and vertigo. Once rupture occurs, the acute pain subsides, since this disruption allows equalization of pressure and the membrane is no longer being stretched. Hearing loss of a temporary nature is present, usually first affecting the lower frequencies. There are initial sensations of "ear fullness" and pain; tinnitus and vertigo are less common unless the membrane has ruptured.

Otoscopic observation demonstrates changes ranging from mild hyperemia to redness and retraction of the entire tympanic membrane. A fluid level frequently can be seen that may appear dark because of blood. Blood in the external canal indicates tympanic membrane rupture.

In divers, there may be pain on descent as external pressure increases (so-called "ear squeeze"). In this case, ascent usually provides rapid relief. The tympanic membrane may rupture on descent if the eustachian tube is blocked, or if descent is too rapid.

Treatment

(1) Nasal vasoconstriction (with Afrin or Neo-Synephrine drops).

(2) Antihistamines (one to two actified tablets every three to four hours).

(3) Attempts at Valsalva maneuver (if the tympanic membrane is still intact).

(4) Inflation of the eustachian tube (politzerization) if such a device is available. Begin pressure at 20 mm. Hg and raise with 5 or 10 mm. increments. However, this is usually ineffective.

(5) Myringotomy. Gross blood should be drained, since, if a clot forms in the middle ear, there is danger of healing with fibrosis and permanent hearing loss.*

(6) Antibiotics may be used, although their efficacy has not been demonstrated. If the purpose is to prevent secondary infection, an antibiotic with good sinus penetration and a broad spectrum (such as ampicillin) should be used. The basic condition, however, is noninfectious initially.

(7) The presence of a ruptured tympanic membrane requires no additional treatment, although the patient should be advised against putting anything in his ear canal, and swimming is interdicted until healing occurs (usually three weeks). In rare instances or with large defects, the membrane may not heal. In large tears of the tympanic membrane, otolaryngologic consultation is necessary and a repair can be performed. However, the morbidity from a chronic perforation may be minimal, and in fact, when there is congenital narrowing of the eustachian tube, a persistent perforation offers sustained relief. This, of course, is the basis for tube insertion in children with chronic otitis media.

---

*See Otolaryngologic Procedures, page 427.

SINUS DISORDERS

AEROSINUSITIS (OR BAROSINUSITIS)

This is caused by the differential in pressure between the sinuses and the external environment when sinus ostia are obstructed, and it usually affects the frontal or maxillary sinuses. Since air cannot leave or enter, pain may occur both on ascent and on descent. Radiographic diagnosis can be made with a Waters view of the maxillary sinus showing an air fluid level in the antrum. Frontal sinusitis also may be seen on this x-ray, and if present requires more vigorous therapy owing to the rare, but lethal, situation of extension of infection and cavernous vein thrombosis. Pre-existing sinus infection commonly is present. Initial symptoms include pain over the sinus and severe headache, often accompanied by increased lacrimation. Occasionally, tooth pain may be the presenting symptom, and sinusitis must be differentiated from barodontalgia in such instances.

Treatment

(1) Use of vaporizer.

(2) Antihistamines.

(3) Nasal vasoconstrictor (Neo-Synephrine or Afrin).

(4) Antibiotics systemically (broad-spectrum).

(5) Control of pain.

If infected fluid persists in the sinus, a drainage procedure is needed and otolaryngologic consultation is necessary.

BARODONTALGIA

This is acute dental pain that occurs more on ascent than descent, and is related to trapped air expanding in the tooth. This symptom indicates pre-existing dental disease. It may occur soon after a filling is inserted, or it may indicate other problems such as a periapical abscess.

Treatment

(1) Analgesia.

(2) Incision and drainage of abscess if present.

(3) Dental consultation.

DISEASES WORSENED BY ALTITUDE CHANGES

Some diseases may be aggravated by altitude and pressure changes, and rapid changes can precipitate a severe life-threatening crisis.

For example, in bullous emphysema, increase in altitude can lead to rupture of a bleb and pneumothorax. After any procedure that allows air into a closed space (e.g., abdominal surgery, pneumoencephalography, cystoscopy, etc.), reduced pressure will cause expansion of the air, with symptoms of pain and signs of distention.

Abdominal cramps are common with ascent because of the expansion of colonic gas. Generally, relief occurs with passage of flatus or redistribution of gas in the colon.

A rare occurrence involves air in a closed space abscess (e.g., amebic), and symptoms are produced by increasing altitude.

ACUTE AIR SICKNESS

Air sickness ("motion sickness," "sea sickness") generally is not due to barometric pressure changes, although it may be worsened by pressure within the ear. The problem stems from the labyrinth, and individual susceptibility is variable.

The best treatment is removal of the stimulus. If this is not possible, a substance such as Dramamine, 50 mg. orally, may be used. Military testing for the space program showed that, in the absence of organic disease, the most effective motion sickness remedy was scopolamine, 0.3 mg. or 0.6 mg., taken with dextroamphetamine, 5 mg. or 10 mg., an hour before flight.

REDUCED PRESSURE DISEASES RELATED TO OXYGEN

Any pulmonary difficulty may be worsened by altitude (even at 5000 or 10,000 feet), and marginally compensated patients can become cyanotic. Treatment is that for acute respiratory failure. Oxygen should be given with caution at low flow (2 to 3 liters per minute by mask). Arterial blood gases are a valuable guide to further use of oxygen. If decompensation is severe, the patient should be transported to a sea level environment accompanied by medical personnel who can provide supplemental oxygen during the trip; when there is insensitivity to carbon dioxide, as in severe chronic lung disease, artificial ventilation may be needed to maintain adequate oxygenation.

References

Association Press: The New Science of Skin and Scuba Diving. Association Press, New York, 1974.

Beard, S. E., et al.: Comparison of helium and nitrogen in production of bends in simulated orbital flights, Aerosp. Med. 38:331, 1961.

Behnke, A. R.: Decompression Sickness Following Exposure to High Pressures. In Fulton, J. G. (ed.): Decompression Sickness. Philadelphia, W. B. Saunders Co., 1951, pp. 53–89.

Burkhardt, W. L., Adler, H., and Thonetz, A. T.: A roentgenographic study of bends and chokes at altitudes. J. Aviation Med. 17:462, 1946.

Clamann, H. G.: Decompression Sickness. In Armstrong, H. G. (ed.): Aerospace Medicine. Baltimore, Williams & Wilkins, Co., 1961, pp. 175–188.

Clay, J. R.: Histopathology of experimental decompression sickness. Aerosp. Med. 34:1107, 1963.

Cryssanthou, C., et al.: Studies on dysbarism influence or bradykinin and bradykinin antagonists on decompression sickness in mice. Aerosp. Med. 35:741, 1964.

Degner, E. A., Ikels, K. G., and Allen, T. H.: Dissolved nitrogen and bends in oxygen-nitrogen mixtures during exercise at decreased pressures. Aerosp. Med. 36:418, 1965.

Dunn, J. E., II, et al.: Experimental animal decompressions to less than 2 mm. Hg absolute (pathologic effects). Aerosp. Med. 36:725, 1965.

Flinn, D. E., and Womack, G. J.: Neurological manifestations of dysbarism: a review and report of a case with multiple episodes. Aerosp. Med. 36:418, 1965.

Gribble, M.De G.: A comparison of the "high altitude" and "high pressure" syndromes of decompression sickness. Br. J. Ind. Med. 17:181, 1960.

Harvey, E. N.: Decompression sickness and bubble formation in blood and tissues. Bull N.Y. Acad. Med. 21:505, 1965.

Haymaker, W., and Johnson, A. D.: Pathology of decompression sickness: a comparison of the lesions in airmen with those in caisson workers and divers. Milit. Med. 117:285, 1965.

Jones, H. B.: Gas Exchange and Blood-tissue Perfusion Factors in Various Body Tissues in Decompression Sickness. In Fulton, J. F. (ed.): Decompression Sickness. Philadelphia, W. B. Saunders Co., 1951, pp. 278–321.

Lewis, S. T.: Decompression sickness in USAF operation flying, 1968–1971. Aerosp. Med. 43:11, 1261, 1972.

Millen, E. J., et al.: Circulatory adaptation to diving in the freshwater turtle. Science 145:591, 1964.

Nims, L. F.: Environmental Factors Affecting Decompression Sickness. In Fulton, J. F. (ed.): Decompression Sickness. Philadelphia, W. B. Saunders Co., 1951, pp. 192–222.

Powell, M. R.: Gas phase separation following decompression in asymptomatic rats. Visual and ultrasound monitoring. Aerosp. Med. 43:1240, 1972.

Rait, W. L.: The etiology of post decompression shock in air-crewmen. Armed Forces Med. J. 10:790, 1959.

Robin, D. E.: Of seals and mitochondria. N. Engl. J. Med. 275:646, 1966.

Roth, E. M.: Space Atmospheres. NASA Sp-117. NASA, Washington, D.C., 1966.

Roth, E. M.: Gas physiology in space operations. N. Engl. J. Med. 275:3, 144, 1966.

Rumbaugh, D. M., and Ternes, J. W.: Learning set performance of squirrel monkeys after rapid decompression to vacuum. Aerosp. Med. 36(1):8, 1965.

Schreiner, H. R., and Kelley, P. L.: Underwater Physiology. *In* Lambertson, C. J. (ed.): Third Symposium on Underwater Physiology, March, 1966. Baltimore, Williams & Wilkins Co., 1967, pp. 275–299.

Strauss, R. H., and Kunkle, T. D.: Isobaric bubble growth: a consequence of altering atmospheric gas. Science *186*:443, 1974.

U.S. Navy Divers' Manual: Navy Department, Washington, D.C., 1973.

Whilten, R. H.: Scotoma as a complication of decompression sickness. Arch. Ophthalmol. *36*:220, 1946.

Womack, G. J.: Evidence for the cerebral vasoconstrictor effects of breathing 100% O$_2$. Aerosp. Med. 32:328, 1961.

H.   TOXIC BITES AND STINGS

Loren A. Johnson

Few subjects in medicine have inspired as many superstitions, phobias, and harmful cures as the bites and stings of venomous animals. Snakes have been regarded as products of satanic transformation, "cursed above every beast" (Genesis 3:14). Along with other venomous land and sea creatures, they have been thought to be endowed with great supernatural power, in aboriginal as well as modern cultures. Only with the development of modern animal toxicology are we able to understand these injuries for what they are, some unique to certain species, and others characteristic of large phylogenic groups.

In his classic survey of county coroners throughout the U.S. between 1950 and 1959, Parrish reported 460 deaths due to venomous animals: 50 per cent from insect stings, 30 per cent from snake bites, 14 per cent from spider bites, and 6 per cent from a variety of others. Proportionate attention is hereby given to the recognition and treatment of bites and stings by endemic species. For injuries by nonendemic species, advice and antivenin can be obtained from research institutions and zoologic gardens through referral by poison control centers.

ARTHROPOD BITES AND STINGS

Spiders, Scorpions, and Centipedes (Class Arachnida); Stinging Insects (Order Hymenoptera); Ectoparasites; and Caterpillars

TYPICAL PRESENTATIONS

A house painter enters the Emergency Department eight hours after being bitten by a plain brown spider. There is a small ischemic plaque with surrounding pain, itching, and erythema.

A middle-aged housewife presents after being bitten on the neck by a black spider. There is right-sided neck pain and swelling, and myalgias and spasms of the abdominal muscles. The blood pressure is 260/140 mm. Hg, and there is no prior history of hypertension.

A child is brought in two hours after being stung on the hand by a scorpion. She has marked local edema, excessive salivation, and opisthotonus.

A hiker with a past history of Hymenoptera allergy presents with facial swelling, stridor, cyanosis, and a blood pressure of 60/40 mm. Hg.

A child enters with multiple wheal formations and retained honey bee stingers.

A gardener walks into the Emergency Department with a swollen hand.

These are some of the widely varying injuries caused by the arthropods, a phylum of "bugs" with multijointed feet, which includes a great variety of venomous forms. Often, the difference between primary toxicity, immediate hypersensitivity, delayed hypersensitivity, and infection may be ill-defined, and the suspect arthropod may go unseen or incorrectly identified. Thus, special attention must be given to its pathogenic habits, to the clinical presentation and pattern of lesions, and to a careful search for retained arthropod parts, before a rational diagnosis can be established.

Arachnid Injuries

BROWN SPIDER BITE

Most spiders are venomous but timid, seldom capable of penetrating the skin with

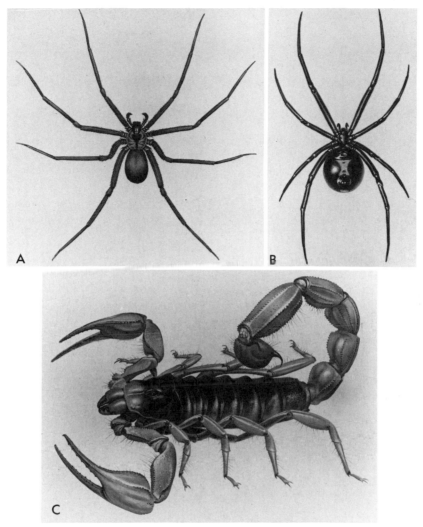

Figure 1. A, Brown recluse spider: *Loxosceles reclusa* (violin on dorsal surface; × 1.5). B, Black widow spider: *Latrodectus mactans* (hour glass on ventral surface; × 1.5). C, Hairy scorpion: *Hadrurus arizonensis* (shown actual size). (Courtesy of Frazier, C. A.; reproduced by permission of Merck Sharp & Dohme, Division of Merck & Co., Inc.)

their fanglike chelicerae, and seldom biting unless squeezed or threatened. Brown spiders (Fig. 1, A) of the genus Loxosceles are common to outbuildings and storage areas throughout the warmer parts of the U.S., and low-grade cases of necrotic arachnidism caused by this group are probably common, owing to the high frequency of exposure. Serious cases are limited to bites by the brown recluse or fiddle-back species (*L. reclusa*), a spindly drab spider with a violin-shaped marking oriented backward on its dorsal cephalothorax, which is endemic to the South Central U.S. and portions of the Southeast. Although the very dangerous

South American brown spider *(L. laeta)* can be found in Southern California, no serious injuries have been reported there.

Loxosceles venom contains several enzyme fractions that cause microvascular injury, microthrombus formation, and necrosis of subcutaneous tissue. Rarely, the underlying fascia, tendons, and muscle may be involved. There is a mild sting with the bite, and pain spreads regionally in a few hours. The wound itches, becomes red with a blanched center, and forms a vesicle. It may stabilize at this stage or show impending necrosis, with central ecchymosis and surrounding blanching, overlying a firmly indurated plaque. There may be extensive erythema and regional lymphangitis, and a scarlatinaform rash can occur. By five days the expanding ecchymosis blackens in a stellate shape, and by two to four weeks the entire necrotic area demarcates and the central eschar sloughs, leaving an indurated ulcer with undermined edges. Areas with a thick subcutaneous fat pad are prone to the formation of large ulcers and microabscess formation and poor healing. Throughout the ischemic period a systemic reaction can occur with headache, fever, weakness, chills, nausea, malaise, purpura, and leukocytosis. Hemolytic reactions may take place within 24 hours and lead to jaundice and renal tubular necrosis. Occasionally, there may be fatal reactions resulting from disseminated intravascular coagulation. Convulsions and heart failure have been reported in children.

Local treatment begins with early excision of the bite focus as soon as an ischemic lesion appears. Indurated subcutaneous tissue also is excised primarily, and within days areas that develop subsequent induration and necrosis are excised secondarily. Such vigorous and thorough débridement limits the spread of venom and ultimately may spare a great deal of tissue. Daily peroxide cleansing and antibiotic ointment help prevent secondary infection, and hyperbaric oxygenation is said to promote healing. Split thickness skin grafting is accomplished within days, once a good granulating base is demonstrated.

In severe cases the patient must rest in bed, and corticosteroids usually are given. They are thought to reduce the pain and the risk of systemic involvement; however, in vitro studies have not demonstrated clearcut effectiveness in limiting necrosis. Thus, steroid therapy probably should be reserved for cases that show systemic toxicity or a rapidly evolving induration, with a plaque growing larger over four hours. A daily dose of triamcinolone, 100 mg., or a comparable dose of another corticosteroid may be given parenterally or orally with phased reduction. Ultimately, injuries that stabilize early and show less than 6 cm. of induration and no necrosis by 48 hours have few complications and probably do not justify corticosteroid therapy. In all cases tetanus immunization is mandatory, and in serious cases bacterial culture and broad spectrum antibiotic coverage are advised.

Many cases of necrotic arachnidism have gone unrecognized as minor necrotic lesions of obscure etiology; however, a new in vitro test makes it possible to confirm the diagnosis by demonstrating the conversion of the victim's lymphocytes to blast forms in the presence of radioactive thymidine and Loxosceles venom. The possibility also is being entertained that active immunity might be achieved in humans, since its discovery in animals and since the development of an effective antivenin for South American brown spider bites.

BLACK WIDOW BITE

The female Black Widow spider (Fig. 1, B) and other female spiders of the genus Latrodectus have a red, yellow, or orange ventral hourglass marking. They are widespread, but more than one-half of bites by the Black Widow itself are reported in California. There is an immediate pinprick sensation, and local dull pain and numbness develop in a few minutes. Redness and swelling may appear around tiny fang marks. After 30 minutes, spasms may occur in abdominal and upper truncal muscles. Anxiety, nausea, vomiting, dizziness, headache, dyspnea, expiratory grunting, dysphagia, ptosis and edema of eyelids, low grade fever, and skin rash are common. Arterial and cerebrospinal fluid pressures may be elevated, especially with head and neck bites, and may lead to hypertensive crisis. Within two days the neurologic dysfunction resolves. Fatalities are rare, and life-threatening reactions usually are seen only in small children, aged persons, and those with unstable medical conditions.

Initial treatment includes topical cleansing, ice application, aspirin, and an opiate analgesic. Hot baths, mild sedation, and bed rest are helpful. For muscle spasms, 10 per cent calcium gluconate given I.V. may be effective; however, better relief of spasms and generalized symptoms is afforded by muscle relaxants such as methocarbamol or orphenadrine, 1 to 2 ml., given parenterally. Hypertensive crisis can be treated with diazoxide, 200 to 300 mg. infused rapidly I.V., with customary precaution. When symptom onset is precipitous and envenomation appears severe, ventilatory support may be required and vital signs should be monitored carefully during the first ten hours. The use of horse serum antivenin (Lyovac) may be justified, particularly in children. One ampule is diluted in up to 50 ml. of saline solution and given I.V. after the appropriate sensitivity testing, in accordance with package insert instructions. Children, hypertensives, and debilitated patients should be hospitalized, and all victims should be covered against tetanus.

SCORPION STING

Scorpions (Fig. 1, C) are nocturnal, and sequester themselves under outbuildings and debris in hot, dry areas. They look crab-like and carry a stinger or telson on the end of a whip-like tail, arched over the back. In Mexico their stings are remarkably toxic; however, death is rare in the U.S., and only the two yellow-backed varieties in and around Arizona, the *Centruroides gertschi* and the *C. sculpturatus*, cause systemic injury by means of their strongly cholinergic venom. Respiratory difficulty; opisthotonos; an itching sensation about the nose, throat, and mouth; dysphasia; drooling; gastric distention; diplopia; transient blindness; nystagmus; urinary and fecal incontinence; penile erection; hypertension; and cardiac dysfunction are all common and may persist for 48 hours. Stings by other domestic species cause only local pain, swelling, and erythema.

Initial treatment includes immobilization and icewater immersion of the involved limb, or topical ice application. A tourniquet is of little benefit. Opiate analgesics are said to potentiate toxicity, and their use should be avoided. Atropine can be used to counter parasympathomimetic effects. Hospitalization is mandatory in very toxic victims, children, or adults with hypertension. Oxygen and supportive ventilation may be required. Antivenin for sculptured scorpion stings can be located through poison control centers in the Southwest. Tetanus prophylaxis is advised.

OTHER ARACHNID INJURIES

Tarantulas (Lycosa) are known to bite when handled carelessly, but none are dangerous. Contact with hair of the animal causes minor inflammation. Centipedes are common in the southern states and may inflict a painful inflammatory bite, with regional lymphadenopathy. Treatment is palliative until pain resolves after a few hours.

Hymenoptera Stings

BEE, WASP, HORNET, AND YELLOWJACKET STINGS

Hymenopterids (Fig. 2, A) are prevalent in all 50 states. Hypersensitivity to their stings occurs in nearly 1 per cent of cases and accounts for the greatest mortality rate from any group of venomous animals in the U.S., with 10 to 30 deaths reported annually. Only 25 per cent of allergic patients have a known history of hypersensitivity, and the severity of reactions increases as a function of repeated exposure.

There are four families of Hymenoptera of special significance to insect allergy. These include the Apidae or honey bees; the Bombidae or bumble bees; the Vespidae or wasps, hornets and yellowjackets; and the Formicidae or ants (discussed in another section). Bumble bees are relatively docile and rarely sting humans. The Vespidae pose the greatest individual danger of hypersensitivity, and, being scavengers, their stings are more likely to cause bacterial infection. The common honey bee accounts for more stings and deaths than any other species, and triggers swarm attacks by releasing an alarm odor, known as a pheromone. It is the only species that leaves its barbed stinger and venom sac in situ. Thus, the presence of the stinger is an accurate diagnostic clue, and its absence makes a specific diagnosis difficult. An aggressive tropical variety of the honey bee, known as the African killer bee, is no more toxic than domestic bees, but is prone to swarm attacks and is expected to expand its range to the Southern. U.S.

Honey bee venom contains basic polypeptides, spreading factors, histamine serotonin, and nonenzymatic proteins, with nine identifiable antigens. Wasp venom is similar and contains large amounts of acetylcholine, serotonin, and kinins, with 12 to 13 identifiable antigens. The quantity of venom injected in single stings is minuscule, and swarm attacks with less than 500 stings rarely are fatal in the absence of hypersensitivity, but they typically cause lethargy, nausea, abdominal cramps, and hypertension, and may cause severe headache, convulsions, fever, and sepsis. Intravenous calcium gluconate provides some relief of symptoms. Parenteral antibiotics may be essential in many situations of infected stings with bacteremia.

Allergic reactions to Hymenoptera

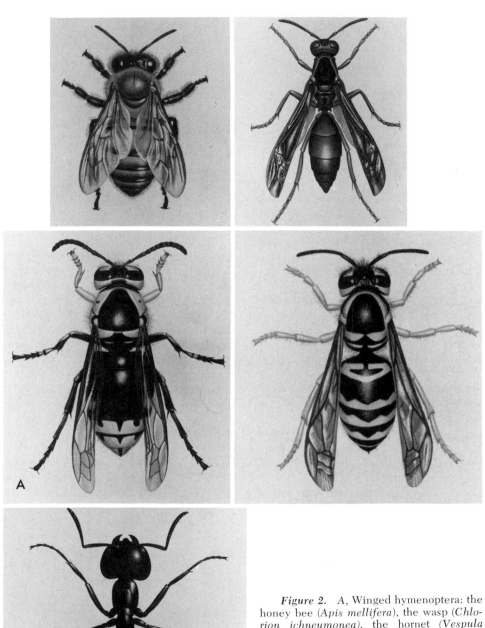

Figure 2. *A,* Winged hymenoptera: the honey bee (*Apis mellifera*), the wasp (*Chlorion ichneumonea*), the hornet (*Vespula maculata*), and the yellowjacket (*Vespula maculiformis*).

B, Fire ant: *Solenopsis invicta* (×6). (*B,* Courtesy of Frazier, C. A.; *A* and *B* reproduced by permission of Merck Sharp & Dohme, Division of Merck & Co., Inc.)

stings may be categorized as: (1) immediate-local, with inordinate local swelling; (2) immediate-mild-generalized, with diffuse swelling or urticaria; (3) immediate-severe-generalized, with anaphylaxis; or (4) delayed, with serum sickness-like reactions and atypical reactions. Generally, the more rapid the onset of the reaction, the more severe it will be, with most fatalities occurring within the first hour from airway obstruction and shock. Stings about the face, neck, and mucous membranes are prone to cause life-threatening swelling around the airway. Delayed allergic reactions usually include arthralgias, gastrointestinal disturbances, and fever; however, unusual responses have occurred, including blood dyscrasias, kidney and liver damage, cerebrovascular accidents, peripheral neuropathy, serum sickness-like reactions, and birth defects. In localized reactions, and even in some generalized reactions, there are no absolute criteria to differentiate a toxic response from an allergic one, and the degree of response to a sting is no index to subsequent degrees of reactivity. Cross-sensitivity exists between all species, especially with Vespidae exposure. Antigens are present in body parts and sensitization can arise by inhalation of wind-borne contaminants, raising the possibility of serious hypersensitivity without a history of prior stings. Indeed, other insects may cause sensitization to unknown degrees of specificity in this manner.

Treatment of Hymenoptera stings begins with nonsqueezing removal by gently scraping the stinger away, taking care that fragments are not retained. The wound is cleansed with soapy water, and ice is applied. Early topical coverage with a paste of meat tenderizer containing papain is soothing and is said to have a detoxifying effect. Allergy-prone patients, or those who manifest the slightest allergic response, should apply a lymph constricting band proximal to the sting and should seek the nearest source of epinephrine and medical attention. In the event of anaphylaxis, aqueous epinephrine in a 1:1000 solution is given subcutaneously. The initial requirement usually is 0.4 to 0.5 cc. and the injection site is massaged vigorously to hasten absorption. For severe anaphylaxis, epinephrine may be given I.V. in a 1:10,000 solution, injected slowly with caution. The patient is observed closely in case a repeated dose is needed in 20 to 30 minutes. If shock occurs, oxygen and intravenous fluid therapy are essential, and if there is severe glottal edema, tracheotomy may be required. Both antihistamines and steroids have delayed effectiveness and are recommended as adjuncts to therapy. Beginning with a daily total dose equivalent to prednisone, 30 mg. initially, oral steroids are given twice daily with phased reduction by 5 mg. each morning over five to seven days. Thereafter, total resolution of symptoms may justify discontinuation of steroid therapy by the second or third day. In all cases, explicit cautionary advice must be given.

For future exposure, hypersensitive patients should be prescribed a sting kit, including a lymph constrictor band, injectible and inhalant forms of epinephrine, an oral antihistamine, and detailed written instructions. They should carry medical identification tags; wear shoes and light, drab, smooth clothing; apply an insect repellant containing diethyltoluamide; and avoid the use of scented toiletries. Outdoor travel and work around endemic areas such as gardens and garbage collection sites should be avoided, especially in the summertime. In addition, the American Academy of Allergy Committee on Insects has recommended that patients who have had systemic or large local reactions be given hyposensitization therapy during risk periods. Ninety-five per cent of individuals so treated have shown lesser reactions when re-stung. Skin testing can be helpful in selecting species-specific hyposensitization mixtures and dose schedules at least three weeks after a previous reaction; however, it is unreliable, potentially sensitizing, and ill-advised for diagnosis, which should rest on the history alone.

ANT STINGS

Stings by most varieties of ants (Fig. 2, B) cause itching and formation of a wheal and vesicle. Occasionally, there is marked swelling and hypersensitivity. Stings by two species of imported fire ants of the Southeast have a unique alkaloidal necrotizing factor that additionally causes intense burning pain, pustule formation, and scarring, and may cause retrosternal pain, dyspnea, hypertension, and hemolysis. Fire ants average about 5 mm. in length and may be brown or black. They are aggressive inhabitants of agricultural areas, and attack humans or livestock in swarms. Treatment consists of early wound cleansing and the application of ice, followed by a topical anti-inflammatory agent. Special attention and full-scale precautionary measures are directed toward the treatment and prophylaxis of hypersensitivity reactions.

Ectoparasite and Miscellaneous Infestations and Injuries

A wide variety of arthropod parasites infest man and act as vectors for the spread of communicable diseases. Discussion here is limited to the diagnosis and treatment of toxic and direct manifestations.

TICK PARALYSIS AND BITES

In addition to being vectors for tularemia and Rocky Mountain spotted fever, all varieties of pregnant female hard ticks (Fig. 3) can cause progressive neurologic impairment through a toxic salivary gland factor that is thought to interfere with synaptic transmission in the spinal cord and peripheral nerves. Rarely, there is brain stem dysfunction. In most cases the tick's attachment in a hair-bearing area has gone unrecognized for several days, while the victim develops ataxia, impaired coordination and areflexia, and ascending motor weakness, similar to that seen with Landry-Guillian-Barré syndrome. The typical occurrence, in a child during summertime, raises suspicion of an-

terior poliomyelitis; however, fever, pain, selective muscle spasms, and spinal fluid abnormalities are absent and the victim is apathetic. In the absence of respiratory embarrassment, the effects are entirely reversible with careful search for and detachment of ticks. Intact removal can be accomplished by smothering the tick with petrolatum or gasoline. In a few minutes, the tick releases its hold and can be extracted whole. Otherwise, mouth parts must be excised.

Bites by the venomous pajaroello tick, common to coastal areas of southern California, may cause vesicle formation necrosis and a painful, superficial ulcer that heals slowly.

MOSQUITO AND FLY BITES

Mosquitos, deer flies, black flies, and sand flies are all blood-sucking insects among the order Diptera, a group responsible for the transmission of several viral, bacterial, and parasitic diseases. Bites cause focal pain, itching, and swelling, and treatment is palliative. In the case of mosquitos, there may be urticaria, lethargy, headache, and nausea, but anaphylaxis and death are rare. In the case of black flies, the bite can be very painful. It should be cleansed, and a topical anti-inflammatory cream should be applied. Oral steroids may be needed for systemic reactions, which are rare. In cases of known allergy, hyposensitization therapy may be justified; however, the application of a diethyltoluamide insect repellent is the best preventive measure.

LOUSE INFESTATION

Lice are small, grey, crablike parasites that are readily transferred through personal and clothing contact. Body lice (*Pediculus humanis linnaeus*) are important vectors of disease, particularly typhus, trench fever, and louse-borne relapsing fever. They cause severe itching, excoriation, pustule formation, and puncta and lichenification along lines of scratching. Head lice (*Pediculus humanis capitus*) are found most commonly in scalp hair of women and children, where they deposit prominent nits or ova. Excoriations, pustule formation, and posterior cervical adenopathy are common, and the hair usually is lusterless and dry. Pubic lice (*Phthirius pubis linnaeus*) infest human

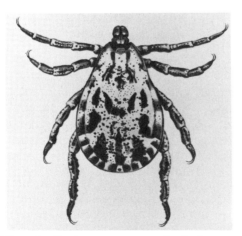

Figure 3. Rocky mountain wood tick: *Dermacentor andersoni* (×6). (Courtesy of Frazier, C. A.; reproduced by permission of Merck Sharp & Dohme, Division of Merck & Co., Inc.)

pubic hair and may migrate to the armpits, eyelashes, and eyebrows, from which they must be meticulously débrided. Recognition usually is delayed until intense itching develops. Small irregular bluish macular eruptions may appear about the trunk and thighs. Treatment of all lice infestation consists of eradication by thorough shampooing and fine combing of the involved areas, and by applying an ectoparasiticide such as gamma benzene hexachloride. The patient should be instructed to boil clothing and to refer sexual partners for treatment.

BED BUG AND REDUVIID BUG BITES

Bed bugs are reddish-brown nocturnal bloodfeeders averaging 4 to 5 mm. in length. They are prevalent throughout the world, and cause itching and erythematous wheals with central red punctae, which may evolve to itching purpuric spots. Local swelling and rare systemic reactions can occur. Bed sheets may show the brown or black spots of blood digested by the bug. Kissing bugs or reduviid bugs are larger blood-sucking arthropods that cause hemorrhagic papules, bullae, and painful urticarial lesions. Treatment is palliative, and prevention requires eradication from sleeping quarters.

MITE INFESTATION

Chigger mites are tiny (0.4 to 0.6 mm.) arthropods, harbored in green vegetation in hot temperate areas, which burrow into the skin of their host in the larval stage, creating papular lesions that itch intensely and occasionally look hemorrhagic. Papules about the waist are common, as the organism may crawl about until it meets the resistance of clothing. Topical astringents, such as camphor and phenol ointment, or a layer of clear fingernail polish, will asphyxiate the mite and reduce itching. Oral antihistamines may be helpful.

Itch mites or scabies cause a similar infestation from indoor sources of contact. Outbreaks can be epidemic, most patients showing typical raised itching puncta of burrows, and some showing a diffuse crusting nonitching rash that resembles exfoliative dermatitis. Gamma benzene hexachloride

is still effective, although there are indications of mild resistance to the drug, which must be applied two or three times initially, and again in one week to cover eggs that may have hatched during the interval. Clothing and bedding must be cleansed thoroughly, and those sharing housing must be referred for treatment.

FLEA BITES

Fleas are small, wingless, blood-sucking insects that infest specific animal hosts, including humans. Bites result in grouped, itching, papular eruptions. Outbreaks are especially common in children in summertime. The patient must be thoroughly bathed, and infested rooms must be decontaminated. Fingernail trimming and antipruritic drugs help prevent excoriations.

IRRITATING CATERPILLAR STINGS

Some caterpillars, such as the gray furry pus caterpillar (*Megalophyte opercularis*), are protected by tiny fragile spines that have an urticating effect on contact, and may cause respiratory irritation on inhalation. There is immediate, intense rhythmic pain that may spread regionally. Local swelling, regional lymphadenopathy, nausea, fever, muscle cramps, headaches, and numbness can occur. A gridlike contact lesion develops rapidly and desquamates within hours or days. Spines can be removed with Scotch tape application. Calcium gluconate given I.V. and antihistamines may provide relief.

BLISTER BEETLES

The extruded hemolymph or the crushed-out coelomic fluid of certain beetles may have a powerful urticating and vesicating effect on the skin and eyes on contact. The toxic substance is cantharidin, sometimes prepared as "Spanish fly," and taken orally under the erroneous assumption that it is an aphrodisiac. In this form it is highly nephrotoxic, and the fatal dose is less than 60 mg. Cutaneous blisters may benefit from topical treatment with magnesium sulfate and methyl alcohol packs.

MARINE ANIMAL BITES AND STINGS

Jellyfish, Stingray, Stinging Fish, Sea Urchins, Stinging Coral, Octopi, and Cone Shells

TYPICAL PRESENTATIONS

A bather enters the Emergency Department with painful, whiplike, urticarial eruptions after contact with a large jellyfish.

A surfer is brought in with a large puncture wound of the calf after stepping on a stingray.

A fisherman enters with pain and slight swelling of his thumb after handling a sculpin.

Only a handful of the world's venomous marine species inhabit U.S. coastal waters, but, in some areas the above mentioned presentations are fairly common. Hundreds of persons each year are injured by stingrays in warmer coastal waters. On the Pacific Coast, sculpin stings requiring treatment are estimated at 300 annually, and jellyfish stings are common among surf bathers and fishermen. In Atlantic and Gulf Coast waters, the Portuguese man-of-war (*Physalia physalis*), a hydroid with trails of tentacles several yards long, poses a significant threat to bathers.

Most venomous marine species are sedentary or slow-swimming, and use their venom apparatus defensively. Injuries arise

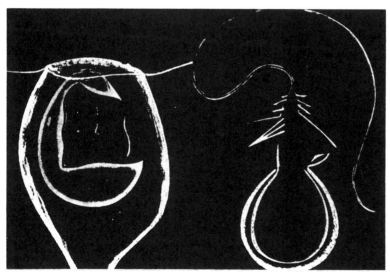

A

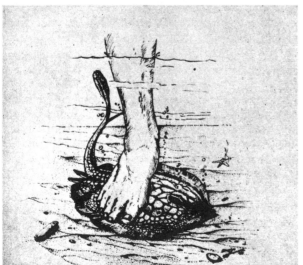

B

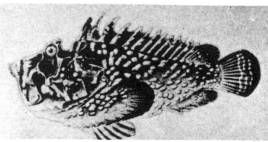

C

Figure 4. A, Diagrammatic sketch of the undischarged and discharged nematocysts of a jellyfish. (From Findlay, E.: Marine toxins and venomous and poisonous marine animals. *In* Russell, F. A. (ed.): Advances in Marine Biology, Vol. 3. New York, Academic Press, 1965, p. 275, Fig. 2; reproduced by permission.)

B, Stinging action of the round stingray.

C, Stonefish: *Synanceja horrida.* (Reprinted by permission. From Halstead, B. W.: Dangerous Marine Animals. Cambridge, Md., Cornell Maritime Press, Inc., 1959.)

from inadvertent contact. Stinging marine vertebrates such as stingrays and spiny fish (including catfish) possess remarkably similar thermolabile venoms; *thus, heat application rather than ice application is the primary mode of therapy.* As a whole, marine animal venoms are simpler and shorter-acting than those of terrestrial animals. Deaths are rare except when due to drowning or anaphylaxis. Although no venomous marine animals have been suspected of harboring tetanus spores, bacterial contamination is not uncommon, and tetanus prophylaxis is therefore advisable.

Jellyfish and Hydroid Stings

Jellyfish and hydroid tentacles (Fig. 4A) carry an abundance of capsular stingers with springlike microscopic barbs that trigger when mechanically or histochemically stimulated. The venom contains a number of quaternary ammonium compounds, histamine and low molecular weight proteins that affect paralysis through cholinergic neurons. Tentacle contact produces localized edema, erythema, vesiculation, itching, and pain in a whiplike urticarial pattern. The pain may spread regionally, and weakness, nausea, headache, truncal muscle spasms, increased lacrimation, perspiration, vertigo, violent twitching, and dyspnea can occur. Collapse and cardiac arrest have been reported. The anaphylaxis phenomenon was discovered during studies with these toxins, and the risk is significant.

Treatment is directed at preventing nematocyst discharge by stabilization fixation, and removal of tentacles. The area should be rinsed with sea water, and large fragments should be teased away. Medicinal alcohol, drinking alcohol, or meat tenderizers can be used as fixatives. Next, a drying agent, such as dry sand, flour, or talc, helps coalesce the tentacles so that they can be scraped away with a blade. Rinsing with a dilute basic solution such as baking soda or ammonium hydroxide helps neutralize the acidic venom. Antihistamines, topical corticosteroids, and opiate analgesics may be needed. Systemic complications are treated symptomatically. One should never stimulate nematocyst discharge by rubbing the area or applying fresh water.

Stingray Injury

Stingrays (Fig. 4B) impale their victims with a sheathed spine, up to 30 cm. in length, carried on the whiplike tail. Most punctures and lacerations occur in the calf when the victim treads on the animal: however, penetrations of the thorax or abdomen can occur. As the sting penetrates the skin, the integumentary sheath is ruptured, releasing the venom. Portions of the sheath and, rarely, portions of the spine remain in the wound. The venom contains thermolabile proteins and serotonin. It depresses respiration and causes reversible repolarization and atrioventricular conduction changes in mammalian hearts. Locally, the intense pain is maximal by 90 minutes and may persist for several hours. Wounds are jagged and may have surrounding discoloration, erythema, and edema, which are slow to resolve. Pain is severe, and weakness, nausea, syncope, sweating, regional muscle cramping, and lymph node pain are common. Severe envenomation may cause vomiting, diarrhea, sweating, respiratory distress, and arrhythmias.

Treatment begins with removal of accessible pieces of the integumentary sheath, and irrigation with salt water. A lymph constricting band is applied intermittently above the wound site, and the extremity is submerged for up to 90 minutes in a bath of water, as hot as the victim will tolerate. This treatment significantly alleviates the pain and systemic complications. The wound then is injected with a local anesthetic and is inspected directly, and with x-ray for evidence of retained material. Débridement, suturing, and systemic analgesia may be required. Individualized antibiotic therapy should be considered, and the patient should be protected against tetanus.

Fish Sting

Pacific Coast sculpins and bullheads, together with the notorious stonefish (Fig. 4, C), of the South Pacific, are members of the scorpionfish family. All are slow-moving bottom dwellers with spines located dorsally, and in the anal and pelvic areas. Integumentary sheaths around some of the dorsal spines form the venom apparatus.

Envenomation arises from shallow

punctures that have a surrounding ischemic appearance and cause excruciating pain, hyperesthesia, paresthesias, swelling, and blister formation. Severe envenomations by the stonefish and other very toxic species may cause dyspnea, hypotension, collapse, and death within one hour. Continuous immersion of the affected part, in water as hot as the patient will tolerate, is clearly the most effective treatment measure. In addition, infiltration of the wound with a solution of emetine hydrochloride is said to be beneficial.

Other stinging fish, including surgeonfishes, toadfishes, ratfishes, weaverfishes, and catfish, cause similar intoxications with their sting. All of their venoms are thermolabile and respond well to the detoxifying effects of hot water immersion.

Sea Urchin Puncture

Both the brittle calcareous spines and the tiny pincer-like pedicellaria of some sea urchins are venomous. Punctures, arising when bathers step on the animal, pose a difficult problem for foreign body removal, and give rise to granulomatous tracts. There is immediate, intense burning pain at the site, and generalized weakness, numbness, paresthesia, muscle atonia, dyspnea, and arrhythmias may occur. Spines of Diadema, a Caribbean genus, may be up to a foot long and may cause dark staining in the puncture tract. For this group, débridement is advised, as spines are not absorbed readily. Spines of most other sea urchins are resorbed within days, and débridement is seldom worthwhile.

Coral Sting

Fire coral and stony coral are tropical species that cause pain, itching, and papular lesions on abrasive contact. Pustules may form and desquamate or ulcerate. Secondary infections are common, and wounds must be scrubbed and soaked thproughly. A commonly used name is "devil's reef." Symptoms are severe within hours and usually clear in 3 days.

Octopus Bite

Octopi, with their powerful jaws shaped like an inverted parrot's beak, can inflict deep punctures, with pain, tingling, itching, and profuse bleeding from the wound. Swelling may be marked. Central nervous system dysfunction and fatalities have been reported from bites by tiny cephalopods, found along Australia's Great Barrier Reef, but those along the Pacific Coast of North America, although among the largest in the world, are relatively docile and less toxic.

Cone Shell Sting

Cone shells, including Californian and Hawaiian coastal varieties, extend the proboscis and impale the victim with a harpoonlike disposable radular tooth. The injury usually occurs when the attractive shell is scraped by an unwary collector. There is immediate intense pain about the ischemic-looking wound, which heals slowly. Numbness, tingling, and muscular irritability are common. Incoordination, aphonia, dysphagia, visual disturbances, chest pain, and coma can occur, and, rarely, there may be death due to cardiac failure or respiratory paralysis.

Sea Snake Bite

Sea snakes inhabit tropical waters across the Indo-Pacific area from the Red Sea to Mexico's Sea of Cortez. Their venom is specifically toxic to striated muscle, releasing myoglobin between 30 minutes and eight hours following the bite. There is marked weakness, ptosis, and muscular rigidity. Pain is excruciating, and death may occur early as a result of cardiac failure, or later as a result of renal tubular necrosis. Treatment is directed at maintaining renal output by means of supporting the blood pressure and alkalinizing the urine.

Nonvenomous Bites

Treatment of shark and other nonvenomous marine bites is straightforward. Wound infections are common, and prophylactic antibiotic therapy and tetanus immunization are advised.

References

Anderson, P. C.: What's new in loxoscelism? Mo. Med. 70(10):711, 1973.

Auer, A. I., and Hershey, F. B.: Surgery for necrotic bites of the brown spider. Arch. Surg. *108*:612, 1974.

Barr, S. E.: Allergy to Hymenoptera stings—review of the world literature: 1953–1970. Ann. Allergy *29(2)*:49, 1971.

Bitseff, E. L., et al.: The management of stingray injuries of the extremities. South. Med. J. *63*:417, 1970.

Dillaha, C. J.: North American loxoscelism. J.A.M.A. *188*:33, 1964.

Feingold, B. F.: Allergic reactions to hymenoptera stings. J. Asthma Res., *9(2)*:55–71, 1971.

Frazier, C. A.: Insect Allergy. St. Louis, Warren H. Green, Inc., 1969.

Frazier, C. A.: Allergic responses to biting and stinging insects. J. Asthma Res. *10(1)*:3, 1972.

Haller, J. S., and Fabara, J. A.: Tick paralysis: case report with emphasis on neurological toxicity. Am. J. Dis. Child. *124*:915, 1972.

Halstead, B. W.: Poisonous and Venomous Marine Animals. Washington, U.S. Government Printing Office, 2 Vols., 1965.

Insect Allergy Committee of the American Academy of Allergy: Insect sting allergy. J.A.M.A. *193*:109, 1965.

Marsden, P. D.: Coleptera (Beetles). *In* Beeson, P. B., and McDermott, W. (eds.): Textbook of Medicine. Philadelphia, W. B. Saunders Co., 1975.

McConnell, J. G., et al.: Alkaloid from fire ant venom. Science *168*:840, 1970.

Parrish, H. M.: Death from bites and stings of venomous animals in the United States. Arch. Intern. Med. *104*:198, 1959.

Passero, M. A., and Dees, S. C.: Allergy to stings from winged things. Am. Fam. Phys. 7:75, 1973.

Pearn, J. H.: Bee stings in operational theatres. Milit. Med. *137*:241, 1972.

Rose, I.: A review of tick paralysis. J. Can. Med. Assoc. 70:175, 1954.

Russel, F. E., Wainschel, J., and Gertsch, W. J.: Bites of Spiders and Other Arthropods. *In* Current Therapy. Philadelphia, W. B. Saunders Co., 1972, pp. 841–843.

Russell, F. E.: Marine Toxins and Venomous and Poisonous Marine Animals. London, Academic Press, 1965.

Russell, F. E.: Pharmacology of Animal Venoms. Clin. Pharmacol. Ther. 8:849, 1967.

Strauss, M. B., and Orris, W. L.: Injuries to divers by marine animals: a simplified approach to recognition and management. Milit. Med. *139*:129, 1974.

Yaron, R.: Scorpion venom: a tutorial review of its effects in men and experimental animals. Clin. Toxicol. *3(4)*:561, 1970.

I. HEAT STRESS DISEASE

Robert P. Proulx

Heat stress disease can be a life threatening emergency, and it is therefore essential that the physician who sees these patients when they are first brought to the hospital be able to assess their condition quickly and accurately. The following typical cases should help.

SOME TYPICAL PATIENTS

HEAT STROKE

On a hot, humid, windless day the ambulance crew brings a young male who has collapsed while jogging. He is not comatose but is irrational and delusional. His skin is hot and dry. His blood pressure is normal and his pulse is elevated. His rectal temperature is 41.8°C. (107°F). He has a grand mal seizure soon after arrival.

On a similar day an elderly patient is brought to the Emergency Department having been found comatose in the park. His skin is warm but slightly moist. His blood pressure is low and his pulse elevated. His rectal temperature is 40.6°C. (105°F.).

Until proved otherwise, both these patients present a medical emergency, *heat stroke,* and need rapid evaluation and therapy to prevent death or prolonged morbidity.

HEAT EXHAUSTION

A fireman fighting a brush fire on a warm day is brought to the Emergency Department because he "does not feel well." He is alert, well oriented, and not at all confused. He complains of dizziness, nausea, and headache. He has warm, moist skin, normal blood pressure and pulse, and a rectal temperature of 38.4°C. (101°F.). This patient probably has *heat exhaustion*—not as serious a condition as heat stroke but one that deserves prompt attention. (However, toxic inhalation must also be considered.)

HEAT CRAMPS

On a summer evening a healthy young male presents himself to the Emergency Department with a complaint of abdominal pain. He works for the road department laying asphalt and has been on the job earlier that day. The day has been hot and the patient has sweated copiously. His vital signs are normal. An abdominal examination reveals visible spasms of the musculature. This patient almost certainly has heat cramps. This is not a life threatening emergency but to the patient his pain certainly *is* an emergency.

These four vignettes describe typical ways patients may present to the Emergency Department with one of the three major heat stress diseases, but to understand how they got that way and what to do about it we must examine some basic principles.

HISTORICAL BACKGROUND

Heat stroke is mentioned in the Bible and has been known for centuries. Well known military campaigns have been influenced by heat disease, and much of the literature on this problem has been generated by military medicine. In civilian life heat disease is often a concern of team physicians. The elderly are another source of civilian cases. Although heat stroke appears infrequently it is as much a medical emergency as shock and must be recognized and treated in the Emergency Department. The literature estimates mortality from heat stroke as 10 to 80 per cent, but untreated heat stroke must approach 100 per cent mortality.

BASIC PHYSICS OF HEAT STRESS

In any animal the core body temperature at any given moment is a result of internal and external factors that increase or lower temperature. In warm-blooded animals internal homeostatic mechanisms are at work to maintain body temperature within relatively narrow limits.

Internal heat production mechanisms are basal metabolism and work. The amount of heat generated by basal metabolism varies, but is in the range of 2000 to 4000 kcal. per day. Heavy work can add up to 600 kcal. per hour, but few people can sustain such effort for prolonged periods. Walking at a brisk pace may add 350 kcal. per hour.

Heat loss is effected by several mechanisms. Radiation of heat through space is a major means of heat loss when ambient temperatures are lower than body temperature. Conversely, if ambient temperatures are higher, body radiation becomes a heat

production mechanism. Convection directly transfers heat as cooler air passes over a warmer object. At times this can be an important means of heat reduction. The evaporation of water or sweat requires energy. As ambient temperatures reach body temperature evaporation is the only effective means of losing heat. As relative humidity approaches 100 per cent evaporation ceases. Exhalation of heated air is not a significant factor in human temperature regulation, but is important in some animals. Heat also can be lost or gained through conduction and can be lost through excretion of urine or feces, but these are insignificant routes of heat dissipation.

Climatic factors are crucial. The sun and ambient temperatures higher than body temperature radiate heat energy to the body. Clothing can decrease significantly the amount of heat absorbed when a person is exposed to direct sunlight. At temperatures lower than body temperature, radiation is the major means of losing body heat.

Wind velocity is important. As relatively cooler and drier masses of air are brought near the body, heat and evaporated sweat are directly transferred. Convection losses are never greater than about 15 per cent of total heat loss.

A hot, humid, windless day is conducive to heat stress disease. These factors have been put into various formulas to obtain an index temperature which can then be correlated with heat disease risk. Assessment of the effect of environment may be made by the following formula:

Index = 70% "wet bulb" temperature + 20% "black globe" temperature + 10% "dry bulb" temperature.

Certain predisposing factors are controllable; others are not (Fig. 1). Drugs may predispose patients to heat stress diseases, particularly the phenothiazines and anticholinergics; in fact, any medication or disease which alters sweating or the thermoregulatory mechanism can accentuate environmental factors and predispose to heat stress disease.

THE PHYSIOLOGY OF HEAT STRESS

Temperature control in human beings is accomplished both in an "acute" manner

FACTORS PREDISPOSING TO HEAT STROKE

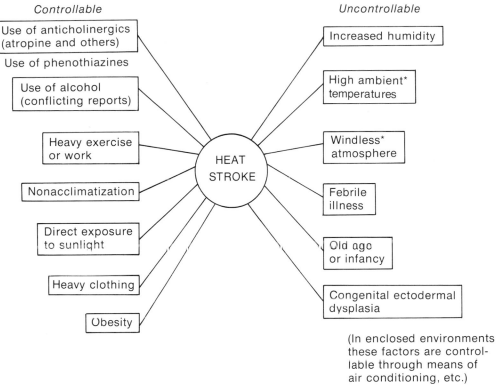

Figure 1. Factors predisposing to heat stroke.

and gradually through acclimatization. As body temperature rises acutely as a result of work and/or climatic factors, blood and skin temperatures rise. Skin sensors plus the direct effect of warmed blood stimulate the hypothalamus, which in turn activates the autonomic nervous system to bring about several changes. Respiratory rate increases to increase heat loss via exhaled air. Cardiac output increases, causing more warm blood to pass through the skin, thereby increasing radiation, convection, and evaporation losses. Skin vasodilation and splanchnic vasoconstriction occur, increasing the amount of blood passing through the skin. Sweat production increases.

Sweat is a hypotonic solution, and in extreme situations up to 12 liters of sweat containing 20 gm. of sodium chloride may be produced per day. In an attempt to restore salt loss and circulating volume the production of antidiuretic hormone and aldosterone is stimulated. Figure 2 illustrates the physiology of temperature control.

Acclimatization occurs over several weeks when a person is exposed to continuing heat stress, allowing a more efficient response to any given heat load. Sweat production can be increased to two and one-half times its previous maximum with a decrease in sodium loss. Increased cardiac output, decreased peripheral vascular resistance, and increased blood volume all occur, thereby allowing more effective heat loss. Endrocrine responses allow enhanced sodium conservation.

DISEASE ENTITIES

Differentiation between the three clinical syndromes (heat cramps, heat exhaustion, and heat stroke) is usually easy (Fig. 3). However, at times more than one condition may be present concomitantly. The three syndromes will be discussed separately here for simplicity, but recognizing the possible overlap and merging of one into another.

HEAT CRAMPS

Although not life threatening, heat cramps are painful. They occur when profuse sweating occurs over a fairly short

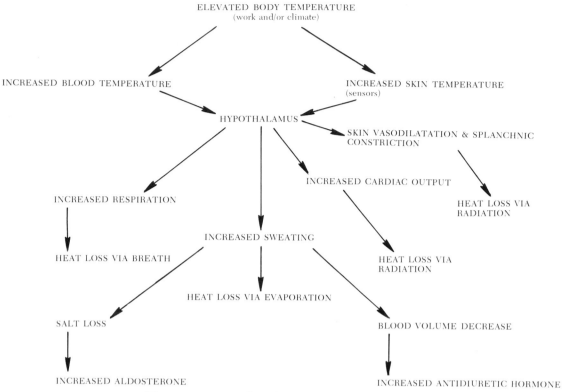

Figure 2. Known physiology of temperature control.

period with adequate water replacement but inadequate salt replacement. This imbalance of sodium hemostasis can precipitate severe skeletal muscle cramps. The leg and abdominal muscles are commonly involved. The rectal temperature will be normal or minimally elevated. The patient will be alert and well oriented with normal blood pressure and pulse. There may be evidence of marked sweating, even though the sweat loss may have occurred hours earlier. Treatment is to replace the salt and other electrolytes if needed. Oral solutions containing 5 cc. (1 teaspoon) of salt per 500 ml. water (1 pint) will work, but intravenous normal saline provides much more rapid and dramatic relief.

After treatment the patient may be released and advised to increase salt intake during periods of marked sweating. Although salt tablets may be used, they often pass through the gastrointestinal tract undigested and may cause vomiting. The best preventive measure is to salt food heavily during risk periods. Laboratory studies are generally unrewarding. Of course other enti-

	Rectal temp.	CNS	Skin	Muscle cramps	Blood pressure	Pulse	Treatment
Heat Stroke	greater than 40°C. (104°F.)	Seizure, psychosis, coma	usually hot and dry	no	normal, high or low	elevated	rapid cooling
Heat Exhaustion	less than 40°C. (104°F.)	headache, dizzy, nausea, other mild symptoms	sweating present	occasionally	normal or low	normal or elevated	replace salt and water
Heat Cramps	less than 40°C. (104°F.)	none	sweating present	yes	normal	normal or elevated	replace salt

Figure 3. Generalizations about heat disease syndromes to aid differentiation.

ties such as hyperventilation, black widow spider bite, and hypokalemia may cause skeletal muscle cramps and must be considered in the differential diagnosis. The patient should not return to work that day.

HEAT EXHAUSTION

This entity comes in two varieties: water-depletion or salt-depletion. Water-depletion heat exhaustion can occur only when the patient is prevented from drinking, e.g., a lost hiker. As dehydration occurs the thirst stimulus is very strong and water will be replaced if made available.

Salt-depletion heat exhaustion is the more common form. Salt loss does not stimulate as strong a subjective demand for salt replacement as thirst does for water replacement. Decreased blood volume will occur if sweat loss is not replaced by drinking water. As salt is lost, perhaps over a period of several days and is not replaced because of poor subjective stimulus, diuresis occurs to normalize tonicity. This also leads to low blood volume. In either type of heat exhaustion the sweating mechanism is preserved. Both patients will have some central nervous system complaint such as headache, nausea, or dizziness with perhaps some mild confusion. Syncope may occur. Rectal temperatures may be elevated or normal, but the severe hyperpyrexia seen with heat stroke never occurs. Blood pressure may be normal or depressed. Rarely, true oligemic shock may exist. The history will identify the water-deprived heat exhaustion patient, who will, of course, be quite thirsty. The salt-depletion heat exhaustion patient may complain of skeletal muscle cramps. Both patients need fluid: hypotonic for the water-depleted victim and isotonic for the salt-depleted patient. Generally the laboratory will not be needed to assist in diagnosis or treatment, but a complete blood count, urinalysis, and tests for electrolytes should be done. Hypernatremia, hyperchloremia, and a highly concentrated urine will be found in water depletion heat exhaustion. Elevation of serum enzymes (SGOT, LDH, CPK) is common. If hypotension exists, a central venous pressure line should be established. Fluid replacement may be oral (5 cc. of salt per 500 ml. of water) or parenteral, depending on the severity of the problem. Severely ill patients should be hospitalized. Salt-deficient patients should be told to liberalize their salt intake during hot periods.

HEAT STROKE

As we have seen, this is a life threatening medical emergency. Without accurate diagnosis and appropriate therapy, death or serious disability will almost certainly occur. In the heat stroke patient, heat stress evokes hypothalamic and/or sweat gland fatigue. It is not known which dominates or whether both play a role. If the ambient temperature is greater than body temperature this lack of sweating leads to an immediate rise in body temperature. As body temperature approaches 42°C. (108°F.) cell death occurs. Certain organs are affected early: the brain, liver, kidney, and heart. Usually the patient collapses suddenly with few or no prodromal symptoms, although in some instances there is a prodromal period of three to five days with symptoms of headache, nausea, or syncope.

The skin will be hot and dry, although some cases have been reported where sweating persisted. Central nervous system damage causes cerebral edema manifested by seizure activity, confusion, delirium, and disorientation. There may be focal neurologic signs and loss of bowel or bladder control. Coma may occur.

Oral temperatures should not be relied upon. Only a rectal temperature will give a valid reading, and in heat stroke usually is 41°C. (106°F.) or greater. It is not unusual to see elevations to 42°C. (108°F.) Cardiac output initially increases to high levels, but if heat stroke is unchecked it will decrease and cardiac failure will ensue. Blood pressure may be normal, elevated, or depressed. Tachycardia will be present. One must rule out seizure disorders, coma of other etiologies, and acute psychosis. Full vital signs will generally be sufficient for differentiation. A spinal tap usually is normal unless a convulsion has occurred. The EEG is not helpful in diagnosis.

Treatment. Treatment must be aimed at rapidly lowering the core body temperature by whatever means available. Physical means include ice bath, ice blanket, and evaporating ice water splashed on the patient with fans. The most reliable and effective method, however, is an ice bath. This is done by immersing the patient in a tub filled with water and ice cubes and massaging the skeletal muscles.

The rectal temperature must be monitored constantly—if possible by a thermocouple left in place. Rectal temperature should not be allowed to fall below 38.8° C. (102° F); otherwise the core body temperature may continue to fall to dangerously low levels. Massage helps to promote circulation, bringing warm blood to the surface for heat transfer. (Pharmacologic means of lowering temperature by using phenothiazines has been advocated but these agents are unreliable and also affect sweating.) While the tub is being readied an intravenous route should be established, preferably a central venous pressure line, for infusion of Ringer's lactate or normal saline. Generally, however, the patient does not need fluid; in fact, pulmonary edema may occur. If hypokalemia is present supplemental potassium should be provided. Severe lactic acidosis has also been seen with heat stroke. There has been some evidence that potassium deficiency might play a major role early in heat stroke — although later, following cellular destruction, hyperkalemia will occur. Early hypocalcemia has been observed in some cases. Oxygen should be administered and a Foley catheter placed. A nasogastric tube is useful.

Most Emergency Departments do not have tubs in their immediate area, but usually one can be borrowed from the Physical Therapy Department and ice can be obtained from the Cafeteria. The Emergency Department should have access to these two areas 24 hours a day just for such emergencies. Shivering may occur in the ice bath and cause an increase in heat output. Some sedation usually is necessary. Phenothiazines such as chlorpromazine in small doses (25 to 50 mg. I.V.) should be given to control shivering and agitation.

Mannitol should be given to decrease cerebral edema and to insure a urine flow adequate to prevent acute tubular necrosis. Over a 60-minute period one or two 12.5 gram ampules followed by one ampule in each liter of fluid may be given. Furosemide can also be used to increase urine output. It is essential to maintain a copious urine flow, since there may be diffuse muscle destruction and myoglobinuria.

While resuscitation is being performed, arterial blood gases, complete blood count, urinalysis, prothrombin time, platelets, electrolytes, and BUN should be tested. Acidosis and electrolyte abnormalities should be corrected as needed. Sodium bicarbonate may be needed to correct acidosis. If seizures occur they may be treated with intravenous diazepam in 5-mg. amounts up to 20 mg. until control is achieved. If shock is present it can best be treated by judicious use of intravenous fluids while monitoring the central venous pressure and by isoproterenol 1 mg. in 500 ml. of 5 per cent dextrose in water intravenously titrated by clinical response. Dopamine also can be used. Heart failure due to either myocardial injury or increased pulmonary resistance may occur. Rapid digitalization may be necessary, particularly in older patients. Many fatal instances of heat stroke have been reported in older people, most of whom have pre-existing heart disease. Caution is needed to avoid possible hypokalemia. Steroids have been recommended but there is no evidence that they are of any value in these patients.

As vital signs stabilize and temperature returns to acceptable levels, the patient may be removed from the ice bath and admitted to the intensive care unit. Subacute problems such as a repeated temperature elevation, acute tubular necrosis, and diffuse intravascular clotting must be watched for by appropriate laboratory and patient monitoring. After the acute problems have been resolved, permanent liver, cardiac, and central nervous system damage may persist. If coma develops, a cuffed endotracheal tube will be needed. If severe renal impairment is present, early dialysis should be performed.

Prehospital Care. Figure 4 illustrates a proposed approach to emergency management of heat stroke. Since it is impractical to achieve rapid cooling in the field, immediate transport is indicated. An intravenous line should be established and oxygen given. Every effort should be made to prevent heat load. The patient should be stripped and air conditioning used if available. Water can be sprinkled on the patient and evaporated by air conditioning or open windows during the ride to the Emergency Department.

In the wilderness environment recognition of the gravity of the situation is important. The victim must be transported as soon as possible to the nearest capable medical facility. In the meantime every effort to reduce heat load must be made. All clothing should be removed and the patient placed in the shade. If water is available, a spray of water and fans to evaporate it should be used. If a cold stream or lake is available, immersion with massage should be done. If shaking chills occur, the patient should be

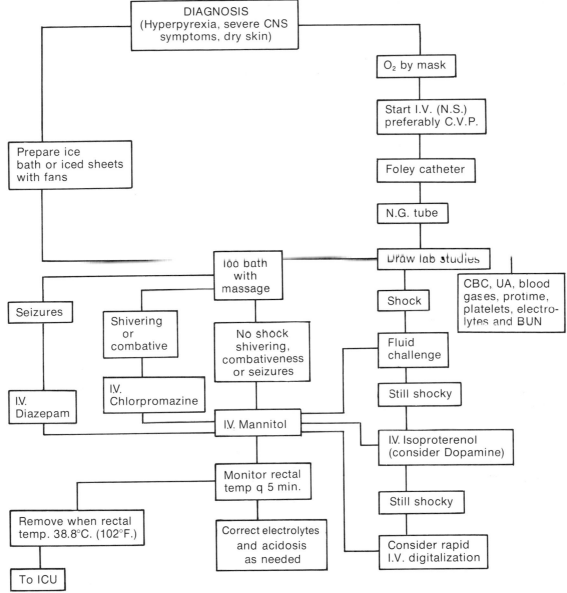

Figure 4.   Proposed plan for management of heat stroke in the Emergency Department.

removed from the water until they stop, then reimmersed. Treatment should be discontinued when central nervous symptoms disappear and the skin temperature appears equal to a normal control (yourself), using the back of the hand as a sensor. When transportation becomes available it should take priority over makeshift cooling meaures. In many situations transport may have to be by stretcher to some point where more rapid transport is available. If a physician is available and has phenothiazines, these should be given parenterally in an attempt to lower temperature.

References

Adam, J. M.: Heat, health and holidays. Practitioner *206*:363, 1971.

Austin, M. G., and Berry, J. W.: Observations on one hundred cases of heatstroke. J.A.M.A. *161*:1525, 1956.

Bass, D. E., et al.: Mechanisms of acclimatization to heat in man. Medicine *34*:323, 1955.

Clowes, G. H. A., Jr., and O'Donnell, T. F.: Current concepts: heat stroke. N. Engl. J. Med. 291:557, 1974.

Darling, R. C.: Heat Exhaustion, Heatstroke and Heat Cramps, A Textbook of Medicine, 9:517, 1955.

Eichler, A. C., McRae, A. S., and Root, H. D.: Heat stroke. Am. J. Surg. 118:855, 1969.

Ferris, E. B., Jr. et al.: Heat stroke: clinical and chemical observations on 44 cases. J. Clin. Invest. 17:245, 1938.

Gauss, H., and Meyer, K. A.: Heat stroke: report of one hundred and fifty-eight cases from Cook County Hospital, Chicago. Am. J. Med. Sci. 154:554, 1917.

Gold, J.: Development of heat pyrexia. J.A.M.A. 173:1175, 1960.

Gottschalk, P. G., and Thomas, J. E.: Heat stroke. Proc. Mayo Clin. 41:470, 1966.

Handbook of Physiology: Sec. 4, Chapter 15, The Temperature Regulation System, 259; Chapter 35, Man in the Desert, 551; Chapter 39, Terrestrial Animals in Humid Heat—Man, 625. Washington, D.C., American Physiological Society, 1964.

Hirsch, E. F., et al.: Biochemical changes observed in heat exhaustion under field conditions. Milit. Med. 135:881, 1970.

Hoagland, R. J., and Bishop, R. H., Jr.: A physiologic treatment of heat stroke. Am. J. Med. Sci. 241:415, 1961.

Kessinger, A., and Rigby, R. G.: Hemorrhage and heat stroke. Geriatrics 25:115, 1970.

Kew, M. C., et al.: The effects of heat stroke on the function and structure of the kidney. Q. J. Med. 36:277, 1967.

Kew, M. C., Abrahams, C., and Seftel, H. C.: Chronic interstitial nephritis as a consequence of heatstroke. Q. J. Med. 39:189, 1970.

Kew, M., et al.: Liver damage in heat stroke. Am. J. Med. 49:192, 1970.

Knochel, J. P.: Environmental heat illness. Arch. Intern. Med. 133:841, 1974.

Koroxenidis, G. T., Shepherd, J. T., and Marshall, R. J.: Cardiovascular response to acute heat stress. J. Appl. Physiol. 16:869, 1961.

Levine, J. A.: Heat stroke in the aged. Am. J. Med. 47:251, 1969.

Malamud, N., Haymaker, W., and Custer, R. P.: Heat stroke: a clinico-pathologic study of 125 fatal cases. Milit. Surg. 99:397, 1946.

Meikle, A. W., and Graybill, J. R.: Fibrinolysis and

hemorrhage in a fatal case of heat stroke. N. Engl. J. Med. 276:911, 1967.

Mehta, A. C., and Baker, R. N.: Persistent neurological deficits in heat stroke. Neurology 20:336, 1970.

O'Donnell, T. F., Jr.: Medical problems of recruit training: a research approach. U.S. Navy Med. 586:28, 1971.

O'Donnell, T. F., and Clowes, G. H. A., Jr.: Circulatory abnormalities of heat stroke. N. Engl. J. Med. 287:734, 1972.

Oechsli, F. W., and Buechley, R. W.: Excess mortality associated with three Los Angeles September hot spells. Environ. Res. 3:277, 1970.

Perchick, J. S., Winkelstein, A., and Shadduch, R. N.: Disseminated intravascular coagulation in heat stroke reponse to heparin therapy. J.A.M.A. 231:5, 480, 1975.

Redfearn, J. A., Jr., and Murphy, R. J.: History of heat stroke in a football trainee. J.A.M.A. 208:699, 1969.

Robey, J. M., Blyth, C. S., and Mueller, F. O.: Athletic injuries, application of epidemiologic methods. J.A.M.A. 217:184, 1971.

Robinson, S., et al.: Rapid acclimatization to work in hot climates. Am. J. Physiol. 140:168, 1943.

Schickele, E.: Environment and fatal heat stroke: an analysis of 157 cases occurring in the army in the U.S. during World War II. Milit. Surg. 100:235, 1947.

Shibolet, S., et al.: Heatstroke: its clinical picture and mechanism in 36 cases. Q. J. Med. 36:526, 1957.

Sohal, R. S., et al.: Heat stroke: an electron microscopic study of endothelial cell damage and disseminated intravascular coagulation. Arch. Intern. Med. 122:43, 1968.

Stefanini, M., and Spicer, D. D.: Hemostatic breakdown, fibrinolysis and acquired hemolytic anemia in a patient with fatal heatstroke: pathogenetic mechanisms. Am. J. Clin. Pathol. 55:180, 1971.

Weber, M. D., and Blakely, J. A.: The hemorrhagic diathesis of heat stroke. Lancet 1:1190, 1969.

Wilkinson, R. T., et al.: Psychological and physiological response to raised body temperature. J. Appl. Physiol. 19:287, 1964.

Wilson, G.: The cardiopathology of heatstroke. J.A.M.A. 114:557, 1940.

Wyndham, C. H., Strydom, N. B., and Morrison, J. F.: Fatigue of the sweat gland response. J. Appl Physiol. 21:107, 1966.

Yudis, M. et al.: Acute renal failure complicating heat stroke—a case report. Milit. Med. 136:884, 1971.

J. THE DIAGNOSIS AND TREATMENT OF SNAKEBITE

James R. Roberts

Snakes are among the most interesting and most feared reptiles on the earth, yet little is known about the mysterious poisons they inject into animals and man, and even less is known about the specific pathophysiology that results from their venoms. Therefore, the medical literature is filled with myths, misunderstandings, folklore, anecdotal treatments, contradictions, and false conclusions about the treatment of poisonous snakebites. A well documented, controlled, projective, double-blind study has yet to be written about the treatment of snakebite in humans. Although the diagnosis and treatment of snakebite is a problem infrequently encountered, it tests the

GENERAL INFORMATION

The number of species of snakes in the world is estimated between 2500 and 3000. Of these, less than 15 per cent are poisonous to man and probably fewer than 200 species are actually dangerous. Snakes range from the Arctic circle to the southern tip of South America, and are found in trees, in deserts, in the ground, in fresh water and in sea water. Only Iceland, Ireland, New Zealand, and a few small islands lack snakes completely. Like other reptiles, snakes are poikilothermic and they seek shelter when temperatures fall below 55°F. and rise above 100°F. Hence, they hibernate in the winter, are often nocturnal, and seek shelter in caves and under logs. They lack external ears and moveable eyelids, have a top crawling speed of 2 to 4 miles per hour, eat their food whole, will commonly eat other snakes, and will attack man only when threatened.

The mysterious flicking tongue of the snake picks up particles from the ground and air. The tiny forked tips are then inserted into pits in the palate which are lined with sensitive cells, called Jacobson's organs, which serve to identify the particles. Snakes have a well developed sense of smell, and can track their prey over terrain that would dumbfound a bloodhound.

DISTRIBUTION

Poisonous snakes are found in America in all the states except Hawaii, Alaska, and Maine, but only two families and four species need concern the practicing physician in the U.S. The coral snakes are members of the family Elapidae. The rattlesnakes, copperheads, and water moccasins (cottonmouth) are members of the family Crotalidae, and are called pit vipers. A pit viper possesses a heat sensing organ, which occupies a pitlike depression on both sides of the head between the eyes and the nostrils. These highly sensitive organs enable snakes to strike a prey with great accuracy, even in total darkness, based on the body heat of the victim.

There are about 30 kinds of rattlesnakes (Genera: *Crotalus* and *Sistrurus*) throughout the United States. They are found mainly in the southwest, Texas, and Florida. The diamondback rattlesnake is considered the most deadly snake in the U.S.

Copperheads (*Agkistrodon contortrix*) are found in the eastern and southern U.S. and into New England, and usually inhabit dry, rocky areas. The moccasins (*Agkistrodon piscivorus*), called "cottonmouth" because of the cotton white interior of their mouths, are semi-aquatic and inhabit the swampy areas in marshes and bayous of the eastern and southeastern states. Two species of brightly colored coral snakes inhabit the U.S. The Eastern coral snake (*Micrurus f. fulvius* and *Micrurus f. tenere*) ranges from coastal North Carolina and Florida to Texas; the less poisonous Arizona coral snake (*Micruroides euryxanthus*) is found in the southwestern U.S.

INCIDENCE AND MORTALITY

Although the actual figures are difficult to obtain, it is estimated that there are about 6000 poisonous snakebites per year in the U.S. Rattlesnakes account for about 55 per cent of these bites, copperheads 34 per cent, cottonmouths 10 per cent, and coral snakes 1 per cent. Less than 1 per cent of these victims die of snakebite poisoning, with rattlesnakes accounting for more than 70 per cent of reported deaths. Only about 14 persons die each year in the U.S. from poisonous snakes. About 70 per cent of these deaths occur in Texas, Georgia, Florida, Alabama, and South Carolina. For example, of the 6680 persons treated for poisonous snakebites in 1959 in the U.S., almost half had suffered copperhead bites. Of these, one possibly died from the copperhead bite, making the mortality rate from bites of this snake very low indeed. About one-half of all copperhead bites result in no systemic symptoms at all, producing only mild local reactions.

Rattlesnake bites are the most destructive, resulting in a much higher incidence of tissue necrosis and in permanent, serious damage to the bitten area. Mortalities from coral snakebites are low. Only about 30 coral snakebites are reported each year throughout the country. In one series (Sowder et al., 1968), there were no deaths in 33 cases of coral snakebites, and in another report (Parrish and Khan, 1967), only one death in 11 cases. The Eastern coral snake is more dangerous than the Arizona variety.

Most bites occur when the victim is within one mile from home, often in his own yard. Those most frequently bitten are children and young adults, and about 55 per cent of all bite victims are under the age of 20; 35 per cent are under the age of 10. Approximately 80 per cent of bites occur between June and October; between December and March they are rare. Peak hours are between 3:00 P.M. and 6:00 P.M., and about 80 per cent of bites occur between 9:00 A.M. and 9:00 P.M. It is not uncommon to be bitten by a poisonous snake after dark. Almost all bites occur on the extremities, approximately one-third on the upper extremities and two-thirds on the lower extremities; the majority are on the hands and fingers, lower legs, and feet. Of the 133 deaths reported by Parrish (1963), approximately 38 per cent occurred in the first 12 hours after the bite, and slightly over 90 per cent in the first 48 hours; delay in treatment was the most important factor contributing to mortality.

IDENTIFICATION OF POISONOUS SNAKES

One can distinguish a poisonous from a nonpoisonous snake by a variety of methods (Fig. 1). If one ventures close enough to a pit viper, a slitlike or elliptical pupil can be seen, and two well developed fangs, up to 1 inch long, will protrude from the maxilla on a hinge mechanism. The undersurface of a pit viper has a single row of subcaudal plates or scales. Nonpoisonous snakes, on the other hand, have round pupils; lack definite fangs, but have small teeth arranged in rows; and possess a double row of ventral scales. Poisonous coral snakes are an exception because they lack pits and have round pupils similar to nonpoisonous snakes.

Venom is produced in glands behind the eye, and muscular contractions force it through the long, hollow fangs, like the action of a hypodermic needle.

CHARACTERISTICS OF THE BITE

Pit vipers produce a characteristic bite when they inject venom into a victim. Most people, however, are bitten by an uniden-

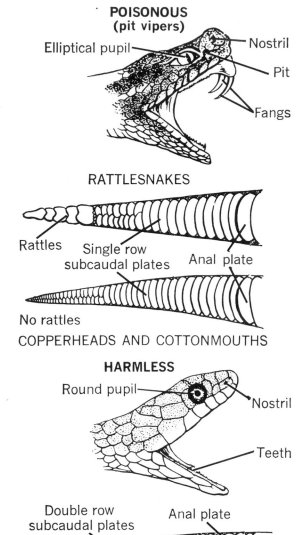

Figure 1. Features of pit vipers and harmless snakes. (From Parrish, H. M., and Carr, C. A.: J.A.M.A. *201*:927, 1967; copyright © 1967, American Medical Association.)

tified snake, usually a nonpoisonous variety. Nonvenomous snakes have four rows of small, curved, needle-like teeth on the upper jaw and two rows on the lower jaw. They produce a bite similar to the one shown in Figure 2. The bite is similar to the scratches made by a blackberry bush. There is little local swelling with only slight discomfort and itching around the teeth marks. A small ooze of blood may be seen but there are no

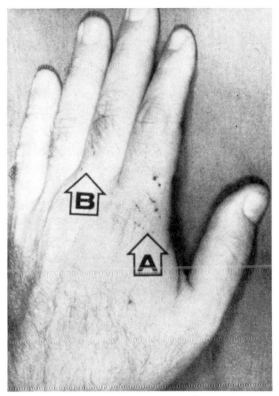

Figure 2. Typical marks on a hand bitten by a nonpoisonous snake. Four rows of teeth marks (A) on the victim's index finger; two rows of teeth marks (B) on the middle finger. (From Parrish, H. M., et al.: South. Med. J. 66:1413, 1973.)

with only minor scratch marks at the site of envenomation. The fangs of coral snakes are less than 6 mm. long and may fail to penetrate the skin, especially if heavy clothing is worn. Coral snakes may strike and hold on to a victim and exert a "chewing" motion, producing more than one wound. A history of a snake retaining its bite for a few seconds suggests a coral snake as culprit.

The amount of venom injected with each bite varies considerably, and probably only two-thirds of bites involve true envenomation. This is an important point, and many patients are subjected to needless treatment in cases in which either the offending snake was nonpoisonous or no actual envenomation occurred. The snake seems able to control the amount of poison released and injects up to three-fourths of its supply per bite. Table 1 gives the estimated number of lethal doses per bite from various snakes. An immediate second strike also may be dangerous. Since one-third of poisonous snakebites involve no venom at all, it is not surprising that the home remedies often employed as treatment, such as mud, chicken fat, and whiskey, are often deemed successful. Basically, the larger and older snakes inject a greater amount of more toxic venom, but even newborn snakes are a threat. Male snakes are probably more toxic than female snakes.

INFLUENCE OF THE BITE LOCATION

The area involved greatly influences the prognosis of a poisonous bite. Direct blood envenomation is probably quite rare and may account for the majority of rapid deaths. Snyder (1968) found that a lethal dose of venom injected directly into a vein in the dog leads to death in less than one minute. Bites of the face and neck are particularly dangerous because of the vascularity of this region. When injected into subcutaneous tissue, venom spreads by lymphatic rather than venous flow.

Since most bites occur in the extremities and actual mortality is low, the main concerns for the emergency physician are: (1) distinguishing a poisonous from a nonpoisonous bite; (2) deciding if envenomation actually has occurred; (3) preventing or limiting severe tissue damage; and (4) life support in cases of severe envenomation.

systemic effects. Proper treatment for nonvenomous snakebites consists of cleansing and tetanus toxoid.

When the bite of a poisonous snake results in envenomation, there will be almost instantaneous excruciating pain in the area bitten. Within a matter of minutes, the injured tissue will become swollen and ecchymotic, and this will lead rapidly to necrosis (Fig. 3). Occasionally, there will be anesthesia around the bite. Systemic symptoms can develop rapidly, often in a matter of minutes, depending on the location of the bite.

Viper bites result in the typical puncture wounds made by the snake's fangs (Fig. 4). Only one puncture may be seen if a glancing blow has occurred, or if the snake has lost a fang. The depth of penetration may be estimated as equal to the distance between the fang marks on the skin.

A coral snakebite, on the other hand, will produce little or no local tissue reaction,

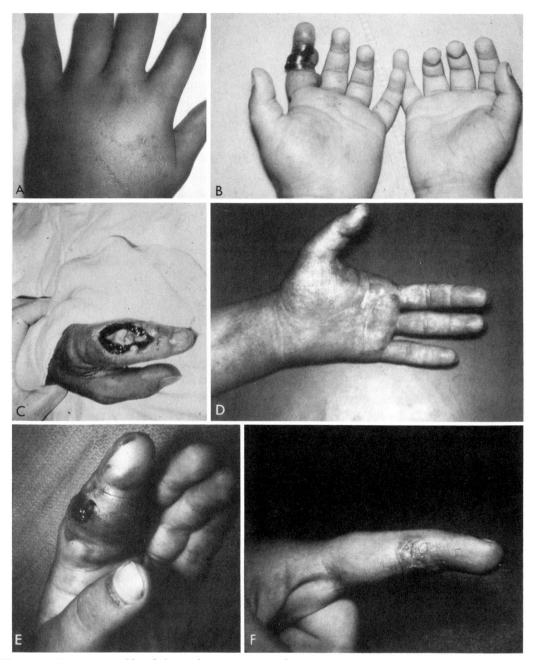

Figure 3. Appearance of hands bitten by poisonous snakes.

A, Snakes rarely bite a person more than once, but this hand was bitten three times (twice on the dorsum of the hand and once on the palmar surface of the index finger) by a pygmy rattlesnake.

B, Left index finger one hour after being bitten by a cottonmouth moccasin. The envenomation has produced asymmetry and edema, hemorrhagic transudate, bleb formation, and early necrosis.

C, Bite of timber rattlesnake three weeks after envenomation. There was loss of extensor tendon and the dorsal capsule of the PIP joint, with complete immobility and anesthesia of the finger.

D, Final result in the patient shown in *C* after filleting the finger and using the available skin over the thumb webspace.

E, Left index finger two hours after rattlesnake bite.

F, Final result of patient shown in *E*, utilizing local surgical treatment.

(From Snyder, C. C., Straight, R., and Glenn, J.: Plast. Reconstr. Surg. *49*:275, 1972; © 1972, The Williams & Wilkins Co., Baltimore.)

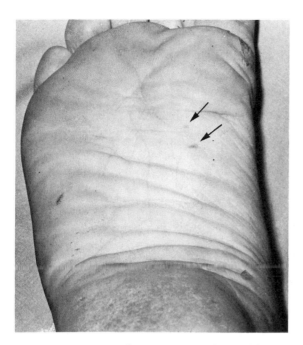

Figure 4. Typical puncture-type fang marks on a foot bitten by a poisonous pit viper. Two fang marks 1 cm. apart were found in the sole of the right foot. The skin around the fang marks was numb to the touch. (From Huang, T. T., et al.: Ann. Surg. *179*:598, 1974, with permission.)

VENOMS AND THEIR EFFECTS

Venom is an extremely complicated substance that varies greatly, not only from species to species, but among different varieties of the same species and even from time to time in the same snake. Dried snake venom is a remarkable substance that may retain its deadly properties up to 26 years when stored under proper conditions. No venom has been analyzed completely, and it is this complexity that has hampered advances in treatment. In general, pit vipers' venom possesses mainly hemotoxins, and coral snakes' mainly neurotoxins, although this is not absolute and may be misleading in some instances, causing errors in clinical judgment. The age, size, and individual sensitivity of the patient will alter responses to envenomation.

Local Reactions

RATTLESNAKES, COPPERHEADS, AND WATER MOCCASINS. At the site of crotalid (pit viper) envenomation, tissue destruction is greatest. There is direct necrosis of tissue almost immediately. Blood and fluid extravasates, and tissue pressure increases and obstructs circulation, producing ischemic dam-

TABLE 1

SNAKE	ESTIMATED MG. OF VENOM YIELDED PER BITE	SUBCUTANEOUS LD$_{50}$ (mg./kg. × 70)	NUMBER OF LETHAL DOSES OF VENOM PER BITE
Copperhead° (*Agkistrodon contortrix*)	52	1792	0.03†
Water moccasin° (*A. piscivorus*)	80–237	1806	0.04–0.12†
Eastern diamondback rattlesnake° (*Crotalus adamanteus*)	410	1015	0.40
Timber rattlesnake° (*C. horridus horridus*)	42–249	1050	0.04–0.24
Pygmy rattlesnake° (*Sistrurus catenatus*)	14–31	350	0.04–0.09†
Eastern coral snake° (*Micrurus fulvius*)	2	91	0.02†
Krait snake (*Bungarus multicinctus*)	11	14	0.80‡
Western diamondback rattlesnake° (*C. atrox*)	253	714	0.36
Taipan (*O. scutalatus*)	100–475	<14	>7.14–33.93‡
Indian cobra (*Naja naja*)	46–325	17.5	2.63–18.57‡

°Indicates snake found in the United States.

†Indicates low mortality expected.

‡Indicates probable high mortality.

age that compounds the direct effects of venom.

Ecchymosis develops rapidly, and blebs and blisters may appear. The skin assumes a gangrenous appearance, and there may be local sloughing. An entire extremity may become swollen in a matterof minutes. Pain is often severe.

CORAL SNAKES. A coral snake may produce only scratch marks or punctures, with little edema. Fatal envenomation may be present without any significant local tissue reaction.

Systemic Manifestations

PIT VIPERS (CROTALIDS). Systemic signs of pit viper envenomation are varied. In mild cases, there may be general weakness, fatigue, anxiety, and nausea. More severe cases exhibit vomiting, sweating, tachycardia, tachypnea, paresthesias, blurred vision, slurred speech, salivation, defecation, epistaxis, hematuria, hematemesis, muscle fasciculations, convulsions, coma, and death. It is difficult to attribute the effects to specific moieties in the venom, although kinins, slow-reacting substance, histamine, phospholipase-A, and serotonin have been implicated. Pit viper venoms have been reported to contain unidentified proteolytic enzymes, nonenzymatic proteins, lecithinase, ATP-ase, DNP-ase, ribonuclease, desoxyribonuclease, L-amino acid oxidase, cholinesterase, and hyaluronidase. A variety of unidentified cardiotoxins, neurotoxins, and hemotoxins abound in venoms, making it a most complex substance to deal with clinically.

CORAL SNAKE. Coral snake venom is different from viper venoms in its effect. It is mainly neurotoxic. Systemic effects of coral snake venom usually occur within one to seven hours, although delays of up to 18 hours have been reported. Paralysis of cranial nerves may occur in two and one-half hours, and complete respiratory paralysis has occurred within four hours of envenomation.

Cardiovascular and Respiratory Effects.

RATTLESNAKE VENOM. Intravenous injection of lethal amounts of rattlesnake venom in dogs produces a precipitous drop in blood pressure and peripheral resistance. This potent vasodilator activity acts directly or indirectly on arterioles or precapillary sphincters. An EKG pattern of myocardial damage or ischemia can be seen, and prema-

ture ventricular contractions and sinus tachycardia are noted. Respiratory activity is decreased, leading to apnea, and intestinal activity is increased, producing vomiting and defecation. There is almost immediate leakage of plasma into the intravascular space, with a rise in the hematocrit. Ownby (1974) noted the direct lysis of endothelial cells and immediate extravasation of blood, and attributes this to the direct action of venom on blood vessels, rather than a secondary effect to necrosis. Clinically, pulmonary edema, vascular collapse, and irreversible shock can occur.

CORAL SNAKE VENOM. Coral snake venom has fewer cardiovascular effects, but the venom does depress myocardial and skeletal muscle. Death usually results from respiratory arrest. The venom has an inhibitory effect on neuromuscular transmission by a blocking action on acetylcholine receptor sites that is not affected by neostigmine or edrophonium. A direct interference of axonal transmission also has been demonstrated (Rosenberg, 1965). Clinically, the first signs of this may be ptosis, strabismus, slurred speech, dilated pupils, dysphagia, and muscle weakness.

Hematologic Effects.

The hematologic effects of crotalid envenomation are most dramatic, and its pathophysiology has been studied in some detail. Clotting abnormalities, red cell morphology, platelet count and function, and bleeding tendencies have all been reported as markedly abnormal, but the literature is quite confusing in many cases. The abnormalities have been attributed to a variety of anticoagulants, procoagulants, fibrinolysins, hemorrhagins, and hemolysins (De Vries and Cohen, 1969).

Disseminated intravascular coagulation (DIC) (defibrination syndrome, consumption coagulopathy, intravascular coagulation–defibrinolysis syndrome), in its strict definition, is probably very rare following envenomation. Wintrobe (1974) feels that the utilization of fibrinogen, platelets, and other clotting factors must be seen for true DIC, and also inherent in the strict definition is the elaboration of thrombin, formation of fibrin, and activation of the fibrinolytic system. Fibrin degradation products also must be produced. This results in diffuse bleeding and vascular occlusion with disastrous systemic complications. The only true case of DIC has been reported in the bite of the Saw scaled viper (*Echis carinatus,* a snake not found in the U.S.). The venom of this snake appears to activate prothrombin directly, convert it to thrombin, and cause platelet aggregation. This syndrome may respond dramatically to heparin treatment when other forms of therapy have failed to correct the hypofibrinogenemia and thrombocytopenia.

Hasiba (1975) has reported a DIC-like syndrome after the bite of the American timber rattlesnake (*Crotalis horridus horridus*). In this case, the patient developed petechiae, gingival bleeding, and ecchymosis with hypofibrinogenemia, thrombocytopenia, and the production of fibrin degradation products, and was treated with heparin. However, in vitro tests suggested that heparin probably had little therapeutic effect.

The documentation of true DIC after the bite of an American snake is lacking in the literature.

Other hematologic syndromes have been reported in snakes not native to the U.S. Among them are: (1) hypofibrinogenemia without thrombocytopenia or fibrinolysis in the Malayan pit viper, (2) hypofibrinogenemia without thrombocytopenia but with fibrinolysis in the Saw scaled viper.

The blood of patients bitten by poisonous snakes has been observed to remain unclotted for days, but with minimal to no hemorrhage. Complete afibrinogenemia has been reported as early as one hour after a bite, and platelet counts lower than 10,000 cu. mm. in less than two hours. Fatal intracerebral hemorrhage has occurred, but bleeding tendencies seem to be related to platelet count and prothrombin time rather than to absolute fibrinogen levels.

Often, prothrombin time is prolonged and platelet count depressed after envenomation. These studies must be ordered, and clinical improvement can be monitored closely with these parameters.

Spherocyte transformation, acanthocytosis, increased red cell osmotic fragility, false-positive direct Coombs' tests, Heinz body formation, intravascular hemolysis, and burring of erythrocytes may occur (see Fig. 5). Venom also interferes with routine procedures in cross-matching blood for transfusions, and cross-matching and typing should be considered early in the management of patients bitten by poisonous snakes.

Renal Complications. Snake venom has a variety of complex nephrotoxic effects, although renal involvement usually occurs in the form of acute renal failure secondary to either tubule necrosis or cortical necrosis. Glomerulonephritis and proliferative nephritis, presumably on a hypersensitive basis, have been reported, as well as nephrotic syndrome and renal infarction.

Hemoglobinuria, probably secondary to intravascular hemolysis, and myoglobinuria may occur. Renal failure is rare following poisonous snakebites.

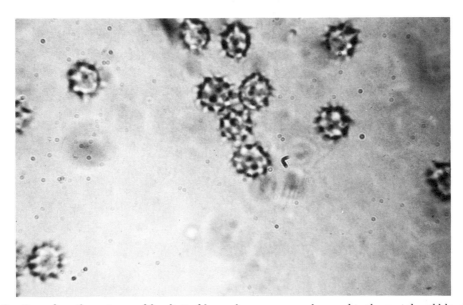

Figure 5. Burred erythrocytes readily elicited by snake venom are observed in the peripheral blood of patients bitten by poisonous snakes. (From Huang, T. T., et al.: Ann. Surg. *179*:598, 1974, with permission.)

Infection. Infection does not seem to be a major complication of snakebites, but it often is difficult to differentiate from envenomation.

Positive cultures have been found for both aerobic and anaerobic organisms in the oral cavity of rattlesnakes. Of the gram-negative bacteria, Aerobacter, Proteus, and Pseudomonas are the most common, and, less frequently, strains of Salmonella. The gram-positive organisms are enterococcus, Streptococcus viridans, and histotoxic Clostridia. In most studies, no *Clostridium tetani*, Bacteroides, or coagulase-positive staphylococci have been isolated. Deaths have been reported from tetanus following snakebites, although the organism has not been cultured in the oral cavity of snakes in the U.S.

TREATMENT

The specific treatment of snakebites is a subject of extreme controversy and conflicting views. This is partly due to the tremendous variation in composition of snake venoms, which lead to a variety of clinical presentations and pathophysiology. Also, there is no well documented study evaluating the different modes of treatment. In general, however, the more rapidly treatment is instituted, the better are the results.

When a patient is suspected of having been bitten by a poisonous snake, it is important to establish if the offending snake truly was poisonous and if envenomation has occurred. The characteristic fang marks and severe local and systemic reactions described can be helpful in deciding. In doubtful cases, observation in the Emergency De-

partment is justified. In confirmed cases, the patient should avoid all unnecessary exercise, such as walking to the hospital, and no alcohol should be consumed. Both will increase the escape of venom from the injection site (see Fig. 6). In cases of severe systemic reactions, first priority must be given to establishing an adequate airway and insuring proper ventilation and cardiovascular integrity.

OBJECTIVES OF TREATMENT

The objectives of treatment are: (1) prevention of the spread of venom; (2) removal of venom; (3) neutralization of venom and general support of the patient; (4) limitation and repair of damage.

Testing for sensitivity to horse serum should be carried out as soon as possible, and antivenin obtained for possible use. The patient should be kept NPO. A large-bore intravenous line should be secured and, if the patient is in a shocklike state (low CVP, small urine output, anxiety, diaphoresis, and weak, thready pulse), he should be placed in Trendelenburg's position and given fluid replacement. Vasopressors may be needed. Equipment for tracheal intubation and a respirator should be placed next to the bedside, and cardiac monitoring instituted. Table 2 represents a reasonable systematic approach to treatment. Pain should be relieved with the appropriate drugs, narcotics if necessary.

TOURNIQUET USE AND IMMOBILIZATION

A tourniquet applied loosely, proximal and distal to the bite, will decrease systemic

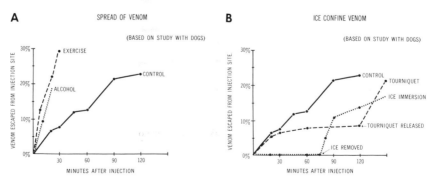

Figure 6. Studies in dogs show (*A*) how alcohol and exercise enhance the spread of venom and (*B*) how well a tourniquet and ice confine venom. (From Snyder, C. C., and Knowles, R. P.: Consultant 3:44, 1963; reproduced with permission of *Consultant*, the Journal of Medical Consultation.)

TABLE 2

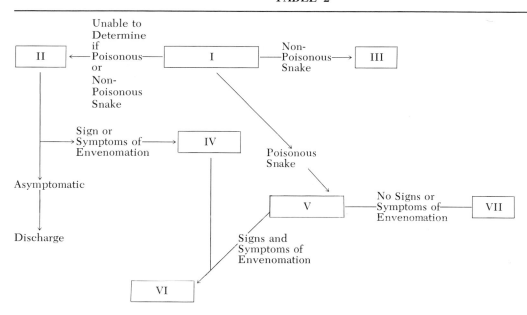

I. Initial evaluation
    (1) Determine if snake was poisonous or nonpoisonous (character of bite, local or systemic reaction, snake identification)
    (2) Initial history and physical examination with attention to underlying medical problems, allergies, circumstances of bite
    (3) Begin record of vital signs
II. (1) NPO/monitor vital signs—strict bed rest—immobilize bitten area
    (2) Large bore IV, bloodwork—draw baselines and hold
    (3) Test for sensitivity to horse serum or antivenin
    (4) Obtain antivenin for possible use
    (5) Tetanus prophylaxis
    (6) Observe in Emergency Department for 4–18 hours
III. (1) Tetanus prophylaxis
    (2) Clean wound
    (3) Check wound in 48–72 hours
IV. (1) Begin EKG monitoring
    (2) Send baseline blood to lab
    (3) Intubation equipment, respirator in room
    (4) Tourniquet, cooling, immobilization
V. (1) NPO/strict bed rest
    (2) Large bore IV
    (3) Draw and send baseline bloodwork
    (4) Monitor vital signs and EKG
    (5) Tetanus prophylaxis
    (6) Obtain antivenin for possible use and test for sensitivity to horse serum immediately
    (7) Intubation equipment and respirator at bedside
    (8) Tourniquet, cooling, immobilization of bitten area
VI. (1) Call for help if available—antivenin immediately if severe or deemed necessary or patient is pregnant
    (2) Reassess airway, breathing, cardiovascular status—admit to intensive care unit
    (3) Surgical excision of envenomated tissue immediately
    (4) Evaluation for early fasciotomy
    (5) CVP or Swan-Ganz catheter
    (6) Foley catheter and urine for studies, forced diuresis if urine positive for hemoglobin or myoglobin
    (7) Medications for relief of pain as needed
    (8) Corticosteroids, antibiotics after aspiration for culture
VII. (1) Observe for 24 hours
    (2) Discharge if asymptomatic

absorption. Venom spreads slowly by lymphatics, unless direct intravascular envenomation has occurred. One should be able to insert a finger under a properly applied tourniquet, which will occlude lymphatic circulation and leave arterial flow intact. A tourniquet that produces ischemia is contraindicated. Most venom remains in the subcutaneous tissues for a considerable time, and a tourniquet, once placed, should not be removed, since this may perpetuate the spread of venom by a milking action.

The tourniquet should be released after two hours or earlier when proper facilities for further treatment are available or if antivenin is administered.

The patient should be kept at strict bed rest, and the bitten area must be completely immobilized.

ICE

The bitten area should be cooled immediately. Dry cold packs will protect the skin from maceration. Extreme cold for extended periods of time, however, may increase pain

---

TABLE 3   *Guide to Sensitivity Testing and the Use of Equine Serum (Antivenin)* [*]

General guidelines: 1. Test *all* patients as soon as possible, regardless of history.
2. A negative history for allergy does not rule out the possibility of a severe reaction or development of serum sickness.
3. Use normal saline as a control when testing.
4. WEIGH THE RISK OF WITHHOLDING ANTIVENIN AGAINST THE RISK OF DEATH FROM ENVENOMATION.

| Negative history | ←————Sensitivity testing————→ | Positive history |

Use 1:10 dilution of horse serum or antivenin.

Use 1:100 dilution of horse serum or antivenin. *Note*: Severe reaction may occur with test dose.

Skin test: 0.02 cc. intracutaneously to raise a wheal. A positive reaction is a wheal with or without erythema or pseudopodia in 5 to 30 minutes.
Conjunctival test: 1 drop in the conjunctival sac. A positive reaction is itching, redness, and possibly edema within 1 to 10 minutes. *Note*: For severe reactions, instill 1 or 2 drops of epinephrine, 1:1000, in eye.

| Negative history and negative sensitivity test | Negative history and questionable or mildly positive sensitivity test | Strongly positive sensitivity test |

Administer antivenin full strength intravenously.

Antivenin contraindicated unless a life-threatening situation exists.

If situation permits, desensitization may be of some value

→If clinically indicated

1. Prepare 1:100, 1:10, and full-strength dilutions of antivenin.
2. Allowing 15 minutes between injections, inject subcutaneously in an extremity, 0.1 cc., 0.2 cc., 0.5 cc. of increasingly concentrated solution until 0.5 cc. of full-strength solution has been injected.
3. If reaction occurs, treat with tourniquet and epinephrine and begin at lower dose.
4. This method *may* be of limited value in "tying-up" antibodies to permit introduction of antigenic substance:

1. Obtain medication and equipment to combat anaphylaxis.
2. *Pretreatment* with epinephrine *may* be of value.
3. Prepare 1:10 dilution of antivenin and administer *slowly* (1 to 2 cc. first 3 minutes) intravenously
4. Continue as clinically indicated, treating complications as necessary.

[*]A national antivenin index is maintained at Oklahoma City Zoo, phone number 405–424–3344, and the Los Angeles County/Southern California Medical Center provides consultation on snake bites for physicians.

and aggravate necrosis. Cooling is only of benefit in the first few hours. Cryotherapy in the form of freezing or extreme low temperatures for more than a few hours only increases tissue destruction and lengthens the period of disability. With ice immersion and a tourniquet, less than one-quarter of the injected venom will be absorbed in the leg of a dog in the first two hours (Snyder and Knowles, 1963).

ANTIVENIN

The most controversial part of therapy is when to use antivenin. Two types are commercially available. The Crotalidae polyvalent antivenin (Wyeth) is active against the venom of rattlesnakes, cottonmouths and copperheads. An antivenin is also available for the Eastern and Texas coral snakes (*Micrurus fulvius*, Wyeth). No antiserum is available against the less virulent Arizona coral snake, *Micruroides euryxanthus*. Antivenin for the exotic snakes found in zoos, e.g., cobras, is not commercially available in the U.S., although some zoos have a supply on hand prepared in foreign countries. The antivenin is supplied in the dry state, which must be reconstituted and used immediately. The unconstituted form has a shelf life of five years, is rarely stocked in hospital pharmacies, and is presently of equine origin only. A 1-cc. vial of one-tenth dilution of horse serum accompanies each vial of antivenin and can be used as an intracutaneous or conjunctival test for sensitivity. Work has been done to develop a goat serum antivenin, but it is unavailable as yet.

Reactions to antivenin are frequent, resulting in close to 100 per cent serum sickness when more than 100 cc. (10 vials) is used. Fatal anaphylactic reactions have occurred. Serum sickness, characterized by skin rashes, fever, malaise, lymphadenopathy, and articular pains, usually appears in seven to 21 days after antivenin has been administered, and a negative sensitivity test does not mean that serum sickness will not develop. Children and small adults need relatively more antivenin than do large

Figure 7. Recommendations for antivenin administration according to grade of envenomation. These criteria are questioned by those advocating early surgical treatment. (From package insert for Antivenin Polyvalent, Wyeth Laboratories)

Grade 0—No evidence of envenomation. History of suspected snakebite. Fang wound(s) may be present. Minimal pain, less than 1 inch of surrounding edema and erythema. No systemic manifestations during first 12 hours following bite.

Grade I—Minimal envenomation. History of suspected snakebite. Fang wound(s) usually present. Moderate pain or throbbing localized at fang wound(s), surrounded by 1 to 5 inches of edema and erythema. No evidence of systemic involvement after 12 hours of observation.

Grade II—Moderate envenomation. The signs and symptoms of Grade I rapidly progress during first 12 hours, with severer and more widely distributed pain; edema spreading toward the trunk; petechiae and ecchymoses limited to area of edema. Nausea, vomiting, giddiness and mild temperature elevation usually present.

Grade III—Severe envenomation. May resemble Grade I or II when brought under observation, but course rapidly progressive. May arrive in shock within a few minutes of bite. Within 12 hours, edema spreads up extremity and may involve part of trunk. Petechiae and ecchymoses may be generalized. Systemic manifestations may include rapid pulse, shock-like state, subnormal temperature.

Grade IV—Very severe envenomation.[6] Seen especially after envenomation by large rattlesnakes. Characterized by sudden pain, rapidly progressive swelling, which may reach and involve trunk within a few hours, with ecchymoses, bleb formation, and necrosis. Systemic manifestations, often commencing within 15 minutes of bite, usually include weakness, nausea and vomiting, vertigo, numbness or tingling of lips or face. Muscle fasciculations, painful muscular cramping, pallor, sweating, cold and clammy skin, rapid and weak pulse, incontinence, convulsions and coma also may be observed; death may occur.

DOSAGE AND ADMINISTRATION

NOTE: Before administration, read sections on precautions to be taken in administration of horse serum and systemic reactions. Since the possibility of a severe immediate reaction (anaphylaxis) always exists whenever horse serum is administered, appropriate therapeutic agents, such as a tourniquet, oxygen supply, epinephrine 1:1000, and another injectable pressor amine, must be ready for immediate use.

SUGGESTED GUIDE
FOR INITIAL DOSAGE OF ANTIVENIN[3-10]

GRADE OF ENVENOMATION	ADMINISTER CONTENTS OF	PREFERABLE ROUTE
0	None	—
I	1 Vial	IM - anterolateral thigh or buttock
II	2 to 4 Vials	At least 50% IV; balance IM
III	At least 5 Vials	IV
IV	10 to 20 Vials, or more	IV

adults. A protocol for the treatment of patients sensitive to antivenin, in cases in which its use is deemed necessary, is found in the drug information insert accompanying each vial of antivenin. A history of sensitivity to horse serum and other allergic conditions should always be sought, and antivenin should be used with extreme caution when the possibility of immediate sensitivity exists. In life-threatening situations, antivenin may be warranted even when a sensitivity by skin testing or history has been shown (see Table 3).

Indications for Antivenin. Figure 7 is a guide for the use of antivenin based on a grading of envenomation. With early surgical débridement, the use of antivenin in Grades I and II envenomation is subject to debate. Large doses (5 to 20 vials) of antivenin are definitely indicated in the early treatment of severe envenomation of life-threatening magnitude, Grades III and IV, and in this instance may be life-saving. If early local treatment is performed, probably only Grades III and IV require antivenin. Specific dosage depends on the clinical course. The actual efficacy of antivenin in preventing local tissue necrosis, myolysis, or hematologic abnormalities has been questioned (Stahnke, 1966), although studies have shown an increased survival rate of dogs when antivenin is used, and there has been evidence that, if given soon enough, it will reduce the amount of local tissue destruction in humans. In mild cases, evidence suggests that surgical treatment, without the routine use of antivenin, yields equally good results (Huang, 1974). The method of grading bites solely on the basis of pain, edema, and ecchymosis is inadequate and misleading and, unless the entire clinical spectrum is considered, may lead to disastrous consequences. The numbering system serves only as a rough approximation of envenomation and is no substitute for careful clinical observation and serial laboratory studies.

If antivenin is used, it should be used as early as possible and given parenterally. The usual route is intravenous. The intramuscular route, and injection around the bite itself, should be discouraged. The absorption of intramuscular antivenin is unpredictable and local injection will only increase swelling. It is important to remember that children need more antivenin than do adults. The clinical course may be precipitous and exaggerated in children.

CORTICOSTEROIDS

The routine use of corticosteroids is controversial. Various steroid preparations have been used for a variety of reasons, and there is little doubt that they decrease the incidence of allergic reactions when antivenin is used. The addition of 100 mg. of hydrocortisone to each vial of diluted antivenin has been suggested to cover possible reactions to horse serum. There is no clear evidence that steroids increase survival, but high doses, the equivalent of 1 to 2 gm. of hydrocortisone every four to six hours for 72 hours, may decrease the swelling and inflammation if used early in the treatment, and may ameliorate some of the toxic symptoms of envenomation. Steroids may be of value in the treatment of the profound hypotension seen after direct intravascular injection of venom, and they should be used in cases in which life-threatening envenomation has occurred.

ANTIHISTAMINES

Antihistamines may be synergistic with snake venom and therefore should not be used.

FLUID THERAPY

Hypotension after a poisonous bite may be severe. In the first hour, it may be due to a direct toxic effect of venom on the myocardium and peripheral vascular system, and may respond to fluids and large doses of steroids. After the first hour, fluid shifts into the area of envenomation may produce a profound hypovolemia. Large amounts of lactated Ringer's solution and whole blood may be required to correct this defect. A central venous pressure reading and a record of hourly urine output can be useful in monitoring fluid balance. If the urine is discolored (hemoglobin or myoglobin), attempts to insure a urine output of at least 1.5 ml./kg./hour in the adult are suggested. In the child over the age of 5, 30 to 50 ml. per hour is suggested; for children aged 2 to 5, 20 to 30 ml. per hour; and for children under 2, 10 to 20 ml. per hour. This urine output may be accomplished with intravenous fluids if the cardiovascular system can handle the fluid load, or with the use of osmotic diuretics such as mannitol. Acute renal failure probably can be prevented and this should be a priority early in the treatment of snakebite. All patients so treated or observed should have a large (No.16–18) intravenous line routinely inserted. For more serious cases, a Swan-Ganz catheter or central venous line is indicated.

ANTIBIOTICS

Although *Clostridium tetani* organisms have not been found in the fangs or mouths of snakes, tetanus prophylaxis is recommended. The value of routine antibiotics is unclear, but secondary infection of necrotic tissue and osteomyelitis of fingers and toes have occurred. Moreover, bacteria have been cultured from snake venom. After aspirating material for Gram stain and aerobic and anaerobic cultures, broad spectrum antibiotics should be started parenterally. Cephalothin at a dose of 1 or 2 gm. intravenously every six hours is a good initial choice. If sepsis occurs, an antibiotic effective against anaerobes (e.g., chloramphenicol or Cleocin) should be added. Tetracyclines should not be used in children, and penicillin alone is probably inadequate.

Blood Products

Packed red blood cells occasionally may be needed to correct the hemolytic anemia associated with snakebite. One should draw blood immediately to type and cross-match, because hemolysis may interfere with subsequent attempts. Although clotting abnormalities often are seen, they usually regress spontaneously. Rarely, fibrinogen or platelets are required for bleeding problems.

Laboratory

A base line complete blood count, fibrinogen level, platelet count, prothrombin time, BUN, and electrolytes should be obtained. These studies should be repeated every two to eight hours, depending on the clinical course. A peripheral smear for the changes in red cell morphology may help in estimating the severity of the bite. In the case of coral snakebites, several arterial blood gas determinations will help monitor pulmonary function, and an intra-arterial catheter should be used routinely in severe cases. Blood lactate level readings may be of value in cases of lactic acidosis accompanying hypotension. The urine should be examined for hemoglobin and myoglobin, and stools should be examined for occult blood.

Surgical Treatment

Early surgical treatment in the Emergency Department may prevent future loss of function and may lessen the amount of tissue destruction following snakebite (Fig. 8). The time-honored incision over the fang marks and suction is of value in removing the venom from the subcutaneous tissues. The early use of incision and prolonged suction can remove 50 per cent of the venom in dogs experimentally treated, and actual surgical excision of the tissue involved, when employed within the first ten minutes, can remove almost 80 per cent. In field conditions, a single vertical incision through and beyond each fang mark may be made to a depth equal to the distance between the fang marks. Continuous mouth suction can be employed. Suction cups are available, although venom will not penetrate the intact mucosa of the mouth and is inactivated in the stomach. Suction should be maintained for 15 to 30 minutes. Cruciate or cross-hatching incisions may lead to necrosis of the skin flaps and may be difficult to revise later. Excellent results have been obtained employing early surgical excision of the ecchymotic, necrotic, and hemorrhagic tissues surrounding the bite, without routine use of antivenin. In the Emergency Department, under local anesthesia, a skin flap is elevated or an elliptical incision made, and the envenomated tissue identified and removed. The major vessels, nerves, and tendons should be left in place, but all subcutaneous tissue and muscle that appears necrotic should be removed. The area may be closed later with the initial skin flap or with grafted tissue. This procedure has proved successful in a series of 54 cases described by Huang (1974) and 84 cases described by Glass (1973). Complications can be necrosis of the skin flaps or loss of the skin graft. Fasciotomy also has gained acceptance as a beneficial surgical treatment, and should be considered early in management when extensive swelling and necrosis are present.

SNAKEBITE DURING PREGNANCY

Little is known about snakebite during pregnancy. Parrish (1966) describes four pregnant patients bitten by pit vipers. Three delivered normal infants; one patient aborted 24 hours after envenomation. Possible mechanisms accounting for abortion may be

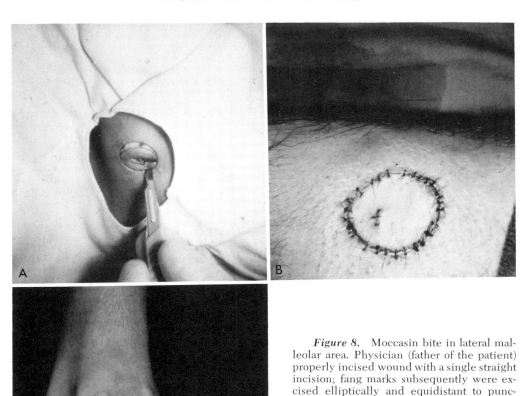

Figure 8. Moccasin bite in lateral malleolar area. Physician (father of the patient) properly incised wound with a single straight incision; fang marks subsequently were excised elliptically and equidistant to punctures (*A*). Three days later the wound was skin-grafted (*B*), and the patient was back in school in ten days (*C*). (From Snyder, C. C., et al.: J. Fla. Med. Assoc. 55:336, 1968.)

(1) anoxia associated with shock, (2) bleeding into the placenta and uterine wall, and (3) uterine contractions initiated by venom. It is advisable to institute aggressive therapy in pregnant patients bitten by poisonous snakes.

IMMUNIZATION

Attempts at producing active immunization by a toxoid have not been successful, mainly because the methods used for detoxifying venom have led to production of a poorly immunogenic substance.

However, encouraging results have been reported recently in this field with the poisonous Habu snake in Japan. Apparent successful immunization in humans has been reported sporadically following multiple injection of small amounts of snake venom in people intimately involved in snake handling.

References

Brown, J. H.: Toxicology and Pharmacology of Venoms from Poisonous Snakes. Springfield, Ill., Charles C Thomas, 1973.

Chavarria, A. P., Villarejos, V. M., and Zomeo, M.: Clinical importance of the prothrombin time determination in snake venom poisoning. Am. J. Trop. Med. Hyg. *19*:342, 1970.

Danzig, L. E., and Abels, G. H.: Hemodialysis of acute renal failure following rattlesnake bite with recovery. J.A.M.A. *175*:136, 1961.

DeVries, A., and Cohen, I.: Hemorrhagic and Blood Coagulation Disturbing Action of Snake Venom. *In* Poller, L. (ed.): Recent Advances in Blood Coagulation. Boston, Little, Brown & Co., 1969.

Dvilansky, A., and Biran, H.: Hypofibrinogenemia after Echis cholorata bite in man. Acta Haematol. Kbh. *49*:123, 1973.

Furtado, M. A., and Lester, I. A.: Myoglobinuria following snakebite. Med. J. Aust. *1*:674, 1968.

Gill, K. A.: The evaluation of cryotherapy in the treatment of snake envenomization. South. Med. J. *63*:552, 1970.

Glass, T. G.: Early débridement in pit viper bite. Surg. Gynecol. Obstet. *136*:774, 1973.

Hasiba, U., et al.: DIC-like syndrome after envenomation by the snake, Crotalus horridus horridus. N. Engl. J. Med. *292*:505, 1975.

Henderson, B. M., and Dujon, E. B.: Snakebites in children. J. Pediatr. Surg. 8:729, 1973.

Huang, T. T., et al.: The use of excisional therapy in the management of snakebite. Ann. Surg. 179:598, 1974.

Jimenez-Porras, J. M.: Biochemistry of snake venoms. Clin. Toxicol. 3:389, 1970.

Ledbetter, E. O., and Kutscher, A. E.: The aerobic and anaerobic flora of rattlesnake fangs and venom. Arch. Environ. Health 19:770, 1969.

Ownby, C. L., et al.: Pathogenesis of hemorrhage induced by rattlesnake venom. Am. J. Pathol. 76:401, 1974.

Parrish, H. M., and Carr, C. A.: Bites by copperheads in the U.S. J.A.M.A. 201:927, 1967.

Parrish, H. M.: Analysis of 460 fatalities from venomous animals in the U.S. Am. J. Med. Sci. 245:129, 1963.

Parrish, H. M., et al.: Clinical features of bites by nonvenomous snakes. South. Med. J. 66:1412, 1973.

Parrish, H. M., and Khan, M. S.: Snakebite during pregnancy. Obstet. Gynecol. 27:468, 1966.

Parrish, H. M., and Khan, M. S.: Bites by coral snakes.

Report of 11 representative cases. Am. J. Med. Sci. 253:561, 1967.

Rosenberg, P.: Effects of venoms on the giant squid. Axon. Toxicon. 3:125, 1965.

Sitprisa, V., et al.: Further observations on renal insufficiency in snakebite. Nephron 13:396, 1974.

Snyder, C. C., and Knowles, R. P.: Snakebite! Consultant (SKF) 3:44, 1963.

Snyder, C. C., Straight, R., and Glenn, J.: The snakebitten hand. Plast. Reconstr. Surg. 49:275, 1972.

Snyder, C. C., et al.: A definitive study of snakebites. J. Fla. Med. Assoc. 55:330, 1968.

Sowder, W. T., and Gehres, G. W.: Snakebite myths and misinformation. J. Fla. Med. Assoc. 55:319, 1968.

Stahnke, H. L.: The Treatment of Venomous Bites and Stings. Tempe, Arizona, Arizona State University Press, 1966.

Weiss, H. J., et al.: Afibrinogenemia in a man following the bite of a rattlesnake (Crotalis adamantus). Am. J. Med. 47:625, 1969.

Wintrobe, M. M., et al.: Clinical Hematology. 7th ed. London, Henry Kimpton, 1974, pp. 1211–1224.

K.   SMOKE INHALATION

Harvey M. Silverman

The problem of smoke inhalation (smoke poisoning, pulmonary burn, respiratory burn) has been generally recognized within the past 15 years, but knowledge in this area is far from complete.

Reports in the 1960s by Phillips (1962), Stone (1967), and others pointed out that respiratory injury is a principal cause of mortality in patients with body surface burns. Moreover, respiratory injury can occur without body surface burns. Zikria et al. (1972) reviewed the autopsies of deaths from fires in New York City over a two-year period and did not find a consistent association of pulmonary pathology with the presence or absence of surface burns.

Smoke inhalation is a significant problem, both in incidence and in morbidity and mortality. It is usually the emergency physician who is called upon to diagnose and to initiate treatment of the victim.

ETIOLOGY

The precise causative factors of the entity of smoke inhalation are not known.

Factors Involved in Producing Inhalation Injury

HEAT AND HUMIDITY

In 1945, noting the uncertainty of the relative roles of thermal and chemical factors, Moritz published the results of investigations to determine the pathologic characteristics of uncomplicated thermal injury of the lungs and air passages and of the temperatures that are necessary for their production. Using, in dogs, an insulated transoral cannula that extended from outside the mouth to below the vocal folds of the larynx, the experimenters were surprised to find that dry air heated to 500° C. was cooled to no more than 50° C. by the time it reached the tracheal bifurcation, and no injury was noted, either of the lower trachea or more distally. It was necessary to force the inhalation of steam to produce significant pulmonary injury. The importance of this experiment was in showing that the upper airway is very efficient in cooling inspired air and that the energy content of hot dry air is not sufficient to produce lower respiratory damage. Thermal burn of the respiratory tract is generally confined to the upper airway, where it occasionally may cause sufficient edema to obstruct the airway.

In 1967, Stone et al. reported the effects of various temperatures and humidities on the survival of experimental rats. Placing rats in drying ovens at various temperatures and standard humidity, they found that mortality for a given time of exposure increased with increased temperature. Keeping the temperature constant and varying humidity, it was found that increased humidity was associated with increased mortality for a given time of exposure.

SMOKE

Smoke generally is considered to be a combination of particulate matter, volatilized products of combustion, and various gases. Smoke particles consist principally of carbon, which may be coated with the condensed products of combustion. The particles vary in size, but many are less than 1 μ and are small enough to be inhaled deeply into the lungs.

In Stone's study (1967), the presence of cotton smoke significantly increased mortality and appeared to be a more important factor than humidity. Zikria et al. (1972) compared the effects of wood smoke and kerosene smoke on dogs. Wood smoke produced significant pulmonary pathology and mortality, but kerosene smoke did not. Analysis of the two types of smoke revealed that wood smoke contained ten times the quantity of carbon monoxide and 20 times the quantity of aldehyde gases. Cotton smoke also was shown to contain large quantities of aldehydes. Wood and cotton, as furniture, mattresses, and clothing, usually are burned in house fires. Newer synthetics can release hydrogen cyanide gas when burned, as well as gases that cause intense respiratory tract irritation.

Although aldehydes cause damage in laboratory conditions, other irritants such as acid anhydrides may be more significant under clinical conditions, because aldehydes tend to condense out of smoke before they are inhaled, whereas the acid anhydrides enter the lungs more readily. Other substances, such as oxides of nitrogen and sulfur, or the products of combustion of plastics, also can produce respiratory irritation.

Toxic substances (e.g., industrial solvents and insecticides) may be released from storage units damaged during fire and thus contribute to the clinical problem.

SOOT

In Zikria's study (1972), kerosene soot and wood soot were blown into the distal trachea by bronchoscopy, and neither produced mortality nor significant pathology. Particulate matter, in and of itself, probably is not significant in the etiology of the clinical problem.

CARBON MONOXIDE

The role of carbon monoxide poisoning in the clinical spectrum of smoke inhalation often has been overlooked until recently. In Zikria's review of autopsy results (1972), he noted that carbon monoxide levels greater than 50 per cent were found in 24 per cent of patients dying within the first 12 hours, making carbon monoxide poisoning the probable primary cause of death. Furthermore, another 34 per cent had carbon monoxide levels between 11 per cent and 49 per cent. Carbon monoxide poisoning was found in 39 per cent of those dying within the first 12 hours who did not have a body surface burn.

Zarem (1973) reported on 13 patients who presented to the Emergency Department with smoke inhalation and had carbon monoxide levels from 8 per cent to 40 per cent. In retrospect, he was able to attribute some of the symptomatology to the carbon monoxide poisoning that had not been diagnosed on clinical grounds.

Carbon monoxide itself is not considered a pulmonary irritant, and clinical problems result from preferential combination with hemoglobin, producing carboxyhemoglobin, which cannot carry oxygen to the tissues. Carboxyhemoglobin levels greater than 50 per cent usually are lethal, and levels greater than 10 per cent are considered significant. Carbon monoxide combines with hemoglobin more than 200 times as readily as does oxygen. Besides decreasing the oxygen-carrying capacity of the blood by virtue of decreasing the amount of hemoglobin available to combine with oxygen, carboxyhemoglobin decreases the delivery of oxygen to tissues because of an effect wherein the dissociation of oxygen from hemoglobin is impaired.

HYPOXIA

Hypoxia is an important contributing factor to the syndrome of smoke inhalation. This appears to be the result of a low oxygen content in the environment secondary to oxygen consumption by the fire, as well as of the presence of carbon monoxide.

In summary, smoke inhalation is a highly lethal clinical condition resulting from irritating products of combustion, carbon monoxide poisoning, and concomitant hypoxia and asphyxiation.

CLASSIFICATION

The inhalation injury may be classified on either anatomic or temporal grounds. Anatomically, the injury may be classified as affecting the upper airway—primarily inflammation and edema of the larynx and trachea—or as affecting areas more distal—primarily inflammation, edema, profuse secretions and debris of the lower airways and disruption of the alveolar capillary membrane.

Smoke inhalation injuries more often are classified on temporal grounds that conform to fairly distinct clinical stages. The classification most commonly referred to is that proposed by Stone, consisting of three clinical stages of which patients will exhibit one or more to varying degrees.

Stage 1: Pulmonary or Respiratory Insufficiency

This stage generally occurs within the first 24 hours and is manifested by respiratory distress, often appearing as though due to upper airway obstruction. An early symptom is pain on deep inspiration.

Stage 2: Pulmonary Edema

This occurs generally eight to 36 hours post-injury, and may be of insidious or acute onset. In addition to being associated with the inhalation injury itself, it also may be related to cardiac disease, tracheostomy, overhydration, or a combination of these factors.

Stage 3: Bacterial Pneumonia

This occurs as early as two days post-injury, or as late as two weeks or more afterward. The earlier the pneumonia occurs, the worse the prognosis. All patients with a significant inhalation injury will have a bacterial pneumonia to some degree.

The recognition that fairly distinct temporal stages occur is of importance to the emergency physician, in that it emphasizes that the patient who initially appears well may develop significant symptomatology. Clinical findings must be correlated with time elapsed since the inhalation.

EVALUATION OF THE PATIENT

HISTORY

An attempt should be made to obtain information concerning the circumstances of the injury. It is important to know the location of the patient, the duration of exposure, the presence of toxic materials, and whether loss of consciousness took place.

The patient in an enclosed area is much more likely to suffer clinically significant smoke inhalation. Duration of exposure is of obvious importance, and many patients with brief exposure hold their breath while escaping, thus avoiding lower respiratory injury. Fires involving toxic substances should alert the emergency physician. Loss of consciousness may be due to anoxia or carbon monoxide toxicity, or might be caused by an anesthetic effect of the substance inhaled.

The physician should also seek evidence of other conditions that might have contributed to exposure, such as head injury, alcohol or drug use, or myocardial infarction. If possible, a brief medical history should be obtained with special emphasis on pre-existent cardiac or pulmonary disease.

Inquiry should be made as to whether the patient took measures to protect his respiratory tract. The three survivors of the well-studied Coconut Grove fire who did not sustain respiratory injury covered their mouths with wet cloths.

SIGNS AND SYMPTOMS

The signs and symptoms of the victim of smoke inhalation who presents to the Emergency Department are quite variable, depending on the nature of the substance inhaled as well as the contribution of hypoxia and carbon monoxide poisoning to the clinical picture. It is worthwhile to repeat that the initial absence of signs and symptoms does not rule out significant pulmonary damage.

Those patients with signs and symptoms may complain of sore throat, hoarseness, dyspnea, or dysphagia. Frequently there is cough which may be productive of carbonaceous sputum that may be blood-tinged. Secretions may be profuse. The patient may complain of headache or dizziness, may be restless and exhibit confused or irritational behavior, or may be comatose. There may be stridorous respirations, nasal flaring, a brassy cough, tachycardia, tachypnea, and suprasternal and intercostal retractions appearing similar to a crouplike state. The patient may be cyanotic or have the "cherry-red appearance" of carbon monoxide poisoning. In most published clinical studies, however, this cherry-red appearance has not been noted or has been overlooked in patients with documented carbon monoxide poisoning. Convulsions may occur.

Patients also may complain of nausea and may vomit, perhaps on the basis of swallowed particulate smoke originally deposited on the oral and nasal mucosa. Gastric dilatation may occur.

The presence of facial burns, particularly about the mouth and nose — especially second- or third-degree burns — often is associated with smoke inhalation injury.

Erythema, or blistering of the nasal and oral mucosa, is associated with an increased incidence of respiratory injury. The presence of singed nasal hairs also is accepted as being associated with a greater likelihood of smoke inhalation injury.

Auscultation of the chest initially may be normal, may reveal diminished breath sounds, or may reveal rales, rhonchi, or wheezes. The presence of the latter, upon admission, is a poor prognostic sign.

LABORATORY DATA

Arterial blood gases and carboxyhemoglobin levels are the most important laboratory determinations, and should be obtained in all patients in whom the diagnosis of smoke inhalation is made or suspected.

The results of arterial blood gas studies are variable, but most often reveal initially a normal or decreased P_{O_2}, a slight decrease in P_{CO_2}, and a near-normal pH. Normal blood gases do not rule out the possibility of future deterioration, consistent with the previously noted latent period seen in many patients. Abnormal blood gases, decreased P_{O_2} being the most common, indicate the need for admission and treatment. An elevated P_{CO_2} usually indicates a more severe injury and a poorer prognosis. The arterial pH may be so low that the administration of bicarbonate will be considered.

Arterial blood gas studies should be obtained to provide baseline values and a guide for initial treatment, and frequent serial determinations are mandatory in management. Carboxyhemoglobin levels should be obtained. This is of major importance in initial diagnosis and therapy. The reported P_{O_2} may well be normal in the face of markedly elevated carboxyhemoglobin levels.

Other laboratory data, although usually less helpful in the early period, should be obtained: i.e., CBC, serum electrolytes, BUN, and glucose. Elevated serum uric acid levels, the cause and significance of which are unclear, have been reported in smoke inhalation patients.

Although early sputum cultures have not been particularly reliable in predicting the pathogens in the pulmonary infections that often follow, one should be obtained initially, particularly if the patient has a productive cough.

OTHER INVESTIGATIONS

The chest x-ray usually does not show acute changes at first and therefore is not helpful in initial diagnosis and treatment; but it should be obtained as a baseline study. The lateral neck x-ray may be useful in helping to assess airway edema.

Myocardial infarction is not an uncommon complication of smoke inhalation, and all adult patients should have an EKG.

Laryngoscopy may be of great help in the early period. An acutely inflamed larynx in a patient with an uncertain diagnosis would be significant information. Repeated laryngoscopy to follow the progress of laryngeal edema may indicate the need for tracheal intubation while it still can be done electively.

Although many patients will have symptoms that appear to be due to acute upper airway obstruction, the cause most often is a tracheobronchitis. These patients, without true upper airway obstruction, will not benefit from and may even deteriorate following, tracheostomy. Laryngoscopy, including transnasal fibroptic laryngoscopy, can indicate which patients have upper airway obstruction and therefore might benefit from tracheal intubation or, perhaps, tracheostomy. In addition, laryngoscopy, being a fairly rapid procedure, may be useful in triage when mass smoke inhalation casualties are involved, indicating which patients are more likely to suffer acute deterioration.

Bronchoscopy may be performed, but is more often a therapeutic procedure performed during the hospital course to remove crusts and debris.

Other diagnostic measures have been employed to some extent, but are of questionable usefulness to the emergency physician at present. Spirometry, done acutely, has shown decreases in vital capacity, forced expiratory volume delivered in one second, and maximum breathing capacity. Measurements made on the second or third day have shown decreased pulmonary compliance, increased respiratory resistance, and increased work of breathing.

Preliminary work with pulmonary cytology has shown a correlation between certain cytologic changes and subsequent clinical diagnosis.

DIAGNOSIS

The diagnosis of smoke inhalation, in any event a matter of controversy, may be difficult at first except in obvious cases. The emergency physician must maintain a high index of suspicion in view of the well documented latent period; if he seriously considers this diagnosis but is still uncertain after a few hours the patient probably should be admitted for observation for 48 hours.

Stone has made the definite diagnosis of smoke inhalation on the basis of the presence of three factors: facial burns; mucosal burns or singed nasal hairs; and a history of burns having been suffered in a closed space. He considered the diagnosis probable if two of these criteria were met.

The diagnosis also should be made if there are wheezes, rales, or rhonchi present; if the patient is in respiratory distress; or if there is a history of unconsciousness not attributable to other causes. Patients with abnormal arterial blood gases with no other apparent explanation, or those with mental status changes, require admission and treatment. Patients with elevated carboxyhemoglobin levels (above 10 per cent) should be admitted even if there are no other signs and symptoms. Patients with initial levels of 15 per cent or higher probably will sustain pulmonary damage due to smoke inhalation. There is a direct correlation between carboxyhemoglobin levels and length of hospitalization.

The presence of significant cough, particularly if productive of copious secretions or carbonaceous material, dysphagia, hoarseness, or changes on the chest x-ray, should indicate admission with the presumptive diagnosis of smoke inhalation.

Reliable patients presenting with minimal symptoms (e.g., mild cough), absence of positive findings, and a questionable history can be observed for a few hours and discharged if there has been no increase in symptoms and changes in findings. All patients not admitted must be clearly warned of the possibility of development of symptoms and strongly advised to return in that event. A baseline chest x-ray should be taken.

FIREFIGHTERS

Firefighters sometimes are patients in the Emergency Department, and their evaluation deserves special mention. They often present with a history of chronic production of carbonaceous sputum, so that its presence is not as significant as in the civilian patient.

Studies have shown that significant concentrations of carbon monoxide may still be present after a fire has been extinguished, or may be present at fires that produce little visible smoke. Firefighters in those circumstances may remove, or fail to wear, protective masks and suffer subclinical carbon monoxide poisoning. Repeat exposure at another fire shortly thereafter may produce a cumulative effect, evident in mental confusion or poor judgment.

Finally, firefighters working in heavy protective garments in the heat produced by the fire may become dehydrated, and this should be borne in mind if such a patient has collapsed at a fire.

TREATMENT

Because there are multiple variables, including density and composition of smoke, length of exposure, severity and clinical stage of injury, presence or absence of body surface burns, even certainty of diagnosis, and because animal models have been difficult to design, the treatment of smoke inhalation is controversial in many respects.

Steam insufflation has been used in rats and dogs to study some types of therapy, on the basis that there is a pathologic similarity with the clinical smoke inhalation injury. In the rat model, therapy with 40 per cent oxygen and high humidity decreased mortality and pulmonary sepsis. Treatment should be individualized, and recognition of the clinical stage is helpful.

Initial therapy in the Emergency Department should be the administration of high humidity and oxygen. Adequate humidity cannot be achieved with the nasal oxygen apparatus and requires more advanced equipment, such as a heated nebulizer or croup tent. Arterial blood gas studies will be helpful in determining the proper oxygen concentration, keeping in mind the possibility of a normal PO_2 with carbon monoxide poisoning. This therapy alone may be sufficient for those patients with mild or moderate distress.

CARBON MONOXIDE POISONING

Carbon monoxide poisoning requires treatment with 100 per cent oxygen, which cannot be achieved with nasal or simple face mask apparatus. The half-life of carbon monoxide in the patient breathing room air is more than four hours, whereas it is less than one hour in a patient breathing 100 per cent oxygen. If readily available, hyperbaric oxygen therapy is the treatment of choice.

BRONCHODILATORS

Should oxygen and humidity not be sufficient for the smoke inhalation patient, further treatment is indicated. Bronchodilators via aerosol and intravenous aminophylline may be given, but are often unsuccessful.

CORTICOSTEROIDS

The indications, dosage, and duration of therapy for the use of steroids are controversial. Patients with respiratory distress who have not responded adequately to oxygen and humidity should be given a large intravenous dose of steroids over a period of one to five minutes. The dose should be no less than 1 gm. of hydrocortisone or an equivalent drug, and larger doses have been recommended by some clinicians, with a repeat dose in eight to 12 hours if needed. This therapy is particularly effective for wheezes that have not responded to the above measures. Maintenance steroids should not be given routinely without clinical indications, since they have been shown to be associated with virulent pulmonary infections. Steroids have been given in the hope of preventing or lessening the pulmonary edema phase, but there is no proof that they are effective. Asymptomatic patients probably should not be given "prophylactic" steroids.

OTHER MEASURES

Good pulmonary toilet is mandatory, with encouragement of deep coughing and proper suctioning as needed. Prophylactic antibiotics should not be given as not only have they been shown to be of no value, but they are associated with pulmonary infections due to resistant organisms. There is no evidence that detergents and proteolytic enzymes are of value. It is usually recommended that analgesia and sedation be used cautiously to avoid respiratory depression, although opiates can be reversed readily with naloxone. A nasogastric tube may be needed for decompression, and antacids may be given for gastric upset and perhaps to help prevent stress ulcers. Reports of elevated histamine levels have led to recommendations by some that antihistamines be given. As noted previously, bronchoscopy may be helpful in removing crusts and debris, but usually is not done acutely. IPPB may help to loosen secretions.

FLUID THERAPY

Fluid therapy should be guided by usual parameters such as urine output and central venous pressure, without blind adherence to formulas. Recommendations have been made both for moderate fluid restriction, to try to lessen pulmonary edema, and for fluid administration based on a consideration of the pulmonary injury as a 10 to 15 per cent body surface burn. It can be helpful to weigh the patient daily.

Smoke inhalation may cause increased pulmonary vascular resistance leading to an increase in central venous pressure. In this case, central venous pressure may not be an accurate guide to fluid administration. In those ill patients in whom accurate fluid administration is vital, pulmonary wedge pressures with the Swan-Ganz catheter may be used as a more accurate guide.

INDICATIONS FOR INTUBATION AND TRACHEOSTOMY

Intubation or tracheostomy may become necessary. True upper airway obstruction, with increasing edema and immobility of the cords seen on repeated laryngoscopy, requires intubation. Other indications are:

(1) Increasing stridor with a dropping PO_2.

(2) Profuse tracheobronchial secretions unmanageable with nasotracheal suction.

(3) Severe burns of the face, mouth, and nares with rapidly increasing edema. (This indication is not absolute if the patient has received large quantities of intravenous fluids free of colloids.)

(4) To prevent aspiration in patients unable to swallow.

(5) The need for ventilatory support.

Orotracheal or nasotracheal intubation is preferable to tracheostomy, and may be employed in the awake patient by the emergency physician, using topical anesthesia and perhaps small doses of intravenous morphine. Tracheostomy should be avoided if possible. It is a procedure that has been strongly criticized because of its complications, particularly life-threatening infections in the acute phase. In addition, pulmonary edema has been noted many times directly following tracheostomy. (It is speculated that this is caused by an acute lowering of intra-alveolar pressure through loss of the glottic barrier.) Although not well documented, tracheal intubation probably also may lead to pulmonary edema.

If tracheostomy is elected, it should be done in the operating room under controlled circumstances, using a cuffed tube with a positive pressure apparatus immediately available.

Stone has reported a marked difference in mortality after some basic therapeutic changes. During the first five-year period, in which tracheostomy was performed almost routinely for the majority of patients suspected of having a pulmonary burn, and antibiotics were administered prophylactically in most cases, mortality was 65 per cent. During the second five-year period, oxygen, humidification, and steroids were used as the main treatment, with 22 per cent mortality.

VENTILATORS

Intermittent positive pressure breathing may be used to administer drugs, for atelectasis, or for pulmonary edema. Caution must be taken to prevent infection of the patient from contaminated apparatus. Patients placed on a respirator should have the benefit of a volume cycle machine, perhaps with expiratory resistance or positive end-expiratory pressure.

TREATMENT OF PULMONARY EDEMA

The treatment of pulmonary edema in the patient with smoke inhalation is dependent upon the cause. In those cases caused by smoke inhalation alone, the most effective treatment is positive pressure ventilation. Digitalis, diuretics, and the other usual treatments for pulmonary edema are not effective. If cardiac disease or overhydration are contributing to the pulmonary edema, the usual therapeutic measures for these conditions should be employed in addition to positive pressure ventilation. The pulmonary edema associated with tracheostomy likewise responds only to positive pressure ventilation.

TREATMENT OF PNEUMONIA

The emergency physician occasionally may be called upon to diagnose and treat the pneumonia phase. Pneumonia that develops early, within the first three days, tends to include microabscess formation and is particularly lethal. There is often poor correlation of sputum culture results with the responsible pathogen in early pneumonia, but blood cultures often are positive and correlate well. The pathogen often is *Staphylococcus aureus* or Pseudomonas. Pneumonias that develop later tend to be less lethal, and have better sputum culture correlation and (usually) negative blood cultures. The pathogens usually are gram-negative bacteria. The pneumonias, early and late, should be treated with specific antibiotics and good bronchopulmonary care.

PROGNOSIS AND COMPLICATIONS

Because of the variability of the severity of smoke inhalation injury, and because of changing therapeutic approaches, the prognosis is unclear. Mortality figures from series of the decade of the 1960s show mortality in the range of 50 per cent. Using strict diagnostic criteria, in the period 1960 to 1969, Stone reported a total mortality of 41 per cent. As noted, however, the figures were significantly improved with a change in therapeutic approach.

Stone's figures indicate that the earlier symptoms occur, the greater the mortality.

For the second five-year period, Stone reported a mortality of 30 per cent for pulmonary insufficiency, 23 per cent for pulmonary edema, and 10 per cent for pneumonia.

In general, it appears that most survivors eventually suffer no long term symptomatology. Various complications have been reported, however, including bronchiectasis, chronic bronchitis, bronchiolitis obliterans, and bronchial and tracheal stenosis.

ON-SITE TREATMENT

On-site treatment is limited by the availability of equipment. The suspected smoke inhalation victim should be moved to a site free of smoke, well away from the fire. Coughing should be encouraged. If available, oxygen should be administered to all suspected victims. Respiratory and cardiac arrest should be treated in the normal fashion, using whatever equipment is at hand. Patients should be removed to an emergency facility as soon as possible.

References

Ambiavagar, M., Chalon, J., and Zargham, I.: Tracheobronchial cytologic changes following lower airway thermal injury. J. Trauma 14:280, 1974.

Beal, D. D., and Conner, G. H.: Respiratory tract injury: a guide to management following thermal and smoke injury. Laryngoscope 80:25, 1970.

Beal, D. D., Lambeth, J. T., and Conner, G. H.: Follow-up studies on patients treated with steroids following pulmonary thermal and acrid smoke injury. Laryngoscope 78:396, 1968.

Bergeaux, G., and Klein, R. C.: Hyperuricemia following smoke inhalation. Am. Rev. Resp. Dis. 109:145, 1974.

Cohn, A. M.: Concepts in management of burns of the respiratory tract. South. Med. J. 66:297, 1973.

DiVincenti, F. C., Pruitt, B. A., Jr., and Reckler, J. M.: Inhalation injuries. J. Trauma 11:109, 1971.

Donnellan, W. L., Poticha, S. M., and Holinger, P. H.: Management and complications of severe pulmonary burn. J.A.M.A. 194:155, 1965.

End, E.: Comment on smoke inhalation. Am. Fam. Physician 8:31, 1973.

Epstein, B. S., et al.: Hypoxemia in the burned patient. Ann. Surg. 158:924, 1963.

Faling, L. J., Medici, T. C., and Chodosh, S.: Sputum cell population measurements in bronchial injury: observations in acute smoke inhalation. Chest 65:56S, 1974.

Garzon, A. A., et al.: Respiratory mechanics in patients with inhalation burns. J. Trauma 10:57, 1970.

Harrison, H. N.: Respiratory tract injury, pathophysiology and response to therapy among burned patients. Ann. N.Y. Acad. Sci. 150:627, 1968.

Harrison, H. N., and Zikria, B. A.: Management of respiratory problems in burned patients. Mod. Treat. 4:1263, 1967.

Landa, J., Avery, W. G., and Sackner, M. A.: Some physiologic observations in smoke inhalation. Chest 61:62, 1972.

Mayer, B. W., Smith, D. S., and Hayden, M. J.: Acute smoke inhalation in children. Am. Fam. Physician 7:80, 1973.

Mintz, A. A., et al.: Pediatric grand rounds: smoke inhalation and respiratory burns. Tex. Med. 68:90, 1972.

Moritz, A. R., Henriques, F. C., and McLean, R.: The effects of inhaled heat on the air passages and lungs. Am. J. Pathol. 21:311, 1945.

Noe, J. M., and Constable, J. D.: A new approach to pulmonary burns: a preliminary report. J. Trauma 13:1015, 1973.

Perez-Guerra, F., Walsh, R. E., and Sagel, S. S.: Bronchiolitis obliterans and tracheal stenosis. J.A.M.A. 218:1568, 1971.

Phillips, A. W., and Cope, O.: Burn therapy. II. The revelation of respiratory tract damage as a principal killer of the burned patient. Ann. Surg. 155:1, 1962.

Phillips, A. W., and Cope, O.: Burn therapy. III. Beware the facial burn! Ann. Surg. 156:759, 1962.

Phillips, A. W., Tanner, J. W., and Cope, O.: Burn therapy. IV. Respiratory tract damage (an account of the clinical, x-ray and postmortem findings) and the meaning of restlessness. Ann. Surg. 158:799, 1963.

Polk, H. C., Jr., King, N., and Weiner, L. J.: Respiratory burn injury (smoke inhalation). D.M. 229:10, 1973.

Polk, H. C., Jr., and Stone, H. H.: Contemporary Burn Management. Boston, Little, Brown & Co., 1971.

Reed, G. F., and Camp, H. L.: Upper airway problems in severely burned patients. Ann. Otol. Rhinol. Laryngol. 78:741, 1969.

Stone, H. H., and Martin, J. D.: Pulmonary injury associated with thermal burns. Surg. Gynecol. Obstet. 129:1242, 1969.

Stone, H. H., Martin, J. D., and Claydon, C. T.: Management of the pulmonary burn. Am. Surg. 33:616, 1967.

Stone, H. H., et al.: Respiratory burns: a correlation of clinical and laboratory results. Ann. Surg. 165:157, 1967.

Taylor, F. W., and Gumbert, J. L.: Cause of death from burns: role of respiratory damage. Ann. Surg. 161:497, 1965.

Thomas, D. M., and Conner, E. H.: Management of the patient "overcome by smoke." J. Ky. Med. Assoc. 66:1051, 1968.

Wanner, A., and Cutchavaree, A.: Early recognition of upper airway obstruction following smoke inhalation. Am. Rev. Resp. Dis. 108:1421, 1973.

Webster, J. R., McCabe, M. M., and Karp, M.: Recognition and management of smoke inhalation. J.A.M.A. 201:287, 1967.

Zarem, H. A., Rattenborg, C. C., and Harmel, M. H.: Carbon monoxide toxicity in human fire victims. Arch. Surg. 107:851, 1973.

Zikria, B. A.: CO level measures smoke injury. Med. World News, p. 17, Sept. 21, 1973.

Zikria, B. A., Ferrer, J. M., and Floch, H. F.: The chemical factors contributing to pulmonary damage in "smoke poisoning." Surgery 71:704, 1972.

Zikria, B. A., et al.: Respiratory tract damage in burns: pathophysiology and therapy. Ann. N.Y. Acad. Sci. 150:618, 1968.

Zikria, B. A., Weston, G. C., and Chodoff, M.: Smoke and carbon monoxide poisoning in fire victims. J. Trauma 12:641, 1972.

L. EMERGENCIES IN SPORTS

James Garrick

THE ATHLETE PATIENT

The injured athlete, regardless of whether he is a professional football player or recreational skier, presents the emergency physician and department with some unique problems. Although definitive care of the ankle sprained winning the high school basketball championship may not differ from that of the ankle sprained on the supermarket steps, the owners of those ankles differ appreciably and so might the way the injuries present. These differences, in a specific number of injuries, are great enough to merit special consideration.

Except for the gross, open trauma seen in wartime or following vehicular accidents, the actual injuries to athletes differ little from those observed in the general population. The frequency of athletic injuries, however, is appreciably different because of the rigors of sports activities and the previous training and experience of the participant. Indeed, athletes *are* different.

Almost by definition, athletes are "healthy." Serious systemic disease is uncommon, not because the athlete is "protected" by his activities, but rather because appreciable systemic disease or gross congenital or acquired abnormalities usually preclude athletic activities. (The alcoholic with cirrhosis may fall down a flight of stairs, sustaining a glenohumeral dislocation, but he won't do it playing competitive football.) Because of this good health, special diagnostic tests, anesthetics, and surgical procedures would be expected to carry fewer risks than in the general—and not so fit—population.

Athletes are often more "body-conscious" than the general population—and well they should be. The lack of 5° of plantar flexion of the ankle means, for the attorney, going up the courthouse steps more slowly, but to the 100-yard sprinter it might mean one second in time—a 10 per cent reduction in speed. For this reason, the athlete often presents with problems that are obscure because they are too "minor" to be of consequence to the nonathlete, and are thus beyond the experience of most physicians.

The athlete wants to get well—indeed, often he wants to get well so badly that he repeatedly compromises healing. There is no "sick leave" from a gymnastics meet, nor is there workman's compensation for the disabled soccer player. Whatever primary or secondary gain that athletes may receive from any sport activity disappears with injury and the inability to participate.

Not only does the athlete want to return to participation as soon as possible—or even sooner—he usually wants to know the exact day this will occur. Most other patients will accept vague answers to questions about the time necessary for healing and return to normal activity, but the athlete is truly different in this regard. This difference presents a problem for many physicians. First, the athlete wishes not to return to "normal" but to supernormal activities, and knowing the demands of these activities requires a thorough knowledge of the sport in question. Most nonparticipants do not have this knowledge, and thus tend to err on the safe side and "overtreat" the athlete.

As regards the problem of estimating the length of time of incapacity, the athlete who demands to know the exact date of return may well merely be repeating the questions presented to him by the coach. Game plans, work-out schedules, and travel arrangements all depend on an exact knowledge of who will be participating, so that coach and athlete have a right to this information regardless of the difficulty it causes for the physician. Unfortunately, here too the tendency is to react with "overtreatment" or overestimates.

Despite some of the problems associated with treating athletes, there are more than enough compensatory benefits. Some of the same characteristics that make athletes "difficult" patients also allow better medicine to be practiced on them.

Often because of the athlete's "body sensitivity," he is able to provide a superb history of the mechanism of injury. Athletes generally know exactly what they were doing at the time of injury and can recreate the circumstance for the examiner. In perhaps one-half to two-thirds of all athletic injuries, a well-taken history will provide a definitive diagnosis.

Athletes often present with injuries early in their course before they become more severe or complicated. The mildly painful, two-day-old Achilles tendinitis is infinitely easier to treat than the ruptured Achilles tendon. One must remember that, in the athletic context, there are few "insignificant" injuries that actually reach the physician, especially the physician in an Emergency Department.

Finally, with the increased medical training of coaches and the more frequent presence of certified athletic trainers,* the athlete often arrives at the Emergency Department having received better initial management than most patients. However, the sprained ankle that has been properly "iced, elevated, and compressed," as is often the case with athletes, may appear different enough on examination actually to pose diagnostic problems. Unfortunately, most physicians are not accustomed to seeing injuries that have received ideal first aid and initial management.

The following discussion does not presume to cover all injuries that might occur during athletic contests. Rather, it is an attempt to cover the idiosyncrasies of injuries that occur with reasonable frequency as a result of athletic or recreational activities.

HEAD AND SPINE

The diagnosis and initial management of trauma to the head and spine are the same for athletes, automobile passengers, or bicycle riders. Head injuries in athletes are almost invariably closed, and in some sports — notably football — they involve forces of a far greater magnitude than most people realize. Even though the present football helmet is a remarkably effective protective device, it is likely that a number in excess of 25 to 30 young men will die each year in the U.S. as a result of closed head injuries that occurred during participation in organized football programs.

Although the football helmet may well decrease appreciably the number of severe head injuries, its use and abuse may coincidentally have increased the frequency of

---

*Certified by the National Athletic Trainers Association.

cervical spine injuries. The use of the helmeted head as an often almost wanton offensive weapon places considerable stress on the cervical spine, especially in the rapidly growing adolescent whose cervical musculature has not developed in concert with his willingness to deliver blows with his helmet. Although cervical spine injuries can occur in any position, hyperflexion is most often the cause.

The wrestler or gymnast presenting with the history and neurologic picture of the typical hyperflexion cervical spine injury poses no "athlete-specific" problem. The football player who arrives at the Emergency Department with his helmet still on presents a very real problem. Some seemingly straightforward observations merit mention.

The helmet need not be removed to provide an airway. In many cases, even the presence of the mask or cage will not preclude introduction of an airway, which can be inserted between the bars, and the angle of the jaw grasped even with the helmet in place. If the mask is in the way, it can be removed safely with bolt cutters (available in most operating rooms) or, with some designs, merely by cutting the side attachments and swinging it cephalad.

One must remember that even a poorly fitted football helmet is extremely difficult to remove by anyone other than the wearer, and labored removal might well further compromise an already injured cervical spine. Admittedly the helmet will have to be removed sometime, but this can easily be accomplished with a cast saw and a little patience. If a cast saw is unavailable, adequate cervical spine films can be obtained with the helmet in place (and stabilized) if necessary.

Although thoracic and lumbar spine injuries occur with some frequency in sports (gymnastics, football, wrestling, weight lifting), these conditions present much as they do in the nonathlete population. Again, one must remember that appreciable forces come to play in the spine and often are presented to a lumbar region in hyperlordosis, as exemplified by the football lineman peering out of his stance.

Lumbar or thoracic spine injuries presenting with neurologic manifestations are uncommon in sports. Indeed, most noncervical spine injuries are either strains or the result of direct blows. The latter may result in transverse or spinous process fractures, and appropriate x-rays should always be obtained.

TRUNK

Trunk injuries in athletes are usually the result of direct blows, or the application of compressive force as in wrestling. Rib fractures are not uncommon and usually occur in the posterior or midaxillary line. Rarely is there any appreciable displacement of these fractures.

Costochondral subluxations/separations are seen rather frequently in athletics. Usually these painful and temporarily disabling injuries are the result of compression of the thoracic cage and are heralded by a painful "snapping" or "popping" sensation. The athlete complains of "something slipping out of place (and back in)." Inspiration—especially deep inspiration—is painful, and breathing becomes shallow for fear of recurrence of the pain. The athlete is usually able to pinpoint the painful area with the tip of a finger. Side-to-side or front-to-back compression of the chest will often reproduce the painful episode and will be resisted by the athlete.

Although the usual treatment for the disrupted costochondral junction is application of a wide (6 in. plus) elasticized rib belt or tightly wrapped elasticized bandage, one must be flexible in the management of this condition. Occasionally, symptoms will increase with compression, and the athlete's response to the treatment must be taken into consideration; if he is most comfortable with no treatment, this is perfectly acceptable.

The subperiosteal hematoma of a rib in the athlete can easily be mistaken for a fracture. The mechanism of injury is usually a direct blow; there often is pain with deep breathing and there is sometimes excruciating point tenderness. Although management is symptomatic in both instances, the athlete with a subperiosteal hematoma will return to participation sooner—often in a few days.

Almost unique in contact sports is the "hip pointer" or iliac crest contusion. A direct blow to the iliac crest delivered by helmet, knee, or shoulder can result not only in subperiosteal hemorrhage, but also either a fracture of the crest or avulsion of the abdominal musculature from its insertion into the crest. Pain is almost immediate, very severe, and may be totally disabling so far as continued sport participation is concerned. The athlete flexes his trunk toward the injury—laterally, anterolaterally, or posterolaterally, depending on the location of the injury. Any attempt at motion, deep breathing, coughing, or sneezing is met with excruciating pain. The abdomen is often rigid, and tenderness, which is initially well localized to the site of injury, may spread to include the entire hemiabdomen. Although some swelling is usually present, the amount is normally less than one would expect to see with symptoms of this magnitude.

Initial management includes the continuous application of ice packs and adequate analgesics. Occasionally, hospitalization will be necessary, as the pain will require injectible analgesics. Local anesthetics, with or without proteolytic enzymes, injected into the area of maximal tenderness will usually give dramatic, if temporary, relief. Rarely can any appreciable portion of the hematoma be aspirated. Sterile precautions are essential if local injection/aspiration is elected, as the hematoma is an ideal potential culture medium.

Trauma to the thoracic or abdominal viscera can occur in sports just as it can with any violent activity. Rupture or contusion of a major viscus presents no differently in the athletic environment than anywhere else. One must be reminded continually of the forces involved in sports, especially those involving body contact, and must remember that the athlete, emotionally involved in the competitive event, may respond inappropriately to questioning in his zeal to continue participation.

UPPER EXTREMITIES

Shoulder

The shoulder girdle is spared by few sports. Direct violence results in the whole spectrum of contusions, fractures, and dislocations. Even noncontact sports, including all throwing activities as well as gymnastics and swimming, result in a host of attritional problems, many of which involve the rotator cuff.

The clavicle itself presents few problems unique to sports, other than the fact that it is often fractured. The relatively high incidence of injuries to the clavicular attachments (to the sternum or acromion) make these almost uniquely athletic injuries.

Sternoclavicular subluxations and dislocations are usually the result of force transmitted through the shoulder: for example, falling on the lateral aspect of the shoulder. Localized pain, tenderness, and swelling—present even in the spontaneously reduced subluxation/dislocation—should lead one to suspect disruption of this small and usually stable joint. Attempts to manipulate the clavicle, such as bringing the 90° abducted arm across the front of the body, are vigorously resisted by the patient.

The posterosuperiorly displaced sternoclavicular dislocation can be serious and even life-threatening with compression of the cervical "viscera," but usually can be reduced by retracting the scapulae and/or grasping the clavicle and lifting it upward. Once reduced, the clavicle must be maintained in an anatomic position until healing has occurred, often accomplished with a figure-8 type dressing.

Acromioclavicular injuries are exceedingly common in sports, especially football, wrestling, and hockey. The forces resulting in this injury are either transmitted—as with a fall on the outstretched arm—or directly applied to the acromion—as when being struck on the anterior portion of the shoulder.

Acromioclavicular sprains ("separations") have been classified into three groups.

(1) Grade I sprains ("shoulder pointers") often are the result of direct blows, entailing some minimal injury to the acromioclavicular ligament but no instability of the joint.

(2) Grade II sprains involve disruption of the acromioclavicular ligament and some minimal upward drift of the lateral end of the clavicle. The guy-wire or tethering effect of the coracoclavicular ligaments, however, prevents upward displacement of more than about 1 cm.—hence the athlete's term, "partial separation."

(3) Grade III sprains of the acromioclavicular joint—"complete separations"—involve disruption of both acromioclavicular and coracoclavicular ligaments, as well as frequent tears of the distal trapezius. The joint in this instance is completely unstable, usually resulting in the distal clavicle being subluxed/dislocated superiorly.

All grades of acromioclavicular sprains have in common the fact that they are usually quite painful. In nearly every instance, the athlete will be able to describe the moment the injury occurred. The more severe grades are usually accompanied by an audible "pop" or "snap" which, coupled with the crepitation palpable in the Grade III sprain, may lead to the erroneous diagnosis of a fractured clavicle.

All grades, especially I and II, present with exquisite pain and tenderness at the acromioclavicular joint. The tenderness and accompanying swelling is well localized initially, but spreads with time, making a definitive determination of the severity of the injury more difficult, since the swelling tends to obscure any deformity present.

Although all grades of sprains are initially managed in a similar fashion with ice, compression, and a sling-and-swath, the ultimate treatment is contingent on differentiating between Grades I/II and Grade III sprains; the latter usually involve surgical intervention.

The history of mechanism of injury and pain offers little in determining whether the sprain is Grade III. Critical in the determination of whether the separation is complete is the instability of the distal clavicle, due to the loss of the tethering effect of the coracoclavicular ligaments. Clinically, if examined early, rupture of the coracoclavicular ligaments is accompanied by tenderness inferior to the clavicle in its distal third—the location of the ligaments. This finding can be present even in the complete sprain that seems to result in no inordinate upward displacement of the clavicle. With time and increased swelling, the finding of coracoclavicular tenderness becomes less reliable.

Upward drift and gross instability of the lateral end of the clavicle is the other diagnostic sign of a "complete separation." This usually is readily apparent early in the post-injury period, but it becomes less so with time and increased swelling. Anteroposterior x-rays of the shoulder may reveal, in this instance, what clinical examination does not—an increased distance between the coracoid process and the inferior surface of the clavicle. With loss of the coracoclavicular ligaments, this finding is often present in routine standing anteroposterior x-rays of the shoulder. If any doubt exists, 10- to 20-lb. weights can be tied to each wrist, and x-rays taken with the patient standing relaxed.

Shoulder dislocations are common in many sports, including football, wrestling, and skiing. From a diagnostic standpoint, the sports-related shoulder dislocation is like any other shoulder dislocation, except that often it will have been reduced before the patient seeks formal medical care. The injury is so common that may coaches and trainers, having seen reductions performed, will attempt them at the time of injury. The establishment of the definitive diagnosis of shoulder dislocation is no less critical if the reduction has already been performed. The three- to four-week period of immobilization after the first dislocation is the only positive factor the athlete has going for him. Whether male or female, the adolescent or young adult athlete has a more than 80 per cent likelihood of recurrence, even if ideally treated. These odds are even worse without proper initial management.

Whether reduced or not, the injured shoulder should be x-rayed in two planes in order to rule out associated injuries. In addition, a complete neurovascular examination is necessary to check for complications not uncommonly associated with this injury.

Although frank dislocations are reasonably commonplace in the general population, the shoulder subluxation is described almost exclusively in athletes. The mechanism of injury—fall on the outstretched hand or elbow, or forced abduction/external rotation—may be similar, although shoulder subluxation also may result from a direct blow or from striking an opponent or object with the flexed arm. Invariably, the athlete who has suffered a subluxation will give a history of "the shoulder coming out (and going back in)" or "opening up." Pain and tenderness may be anterior or posterior, and, if it is the initial injury, the range of active or passive motion will be appreciably limited by pain. Attempts to recreate the mechanism of injury by passively abducting and externally rotating the shoulder will usually be met by extreme apprehension and guarding. An accompaniment of a "snap" or momentary change in position of the shoulder is not uncommon during these maneuvers, the athlete observing "that's what happened." Should this occur, the diagnosis has been established.

The initial shoulder subluxation is treated exactly like a frank dislocation. As is also true with the latter, subsequent episodes are harbingers of an increased likelihood of future recurrence, and usually are treated symptomatically.

Elbow

Sport-specific elbow injuries are usually of the overuse variety, and can be serious when present in children with open epiphyses. Children engaged in throwing sports who present with elbow or shoulder pain must be deemed to have significant injuries until it is proved otherwise. One must remember that a child's elbow is largely composed of articular cartilage, so that "normal" x-rays or x-rays showing "minimal" bony abnormalities may coexist with appreciable injuries.

It is sufficient to say that the sudden onset of elbow or shoulder pain in an athlete, especially a child, whether or not it is accompanied by the usual painful limitation of motion, merits thorough investigation and consultation. The extremity must be placed at rest (sling) until the investigation is complete.

The gradual onset of elbow or shoulder pain in the skeletally immature child cannot be ignored. "Little League elbow" in all its forms, and with its potential for permanent disability, often has an insidious onset and may appear similar to the various "overuse" syndromes seen in adults. Although adult elbow or shoulder pain from throwing or racquet sports is often self-limited and benign, requiring only symptomatic treatment, one can never assume such to be the case with children.

Wrist

Wrist injuries in the athlete population are commonplace, not only as a result of falling on the outstretched hand (wrestling, basketball, and gymnastics), but also from striking an opponent with the palm of the dorsiflexed hand (football and martial arts). The adage "an athlete has never 'sprained' his wrist until a navicular fracture has been ruled out" is, unfortunately, very true. Painful limitation of wrist motion following a hyperdorsiflexion injury, and the presence of pain over the carpal navicular ("snuff box"), should be evaluated by at least biplane x-rays of the navicular. If negative, the wrist should be splinted in a position of function and the x-rays repeated in two to three weeks. Such a regimen not only definitively treats the sprain, but also protects the carpal navicular in the interim in case a fracture line appears on the repeat x-rays.

LOWER EXTREMITIES

Almost regardless of the athletic activity, the lower extremities are involved more often in athletic injuries than the whole of the rest of the body combined. Lower extremity injuries present appreciable diagnostic problems, complicated by the fact that only rarely are bony abnormalities present; thus, x-rays although appropriate in order to rule out other problems, often are of little help.

Hip and Thigh

Athletic injuries to the hip and thigh rarely involve neurovascular structures or bone. Femoral fractures, sciatic nerve injuries, and femoral artery lacerations are not unheard of in athletics, but are of minor numerical importance when compared to injuries of the thigh musculature. Thus, almost all hip and thigh injuries are contusions and strains.

Thigh contusions of medical significance nearly always involve the quadriceps muscle ("charley horse"). Encircling and originating from almost three-quarters of the circumference of the length of the femur, the highly developed quadriceps muscle of the athlete presents a large target for direct blows. Although usually the result of a blow from a helmet or shoulder (in football), the quadriceps contusion can result from being struck by the knee, foot, or an item of equipment (hockey stick, bat, etc.), or simply from being stepped on by a shoe or boot.

Generally, the more significant quadriceps contusion is the result of greater forces applied to the muscle during active contraction. Often, effective function of the muscle is immediately lost, so that continued participation is precluded. Unless effective compression is instituted immediately, bleeding of the contused area into the substance of the muscle can be appreciable, resulting in an exceedingly painful, tensely swollen, tender ecchymotic anterior thigh. In this in-

stance, even antigravity function of the muscle is lost and a gross "quadriceps lag" is readily apparent.

The spectacular thigh contusion described above is generally not the problem injury. When an athlete is unable to extend the knee and has an area of swelling growing larger almost by the minute, it is at once obvious that he has been injured and requires care. The slightly less severe thigh contusion presents the greater recognition/management problem. In these cases, the quadriceps continue to retain some function, albeit sluggish. More often than not the athlete attempts to "run if off," and succeeds only in actively pumping more and more blood into the substance of the muscle. Often this injury is seen late at night or on the following day when the athlete seeks aid because of increasingly severe pain, the presence of a large and often spectacular area of ecchymosis, or the discovery upon awakening that he is unable to bend the knee.

Recognition/diagnosis in either of the above instances is reasonably straightforward at the time that medical aid is sought. Some additional measure of severity can be established by determining the amount of *painless* passive flexion present at the knee. With the patient prone, the ankle is gently grasped and the knee passively flexed. Generally, if less than 70 to 80° of painless flexion is present, the injury must be regarded as potentially serious.

Initial management consists of complete rest of the quadriceps (often in bed), elevation, and the application of cold and compression. As is true with all quadriceps contusions, activity should be limited to only that which can be accomplished painlessly—a difficult, but essential order for the young athlete eager to return to participation and often the target of peer or coach abuse for "being laid up by a bruised thigh."

The problem with the quadriceps contusion is not the contused muscle per se, but rather one of the complications of the injury—myositis ossificans. The development of this condition, frequently visible on x-rays as early as two to three weeks post-injury, often means the end of the athlete's career. Once established, the new bone formation will continue as long as the muscle is abused. "Abuse" in this instance can consist of massage, painful walking, running, exercises, or other activities—indeed, the same abuses that well may have prompted the new bone formation in the first place. Once present, myositis ossificans is a condition for which treatment and rehabilitation times are measured in months and even years. Prevention, by proper conservative initial management, is obviously preferable.

The other major injury category in the hip and thigh also involves the musculature, but in a dynamic manner, by no means limited to violent contact sports. Indeed, strains ("muscle pulls") cross almost all sport boundaries.

Although virtually every muscle in the thigh can be strained, the vast majority of injuries involve the hamstrings and the rectus femoris portion of the quadriceps. Regardless of the muscle involved, all strains are classified in a similar fashion and have generally common mechanisms of injury. Strains (like sprains) are classified as mild (I), moderate (II), or severe (III), and can involve any portion of the musculotendinous mechanism or its attachments to bone. In adolescents and children, the more severe injuries often involve the tendinous insertion into bone; in young adults, the muscle belly or musculotendinous portion; and in older adults, the tendon itself.

The mechanism of injury in most strains is overload of a contracting musculotendinous unit. Although passive stretching (especially ballistic or "bounce" stretching) can result in strains, such is not usually the case. The injuries occur at the time of maximum activity, acceleration, or overload.

An exacting history of the moment of injury is absolutely essential because, more often than not, it alone may allow classification by severity. A detailed history is especially important in sports, as, not infrequently, the athlete will attempt to continue participation ("run it off"), or "wait to see how it gets along" for a day or days, thus allowing the "golden period" for diagnosis—that time, minutes to hours after the injury was sustained—to slip by and obscure many of the physical findings.

Generally, those injuries having the most dramatic and sudden onset are the most severe. Thus, the athlete who hears or feels a load "snap" or "pop," and thinks he has been "shot" or struck, has a Grade III strain until it is proved otherwise. If a bystander or fellow competitor also hears a "snap," the likelihood of a severe injury is even greater. Likewise, an injury resulting in sudden disability (e.g., inability to actively extend the knee) should be considered severe until proved otherwise.

At the other end of the severity spectrum is the grade I or mild strain, heralded by a "tightening-up" or "bunching-up" of the muscle over two or three steps. If the athlete ignores the symptoms and continues the activity, this may progress to major injury, but generally he will stop with the "tightening" sensation.

Determination of the exact site of injury—portion of the musculotendinous unit involved—is important, because this often determines whether the Grade III strain will be managed surgically. Tendon avulsion, with or without a large fragment of bone or complete musculotendinous junction disruptions, requires urgent surgical repair. Tears within the belly of a muscle are less likely to require operative intervention. In the former instance (tendinous avulsions from bone), x-rays may be helpful in establishing severity. Generally, however, a knowledge of anatomy is necessary for a definitive diagnosis.

Examination immediately post-injury often will reveal the severely strained muscle to possess a palpable defect, an abnormal contour ("bulge") when contracted, or flaccidity with attempts at contraction. Should the rupture occur at the muscle belly or the musculotendinous junction, a palpable hematoma will be present. Pain with attempts at contraction may or may not be severe, and in any case may not parallel the severity of the injury.

The signs that permit an early definitive diagnosis often present differently with passing time or subsequent activity. The initially palpable defect may fill with blood and become less obvious. The initially soft hematoma may become more firm, and differ by palpation from the surrounding muscle only because it cannot be felt actively to contract. The well-defined initial hematoma may diffuse into surrounding soft tissue and present only as an area of ecchymosis—a critical finding in strains, because, as a general rule, those that result in ecchymosis should be considered severe until proved otherwise.

The hematoma and reflex muscle spasm following moderate or severe strains results in another important hallmark: painful resistance to passive stretching. Thus, the strained rectus femoris will not allow passive simultaneous knee flexion and hip extension, and the strained hamstring will painfully limit straight leg raising.

Save those severe strains that require surgical repair, the initial management of musculotendinous injuries differs little with regard to the muscle involved or the severity. Ice, compression, and rest in a position of relaxation (e.g., knee flexion for the hamstring injury) all decrease bleeding and theoretically decrease the ultimate amount of motion-limiting fibrosis with healing. Initially, comfort is the watchword, and activities that are painful (even walking) should be prohibited.

Knee

The knee is the most frequently and diversely injured area of the athlete's body. Definitive management of knee injuries often requires multiple examinations and a myriad of special diagnostic procedures (routine and special x-rays, arthrography, tomography, and arthroscopy) and is the subject of entire volumes. Emergency management of knee injuries, on the other hand, requires but a few, straightforward, and usually objective decisions, and for athletes can be placed in three categories: emergent, urgent, and routine. Emergent injuries require some definitive procedure within hours, if not minutes. Urgent injuries require definitive special diagnostic tests, consultation, or surgical procedures within a few days. Routine knee injuries require symptomatic care, protection, and re-evaluation.

Fortunately, knee injuries in athletes only rarely require "emergency" management. With the exception of injuries complicated by open wounds, nearly all conditions in this group are so placed by virtue of potential or present neurovascular involvement. As a general rule, if the skin is intact, the circulation and neurologic function of the extremity normal, and no deformity is present on x-ray or gross examination, the injury does not fall into the emergent category. The examiner must bear in mind while performing this screening examination that the posture of the extremity being examined is not necessarily that present immediately following the injury. Indeed, the reduced but previously frankly dislocated knee may appear normal to casual inspection and x-ray examination, and yet be totally unstable. Thus, the grossly unstable knee should be closely observed for the complications not uncommonly seen in a reduced dislocation, e.g., vascular injury in the popliteal space, which can result in amputation.

Displaced epiphyseal fractures and other major intra-articular fractures or disruptions of the quadriceps mechanism, although not truly emergent by the above definition, carry with them a greater degree of urgency than those other injuries classified as "urgent."

Although the urgent management category contains a host of specific injuries (Grade III sprains of collateral and/or cruciate ligaments, patellar fractures and/or dislocations, meniscus injuries with displaced fragments, etc.), there exist some common denominators in the decision-making process. The following indicate significant problems until the specific injuries can be ruled out.

HISTORY

(1) An audible "snap," "pop," or "ripping" signifies collateral or cruciate rupture, dislocation of the patella, or patellar/quadriceps tendon rupture. If someone other than the patient hears a "pop," isolated cruciate rupture is indicated; if a "tearing" or "ripping," patellar dislocation is likely.

(2) The sensation of "something slipping out of place (and back in)" signifies patellar dislocation/subluxation or meniscus injury.

(3) Unwillingness to attempt weight bearing suggest patellar dislocation, meniscus injury, or intra-articular fracture.

(4) Inability to bear weight suggests meniscus injury with displaced fragment or intra-articular fracture.

(5) Initial pain relief (partial or complete) with knee flexion suggests meniscus injury; with extension, dislocated patella.

(6) A sensation of the "joint opening" or coming apart suggests collateral ligament rupture or some form of rotary instability.

(7) Initial pain lasting 5 to 60 seconds, followed by pain-free motion and/or weight bearing and/or ambulaion, suggests rupture (complete) of collateral liagment.

(8) Obvious, rapid swelling (within six hours) suggests hemarthrosis from cruciate

or meniscus injury or patellar dislocation. The latter often results in the largest and most rapidly occurring hemarthrosis.

(9) Sensation of instability, often expressed as "bends the wrong way" or "wobbles," suggests collateral ligament rupture (complete).

INSPECTION

(1) Gross, tense effusion (hemarthrosis) suggests dislocated patella, cruciate injury, or possible meniscus injury.

(2) Ecchymosis (medial or anteromedial) suggests dislocated patella or medial collateral ligament rupture.

EXAMINATION

(1) Medial or lateral instability, which may as often as not be *painless*, suggests rupture (complete) of collateral ligament.

(2) Tenderness at medial border of patella and/or proximal portion of adductor tubercle suggests dislocated patella.

(3) Grossly bloody effusion suggests dislocated patella, cruciate rupture, intra-articular fracture—some meniscus injuries, some medial collateral ligament injuries.

(4) Grossly bloody effusion with floating fat globules suggests intra-articular fracture.

It is most important in the emergency management of knee injuries in athletes that the severe, or potentially severe, problem should not be ignored simply because it may present in a seemingly aberrant manner. The Grade III sprain (complete rupture) of the medial collateral liagment is the best example. Almost without exception, the athlete will attempt—often successfully—to continue participation after the injury. Although the injury is a severe one, usually requiring operative repair, it is commonly painless for the first few hours. Indeed, on examination, valgus stressing of the knee will reveal gross instability, but, if examined early, anesthesia/analgesia is unnecessary because of the absence of pain.

As with virtually all other sports injuries, ice, compression, and rest (immobilization) constitute early management. Immobilization is best obtained by the use of a commercially available canvas knee splint/corset with semi-rigid stays. This appliance offers easy removal for re-examination, and can be loosened at home by the patient should appreciable swelling occur. A posterior splint also offers these advantages. The use of a cylinder cast as "emergency treatment" offers two problems: that of limb constriction with swelling and, more important, the reluctance on the part of many physicians to remove it to re-examine the patient.

Leg

Although leg injuries are reasonably common in running and jumping sports, only three merit special attention in the athletic context—musculotendinous injuries to the Achilles mechanism; shin splints; and stress fractures.

As with the thigh, calf injuries are the result of direct blows or dynamic overload. Calf or leg contusions carry with them an additional risk, that of pressure ischemia/necrosis. Thus, early vigorous management (ice, elevation, and rest) and careful observation for the signs of compartment syndromes must be undertaken. Sensory disturbances, increase in pain, or circulatory alterations cannot be ignored. One must be ever mindful that entire anatomic regions can undergo necrosis concurrent with no change in distal pulses, and occasionally with only subtle neurologic evidence.

Strains of the Achilles mechanism are commonplace and generally follow the rules presented in the discussion of thigh injuries. The young athlete most often injures the muscle belly or musculotendinous junction, and, although these injuries often result in appreciable pain, swelling, and ecchymosis, they usually can be managed conservatively with ice, compression, elevation, and rest (bed rest or crutches).

The older athlete (fourth and fifth decades) may present with a slightly different problem: rupture of the Achilles tendon. Acute rupture of this tendon usually occurs as a result of activity/overload, is accompanied by a loud "snap" or "pop" and the sensation of being struck in the posterodistal leg, and, more often than not, is relatively or absolutely painless. The athlete may think he has sprained his ankle, is often bewildered by the fact that so dramatic an occurrence does not result in pain on ambulation, and thus may not seek immediate care.

In the immediate post-injury period, the diagnosis should be obvious. Indeed, the above history all but makes the diagnosis. A palpable gap in the tendon is usually present and often is not obliterated by a hematoma for a day or two. Although active plantar flexion may be retained, the athlete will be unable to stand unsupported on the toe of the involved side. With the patient prone, and the knee flexed to 90°, a brisk squeeze of the gastrocnemius–soleus muscle belly will result in the ankle reflexly dipping into plantar flexion only if continuity of the Achilles mechanism remains.

Whether or not one opts to treat the ruptured Achilles tendon surgically is not critical in initial management. Either way, a compression dressing should be applied from the knee to the toes, utilizing plaster splints to place the ankle in plantar flexion. Weight bearing is not permitted.

Although the host of overuse syndromes present in the leg (e.g., shin splints, stress fractures, etc.) rarely present as emergencies, one must bear in mind the significant sequelae that might result from these conditions.

Stress fractures of the tibia or fibula usually present with the insidious onset of activity-related pain, often the result of some "change." The "change" may be in length or character of work-outs, the field or running surface, or the shoes. Although the pain may be rather generalized, tenderness—and occasional swelling—usually is well localized in the bone involved. Although x-rays should be obtained, more often than not they will show nothing during the first two to three weeks. Management usually consists of decreasing the precipitating activity and re-examination. Stress fractures (real or potential) should not be ignored, as continuation of the activity may result in conversion to an overt complete fracture.

Shin splints—activity-related anterior leg pain—usually do not result in focal bone tenderness, and are unaccompanied by neurologic or vascular changes. The condition is poorly understood, difficult to manage, and noted here only to call attention to the fact that anterior pain also may signify the onset of a compartment syndrome. Thus, a thorough sensory examination is always indicated.

Ankle

Ankle injuries are among the most common injuries in athletics. Over 75 per cent are sprains, and most of these are of the inversion variety. The mechanism of injury involves inversion, plantar flexion, and internal rotation (of the foot), and usually is the result of stepping on an irregular surface (poorly maintained field or another player's foot) or a "cutting" (turning) maneuver. The athlete describes the ankle as "rolling under," "turning over," or "twisting." The history of a "snap" or "tearing sensation" usually means appreciable ligamentous damage.

The rapid occurrence of swelling or the presence of ecchymosis, although common, may be meaningless in ascertaining the severity of the injury. The presence of a pathologic anterior drawer sign means rupture of the anterior talofibular ligament, the first structure to be torn in the classic inversion sprain. Talar tilt (either seen clinically or in stress x-rays) indicates loss of both anterior talofibular and fibulocalcaneal ligaments and a grossly unstable ankle.

Because of the tendency for severe swelling and the frequent necessity for re-examination, the fresh ankle sprain initially should be immobilized in a soft compression dressing or posterior splint, rather than a short leg cast. Elevation and rest (crutches) are extremely important in the initial management of most ankle sprains, regardless of the ultimate definitive management. Accurate diagnosis, with stress x-ray confirmation, is of utmost importance to athletes anxious to return to their sport as soon as possible.

Not uncommon in skiing and vigorous contact sports is dislocation of the peroneal tendons, a condition often misdiagnosed as a lateral ankle sprain. The mechanism of injury, however, is considerably different from the usual ankle sprain, and usually is the result of hyperdorsiflexion of the ankle while weight bearing (e.g., falling over the tip of one's skis).

The athlete often reports the sensation of "something slipping out place," an historical feature not characteristic of an ankle sprain. Although the peroneal tendons usually spontaneously reduce, they leave behind evidence of their sojourn: tenderness and ecchymosis extending as far as 6 inches proximally from the fibular tip posteriorly, and, in over one-third of the cases, a tiny fleck of bone just lateral to the lateral malleolus in AP or mortise-view x-rays. Diagnosis of this condition is important, as it is prone to recur unless correctly managed initially (by surgery or proper cast immobilization).

INDEX

Numbers in *italics* refer to illustrations;
those followed by (t) refer to tables.